Medical Pharmacology and Therapeutics

SECOND EDITION

Dedication:

To our families

Commissioning Editor: Timothy Horne
Development Editor: Hannah Kenner
Project Manager: Frances Affleck
Designer: Sarah Russell
Illustration Manager: Bruce Hogarth

Medical Pharmacology and Therapeutics

SECOND EDITION

Derek G. Waller BSc (Hons), DM, MBBS (Hons), FRCP

Consultant Physician and Senior Lecturer in Medicine and Clinical Pharmacology
Southampton University Hospitals Trust

Andrew G. Renwick OBE, BSc, PhD, DSc

Emeritus Professor of Biochemical Pharmacology
School of Medicine
University of Southampton

Keith Hillier BSc, PhD, DSc

Senior Lecturer in Pharmacology
School of Medicine
Clinical Pharmacology and Division of Education
University of Southampton

Illustrations by Hardlines, Oxford and Ian Ramsden

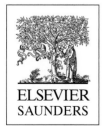

ELSEVIER
SAUNDERS

Edinburgh · London · New York · Oxford · Philadelphia · St Louis · Sydney · Toronto 2005

ELSEVIER
SAUNDERS

© Harcourt Publishers Limited 2001
© 2005, Elsevier Limited. All rights reserved.

The right of Derek G. Waller, Andrew G. Renwick and Keith Hillier to be identified as authors of this work has been asserted by them in accordance with the Copyright, Designs and Patents Act 1988

No part of this publication may be reproduced, stored in a retrieval system, or transmitted in any form or by any means, electronic, mechanical, photocopying, recording or otherwise, without either the prior permission of the publishers or a licence permitting restricted copying in the United Kingdom issued by the Copyright Licensing Agency, 90 Tottenham Court Road, London W1T 4LP. Permissions may be sought directly from Elsevier's Health Sciences Rights Department in Philadelphia, USA: phone: (+1) 215 239 3804, fax: (+1) 215 239 3805, e-mail: healthpermissions@elsevier.com. You may also complete your request on-line via the Elsevier homepage (http://www.elsevier.com), by selecting 'Support and contact' and then 'Copyright and Permission'.

First edition 2001
This edition 2005
  Reprinted 2006, 2007

ISBN-13: 978 0 7020 2754 3
ISBN-10: 0 7020 2754 5

British Library Cataloguing in Publication Data
A catalogue record for this book is available from the British Library

Library of Congress Cataloging in Publication Data
A catalog record for this book is available from the Library of Congress

Working together to grow
libraries in developing countries

www.elsevier.com | www.bookaid.org | www.sabre.org

ELSEVIER   BOOK AID International   Sabre Foundation

ELSEVIER your source for books, journals and multimedia in the health sciences

www.elsevierhealth.com

The publisher's policy is to use **paper manufactured from sustainable forests**

Printed in China

Contents

Preface

Medical Pharmacology and Therapeutics, Second Edition, has been thoroughly revised and expanded while preserving the basic approach of the first edition, which has remained widely popular.

The aim of *Medical Pharmacology and Therapeutics, Second Edition*, is to explain clinical pharmacology and therapeutics within the context of principles for the management of common diseases. Thus the chapters that deal with major disease contain:

- An outline of the major pathogenic mechanisms of the disease and consequent clinical symptoms and signs, helping the reader to put into context the actions of drugs and the consequences of their therapeutic use.
- A comprehensive review of major drug classes relevant to the management of the diseases in question. Example drugs are used to illustrate pharmacological principles and to introduce the reader to drugs currently in widespread clinical use. The mechanisms of drug action, key pharmacokinetic properties and important unwanted effects associated with their use are explained.
- A structured approach to the principles of disease management, outlining core principles of drug choice and planning a therapeutic regimen for many common diseases.
- A drug compendium which gives further details on most of the drugs available in the classes are included in each relevant chapter. For easy reference these tables set out key similarities and differences among drugs and complement the information in the main chapter.

- Self-assessment exercises and case studies to enable the reader to test their understanding of the principles covered in each chapter.
- Other chapters in the book deal with generic concepts of pharmacology and therapeutics including: chapters about how drugs work at a cellular level, drug development, the autonomic nervous system, drug toxicity and drug prescribing. Where relevant these chapters have been improved and information about genetic variations in both drug handling in the body and drug responses have been included.

This overall approach in *Medical Pharmacology and Therapeutics, Second Edition*, reflects the ways in which drugs are generally used in clinical practice and follows the recent developments in healthcare education. This approach should appeal to all healthcare professionals who need to be knowledgeable about the effective and safe use of medicines.

It is our intention that the new edition of this book will encourage readers to develop a deeper understanding of the principles of drug usage that will help them to become rational, safe and effective prescribers. As medical science advances these principles should underpin the life-long learning essential for the maintenance of these skills.

DGW
AGR
KH

Acknowledgements

Grateful thanks to the following specialist physicians who commented on chapters.

Ray Armstrong
Chris Canning
Pamela Crawford
John Cumming
Louise Dubras
David Firie
Jonathon Frankel
Tony Frew
Peter Friedmann
Richard Holt
John Iredale
Kim Orchard
Tom Pearce
Martin Prevett
Derek Sandeman
Cliff Shearman
Malvena Stewart-Taylor
Jane Wilkinson

Drug dosage and nomenclature

Drug nomenclature

In the past, the non-proprietary (generic) names of some drugs have varied from country to country, leading to potential confusion. Progressively, international agreement has been reached to rationalise these variations in names and a single recommended International Non- proprietary Name (rINN) given to all drugs.

Where the previously given British Approved Name (BAN) and the rINN have differed, the rINN is now the accepted name and is used through this book.

A source of minor irritation, however, is that in most authoritative publications issuing from the UK the internationally accepted name is still being called its BAN or new BAN, and this is likely to continue. For full information on this, the reader is referred to:

http://medicines.mhra.gov.uk/inforesources/ productinfo/banrinn.htm

A special case has been made for two medicinal substances: adrenaline (rINN – epinephrine) and noradrenaline (rINN – norepinephrine). Because of the clinical importance of these substances and the widespread European use and understanding of the terms adrenaline and noradrenaline, manufacturers have been asked to continue to dual-label products adrenaline (epinephrine) and noradrenaline (norephinephrine). In this book where the use of these agents as administered drugs is being described dual names are given. In keeping with European convention, however, adrenaline and noradrenaline alone are used when referring to the physiological effects of the naturally occurring substances.

Drug dosages

Medical knowledge is constantly changing. As new information becomes available, changes in treatment, procedures, equipment and the use of drugs become necessary. The authors and the publishers have taken care to ensure that the information given in the text is accurate and up to date. However, readers are strongly advised to confirm that the information, especially with regard to drug usage, complies with the latest legislation and standards of practice.

General principles

1

Sites and mechanisms of drug action

Modern clinical and biological sciences have provided a detailed understanding of the interaction of many therapeutic drugs with biological systems at a molecular level. Many medical students find it difficult to evaluate the depth of information necessary for them to understand the effective use of drugs and to become competent as safe and effective prescribers. The depth of knowledge can range from the general (e.g. it paralyses the patient) to the highly specific (e.g. it alters the tertiary structure of the receptor protein by interfering with the hydrogen bonding between certain specific amino acids). The former is totally inadequate because it allows no possibility of predicting any problems, while the latter is excessive (but may be fascinating, e.g. such detailed information could explain why some individuals show abnormal responses). The appropriate depth of understanding is that which provides:

- a suitable framework to allow comparison of the relative benefits and risks of alternative drugs (drug selection)
- an ability to predict possible problems in a particular individual owing to other disease processes, other medicines, etc.
- the acquisition of the skills of numeracy for accurately calculating drug doses and dilutions.

Sites of drug action

The actions of drugs can be divided into those occurring at specific sites and those that are non-specific.

Non-specific effects. The response is mediated via a generalised effect in many organs, such as an osmotic effect, and the response observed depends on the distribution of the drug, with the main response in the organ(s) with the highest concentrations. Such effects offer little prospect of developing a number of drugs that are highly selective for particular organs or diseases. However, all is not lost, as even such a general example as an osmotic effect can be harnessed for specialised use, such as an osmotic diuretic (Ch. 14).

Specific sites. The effect is produced by interaction of the drug with a specific site(s) either on the cell membrane or inside the cell. In some cases, the site of action may involve one (or more) members of a group, or a family, of receptors. Under such circumstances, the drug may interact preferentially with one member of a family of receptors and it is said to be *selective*; for example, in considering drugs that act on the family of adrenergic receptors (adrenoceptors), a drug that has a higher affinity for β-adrenoceptors (β-adrenergic receptors) than for α-adrenoceptors would be *relatively* selective for β-adrenoceptors. Alternatively, the drug may show a similar affinity for all adrenoceptors and would be described as *non-selective* within the adrenoceptor family; however, if it does not act on other receptor families, it could be described as being selective *for* adrenoceptors as a whole. Selectivity may be further contextualised; for example, drugs that may be selective for β-adrenoceptors compared with a-adrenoceptors, could also exhibit a further level of selectivity among β-adrenoceptors, being selective for β_1-adrenoceptors compared with β_2-adrenoceptors. Such drugs are widely used in medicine.

Specific sites of action

The activities of most cellular processes are controlled in order to optimise homeostatic conditions for the cell in relation to the prevailing physiological and metabolic requirements. For example, the heart rate and force of contraction increase during exercise, and this is accompanied by modification of energy sources. Such reflex actions require the appropriate response of different cells in the body to a signal (or signals) produced as a result of the altered physiological state. The signals typically take the form of specific chemicals (such as noradrenaline), which are either released into the circulation or released locally and which are recognised by the cell. Therefore, homeostasis is dependent on:

- the generation of a signal

3

- the recognition of specific signals
- the production of appropriate cellular changes as a consequence of signal recognition.

Each of these three steps provides important targets for drug action.

Receptor-mediated mechanisms

Recognition of the signal involves the chemical signal binding to a specific and specialised macromolecule of the cell, and it is this binding that triggers the cellular response. The chemical forming the signal is termed a *ligand*, because it ligates to (ties itself to) the specialised cellular macromolecule. The cellular macromolecule is termed a *receptor*, because it receives the ligand.

Receptors may be either in the cell membrane, in order to react with extracellular ligands that cannot readily cross the cell membrane (such as peptides), or in the cytoplasm, for lipid-soluble ligands that can cross the cell membrane. The binding of the ligand to the receptor results in a ligand–receptor complex, which triggers the intracellular changes. These changes may be brought about:

- directly, for example by inhibiting a process
- indirectly, by the primary signal altering a secondary intracellular control process (a *'second messenger'*), which then brings about the overall cellular event
- indirectly, by interacting with DNA to alter the synthesis of the enzymes etc. involved in the process.

Interaction of a drug with a specific receptor may have one of two types of effect on receptor function. The drug may:

- mimic the normal endogenous ligand and produce the same cellular response: such drugs have a 'positive' effect and are called *agonists*
- block the binding and actions of the normal receptor ligand: such drugs are called *antagonists*.

Properties of receptors

Receptor binding
The binding of the ligand to the receptor is normally reversible; consequently, the intensity and duration of the intracellular changes are dependent on the continuing presence of the ligand. The interaction between the ligand and its receptor does not usually involve permanent covalent chemical bonds but weaker, reversible forces such as:

- ionic bonding between ionisable groups in the ligand (e.g. $-NH_3^+$) and in the receptor (e.g. $-COO^-$)
- hydrogen bonding between amino-, hydroxyl-, keto-functions, etc. in the drug and the receptor

- hydrophobic interactions between lipid-soluble sites in the ligand and receptor
- van der Waals forces, which are very weak interatomic attractions.

Receptor specificity
There are numerous possible extracellular and intracellular chemical signals produced in the body, which can affect different processes. Therefore, a fundamental property of a receptor is its *specificity*, i.e. the extent to which it can recognise and respond to only one ligand (or group of related ligands, such as adrenaline and noradrenaline). Some receptors show high specificity and bind a single endogenous ligand (e.g. acetylcholine is the only endogenous ligand that binds to N_1 nicotinic receptors; see Ch. 4), whereas other receptors are less specific and will bind a number of related endogenous ligands (e.g. the β_1-adrenoceptors on the heart will bind noradrenaline, adrenaline and to some extent dopamine, which are all catecholamines).

The ability of receptors to recognise and bind the correct ligand depends on an interaction between the receptor molecule and certain specific characteristics of the chemical structure of the ligand. The formulae of representative endogenous ligands that bind primarily to different receptors are shown in Figure 1.1, and it is clear that the differences between them may be subtle. Receptor specificity occurs because the specific three-dimensional organisation of the different sites for reversible binding interactions (such as anion and cation sites, lipid centres and hydrogen bonding sites; see above) corresponds to the three-dimensional structure of the endogenous ligand. Receptors are proteins that are folded into a tertiary structure such that the necessary specific arrangement of bonding centres is brought together within a small volume – the receptor site (Fig. 1.2).

Three-dimensional aspects
Receptors have a three-dimensional organisation in space and, therefore, the ligand has to be presented to the receptor in the correct configuration (rather like fitting a hand into the correct glove). Because some drugs are a mixture of stereoisomers (the same chemical structures but with different three-dimensional configurations), the different isomers may show very different binding characteristics and biological properties. For example, the different stereoisomers of the α- and β-adrenoceptor antagonist drug labetalol bind to different types of receptor. A drug that is an equal mixture of *levo-* and *dextro*-isomers (or S- and R- forms; a racemate) could be a mixture of 50% active compound plus 50% inactive, or in some cases, a mixture of 50% therapeutic drug and 50% inactive but toxic compound. In consequence, there has been a trend in recent years for the development of single isomers for therapeutic uses; one of the earliest examples was the use of levodopa (the *levo*-isomer of dopa) in Parkinson's disease (Ch. 23).

(a)

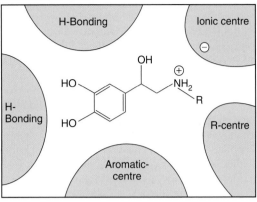

Dopamine

Noradrenaline

5-Hydroxytryptamine (5HT)

Histamine

ADRENOCEPTOR

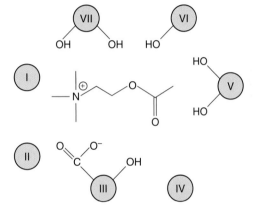

MUSCARINIC RECEPTOR

Fig. 1.2
Receptor ligand-binding sites. The coloured areas are schematic cross-sections of the transmembrane segments of the receptor protein. Different segments provide different properties (hydrogen bonding, anionic site, etc.) to make up the active site.

(b)

Glycine

Glutamate

Aspartate

γ-Aminobutyrate (GABA)

(c)

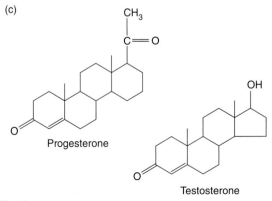

Progesterone

Testosterone

Fig. 1.1
Groups of chemicals that show preference for different receptors in spite of similar structure. (a) Biogenic amines; (b) amino acids; (c) steroids.

Receptor types and subtypes

Different types of receptor recognise different ligands; for example, there are receptors that bind catecholamines, such as noradrenaline and adrenaline, but do not bind acetylcholine (see receptor specificity above). There may be a number of subtypes of a receptor each of which specifically recognises or binds the same ligand. For example, α_1, α_2, β_1, β_2 and β_3 adrenoceptors all bind adrenaline, but they occur to a different extent in different tissues, and produce different intracellular changes when stimulated or blocked (see below). The different characteristics of the receptor subtypes allow a drug (or natural hormone) with a particular three-dimensional structure to show selective actions by recognising and then acting preferentially on one particular receptor, with fewer unwanted effects from stimulation of related receptors. It should be noted that although the drug may prefer one receptor subtype, this is never absolute. For example, the neurotransmitter acetylcholine acts without preference via different receptors on ganglia (nicotinic N_1 receptor subtype), the neuromuscular junction of skeletal muscle (nicotinic N_2 receptor subtype) and at smooth muscle (muscarinic receptor subtype); however, drugs have been produced which act with relative preference (selectivity) on these different receptors and are used for different clinical purposes. This aspect is discussed in detail in Chapter 4. Until recently, receptor subtypes were 'discovered' when a pharmaceutical company developed a new agonist or antagonist that was found to alter some, but not all, of the activities of a currently known receptor class. Recent developments in molecular biology have enhanced our abilities to detect receptor subtypes. Based on genetic information it is now recognised that there are multiple types of most receptors, and also that there is genetic variation between individuals (pharmacogenetics – see Chs 2 and 4). The recognition and cloning of subtypes of receptors is important in that it should facilitate the development of drugs showing greater selectivity and hopefully fewer unwanted effects. Greater understanding of genetic differences underlying human variability in drug responses offers the potential for individualisation of the mode of treatment and selection of the correct drug and dosage.

Receptor numbers

The number of receptors present in a cell is not static, and there is a high turnover of receptors which are being formed and removed continuously. The numbers of receptors within the cell membrane may be altered during repeated drug treatment, with either an increase (*upregulation*) or a decrease (*downregulation*) in receptor numbers. Changes in receptor numbers following treatment with some drugs can be an important part of the therapeutic response. A well-recognised example is the therapeutic benefit of tricyclic antidepressants, which, on administration, increase the availability of monoamine neurotransmitters within hours; however, it is the subsequent relatively slow adaptive downregulation in monoamine receptor numbers that occurs over many days or weeks which is associated with the time taken to produce a therapeutic response. Tolerance to the effects of some drugs (e.g. opioids) may arise from downregulation of opioid receptor numbers; as a result, there is the need for increased doses to produce the same activity (Ch. 19).

Transmembrane ion channels

The intracellular concentrations of ions such as Na^+, K^+, Ca^{2+} and Cl^- are controlled by a combination of ion pumps, which transport specific ions from one side of the membrane to the other, and ion channels (or gates), which open to allow the selective transfer of ions down their concentration gradients. Based on concentration gradients across the cell membrane, both Na^+ and Ca^{2+} will diffuse into the cell if the channels are open, making the cytosol more positive and causing depolarisation of excitable tissues; K^+ will diffuse out of a cell, making the cytosol more negative and inhibiting depolarisation; Cl^- diffuses into the cell, making the cytosol more negative and inhibiting depolarisation.

Some ion channels show voltage-dependent opening, i.e. they will open and close depending upon the voltage across the membrane (e.g. many of the channels that control excitability of the heart; see Ch. 8), while others open in response to the presence of a ligand (e.g. the Na^+ channel linked to acetylcholine stimulation of the nicotinic receptor and Cl^- channels linked to gamma-aminobutyric acid [GABA] receptors; see Ch. 4). Voltage-dependent and ligand-operated channels can be intimately linked in the movement of ions and in maintaining cellular homeostasis.

Voltage-gated ion channels consist of a number of subunits (Fig. 1.3) each of which is a transmembrane protein that crosses the membrane in a number of loops. The central unit contains the pore through which the ions pass and is largely responsible for the specificity of the channel for a particular ion. Ion specificity is determined by the amino acid composition of a short segment of the pore, which is different for each type of ion channel. Both Na^+ and K^+ channels show fast inactivation after opening; this is produced by an intracellular loop of the channel, which blocks the open channel from the intracellular end (Fig. 1.3). The activity of voltage-gated channels may be modulated by drugs, either *indirectly* via intracellular events, such as second messenger-mediated changes, or *directly*, for example local anaesthetics (Ch. 18) binding to and blocking activated Na^+ channels.

There are a number of different subtypes for each of the main types of cation channels (Na^+, K^+ and Ca^{2+}). These subtypes have different characteristics, and this allows the possibility of selective drug actions. There are at least five different voltage-gated Ca^{2+} channels (L, N, P/Q, R and T). The differences arise from the nature of the α_1-subunits, and that for L-type channels has three high-affinity, stereoselective binding sites for dihydropyridines, verapamil and diltiazem-type calcium channel antagonists. The different types of Ca^{2+} and K^+ channels are described in Chapter 5 in relation to the clinical uses of selective drugs. Sodium channels are of vital importance in excitable tissues, and different types of channel are present in the membrane of the axon of nerves (Ch. 18), and at the neuromuscular junction (Ch. 27). Chloride channels are described in Chapter 20.

Ligand-gated channels are often complex in nature and may consist of a number of transmembrane subunits, which cluster around a central channel. Each peptide subunit is orientated so that hydrophilic chains face towards the channel and hydrophobic chains towards the membrane lipid bilayer. The ligand-binding domain is usually present on one of the subunits or is produced by the juxtaposition of subunits. The nicotinic acetylcholine receptor is a good example of this type of structure since it comprises five transmembrane subunits

(a) Sodium channel

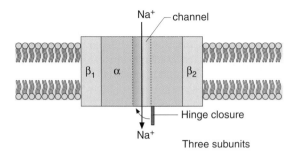

(b) Calcium channel

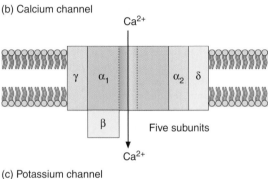

(c) Potassium channel

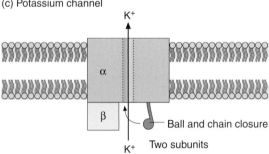

Fig. 1.3
Typical transmembrane ion channels. (The different subunits [α, β, γ] in different channels are not the same peptide sequences.) Ions diffuse down their concentration gradients when the channel is open. Two types of inactivation of open channels have been described (hinged, and ball and chain), which involve an intracellular loop of the channel. The ligand-gated GABA-linked Cl⁻ channel is shown in Figure 20.1.

and requires the binding of two molecules of acetylcholine for channel opening. Channel opening is a very rapid process, lasting only milliseconds, and is usually short-lived, because the ligand is rapidly inactivated (Ch. 4). Pharmacologically induced prolonged occupancy of the ligand-binding site by an agonist such as suxamethonium (succinylcholine) actually leads to a reduction in channel opening owing to a further conformational change in the receptor protein, which is associated with both receptor occupancy and a closed channel (see muscle relaxants; Ch. 27). Other ligand-gated ion channels that mediate fast synaptic transmission are linked to $GABA_A$ receptors, glycine receptors and 5-hydroxytryptamine type 3 ($5HT_3$) receptors.

Ion channels may be influenced by transmembrane receptors linked to guanosine-binding proteins (G-proteins) (see below) in two ways:

- indirectly, via the second messenger system affecting the status of the channel
- directly, via the G-protein subunits (α or βγ, see below) interacting with the channel.

G-protein-linked transmembrane receptors and second messenger systems

The structure of a hypothetical G-protein-linked transmembrane receptor is shown in Figure 1.4. Most transmembrane receptors have the N-terminals on the extracellular side and cross the membrane seven times with helical segments (heptahelical), so that the C-terminal is on the inside of the cell. The outer loops produce the active site for ligand binding and the inner loops are involved in coupling to the second messenger system, usually via a G-protein. The binding of an appropriate agonist (natural ligand or agonist drug) to the ligand-binding site, on the extracellular side of the membrane, alters the three-dimensional conformation of the receptor protein. The consequences of the change in conformation depend on the nature of the receptor, and the intracellular enzymes and other systems to which it is linked. The intracellular enzyme systems produce an

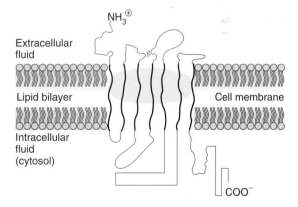

Fig. 1.4
Hypothetical transmembrane receptor based on the β-adrenoceptor. The receptor is a glycoprotein in which sites of glycosylation are indicated by a straight line. The orientation of the receptor within the membrane is achieved by folding of the polypeptide chain plus the presence of hydrophilic centres (such as the extracellular polysaccharide chain) and the transmembrane segments (shown as thick regions), which orientate the peptide within the cell membrane. The receptor is stabilised across the membrane by the presence of polar amino groups where the chains leave the lipid bilayer, which can interact with the phospholipid end of the bilayer. The ligand-binding site (Fig. 1.2) represents a small volume in space (coloured pink in this diagram) in which the parts of the polypeptide are orientated in such a way as to bind specific ligands only. Other possible ligands may be too large for the site or may show much weaker binding characteristics.

intracellular signal, the second messenger, which alters the functioning of the cell.

Second messenger systems

There are two complementary second messenger systems (Fig. 1.5).

Cyclic nucleotide system. One system is based on cyclic nucleotides such as cyclic adenosine monophosphate (cAMP), which is synthesised from adenosine triphosphate (ATP) via the enzyme adenyl (adenylyl adenylate) cyclase, and cyclic guanosine monophosphate (cGMP), which is synthesised from guanosine triphosphate (GTP) via guanyl (guanylyl guanylate) cyclase. There are many isoforms of adenylate cyclase; these show different tissue distributions and could be important selective sites of drug action in the future. The cyclic nucleotide second messenger is inactivated by hydrolysis by phosphodiesterase enzymes to give AMP or GMP, and the isoforms of phosphodiesterase provide another potential site for selective drug action (see sildenafil – Ch. 16).

The phosphatidylinositol system. The other system is based on inositol 1,4,5-trisphosphate (IP_3) and diacylglycerol (DAG), which are synthesised from the membrane phospholipid phosphatidylinositol 4,5-bisphosphate (PIP_2) by the enzyme phospholipase C_β (Fig. 1.5). There are a number of isoenzymes of phospholipase C, and these may be activated by the α-subunits of G-proteins (phospholipase $C_{\beta1}$) or the βγ-subunits of G-proteins (phospholipase $C_{\beta2}$) (see below). The second messengers produced by phospholipase C (IP_3 and DAG) are inactivated and then converted back to PIP_2.

The G-protein system

The G-protein system (Fig. 1.6) consists of three different subunits (i.e. it is a heterotrimer).

- **The α-subunit.** Twenty-three different types have been identified that belong to four families (α_s, α_i, α_q and α_{12}). The α-subunit is important because it binds GDP/GTP; it also has GTPase activity, which is involved in terminating the activity. When an agonist binds to the receptor, GDP (which is normally present) is replaced by GTP and the α-subunit dissociates from the βγ-subunits. The α-subunit/GTP complex is active while GTP is bound to it, but it is inactivated when the GTP is hydrolysed to GDP.
- **The β-subunit.** Five closely related forms have been identified. The β-subunit remains associated with the γ-subunit when the receptor is occupied and the combined βγ-subunit may activate cellular enzymes, such as phospholipase C.
- **The γ-subunit.** Ten different forms are known. The γ-subunit remains associated with the β-subunit when the receptor is occupied.

The sequence from receptor binding to activation of second messenger systems is illustrated in Figure 1.6. Binding of an agonist to the receptor results in the replacement of GDP by GTP, and the α- and βγ-subunits of the G-protein are activated. GDP binds more strongly than GTP to the non-activated receptor, but the reverse is true once the ligand binds to the receptor. The subunits dissociate from the receptor protein and exert their intracellular effects via activation of second messenger systems. The α-subunit has GTPase activity, which

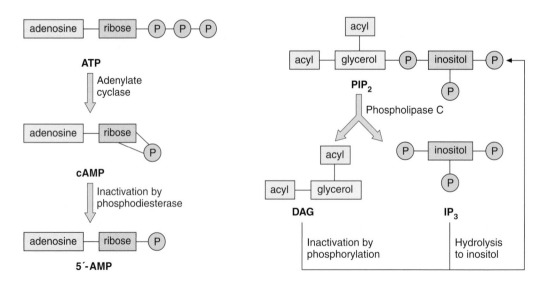

Fig. 1.5

Second messenger systems. The transmembrane receptor (see Fig. 1.4) produces intracellular changes normally by either activating or inhibiting the formation of intracellular second messengers such as cAMP (produced from ATP via the enzyme adenylate cyclase), cGMP (produced from GTP via the enzyme guanylate cyclase) or diacylglycerol (DAG) and inositol trisphosphate (IP_3) (produced from membrane phospholipid by phospholipase C). The receptor acts on the enzymes in the cell membrane via G-proteins (see Fig. 1.6).

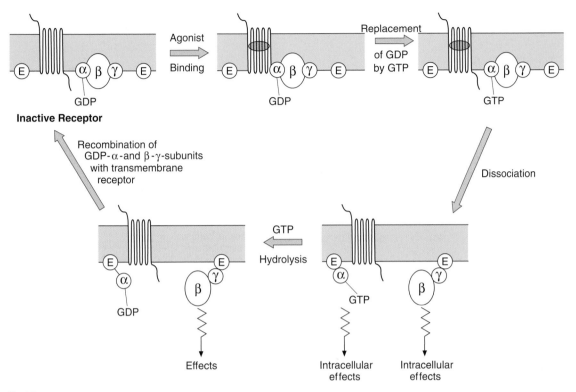

Fig. 1.6
The functioning of G-protein subunits. Ligand binding results in replacement of GDP on the α-subunit by GTP and this is followed by dissociation of the α- and βγ-subunits, which affect a range of intracellular systems (shown as E on the figure) such as second messenger systems (e.g. adenylate cyclase and phospholipase C), other enzymes and ion channels (see Fig. 1.5). Hydrolysis of GTP inactivates the α-subunit, which then reforms the inactive transmembrane receptor.

converts the active α-subunit/GTP complex to an inactive α-subunit/GDP complex; the GTPase activity is regulated by a family of proteins, which may provide additional future sites for selective drug actions. The GDP-α- and βγ-subunits recombine with the receptor protein to give the inactive form of the receptor/G-protein complex.

There are three main types of G-proteins, the properties of which are largely determined by the nature of the α-subunit:

- G_s: stimulates membrane-bound adenyl cyclase to increase cAMP
- G_i (and G_o): inhibits adenyl cyclase to decrease cAMP
- G_q (and G_{12}): activates phospholipase C.

Activation of the receptor/G-protein complex can produce a number of intracellular events (Fig. 1.7) which affect many cellular processes such as enzyme activity (via the enzyme protein *per se* or via gene transcription), contractile proteins, ion channels (affecting depolarisation of the cell) and cytokine production. The intracellular effects are mediated by the GTP-α-subunit or the βγ-subunit. Depending on the type of G-protein, the GTP-α-subunit may close K^+ channels, activate phospholipase C or activate adenyl cyclase, while the βγ-subunit may open K^+ channels, close Ca^{2+} channels, activate phospholipase A or C, activate or inhibit adenylate cyclase, activate receptor kinases or activate the transmembrane Ca^{2+} pump. The effects on ion channels may be direct – for example, the βγ-subunit of the acetylcholine muscarinic receptor acts directly to open K^+ channels in the sinoatrial node to hyperpolarise the cell. In other cases, the opening of a K^+ channel may be produced indirectly via phosphorylation of channels through cAMP-mediated activation of protein kinase A.

The intracellular concentration of Ca^{2+} is important for many processes and this is affected by G_i and G_o proteins, which inhibit N and P/Q type Ca^{2+} channels, G_s proteins, which stimulate L and P/Q channels, and G_q and G_{12} proteins, which release Ca^{2+} from intracellular stores via the action of IP_3 on its receptors on the endoplasmic reticulum.

Examples of G-protein-coupled receptors are given in Table 1.1.

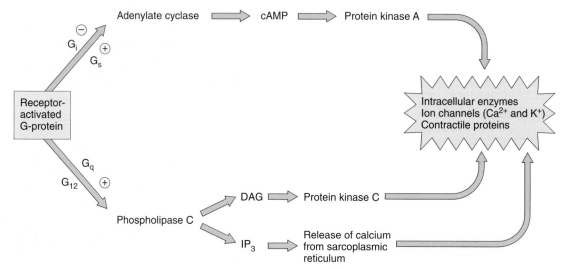

Fig. 1.7
The intracellular consequences of receptor activation and G-protein dissociation. The G-proteins affect the second messenger systems (Fig. 1.5) and the changes in cAMP, cGMP, diacylglycerol (DAG) and inositol trisphosphate (IP_3) produce a number of intracellular changes either directly, indirectly via actions on protein kinases (which change the activities of other proteins by phosphorylation) or by actions on ion channels, which alter the internal environment.

Kinase-linked transmembrane receptors

Kinase-linked transmembrane receptors are similar to the G-protein-linked receptors in that they have a ligand-binding domain on the surface of the cell membrane, traverse the membrane and have an intracellular 'effector' region (Fig. 1.8). However, they differ in a number of important respects:

- the extracellular region associated with the ligand-binding domain is very large; this is related to the size of the endogenous ligands, which are peptides such as insulin and cytokines
- there is a single transmembrane helical region
- the intracellular region possesses tyrosine kinase activity; different receptors have different intracellular effector regions.

Table 1.1
Examples of receptors linked to G-proteins

Ligand	Receptor	Type of G-protein
Noradrenaline	α_1	G_q
	α_2	G_i
	$\beta_1, \beta_2, \beta_3$	G_s
Acetylcholine (muscarinic)	M_1, M_3, M_5	G_q
	M_2, M_4	G_i
5-Hydroxytryptamine (5HT)	$5HT_1$ ($5HT_{1A}, 5HT_{1B}, 5HT_{1D}$)	G_i (+G_q?)
	$5HT_2$ ($5HT_2, 5HT_{1C}$)	G_q
	$5HT_3$	(ligand-gated ion channel)
	$5HT_4$	G_s
Dopamine	D_1	G_s
	D_2	G_i
Adenosine	A_1	G_i
	A_{2a}	G_s

G_s increases cAMP; G_i decreases cAMP and G_q activates phospholipase.

Intracellular hormone receptors

Many hormones produce long-term changes in cellular activity by altering the genetic expression of enzymes, cytokines or receptor proteins. Such actions on DNA expression are mediated by interactions with intracellular receptors. The sequence of hormone binding and actions are shown in Figure 1.9. The cytosolic hormone receptor is usually in an inactive form linked to a protein called heat shock protein (HSP). Binding of the hormone causes dissociation of the HSP and the hormone binds to its receptor. The hormone/receptor complex passes through pores in the nuclear membrane and interacts with *hormone response elements* on the genome to modify the expression of downstream genes. The translocation and binding involves a variety of different chaperone proteins, and the system is considerably more complex than indicated in Figure 1.9. Binding of the hormone/receptor to the hormone response element usually activates genes, but binding sometimes silences gene expression and results in a decrease in mRNA synthesis (Fig. 1.9). Steroid hormones (and some other hormones) are recognised by specific members of the steroid/thyroid receptor superfamily (Box 1.1).

Steroids, and synthetic steroid analogues, show specificity for different receptors, which then determines the spectrum of DNA gene expression that is affected. Frequently, the hormone response element needs two hormone/receptor complexes to form a dimer in order to alter gene expression. Some steroid hormone/receptor complexes (e.g. involving ER, PR, AR, GR and MR – see Box 1.1) form homodimers (e.g. ER–ER) while

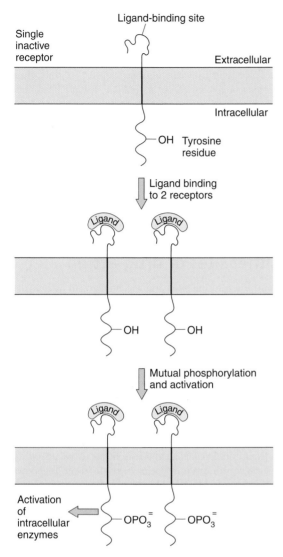

Fig. 1.8
Kinase-linked transmembrane receptor. The receptor has a large extracellular domain, a single transmembrane segment and an intracellular tyrosine kinase domain, which is responsible for intracellular effects (see text for details).

Ligand binding is accompanied by dimerisation of two kinase-linked receptors, and these phosphorylate each other. This activated 'pair of receptors' then phosphorylates specific intracellular protein(s). The phosphorylated intracellular proteins are active enzymes, such as kinases or phospholipases, which can then bring about the relevant intracellular changes appropriate to the biological activities of the extracellular ligand. These intracellular enzymes can either act directly on metabolising enzymes or alter the gene transcription of enzymes.

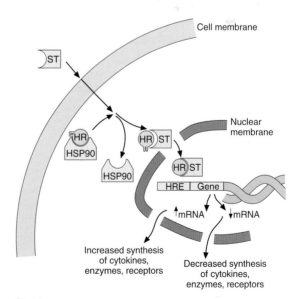

Fig. 1.9
The activation of intracellular hormone receptors. Steroid hormones (ST) are lipid-soluble compounds which readily cross membranes and bind to intracellular receptors (HR). This binding displaces a protein called heat shock protein (HSP90) and the hormone/receptor complex enters the nucleus, where it can either increase or decrease gene expression by binding to hormone response elements (HRE) on DNA.

Box 1.1

The steroid/thyroid superfamily of receptors

Oestrogen receptor	ER
Progesterone receptor	PR
Androgen receptor	AR
Glucocorticoid receptor	GR
Mineralcorticoid receptor	MR
Thyroid hormone receptor	TR
Vitamin D receptor	VDR
Retinoic acid receptor	RAR
9-*cis*-Retinoic acid receptor	RXR

---

the others (TR, VDR, RAR and RXR) form heterodimers (e.g. RAR–RXR).

The steroid receptor is made up of five regions with different functions (Table 1.2). The different regions are involved in hormone recognition, DNA binding and DNA modulation.

Hormone drugs act primarily by mimicking the endogenous hormone (i.e. as an agonist) but often the drug has a longer half-life (Ch. 2) than the endogenous ligand and produces a long-term change. Some drugs act as antagonists by blocking the binding of the normal ligand.

Protease-activated receptors

Protease-activated receptors (also called proteinase-activated receptors) are recently identified transmembrane, G-protein-coupled receptors, which are stimulated by cleavage of the N-terminus of the receptor by a serine protease, rather than by the usual receptor occupancy (as described above). Proteolysis produces a new N-terminal sequence of the receptor protein that can act as a ligand, which becomes 'tethered' back onto the receptor within extracellular loop-2. To date, four protease-activated receptors (PAR 1–4) have been identified, each with distinct N-terminal cleavage sites and different tethered ligands. The receptors appear to play roles in platelet activation and clotting (Ch. 11), inflammation and tissue repair, and possibly also in detecting noxious stimuli at sensory nerve endings. The processes of receptor inactivation and intracellular events are not defined, and clinically useful and selective drugs for these receptors await development.

Other sites of drug action

In addition to the sites and mechanisms of actions discussed above, drugs may also bind to and either activate or inhibit other specific sites.

- **Specific cell membrane ion pumps**. For example, Na^+/K^+-ATPase in the brain is activated by the anticonvulsant phenytoin whereas that in cardiac tissue is inhibited by digoxin; K^+/H^+-ATPase in gastric parietal cells is inhibited by proton pump inhibitors (e.g. omeprazole, Ch. 33).
- **Specific enzymes**. For example, a number of anticancer drugs inhibit enzymes involved in purine, pyrimidine or DNA synthesis. Some drugs act on the enzymes that synthesise or degrade the endogenous ligands for extracellular or intracellular receptors.
- **Specific organelles**. For example, some antibiotics interfere with the functioning of the bacterial ribosome.
- **Specific transport proteins**. For example, diuretics affect Na^+ transport in the renal tubules, and probenecid inhibits renal tubular secretion of anions.

Table 1.2
The structure of steroid hormone receptors

Region	Action	Role
N-terminus		
A/B	Transactivation	Activates target genes and gives the specificity of the receptor response
C	DNA binding and dimerisation	Binds receptor to DNA by two zinc finger regions
D	Nuclear localisation	Hinge region to allow correct conformation
E	Ligand binding	Ligand specificity of receptor; a large complex region; this region also binds heat shock protein
F	Unknown	Deletion of this region does not alter functioning
C-terminus		

Types of drug action

Drug actions can show a number of important properties:

- specificity
- selectivity
- potency
- efficacy.

Specificity
The ideal drug would be 100% specific, acting only on one type of receptor. The less specific the drug action, the wider variety of adverse effects that are possible (see, for example, tricyclic antidepressants, Ch. 22).

Selectivity
Many drugs may act preferentially on particular receptor types or subtypes, such as β_1- and β_2-adrenoceptors, to different extents (see above). For such drugs it is possible to determine dose–response relationships at each receptor subtype. The selectivity of the drug is the measure of the separation of the dose–response curves for different receptor subtypes. The maintenance of drug selectivity is dependent on the dose and on the concentration at the receptors, since high concentrations will give

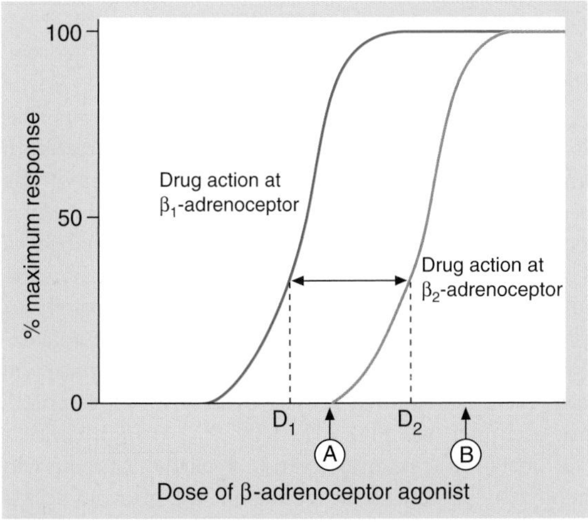

Fig. 1.10
Effect of dosage on the selectivity of a β-adrenoceptor agonist.
This illustrates that selectivity of drug action depends critically on the use of correct doses. The theoretical drug is administered at progressively increasing concentrations. The drug shows β_1-adrenoceptor selectivity, because at doses of A or less it produces dose-related β_1-adrenoceptor stimulation with little effect on β_2-adrenoceptors. This selectivity diminishes as the dose is increased progressively above A and is completely lost at dose B (which produces a maximum response of the drug on both β_1- and β_2-adrenoceptors). The extent of selectivity is given by the comparative potencies at each receptor type (i.e. it is the degree of separation of the two curves) calculated at doses giving similar responses, e.g. the ratio of D_1 to D_2 in the diagram.

a maximal stimulation at both receptor subtypes (Fig. 1.10).

Potency
The potency of a drug in vitro is determined by the strength of its binding to the receptor, which is a reflection of the receptor affinity. The more potent a drug, the lower will be the concentration needed to bind to the receptor and to give a response for an agonist, or to block a response for an antagonist. Potencies of different drugs are compared using the ratio of the doses required to produce (or block) the same response. Because dose–response curves are usually parallel (for drugs that share a common mechanism of action), the ratio is the same at different response values, e.g. 10%, 20% or 50% response. (Figure 1.10 can be used to compare the potency of the drug on β_1- and β_2-adrenoceptors.) Potencies cannot be determined by comparing the responses to similar doses because the difference between drugs will vary with the dose. Drugs that show the highest receptor affinities are the most potent in vitro; however, the dose–response relationship in vivo depends also on the delivery of the drug to its site of action, and this can be affected by absorption, distribution and elimination (pharmacokinetics – Ch. 2). Therefore, the in vivo potencies of a series of related drugs may not reflect their in vitro receptor-binding properties.

Efficacy
The efficacy of a drug is its ability to produce the maximal response possible. For example, agonists can be divided into two groups:

- *full agonists*, which give an increase in response with increase in concentration until the maximum possible response is obtained
- *partial agonists*, which also give an increase in response with increase in concentration but cannot produce the maximum possible response (Fig. 1.11, see later).

Classification of drug action

Specific types of drug action will be introduced throughout this book. They can be classified as:

- agonists
- antagonists
- partial agonists
- inverse agonists
- allosteric modulators
- enzyme inhibitors/activators
- non-specific.

Agonists
An agonist binds to the receptor or site of action and produces a conformational change in the receptor that

13

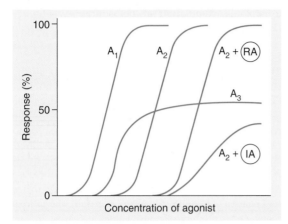

Fig. 1.11
Dose–response curves for agonists in the absence or presence of reversible (competitive) or irreversible (non-competitive) antagonists. A_1, A_2, two different agonists (A_1 more potent than A_2); A_3, partial agonist; RA, reversible antagonist; IA, irreversible antagonist.

mimics the action of the normal ligand. The action of the compound will be additive with the natural ligand at low concentrations of drug. Drugs may differ in their affinity (or strength of binding) for the receptor and the rate of association/dissociation.

The affinity or strength of binding of the drug to the receptor. This determines the concentration necessary to produce a response and, therefore, is directly related to the potency of the drug. In the examples in Figure 1.11, drug A_1 is more potent than drug A_2, but both are capable of giving a maximal response. For some compounds a maximal response may require all of the receptors to be occupied, but for most drugs/receptors the maximal response is produced while some receptors remain unoccupied, that is, there may be spare receptors. The presence of spare receptors becomes important when considering changes in receptor numbers owing to adaptive responses during chronic treatment (tolerance) or caused by irreversible binding of an antagonist (see below).

The rate of binding/dissociation. This is usually of negligible importance in determining the rates of onset or termination of effect in vivo, because these depend mainly on the rates of delivery to and removal from the target organ, that is, on the overall absorption or elimination rate of the drug from the body (see Ch. 2).

Changes in the number of receptors. The effect of changes in the numbers of receptors on dose–response relationships is complex. With downregulation of receptors, the response obtained depends upon the extent of downregulation and also on the extent of occupancy that is necessary to produce a maximal response. In practice, maximal drug effects are normally produced at concentrations that do not give 100% receptor occupancy; with downregulation, the same maximal response

may be produced but only with higher percentage occupancy of the reduced number of receptors.

Antagonists

An antagonist binds to the receptor but does not cause the necessary conformational change that activates the receptor. The compound will block access to the receptor-binding site by the normal ligand. The drug effect may only be detectable when the natural agonist is present (e.g. β-adrenoceptor antagonists lower heart rate, particularly when the rate is increased by stimulation of the sympathetic nervous system). The binding of most clinically useful antagonists is reversible and competitive; in consequence, the receptor blockade can be overcome by an increase in the concentration of the natural receptor ligand or by the administration of an agonist drug. Therefore, reversible antagonist drugs move the dose–response curve for an agonist to the right but do not alter the maximum possible response (as shown in curve A_2+RA in Fig. 1.11). Antagonists also exhibit selectivity of action. For example, the β-adrenoceptor antagonist propranolol is a non-selective antagonist acting equally on β_1- and β_2-adrenoceptors, whereas atenolol shows selectivity towards β_1-adrenoceptors and has less effect on β_2-adrenoceptors.

Irreversible antagonists, such as phenoxybenzamine, bind covalently to their site of action, and a full response cannot be achieved even by a very large increase in agonist concentration (as shown in curve A_2+IA in Fig. 1.11).

Partial agonists

A drug showing both agonist and antagonist properties is known as a partial agonist: the activity expressed at any time is dependent on the concentration of the natural ligand or agonist. Even maximal binding of a partial agonist to all available receptors produces a submaximal response, possibly because of incomplete amplification of the receptor signal via the G-proteins. A partial agonist will show agonist activity at low concentrations of the natural ligand, but the dose–response will not reach the maximal activity even when all receptors are occupied (see Fig. 1.11, drug A_3). At high concentrations of the natural ligand, a partial agonist will behave as an antagonist, because it will prevent access of the natural ligand to the receptor and thereby result in a submaximal response.

Inverse agonists

The concept of an inverse agonist arose because some compounds were found to show 'negative efficacy' – in other words, they acted on receptors to produce a change opposite to that caused by an agonist. This discovery gave rise to the concept that receptors exist as an equilibrium between inactive and active forms in the absence of an agonist ligand. The presence of an agonist will increase the proportion of active receptors. The presence of an inverse agonist will shift the balance towards more inactive receptors, thereby reducing the level of basal activity and actions. Antagonists (see above) bind to the receptor and block the activity of both agonists and inverse agonists. The concept of a degree of receptor activation in the absence of an agonist ligand is supported by observations that cell lines which express increased numbers of β_2-adrenoceptors show increased basal adenylate cyclase activity (in the absence of an agonist signal). The mechanism of action of inverse agonists is not well characterised, but they may destabilise the receptor/G-protein coupling, or they may preferentially bind to the inactivated form of the receptor, thereby shifting the equilibrium away from the active form. A final complication, which awaits resolution, is that some drugs, for example β-adrenoceptor antagonists, that are normal antagonists at some tissue receptors may be inverse agonists when the receptor is expressed on a different tissue. The role of inverse agonist activity in the therapeutic effects of drugs remains to be fully elucidated.

Allosteric modulators

An allosteric modulator does not act directly on the ligand/receptor site but may bind elsewhere on the receptor to enhance or decrease the binding of the natural ligand to its receptor. An example is the benzodiazepine drugs, which alter the affinity of Cl^- channels for the neurotransmitter GABA (Ch. 20).

Enzyme inhibitors/activators

Some drugs have a site of action that is an enzyme; the drug acts either on the catalytic site or at an allosteric site. An example is the anticholinesterase group of drugs (see Ch. 4).

Non-specific actions

Some compounds produce their desired therapeutic outcome without interaction with a specific site of action on a protein. Examples are the modulation of neuronal cell membrane fluidity by general anaesthetics (which also act on benzodiazepine receptors – see Ch. 17), and the action of osmotic diuretics on the kidney.

Tolerance to drug effects

Tolerance to drug effects is characterised by a decrease in response with repeated doses. Tolerance may occur through:

- a decrease in the concentrations of drug at the receptor
- a decrease in response produced by the receptor to the same concentration of drug

- a decrease in the number of receptors (so that an increased % occupancy is necessary to produce the same response).

The relationship between drug dosage and the concentrations delivered to the receptor is discussed in Chapter 2: some drugs stimulate their own metabolism and, as a result, they are eliminated more rapidly on repeated dosage and less drug is available to produce a response. However, most clinically important examples of tolerance arise from changes in receptor numbers and concentration–response relationships.

Desensitisation is used to describe both long-term and short-term changes in dose–response relationships arising from a decrease in response of the receptor. Desensitisation can occur by a number of mechanisms:

- decreased receptor numbers (downregulation): a slow process taking hours or days
- decreased receptor binding affinity
- decreased G-protein coupling
- modulation of the downstream response to the initial signal.

Extracellular receptors coupled to G-proteins show rapid desensitisation (within minutes) during continued activation, which occurs through three mechanisms.

- **Homologous desensitisation**. The enzymes activated following ligand binding to a receptor/G-protein complex include *G-protein-coupled receptor kinases* (GRKs); these interact with the $\beta\gamma$-subunit of the G-protein and inactivate the occupied receptor protein by phosphorylation (a related peptide [β-arrestin] enhances the GRK-mediated desensitisation).
- **Heterologous desensitisation**. The receptor (whether occupied or not) is inactivated through phosphorylation by a cAMP-dependent kinase (protein kinase A or protein kinase C), which causes uncoupling of the G-protein and can be switched on by a variety of signals that increase cAMP.
- **Receptor internalisation**. Endocytosis of the agonist-coupled receptor can occur within minutes of constant activation of G-protein-coupled receptors and makes the receptor unavailable for further agonist actions by uncoupling the G-protein from the receptor. The phosphorylated receptor protein may then be internalised and undergo intracellular dephosphorylation prior to re-entering the cytoplasmic membrane.

Downstream modulation of the signal may also occur through feedback mechanisms or simply through depletion of some essential cofactor. An example of the latter is the chronic administration of organic nitrates, which may deplete the SH groups necessary for the generation of nitric oxide (see angina, Ch. 5); high doses of indirectly acting sympathomimetic amines may cause depletion of neuronal noradrenaline, which is necessary for their activity (see Ch. 4).

Conclusions

The specificity and selectivity of drugs arise from their ability to interact with and affect certain target sites within a cell. In principle, high selectivity should result in safer drugs with fewer adverse effects. Our increasing knowledge of the complexity of receptor pharmacology offers the promise of safer drugs in the future, especially when genetic differences in pharmacokinetics (Ch. 2) and receptors (Ch. 4) can be taken into account using individual genetic information, prior to the subject being administered any drug. However, it should be remembered that:

- not all effects seen following drug administration are caused by the drug (a 'placebo effect' can be produced just by a clinical consultation)
- nearly all drugs show multiple effects no matter how receptor-selective they are
- not all effects produced by a drug will be therapeutically beneficial.

FURTHER READING

Ackerman MJ, Clapham DE (1997) Ion-channels – basic science and clinical disease. *N Engl J Med* 336, 1575–1586

Bourguet W, Germain P, Gronemeyer H (2000) Nuclear receptor ligand-binding domains: three-dimensional structures, molecular interactions and pharmacological implications. *Trends Pharmacol Sci* 21, 381–388

Catterall WA (1995) Structure and function of voltage-gated ion channels. *Annu Rev Biochem* 64, 493–531

Catterell WA, Goldin AL, Waxman SG (2003) International Union of Pharmacology. XL. Compendium of voltage-gated ion channels: sodium channels. *Pharmacol Rev* 55, 575–578

Catterall WA, Striessnig J, Snutch TP et al (2003) International Union of Pharmacology. XL. Compendium of voltage-gated ion channels: calcium channels. *Pharmacol Rev* 55, 579–581

Chuang TT, Iacovelli L, Sallese M, de Blasi A (1996) G protein-coupled receptors: heterologous regulation of homologous desensitization and its implications. *Trends Pharmacol Sci* 17, 416–421

Dohlman HG, Thomer J, Caron MG, Lefkowitz RJ (1991) Model systems for the study of seven-transmembrane-segment receptors. *Annu Rev Biochem* 60, 653–688

Dolphin A (2003) International Union of Pharmacology. XL. Compendium of voltage-gated ion channels: G protein modulation of voltage-gated calcium channels. *Pharmacol Rev* 55, 607–627

Ferguson FFG (2001) Evolving concepts in G protein-coupled receptor endocytosis: the role in receptor desensitization and signaling. *Pharmacol Rev* 53, 1–24

Fredholm BB, IJzerman AP, Jacobson KA, Klotz KN, Linden J (2001) International Union of Pharmacology. XXV. Nomenclature and classification of adenosine receptors. *Pharmacol Rev* 53, 527–552

Gudermann T, Kalkbrenner F, Schultz G (1996) Diversity and selectivity of receptor–G-protein interaction. *Annu Rev Pharmacol Toxicol* 36, 429–459

Gutman GA, Chandy KG, Adelman JP et al (2003) International Union of Pharmacology. XL. Compendium of voltage-gated ion channels: potassium channels. *Pharmacol Rev* 55, 583–586

Hanoune J, Defer N (2001) Regulation and role of adenylyl cyclase isoforms. *Annu Rev Pharmacol Toxicol* 41, 145–174

Hofmann F, Biel M, Kaupp UB (2003) International Union of Pharmacology. XL. Compendiumof voltage-gated ion channels: cyclic nucleotide modulated channels. *Pharmacol Rev* 55, 587–589

Hollinger S, Hepler JR (2002) Cellular regulation of RGS proteins: modulators and integrators of G protein signaling. *Pharmacol Rev* 54, 527–559

IUPHAR committee on receptor nomenclature and drug database. **http://iuphar-db.org/iuphar-rd/index.html** (accessed September 2004; this gives a very full appraisal of the important receptor subtypes and channels and details of selective agonists and antagonists)

Koenig JA, Edwardson JM (1997) Endocytosis and recycling of G protein-coupled receptors. *Trends Pharmacol Sci* 18, 276–287

Lucas KA, Pitari GM, Kazerounian S, Ruiz-Stewart I, Park J, Schulz S et al (2000) Guanylyl cyclases and signaling by cyclic GMP. *Pharmacol Rev* 52, 375–413

Milligan G, Bond RA, Lee M (1995) Inverse agonism: pharmacological curiosity or potential therapeutic strategy? *Trends Pharmacol Sci* 16, 10–13

Polson JB (1996) Cyclic nucleotide phosphodiesterases and vascular smooth muscle. *Annu Rev Pharmacol Toxicol* 36, 403–427

Privalsky ML (2004) The role of corepressors in transcriptional regulation by nuclear hormone receptors. *Annu Rev Physiol* 66, 315–360

Simon MI, Strathmann MP, Gautam N (1991) Diversity of G proteins in signal transduction. *Science* 252, 802–808

Strader CD, Fong TM, Tota MR, Underwood D, Dixon RAF (1994) Structure and function of G-protein-coupled receptors. *Annu Rev Biochem* 63, 101–132

Strange PG (2003) Mechanisms of inverse agonism at G-protein-coupled receptors. *Trends Pharmacol Sci* 23, 89–95

Sunahara RK, Dessauer CW, Gilman AG (1996) Complexity and diversity of mammalian adenylyl cyclases. *Annu Rev Pharmacol Toxicol* 36, 461–480

Tsai M-J, O'Malley BW (1994) Molecular mechanisms of action of steroid/thyroid receptor superfamily members. *Annu Rev Biochem* 63, 451–486

Wei LN (2003) Retinoid receptors and their coregulators. *Annu Rev Pharmacol Toxicol* 43, 47–72

Wess J (1993) Molecular basis of muscarinic acetylcholine receptor function. *Trends Pharmacol Sci* 14, 308–313

2 Pharmacokinetics

The nature of the response of an individual to a particular drug, for example a decrease in blood pressure, depends on the inherent pharmacological properties of the drug at its site of action. However, the time delay between drug administration and response, and the intensity and duration of response, usually depend on the rate and extent of uptake from the site of administration, the distribution to different tissues, including the site of action, and the rate of elimination from the body: in summary, the response of the patient represents a combination of the effects of the drug at its site of action in the body (*pharmacodynamics*) and the effects of the body on drug delivery to its site of action (*pharmacokinetics*) (Fig. 2.1). Both pharmacodynamic and pharmacokinetic aspects are subject to a number of variables (Fig. 2.1), which affect the dose–response relationship. Pharmacodynamic aspects are determined by processes such as drug–receptor interaction and are specific to the class of the drug, e.g. β-adrenoceptor antagonists. Pharmacokinetic aspects are determined by general processes, such as transfer across membranes, xenobiotic (foreign compound) metabolism and renal elimination, which apply irrespective of the pharmacodynamic properties.

Pharmacokinetics may be divided into three basic processes:

- **absorption:** the transfer of the drug from the site of administration to the general circulation

- **distribution:** the transfer of the drug from the general circulation into the different organs of the body
- **elimination:** the removal of the drug from the body, which may involve either excretion or metabolism.

Each of these can be described in terms of chemical, biochemical and physiological processes and also in mathematical terms. The mathematical description of pharmacokinetic processes determines many of the quantitative aspects of drug prescribing:

- why oral and intravenous treatments may require different doses
- the interval between doses during chronic therapy
- the dosage adjustment that may be necessary in hepatic and renal disease
- the calculation of dosages for the very young and the elderly.

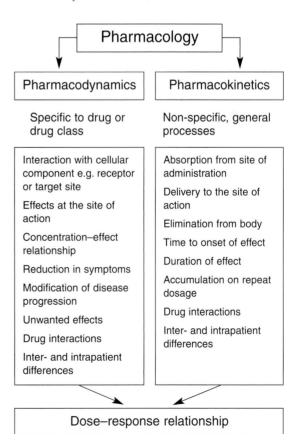

Fig. 2.1
Factors determining the response of a patient to a drug.

17

The biological basis of pharmacokinetics

Drug structures bear little resemblance to normal dietary constituents such as carbohydrates, fats and proteins, and they are handled in the body by different processes. Drugs that bind to the receptor for a specific endogenous neurotransmitter rarely resemble the natural ligand in chemical structure, and they do not usually share the same carrier processes or metabolising enzymes with the natural ligand. Consequently, the movement of drugs around the body is mostly by simple passive diffusion rather than by specific transporters, while metabolism is usually by 'drug-metabolising enzymes', which have a low substrate specificity and can handle a wide variety of drug substrates.

General considerations

Passage across membranes

With the exception of direct intravenous or intra-arterial injections, a drug must cross at least one membrane in its movement from the site of administration into the general circulation. Drugs acting at intracellular sites must also cross the cell membrane to exert an effect. The main mechanisms by which drugs can cross membranes (Fig. 2.2) are:

- passive diffusion
- carrier-mediated processes: facilitated diffusion and active transport
- through pores or ion channels
- by pinocytosis.

Passive diffusion. Passive movement down a concentration gradient occurs for all drugs. To cross a membrane, the drug must pass into the phospholipid bilayer (Fig. 2.2) and therefore has to have a degree of lipid solubility. Eventually a state of equilibrium will be reached in which equal concentrations of the diffusible form of the drug are present in solution on each side of the membrane.

Carrier-mediated processes. In *facilitated diffusion*, energy is not consumed and the drug cannot be transported against a concentration gradient; by comparison, *active transport* is an energy-dependent mechanism resulting in accumulation of the drug on one side of the membrane. In each case the drug or its metabolite resembles the natural ligand for the carrier process sufficiently to bind to the carrier macromolecule. Examples of drugs transported into cells via specific carriers that are used for nutrients include levodopa (Ch. 24), which crosses the blood–brain barrier by facilitated diffusion, and base analogues such as 5-fluorouracil (Ch. 52), which undergoes active uptake. There are a number of relatively non-specific carriers which can transport drugs out of cells, such as P-glycoprotein (PGP), organic anion transporters (OAT1 to OAT4) and organic cation transporters (OCT1 and OCT2). PGP is of most importance in the gut, blood–brain barrier and kidneys, and also in cells that develop resistance to anticancer drugs (Ch. 52), while the others are most important in the brain and kidneys (see later). Drugs that bind to carrier proteins but are released only slowly act as inhibitors of the carrier; for example, probenecid inhibits the secretion of anions, such as penicillins, by the renal tubule (Ch. 51).

Passage through membrane pores or ion channels. Movement occurs down a concentration gradient and can only occur for extremely small water-soluble molecules (<100 Da). This is applicable to therapeutic ions such as lithium and radioactive iodide.

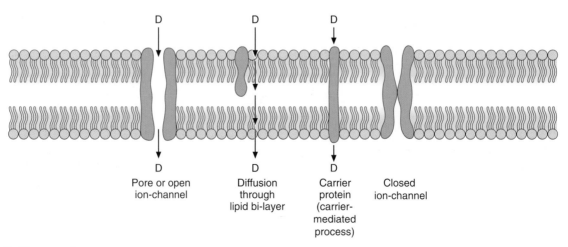

Fig. 2.2
The passage of drugs (D) across membrane bilayers.

Pinocytosis. This can be regarded as a form of carrier-mediated entry into the cell cytoplasm. Pinocytosis is normally concerned with the uptake of macromolecules; however, successful attempts have been made to utilise it for targeted drug uptake by incorporating the drug into a lipid vesicle or liposome (e.g. amphotericin and doxorubicin – Ch. 51).

A number of reversible and irreversible processes can influence the total concentration of drug present on each side of the membrane (Fig. 2.3). Ionisation is a fundamental property of most drugs and will occur whenever the drug is in solution. The majority of drugs are either weak acids, such as aspirin, or weak bases, such as propranolol. The presence of an ionisable group(s) is essential for the mechanism of action of most drugs, because ionic forces represent a key part of ligand–receptor interactions. Drug receptors are formed by the three-dimensional arrangement of a protein (Ch. 1), and drug binding requires both lipid- and water-soluble sites within the drug molecule; the latter are usually produced by an ionisable functional group.

The overall polarity of the drug and its extent of ionisation determine the extent of distribution (for example, entry into the brain), accumulation in adipose tissue, and mechanism and route of elimination from the body. Ionisation is a fundamental property and occurs when drugs containing acidic or basic groups dissolve in an aqueous body fluid.

$$[\text{Acidic drug}] \rightleftharpoons [\text{Acidic drug}]^- + H^+$$

$$[\text{Basic drug}] + H^+ \rightleftharpoons [\text{Basic drug} - H]^+$$

In general terms, the ionised form of the molecule can be regarded as the water-soluble form and the un-ionised form as the lipid-soluble form. Drugs with ionisable groups exist as an equilibrium between charged and uncharged forms. The extent of ionisation can affect both the pharmacodynamics (for example, the affinity for the receptor) and the pharmacokinetics (for example, the extent of uptake by adipose tissue and the route of elimination). The ease with which a drug can enter and cross a lipid bilayer is determined by the lipid solubility of its un-ionised form. Drugs that are fixed in their ionised form at all pH values, such as the quaternary amines, cross membranes extremely slowly or not at all; they have limited effects on the brain (because of lack of entry) and are given by injection (because of lack of absorption from the intestine).

The extent of ionisation of a drug depends on the strength of the ionisable group and the pH of the solution. The extent of ionisation is given by the acid dissociation constant K_a.

$$\text{Conjugate acid} \rightleftharpoons \text{Conjugate base} + H^+$$

$$K_a = \frac{[\text{conjugate base}]\,[H^+]}{[\text{conjugate acid}]} \qquad (2.1)$$

The term conjugate acid refers to a form of the drug able to release a proton, such as an un-ionised acidic drug (Drug–COOH) or an ionised basic drug (Drug–NH_3^+). The conjugate base is the corresponding equilibrium form of the drug that has lost the proton, such as an ionised acidic drug (Drug–COO^-) or an un-ionised basic drug (Drug–NH_2).

For acidic drugs, the value of K_a is normally low (e.g. 10^{-5}) and therefore it is easier to compare compounds using the negative logarithm of the K_a, which is called the pK_a (e.g. 5).

For acidic functional groups, a strong acid will have a high tendency to dissociate to give H^+; this results in a high value for K_a (e.g. 10^{-1} or 10^{-2}) and numerically a low pK_a (e.g. 1 or 2). Thus, strongly acidic groups (such as Drug–SO_3H) have a pK_a of 1–2, while weakly acidic groups (such as a phenolic–OH) have a pK_a of 9–10. In contrast, for basic functional groups, the stronger the base, the greater will be its ability to retain the H^+ as a conjugate acid – resulting in a low K_a and a high pK_a. Thus, strongly basic groups (such as R–NH_2 where R is an alkyl group) have a pK_a of 10–11, while weakly basic groups (such as R_3N) have a pK_a of 2–3.

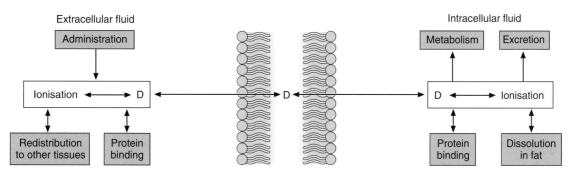

Fig. 2.3
Passive diffusion and the factors that affect the concentrations of drug freely available in solution (as an equilibrium between un-ionised and ionised forms).

The pH of body fluids is controlled by the buffering capacity of the ionic groups present in endogenous molecules such as phosphate ions and proteins. When the fluids on each side of a membrane (see Fig. 2.3) have the same pH values, there will be equal concentrations of both the diffusible, un-ionised form and the polar ionised form of the drug on each side of the membrane at equilibrium. When the fluids on each side of a membrane are at different pH values, the concentration of ionised drug in equilibrium with the un-ionised will be determined by the pH of the solution and the pK_a of the drug. This results in pH-dependent differences in drug concentration on each side of a membrane (pH partitioning). The pH differences between plasma (pH 7.4) and stomach contents (pH 1–2) and urine (pH 5–7) can influence drug absorption and drug elimination.

Drugs are 50% ionised when the pH of the solution equals the pK_a of the drug. Acidic drugs are most ionised when the pH of the solution exceeds the pK_a, whereas basic drugs are most ionised when the pH is lower than the pK_a (Fig. 2.4). The practical importance is that the total concentration of drug will be higher on the side of the membrane where it is most ionised (Fig. 2.5), which has implications for drug absorption from the stomach and the renal elimination of some drugs. In drug overdose, increasing the pH of the urine can enhance the renal elimination of acidic drugs, such as aspirin, by retaining the ionised drug in the urine (see below), whereas a decrease in urine pH can be useful for basic drugs, such as dexamfetamine. It is important to realise that changing urine pH in the wrong direction for the type of drug taken in overdose will make matters worse and could kill the person!

The low pH of the stomach contents (usually pH 1–2) means that most acidic drugs are present largely in their un-ionised (proton-associated) form and pH partitioning allows the drug to pass into plasma (pH 7.4) where it is more ionised. In contrast, basic drugs are highly ionised in the stomach and absorption is negligible until

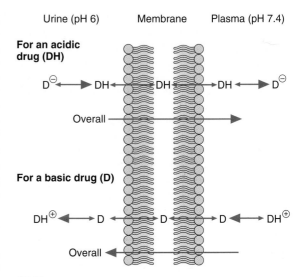

Fig. 2.5
Partitioning of acidic and basic drugs across a pH gradient.

the stomach empties and the drug can be absorbed from the lumen of the duodenum (pH about 8).

Absorption

Absorption is the process of transfer of the drug from the site of administration into the general or systemic circulation.

Absorption from the gut

The easiest and most convenient route of administration of medicines is orally by tablets, capsules or syrups; however, this route presents the greatest number of barriers for the drug prior to reaching the systemic circulation. A number of factors can affect the rate and extent to which a drug can pass from the gut lumen into the general circulation.

Drug structure

Drug structure is a major determinant of absorption, distribution and elimination. Drugs need to be lipid soluble to be absorbed from the gut. Therefore, highly polar acids and bases tend to be absorbed only slowly and incompletely, with much of the dose not absorbed but voided in the faeces. High polarity may be useful for delivery of the drug to the lower bowel (see Ch. 34). The structure of some drugs can make them unstable either at the low pH of the stomach, for example penicillin G, or in the presence of digestive enzymes, for example insulin. Such compounds have to be given by injection, but other routes of delivery may be possible (e.g. inhalation for insulin).

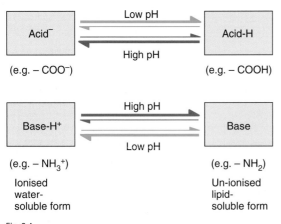

Fig. 2.4
The effect of pH on drug ionisation.

Drugs that are weak acids or bases may undergo pH partitioning between the gut lumen and mucosal cells. Acidic drugs will be least ionised in the stomach lumen, and most absorption would be expected at this site. However, the potential for absorption in the stomach is decreased by its low surface area and the presence of a zone at neutral pH on the immediate surface of the gastric mucosal cells (the mucosal bicarbonate layer). In consequence, even weak acids, such as aspirin, tend to be absorbed mainly from the small intestine. Basic drugs are highly ionised in the stomach; as a result, absorption does not occur until the drug has passed from the stomach to the small intestine.

Formulation

Drugs cannot be absorbed until the administered tablet/ capsule disintegrates and the drug is dissolved in the gastrointestinal contents to form a molecular solution. Most tablets disintegrate and dissolve rapidly and completely and all of the dose is rapidly available for absorption. However, some formulations are produced that disintegrate slowly so that the rate at which the drug is absorbed is limited by the rate of release and dissolution of drug from the formulation, rather than by the transfer of the dissolved drug across the gut wall. This is the basis for *modified-release formulations* (e.g. slow-release) in which the drug either is incorporated into a complex matrix from which it diffuses, or is administered in a crystallised form that dissolves only slowly. Dissolution of a tablet in the stomach can be prevented by coating it in an acid-insoluble layer, producing an *enteric-coated formulation*, for example omeprazole and aspirin. This allows delivery of intact drug to the duodenum.

Gastric emptying

The rate of gastric emptying determines the rate at which a drug is delivered to the small intestine, which is the major site of absorption. A delay between dose administration and the detection of the drug in the circulation is seen frequently after oral dosing, and is usually caused by delayed gastric emptying. The co-administration of drugs that slow gastric emptying, for example antimuscarinics, can alter the rate of drug absorption.

Food has a complex effect on drug absorption since it reduces the rate of gastric emptying and delays absorption, but it can also alter the total amount of drug absorbed.

First-pass metabolism

Metabolism of drugs (see below) can occur prior to and during absorption, and this can limit the amount of parent compound reaching the general circulation. Drugs taken orally have to pass four major metabolic barriers before they reach the general circulation.

Intestinal lumen. This contains digestive enzymes secreted by the mucosal cells and pancreas that are able to split amide, ester and glycosidic bonds. Intestinal proteases prevent the oral administration of peptides, which are the usual products derived from molecular biological approaches to drug development. In addition, the lower bowel contains large numbers of aerobic and anaerobic bacteria, which are capable of performing a range of metabolic reactions, especially hydrolysis and reduction.

Intestinal wall. The cells of the wall are rich in enzymes such as monoamine oxidase (MAO), L-aromatic amino acid decarboxylase, CYP3A4 (see below) and the enzymes responsible for the phase 2 conjugation reactions (see below). In addition, the luminal membrane of the intestinal cells contains the efflux transporter PGP, which transfers some drugs that have entered the cell back into the intestinal lumen. Drug molecules that enter the enterocyte may undergo three possible fates – i.e. diffuse into the hepatic portal circulation, undergo metabolism within the cell, or be transported back into the gut lumen by PGP. There are overlapping substrate specificities of CYP3A4 and PGP, and for common substrates the combined actions can prevent the majority of an oral dose reaching the portal circulation.

Liver. Blood from the intestine is delivered directly to the liver, which is the major site of drug metabolism in the body (see metabolism, below).

Lung. Cells of the lung have high affinity for many basic drugs and are the main site of metabolism for many local hormones via MAO or peptidase activity.

If there is extensive metabolism at one or more of these sites, only a fraction of the administered oral dose may reach the general circulation. This process is known as *first-pass metabolism* because it occurs at the first passage through these organs. The liver is generally the most important site of first-pass metabolism. Hepatic metabolism can be avoided by administration of the drug to a region of the gut from which the blood does not drain into the hepatic portal vein, for example the buccal cavity and rectum. A good example of avoiding hepatic first-pass metabolism is the buccal administration of glyceryl trinitrate (Ch. 5).

Absorption from other routes

Percutaneous (transcutaneous) administration

The human epidermis (especially the stratum corneum) represents an effective permeability barrier to water loss and to the transfer of water-soluble compounds. Although lipid-soluble drugs are able to cross this barrier, the rate and extent of entry are very limited. In consequence, this route is only really effective for use with potent non-irritant drugs, such as glyceryl trinitrate, or to produce a local effect. The slow and continued absorption from dermal administration (e.g. via adhesive patches) can be used to produce low, but relatively constant, blood concentrations, e.g. the use of nicotine patches.

Intradermal and subcutaneous injection

Intradermal or subcutaneous injection avoids the barrier presented by the stratum corneum, and entry into the general circulation is limited largely by the blood flow to the site of injection. However, these sites only allow the administration of small volumes of drug and tend to be used for local effects, such as local anaesthesia, or to limit the rate of drug absorption, for example insulin. Slow uptake from the site of injection, as seen with some insulin preparations, can result in an increased duration of action.

Intramuscular injection

The rate of absorption from an intramuscular injection depends on two variables: the local blood flow and the water solubility of the drug, both of which enhance the rate of removal from the injection site. Absorption of drugs from the injection site can be prolonged intentionally either by incorporation of the drug into a lipid vehicle or by formation of a sparingly soluble salt, such as procaine benzylpenicillin, thereby creating a depot formulation.

Intranasal administration

The nasal mucosa provides a good surface area for absorption, combined with lower levels of proteases and drug-metabolising enzymes compared with the gastrointestinal tract. In consequence, intranasal administration is used for the administration of some potent peptides, such as desmopressin (Ch. 43), as well as for drugs that are designed to produce local effects, such as nasal decongestants.

Inhalation

Although the lungs possess the characteristics of a good site for drug absorption (a large surface area and extensive blood flow), inhalation is rarely used to produce systemic effects. The principal reason for this is the difficulty of delivering non-volatile drugs to the alveoli. Therefore, drug administration by inhalation is largely restricted to:

• volatile compounds, such as general anaesthetics
• locally acting drugs, such as bronchodilators used in asthma
• potent agents, such as ergotamine for migraine, since this route avoids the gastric stasis that is a common feature of a migraine attack.

The last two groups present technical problems for administration because the drugs are not volatile and have to be given either as aerosols containing the drug or as fine particles of the solid drug. Particles greater than 10 μm in diameter settle out in the upper airways, which are poor sites for absorption, and the drug then passes back up the airways via ciliary motion and is eventually swallowed. The optimum particle size for airways deposition is 2–5 μm. It has been estimated that only 5–10% of the dose may be absorbed from the airways, even when the administration technique generates mostly small particles (i.e. 5 μm or less). Particles less than 1 μm in diameter are not deposited in the airways and are exhaled.

Minor routes

Although drugs may be applied to all body surfaces and orifices, this is usually to produce a local and not a systemic effect. However, absorption from the site of administration may be important in limiting the duration of action and in producing unwanted systemic actions.

Distribution

Distribution is the process by which the drug is transferred reversibly from the general circulation into the tissues as the concentrations in blood increase, and from tissues into blood when the blood concentrations decrease. For most drugs this occurs by simple diffusion of the un-ionised form across cell membranes until equilibrium is reached (Fig. 2.3). At equilibrium, any process that removes the drug from one side of the membrane results in movement of drug across the membrane to re-establish the equilibrium (Fig. 2.3).

After an intravenous injection, there is a high initial plasma concentration, and the drug may rapidly enter and equilibrate with well-perfused tissues such as the brain, liver and lungs (Table 2.1), giving relatively high concentrations in these tissues. However, the drug will continue to enter poorly perfused tissues, and this will lower the plasma concentration. The high concentrations in the rapidly perfused tissues then decrease in parallel with the decreasing plasma concentrations, which results in a transfer of drug back from those tissues into the plasma (Fig. 2.6). In most cases, the uptake into well-perfused tissues is so rapid that these tissues may be assumed to equilibrate instantaneously with plasma and represent part of the 'central' compartment (see below). Redistribution from well-perfused to poorly perfused tissues is of clinical importance for terminating the action of some drugs that are given as a rapid intravenous injection or bolus. For example, thiopental produces rapid anaesthesia after intravenous dosage, but this is short lived because continued uptake into muscle lowers the concentrations in the blood and in the brain (section A to B in Fig. 2.6; see also Fig.17.2).

The processes of elimination (such as metabolism and excretion) are of major importance and are discussed in detail below. Elimination processes lower the concentration of the drug within the cells of the organ that eliminates the drug; this results in a transfer from plasma into the drug-eliminating cells in order to

Table 2.1
Relative organ perfusion rates in humans[a]

Organ	Cardiac output (%)	Blood flow (ml min^{-1} 100 g^{-1} tissue)
Well-perfused organs		
Lung	100	1000
Adrenals	1	550
Kidneys	23	450
Thyroid	2	400
Liver	25	75
Heart	5	70
Intestines	20	60
Brain	15	55
Placenta (full term)	–	10–15
Poorly perfused organs		
Skin	9	5
Skeletal muscle	16	3
Connective tissue	–	1
Fat	2	1

[a]Except for the placenta, the data are for an adult male under resting conditions.

maintain the equilibrium. The resultant fall in the concentration of drug in plasma results in drug transfer from other tissues into plasma in order to maintain their equilibria. Thus, there is a net transfer from other tissues to the organ of elimination. Figure 2.6 illustrates how elimination (shown as a dashed line) produces a parallel

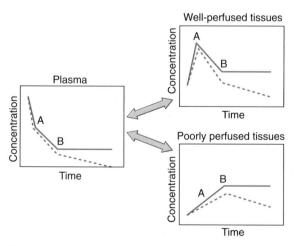

Fig. 2.6
A simplified scheme for the redistribution of drugs between tissues. The initial decrease in plasma concentrations results from uptake into well-perfused tissues, which essentially reaches equilibrium at point A. Between points A and B, the drug continues to enter poorly perfused tissues, which results in a decrease in the concentrations in both plasma and well-perfused tissues. At point B, all tissues are in equilibrium. N.B. The scheme has been simplified by representing the phases as discrete linear steps and also by the omission of any removal process. The presence of a removal process would produce a parallel decrease in all tissues from point B (shown as ----).

decrease in drug concentrations in both plasma and tissues.

Reversible protein binding

Many drugs show an affinity for specific sites on proteins, which results in a reversible association or binding:

$$\text{Drug} + \text{protein} \rightleftharpoons \text{Drug–protein complex}$$

The drug–protein complex is not biologically active.

Binding sites occur with circulating proteins such as albumin and α_1-acid glycoprotein (Table 2.2) and with intracellular proteins (Fig. 2.3). The drug–protein binding interaction resembles the drug–receptor interaction since it is an extremely rapid, reversible and saturable process and different ligands can compete for the same site. However, it differs in two extremely important respects:

- drug–protein binding is of low specificity and does not result in any pharmacological effect but serves simply to lower the concentration of free drug in solution; such protein binding lowers the concentration of drug available to act at the receptor
- large amounts of drug may be present in the body bound to proteins such as albumin; in contrast, the amount of drug actually bound to receptors at the site of pharmacological activity is only a minute fraction of the total body load (but is in equilibrium with the total body load – see later).

The rapidly reversible nature of protein binding is important because protein-bound drug can act as a depot. If the intracellular concentration of unbound drug decreases, for example through metabolism, then this will affect all the equilibria shown in Figure 2.3.

Table 2.2
Examples of drugs that undergo extensive plasma protein binding and may show therapeutically important interactions

Bound to albumin	Bound to α_1-acid glycoprotein
Clofibrate	Chlorpromazine
Digitoxin	Propranolol
Furosemide	Quinidine
Ibuprofen	Tricyclic antidepressants
Indometacin	Lidocaine
Phenytoin	
Salicylates	
Sulphonamides	
Thiazides	
Tolbutamide	
Warfarin	

Drug will dissociate from intracellular protein-binding sites, and some will transfer across the membrane from plasma until the intracellular equilibria are re-established. As a result, the extracellular (plasma) concentration of unbound drug will decrease, and drug will dissociate from plasma protein-binding sites. The ratio of the total amount of drug in the extracellular and intracellular compartments is determined by the relative affinity of the intra- and extracellular binding proteins.

Competition for protein binding can occur between different drugs (drug interaction; see Ch. 56), and also between drugs and natural, endogenous ligands. Administration of a highly protein-bound drug (such as aspirin) to an individual who is already receiving maintenance therapy with a drug that binds reversibly to plasma proteins (such as warfarin; see Ch. 11) will result in displacement of the initial drug from its binding sites; this increases the unbound concentration and therefore the biological activity. In practice, such protein-binding interactions are frequently of limited duration because the extra free drug is removed by metabolism or excretion.

An important interaction involving the displacement of an endogenous compound occurs in infants given drugs such as sulphonamides: drugs that compete for the same albumin binding sites as endogenous bilirubin can displace the bilirubin and cause a potentially dangerous increase in its plasma concentration.

Irreversible protein binding

Certain drugs, because of their chemical reactivity, undergo covalent binding to plasma or tissue components, such as proteins or nucleic acids. When the binding is irreversible, as for example the interaction of some cytotoxic agents with DNA, then this should be considered as an elimination process (because the parent drug cannot re-enter the circulation, as occurs after simple distribution to tissues). In contrast, the covalent binding of thiol-containing drugs, such as captopril (Ch. 6), to proteins, via the formation of a disulphide bridge, may be slowly reversible. In such cases, the covalently bound drug will not dissociate in response to a rapid decrease in the concentration of unbound drug and such binding represents a slowly equilibrating reservoir of drug.

Distribution to specific organs

Although the distribution of drugs to all organs is covered by the general considerations discussed above, two systems require more detailed consideration: the brain, because of the difficulty of drug entry, and the fetus, because of the potential for toxicity.

Brain

Lipid-soluble drugs, such as the anaesthetic thiopental, readily pass from the blood into the brain, and for such drugs the brain represents a typical well-perfused tissue (see Fig. 2.6, Table 2.1). In contrast, the entry of water-soluble drugs into the brain is much slower than into other well-perfused tissues, and this has given rise to the concept of a blood–brain barrier. The functional basis of the barrier (Fig. 2.7) is reduced capillary permeability owing to:

- tight junctions between adjacent endothelial cells (the capillaries are composed of an endothelial cell layer without smooth muscle)
- a decrease in the size and number of pores in the endothelial cell membranes
- the presence of a surrounding layer of astrocytes.

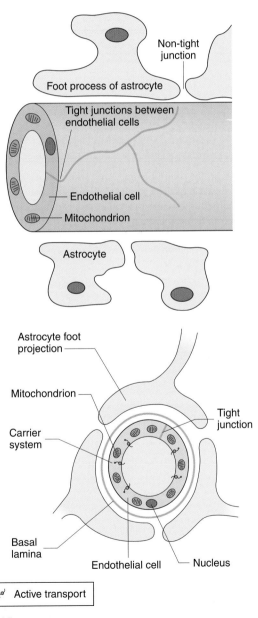

Fig. 2.7
The blood–brain barrier.

Therefore, only lipid-soluble compounds can readily enter the brain. Water-soluble endogenous compounds needed for normal brain functioning, such as carbohydrates and amino acids, enter the brain via specific transport processes. Some drugs, for example levodopa, may enter the brain using these transport processes, and in such cases the rate of transport of the drug will be influenced by the concentrations of competitive endogenous substrates.

There is limited drug-metabolising ability in the brain and drugs leave by diffusion back into plasma, by active transport processes in the choroid plexus, or by elimination in the cerebrospinal fluid. Transporters, such as PGP, in the endothelial cells are an important part of the blood–brain barrier, and serve to return drug molecules that have entered the cell back into the circulation, thereby preventing their entry into the brain and reducing any effects in the central nervous system. Organic acid transporters are important in removing polar neurotransmitter metabolites from the brain.

Fetus

Lipid-soluble drugs can readily cross the placenta and enter the fetus. The placental blood flow is low compared with that in the liver, lung and spleen (Table 2.1); consequently, the fetal concentrations equilibrate slowly with the maternal circulation. Highly polar and large molecules (such as heparin; see Ch. 11) do not readily cross the placenta. The fetal liver has only low levels of drug-metabolising enzymes. It is maternal elimination processes that predominantly control fetal concentrations of drug; lowering of maternal concentrations allows drug to diffuse back across the placenta from fetal to maternal circulation.

After delivery, the baby may show effects from drugs given to the mother close to delivery (such as pethidine for pain control; see Ch. 19): such effects may be prolonged because the infant now has to rely on his or her own immature elimination processes (Ch. 54).

Elimination

Elimination is the removal of drug from the body and may involve *metabolism*, in which the drug molecule is transformed into a different molecule, and/or *excretion*, in which the drug molecule is expelled in the body's liquid, solid or gaseous 'waste'.

Metabolism

Lipid solubility is an essential property of most drugs, since it allows the compound to cross lipid barriers and hence to be given via the oral route. Metabolism is essential for the elimination of lipid-soluble chemicals from the body, because it converts a lipid-soluble molecule (which would be reabsorbed from urine in the kidney tubule) into a water-soluble species (which is capable of rapid elimination in the urine). The drug itself is eliminated as soon as metabolism converts it into a different chemical structure. However, the elimination of the unwanted carbon skeleton of the drug may involve a complex series of biotransformation reactions (see below).

Metabolism of the parent drug produces a new chemical entity, which may show different pharmacological properties:

● complete loss of biological activity, which is the usual result of drug metabolism; this can increase polarity (especially phase 2 metabolism – see below) and prevent receptor binding
● decrease in activity, when the metabolite retains some activity
● increase in activity, when the metabolite is more potent than the parent drug
● change in activity, when the metabolite shows different pharmacological properties which can be less active or more toxic.

The various steps of drug metabolism can be divided into two phases (Fig. 2.8). Although many compounds undergo both phases of metabolism, it is possible for a chemical to undergo only a phase 1 or a phase 2 reaction. Phase 1 metabolism (oxidation, reduction and hydrolysis) is usually described as *preconjugation*, because it produces a molecule that is a suitable substrate for a phase 2 or *conjugation* reaction. The enzymes involved in these reactions have low substrate specificities and can metabolise a vast range of drug substrates (as well as most environmental pollutants). In this section, drug metabolism is discussed in terms of the functional groups that may be found in different drugs, rather than individual specific compounds. (In the following tables, R refers to an aliphatic or aromatic group and Ar refers specifically to an aromatic group.)

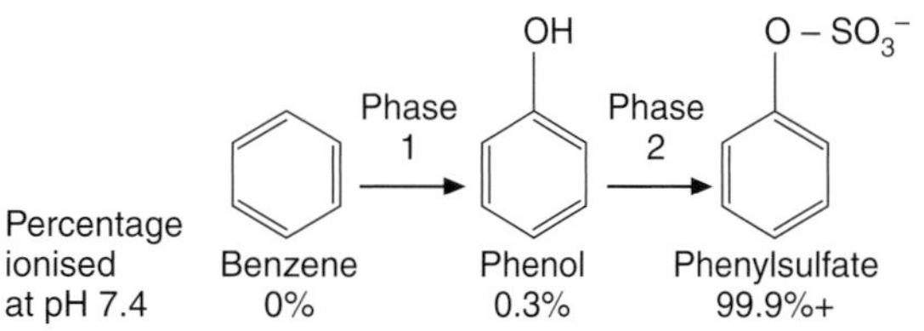

	Benzene	Phenol	Phenylsulfate
Percentage ionised at pH 7.4	0%	0.3%	99.9%+

Fig. 2.8
The two phases of drug metabolism.

Phase 1

Oxidation is by far the most important of the phase 1 reactions and can occur at carbon, nitrogen or sulphur atoms (Table 2.3). In most cases, an oxygen atom is retained in the metabolite, although some reactions, such as dealkylation, result in loss of the oxygen atom in a small fragment of the original molecule.

Table 2.3
Oxidation reactions

Oxidation at carbon atoms

Aromatic	$ArH \rightarrow ArOH$
Alkyl	$RCH_3 \rightarrow RCH_2OH \rightarrow RCHO \rightarrow RCOOH$
Dealkylation	$ROCH_3 \rightarrow ROH + HCHO$
	$RNHCH_3 \rightarrow RNH_2 + HCHO$
Deamination	$RCH_2NH_2 \rightarrow RCHO + NH_3$
	$RCH(CH_3)NH_2 \rightarrow RCO(CH_3) + NH$

Oxidation at nitrogen atoms

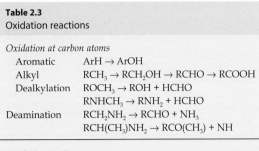

Secondary amines	$R'-N-R \rightarrow R'-N-R$
Tertiary amines	$R_3N \rightarrow R_3N \rightarrow O$

Oxidation at sulphur atoms

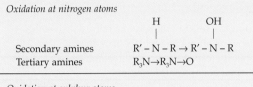

Thioethers	$R–S–R \rightarrow R–S–R$

R, aliphatic or aromatic group; Ar, aromatic group.

Oxidation reactions are catalysed by a diverse group of enzymes, of which the cytochrome P450 system is the most important. Cytochrome P450 is a superfamily of membrane-bound enzymes (Table 2.4) which are present in the smooth endoplasmic reticulum of cells (Fig. 2.9). The liver is the major site of drug oxidation. The amounts of cytochrome P450 in extrahepatic tissues are low compared with those in liver.

Cytochrome P450 is a haemoprotein that can bind both the drug and molecular oxygen (Fig. 2.10). It catalyses the transfer of one oxygen atom to the substrate while the other oxygen atom is reduced to water:

$$RH + O_2 + NADPH + H^+ \rightarrow ROH + H_2O + NADP^+$$

The reaction involves initial binding of the drug substrate to the ferric (Fe^{3+}) form of cytochrome P450 (Fig.

2.10), followed by reduction (via a specific cytochrome P450 reductase) and then binding of molecular oxygen. Further reduction is followed by molecular rearrangement, with release of the reaction products and regeneration of ferric cytochrome P450.

Oxidations at nitrogen and sulphur atoms are frequently performed by a second enzyme of the endoplasmic reticulum, the flavin-containing mono-oxygenase, which also requires molecular oxygen and NADPH. A number of other enzymes, such as alcohol dehydrogenase, aldehyde oxidase and MAO, may be involved in the oxidation of specific functional groups.

Reduction can occur at unsaturated carbon atoms and at nitrogen and sulphur centres (Table 2.5); such reactions are less common than oxidation. Reduction reactions can be performed both by the body tissues and also by the intestinal microflora. The tissue enzymes include cytochrome P450 and cytochrome P450 reductase.

Hydrolysis and *hydration* reactions (Table 2.6) involve addition of water to the drug molecule. In hydrolysis, the drug molecule is split by the addition of water. A number of enzymes present in many tissues are able to hydrolyse ester and amide bonds in drugs. The intestinal flora are also important for the hydrolysis of esters and amides and of drug conjugates eliminated in the bile (see below). In hydration reactions, the water molecule is retained in the drug metabolite. The hydration of the epoxide ring to produce a dihydrodiol (Table 2.6) is performed by a microsomal enzyme, epoxide hydrolase. This is an important reaction in the metabolism and toxicity of a number of aromatic compounds, for example the drug carbamazepine (Ch. 23).

Phase 2

Phase 2 or conjugation reactions involve the synthesis of a covalent bond between the drug, or its phase 1 metabolite, and a normal body constituent (endogenous substrate). Energy to synthesise the bond is supplied by activation of either the endogenous substrate or the drug. The types of phase 2 reactions are listed in

Table 2.4
The cytochrome P450 superfamily

Isoenzyme	Typical substrate	Comments
CYP1A	Theophylline	Induced by smoking
CYP2A	Testosterone	Induced by polycyclic hydrocarbons (e.g. smoking)
CYP2B	Numerous	Induced by phenobarbital
CYP2C	Numerous	Constitutive; 2C19 shows genetic polymorphism
CYP2D	Debrisoquine/sparteine	Constitutive; 2D6 shows genetic polymorphism
CYP2E	Nitrosamines	Induced by alcohol
CYP3A	Nifedipine/ciclosporin	Main constitutive enzyme induced by carbamazepine
CYP4	Fatty acids	Induced by clofibrate

Human liver contains at least 20 isoenzymes of cytochrome P450.
Families 1–4 are related to drugs and their metabolism; families 17, 19, 21 and 22 are related to steroid biosynthesis.

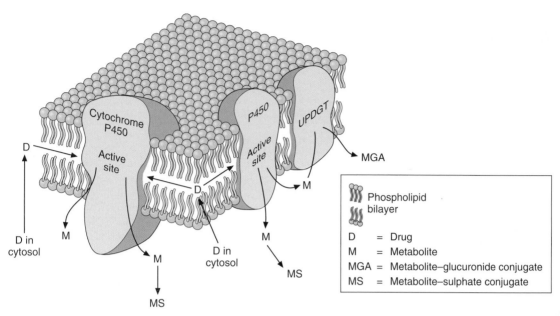

Fig. 2.9
Drug metabolism in the smooth endoplasmic reticulum. The lipid-soluble drug (D) partitions into the lipid bilayer of the endoplasmic reticulum. The cytochrome P450 oxidises the drug to a metabolite (M) that is more water soluble and diffuses out of the lipid layer. The metabolite may undergo a phase 2 (conjugation) reaction with UDP-glucuronyl transferase (UDPGT) in the endoplasmic reticulum or sulphate in the cytosol, to give a glucuronide conjugate (MGA) or a sulphate conjugate (MS), respectively.

Table 2.7, which shows the functional group necessary in the drug molecule and the activated species for the reaction. In most cases, the reaction involves an activated endogenous substrate. The products of conjugation reactions are usually highly water soluble and without biological activity.

The activated endogenous substrate for *glucuronide* synthesis is uridine-diphosphate glucuronic acid (UDPGA), which is synthesised from UDP-glucose. The enzymes that transfer the glucuronic acid moiety to the drug (UDP-glucuronyl transferases) occur in the endoplasmic reticulum close to the cytochrome P450 system, the products of which frequently undergo glucuronidation (Fig. 2.9). Glucuronide synthesis occurs in many

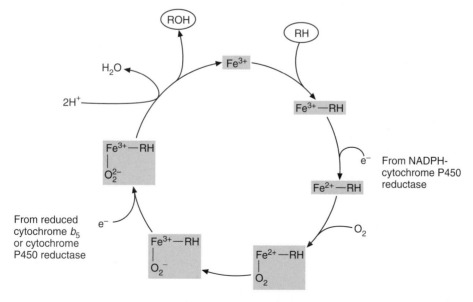

Fig. 2.10
The oxidation of substrate (RH) by cytochrome P450. Fe^{3+}, the active site of cytochrome P450 in its ferric state; RH, drug substrate; ROH, oxidised metabolite. Cytochrome b_5 is present in the endoplasmic reticulum and can transfer an electron to cytochrome P450 as part of its redox reactions.

Table 2.5
Reduction reactions

Reduction at carbon atoms

Aldehydes	$RCHO \rightarrow RCH_2OH$
Ketones	$RCOR \rightarrow RCHOHR$

Reduction at nitrogen atoms

Nitro groups	$ArNO_2 \rightarrow ArNO \rightarrow ArNHOH \rightarrow ArNH_2$
Azo group	$ArN=NAr' \rightarrow ArNH_2 + H_2NAr'$

Reduction at sulphur atoms

Sulphoxides	$R\text{–}\overset{\overset{O}{\uparrow}}{S}\text{–}R \rightarrow R\text{–}S\text{–}R$
Disulphides	$R\text{–}S\text{–}S\text{–}R' \rightarrow RSH + HSR'$

R, aliphatic or aromatic group; Ar, aromatic group.

Table 2.6
Hydrolysis and hydration reactions

Hydrolysis reactions

Esters	$RCO.OR' \rightarrow RCOOH + HOR'$
Amides	$RCO.NHR' \rightarrow RCOH + H_2NR'$

Hydration reactions

Epoxides

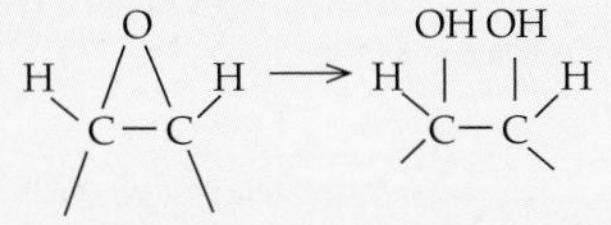

R, R′, different aliphatic/aromatic groups.

tissues, especially the gut wall and liver, where it may contribute significantly to the first-pass metabolism of substrates such as simple phenols.

In contrast, *sulphate* conjugation is performed by a cytosolic enzyme, which utilises high-energy sulphate (3′-phosphoadenosine-5′-phosphosulphate or PAPS) as the endogenous substrate. The capacity for sulphate conjugation is limited by the availability of PAPS, rather than the transferase enzyme. Sulphate conjugation is highly dose-dependent, and saturation of sulphate conjugation contributes to the metabolic events involved in the liver toxicity seen in paracetamol (acetaminophen in the USA) overdose (see Ch. 53).

The reactions of *acetylation* and *methylation* frequently decrease, rather than increase, polarity, because they block an ionisable functional group. These reactions mask potentially active functional groups such as amino and catechol moieties, and the enzymes are primarily involved in the inactivation of neurotransmitters such as noradrenaline or of local hormones such as histamine.

The conjugation of drug carboxylic acid groups with *amino acids* is unusual because the drug is converted to a high-energy form (a CoA derivative) prior to the formation of the conjugate bond. The enzymes involved in the formation of the drug CoA derivatives are involved in the metabolism of intermediate-chain-length fatty acids. Conjugation of the drug CoA derivative with an amino acid is catalysed by transferase enzymes.

Conjugation with the tripeptide *glutathione* (L-α-glutamyl-L-cysteinylglycine) is important in drug toxicity. This reaction is catalysed by a family of transferase enzymes and the product has a covalent bond between the drug, or its metabolite, and the thiol group in the cysteine (Fig. 2.11). The substrates are often

Table 2.7
Major conjugation reactions

Reaction	Functional group	Activated species	Product
Glucuronidation	–OH –COOH –NH$_2$	UDPGA (uridine diphosphate glucuronic acid)	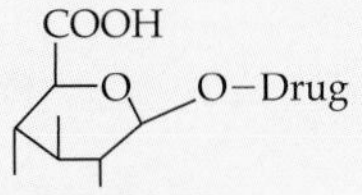
Sulphation	–OH –NH$_3$	PAPS (3′-phosphoadenosine 5′-phosphosulfate)	–O–SO$_3$H –NH–SO$_3$H
Acetylation	–NH$_2$ –NHNH$_2$	Acetyl-CoA	–NH–COCH$_3$ – NHNH–COCH$_3$
Methylation	–OH –NH$_2$ –SH	S-Adenosyl methionine	–OCH$_3$ –NHCH$_3$ –SCH$_3$
Amino acid	–COOH	Drug-CoA	CO-NHCHRCOOH
Glutathione	Various	–	Glutathione conjugate

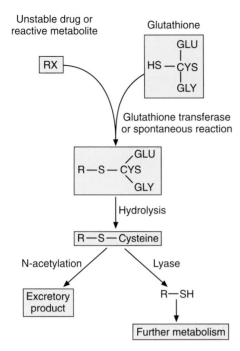

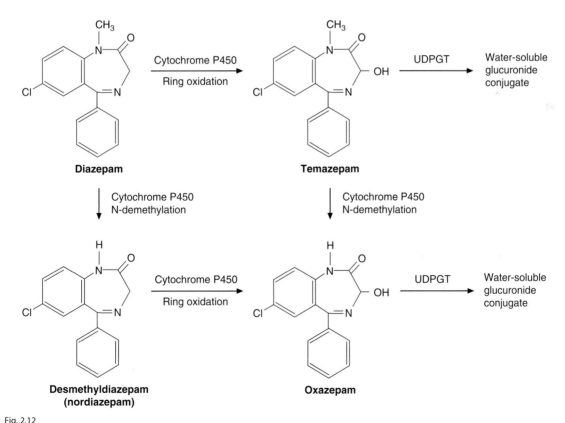

Fig. 2.11
The formation and further metabolism of glutathione conjugates.

reactive drugs or activated metabolites, which are inherently unstable (see Ch. 53), and the reaction can also occur non-enzymatically. Glutathione conjugation is a detoxication reaction in which glutathione acts as a scavenging agent to protect the cell from toxic damage. The initial glutathione conjugate undergoes a series of subsequent metabolic reactions, which illustrates the complexity of drug metabolism (Fig. 2.11).

A good example of a drug that undergoes a complex array of biotransformation reactions is diazepam (Fig. 2.12). Cytochrome P450-mediated oxidation and removal of the N-methyl group (see Table 2.3) produces N-desmethyldiazepam, which retains biological activity at $GABA_A$ receptors. Both diazepam and N-desmethyldiazepam undergo ring oxidation, giving temazepam and oxazepam, respectively, which are also used as anxiolytics and sedatives (see Ch. 20). Oxazepam and temazepam contain an aliphatic hydroxyl group, which is conjugated with glucuronic acid, giving an inactive, water-soluble excretory product. In addition, temazepam can undergo N-demethylation to give oxazepam.

Fig. 2.12
The pathways of metabolism of diazepam in humans. This figure illustrates that a single drug may generate a number of metabolites, which may possess similar pharmacological properties. UDP-glucuronyl transferase (UDPGT) is the enzyme that transfers glucuronic acid from UDPGA to the alicyclic OH group.

Factors affecting drug metabolism

The ability of individuals to metabolise drugs is determined by their genetic constitution, their environment and their physiological status.

Genetic constitution

This is an increasingly important area of pharmacology and is presented at the end of this chapter under **Pharmacogenomics, pharmacogenetics and drug responses**.

Environmental influences

The activity of drug-metabolising enzymes, especially the cytochrome P450 system, can be increased or inhibited by foreign compounds such as environmental contaminants and therapeutic drugs. Induction of cytochrome P450 results in increased synthesis of the haemoprotein following exposure to the inducing agent. Environmental contaminants such as organochlorine pesticides (e.g. DDT) and polycyclic aromatic hydrocarbons (e.g. benzo[a]pyrene in cigarette smoke) induce the CYP1A and CYP2A isoenzymes (Table 2.4). Therapeutic drugs can induce members of the CYP2, CYP3 and CYP4 families (Table 2.8). Chronic consumption of alcohol induces CYP2E. Induction of cytochrome P450 isoenzymes occurs over a period of a few days, during which the inducer interacts with nuclear receptors to increase the transcription of the mRNA, following which the additional enzyme is synthesised. The increased amounts of the enzyme last for a few days after the removal of the inducing agent, during which the extra enzyme is removed by normal protein turnover. In contrast, inhibition of drug-metabolising enzymes is by direct reversible competition for the enzyme site and the time course follows closely the absorption and elimination of the inhibitor substance. A number of drugs (Table 2.8) can produce clinically significant drug interactions because of their induction or inhibition of cytochrome P450 enzymes. Such changes in hepatic metabolism can affect both the bioavailability and clearance of drugs undergoing hepatic elimination (see below).

Physiological status

The functional capacity of the drug-metabolising enzymes is dependent on both the intrinsic enzyme activity and the delivery of drug to the site of metabolism via the circulation. Drug metabolism, and hence clearance and half-life (see below), for most drugs, is affected significantly by age (the very young and the elderly) and by liver disease. This is discussed in detail in Chapter 56.

Excretion

Drugs and their metabolites may be eliminated from the circulation by various routes:

- **in fluids (urine, bile, sweat, tears, milk, etc.)**: these routes are most important for low-molecular-weight polar compounds, and the urine is the major route; milk is important because of the potential for exposure of the breastfed infant
- **in solids (faeces, hair, etc.)**: drugs enter the gastrointestinal tract by various mechanisms (see below) and faecal elimination is most important for high-molecular-weight compounds; the sequestration of foreign compounds into hair is not of quantitative importance, because of the slow growth of hair, but distribution of a drug along the hair can be used to indicate the history of drug intake during the preceding weeks
- **in gases (expired air)**: this route is only of importance for volatile compounds.

Excretion via the urine

There are three processes involved in the handling of drugs and their metabolites in the kidney: glomerular filtration, reabsorption and tubular secretion. The total urinary excretion of a drug depends on the balance of these three processes: total excretion equals glomerular filtration plus tubular secretion minus any reabsorption.

Glomerular filtration. All molecules less than about 20 kDa undergo filtration under positive hydrostatic pressure through the pores of 7–8 nm in the glomerular membrane. The glomerular filtrate contains about 20% of the plasma volume delivered to the glomerulus, and about 20% of water-soluble, low-molecular-weight compounds in plasma, including non-protein-bound drugs, enter the filtrate. Plasma proteins and protein-bound drug are not filtered; therefore, the efficiency of glomerular filtration for a drug is influenced by the extent of plasma-protein binding.

Reabsorption. The glomerular filtrate contains numerous constituents that the body cannot afford to lose. There are specific tubular uptake processes for carbohydrates, amino acids, vitamins, etc. and most of the water is also reabsorbed. Drugs may pass back from the tubule into the plasma if they are substrates for these specific uptake processes (very rare) or if they are lipid

Table 2.8
Common inducers and inhibitors of cytochrome P450

Inducers	Inhibitors
Barbiturates (esp. phenobarbital)	Cimetidine
Phenytoin	Allopurinol
Carbamazepine	Isoniazid
Grisofulvin	Chloramphenicol
Rifampicin (rifampin)	Disulfiram
Glutethimide	Quinine
	Erythromycin

soluble. The urine is concentrated on its passage down the renal tubule and the tubule-to-plasma concentration gradient increases, so that only the most polar and least diffusible molecules will remain in the urine. Because of extensive reabsorption, lipid-soluble drugs are not eliminated via the urine, and are retained in the circulation until they are metabolised to water-soluble products (see above), which are efficiently removed from the body. The pH of urine is usually less than that of plasma; consequently, pH partitioning, between urine (pH 5–6) and plasma (pH 7.4), may either increase or decrease the tendency of the compound to be reabsorbed (see above).

Tubular secretion. The renal tubule has secretory transporters on both the basolateral and apical membranes for compounds that are acidic (organic anion transporters – OATs 1–4) or basic (organic cation transporters – OCTs 1–3). In addition, there are multidrug resistance-associated proteins (MRPs), which were originally identified in a cell line resistant to anticancer drugs but have since been found as important transporters in various tissues. Drugs and their metabolites (especially the glucuronic acid and sulphate conjugates) may undergo an active carrier-mediated elimination, primarily by OATs but also by MRPs. Because secretion lowers the plasma concentration of unbound drug by an active process, there will be a rapid dissociation of any drug–protein complex; as a result, even highly protein-bound drugs may be cleared almost completely from the blood in a single passage through the kidney.

Excretion via the faeces

Uptake into hepatocytes and subsequent elimination in bile is the principal route of elimination of larger molecules (those with a molecular weight greater than about 500 Da). Conjugation with glucuronic acid increases the molecular weight of the substrate by almost 200 Da, and therefore bile can be an important route for the elimination of glucuronide conjugates. Once the drug, or its conjugate, has entered the intestinal lumen via the bile, it passes down the gut and eventually may be eliminated in the faeces. However, some drugs may be reabsorbed from the lumen of the gut and re-enter the hepatic portal vein. As a result, the drug is recycled between the liver, bile, gut lumen and hepatic portal vein. This is described as an enterohepatic circulation (Fig. 2.13); it can maintain the drug concentrations in the general circulation, because some of the reabsorbed drug will escape hepatic extraction and pass through the sinusoids from the hepatic portal vein into the hepatic vein. Highly polar glucuronide conjugates of drugs, or their oxidised metabolites, that are excreted into the bile undergo little reabsorption in the upper intestine, but the bacterial flora of the lower intestine can hydrolyse the conjugate back to the original drug, or its oxidised metabolite, and glucuronic acid. The original drug, or its primary metabolite, will

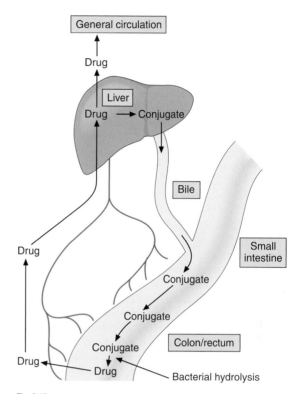

Fig. 2.13
Enterohepatic circulation of drugs.

have a greater lipid solubility than the glucuronic acid conjugate and will be absorbed from the gut lumen and enter the hepatic portal vein (Fig. 2.13).

The mathematical basis of pharmacokinetics

The use of mathematics to describe the fate of a drug in the body can be complex and rather daunting for undergraduates. Nevertheless, a basic understanding is essential for an appreciation of many aspects of drug handling and for the rational prescribing of drugs. The following account gives the mathematics for the absorption, distribution and elimination of a single dose of a drug, before brief consideration of chronic (repeat-dose) administration and the factors that can affect pharmacokinetic processes.

General considerations

Two different but complementary approaches can be used to describe pharmacokinetics.

- **Compartmental model analysis**. Plasma concentration–time curves are described by an equation containing one or more exponential functions. This approach gives a precise mathematical description of the concentration–time curve and can be used to predict the concentration of drug at any time after a dose. However, it is difficult to relate the mathematical values to the physiological disposition of the compound.
- **Model-independent analysis**. This approach may be related more closely to the physiological processes governing the disposition of the chemical. It is more useful in predicting the influence of variables such as disease, age and the administration of other compounds on the concentrations of the drug.

Some undergraduate texts provide details of compartmental analysis, but the model-independent methods are of greater potential value to medical undergraduates and are the basis of the following account.

The three basic processes that need to be described mathematically are absorption, distribution and elimination. For each process, it is important to know the *rate* or speed with which the drug is processed and the *extent* of the process, i.e. the amount or proportion of drug that undergoes that process.

For nearly all physiological and metabolic processes, the rate of reaction is proportional to the amount of substrate (drug) available: this is described as a *first-order reaction*. Diffusion down a concentration gradient and glomerular filtration are examples of first-order reactions. Protein-mediated reactions, such as metabolism and active transport, are also first-order at low concentrations because if the concentration of the substate is doubled, then the formation of product is doubled. However, as the substrate concentration increases, the enzyme or transporter can become saturated with substrate and the rate of reaction cannot increase in response to a further increase in concentration. The process then occurs at a fixed maximum rate that is independent of substrate concentration, and the reaction is described as a *zero-order reaction*; examples are the metabolism of ethanol (Ch. 54) and phenytoin (Ch. 23). When the substrate concentration has decreased sufficiently for protein sites to become available again, then the change in concentration will proceed at a rate proportional to the concentration available – in other words, the reaction will revert to first-order.

Zero-order reactions

If a drug is being processed (absorbed, distributed or eliminated) according to zero-order kinetics, then the change in concentration with time (dC/dt) is a fixed amount per time – independent of concentration:

$$\frac{dC}{dt} = -k \tag{2.2}$$

The units of k (the reaction rate constant) will be an amount per unit time (e.g. mg min^{-1}). A graph of concentration against time will produce a straight line with a slope of $-k$ (Fig. 2.14a).

First-order reactions

In first-order reactions, the change in concentration at any time (dC/dt) is proportional to the concentration present at that time:

$$\frac{dC}{dt} = -kC \tag{2.3}$$

The units of the rate constant, k, are time^{-1} (e.g. h^{-1}), and k may be regarded as the proportional change per unit of time. The rate of change will be high at high concentrations but low at low concentrations (Fig. 2.14b), and a graph of concentration against time will produce an exponential decrease. Such a curve can be described by an exponential equation:

$$C = C_0 e^{-kt} \tag{2.4}$$

where C is the concentration at time t and C_0 is the initial concentration (when time = 0). This equation may be written more simply by taking natural logarithms:

$$\ln C = \ln C_0 - kt \tag{2.5}$$

and a graph of $\ln C$ against time will produce a straight line with a slope of $-k$ and an intercept of $\ln C_0$ (Fig. 2.14c).

The units of k (which are time^{-1}, e.g. h^{-1}) are difficult to use practically, and therefore the rate of a first-order reaction is usually described in terms of its half-life (which has units of time). The half-life is the time taken for a concentration to decrease to one-half. The half-life is independent of concentration (Fig. 2.15) and is a characteristic for that particular first-order process and that particular drug. The decrease in plasma concentration after an intravenous bolus dose is shown in Figure 2.15, which has been plotted such that the concentration is halved every hour.

The relationship between the half-life and the rate constant is derived by substituting $C_0 = 2$ and $C = 1$ into the above equation, when the time interval t will be one half-life ($t_{1/2}$).

$$\ln 1 = \ln 2 - kt_{1/2} \tag{2.6}$$

$$0 = 0.693 - kt_{1/2}$$

$$t_{1/2} = \frac{0.693}{k}$$

A half-life can be calculated for any first-order process (e.g. for absorption, distribution or elimination); in practice, the 'half-life' reported for a drug is the half-life

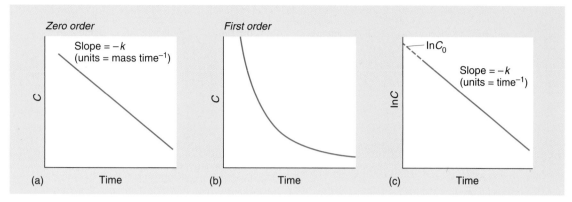

Fig. 2.14
Zero- and first-order kinetics. C, concentration; k, rate constant.

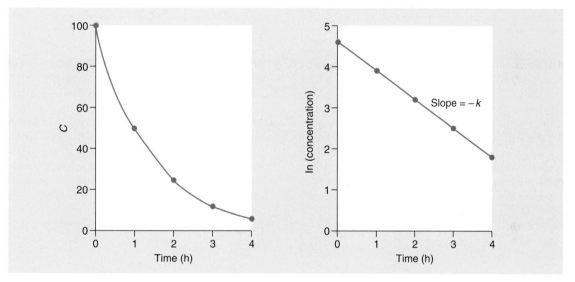

Fig. 2.15
The elimination half-life of a drug in plasma. Here the concentration (C) decreases by 50% every hour, i.e. the half-life is 1 h.

for the elimination rate (i.e. the slowest, terminal phase of the plasma concentration–time curve; see below).

Absorption

The mathematics of absorption apply to all 'non-intravenous' routes – for example, oral, inhalation, percutaneous, etc. – and are illustrated by absorption from the gut lumen.

Rate of absorption

For some drugs, it is possible to see three distinct phases in the plasma concentration–time curve that reflect absorption, distribution and elimination (Fig. 2.16a). However, for most drugs, the distribution phase is not seen after oral dosage (Fig 2.16b). The rate of absorption after oral administration is determined by the rate at which the drug is able to pass from the gut lumen into the systemic circulation. The rate of absorption influences the shape of the plasma concentration–time curve after an oral dose, as shown in Figure 2.17. For lipid-soluble drugs, there is an initial steep increase, from which the absorption rate constant (k_a) can be calculated, and a slower decrease, from which the elimination rate constant (k) can be calculated. In Figure 2.17a, the absorption is essentially complete by point B since the subsequent data are fitted by a single exponential rate constant (the elimination rate) (see below).

A number of factors can affect this apparently simple pattern.

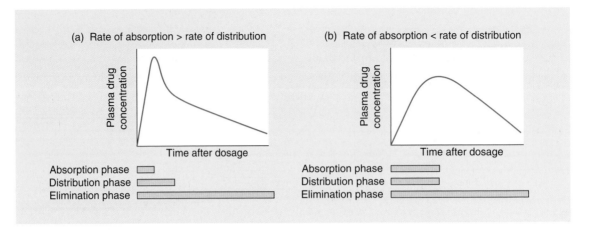

Fig. 2.16
Plasma concentration–time profiles after oral administration. The processes of distribution and elimination start as soon as some of the drug has entered the general circulation. A clear distribution phase is seen if the rate of absorption is extremely rapid, so that absorption is complete before distribution is finished (Fig. 2.16a). For most drugs, the rate of absorption is slow compared with the rate of distribution, and distribution occurs as rapidly as the drug is absorbed; therefore, distribution is complete when absorption is complete, and a clear distribution phase is not seen (Fig 2.16b).

- **Gastric emptying**. Basic drugs undergo negligible absorption from the stomach (see above). In consequence, there can be a delay of up to an hour between drug administration and the detection of drug in the general circulation (Fig. 2.17b).
- **Food**. The pattern of absorption can be affected by changes in gastric emptying (Fig. 2.17b) and food can alter the absorption rate, i.e. value of k_a (Fig. 2.17c).
- **Decomposition or first-pass metabolism prior to or during absorption**. This will reduce the amount of

drug that reaches the general circulation but will not affect the rate of absorption (which is usually determined by lipid solubility). Therefore, the curve is parallel but at lower concentrations (Fig. 2.17d).
- **Modified-release formulation**. If a drug is eliminated rapidly, the plasma concentrations will show rapid fluctuations during regular oral dosing, and patients may have to take the drug at very frequent intervals. This can be avoided by giving a tablet that releases drug at a slow and predictable rate over many

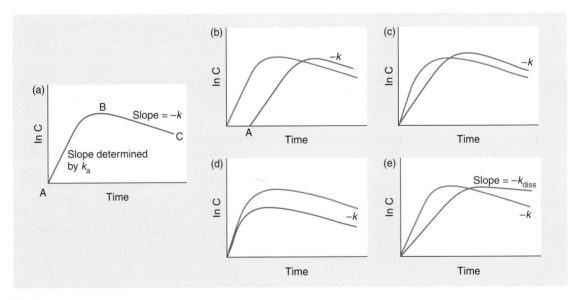

Fig. 2.17
Plasma concentration–time curves following oral administration. (a) General profile (A, start of absorption; B, end of absorption; B–C, elimination [rate = k]) (this 'normal' profile is repeated as a green line in panels b–e). (b) Influence of gastric emptying: there is a delay between $t = 0$ and A. (c) Influence of food: slower absorption results in a reduction in the absorption rate constant (k_a) derived from A–B. (d) Decrease in bioavailability (owing to incomplete dissolution of formulation, decomposition, increased first-pass metabolism). (e) Slow-release formulation: the rate at which the drug can be eliminated is limited by the rate at which the formulation disintegrates (k_{diss}).

hours: a modified-release formulation. The profile is affected by continuing absorption from the intestine, and the terminal slope of the concentration–time curve is then determined by the dissolution rate of the oral formulation, not by the elimination of the drug from the circulation (Fig. 2.17e).

Extent of absorption

The parameter that measures the extent of absorption is termed the *bioavailability* (*F*). This is defined as *the fraction of the administered dose that reaches the systemic circulation as the parent drug* (not as metabolites). For oral administration, incomplete bioavailability (*F*<1) may result from:

- incomplete absorption and loss in the faeces, either because the molecule is too polar to be absorbed or because the tablet did not release all of its contents
- first-pass metabolism, in the gut lumen, during passage across the gut wall or by the liver prior to the drug reaching the systemic circulation.

The bioavailability of a drug has important therapeutic implications, because it is the major factor determining the dosage requirements for different routes of administration. For example, if a drug has an oral bioavailability of 0.1, the oral dose needed for therapeutic effectiveness will need to be 10 times higher than the corresponding intravenous dose.

The bioavailability of a drug is normally determined by comparison of plasma concentration data obtained after oral administration (when the fraction *F* enters the general circulation as the parent drug) with data following intravenous administration (when, by definition, 100% enters the general circulation as the parent drug). The amount in the circulation cannot be compared at only one time point, because intravenous and oral dosing show different concentration–time profiles. This is avoided by using the total area under the plasma concentration–time curve (AUC) from $t = 0$ to $t =$ infinity (which is a reflection of the total amount of drug that has entered the general circulation):

$$F = \frac{AUC_{oral}}{AUC_{iv}} \tag{2.7}$$

if the oral and intravenous (iv) doses are equal or

$$F = \frac{AUC_{oral} \times Dose_{iv}}{AUC_{iv} \times Dose_{oral}} \tag{2.8}$$

if different doses are used.

This calculation assumes that the elimination (clearance – see below) is first-order. The AUC is a reflection of overall body exposure and is discussed below under clearance.

An alternative method to calculate *F* is to measure the total urinary excretion *of the parent drug* (Aex) following oral and intravenous doses (even in situations where the urine is a minor route of elimination), and:

$$F = \frac{Aex_{oral}}{Aex_{iv}} \tag{2.9}$$

for two equal doses.

Distribution

Distribution of a drug is the reversible movement of the parent drug from the blood into the tissues during administration and its re-entry from tissue into blood *as the parent drug* during elimination.

Rate of distribution

Because distribution is usually more rapid than absorption from the intestine (Fig. 2.16b), the rate of distribution can be measured reliably only following an intravenous bolus dose. Some drugs reach equilibrium between blood/plasma and tissues very rapidly and a distinct distribution phase is not apparent, and only the terminal elimination phase is seen after an intravenous injection (Fig. 2.18a). Most drugs take a finite time to distribute into, and equilibrate with, the tissues, which results in a rapid distribution phase (Slope A–B in Fig. 2.18b, which has a high rate constant), prior to the slower terminal elimination phase (slope B–C in Fig. 2.18b, which has a lower rate constant). In Figure 2.18b, the processes of distribution are complete by point B. The concentration–time curve in Figure 2.18b cannot be described by a single exponential term, and two first-order rates occur. By convention, the faster (distribution) rate is termed α and the slower (elimination) rate β. The distribution rate constant (α) cannot be derived directly from the slope A–B, because both distribution and elimination start as soon as the drug enters the body and A–B represents the summation of both processes. Back extrapolation of the terminal (β) phase gives an initial concentration at point D, which is the value that would have been obtained if distribution had been instantaneous. In practice, the distribution rate (α) is calculated for the difference between the line D–B for each time point and the actual concentration measured (given by the line A–B in Fig. 2.18b). The rate of distribution is only occasionally of clinical relevance. The time delay between an intravenous bolus dose and the response may be caused by the time taken for distribution to the site of action. Redistribution of intravenous drugs, such as thiopental (Ch. 17), may limit the duration of action (see Fig. 2.6).

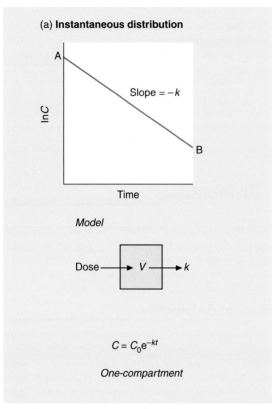

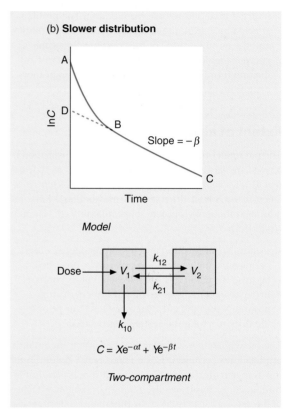

Fig. 2.18

Plasma concentration–time curves for the distribution of drugs into one- and two-compartment models. The terms k, α, β, k_{10}, k_{12}, k_{21}, are rate constants; α and β are composite rate constants which define the distribution and elimination rates. The terms α and β relate to distribution (k_{12} or k_{21}) and elimination (k_{10}) processes and are determined by k_{10}, k_{12}, and k_{21}. V are volumes of distribution, and X and Y are constants. (Note: the equation for a two-compartment system is usually written as $C = Ae^{-\alpha t} + Be^{-\beta t}$, where A and B are constants equivalent to X and Y; X and Y were used to avoid confusion with points A and B on the graph.)

Instantaneous and slow distributions are described by different mathematical models: the former is described as a *one-compartment model* (Fig. 2.18a), in which all tissues are in equilibrium instantaneously; the latter is described as a *two-compartment model* (Fig. 2.18b), in which the drug initially enters and reaches instantaneous equilibrium with one compartment (blood and possibly well-perfused tissues) prior to equilibrating more slowly with a second compartment (possibly poorly perfused tissues; refer back to Fig. 2.6). This is shown schematically in Figure 2.19.

The rate of distribution is dependent on two main variables:

- for *water-soluble drugs*, the rate of distribution depends on the rate of passage across membranes, i.e. the diffusion characteristics of the drug
- for *lipid-soluble drugs*, the rate of distribution depends on the rate of delivery (the blood flow) to those tissues, such as adipose, that accumulate the drug.

For some drugs, the natural logarithm of the plasma concentration–time curve shows three distinct phases; such curves require three exponential rates and represent a *three-compartment model*. Although two- or three-compartment models may be necessary to give a mathematical description of the data, they are of limited practical value.

Extent of distribution

The extent of distribution of a drug from plasma into tissues is of clinical importance because it determines the relationship between the measurable plasma concentration and the total amount of drug in the body (body burden). In consequence, the extent of distribution determines the amount of a drug that has to be administered in order to produce a particular plasma concentration (see below).

The extent of distribution of a drug from blood or plasma into tissues can be determined in animals by measuring concentrations in both blood and all the

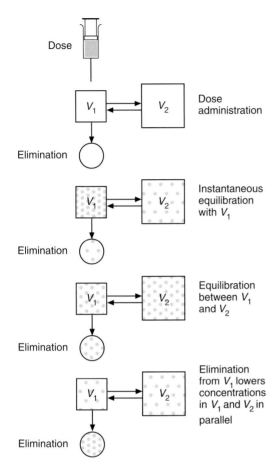

Fig. 2.19
Schematic diagram of drug distribution. (Note, at equilibrium, the total concentrations in V_1 and V_2 may be different, because of protein binding, etc.)

Dose administration

Instantaneous equilibration with V_1

Equilibration between V_1 and V_2

Elimination from V_1 lowers concentrations in V_1 and V_2 in parallel

tissues of the body. However, in humans, only the concentration in blood or plasma can be measured, and therefore the extent of distribution has to be estimated from the amount remaining in blood, or more usually plasma, after completion of distribution.

The parameter that describes the extent of distribution is the *apparent volume of distribution* (V), where:

$$V = \frac{\text{Total amount of drug in the body}}{\text{Plasma concentration}} \qquad (2.10)$$

The apparent volume of distribution is a characteristic property of the drug that, like half-life, bioavailability and clearance, is independent of dose. In the simple example shown by Figure 2.18a, if a dose of 50 mg of a particular drug is injected, this will mix instantaneously into the apparent volume of distribution V. If the initial plasma concentration is 1 µg ml⁻¹ (equivalent to point A on Fig. 2.18a), then the apparent volume of distribution will be given by:

$$V = \frac{\text{Total amount (dose)}}{\text{Plasma concentration}} = \frac{50\,000\ \mu g}{1\ \mu g\ ml^{-1}} = 50\,000\ ml = 50\ l$$

In other words, after giving the dose, it appears that the drug has been dissolved in 50 litres of plasma. However, plasma volume is only 3 litres and, therefore, much of the drug must have left the plasma and entered tissues, in order to give the low concentration present (1 µg ml⁻¹). The clinical relevance of V is shown when a physician needs to calculate how much drug should be given to a patient in order to produce a specific desired plasma concentration. If an initial plasma concentration of 2.5 µg ml⁻¹ of the same drug were needed for a clinical effect, this would be produced by giving a dose of [plasma concentration × V] or [2.5 µg ml⁻¹ × 50 000 ml] – that is, 125 000 µg or 125 mg.

In the more complex example shown in Figure 2.18b, the dose of 50 mg will distribute instantaneously only into V_1, which is usually termed the central compartment, and will usually comprise plasma and well-perfused tissues. Measurement of the initial concentration (point A in Fig. 2.18b) will not represent distribution into V_2 and the volume calculated using point A will under-represent the true extent of distribution (see Fig. 2.19). Distribution into V_2, which is usually termed the peripheral compartment and will usually comprise poorly perfused tissues, is not complete until point B in Figure 2.18b. However, by the time point B is reached, there will have been considerable elimination, and so the total amount of drug in the body is no longer known. This can be overcome by using the elimination phase (B–C in Fig. 2.18b) to back-extrapolate to the intercept (point D), which is the concentration that would have been obtained if distribution into V_2 had been instantaneous (see Equation 2.10):

$$V = \frac{\text{Dose}}{\text{Concentration at point D}} \qquad (2.11)$$

Alternative equations for the calculation of V are presented below.

V is not a physiological volume but simply a reflection of the amount of drug remaining in the blood or plasma after distribution and provides no information on where the drug has been taken up. Thus, a high value for V could result from either reversible accumulation in adipose tissue (owing to dissolution in fat) or reversible accumulation in liver and lung (owing to high intracellular protein binding). The actual tissue distribution can be determined only by measurement of tissue concentrations.

The value of V is usually calculated using the total concentration in plasma – that is, free (unbound) drug plus protein-bound drug. A low value for V can result if a drug is highly bound to plasma proteins but not to tissue proteins; if the drug shows an even higher affinity for tissue (lipid or protein; see Fig. 2.3), then it will have a high value for *V*. The term *V* reflects the *relative* affinity of plasma and tissues for a drug, and there is no simple relationship between plasma-protein binding and *V* (Table 2.9).

If the tissues have a very high affinity for the drug, the value of *V* will be extremely high and may greatly exceed the bodyweight. Chloroquine is a good example of such a drug (Table 2.9) and the value illustrates clearly that *V* should be regarded as a mathematical ratio (not as an indication of physiological distribution to an actual volume of plasma!).

The term *V* represents the volume of plasma that has to be cleared of drug by the organs of elimination, such as the liver and kidneys, which extract the drug from the plasma and remove it from the body by metabolism or excretion. It is independent of dose or concentration. Because *V* is constant, a twofold increase in plasma concentration will be accompanied by a twofold increase in the total amount of drug in the body (Equation 2.10). Although apparent volume of distribution may seem a rather abstract (and possibly even irrelevant) parameter, it is important for two reasons. Firstly, it is the parameter that relates the total body drug load present at any time to the plasma concentration. Secondly, together with clearance, it determines the overall elimination rate constant (*k*) and therefore the half-life. The half-life determines the duration of action of a single dose, the time interval between doses on repeated dosage and the potential for accumulation (see below).

Elimination

Elimination can also be described in terms of both *rate* and *extent*. The rate at which the drug is eliminated is important because it usually determines the duration of response, the time interval between doses, and the time to reach equilibrium during repeated dosing. The extent of elimination is eventually 100%. The *route* of elimination is important because it can determine the effects of renal/liver disease, age and drug interactions.

Table 2.9
The apparent volume of distribution (*V*) and plasma-protein binding of selected drugs

Drug	*V* (ℓ kg^{-1})	Binding (%)
Warfarin and furosemide	0.1	99
Aspirin	0.2	49
Gentamicin	0.3	<10
Propranolol	3.9	93
Nortriptyline	18.5	95
Chloroquine	185.7	61

Note: *V* is given in ℓ/kg body weight; therefore, for chloroquine, the total volume of distribution will be 13 000 ℓ per 70 kg patient.

Rate of elimination

The rate of elimination is usually indicated by the terminal half-life – that is, the half-life for the final (slowest) rate (*k* in Fig. 2.18a; *β* in Fig. 2.18b). The elimination half-lives of drugs range from a few minutes to many days (and, in rare cases, weeks). Precise knowledge about the half-life of every drug is not necessary and, therefore, in this book we have used the descriptive terms given in Table 2.10 to indicate the approximate half-life and the influence this would have on clinical use of the drug.

The rate at which a drug can be eliminated from the body, and therefore the half-life, is determined by two independent, biologically-determined variables: the activity of the mechanisms metabolising/excreting the drug and the extent of movement of drug from the blood into tissues.

The activity of the metabolising enzymes or excretory mechanisms. The organs of elimination (usually liver and kidneys) remove drug that is brought to them via the blood. Providing that first-order kinetics apply (in other words, the process is not saturated), a constant proportion of the drug carried in the blood will be removed on each passage through the organ of elimination, independent of the concentration in the blood. In

Table 2.10
Half-life descriptions used in this book

Description	Half-life (h)	Doses per day for chronic treatment	Comment
Very short	<1	–	A modified-release formulation may be preferred
Short	1–6	3–4	A modified-release formulation may be preferred
Intermediate	6–12	1–2	
Long	12–24	1	Once-daily dosage may be adequate
Very long	>24	1	Potential for accumulation

effect, this is equivalent to a constant proportion of the blood flow to the organ *being cleared of drug*. The more active the process (e.g. hepatic metabolism), the greater will be the proportion of the blood flow cleared of drug on one passage through the organ. For example, if 10% of the drug carried to the liver by the plasma (at a flow rate of 800 ml min^{-1}) is cleared, by uptake and metabolism, this is equivalent to a clearance of 10% of the plasma flow (80 ml min^{-1}); if 20% of the drug is cleared, this gives a clearance of 160 ml min^{-1}. The proportion of the blood flow cleared of drug will have units of volume per time (e.g. ml min^{-1}). The *plasma clearance* (CL) of the drug is the sum of all clearance processes (metabolism + renal + bile + exhalation + etc.) and is the volume of plasma cleared of drug per unit time; it is the best indication of the overall activity of the elimination processes.

$$CL = \frac{\text{Rate of elimination from the body}}{\text{Plasma concentration}} \qquad (2.12)$$

For example $\dfrac{\mu g\ min^{-1}}{\mu g\ ml^{-1}} = ml\ min^{-1}$

The plasma clearance is a characteristic value for a particular drug (see Table 2.11), is a constant for first-order (non-saturated) reactions, and is independent of dose or concentration. Because clearance is constant (Equation 2.12), a twofold increase in plasma concentration will be accompanied by a twofold increase in the rate of elimination. The greater the value of plasma clearance, the greater will be the rate at which the drug will be removed from the body, i.e. the elimination rate constant (k) is proportional to plasma clearance.

Reversible passage of drug from the blood into tissues. The organs of elimination can only act on drug that is delivered to them via the blood supply. If, after

equilibration with tissues, the blood or plasma concentration is very low, then V is very high. The low plasma concentration will result in a low rate of elimination from the body; in other words, the rate at which the drug can be eliminated will be limited by the extent of tissue distribution. Therefore, the elimination rate constant (k) is inversely proportional to the apparent volume of distribution.

$$k \propto \frac{1}{V} \qquad (2.13)$$

Plasma clearance

The overall rate of elimination is dependent on the two variables, the volume of plasma cleared per minute (CL) and the total apparent volume of plasma that has to be cleared (V):

$$k = \frac{CL}{V} \qquad (2.14)$$

or

$$t_{1/2} = \frac{0.693\,V}{CL} \quad \text{since } t_{1/2} = \frac{0.693}{k}$$

This is illustrated in Figure 2.20 and Table 2.11. The elimination rate constant (or half-life) is the best indication of changes in drug concentration with time, and for many drugs this will relate to changes in therapeutic activity following a *single dose*. Clearance is the best measurement of the ability of the organs of elimination to remove the drug and determines the average plasma concentrations (and therefore therapeutic activity) at *steady state* (see below). Clearance is usually determined using the area under the concentration–time curve (AUC).

Table 2.11
Pharmacokinetic parameters of selected drugs

	Clearance (ml min^{-1})	Apparent volume of distribution (ℓ per 70 kg)	Half-life (h)
Warfarin	3	8	37
Digitoxin	4	38	161
Diazepam	27	77	43
Valproic acid	76	27	5.6
Digoxin	130	640	39
Ampicillin	270	20	1.3
Amlodipine	333	1470	36
Nifedipine	500	80	1.8
Lidocaine	640	77	1.8
Propranolol	840	270	3.9
Imipramine	1050	1600	18

Note: The drugs are arranged in order of increasing plasma clearance. A long half-life may result from a low clearance (e.g. digitoxin), a high apparent volume of distribution (e.g. amlodipine) or both.

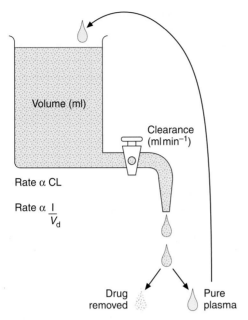

Fig. 2.20
The relationship between clearance, apparent volume of distribution and overall elimination rate. The drug is eliminated by the clearance process, which removes drug from a fixed volume of plasma per unit time. The drug is then separated and the pure plasma added back to the tank to maintain a constant volume (the apparent volume of distribution, V). The fluid, therefore, continuously recycles via the clearance process and the concentration of drug decreases exponentially. The time taken for one cycle is equal to the volume divided by the clearance (the greater the volume, the greater the time needed; however, the greater the clearance, the shorter the time).

$$CL = \frac{Dose}{AUC} \tag{2.15}$$

This simple equation is used to calculate clearance (one of the most important pharmacokinetic parameters) under the following conditions:

1. The dose must be given intravenously so that it is all available to the organs of elimination (i.e. $CL = Dose/AUC_{iv}$). For the oral route, only a fraction (F; see above) may reach the general circulation and therefore the dose used in the calculation should be the corrected dose (the administered dose $\times F$, as applied in Equation 2.8). Equation 2.8 is based on the fact that the clearance processes reflect what happens to the drug once it is in the general circulation and do not depend on the route of administration, and is a rearrangement of

$$CL = \frac{Dose_{iv}}{AUC_{iv}} = F \times \frac{Dose_{oral}}{AUC_{oral}}$$

2. The AUC should be the area under the concentration–time curve, not the logarithm of the concentration–time curve.

3. The AUC should be extrapolated to infinity.

Using Equations 2.14 and 2.15, V can be calculated and is more reliable than the extrapolation method given in Figure 2.18b:

$$CL = \frac{Dose}{AUC} = kV$$

$$V = \frac{Dose}{AUC \times k} \quad or \quad \frac{Dose}{AUC \times \beta} \tag{2.16}$$

Plasma clearance, as defined above, is the sum of all clearance processes and is the best measure of the functional status of the total body elimination. Measurement of specific processes such as metabolic clearance or renal clearance would require specific measurement of the rate of elimination by that process. In practice, this is only really possible for *renal clearance* (CL_r).

Renal clearance can be calculated from the rate of excretion in urine (*as the parent drug*) during a urine collection and the mid-point plasma concentration:

$$CL_r = \frac{\begin{array}{c}Rate\ of\ excretion\ in\ urine\\(as\ the\ parent\ drug)\end{array}}{Plasma\ concentration\ (mid-point)} \tag{2.17}$$

$$\frac{\mu g\ min^{-1}}{\mu g\ ml^{-1}} = ml\ min^{-1}$$

Alternatively, CL_r can be measured from the amount of parent drug excreted in urine over a known time interval (for example 48 h), divided by the AUC for the same time interval:

$$CL_r = \frac{Total\ amount\ of\ parent\ drug\ in\ urine_{(0-t)}}{AUC_{(0-t)}} \tag{2.18}$$

Measurement of renal clearance can be useful in a number of ways.

- Comparison of renal clearance with plasma clearance will show the importance of the kidney in the overall elimination of the compound; this can be of value in predicting the potential impact of renal disease.
- The difference between plasma and renal clearance is normally equivalent to **metabolic clearance** (which cannot be measured directly), and this can be of value in predicting the potential impact of liver disease.
- Comparison of renal clearance with the glomerular filtration rate (GFR), after allowance for protein binding, provides an estimate of the extent of either reabsorption (if clearance is less than GFR) or active secretion (if clearance is greater than GFR).
- Renal clearance can be changed by altering kidney function, for example by changing the urine pH, which can be useful in treating drug overdose (see Ch. 53).

Biliary clearance of a drug can be measured using the above approach, but in practice is seldom done, because of the difficulty of collecting bile samples.

Extent of elimination

The extent of elimination is of limited value because eventually all the drug will be removed from the body. Measurement of total elimination in urine, faeces and expired air as parent drug and metabolites can give useful insights into the extent of absorption, metabolism, and renal and biliary elimination.

Chronic administration

Long-term or chronic drug therapy is designed to maintain a constant concentration of the drug in blood, with an equilibrium (steady state) established between blood and all tissues of the body, including the site of action. In practice, a constant concentration can only be achieved by an intravenous infusion that has continued long enough to reach steady state (Fig. 2.21).

Time to reach steady state

During constant infusion, the time to reach steady state is dependent on the elimination half-life, and steady state is approached after four or five half-lives. Intuitively, it may seem peculiar that the elimination half-life determines the time required to reach equilibrium during

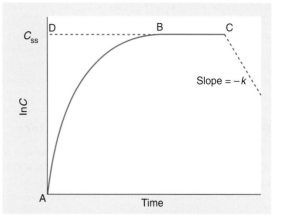

Fig. 2.21 **Constant intravenous infusion (between points A and C).** Steady state is reached at point B and the steady-state concentration (C_{ss}; given by D) can be used to calculate clearance: CL = rate of infusion/C_{ss} (see text). Clearance can also be calculated from the area under the total curve (AUC) and the total dose infused between A and C. The slope on cessation of infusion is the terminal elimination phase (k or β). The distribution phase is not usually detected because distribution is occurring throughout the period A to C. The apparent volume of distribution can be calculated as: V = Dose/(AUC × k). The *increase* to steady state is determined by the *elimination* rate constant and it takes approximately four to five half-lives to reach steady state.

constant input. The relationship is more readily understood if plasma concentrations following both increases and decreases in dose rate are considered (Table 2.12). The plasma concentration at steady state (C_{ss}) is directly proportional to the infusion rate; plasma concentrations reach 95% of the new steady-state conditions by four or five half-lives after a change in infusion rate.

Table 2.12
Plasma concentrations following a change in dosage[a]

	Drug concentration in plasma (ng ml^{-1}) after a change in dose rate (mg h^{-1})					Percentage change A-E
	A	B	C	D	E	
	(1 to 0)	(1 to 0.5)	(1 to 2)	(0 to 1)	(0 to 2)	
Initial concentration	100	100	100	0	0	0
After 1 half-life	50	75	150	50	100	50
After 2 half-lives	25	62.5	175	75	150	75
After 3 half-lives	12.5	56.25	187.5	87.5	175	87.5
After 4 half-lives	6.25	53.125	193.75	93.75	187.5	93.75
After 5 half-lives	3.125	51.5625	196.875	96.875	193.75	96.875
At infinity	0	50	200	100	200	100

[a]Theoretical changes in plasma concentrations of a drug that has been given by continuous intravenous infusion.
Notes:
The steady-state concentrations (initial and infinity) are directly proportional to the infusion rate.
The percentage changes (from initial conditions to infinity) are identical and independent of the rate of infusion.
After four or five half-lives, the change in concentration represents about 95% of the overall change to infinity (the new steady state).
Clearance = *rate of infusion*/C_{ss} = 1 000 000 ng h^{-1}/100 ng ml^{-1} = 167 ml min.$^{-1}$

Since the elimination half-life is dependent on both CL and V, each of these can contribute to any delay in achieving steady state. A drug with a large V will have a long half-life and, therefore, it will take a longer time to reach steady state. It is easy to envisage the slow filling of such a high volume of distribution during regular administration.

Plasma concentration at steady state

Once steady state has been reached, the plasma and tissues are in equilibrium, and the distribution rate constant and V will not affect the plasma concentration. The value of C_{ss} is determined solely by the balance between the rate of infusion and the rate of elimination (or clearance): from Equation 2.12, the rate of elimination equals $CL \times C_{ss}$, so that $CL \times C_{ss}$ = Rate of infusion or

$$C_{ss} = \frac{\text{Rate of infusion}}{CL} \qquad (2.19)$$

This relationship for an intravenous infusion can be used to calculate plasma clearance:

$$CL = \frac{\text{Rate of infusion}}{C_{ss}} \qquad (2.20)$$

Clearance and volume of distribution can also be calculated using the AUC between zero and infinity and the terminal slope after cessation of the infusion (see Fig. 2.21).

Oral administration

Most chronic administration is via the oral route, and the rate and extent of absorption need to be considered. Also, oral therapy is by intermittent doses and therefore there will be a series of peaks and troughs between doses (Fig. 2.22).

The *rate of absorption* will influence the interdose profile, since very rapid absorption will exaggerate fluctuations, while slow absorption will dampen down the peak.

The *extent of absorption*, or bioavailability (F), will influence the average steady-state concentration, because it determines the dose entering the circulation. The rate of input during chronic oral therapy is given by:

$$\frac{D \times F}{t} \qquad (2.21)$$

where D is the administered dose, F is bioavailability, and t is the interval between doses. At steady state, the rate of input is balanced by the rate of elimination, that is:

$$\frac{D \times F}{t} = CL \times C_{ss} \qquad (2.22)$$

Therefore:

$$C_{ss} = \frac{D \times F}{t \times CL} \qquad (2.23)$$

This is an important equation and reflects the balance between input and output, which is, in reality, a balance between the prescriber and the person taking the drug:

- The input of drug is determined by the prescriber, who can change C_{ss} by altering either the dose or the dose interval (and sometimes the bioavailability of the drug formulation).
- The removal of drug is determined by the characteristics of the individual taking the drug: metabolism/renal function can change C_{ss} by altering bioavailability and/or clearance.

Loading dose

A therapeutic problem may arise when a rapid effect is required for a drug that has a long or very long half-life; for example, the steady-state conditions will not be reached until 2–4 days if the half-life is 12–24 h, or over 4 or 5 weeks if the half-life is 1 week. Increasing the dose rate (for example, column E compared with column D in Table 2.12) does not reduce the time to reach steady state. A higher dose rate will reduce the time taken to reach any particular concentration, but plasma concentrations will continue to increase to give a higher steady-state level (after the same time interval of about four or five half-lives).

Any delay between the initiation of treatment and the attainment of steady state may be avoided by the administration of a *loading dose*. A loading dose is a high

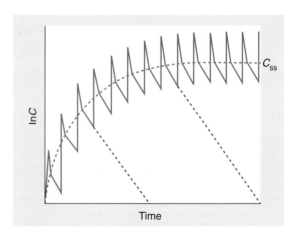

Fig. 2.22
Chronic oral therapy (——) compared with intravenous (----) infusion at the same dosage rate. The oral dose shows very rapid absorption and distribution followed by a more slow elimination phase within each dose interval. Cessation of therapy after any dose would produce the line shown in blue.

initial or first dose that, as the name implies, is designed to 'load up' the body. In principle, this is done by giving a first dose that is equivalent to the total steady-state body load which would be produced by the intended chronic dosage regimen. This will avoid the slow build-up to steady state, and the steady-state body load can then be maintained by giving the dosage regimen that would eventually have resulted in the same steady-state concentration. The amount of drug equivalent to the steady-state body load is the target C_{ss} multiplied by V (see Equation 2.10).

$$\text{Loading dose} = C_{ss} \times V \quad (2.24)$$

In cases where C_{ss} or V are not known, the loading dose can be calculated based on the proposed maintenance regimen by replacing C_{ss} with Equation 2.24 and V by CL/k (Equation 2.14):

$$\begin{aligned}\text{Loading dose} &= \frac{D \times F}{t \times CL} \times \frac{CL}{k} \\ &= \frac{D \times F}{t \times k} \\ &= \frac{D \times F \times 1.44 \times t_{1/2}}{t} \quad (2.25)\end{aligned}$$

It is clear from this last equation that the magnitude of any loading dose compared with the maintenance dose is proportional to the half-life.

Good examples of drugs that may require a loading dose are the cardiac glycosides digoxin and digitoxin, which are compared in Table 2.13. The values given in Table 2.13 are to illustrate the concept of a loading dose: the doses used clinically should take into account body-weight, age, and the presence of severe renal or liver impairment.

Loading doses may need to be given in two or three fractions over a period of about 24–36 h. The reason is that during tissue distribution of the loading dose, there are higher (non-steady-state) concentrations in the blood and rapidly equilibrating tissues, and lower (non-steady-

state) concentrations in the slowly equilibrating tissues (see Fig. 2.6). The excessive concentrations in rapidly equilibrating tissues may give rise to toxicity. This can be minimised by giving the loading dose in fractions, which would allow distribution of one fraction before the next was given. The fractional loading doses should be given within the period of the normal dose interval.

Factors affecting pharmacokinetics

A number of factors can affect the physiological processes of absorption, distribution and elimination. Aspects such as pregnancy, age, and diseases of the organs of elimination are discussed in Chapter 56. Clinically important variability arises from differences in bioavailability, V and CL:

- **drug interactions**: see Chapter 56, and the induction and inhibition of P450 discussed above
- **age**: see Chapter 56
- **diseases**, especially of the liver and kidneys: see Chapter 56
- **environmental factors**, for example alcohol and smoking
- **genetics**: this is becoming an increasingly important area and is discussed in detail below in relation to pharmacokinetics and in Chapter 4 in relation to receptors.

Pharmacogenomics, pharmacogenetics and drug responses

There are person-to-person variations for any biological property, including the responses to drug administra-

Table 2-13
Pharmacokinetics and dosage for digoxin and digitoxin

	Digoxin	Digitoxin
Elimination half-life (days)	1.6	7
Time to steady state (days; $4 \times t_{1/2}$)	6	28
'Therapeutic' plasma concentrations (ng ml^{-1} or µg l^{-1})	0.5–2.0	10–35
Volume of distribution (1/70 kg)	600	40
Typical loading dose ($C_{ss} \times V$) (mg)	up to 1.2	up to 1.4
Bioavailability (F)	0.75	>0.9
Normal oral maintenance dose (Dose $\times F/t$; mg per day)	0.125–0.5	0.05–0.2
Typical loading dose (maintenance dose $\times 1.44 \times t_{1/2}$) (mg)	0.3–1.2	0.5–2.0

tion. The nature of the response is usually similar in all individuals, because they share the same underlying biology, but the magnitude of the response to the same dose of a drug can differ markedly within a group of individuals. For many responses, this variation is reflected in a single Gaussian distribution (Fig. 2.23a), and such variability is an inherent part of the need to individualise dosage for the person. The presence of a polymorphism (Fig. 2.23b) can give rise to much wider person-to-person variation in response, such that some individuals may show no response, while others show toxicity at the same dose. The genetic origins of many polymorphisms is of increasing importance both in relation to drug development (see Ch. 3) and also because it allows the possibility in the future for genetic screening to be used to individualise drug and dosage selection.

Pharmacogenetics relates to how genetic differences between individuals affect the fate of a drug or the response to a drug. Pharmacogenetic research has been undertaken for more than four decades, largely in relation to in vivo variability, and has often used classic genetic techniques such as studies in twins and patterns of inheritance.

Pharmacogenomics relates to genome-wide approaches that define the presence of single-nucleotide polymorphisms (SNPs) in the genes which affect the activity of the gene product. Molecular biological techniques have allowed recognition of more than 1.4 million SNPs in the human genome. SNPs can be:

- in the upstream regulatory sequence of a coding gene, which can result in increased or decreased expression of the gene in response to the regulatory transcription factors that control that gene product; the gene product will be the same as the normal or 'wild' type of gene product
- in the coding region of the gene, which will result in a gene product with an altered amino acid sequence that may have higher activity (although this is unlikely), similar activity, lower activity or no activity at all.

In addition, there can be other inactive SNPs because they are in non-coding or silent regions of the genome, or because the base change does not alter the amino acid encoded (although this can result in altered expresson – see PGP below). In consequence, a major challenge for the future is not in identifying SNPs and the presence of genotypic differences, but rather in defining the functional consequences of the genetic difference and the magnitude of phenotypic differences. Future research will also focus on the importance of different combinations of genetic variants (haplotypes) rather than on single gene differences.

The rapid advances in molecular biology have allowed analysis of person-to-person differences in the sequences of the genes involved in drug metabolism and drug transport (pharmacokinetics) and receptors (pharmacodynamics). The earliest studies on pharmacogenetics were performed in relation to enzymes involved in drug metabolism. N-Acetyltransferase was one of the first drug metabolism pathways to be shown to have a genetic influence on both plasma concentrations of a drug (isoniazid) and the therapeutic

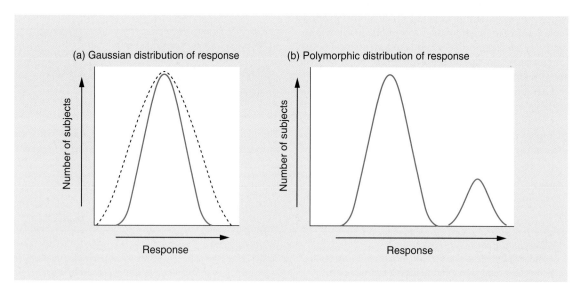

Fig. 2.23
Inter-individual variation in response to a single dose. The graphs show the numbers of individuals in a population showing a particular level of response to a single dose of a drug against the magnitude of the response. In Figure 2.23a, most individuals show the average response and the overall shape is a normal distribution. In a normal monomorphic distribution (Fig. 2.23a), the magnitude of inter-individual variability is indicated by the coefficient of variation (the dotted line in Figure 2.23a is for a response showing wider inter-individual variation). Both the coefficient of variation and the magnitude of the difference between phenotypes affect the variation in a polymorphic distribution (Fig. 2.23b).

response. Individuals with low enzyme activity, so-called 'slow acetylators', had higher blood concentrations of isoniazid and a better response but a greater risk of toxicity than did 'fast acetylators'. Because N-acetylation is a minor pathway of drug metabolism, pharmacogenetics remained of largely academic interest until the late 1970s, when it was found that CYP2D6 – one of the isoforms of cytochrome P450, the major drug-metabolising enzyme – showed a functionally important genetic polymorphism that could affect a wide

Table 2-14
Pharmacogenetic differences in drug-metabolising enzymes

Enzyme	Incidence of deficiency or slow-metaboliser status[a]	Typical substrates	Consequences of deficiency or slow-metaboliser status
Phase I reactions			
Plasma pseudocholinesterase	1 in 3000	Suxamethonium (succinylcholine)	Prolonged paralysis
Alcohol dehydrogenase	5–10% (approx. 90% in Asians)	Ethanol	Profound vasodilation on ingestion of alcohol
CYP2A6	?	Nicotine	Reduced nicotine metabolism
CYP2B6	?	Anticancer drugs?	Reduced metabolism – but functional importance is unclear
CYP2C9	About 3% (UK)	Tolbutamide, diazepam, warfarin	Increased response if parent drug is active
CYP2C19	5% (about 20% in Asians)	S-mephenytoin, omeprazole	Increased response if parent drug is active
CYP2D6	5–10%	Nortriptyline, codeine	Increased response if parent drug is active, but reduced response if oxidation produces the active form, e.g. codeine
Dihydropyrimidine dehydrogenase	1% are heterozygous	Fluorouracil	Enhanced drug response
Phase II reactions			
N-Acetyltransferase	50% (10–20% in Asians)	Isoniazid, hydralazine, procainamide	Enhanced drug response in slow acetylators
Glucuronyl-transferase 1A1	10% (1–4% in Asians)	Irinotecan (bilirubin)	Enhanced effect (Gilbert's syndrome)
Thiopurine S-methyl transferase	0.3%	Mercaptopurine, azathioprine	Increased risk of toxicity (because the doses normally used are close to toxic)
Catechol O-methyltransferase	25%	Levodopa	Slightly enhanced drug effect
Transporters			
PGP	A number of SNPs have been identified, the incidences of which vary with ethnic origins	Digoxin, anti-cancer drugs, dihydropyridines	Possibly higher drug levels with some SNPs, but lower drug levels due to increased activity with other SNPs

[a] Incidence for Caucasians
PGP, P-glycoprotein; SNP, single-nucleotide polymorphism

variety of different drugs. It is now known that the basic genotypic difference relates to the coding of an inactive enzyme in those without appreciable CYP2D6 activity – 'poor metabolisers' – but that 75 different alleles have been described and also there are variations in the number of copies of the coding region, with normal 'extensive metabolisers' having one copy of the normal gene, although individuals with up to 13 copies have been been identified. Cytochrome P450 was one of the earliest enzyme systems to be a focus of research on human genomics.

Knowledge of the precise nature of the differences (SNPs) for genetic polymorphisms is beyond the scope of an undergraduate text, and is not necessary to understand or appreciate either the current position or possible future developments in the area of pharmacogenomics. There is a well-established database on genetic differences in many of the major pathways of foreign compound metabolism (Table 2.14), and the functional consequences are outlined. Ethnic origins can affect the proportion of the population showing a genetic deficiency or polymorphism (see Table 2.14). In addition, the extent of metabolism in the general

population may be different; for example, subjects from the Indian subcontinent show a two- to threefold lower systemic clearance of nifedipine (a CYP3A substrate) compared with Caucasians, and this probably has a genetic basis in the control of enzyme expression.

There is an increasing interest in pharmacogenetics of transporter proteins. Although in its infancy, compared with pharmacogenetics of drug metabolism, the available data indicate that there are functionally important polymorphisms in some adenosine triphosphate (ATP)-binding transporter proteins. A number of SNPs have been identified in the *MDR1* gene, which codes for PGP, although the consequences of this for drug transport and for the aetiology of diseases are not clear. There are splice variants for the OAT transporters in the kidneys, but, again, the incidence and consequences of these for humans have not been defined.

Information on genetic polymorphisms and genetic variants of the enzymes and transporters involved in drug metabolism and biodisposition can be found on the OMIM™ (Online Mendelian Inheritance in Man™; John Hopkins University) database (**http://www.ncbi. nlm.nih.gov/entrez/dispomim.cgi?id=235200**).

FURTHER READING

Abdel-Rahman SM, Kauffman RE (2004) The integration of pharmacokinetics and pharmacodynamics: understanding dose–response. *Annu Rev Pharmacol Toxicol* 44, 111–136

Aweeka F, Greenblatt RM, Blaschke TF (2004) Sex differences in pharmacokinetics and pharmacodynamics. *Annu Rev Pharmacol Toxicol* 44, 499–523

Burckhardt BC, Burckhardt G (2003) Transport of organic anions across the basolateral membrane of proximal tubule cells. *Rev Physiol Biochem Pharmacol* 146, 95–158

Cholerton S, Daly AK, Idle JR (1992) The role of individual human cytochromes P450 in drug metabolism and clinical response. *Trends Pharmacol Sci* 13, 434–439

Daly AK (2003) Pharmacogenetics of the major polymorphic metabolizing enzymes. *Fundam Clin Pharmacol* 17, 27–41

de Boer AG, van der Sandt ICJ, Gaillard PJ (2003) The role of drug transporters at the blood–brain barrier. *Annu Rev Pharmacol Toxicol* 43, 629–656

Evans WE, McLeod HL (2003) Pharmacogenomics – drug disposition, drug targets, and side effects. *N Engl J Med* 348, 538–549

Fromm MF (2004) Importance of P-glycoprotein at blood–tissue barriers. *Trends Pharmacol Sci* 25, 423–429

Gonzalez TJ (1992) Human cytochromes P450: problems and prospects. *Trends Pharmacol Sci* 13, 346–352

Gurwitz D, Weizman A, Rehavi M (2003) Education: teaching pharmacogenomics to prepare future physicians and researchers for personalized medicine. *Trends Pharmacol Sci* 24, 122–125

Handschin C, Meyer UA (2003) Induction of drug metabolism: the role of nuclear receptors. *Pharmacol Rev* 55, 649–673

Lee G, Dallas S, Hong M, Bendayan R (2001) Drug transporters in the central nervous system: brain barriers and brain parenchyma considerations. *Pharmacol Rev* 53, 569–596

Lee W, Kim RB (2004) Transporters and renal drug elimination *Annu Rev Pharmacol Toxicol* 44, 137–166

Lin JH, Lu AY (2001) Interindividual variability in inhibition and induction of cytochrome P450 enzymes. *Annu Rev Pharmacol Toxicol* 41, 535–567

Marzolini C, Paus E, Buclin T, Kim RB (2004) Polymorphisms in human MDR1 (P-glycoprotein): recent advances and clinical relevance. *Clin Pharmacol Ther* 75, 13–33

Pirmohamed M, Park BK (2001) Genetic susceptibility to adverse drug reactions. *Trends Pharmacol Sci* 22, 298–305

Schwab M, Eichelbaum M, Fromm MF (2003) Genetic polymorphisms of the human *MDR1* drug transporter. *Annu Rev Pharmacol Toxicol* 43, 285–307

Tukey RH, Strassburg CP (2000) Human UDP-glucuronosyltransferases: metabolism, expression, and disease. *Annu Rev Pharmacol Toxicol* 40, 581–616

Weinshilboum R (2003) Inheritance and drug response. *N Engl J Med* 348, 529–537

Xie H-G, Kim RB, Wood AJJ, Stein MC (2001) Molecular basis of ethnic differences in drug disposition and response. *Annu Rev Pharmacol Toxicol* 41, 815–850

Self-assessment

1. The following statements describe drug pharmacokinetics. Are they true or false?

    a. The plasma clearance of a drug usually decreases with increase in the dose prescribed.
    b. First-pass metabolism may limit the bioavailability of orally administered drugs.
    c. Drugs that show high first-pass metabolism in the liver also have a high systemic clearance.
    d. The half-life of many drugs is longer in infants than in children or adults.
    e. A decrease in renal function may affect both systemic clearance and oral bioavailability.
    f. Benzathine benzylpenicillin has a prolonged half-life because the renal extraction of penicillin is reduced.
    g. Nifedipine is eliminated more rapidly in cigarette smokers.
    h. Chronic treatment with phenobarbital can increase the systemic clearance and oral bioavailability of co-administered drugs.
    i. A loading dose is not necessary for drugs that have short half-lives.
    j. An obese person is likely to show an increased volume of distribution and decreased clearance of prescribed drugs.
    k. Drugs are always taken with meals in order to reduce unwanted effects.

2. Figure 2.24 shows the changes in plasma levels of two drugs, A and B, given as 10-mg doses by oral and intravenous routes. From the plasma concentration–time curves, compare the two drugs for the following properties (do not perform detailed calculations):

    a. Absorption from the gut.
    b. Oral bioavailability.
    c. Distribution to tissues.
    d. Elimination half-life.
    e. Extent of accumulation during daily administration of each drug.

3. The pharmacokinetics of three drugs, A, B and C, were studied in the blood and urine of a healthy adult male volunteer (70 kg) following both oral and intravenous administration of 20-mg doses (Table 2.15). From the data given, compare:

    a. The extent of absorption (bioavailability, F) (you cannot calculate the rate of absorption from these data).
    b. The apparent volume of distribution (V) (you cannot calculate the rate of distribution from these data).

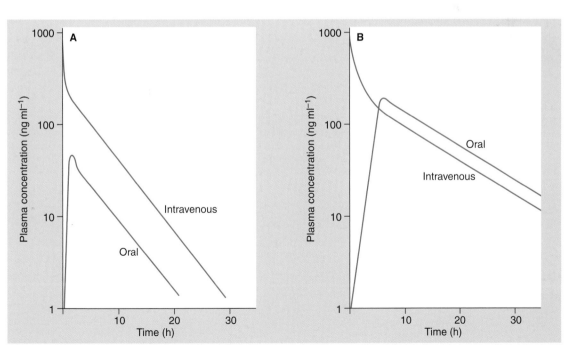

Fig. 2.24
Plasma concentration–time curves for two drugs.

Table 2.15
Data for question 3

Parameter	A		B		C	
	Intravenous	Oral	Intravenous	Oral	Intravenous	Oral
AUC (μg ml^{-1} min)	16	2	1000	995	40	26
Terminal slope (min^{-1})	0.0063	0.0063	0.00022	0.00022	0.014	0.003
Percentage of dose in urine (unchanged)	0		5		98	
Percentage of dose in urine as metabolites	100		95		0	

AUC, total area under the plasma concentration-time curve.

c. The elimination of these drugs (half-life, $t_{1/2}$) and clearance (CL, and route).

d. Their potential for accumulation during chronic dosage (related to half-life and interval between doses).

e. List genetic and environmental factors that may affect the disposition of these drugs (A, B, C,) in different individuals.

The answers are provided on pages 703–706.

3

Drug discovery, evaluation and safety

One of the features which is thought to distinguish man from other animals is his desire to take medicines

(Sir William Osler, 1849–1919)

Initially, most medicines were of botanical or zoological origin; however, since the 1950s, there has been an enormous increase in the use of synthetic organic chemicals. The recent introduction of molecules produced by recombinant DNA technology has extended this to agents identical to those of human origin: examples include epoetin (recombinant erythropoietin) and human insulins. The major benefit of drugs for the treatment of disease is illustrated most dramatically with antimicrobial chemotherapy. Antimicrobial chemotherapy has revolutionised the chances of patients surviving severe infections such as lobar pneumonia, the mortality of which was 27% in the pre-antibiotic era but fell to 8% (and subsequently less) following the introduction of sulphonamides and, subsequently, penicillins.

Early agents were often naturally occurring inorganic salts such as mercury compounds or plant extracts, often containing a mixture of complex organic compounds, more than one of which may have been the active constituent. The active constituents of many plant-derived preparations are nitrogen-containing organic molecules, which are also known as alkaloids; for example, laudanum is an alcohol extract of opium which contains high concentrations of the alkaloid morphine. Early therapeutic successes included the use of foxgloves (which contain cardiac glycosides) for the treatment of 'dropsy' (fluid retention); however, there was also considerable toxicity, because the plant preparations contained variable amounts of the active glycoside and such compounds have a narrow therapeutic index (Ch. 7).

A major advance in the development of safe medicines derived from natural sources was the isolation, purification and chemical characterisation of the active component. This had three main advantages:

- The administration of controlled amounts of the active compound removed any biological variability

in potency of the plant preparation, for example due to climatic or soil conditions where the plant grew.
- The active component with the desired effect could be given without also administering a cocktail of other unnecessary natural components; other components may have interfered with therapy by producing unrelated and unwanted effects or possibly reduced the desired effect by blocking the mechanism of action.
- The identification and isolation of the active component allowed the mechanism of action to be defined, leading to the synthesis and development of improved agents with the same action but with greater potency, greater selectivity, fewer unwanted effects, altered duration of action, greater absorption, etc.

Thus, although drug therapy has natural and humble origins, it is the application of scientific principles which has given rise to the clinical safety and efficacy of modern medicines.

A major advantage of modern drugs is their ability to act selectively, that is, to affect only certain specific body systems or processes. For example, a drug which both lowered blood glucose and reduced blood pressure would not be suitable for the treatment of someone with diabetes (because of unwanted hypotensive effects) or a person with hypertension (because of unwanted hypoglycaemic effects) or even those with both conditions (because different doses may be needed for each effect).

Drug discovery

The discovery of a new drug can be achieved in several different ways (Fig. 3.1). The simplest and crudest method is to subject new chemical entities (novel chemicals not previously synthesised) to a battery of screening tests that are designed to detect different types of biological activity. These include in vitro studies on isolated tissues, as well as in vivo studies of complex and integrated systems, such as animal behaviour. Chemicals for screening may be produced by direct chemical synthesis or may be isolated from biological sources, such as plants, and then purified and characterised. In general, this is not an efficient type of research, because, on average, several thousand chemicals are screened for each compound that eventually is marketed as a medicine.

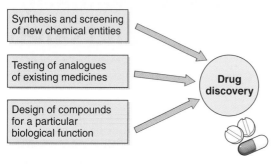

Fig. 3.1
Approaches to drug discovery.

A second approach involves the synthesis and testing of chemical analogues of existing medicines, but the products of this research usually show only minor advances in absorption, potency or a more selective action. However, unexpected additional properties may become evident when the compound is tried in humans; for example, minor modifications of the sulphanilamide antibiotic molecule gave rise to the thiazide diuretics and the sulphonylurea hypoglycaemics.

More recently, attempts have been made to design substances to fulfil a particular biological role, which may entail the synthesis of a naturally occurring substance (or a structural analogue), its precursor or an antagonist. Good examples include levodopa, used in the treatment of Parkinson's disease, the histamine H_2 receptor antagonists, and omeprazole, the first proton pump inhibitor. Logical drug development of this type depends on a detailed understanding of human physiology both in health and disease. Most recently, the modelling of receptor binding sites has facilitated the development of ligands with high binding affinities and, often, high selectivity.

The recent phenomenal advances in molecular biology and the unravelling of the human genome have led to the increasing use of genomic techniques, both to identify genes associated with pathological conditions and to develop compounds that can either mimic or interfere with the activity of the gene product. Such compounds are often proteins, which gives rise to problems of drug delivery to the relevant tissue and to the site of action, which may be intracellular. The potential of genomic research is enormous but currently under-exploited in relation to the development of marketed drugs. However, given the time and cost involved in getting a new drug approved (see below) it can be anticipated that we are currently seeing only the tip of the iceberg of drugs that will be developed based on these methods. A good example of the potential of genomic research is the drug imatinib (Ch. 52), which was developed to inhibit the enzyme Bcr-Abl tyrosine protein kinase, which was identified in chronic myelogenous leukaemia by molecular biological methods; Imatinib is a typical non-protein

organic molecule with a high oral bioavailability, and is eliminated by CYP3A4-mediated metabolism.

Information on genetic polymorphisms and genetic variants in possible targets for drug action can be found on the OMIM™ (Online Mendelian Inheritance in Man™; John Hopkins University) database (**http://www.ncbi.nlm.nih.gov/entrez/dispomim.cgi?id=235200**).

Drug approval

Each year, a vast number of synthetic novel compounds (new chemical entities) and pure compounds isolated from plant sources are screened for useful and/or novel pharmacological activities. Potentially valuable compounds are then subjected to a sequence of in vitro and in vivo animal studies and clinical trials, which provide essential information on safety and therapeutic benefit (Fig. 3.2).

All drugs and formulations licensed for sale in the UK have to pass a rigorous evaluation of:

- safety
- quality
- efficacy.

The UK Committee on Safety of Medicines (CSM – **http://www.mca.gov.uk/aboutagency/regframework/csm/csmhomemain.htm**) is one of a number of committees established under the Medicines Act (1968) to advise the Secretary of State for Health, via the Medicines and Healthcare products Regulatory Agency (MHRA – **http://www.mca.gov.uk/home.htm**), on the quality, safety and efficacy of all products licensed for medicinal use in the UK.

Harmonisation of drug regulation in the European Union (EU) has resulted in the establishment of a central organisation, in addition to national bodies. The European Agency for the Evaluation of Medicinal Products (EMEA – **http://www.emea.eu.int/index/indexh1.htm**) is responsible for medicines in the EU and receives advice from the Committee on Proprietary Medical Products (CPMP), which is a body of international experts equivalent to the CSM. Under the current systems, new drugs are evaluated by the CPMP, and national advisory bodies such as the CSM have an opportunity to assess the data before a final CPMP conclusion is reached.

Safety

Historically, the introduction of new drugs has been bought at a price of significant toxicity, and regulatory systems have arisen as much to protect patients from toxicity as to ensure benefit. The establishment of the Food and Drugs Administration (FDA – **http://www.fda.gov/cder/index.html**) in the USA followed a dramatic

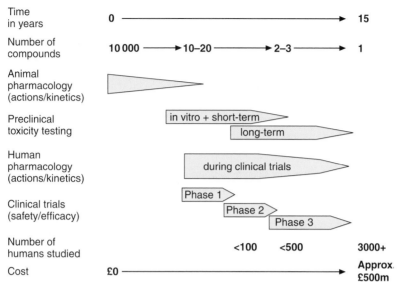

Fig. 3.2
The development of a new drug to the point at which a licence is approved. Postmarketing surveillance will continue to add data on safety and efficacy.

incident in 1937, when 76 people died of renal failure after taking an elixir of sulphanilamide which contained the solvent diethylene glycol. Similarly, some 30 years later, the occurrence of limb malformations (phocomelia) and cardiac defects in infants born to mothers who had taken thalidomide for the treatment of nausea in the first trimester of pregnancy led to the establishment of the precursor of the UK CSM.

Today, major tragedies are avoided by a combination of in vitro studies and animal toxicity tests (preclinical testing) and careful observation during clinical studies on new drugs (see below). The development and continuing refinement of preclinical toxicity testing has increased the likelihood of identifying chemicals with direct organ toxicity. During clinical trials, such adverse actions and immunologically-mediated effects are likely to be seen at the lower end of the dose range that are used in clinical trials (see Ch. 53).

Quality

An important function of regulatory bodies is to ensure the consistency of prescribed medicines. Drugs have to comply with defined criteria for purity, and limits are set on the content of any potentially toxic impurities. The stability – and, if necessary, sterility – of the drug also has to be established. Similarly, licensed formulations have to contain a defined, and approved, amount of the active drug, which has to be released at a specified rate. There have been a number of cases in the past where a simple change to the manufactured formulation has affected tablet disintegration, the release of drug and the therapeutic response. The quality of drugs for

human use is defined by the specifications in the British Pharmacopoeia and European Pharmacopoeia.

Efficacy

All medicines, apart from homeopathic products, must have evidence of efficacy for their licensed indications. Efficacy can be established only by trials in the patients for whom the medicine is intended, and therefore the demonstration of efficacy is a major aim of the later phases of clinical research (Fig. 3.2).

Establishing safety and efficacy

Regulatory bodies such as the CSM and CPMP require supporting data from in vitro studies, animal studies and clinical investigations before a new drug is approved. Although there is some overlap, the basic aims and goals are:

- **preclinical studies**: to establish the basic pharmacology, pharmacokinetics and toxicological profile of the drug and its metabolites, using animals and in vitro systems
- **phase I clinical studies**: to establish the human pharmacology and pharmacokinetics, together with a simple safety profile
- **phase II clinical studies**: to establish the dose–reponse and to develop the dosage protocol for clinical use, together with more extensive safety data

- **phase III clinical studies**: to establish the efficacy and safety profile of the drug in people with the proposed disease for which the drug will be indicated
- **pharmacovigilance**: to monitor adverse events following approval and the more widespread use of the drug.

Preclinical studies

Preclinical studies must be carried out before a compound can be given to humans. These studies investigate three areas:

- **pharmacological effects**: in vitro effects using isolated cells/organs; receptor binding characteristics; in vivo effects in animals and/or animal models of human diseases; prediction of potential therapeutic use
- **pharmacokinetics**: identification of metabolites (since these may be the active form of the compound); evidence of bioavailability (to assist with the design of both clinical trials and in vivo animal toxicity studies); establishment of principal route and rate of elimination
- **toxicological effects**: a battery of in vitro and in vivo studies undertaken with the aim of identifying toxicity as early as possible, and before there is extensive in vivo exposure of animals or, subsequently, of humans.

Toxicity testing

Toxicity testing has two primary goals: recognition of hazards and prediction of the likely risk of that hazard occurring in humans receiving therapeutic doses. A wide range of doses is studied; high doses are required to increase the ability to detect hazards, and lower doses are needed to predict the risk at doses producing the anticipated therapeutic effect. Toxicity tests include the following:

- **Mutagenicity**: a variety of in vitro tests using bacteria and mammalian cell lines are employed at an early stage to define any potential damage to DNA that may be linked to carcinogenicity or teratogenicity.
- **Acute toxicity**: a single dose is given by the route proposed for human use; this may reveal a likely site for toxicity and is essential in defining the initial dose for human studies. Acute toxicity data are essential for safe manufacture; the LD_{50} (a precise estimate of the dose required to kill 50% of an animal population) has been replaced by simpler and more humane methods that define the dose range associated with acute toxicity.
- **Subacute toxicity**: repeated doses are given for 14 or 28 days; this will usually reveal the target for toxic

effects, and comparison with single-dose data may indicate any potential for accumulation.
- **Chronic toxicity**: repeated doses are given for up to 6 months; this reveals the target for toxicity (except cancer). The aim is to define dose regimens associated with adverse effects and a no-observed adverse effect level ('safe' dose).
- **Carcinogenicity**: repeated doses are given throughout the lifetime of the animal (usually 2 years in a rodent bioassay).
- **Reproductive toxicity**: repeated doses are given from prior to mating and throughout gestation to assess any effect on fertility, implantation, fetal growth, the production of fetal abnormalities (teratogenicity) and neonatal growth.

The extent of animal toxicity testing required prior to the first administration to humans is related to the proposed duration of human exposure and the population to be treated. All drugs are subjected to an initial in vitro screen for mutagenic potential: if satisfactory, this is followed by acute and subacute studies for up to 14 days of administration to two animal species.

An international review of the extent of in vivo animal testing necessary prior to phase I and phase II clinical trials has concluded that the duration of animal toxicity tests should be the same as proposed human exposure (Table 3.1). The same advice applies for phase III studies in Japan and the USA, but the EU recommends more extensive animal studies, i.e. 1-month studies in rodents and non-rodents for a 2-week phase III human trial, 3 months in animals for a 1-month phase III study in humans, and 6 months in rodents and 3 months in non-rodents for a 3-month phase III human trial. Dogs are the 'non-rodent species' usually studied.

Table 3.1

European Medicines Evaluation Agency (EMEA) guidelines for the length of animal toxicity studies necessary to support phase I and phase II studies in humans.

Duration of clinical trial	Minimum duration of repeat-dose animal toxicity studies	
	Rodents	**Non-rodents**
Single dose	2 weeks	2 weeks
Up to 2 weeks	2 weeks	2 weeks
Up to 1 month	1 month	1 month
Up to 3 months	3 months	3 months
More than 3 months	6 months	6 months

Adapted from EMEA guidance at
http://www.emea.eu.int/pdfs/human/ich/028695en.pdf

Teratogenicity and reproductive toxicity studies are required if the drug is to be given to women of child-bearing age; rabbits have been used for teratogenicity studies since the thalidomide tragedy, because, unlike rodents, they show fetal abnormalities when treated with thalidomide. Carcinogenicity testing is necessary for drugs that may be used for long periods, for example over 1 year.

The use of animals for the establishment of chemical safety is an emotive issue, and there is extensive current research to replace in vivo animal studies with in vitro tests based on known mechanisms of toxicity. Despite these advances, toxicology as a predictive science is still in its infancy, and at present it is impossible to replicate the complexity of mammalian physiology and biochemistry by in vitro systems. In vivo studies remain essential to investigate both interference with integrative functions and complex homeostatic mechanisms. Carefully controlled safety studies in animals are an essential part of the current procedures adopted to prevent extensive human toxicity, which would inevitably result from the use of untested compounds. Although toxicology has failed in the past to prevent some tragedies (see above), these have led to improvements in methods, and current tests provide an effective predictive screen. However, it is worth noting that, even recently, there are examples of approved drugs which have had to be withdrawn because of severe reactions that were not detected in preclinical studies. Examples are rofecoxib (p. 364) and the 'statin' cerivastatin.

Students should be aware that not all hazards detected at very high doses in experimental animals are of relevance to human health. An important function of expert advisory bodies such as the CSM and the CPMP is to assess the relevance to human health of effects detected in experimental animals at doses that may be two orders of magnitude (or more) above human exposures. Many 'chemical scare' stories in the media are based on a hazard detected at high experimental doses in animals rather than the relevant risk estimated for human exposures.

Premarketing clinical studies: phases I–III

The purposes of premarketing clinical studies are:

- to establish that the drug has a useful action in humans
- to define any toxicity at therapeutic doses in humans
- to establish the nature of common (type A) unwanted effects (see Ch. 53).

Traditionally, premarketing clinical studies have been subdivided into three phases, but the distinction between these is blurred and there are differences of opinion about the classification system that follows.

Phase I studies

Phase I is the term used to describe the first few administrations of a new drug to humans. A principal aim of these studies is to define basic properties, such as route of administration, pharmacokinetics and metabolism, and tolerability. The studies are usually carried out by the pharmaceutical company, often using a specialised contract research organisation. Subjects taking part in phase I studies are often healthy volunteers recruited by open advertisement, especially when the compound is of low toxicity and has wide potential use, for example an antihistamine. In some cases, people suffering from the condition in which the drug will be used may be studied, for example cytotoxic agents used for cancer chemotherapy.

The first few administrations are usually by mouth in a dose that may be as low as one-fiftieth of the minimum required to produce a pharmacological effect in animals (after scaling for differences in bodyweight). Depending upon what is found, the dose may be then built up, either in small increments or by doubling, until a pharmacological effect is observed or an unwanted action occurs. During these studies, toxic effects are looked for by means of routine haematology and biochemical investigations of liver and renal function; other tests, including an electrocardiogram, will be performed as appropriate. It is also usual to study the disposition, metabolism and main pathways of elimination of the new drug in humans at this stage. Such studies help to identify not only the most suitable dose and route of administration for future clinical studies but also the choice of appropriate animal species for further toxicity studies. Investigations of drug metabolism and pharmacokinetics often necessitate the use of radioactively labelled compounds containing carbon-14 or tritium (^{3}H) as part of the drug molecule.

Phase II studies

During phase II studies, the detailed clinical pharmacology of the new compound is determined, by skilled investigators, in people with the intended clinical condition. A principal aim of these studies is to define the relationship between dose and pharmacological and/or therapeutic response in humans. Evidence of a beneficial effect will normally emerge during phase II studies. However, the large subjective element in human illness may make it difficult to distinguish between pharmacological and placebo effects. Additional studies may be undertaken at this stage in special groups: for example, elderly people, if it is intended that the drug will be used in that population. Other studies may investigate the mechanism of action or test for potential interactions with other drugs. The optimum dosage regimen should be defined in the phase II studies, and this is then used in large clinical trials, which aim to demonstrate the efficacy and safety of the drug.

Phase III studies

The phase III studies are the main clinical trials and usually involve comparison with a placebo that looks (and tastes) similar to the active compound. However, it is difficult to justify the use of a placebo once an effective form of treatment has been established for a condition, and lack of treatment may result in risk to the individual. It is normal to establish the advantages and disadvantages of the new compound by comparison with the best available treatment or the leading drug in the class. In these trials, the drug under evaluation may be used alone or given with other established treatment for the disease being treated. In some circumstances (e.g. cancer chemotherapy), the new agent or placebo is added to the best available current treatment.

Clinical trials are of two main types (Fig. 3.3): within-subject and between-subject comparisons. In within-subject trials, an individual is randomly allocated to commence treatment with either the new compound or its comparator before 'crossing over' to the alternative therapy. By contrast, between-subject comparisons involve randomisation to receive one or other of two (or more) treatments.

Within-subject comparisons can usually be performed on a smaller number of subjects (about half that required for between-subject studies), since the individual acts as his or her own control and most other variables are, therefore, eliminated. However, such studies often require longer involvement of each individual and there may be carry-over effects from one treatment that affect the apparent efficacy of the alternative therapy. Studies of this type may be difficult to interpret when there is a pronounced seasonal variation in the severity of a condition, such as Raynaud's phenomenon or hayfever. Crossover studies (Fig. 3.3) cannot be used if the treatment is curative, for example, an antibiotic for treating acute infections.

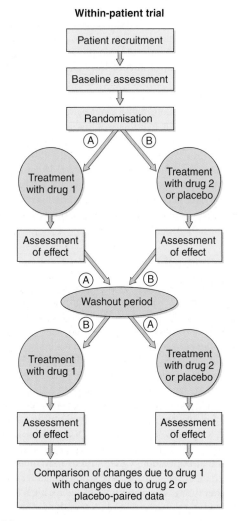

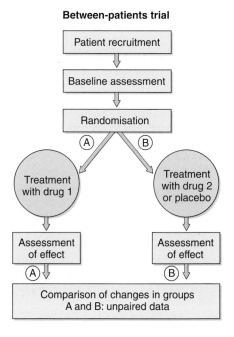

Fig. 3.3
The design of clinical trials. Subjects are randomly allocated to group A or group B.

Between-subject comparisons require roughly twice as many participants but have the advantages that each subject will usually be studied for shorter periods of time and carry-over effects are avoided. Although it is not possible to provide a perfect match between subjects entering the two (or more) different treatment groups, this approach to the evaluation of new drugs is preferred by many drug regulatory authorities.

Whichever form of comparison is made, measurements of benefit (and adverse effects) are made at regular intervals using a combination of objective and subjective techniques (Table 3.2). Throughout these studies, careful attention is paid to the detection and reporting of both unwanted effects (type A reactions) and other unpredictable type B reactions (Ch. 53). However, the majority of the latter are not seen prior to the marketing of a new drug, because they may occur only once in every 1000–10 000 or more individuals treated with the drug. It is salutary to note that, by the time a new medicine is marketed, only 2000–3000 people may have taken the drug, usually for short periods. Only a few hundred people may have 6 months or more of exposure to the new compound and the total experience may amount to no more than 500 patient-years (1000 patients taking the drug for 6 months is 500 patient-years).

Postmarketing surveillance: phase IV

Phase IV studies involve pharmacovigilance (postmarketing surveillance) and further postmarketing studies of efficacy, sometimes for additional indications to those licensed. The full spectrum of benefits and risks of medicines may not become clear until after marketing. Reasons for this include the low frequency of certain adverse drug reactions, and the tendency to avoid the inclusion of children, the elderly and women of childbearing age in premarketing clinical studies. Another factor is the widespread use of other medicines in normal clinical practice, which could produce an unexpected interaction with the new drug.

Two main systems of pharmacovigilance, or postmarketing surveillance, are in use in the UK. The first and most important is known as the yellow card system; it depends upon doctors reporting suspected serious adverse reactions directly to the MHRA using postage prepaid cards (available in the British National Formulary [BNF], GP prescribing pads and the Monthly Index of Medical Specialties [MIMS]). In addition to reporting suspected serious adverse effects of established drugs, doctors are asked to supply information about all unwanted effects of medicines that have been marketed recently. These products are identified by the use of inverted black triangles in the BNF, MIMS and summary of product characteristics. Each year, the MHRA receives some 20 000 yellow cards/slips. In return for their efforts, doctors are supplied at regular intervals with an information circular about current drug-related problems.

The second form of pharmacovigilance involves systematic postmarketing surveillance of recently marketed medicines. This may be organised by the pharmaceutical company responsible for the manufacture of the new drug (companies also receive information via their representatives).

Prescription event monitoring (PEM) provides a method for the detailed further study of observations or possible associations provided by pharmacovigilance programmes. This involves the identification by the Prescription Pricing Authority of individuals who have been prescribed a drug of interest, and the subsequent distribution of 'green cards' to the individuals' GPs, with a request that they complete all details about the person and events that occurred. The cards are then returned to the coordinating unit in Southampton, where the data are analysed. PEM has the advantage that it does not require doctors to make a value judgement concerning a link between the prescription of a drug and any medical event that occurs in the subject while receiving the drug. At first sight, a broken leg may be thought an unlikely drug adverse effect, but it could be the result of drug-related hypotension, ataxia or metabolic bone disease.

Finally, detailed monitoring of adverse reactions to drug therapy takes place in certain hospitals. These data contribute further to our overall knowledge. The future computerisation of medical records, including drug prescribing, offers the promise of more rapid identification of adverse events and a greater ability to investigate possible associations between prescription and adverse events.

Recent developments in information about the beneficial and adverse effects of drugs have been:

- the use of systematic meta-analyses of clinical trials' data

Table 3.2
Examples of response measurements during clinical trials

New drug type	Measurement techniques	
	Objective	Subjective*
Antianginal	Exercise tolerance	Fatigue
	Blood pressure	Frequency of anginal
	Heart rate	attacks
	GTN use	Pain intensity
Antiarthritic	Grip strength	Duration of morning
	Joint size	stiffness
	Paracetamol use	Pain intensity

*Subjective effects are often quantified by the use of a 10 cm visual analogue scale, e.g. 0 cm = no pain at all; 10 cm = the worst pain I have ever had.
GTN, glyceryl trinitrate.

- the establishment in the UK of the National Institute for Clinical Excellence (NICE).

Combining the data from a number of similar clinical trials can provide an overview of the validity and reproducibility of clinical findings. The statistical method used, meta-analysis, is complex and only trials of a similar design, including outcome measures, sensitivity, duration, etc., should be combined. The Cochrane database (**http://www.update-software.com/cochrane/**) provides a regularly updated collection of evidence-based medicine; the abstracts in the database can be searched without charge.

NICE (**http://www.nice.org.uk/**) was established in 1999 as an independent organisation responsible for providing national guidance on treatments and care for people using the NHS in England and Wales. It provides advice on the clinical value and cost-effectiveness of new treatments, but also on existing treatments if there is uncertainty about their use. Their information leaflet states that NICE produces guidance on:

- the use of new and existing medicines and treatments within the NHS in England and Wales (technology appraisals)
- the appropriate treatment and care of people with specific diseases and conditions within the NHS in England and Wales (clinical guidelines)
- whether interventional procedures used for diagnosis or treatment are safe and work well enough for routine use (interventional procedures).

Reference is made to NICE guidance in this book in those cases where a drug has limited recommended uses in the UK, despite having a full entry in the BNF.

FURTHER READING

Austin CP (2004) The impact of the completed human genome sequence on the development of novel therapeutics for human disease. *Annu Rev Med* 55, 1–13

Dollery C (2003) The clinical pharmacologist's view; drug discovery and early development. In: Wilkins MR (ed) *Experimental therapeutics*. London: Martin Dunitz, Taylor and Francis; pp 3–24

Kerwin R (2004) The National Institute for Clinical Excellence and its relevance to pharmacology. *Trends Pharmacol Sci* 25, 346–348

Lynch A, Connelly J (2003) The toxicologist's view; non-clinical safety assessment. In: Wilkins MR (ed) Experimental Therapeutics. London: Martin Dunitz, Taylor and Francis; pp 25–50

McLeod HL, Evans WE (2001) Pharmacogenomics: unlocking the human genome for better drug therapy. *Annu Rev Pharmacol Toxicol* 41, 101–121

Shah RR, Branch SK, Steele C (2003) The regulator's view; regulatory requirements for marketing authorizations for new medicinal products in the European Union. In: Wilkins MR (ed) Experimental Therapeutics. London: Martin Dunitz, Taylor and Francis; pp 51–75

The nervous system, neurotransmission and the peripheral autonomic nervous system

There are two principal, interrelated neuronal systems in the body:

- the central nervous system (CNS), which comprises the brain and spinal cord
- the peripheral nervous system, which connects the CNS to the organs of the body; it includes afferent nerves from the peripheral tissues to the CNS, efferent nerves to involuntary muscles and other tissues (the autonomic nervous system [ANS] – see Fig. 4.8), and efferent nerves from the CNS to voluntary muscles via the neuromuscular junction (the somatic nervous system – see Ch. 27).

The CNS, therefore, has an integrating role:

- receiving information via visceral afferents (e.g. from viscera, smooth muscle and cardiac muscle) and somatic afferents (from skeletal muscle, joints and skin)
- sending instructions via the autonomic efferents (to glands, smooth muscle and cardiac muscle) and somatic motor efferents (to skeletal muscle) (Fig. 4.1).

The basic unit of the nervous system is the neuron, which usually consists of a cell body (or soma), an axon (which transmits the impulse to another nerve or an effector organ) and dendrites (which receive impulses from other nerves). Both axons and dendrites may show

numerous branches. The interconnections between neurons are known as synapses.

The human brain contains approximately 10^{12} neurons, each of which may connect via synapses with hundreds or even thousands of other neurons. The neurons and interconnections may occur in well-defined areas or tracts and control specific functions or activities, but some areas of the brain represent a more diffuse network, for example the cerebral cortex. In the peripheral nervous system, the axons tend to be longer and less branched than those in the CNS.

There are three main types of neuron–neuron synapse (Fig. 4.2):

- axo-dendritic: the axon of the transmitting (innervating) cell forms a synaptic knob with the dendrite of the receiving (innervated) cell; this type accounts for 98% of synapses in the cortex
- axo-somatic: the axon of the innervating cell makes a synapse on the cell body of the innervated cell
- axo-axonal: the synapse with the axon of the innervating cell is on the axon of the innervated cell; this type usually serves to alter the local release of neurotransmitter from the receiving cell (for example, see opioid analgesics, Ch. 19).

Synapses and interconnections are so numerous in the brain that about 50% of the total surface area of neuronal cells, and their processes, is covered by synapses. The

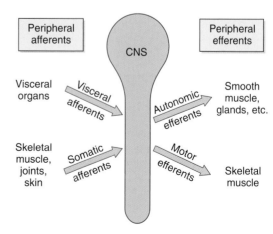

Fig. 4.1
The major neuronal connections of the central nervous system (CNS).

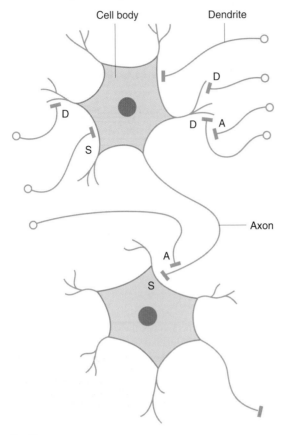

Fig. 4.2
Types of interneuronal synapses in the central nervous system.
D, axo-dendritic; S, axo-somatic; A, axo-axonal.

CNS shows a far greater range of types of interneuronal junction compared with the peripheral nervous system.

Neurotransmission

The synapse

The action potential in a nerve represents a wave of depolarisation in which the normally electronegative cytosol becomes positive owing to the opening of voltage-gated Na^+ channels and the influx of Na^+. This influx causes slight depolarisation further along the axon, and the adjacent Na^+ channels open, causing full depolarisation, thereby propagating or conducting the action potential along the axon. The propagation along nerves is fast and conduction velocities range from 1 to 100 m s^{-1}, depending on the type of nerve fibre (see Ch. 18).

Depolarisation is propagated along the axon to its end, until the synaptic knob is reached.

The synapse is responsible for transfer of the signal, represented by the action potential, to the adjoining innervated nerve (via one of the connections shown in Fig. 4.2). In mammals, the signal is transferred in the form of a 'chemical message'; the chemical that is released is called a *neurotransmitter*. There are a large number of different neurotransmitters, and each transmitter has its own specific processes for synthesis, storage, release, reuptake and inactivation, as well as its own family of receptors. In consequence, neurotransmission is a particularly fertile area for drug action, affecting the CNS and the peripheral somatic and autonomic systems. A schematic for 'typical' neurotransmission is given in Figure 4.3.

The typical neurotransmitter is either synthesised in the soma and transferred to the nerve terminal (e.g. peptides), or synthesised locally in the presynaptic nerve terminal by enzymes that are produced by protein synthesis in the cell soma and transported along the axon to the nerve terminal (e.g. acetylcholine and noradrenaline).

The neurotransmitter is taken up from the cytosol within the nerve ending and enclosed within membrane vesicles using a specific transporter (Fig. 4.3). This results in a low concentration of neurotransmitter free in the cytoplasm, which allows the synthesising enzyme to make large amounts of the neurotransmitter, without a build-up of the product switching off further synthesis (end-product inhibition). The transmitter within the vesicle may form a complex; for example, noradrenaline forms a complex with adenosine triphosphate (ATP), which reduces the free concentration of noradrenaline within the vesicle. When the action potential, associated with the opening of Na^+ channels, reaches the presynaptic nerve terminal, it causes the opening of voltage-gated Ca^{2+} channels (Ch. 1). The influx of Ca^{2+} causes the membranes of the vesicles to fuse with the presynaptic cell membrane and release the neurotransmitter into the synapse. The membrane of the vesicle is recovered by endocytosis and 'refilled' for later use. The neurotransmitter binds to the receptors on the pre- or postsynaptic membrane and thereby transmits the signal to the innervated cell, via its action at the receptor (see Ch. 1 for the characteristics of different types of receptor).

There is an equilibrium established between neurotransmitter (NT) free in the synapse, the receptors (R) and the neurotransmitter–receptor complex (NTR).

$$[NT] + [R] \rightleftharpoons [NTR]$$

The higher the concentration of neurotransmitter, the greater the number of receptors that will be occupied and the greater the likelihood of postsynaptic depolarisation and hence transmission of the impulse to the innervated neuron, or of postsynaptic changes at a neuroeffector junction (such as smooth muscle contraction).

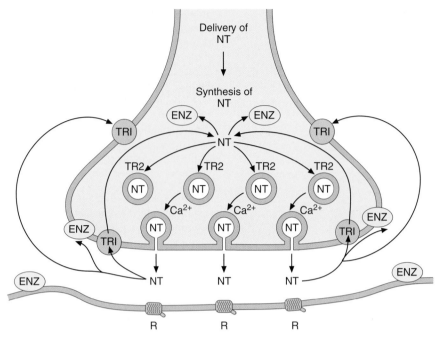

Fig. 4.3
Generalised scheme for synaptic transmission. NT, neurotransmitter (which is either synthesised in the soma and delivered to the nerve terminal [e.g. peptides] or synthesised locally in the nerve terminal [e.g. catecholamines and acetylcholine]); ENZ, enzyme that metabolises NT to inactive products; TR1, specific transporter that carries NT from the synaptic cleft into the cytoplasm of the presynaptic axon; TR2, specific transporter that carries NT from the cytoplasm into the vesicles; R, receptor on postsynaptic membrane, which binds NT and produces the appropriate change in the postsynaptic cell (there are also presynaptic receptors; see text for details). Ca^{2+}, involved in transmitting the signal (see text for details).

The association of the neurotransmitter and the postsynaptic receptor is only transient, because the concentration of transmitter within the synapse decreases very rapidly. Two main processes can be involved in lowering the concentration of neurotransmitter:

- specific carriers can transport the neurotransmitter back into the presynaptic nerve ending
- inactivating enzymes around the synapse can metabolise the neurotransmitter.

As the concentration of neurotransmitter decreases, so the neurotransmitter–receptor complex will dissociate to re-establish the equilibrium, thereby reducing receptor occupancy and stopping the signal on the postsynaptic cell.

The release of the neurotransmitter can be 'fine-tuned' by axo-axonic connection and by presynaptic receptors (which are discussed below).

Electrophysiological consequences of neurotransmission

Binding of the neurotransmitter to the receptor on the postsynaptic membrane may result in a range of pos-

sible effects, depending on the type of the receptor and the system to which it is coupled (see Ch. 1). Receptor binding can either activate (excite) or inhibit the innervated neuron or cell.

Excitatory effects

With excitatory transmission, binding of the neurotransmitter to a sufficient number of receptors on the postsynaptic membrane causes depolarisation of the membrane, giving rise to an excitatory postsynaptic potential (EPSP). The current inflow caused by the release of small numbers of synaptic vesicles is insufficient to cause generalised depolarisation, which only occurs when a threshold potential is reached (see Ch. 8); the release of small numbers of vesicles serves to increase the excitability of the innervated neuron. EPSPs decay rapidly because the resting potential is maintained by the activity of a range of ion channels and Na^+/K^+-ATPase, which maintains the concentration gradients of Na^+ (high outside the cell) and K^+ (high inside cell) (Fig. 4.4). These homeostatic processes reverse changes in ion concentrations across the membrane. Summation of the effects of the release of a large number of synaptic vesicles within a short time (a few milliseconds), giving a period of high receptor occupancy, is necessary to reach the threshold potential, above which an action potential will occur in the innervated neuron. The main ionic mechanism for an EPSP is the opening of a Na^+ channel

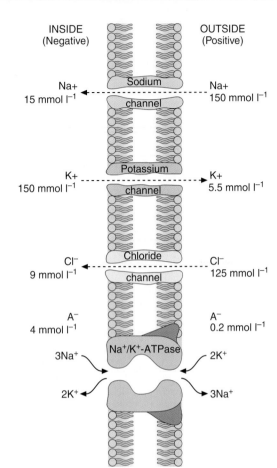

INSIDE
(Negative)

OUTSIDE
(Positive)

Na+
15 mmol l⁻¹

Sodium
channel

Na+
150 mmol l⁻¹

K+
150 mmol l⁻¹

Potassium
channel

K+
5.5 mmol l⁻¹

Cl⁻
9 mmol l⁻¹

Chloride
channel

Cl⁻
125 mmol l⁻¹

A⁻
4 mmol l⁻¹

A⁻
0.2 mmol l⁻¹

3Na⁺

Na⁺/K⁺-ATPase

2K⁺

2K⁺

3Na⁺

Fig. 4.4
Factors influencing the resting potential. The inside of the resting cell membrane is negative with respect to the outside because the diffusion of K^+ down its concentration gradient (out of the cell) exceeds that of Na^+ (into the cell). The concentration gradients are maintained by the Na^+/K^+-ATPase. Hyperpolarisation of the cell may arise from the opening of K^+ or Cl^- channels or from the activation of the Na^+/K^+-ATPase. A^-, negatively charged anionic groups on proteins.

(Ch. 1) but the closing of a K^+ channel will also cause an EPSP (see Fig. 4.4). Nicotinic acetylcholine (ACh) receptors, for example, are associated directly with Na^+ channels, and the binding of two molecules of ACh causes channel opening, thereby initiating a wave of depolarisation in the innervated nerve.

Inhibitory effects

With inhibitory transmission, binding of the neurotransmitter to the postsynaptic receptor hyperpolarises the innervated neuron and thereby reduces its excitability, i.e. it causes an inhibitory postsynaptic potential (IPSP). The main ionic mechanism for an IPSP is the opening of chloride (Cl^-) channels, so that Cl^- diffuses down its concentration gradient into the cell; the opening of a K^+ channel (outward flow) will also cause an IPSP. Enhancing the opening of Cl^- channels is an important mechanism of action of a number of anxiolytics (Ch. 20) and

antiepileptic drugs (Ch. 23). Axo-axonal synapses frequently inhibit neurotransmitter release by the generation of an IPSP (see opioid analgesics, Ch. 19).

Neurotransmitters

There are numerous neurotransmitters, and modulators of neurotransmission; these may be divided into five major classes based on their chemical structure:

● **esters**, e.g. ACh
● **amines**, e.g. noradrenaline, dopamine, histamine, 5-hydroxytryptamine (5HT)
● **amino acids**, e.g. glutamate, glycine, gamma-aminobutyric acid (GABA)
● **peptides**, e.g. opioids, substance P
● **purines**, e.g. adenosine, ATP.

The principal neurotransmitters within the central and peripheral nervous systems are described based on the processes given in schematic form in Figure 4.3. A table of drug receptor types is provided at the end of this chapter.

Esters

Acetylcholine

Synthesis

Acetylcholine (ACh) $[(CH_3)_3N^+CH_2CH_2OCOCH_3]$ is synthesised within the cytosol of the neuron from choline $[(CH_3)_3N^+CH_2CH_2OH]$ and acetyl-CoA. Choline is a highly polar, quaternary amino compound that is also present in phospholipids (e.g. phosphatidylcholine) and which is obtained largely from the diet. Because of its fixed positive charge, it does not really cross membranes and there are specific transporters to allow uptake from the gastrointestinal tract and across the blood–brain barrier (Ch. 2), as well as across the neuronal membrane (TR1 in Fig. 4.3, which transports choline rather than ACh; see below). Acetylation of the hydroxyl group of choline to form ACh is catalysed by the enzyme choline acetyltransferase. The rate of synthesis of ACh is controlled closely and is related to ACh turnover, so that rapid release of ACh stores is associated with enhanced synthesis.

Storage

The cytosolic ACh is taken up into membrane vesicles by a specific transmembrane transporter and is stored in the vesicles in association with ATP and acidic proteoglycans (which are also released on exocytosis of the vesicles). Each vesicle contains 1000 to 50 000 ACh molecules and neuromuscular junctions contain about 300 000 vesicles.

Release

Release occurs by Ca^{2+}-mediated fusion of the vesicle membrane with the cytoplasmic membrane and exocytosis (as shown in Fig. 4.3). This process can be inhibited by botulinum toxin and stimulated by the toxin from the black widow spider. The numbers of vesicles released depends on the site of the synapse, with between 30 and 300 vesicles undergoing exocytosis, releasing from 30 000 to over 3 million ACh molecules into the synaptic cleft. Neurons within the CNS are more sensitive to ACh release and require fewer ACh molecules to cause an EPSP compared with the neuromuscular junction, which requires millions of molecules to be released.

Removal of activity

Released ACh is very rapidly hydrolysed within the synaptic cleft to give choline and acetate, neither of which binds to the postsynaptic receptors. Both presynaptic and postsynaptic membranes are rich in *acetylcholine esterase* (AChE), and the released ACh is hydrolysed very rapidly (usually <1 ms). This rapid hydrolysis, and the rapid equilibration between ACh bound to the receptor and free in the synapse, means that the 'receptor phase' of the transmission process only lasts for 1–2 ms (the postsynaptic changes may be more prolonged; see below).

The active site of the esterase enzyme has two critical features (Fig. 4.5):

- an anionic site, which forms an ionic bond to the quaternary nitrogen of the choline part of ACh
- a hydrolytic site, which contains a serine moiety; the hydroxyl group of the serine accepts the acetyl group (CH₃CO-) from ACh and very rapidly transfers it to water to complete the hydrolysis reaction.

Inhibition of AChE will prevent the breakdown of ACh and lead to prolonged receptor occupancy, the consequences of which depend on the nature of the receptor and the innervated cell/tissue. AChE inhibitors can be divided into three types.

- **Inhibitors that bind to the anionic site**. The enzyme can be inhibited by an agent binding reversibly to the anionic site, for example edrophonium (Ch. 28).
- **Inhibitors that carbamylate the serine group**. Some inhibitors bind to the anionic site and transfer a carbamoyl group [(CH₃)₂NCO-] instead of an acetyl group (CH₃CO-) from the drug to the serine hydroxyl group. The carbamoyl group is hydrolysed more slowly from the serine than is an acetyl group

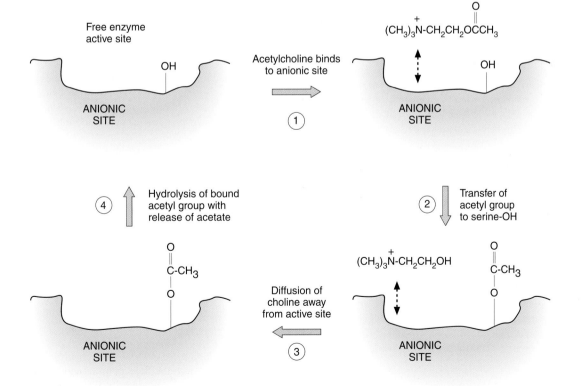

Fig. 4.5
The hydrolysis of acetylcholine by acetylcholine esterase. (Steps 3 and 4 would occur simultaneously.)

and, as a result, prolonged and profound (but reversible) inhibition of the enzyme occurs; this occurs, for example, with neostigmine and pyridostigmine These are used in treating myasthenia gravis and reversing neuromuscular block by non-depolarising blockers (Chs 27 and 28).

- **Inhibitors that phosphorylate the serine hydroxyl group**. Some inhibitors react with the serine hydroxyl group (with or without binding to the anionic site) to produce a phosphorylated enzyme. The phosphorylated enzyme is stable to hydrolysis and, therefore, inhibitors such as the organophosphates, which inhibit AChE in this way, cause irreversible inhibition of the enzyme (or very slowly and only partially reversible inhibition). Such permanent changes in enzyme activity are of limited clinical use. Compounds in this group may be encountered clinically in subjects suffering accidental or intentional poisoning. Organophosphates are important environmental chemicals due to their use as pesticides, and there has been concern in recent years over the exposure of agricultural workers to such compounds, for example in sheep dips. Organophosphates have also been used as nerve gases for chemical warfare. The active serine hydroxyl group may be regenerated by administration of pralidoxime, which is an antidote to organophosphate poisoning. The drug ecothiopate acts via phosphorylation of AChE and has limited clinical use in ophthalmology.

It should be appreciated that AChE inhibitors increase the concentrations of ACh at all nicotinic and muscarinic receptor sites (Ch. 1 and see below), and therefore produce a diverse array of effects. For example, when an AChE inhibitor is used to overcome reversible neuromuscular blockade (see Ch. 27), it increases ACh-mediated effects in the parasympathetic nervous system, for example on the gastrointestinal tract and heart. These unwanted effects of ACh can be blocked by co-administration of an antimuscarinic agent (see drug receptor table at the end of this chapter).

Unlike many other neurotransmitters, ACh is not inactivated by a specific reuptake process, but because choline is a limited resource, there is a specific reuptake mechanism to allow choline to re-enter the presynaptic neuron rather than simply diffuse away. No such process occurs for acetate because it is readily available from intermediary metabolism. Presynaptic uptake of choline can be inhibited by structural analogues, such as hemicholinium, but such drugs are not useful clinically because of the widespread and non-specific consequences of impairment of ACh uptake, synthesis and release.

Acetylcholine receptors

There are three main types of cholinergic ACh receptors, which show different distribution and agonist/antagonist specificities (see drug receptor table at the end of this chapter). The receptors were named after nitrogen-containing basic compounds (alkaloids) present in plants (nicotine) or fungae (muscarine).

Nicotinic (N_1) receptors. These occur within the CNS and on the postsynaptic membranes of all ganglia of both the sympathetic and parasympathetic branches of the ANS.

Nicotinic (N_2) receptors. These occur at the junction between the somatic motor nerves and somatic muscles (the neuromuscular junction; see Ch. 27).

The nicotinic receptor is a pentamer of five subunits, with disulphide cross-linking between adjacent subunits; there are different types of subunit (α, β, γ and δ), and different combinations give rise to neuronal N_1 receptors compared with the neuromuscular junction N_2 receptor. The differences between N_2 and N_1 receptors in their agonist/antagonist ligand-binding characteristics are clinically very important, because they allow neuromuscular blockade (paralysis) without major effects on the ANS.

Muscarinic (M) receptors. These occur within the CNS and postganglionic fibre/effector organ junctions of the parasympathetic branch of the ANS. These receptors are also present on most sweat glands (but not on the palms of the hands), which are innervated by the sympathetic branch of the ANS. Application of molecular biology has identified five subtypes of muscarinic receptor. Experimental studies have demonstrated that at least three of these show different antagonist specificities and, as a result, there is the potential for selective drug activity (see drug receptor table at the end of this chapter).

In addition to occurring on postsynaptic sites, N_1 and M receptors are also found presynaptically (see below) and recent data suggest that the main role of N_1 receptors in the CNS may be as presynaptic neuromodulators.

Amines

Noradrenaline

Noradrenaline is a member of a group of amine transmitters called catecholamines (a catechol is a benzene ring with two adjacent hydroxyl groups; Fig. 4.6a).

Both the catechol and amino groups are important for receptor binding, and the catecholamines in Figure 4.6a are interrelated metabolically. Noradrenaline, adrenaline and dopamine may be used therapeutically. The approved names of noradrenaline and adrenaline *when used as medicines* are *norepinephrine* and *epinephrine*, respectively. In the USA, these alternative 'epinephric' names are used also to describe their neurotransmitter roles, but the receptors are still described by the 'adrenal' nomenclature; hence, US texts describe epinephrine activity on adrenoceptors. To avoid this confusion (and

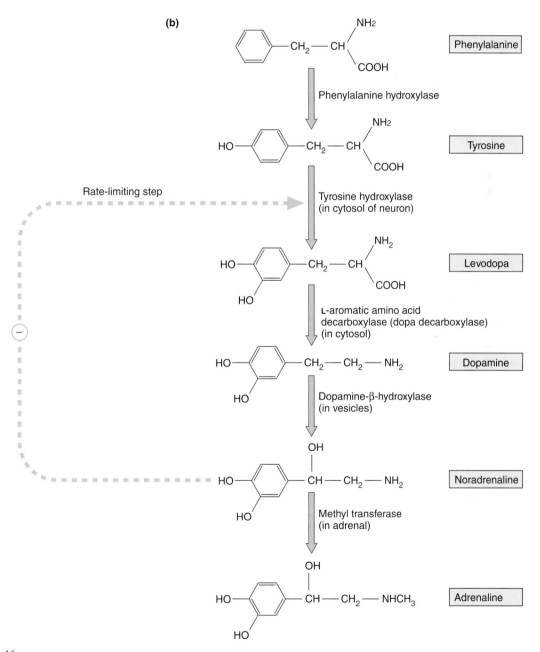

Fig. 4.6
The structure of the main physiological catecholamines (a) and their synthesis from amino acid precursors (b).

to avoid the term 'norepinphrinergic receptors'), we have kept the 'adrenal' nomenclature where hormones are formulated and administered as drugs.

Synthesis

Catecholamine neurotransmitters are synthesised from inactive precursors (Fig. 4.6b). The basic carbon skeleton of catecholamines is derived from phenylalanine or tyrosine, which are aromatic amino acids. Phenylalanine has an unsubstituted benzene ring, while tyrosine has a 4-hydroxyl (phenolic) group. Both phenylalanine and tyrosine are used in protein synthesis. To convert tyrosine to a catecholamine requires oxidation at the aromatic ring (to produce a catechol) and decarboxylation at the amino acid end to produce an amine.

The sequence of synthesis of adrenaline (via dopamine and noradrenaline) is given in Figure 4.6b. The oxidation of tyrosine to levodopa by *tyrosine hydroxylase* within the neuron commits the molecule to become a neurotransmitter, because levodopa is not used in protein synthesis (there is no tRNA). This is the rate-limiting step, and it is subject to negative feedback by the subsequent catecholamines, thereby regulating supply. Tyrosine hydroxylase is activated by cyclic adenosine monophosphate (cAMP)-dependent protein kinases, and this may be involved in the presynaptic regulation of transmitter synthesis (via presynaptic receptors; see below).

Conversion of levodopa to dopamine is catalysed by a cytosolic enzyme, *L-aromatic amino acid decarboxylase* (usually known as dopa decarboxylase), which is able to decarboxylate a range of aromatic amino acids. The amine product, dopamine, is then taken up by vesicles via a specific transporter. In dopaminergic neurons, this is the end of the synthetic pathway.

The vesicles of noradrenergic neurons contain the enzyme *dopamine-β-hydroxylase*, which oxidises the β-carbon (i.e. that next to the CH_2NH_2 group). This enzyme is largely present in the membranes of the vesicles, but on exocytosis some is lost into the synapse, following which it diffuses into the bloodstream and is slowly cleared. Dopamine-β-hydroxylase in blood can be used as a reflection of peripheral noradrenaline release. In noradrenergic neurons, this is the end of the synthetic pathway.

The adrenal medulla contains an additional enzyme (*phenylethanolamine-N-methyl transferase*), which converts noradrenaline to adrenaline by the addition of a methyl group to the nitrogen atom (Fig. 4.6b).

Administration of levodopa directly (see Parkinson's disease; Ch. 24) bypasses the rate-limiting step and, therefore, results in increased formation of dopamine. This treatment can remain effective so long as there is sufficient dopa decarboxylase to convert the catechol amino acid to the catecholamine.

The recognition of this synthetic sequence led to the development of α-methyldopa (an analogue of levodopa with a -CH₃ group in addition to the -NH₂ and -COOH groups on the α-carbon) as a false substrate/inhibitor of dopa decarboxylase. For many years it was thought that the hypotensive effect of α-methyldopa was a result of a decrease in noradrenaline synthesis. It is now realised that it is a substrate for dopa decarboxylase and that the products (α-methyldopamine and α-methylnoradrenaline) act on α₂-adrenoceptors in the medulla to reduce sympathetic output (Ch. 6).

Storage

Noradrenaline (or dopamine) is stored in the vesicles as a complex with ATP and proteoglycans. Formation of the complex reduces the osmotic pressure that would result from a similar amount of noradrenaline in solution. There is a specific catecholamine transporter (TR2 in Fig. 4.3) that transfers noradrenaline (or dopamine) from the cytoplasm into the vesicles. The transporter can be inhibited by the drug reserpine, which was used to lower blood pressure but is no longer used because of unacceptable unwanted effects arising from its non-specificity.

Release

Release, in response to a nerve impulse, occurs by Ca^{2+}-mediated fusion of the noradrenaline vesicle with the cytoplasmic membrane.

Noradrenaline present in the cytoplasm may also be released by certain low-molecular-weight basic compounds – for example, food constituents (such as tyramine), therapeutic drugs (such as ephedrine) and some drugs of abuse (such as amfetamines and metamfetamine). Such compounds are taken into the synapse cytosol by uptake 1 (see below – TR1 in Fig. 4.3) and into the vesicles, from which they displace noradrenaline. The increased noradrenaline in the cytoplasm is either degraded by monoamine oxidase (MAO; see below) or exchanges with dexamfetamine via the uptake-1 transporter (TR1 in Fig. 4.3) and is transported out of the cell into the synapse. This releases noradrenaline into the synapse, which is responsible for the effects produced by compounds like tyramine. Such compounds, therefore, are called '*indirectly acting sympathomimetic amines*'.

Adrenergic neuron-blocking drugs also exert their principal action presynaptically on noradrenaline release. Drugs such as bretylium, guanethidine and debrisoquine (discontinued) are taken into the neuron by uptake 1 (see below; TR1 in Fig. 4.3) and then bind to the vesicle and block its exocytosis in response to a nerve stimulation. Such drugs lower blood pressure but are of little clinical use because of unwanted effects, which can include an initial hypertension as the drug enters the cytoplasm and displaces noradrenaline.

Removal of activity

The principal mechanism for the removal of noradrenaline from the synapse is reuptake into the presynaptic neuron via a specific carrier called uptake 1 (TR1 in Fig. 4.3) (uptake 2 is a low-affinity transporter into non-neuronal tissue, but this process does not seem to be critical). The uptake-1 transporter protein varies with the neurotransmitter type released from the neuron, e.g. noradrenaline, dopamine or 5HT. Newer therapeutic agents are able to exploit the differences between transporters, e.g. the selective serotonin (5HT) reuptake inhibitors (SSRIs) used for treating depression (Ch. 22). Blockade of noradrenaline reuptake, by drugs such as tricyclic antidepressants (Ch. 22) and cocaine (Ch. 18), increases the concentrations of noradrenaline in the synapse and, therefore, increases the activity at the postsynaptic receptor.

Metabolism is important in the elimination of noradrenaline but plays only a minor role in the termination of its action in the synapse, which is by reuptake. There are two main enzymes involved in noradrenaline metabolism: MAO and catechol-*O*-methyltransferase (COMT).

Monoamine oxidase. MAO is present inside the cell on the surface of the mitochondria and is primarily responsible for degradation of intracellular noradrenaline. Oxidative removal of the amino group on noradrenaline (see Fig. 4.6b) via MAO is the major pathway of metabolism of noradrenaline and other aminergic neurotransmitters, and converts the primary amino group ($-CH_2NH_2$; see Fig. 4.6b) into an aldehyde ($-CHO$); loss of the amino group prevents binding to the postsynaptic receptor. In the periphery, the aldehyde is oxidised to an acid ($-COOH$), which is excreted in the urine, whereas in the CNS, the aldehyde is reduced to an alcohol ($-CH_2OH$), which is conjugated with sulphate (see Ch. 2) before being excreted in the urine. There are two main forms of MAO (Table 4.1), which differ in their organ distribution and substrate affinities. MAO inhibitors that are selective for one of the isoenzymes are able to exploit these differences and minimise unwanted effects (see Ch. 22). MAO inhibitors are used mainly for their effects on aminergic transmitters within the CNS rather than in the peripheral sympathetic nervous system and are discussed in the sections on antidepressants (Ch. 22) and Parkinson's disease (Ch. 24).

Catechol-*O*-methyltransferase. COMT is a membrane-bound enzyme present around the synapse and within the presynaptic neuron. The enzyme catalyses the transfer of a methyl group onto the phenolic group at position 3 of the aromatic ring (see Fig. 4.6b) to convert the -OH group into $-OCH_3$. This removes the catechol centre and prevents binding to the postsynaptic receptor. COMT is a minor route of inactivation of both dopamine and noradrenaline. Inhibitors of COMT are used as an adjunct to levodopa therapy for Parkinson's disease (Ch. 24).

Metabolites of noradrenaline. The main metabolites of noradrenaline excreted in urine are:

- 3,4-dihydroxymandelic acid (formed by oxidation of the $-CH_2NH_2$ into $-COOH$) and vanillylmandelic acid (its 3-O-methyl analogue)
- 3,4-dihydroxyphenylglycol (formed by replacement of $-CH_2NH_2$ by CH_2OH), 3-methoxy-4-hydroxyphenylglycol (its 3-O-methyl analogue) and their sulphate conjugates.

Receptors

Noradrenaline and adrenaline receptors (adrenoceptors) were originally divided into two types, α and β, based on pharmacological responses, but it was soon recognised that there were two main α-subtypes (α_1 and α_2) and three main β-subtypes (β_1, β_2 and β_3) (see drug receptor table at the end of this chapter). Adrenoceptors occur in the CNS and in the periphery, particularly at the junction between the postganglionic nerve and the effector organ of the sympathetic branch of the ANS. The clinical uses of drugs that act on these receptors are discussed in later chapters. In addition, it is now realised that there are multiple forms of some of these main subtypes (i.e α_{1A}, α_{1B} and α_{1D}, and α_{2A}, α_{2B} and α_{2C}). The different receptor subtypes (see drug receptor table at the end of this chapter) show different affinities for the endogenous catecholamines noradrenaline and adrenaline:

Table 4.1
Monoamine oxidase (MAO) and its inhibitors

Isoenzyme	Location in human tissues	Main substrates	Examples of inhibitors	
			Irreversible	Reversible
MAO-A	Gastrointestinal tract, placenta	5-Hydroxytryptamine, noradrenaline	Clorgiline	Moclobemide
MAO-B	Brain,[a] liver,[a] platelets	Phenylethylamine, tyramine	Selegiline	Lazabemide
MAO-A or MAO-B		Tyramine, dopamine, adrenaline	Iproniazid, tranylcypromine, pargyline, phenelzine	

[a]Both isoenzymes are present, but in humans the amount of MAO-B exceeds that of MAO-A.

α_1, α_{2A}, α_{2C}, β_2: adrenaline $\geq$ noradrenaline
β_1: adrenaline = noradrenaline
α_{2B}, β_3: noradrenaline > adrenaline.

Dopamine

Dopamine is a neurotransmitter in its own right both within the CNS and in the periphery (Fig. 4.6a).

Synthesis

Synthesis has been described above with noradrenaline.

Storage

Storage has been described above with noradrenaline.

Release

Nerve stimulation causes release of dopamine present in vesicles (see noradrenaline). Dopaminergic neurons are not important in the clinical responses to indirectly acting sympathomimetics and adrenergic neuron-blocking drugs (see above), although certain behavioural responses to amfetamines in rats are linked to dopamine D_2 receptor activity. The antiviral drug amantadine, which is of some value in Parkinson's disease, causes release of dopamine.

Removal of activity

Dopamine is removed by similar mechanisms to those seen with noradrenaline, with reuptake representing the major pathway. Metabolism yields primarily 3,4-dihydroxyphenylacetic acid and its 3-methyl analogue (homovanillic acid).

Receptors

It is now recognised that there are a number of types of dopamine receptors, although selective therapeutic agents are not available for some of these (see drug receptor table at the end of this chapter). The original classification was into D_1 (which increase cAMP) and D_2 (which decrease cAMP). The latter are more closely linked to schizophrenia. This subdivision has now been revised into D_1 and D_5 (which increase cAMP) and D_2, D_3 and D_4 (which decrease cAMP). The D_4 receptor shows polymorphic expression; hopes that this subtype may be the key to schizophrenia have not been fulfilled, although clozapine, a selective D_4 receptor antagonist, is a valuable antipsychotic drug (Ch. 21).

5-Hydroxytryptamine

5HT (or serotonin; Fig. 4.7a) is a neurotransmitter in the CNS and periphery that shows characteristics similar to the catecholamines.

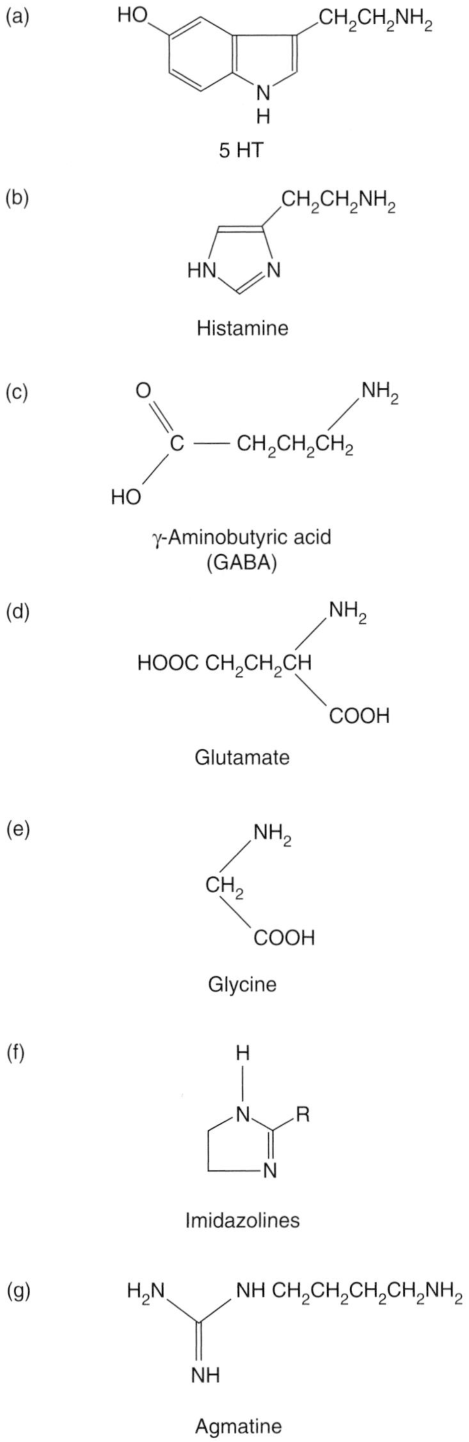

Synthesis

5HT is synthesised from the amino acid tryptophan, by two reactions that are similar to those used in the conversion of tyrosine to dopamine. The first reaction is

(a) 5 HT

(b) Histamine

(c) γ-Aminobutyric acid (GABA)

(d) Glutamate

(e) Glycine

(f) Imidazolines

(g) Agmatine

Fig. 4.7
The structures of some of the diverse amine, amino acid and imidazoline neurotransmitters.

oxidation of the benzene ring of tryptophan to form 5-hydroxytryptophan, which is catalysed by the enzyme *tryptophan hydroxylase* (which is the rate-limiting step and is only found in 5HT-producing cells). Conversion of the amino acid function to an amine is catalysed by aromatic amino acid decarboxylase (see noradrenaline synthesis).

5HT is present in the diet but undergoes essentially complete first-pass metabolism by MAO in the gut wall and liver. 5HT is not synthesised by blood platelets, but they have a very efficient transporter, which allows them to accumulate high concentrations of 5HT from the circulation.

Storage
The major sites of 5HT storage in the body are the enterochromaffin cells of the gastrointestinal tract and platelets, with less than 10% in the brain. 5HT is stored in vesicles as a complex with ATP. There is an active uptake process, which is similar to that in adrenergic neurons and which can be inhibited by reserpine.

Release
The release of 5HT vesicles is by Ca^{2+}-mediated exocytosis. A rise in intraluminal pressure in the gastrointestinal tract stimulates the release of 5HT from the chromaffin cells. Release of 5HT from chromaffin cells contributes to nausea following cancer chemotherapy with cytotoxic drugs, both locally and via an action on the chemoreceptor trigger zone. There is a significant release of platelet 5HT in migraine.

Removal of activity
The principal mechanism of inactivation of released 5HT is via its reuptake into the presynaptic nerve. The process shows a high affinity for 5HT, and is different from that on adrenergic neurons, which has allowed selective inhibitors to be developed. Selective serotonin reuptake inhibitors (SSRIs) are useful antidepressants (Ch. 22).

Metabolism within the neuron is by MAO, which converts the $-CH_2NH_2$ group to an aldehyde (-CHO), which is then oxidised to a carboxylic acid (-COOH), producing the excretory product 5-hydroxyindoleacetic acid (5-HIAA). There is a considerable turnover of 5HT in the chromaffin and nerve cells, and 5-HIAA is a normal constituent of human urine.

Receptors
There is a family of 5HT receptors, which has allowed the development of selective drugs (see drug receptor table at the end of this chapter). Thus far, the different 5HT receptors comprise 13 different heptahelical, G-protein-coupled receptors and one ligand-gated ion channel, which are divided into seven classes ($5HT_1$ to $5HT_7$) on the basis of their structural and operational characteristics. Not all of the subtypes of receptors have recognised physiological roles. The $5HT_1$ group are mostly presynaptic and inhibit adenylate cyclase, whereas the $5HT_2$ group are mostly postsynaptic in the periphery and activate phospholipase C.

Histamine
Histamine (Fig. 4.7b) is an important transmitter both in the CNS and in the periphery, as well as being a mediator released from mast cells and basophils.

Synthesis
The amino acid histidine is converted to histamine through decarboxylation by *histidine decarboxylase*. In addition to the synthesis and storage of histamine by mast cells and basophils, there is continual synthesis, release and metabolic inactivation by growing tissues and in wound healing.

Storage
Most attention has focused on the storage of histamine in mediator-releasing cells, such as mast cells and basophils. In such cells, it is present in granules, associated with heparin. The presence of histidine decarboxylase and the storage of histamine in neurons in the CNS and periphery have not been clearly demonstrated.

Release
The release of histamine from mast cells and basophils has been studied extensively in relation to allergic reactions (Chs 12 and 39). The release of histamine from neurons may be similar to the release of other amine neurotransmitters, but this has not been demonstrated unequivocally.

Removal of activity
Histamine is rapidly inactivated by oxidation of the amino group ($-CH_2NH_2$) to an aldehyde and then an acid (-COOH), imidazoleacetic acid. Histamine is not a substrate for MAO and the oxidation is catalysed by *diamine oxidase* (or histaminase). A second, minor route of metabolism is methylation of the cyclic -NH group by *histamine-N-methyltransferase*, and the product is then a substrate for MAO, producing *N*-methylimidazoleacetic acid. Histamine is also eliminated as an *N*-acetyl conjugate.

Receptors
There are four receptors for histamine (see drug receptor table at the end of this chapter). H_1 receptors have been studied extensively in relation to inflammation and allergy (Chs 12 and 39). The discovery of H_2 receptors affecting the release of gastric acid led to the development of an important treatment for peptic ulcer disease (Ch. 33). Histamine-containing neurons are found in the brain, particularly in the brainstem, with pathways projecting into the cerebral cortex. H_1 receptors are probably important in these pathways, because sedation is a serious problem with H_1 receptor antagonists (Ch. 39) that are able to cross the blood–brain barrier (Ch. 2). The so-called second-generation antihistamines produce less sedation. H_1 receptors are also involved in emesis (Ch. 32). H_2 receptors are present in

the brain and are probably responsible for the confusional state associated with the use of the H_2 receptor antagonist cimetidine (Ch. 33).

Amino acids

Gamma-aminobutyric acid

GABA ($HOOCCH_2CH_2CH_2NH_2$) is an important inhibitory neurotransmitter responsible for about 40% of all inhibitory activity in the CNS (Fig. 4.7c).

Synthesis
GABA is formed by the decarboxylation of glutamate via the enzyme *glutamate decarboxylase*, which is present in GABAergic neurons.

Storage
GABA is stored in membrane vesicles in the brain and in interneurons within the spinal cord (particularly laminae II and III).

Release
GABA is released by Ca^{2+}-mediated exocytosis. Cotransmitters, such as glycine, metenkephalin and neuropeptide Y, are stored in GABA vesicles and released with GABA.

Removal of activity
Uptake is the principal mechanism for the removal of GABA from the synaptic cleft. The antiepileptic drug tiagabine may act as a specific inhibitor of GABA uptake.

GABA is metabolised by transamination with α-ketoglutarate, which forms the corresponding aldehyde (succinic semialdehyde) and amino acid (glutamic acid). The antiepileptic drug vigabatrine inhibits GABA transamination.

Receptors
There are two main GABA receptors, with different mechanisms of action (see drug receptor table at the end of this chapter). Both mechanisms inhibit depolarisation, with $GABA_A$ causing rapid inhibition and $GABA_B$ giving a slower and more prolonged response. The $GABA_A$ receptor comprises four subunits (α, β, γ and δ). There are multiple forms of each subunit and numerous possible combinations (see Fig. 20.1); consequently, the $GABA_A$ receptor should be regarded as a family of receptors. $GABA_B$ receptors are G-protein-linked receptors that hyperpolarise the cell by closing Ca^{2+} channels and opening K^+ channels. In addition, there is a third receptor, $GABA_C$, which is linked to changes in Cl^- conductance associated with retinal function, but its physiological and clinical significance remains unclear. Both $GABA_A$ and $GABA_B$ receptors are found presynaptically and inhibit neurotransmitter release by hyperpolarising the cell (via opening Cl^- or K^+ channels) and reducing release of the vesicles of the innervating cell (via closing Ca^{2+} channels). Many important drugs act by altering GABA breakdown or by enhancing GABA activity at its receptor (Chs 20 and 23).

Glutamate

Glutamate (Fig. 4.7d) is an important excitatory amino acid neurotransmitter that acts on receptors in the CNS. Aspartate (which is similar to glutamate but has only one CH_2 group) acts at the same receptors. Administration of glutamate or aspartate causes CNS excitation, tachycardia, nausea and headache, and convulsions at very high doses. Hyperactivity at glutamate receptors has been proposed as a factor in the generation of epilepsy (Ch. 23).

Synthesis
Glutamate (glutamic acid) is a normal endogenous amino acid that is formed in most cells and is widely distributed within the CNS.

Storage
Glutamate is stored in presynaptic vesicles in the neurons.

Release
Exocytosis of vesicles is mediated via the influx of Ca^{2+} into the presynaptic nerve terminal, as occurs for other neurotransmitters. Some antiepilepsy drugs, for example lamotrigine and valproate (Ch. 23), inhibit glutamate release.

Removal of activity
The action of glutamate in the synapse is terminated by a specific carrier, which transports glutamate into the neuron and surrounding glial cells.

Receptors
Glutamate receptors are described by names rather than symbols such as G_1, G_2 etc. (see drug receptor table at the end of this chapter).

Glycine

Glycine (Fig. 4.7e) is a widely available amino acid that acts as an inhibitory neurotransmitter. It is released in response to nerve stimulation and acts in the spine, lower brainstem and retina.

Synthesis
Glycine is present in all cells and is accumulated by neurons.

Storage
Glycine is stored within neurons in vesicles; few details are available.

Release

Vesicle release accompanies an action potential, as described above for other neurotransmitters. Tetanus toxin prevents glycine release, and the decrease in glycine-mediated inhibition results in reflex hyperexcitability.

Removal of activity

Released glycine is inactivated by a high-affinity uptake process.

Receptors

Glycine receptors are ligand-gated Cl^- channels similar in structure to $GABA_A$ channels: they are present mainly on interneurons in the spinal cord. Strychnine produces convulsions through the blockade of glycine receptors. (Glycine is important for the activity of NMDA [N-methyl-D-aspartate] receptors; see drug receptor table at the end of this chapter.)

Peptides

The importance of peptides as neurotransmitters has been appreciated in recent years, largely because of the development of highly specific and sensitive probes, combined with histochemical techniques, that allow their detection and measurement. Unlike other classes of neurotransmitter, peptides are synthesised in the cell body as a precursor, which is transported down the axon to its site of storage. There are specific receptors for different peptides (see drug receptor table at the end of this chapter). An action potential causes the release of the peptide from its precursor; inactivation is probably via hydrolysis by a local peptidase.

Peptide neurotransmitters are often found stored in the same nerve endings as other transmitters (described above) and undergo simultaneous release (cotransmission).

Peptides do not cross the blood–brain barrier readily. A major problem for exploiting our increasing knowledge of the importance of peptides is delivering the novel products of molecular biology to the sites within the brain where they can have an effect.

Substance P is released from C-fibres (Ch. 19) by a Ca^{2+}-linked mechanism and is the principal neurotransmitter for sensory afferents in the dorsal horn. It is also present in the substantia nigra, associated with dopaminergic neurons, and may be involved in the control of movement.

Opioid peptides are a range of peptides that are the natural ligands for opioid receptors (known formerly as the 'morphine' receptor); the receptor was recognised in the brain and gastrointestinal tract for many years before the natural ligand was identified. These are discussed in Chapter 19.

A number of other peptides are detectable in the CNS and produce physiological effects if given by intrathecal injection. A number of these peptides in the brain are also present in high concentrations in the hypothalamus and/or pituitary gland (e.g. neurotensin, oxytocin, somatostatin, vasopressin; see Chapters 43 and 45) or in the gastrointestinal tract (e.g. cholecystokinin and vasoactive intestinal peptide).

Low-molecular-weight peptides frequently act via G-protein-linked receptors. The principal peptide receptors and their effects are given in the drug receptor table at the end of this chapter.

Purines

Adenosine and guanosine are endogenous purines and exist in the body as such, attached to ribose or deoxyribose (as nucleosides) and as mono-, bi- or triphosphorylated nucleotides. The nucleotides are the usual intracellular form and are involved in the energetics of biochemical processes (for example ATP) and as intracellular signals (cAMP and cGMP) as well as being involved in the synthesis of RNA and DNA. ATP is present in the presynaptic vesicles of some other neurotransmitters and is released along with the primary neurotransmitter, following which it may act on postsynaptic receptors (cotransmission). Extracellular ATP is rapidly hydrolysed via adenosine diphosphate (ADP) to form adenosine. Adenosine itself is very rapidly metabolised and inactivated.

There is a family of purine receptors that show high selectivity (almost specificity) for different purines and give different responses (see drug receptor table at the end of this chapter). The adenosine receptors $(A_1–A_3)$ show very high selectivity for adenosine itself and are specific under physiological conditions. In contrast, purinergic receptors (P_2) are specific for the adenosine triphosphates.

Imidazolines

The realisation that there may be an additional, unrecognised group of neurotransmitters/receptors involved in the control of blood pressure arose from studies on α_2-adrenoceptor agonists. The unwanted effects produced by the drug clonidine, an early imidazoline α_2-adrenoceptor agonist, led to the development of moxonidine and rilmenidine. These imidazolines possessed fewer unwanted effects, but not all of their actions could be interpreted in relation to the α_2-adrenoceptor. A specific imidazoline-binding site was identified in the rostral ventrolateral medulla, and an endogenous 'ligand' that would displace clonidine from this site was proposed (see Ch. 6).

This led to the suggestion that there is an imidazoline receptor that has a high affinity for imidazoline compounds (Fig. 4.7f). It was subsequently suggested that there are three imidazoline receptors (I_1, I_2 and I_3) and that agmatine (Fig. 4.7g), which is a metabolite of arginine, is an endogenous ligand. This compound occurs in synaptosomes and is a postulated natural transmitter.

Binding sites of the I_1 type are present in the brainstem and kidney, liver and prostate. However, there are still considerable doubts about the validity of these binding sites as receptors for neurotransmission. The role of the I_1 receptor in controlling blood pressure is not clearly established. In contrast to the uncertainties about the I_1 site, the I_2 binding site has been established as being associated with MAO and is an allosteric modulating region on the enzyme, not a neurotransmitter receptor. The I_3 site appears to modulate the action of K^+_{ATP} channels and to be linked to insulin release from the pancreas.

Presynaptic receptors

An important neuronal characteristic not shown in the schematic for synaptic neurotransmission (Fig. 4.3) is the presence of presynaptic receptors. Presynaptic receptors may either increase or decrease the release of the neurotransmitter and are described as facilitatory and inhibitory, respectively. There are two main sources of ligands for presynaptic receptors:

- neurotransmitter released from the vesicles that can act presynaptically (autoreceptors)
- neurotransmitter released from other neurons, usually by axo-axonal synapses, involving a different neurotransmitter to that released by the neuron itself (heteroreceptors).

The first recognition of a clinically important presynaptic receptor was the discovery that the α-agonist clonidine decreased blood pressure (rather than increasing it via α_1-adrenoceptors) and it was shown to act via presynaptic α_2-adrenoceptors, which inhibit the release of noradrenaline. Presynaptic receptors (Table 4.2) are increasingly being recognised as having important roles in the clinical effects produced by many drugs.

Pharmacogenomics, pharmacogenetics and drug responses

Genetic polymorphisms in receptors and second messenger systems are likely to be of increasing importance in the future. While polymorphisms in pharmacokinetics (see Ch. 2) are likely to have an important impact on dosage selection, polymorphisms in receptors may be more important for drug selection. For example, discovery of a major polymorphism that caused a functional deficit in the angiotensin (AT_2) receptor would mean that neither an angiotensin-converting enzyme (ACE) inhibitor (Ch. 6) nor an AT_2 receptor antagonist would be a good choice to lower blood pressure in such subjects, whereas a β-adrenoceptor antagonist would still be effective. In contrast, a functional deficit in the β_1-adrenoceptor could make an ACE inhibitor a better choice than a β-adrenoceptor antagonist for treating cardiovascular conditions.

Genetic polymorphisms have been reported in each of the main adrenergic receptors, and these are a major focus of research in relation to the aetiology of cardiovascular and respiratory diseases. To date, few studies have been performed on the influence of genetic differences in receptor structure on drug responses. Nine polymorphisms have been identified in the β_2-adrenoceptor, and certain genetic variants have been associated with different asthma phenotypes and also with differences in drug responses. In contrast, identified polymorphisms in the α_1-adrenoceptor have not been associated with risk of hypertension or altered responses to drugs.

Pharmacogenetic variability will be increasingly important to optimise drug responses and to minimise adverse effects in individuals. Exploitation of genetic differences will require specific individual genetic information. Until such information is available routinely, careful monitoring of the subject's response will remain the best guide to successful treatment.

Information on genetic polymorphisms in different receptors can be found on the OMIM™ (Online Mendelian Inheritance in Man™; John Hopkins University) database (**http://www.ncbi.nlm.nih.gov/entrez/dispomim. cgi?id=235200**).

The central and peripheral nervous systems

The central nervous system

The CNS is the site of action for the drugs discussed in many later chapters. The CNS contains many different neurotransmitters, which produce a variety of effects in different brain regions. The greatest opportunities for selective therapeutic intervention occur when specific activities or functions are associated with a specific neurotransmitter. However, this is rare, and modification of the activity of a neurotransmitter within the CNS will usually affect a number of functions either directly controlled by that neurotransmitter or indirectly linked to its activity.

Table 4.2
Presynaptic receptors and the release of neurotransmitters

Neurotransmitter	Autoreceptor		Heteroreceptor	
	Inhibitory	Facilitatory	Inhibitory	Facilitatory
Acetylcholine	M_2	N_1	α_2, D_2/D_3, $5HT_3$	NMDA
Dopamine	D_2/D_3	–	M_2	N_1, NMDA
Gamma-aminobutyric acid (GABA)	$GABA_B$	–	–	–
Histamine	H_3	–	–	–
5-Hydroxytryptamine (5HT)	$5HT_{1D}$	$5HT_3$	α_2	–
Noradrenaline	α_2	β_2	H_3, M_2, D_2, opioid	N_1, angiotensin II

NMDA, N-methyl-d-aspartate.

In many cases, the unwanted effects of a drug can be anticipated from the roles of the neurotransmitter affected. Selectivity of therapeutic effect may be possible if the dose is adjusted carefully to correct an underlying pathophysiological imbalance in one part of the brain, while at the same time not creating an imbalance elsewhere within normally functioning tracts. However, in many cases, the dose–response relationships for therapeutic and unwanted effects are very close and toxicity is inevitable to some degree, in at least a proportion of people (see Ch. 53). These concepts are illustrated well by the example of dopamine, because psychotic changes and nausea may accompany attempts to increase dopaminergic activity to treat Parkinson's disease (Ch. 24), while parkinsonism-like unwanted effects are frequently encountered when dopamine antagonists are used in the treatment of psychotic disorders (Ch. 21) or given as antiemetics (Ch. 32).

The composition of the 'internal environment' of the brain is controlled by the blood–brain barrier (Ch. 2), which limits the entry of potentially neuroactive, polar compounds such as catecholamines, amino acids and peptides, as well as polar therapeutic drugs.

The peripheral autonomic nervous system

The ANS is an important site for drug action because:

- the ANS either controls or contributes to the control of the functioning of nearly all of the major organ systems of the body
- ANS dysfunction is present in many diseases
- the ANS utilises two major different neurotransmitters and a number of receptor subtypes, providing a number of sites for drug action (Box 4.1), which allows the activity of different organs to be modified selectively and independently.

The peripheral ANS is subdivided into two main branches:

- *parasympathetic nervous system*, which utilises ACh as the final transmitter at muscarinic receptors on the effector organs
- *sympathetic nervous system*, which utilises noradrenaline as the transmitter at adrenoceptors on most, but not all, effector organs.

Anatomically, in both branches of the ANS, the efferent neurons innervating effector organs are linked to neurons in the CNS via ganglia (Fig. 4.8 and Box 4.2). The distribution and neuronal interconnections differ between the two branches.

- The parasympathetic efferents give discrete innervations of organs, and the ganglia are close to the innervated organs; there are few or no interconnections between ganglia; consequently, organs can be affected individually and independently.
- The sympathetic efferents are involved in the 'flight or fight' response and affect multiorgan systems simultaneously. Many of the ganglia are close to the spinal column, lying in the paravertebral sympathetic ganglion chain, and have broad

---

Box 4.1

Sites of drug action within the ANS

Postsynaptic receptors in ganglion (nicotinic N_1)
Muscarinic receptors at neuroeffector synapses (M subtypes)
Noradrenergic receptors at neuroeffector synapses (α- and β-subtypes)
Presynaptic receptors
Release, storage, synthesis and inactivation of acetylcholine
Release, storage, synthesis and inactivation of noradrenaline

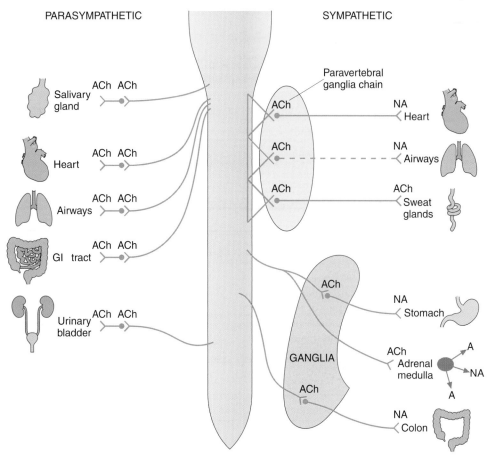

Fig. 4.8
Schematic diagram of the autonomic nervous system, illustrating the types of organisation occurring. ACh, acetylcholine; NA, noradrenaline; A, adrenaline; GI, gastrointestinal. The ganglia innervating some organs are not part of the paravertebral chain but are grouped together to form the coeliac, superior mesenteric and inferior mesenteric ganglia. Airways have sparse sympathetic innervation and dilation is mainly a result of circulating adrenaline.

Box 4.2

Organisation of the autonomic nervous system

Both parasympathetic and sympathetic efferent nerves are connected to the CNS via ganglia

Acetylcholine and noradrenaline are the principal neurotransmitters in the ANS

Stimulation of the sympathetic nervous system has a global effect in the body whereas the parasympathetic nervous system is more organ-specific (Fig. 4.8)

The neurotransmitters are synthesised in the presynaptic neuron, stored, and released into the synapse in response to depolarisation

At all ganglia, the neurotransmitter is acetylcholine acting on nicotinic N_1 acetylcholine receptors

Parasympathetic efferents have muscarinic receptors at neuroeffector synapses

Most sympathetic efferents have noradrenergic receptors at neuroffector synapses

Adrenaline and noradrenaline are synthesised and released in the adrenal medulla in response to sympathetic stimulation

interconnections. The whole system can be activated simultaneously because the nerve fibres leaving the spinal column interconnect with more than one ganglion and because a preganglionic nerve can give rise to a large number of postganglionic fibres. Some sympathetic nerves (e.g. those involved in the emptying of the bladder or rectum) have long preganglionic sympathetic fibres and the ganglia are not part of a paravertebral chain but occur in more distal sites, such as the coeliac ganglia (Fig. 4.8).

The ANS is important in pharmacology because of its potential to be modulated by therapeutic drugs and the ability of receptor subtypes to produce specific effects. The structures of the transmembrane ACh and noradrenaline receptors, together with their related second

Table 4.3
Autonomic nervous system innervation of the major organ system.

Organ system	Parasympathetic NS		Sympathetic NS	
	Effect	Receptor type[a]	Effect	Receptor type[a]
Heart				
Rate	↓	M	↑	β_1, β_2
Contractility	↓ in atria	M	↑	β_1
Vascular smooth muscle				
In skin/gut	(Dilate)	(M)	Constrict	α_1
In skeletal muscle	(Dilate)	(M)	Dilate	β_2[b]
Bronchial smooth muscle	Constrict	M	Dilate	β_2[b]
Gastrointestinal tract				
Motility	↑	M	↓	α_1, β_2
Sphincter tone	↓	M	↑	α_1
Secretions	↑	M	(↓)	?
Uterine smooth muscle	–	–	↑	α_1
tone in pregnancy	–	–	↓	β_2
Urinary bladder				
Detrusor	↑	M	(↓)	β_2
Sphincter	↓	M	↑	α_1
Penis	Erection	M	Ejaculation	α_1
Skin				
Pilomotor muscles	–	–	↑	α_1
Sweat glands	–	–	Secretion	M
			Local secretion	α_1
Eye				
Radial muscle	–	–	↑	α_1
Sphincter muscle	↑	M	–	–
Ciliary muscle	↑ near vision	M	(↓ far vision)	β_2
Metabolic functions				
Hepatic glycogenolysis	–	–	↑	β_2, α
Skeletal muscle glycogenolysis	–	–	↑	β_2[b]
Fat cell lipolysis	–	–	↑	$\beta_1; \alpha; \beta_3$[b]
Pancreas insulin secretion	↑	M	↓	α

Functions in parentheses are of doubtful physiological significance. M, muscarinic receptor; α and β, adrenoceptors; ↑ *or* ↓ increase *or* decrease: contraction *or* relaxation.
[a]Only the principal receptor types are shown.
[b]Respond to circulating adrenaline; no noradrenergic innervation.

messenger systems, have been described above and in Chapter 1.

Many organs are innervated by both the parasympathetic and sympathetic nervous systems, which frequently have opposite effects on the organ function; this has given rise to the concept (albeit imperfect) of *physiological antagonism* between the two branches of the ANS. Table 4.3 shows the principal organ systems, their efferent ANS innervation, their response to parasympathetic and sympathetic stimulation, and the principal neurotransmitter receptor at postganglionic fibre/effector organ junctions.

ACh is the neurotransmitter at all ANS ganglia. The postsynaptic ACh receptors of ganglia are nicotinic N_1 receptors (Ch. 1), which cause a fast EPSP mediated by the opening of Na^+ channels. Ganglia also contain M_2 receptors, which inhibit depolarisation (IPSP) through an increase in K^+ conductance; in addition, a more prolonged EPSP may be produced via M_3 receptors (up to 10 s), which close K^+ channels, and this EPSP may also be extended via a peptide-mediated action.

Ganglion-blocking drugs were one of the earliest class of drug found to affect the ANS. As their name implies, they are able to block the N_1 ACh receptors in the postsynaptic membrane of the ganglia of both branches of the ANS. Because they produce both sympathetic effects (lowering blood pressure) and parasympathetic effects (producing numerous effects – see Table 4.3), they have very restricted clinical use. The effects of ganglion-blocking drugs illustrate the balance of sympathetic and parasympathetic drives in the control of different body systems under resting conditions (see Table 4.4). Under resting conditions, most organs are under a parasympathetic drive, but this will be affected by activities that produce an increase in sympathetic drive, for example exercise or a 'flight or fight' response, which releases adrenaline from the adrenal medulla.

Physiological functions may require coordination of sympathetic and parasympathetic activities; for example, urination is brought about by a decreased adrenergic drive to the sphincter muscle and an increased muscarinic drive to the detrusor muscle (see urinary bladder; Table 4.3).

Students should familiarise themselves with the ANS and the possible sites of drug action (Table 4.3). Such knowledge is fundamental to understanding both the principal mechanisms of action for some drugs and the source of unwanted effects for others.

Table 4.4
The effects of ganglion blockade in a resting subject

Organ	Effect of ganglion blockade	Predominant system
Heart	Increased rate	PNS
Vascular smooth muscle	Decreased tone/dilation	SNS
Bronchial smooth muscle	Little effect/slight dilation	PNS
Gastrointestinal tract	Decreased motility	PNS
Urinary bladder	Urinary retention	PNS
Penis	Blocked erection and ejaculation	PNS/SNS
Sweat glands	Blocked secretion	SNS
Eye	Dilation of pupil	PNS
	Loss of accommodation	PNS

PNS and SNS, parasympathetic and sympathetic nervous systems, respectively.

FURTHER READING

Barnes NM, Sharp T (1999) A review of central 5-HT receptors and their function. *Neuropharmacology* 38, 1083–1152

Berg KA, Maayani S, Clarke WP (1998) Interactions between effectors linked to serotonin receptors. *Ann NY Acad Sci* 861, 111–120

Bloom FE, Morales M (1998) The central 5-HT₃ receptor in CNS disorders. *Neurochem Res* 23, 653–659

Bousquet P, Dontenwill M, Greney H, Feldman J (1998) II-Imidazoline receptors: an update. *J Hypertens* 16 (suppl), S1–S5

Bousquet P, Monassier L, Feldman J (1998) Autonomic nervous system as a target for cardiovascular drugs. *Clin Exp Pharmacol Physiol* 25, 446–448

Bowery NG, Bettler B, Froestl W et al (2002) International Union of Pharmacology. XXXIII. Mammalian gamma-aminobutyric acid(B) receptors: structure and function. *Pharmacol Rev* 54, 247–264

Buckley NJ, Bachfischer U, Canut M et al (1999) Repression and activation of muscarinic receptor genes. *Life Sci* 64, 495–499

Burgen AS (2000) Targets of drug action. *Annu Rev Pharmacol Toxicol* 40, 1–16

Buscher R, Herrmann V, Insel PA (1999) Human adrenoceptor polymorphisms: evolving recognition of clinical importance. *Trends Pharmacol Sci* 20, 94–99

Cartmell J, Schoepp DD (2000) Regulation of neurotransmitter release by metabotropic glutamate receptors. *J Neurochem* 75, 889–907

Dajas-Bailador F, Wonnacott S (2004) Nicotinic acetylcholine receptors and the regulation of neuronal signalling. *Trends Pharmacol Sci* 25, 317–324

Docherty JR (1998) Subtypes of functional alpha 1- and alpha 2-adrenoceptors. *Eur J Pharmacol* 361, 1–15

Eglen RM, Reddy H, Watson N, Challiss RAJ (1994) Muscarinic acetylcholine receptor subtypes in smooth muscle. *Trends Pharmacol Sci* 15, 114–119

Eglen RM, Choppin A, Dillon MP, Hegde S (1999) Muscarinic receptor ligands and their therapeutic potential. *Curr Opin Chem Biol* 3, 426–432

Frishman WH, Kotob F (1999) Alpha-adrenergic blocking drugs in clinical medicine. *J Clin Pharmacol* 39, 7–16

Grace AA, Gerfen CR, Aston-Jones G (1998) Catecholamines in the central nervous system. Overview. *Adv Pharmacol* 42, 655–670

Green AR, Hainsworth AH, Jackson DM (2000) GABA potentiation: a logical pharmacological approach for the treatment of acute ischaemic stroke. *Neuropharmacology* 39, 1483–1494

Hieble JP (2000) Adrenoceptor subclassification: an approach to improved cardiovascular therapeutics. *Pharm Acta Helv* 74, 163–171

Hoyer D, Hannon JP, Martin GR (2002) Molecular, pharmacological and functional diversity of 5-HT receptors. *Pharmacol Biochem Behav* 71, 533–554

Insel PA (1996) Adrenoceptors – evolving concepts and clinical implications. *N Engl J Med* 334, 580–585

Kennedy C (2000) The discovery and development of P2 receptor subtypes. *J Auton Nerv Syst* 81, 158–163

Kirstein SL, Insel PA (2004) Autonomic nervous system pharmacogenomics: a progress report. *Pharmacol Rev* 56, 31–52

Mackinnon AC, Spedding M, Brown CM (1994) α_2-Adrenoceptors: more subtypes but fewer functional differences. *Trends Pharmacol Sci* 15, 119–123

Mayersohn M, Guentert TW (1995) Clinical pharmacokinetics of the monoamine oxidase-A inhibitor moclobemide. *Clin Pharmacokinet* 29, 292–332

Minneman KP, Esbenshade TA (1994) α_1-Adrenergic receptor subtypes. *Annu Rev Pharmacol Toxicol* 34, 117–133

Noll G, Wenzel RR, Binggeli C, Corti C, Luscher TF (1998) Role of sympathetic nervous system in hypertension and effects of cardiovascular drugs. *Eur Heart J* 19(suppl), F32–F38

Piascik MT, Perez DM (2001) Alpha1-adrenergic receptors: new insights and directions. *J Pharmacol Exp Ther* 298, 403–410

Rana BK, Shiina T, Insel PA (2001) Genetic variations and polymorphisms of G protein-coupled receptors: functional and therapeutic implications. *Annu Rev Pharmacol Toxicol* 41, 593–624

Rangachari PK (1998) The fate of released histamine: reception, response and termination. *Yale J Biol Med* 71, 173–182

Robidoux J, Martin TL, Collins S (2004) Beta-adrenergic receptors and regulation of energy expenditure: a family affair. *Annu Rev Pharmacol Toxicol* 44, 297–323

Romanelli MN, Gualtieri F (2003) Cholinergic nicotinic receptors: competitive ligands, allosteric modulators, and their potential applications. *Med Res Rev* 23, 393–426

Rudolph U, Crestani F, Möhler H (2001) $GABA_A$ receptor subtypes: dissecting their pharmacological functions. *Trends Pharmacol Sci* 22, 188–194

Satchell D (2000) Purinergic nerves and purinoceptors: early perspectives. *J Auton Nerv Syst* 81, 212–217

Shaikh S, Kerwin RW (2002) Receptor pharmacogenetics: relevance to CNS syndromes. *Br J Clin Pharmacol* 54, 344–348

Sherwin AL (1999) Neuroactive amino acids in focally epileptic human brain: a review. *Neurochem Res* 24, 1387–1395

Simons FE, Simons KJ (1999) Clinical pharmacology of new histamine H_1 receptor antagonists. *Clin Pharmacokinet* 36, 329–352

Small KM, McGraw DW, Liggett SB (2003) Pharmacology and physiology of human adrenergic receptor polymorphisms. *Annu Rev Pharmacol Toxicol* 43, 381–411

Strosberg AD, Pietri-Rouxel F (1996) Function and regulation of the β_3-adrenoceptor. *Trends Pharmacol Sci* 17, 373–381

Takana K (2000) Functions of glutamate transporters in the brain. *Neurosci Res* 37, 15–19

Thibonnier M, Coles P, Thibonnier A, Shoham M (2001) The basic and clinical pharmacology of nonpeptide vasopressin receptor antagonists. *Annu Rev Pharmacol Toxicol* 41, 175–202

Torphy TJ (1994) β-Adrenoceptors, cAMP and airway smooth muscle relaxation: challenges to dogma. *Trends Pharmacol Sci* 15, 370–374

Vanden Broeck J, Torfs H, Poels J et al (1999) Tachykinin-like peptides and their receptors. A review. *Ann NY Acad Sci* 897, 374–387

Waagepetersen HS, Sonnewald U, Schousboe A (1999) The GABA paradox: multiple roles as metabolite, neurotransmitter, and neurodifferentiative agent. *J Neurochem* 73, 1335–1342

Wallukat G (2002) The beta-adrenergic receptors. *Herz* 27, 683–690

Williams M (2000) Purines: from premise to promise. *J Auton Nerv Syst* 81, 285–288

Zhang D, Pan Z-H, Awobuluyi M, Lipton SA (2001) Structure and function of $GABA_C$ receptors: a comparison of native versus recombinant receptors. *Trends Pharmacol Sci* 22, 121–132

Self-assessment

In the following questions, the first statement, in italics, is true. Is the accompanying statement also true?

1. *The autonomic nervous system (ANS) is only one of the neuronal systems controlling bodily functions.* The sympathetic division of the ANS utilises adrenaline as its primary transmitter substance.

2. *Drugs acting at the ganglia affect both sympathetic and parasympathetic nervous systems.* Ganglion-blocking drugs also block the neuromuscular junction.

3. *Acetylcholine is metabolised extremely rapidly by acetylcholinesterase in the synaptic cleft.* Acetylcholine esterase is not the only enzyme in the body that breaks down acetylcholine.

4. *Dopamine and noradrenaline are synthesised from the intermediate precursor levodopa.* Dopamine is a transmitter in the peripheral autonomic nervous system.

5. *There are two major monoamine oxidase isoenzymes, MAO-A and MAO-B.* Both isoenzymes metabolise tyramine.

6. *The differentiation of adrenoceptors into several subtypes is of clinical importance.* Both α_1- and α_2-adrenoceptor antagonists can be used to lower blood pressure.

7. *Botulism periodically causes fatalities and is caused by poisoning by the bacterial toxin from Clostridium botulinum.* Botulinum toxin enhances acetylcholine release from cholinergic neurons.

8. *There are three major types of β-adrenoceptor: β_1, β_2 and β_3.* The β_3-adrenoceptor is most widespread.

9. *Stimulation of presynaptic adrenoceptors controls noradrenaline release.* Propranolol inhibits noradrenaline release.

10. *The major route by which the action of synaptic noradrenaline and 5HT is curtailed is by reuptake into presynaptic neurons by an uptake mechanism.* The reuptake of noradrenaline and 5HT can be selectively controlled.

11. *The parasympathetic and sympathetic nervous systems often have opposite effects in an organ.* Sympathetic nervous stimulation to the gut inhibits gut motility and sphincter tone.

12. *The vagal cranial nerve to the eye decreases pupil size and limits accommodation to near vision.* Adrenaline (epinephrine) decreases pupil size.

The answers are provided on pages 706–707.

Types of receptors and examples of agonists and antagonists

Receptor type	Principal location(s)	Mechanism	Main effects	Agonists	Antagonists
Acetylcholine					
Muscarinic[a]					
M_1	CNS and autonomic ganglia (minor role)	G_q: ↑ phospholipase C	Neurotransmission in CNS	Oxotremorine	Pirenzepine
M_2	Heart	G_i: ↓ adenylate cyclase	Bradycardia		
M_3	Smooth muscles, secretory glands	G_q: ↑ phospholipase C	Contraction, secretion		
$M_1 + M_2 + M_3$				Bethanecol, pilocarpine, carbachol	Atropine, hyoscine, propantheline, ipratropium
Nicotinic					
N_1	Autonomic ganglia	Ligand-gated ion channel	Postganglionic activation	Carbachol, nicotine	Trimetaphan, mecamylamine
N_2	Neuromuscular junction	Ligand-gated ion channel	Muscle contraction	Nicotine	Gallamine, vecuronium
Adrenergic					
α-Adrenoceptors[b]					
α_1	CNS and postsynaptic in sympathetic nervous system	G_q: ↑ phospholipase C	Contraction of arterial smooth muscle, decrease in contractions of gut	Phenylephrine, oxymetazoline	Prazosin, indoramin
α_2	Presynaptic (in both α- and β-adrenergic neurons)	Gi: ↓ adenylate cyclase	Decreased noradrenaline release	Clonidine	Yohimbine
$\alpha_1 + \alpha_2$				Noradrenaline, adrenaline	Phenoxybenzamine, phentolamine
β-Adrenoceptors[c]					
β_1	CNS and heart (nodes and myocardium)	G_s: ↑ adenylate cyclase	Increased force and rate of cardiac contraction	Dobutamine	Atenolol, metoprolol

continued

Drug receptors

Drug receptors

Types of receptors and examples of agonists and antagonists *(continued)*

Receptor type	Principal location(s)	Mechanism	Main effects	Agonists	Antagonists
β-*Adrenoceptors*[c] *(continued)*					
β_2	Widespread	G_s; ↑ adenylate cyclase	Bronchial dilation, decrease in contraction of gut, metabolic effects	Salbutamol, terbutaline	Butoxamine
β_3	Adipocytes	G_s; ↑ adenylate cyclase	Mobilisation of fat stores	–	–
$\beta_1 + \beta_2$				Adrenaline, isoprenaline	Propranolol, oxprenolol
Dopamine					
D_1	CNS (N, O, P, S), kidney,[d] heart[d]	G_s; ↑ adenylate cyclase	Vasodilation in kidney (see notes)	Fenoldopam	
D_2	CNS (C, N, O, SN), pituitary gland, chemoreceptor trigger zone gastrointestinal tract	G_i; ↓ adenylate cyclase, ↑ K^+ channels, ↓ Ca^{2+} channels	Linked to schizophrenia, prolactin secretion, movement control, memory	Bromocriptine, pergolide	Butyrophenones, sulpiride, renoxipride
D_3	CNS (F, Me, Mi) (limbic system)	G_i; ↓ adenylate cyclase	Cognition emotion		Sulpiride
D_4	CNS, heart	G_i ↓ adenylate cyclase	Linked to schizophrenia		Clozapine
D_5	CNS (Hi, Hy)	G_s; ↑ adenylate cyclase			
$D_1 + D_2$					Phenothiazines
5-Hydroxytryptamine (5HT), serotonin[e]					
$5HT_{1A}$	CNS (Hi, R)	G_i; ↓ cAMP	Autoregulation, anxiety	Buspirone	
$5HT_{1B}$	CNS (B, G, S), blood vessels	G_i ↓ cAMP	Autoregulation, vasoconstriction	Sumatriptan	
$5HT_{1D}$	CNS, blood vessels	G_i; ↓ cAMP	Vasoconstriction	Sumatriptan	Metergoline
$5HT_{1E}$	CNS (Co. P)	G_i; ↓ cAMP			
$5HT_{1F}$	CNS (Co. Hi)	G_i; ↓ cAMP		Sumatriptan	
$5HT_{2A}$	CNS (Co), platelets, smooth muscle	G_q; ↑ IP_3	Schizophrenia, platelet aggregation, vasodilation		Ketanserin, trazodone, mianserin, clozapine

continued

Types of receptors and examples of agonists and antagonists *(continued)*

Receptor type	Principal location(s)	Mechanism	Main effects	Agonists	Antagonists
5-Hydroxytryptamine (5HT), serotonin)[e] *(continued)*					
$5HT_{2B}$	Stomach	$G_q; \uparrow IP_3$	Contraction, morphogenesis		
$5HT_{2C}$	CNS (Ch, Hi, SN)	$G_q; \uparrow IP_3$	Satiety		
$5HT_3$	CNS (A), enteric nerves, sensory nerves	Ligand-gated Na^+/K^+ channels	Emesis		Granisetron, ondansetron
$5HT_4$	CNS, myenteric plexus, smooth muscle	$G_s; \uparrow cAMP$	Anxiety, memory	Metoclopramide, renzapride, cisapride	
$5HT_{5A}$	CNS	$G_i; \downarrow cAMP$			
$5HT_{5B}$	CNS	?			
$5HT_6$	CNS	$G_s; \uparrow cAMP$			
$5HT_7$	CNS	$G_s; \uparrow cAMP$			Clozapine
Histamine					
H_1	CNS, endothelium, smooth muscle	$G_q; \uparrow$ phospholipase C, $\uparrow IP_3$	Sedation, sleep		Mepyramine
H_2	CNS, cardiac muscle, stomach	$G_s; \uparrow cAMP$	Gastric acid secretion	Dimaprit	Cimetidine, ranitidine
H_3	CNS (presynaptic), myenteric plexus	?	Appetite, cognition		Thioperamide
H_4	Eosinophils, basophils, mast cells	G-protein?			
Gamma-aminobutyric acid (GABA)[f]					
$GABA_A$	Brain neurons, spinal motor neurons and interneurons	Ligand-gated Cl^- channel (open)[g]	Widespread reduction of impulse transmission in CNS, inhibition of sensory signals at spinal level	Muscimol (benzodiazepines) (zolpidem)	(Picrotoxin) (flumazenil)

continued

Drug receptors

Types of receptors and examples of agonists and antagonists *(continued)*

Receptor type	Principal location(s)	Mechanism	Main effects	Agonists	Antagonists
Gamma-aminobutyric acid (GABA)[f] *(continued)*					
GABA$_B$	Brain neurons, glial cells, spinal motor neurons and interneurons	G-protein effects on Ca^{2+} channel (closes) and K$^+$ channel (opens)	Widespread reduction of impulse transmission in CNS, suppression of polysynaptic reflexes in spine, generation of spike and wave discharges in absence epilepsy	Baclofen	
Glutamate[h]					
N-Methyl D-aspartate(NMDA)[i]	CNS (B, C, sensory pathways)	Ligand-gated Ca^{2+} channel (slow)	Learning		Ketamine, phenyclidine (inhibit Ca^{2+} flux)
Kainate	CNS (Hi)	Ligand-gated Ca^{2+} channel (fast)		Kainate	
AMPA	CNS (similar to NMDA receptors)	Ligand-gated Ca^{2+} channel (fast)			
Metabotropic Group I (mglu$_1$ and mglu$_5$) Group II (mglu$_2$ and mglu$_3$) Group III (mglu$_4$, mglu$_6$, mglu$_7$, and mglu$_8$)	CNS (Hi, S, T)	G$_q$: ↑ phospholipase C ↑ IP$_3$ G$_i$: ↓cAMP G$_i$: ↓cAMP	Increased attentiveness		
Peptides					
Angiotensin					
AT$_1$		G$_q$: ↑phospholipase C G$_i$: ↓cAMP	Vasoconstriction, salt retention		Losartan
AT$_2$		G$_i$: ↓cAMP	Weak vasodilation, fetal development, vascular growth		
Bradykinin					
B$_1$		G$_q$: ↑ phospholipase C	Inflammation		

continued

Types of receptors and examples of agonists and antagonists *(continued)*

Receptor type	Principal location(s)	Mechanism	Main effects	Agonists	Antagonists
Bradykinin (continued)					
B_2		G-protein; multiple signals, may be multiple receptors	Most actions of kinins, vasodilation, pain response		
Endothelins					
ET_A		G_q: ↑ phospholipase C: ↑ Ca^{2+} via IP_3	Vasoconstriction		
ET_B		G_q: ↑ phospholipase C	Release of nitric oxide, vasodilation		
Natriuretic peptides					
ANP_A		G-protein, guanylate cyclase			
ANP_B		G-protein, guanylate cyclase			
Neurokinins (tachykinins)					
NK_1		G_q: slow build-up of response	Nociception (substance P)		
NK_2		G_q: slow build-up of response	Nociception (neurokinin A)		
NK_3		G_q	(Neurokinin B)		
Opioids					
δ, κ, μ		G_i: ↓ Camp	See Chapter 19 for details		
Vasopressin					
V_1		G_q: ↑ phospholipase C, ↑ IP_3, ↑ Ca^{2+}	Vasoconstriction		
V_2		G_s: ↑ adenylate cyclase	Antidiuretic effect on collecting duct and ascending limb of loop of Henle		
V_3 or V_{1b}	Pituitary	G_q plus G_i (depending on occupancy)	Modulates ACTH secretion		

continued

Drug receptors

Drug receptors

Types of receptors and examples of agonists and antagonists *(continued)*

Receptor type	Principal location(s)	Mechanism	Main effects	Agonists	Antagonists
Purines					
Adenosine[j]					
A_1		G_i: $\downarrow$ adenylate cyclase, $\uparrow K^+$ conduction in heart	Decreased glomerular filtration rate, cardiac depression, vasoconstriction, decreased CNS activity, bronchoconstriction	–	Methylxanthines[k]
A_{2A}		G_s: $\uparrow$ adenylate cyclase	Vasodilation, decreased CNS activity, inhibition of platelet aggregation, bronchodilation		
A_{2B}		G_q: $\uparrow$ phospholipase C	Action on intestine and bladder	–	Enprofylline[l]
		G_s: $\uparrow$ cAMP: Ca^{2+} influx	Release of mediators from mast cells?		
A_3		G_i: $\downarrow$ cAMP	Wide tissue distribution; release of mediators from mast cells		
ATP					
P2X (P2Y$_\alpha$ in brain)		Ligand-gated ion channels (Na^+, Ca^{2+} and K^+)	Neuronal depolarisation, influx of Na^+ and Ca^{2+} > efflux of K^+		
P2Y$_\beta$ in brain		G-protein, closes K^+ channel			

continued

82

Drug receptors

Types of receptors and examples of agonists and antagonists *(continued)*

Receptor type	Principal location(s)	Mechanism	Main effects	Agonists	Antagonists
ADP					
P2Y$_1$		G$_q$: ↑ phospholipase C	Change of platelet shape,[m] activation of nitric oxide synthetase[m]		
P2$_{ADP}$		G$_i$: ↓ cAMP	Platelet aggregation[m]		
UTP or ATP					
P2Y$_2$		G$_q$: ↑ phospholipase C	Vasoconstriction[m]		

[a]Additional muscarinic receptors (M$_4$ (G$_i$) and M$_5$ (G$_q$)) have been identified recently but their physiological importance is not defined.

[b]Three α$_1$-adrenoceptors have been identified (α$_{1A}$, α$_{1B}$, α$_{1C}$) all of which act via G$_q$ proteins: α$_{1A}$ adrenoceptors have a higher affinity for noradrenaline than for adrenaline, α$_{1B}$ and α$_{1C}$ adrenoceptors do not show selectivity.

[c]The β-adrenoceptors differ in their affinities for noradrenaline (NA) and adrenaline (A): β$_1$, A ≥ NA; β$_2$, A > NA: β$_3$, NA > A.

[d]The mRNA for D$_5$ receptors has not been found in heart and kidneys and, therefore, the type of receptor in these organs remains questionable (it could be D$_1$). CNS areas: A, area postrema; B, basal ganglia; C, caudate putamen; Ch, choroid; Co, cortex; F, frontal cortex ; G, globus pallidus; Hi, hippocampus; Hy, hypothalamus; Me, medulla; Mi, midbrain; N, nucleus accumbens; 0, olfactory tubercle; P, putamen; R raphe nucleus; S, striatum; SN, substantia nigra; T, thalamus.

[e]There are many experimental drugs that are selective agonists and antagonists for receptors subtypes and some are undergoing clinical trials for various conditions. Only clinically useful examples are given. The identification and classification of 5HT receptors is a complex and rapidly changing field (for example, four variants of the 5HT$_7$ receptor have been recognised, three of which occur in humans). 5HT$_{1C}$ was the first 5HT receptor sequence to be cloned but was reclassified as 5HT$_{2C}$ when it was found to alter IP$_3$ not cAMP. 5HT is involved in numerous pathways within the CNS and the roles of the different receptor types has not been fully characterised. Effects associated with the different receptors are not well established, with the exception of 5HT$_3$ and emesis. Ergotamine is a selective antagonist (and partial agonist) for the 5HT$_1$ subgroup; methysergide is a selective antagonist (and partial agonist) for the 5HT$_2$ subgroup.

[f]GABA produces inhibition of neurotransmission widely throughout the brain.

[g]The GABA$_A$ receptor Cl$^-$ channel has a binding site for GABA and also adjacent binding sites for benzodiazepines (which affect the response to GABA), barbiturates, picrotoxin and steroids.

[h]Glutamate produces increased neuronal activity in many regions of the CNS; the different receptors are formed from subunits that can exist in different isoforms; a number of variants have been demonstrated for each.

[i]A low concentration of glycine (below endogenous levels) is necessary for NMDA receptors to open; endogenous amines such as spermidine also facilitate opening. Alcohol inhibits NMDA receptors and tolerance to alcohol is linked to upregulation of NMDA receptors associated with hyperexcitability on withdrawal (see Ch. 54).

[j]A$_1$–A$_3$ receptors used to be called P$_1$ receptors: A$_3$ receptors have been identified on rat mast cells and A$_{2B}$ on human mast cells.

[k]Methylxanthines increase alertness by blocking A$_1$/A$_2$ receptors.

[l]An anti-asthma drug that is a selective antagonist of A$_{2B}$ receptors.

[m]Part of response to vascular damage.

The cardiovascular system

5

Ischaemic heart disease

The heart receives about 5% of cardiac output at rest, and extracts about 75% of the oxygen from the perfusing blood. Coronary artery blood flow increases three- to four-fold with exercise, to cope with the increase in myocardial oxygen demand. Ischaemic heart disease most frequently occurs as a result of restriction of blood flow by atheroma in large epicardial coronary arteries. Atheromatous plaques tend to form in areas of flow disturbance, such as bends in the vessels or near branching vessels. The plaques are often localised, but atheroma can diffusely involve a long segment of the vessel. When localised, plaques are frequently eccentric, leaving a portion of the arterial wall free of significant disease and still able to respond to vasoconstrictor and vasodilator influences. These segments of artery are particularly prone to vasospasm, since flow disturbances impair endothelial function in areas affected by atheroma, and reduce shear stress-mediated local generation of the vasodilator substance nitric oxide (EDRF, endothelium-derived relaxing factor). If the coronary artery disease is longstanding, then smaller collateral vessels can develop, and improve perfusion beyond the atheromatous narrowing.

In people who smoke, who have hypertension or who have hypercholesterolaemia, coronary artery atheroma, in common with atheroma in other parts of the vascular tree, occurs at a younger age and more extensively. Some atheromatous plaques have a lipid-rich core, with a substantial inflammatory cell infiltration and a thin fibrous cap; such plaques are relatively unstable. Other plaques are more fibrotic, with a thick fibrous cap, and are stable. These properties are important in determining progression to an acute coronary syndrome, since unstable plaques are more prone to disruption (see below).

Myocardial ischaemia can also arise in the presence of normal epicardial coronary arteries. In this situation, it arises either from abnormal regulation of the microvascular circulation, or from intense epicardial vasoconstriction (coronary vasospasm).

Angina

Stable angina

Angina pectoris is a symptom of reversible myocardial ischaemia and is most frequently experienced as chest pain on exertion that is relieved by rest. Reversible myocardial ischaemia can also present with shortness of breath, or occur without symptoms (silent ischaemia). The symptoms are the consequence of an imbalance between oxygen supply and oxygen demand in the ischaemic area of myocardium (Fig. 5.1). This results from an inability of the coronary blood flow to increase sufficiently to meet the metabolic demands of the heart, usually because of a fixed atheromatous narrowing of a coronary artery. Coronary artery vasospasm often accentuates the reduction in flow produced by fixed obstructions, and when it is present angina occurs at a lower work load.

Acute coronary syndromes

These cover the spectrum from unstable angina to myocardial infarction and sudden death, and have a common pathophysiological origin in an unstable coronary artery atheromatous plaque. Disruption of unstable plaques can be precipitated by sudden stresses on the fibrous cap of the plaque produced by local disturbance of blood flow, or by vasospasm. The resultant fissuring or ulceration of the surface of the plaque promotes platelet aggregation (Ch. 11), thrombus formation and local vasospasm. Platelet–thrombin microemboli can break off and impact in small distal vessels.

If vessel occlusion is incomplete, angina occurs on minimal exertion; if the vessel is almost completely occluded, then angina occurs at rest. In unstable angina, spontaneous lysis of the thrombus and reduction in local vasospasm takes place within about 20 min; reperfusion of the ischaemic tissue then occurs, without lasting damage. More prolonged occlusion leads to myocardial infarction.

Myocardial infarction and sudden cardiac death
Myocardial infarction most commonly arises from complete coronary artery occlusion, following disruption of an unstable atheromatous plaque (see unstable angina above). Occlusion often occurs at the site of an atheromatous lesion that previously was only mildly or mod-

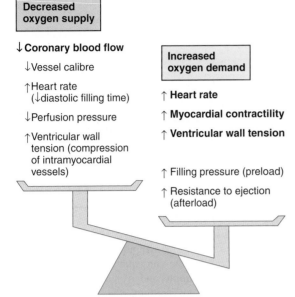

Decreased oxygen supply

↓ **Coronary blood flow**

↓ Vessel calibre

↑ Heart rate
(↓ diastolic filling time)

↓ Perfusion pressure

↑ Ventricular wall
tension (compression
of intramyocardial
vessels)

Increased oxygen demand

↑ **Heart rate**

↑ **Myocardial contractility**

↑ **Ventricular wall tension**

↑ Filling pressure (preload)

↑ Resistance to ejection
(afterload)

Fig. 5.1
Factors affecting the balance of oxygen supply and demand in angina.

erately stenotic and may not have caused symptoms prior to disruption. If the occlusion lasts for longer than 20–30 min, muscle necrosis begins subendocardially and then extends transmurally over the next few hours. If early reperfusion occurs, this results in a subendocardial infarction (more usually called a non-ST-elevation infarction, because of the absence of characteristic ST segment changes on the electrocardiograph [ECG]). More prolonged occlusion produces an ST elevation infarction. Diagnosis of acute myocardial infarction requires a rise in sensitive cardiac markers, such as troponin I or T, or characteristic ST-segment elevation on the ECG in the early stages, before the cardiac markers have had time to increase. Activation of endogenous thrombolysis (Ch. 11) and the presence of a good collateral circulation are factors that naturally limit the size of the infarct.

Sudden cardiac death results when fatal ventricular arrhythmias arise from ischaemic tissue, often following complete coronary artery occlusion.

Drug treatment of angina

Drug treatment for angina is directed either:

- to increase oxygen supply by improving coronary blood flow, or
- to reduce oxygen demand by decreasing cardiac work.

Drugs can be taken to relieve the ischaemia rapidly during an acute attack or as regular prophylaxis to reduce the risk of subsequent episodes. Four major classes of drug are used to treat angina:

- nitrovasodilators (especially organic nitrates)
- β-adrenoceptor antagonists (β-blockers)
- calcium channel antagonists (calcium antagonists)
- potassium channel openers.

Organic nitrates

Examples: glyceryl trinitrate, isosorbide dinitrate, isosorbide mononitrate

Mechanism of action and effects
The organic nitrates are vasodilators that relax vascular smooth muscle by mimicking the effects of endogenous nitric oxide. Enzymatic degradation of the nitrate releases nitric oxide, which combines with thiol groups in vascular endothelium to form nitrosothiols. Nitric oxide and nitrosothiols activate guanylate cyclase and lead to generation of cyclic guanosine monophosphate (cGMP, Fig. 5.2). This, in turn, reduces the availability of intracellular Ca^{2+} to the contractile mechanism of vascular smooth muscle, causing relaxation. Vasodilation is produced in three main vascular beds.

- **Venous capacitance vessels**, leading to peripheral pooling of blood and reduced venous return to the heart: this lowers left ventricular filling pressure (preload), decreases ventricular wall tension, and, therefore, reduces myocardial oxygen demand. Venous dilation is produced at moderate plasma nitrate concentrations; tolerance to this action occurs rapidly during continued treatment.
- **Arterial resistance vessels (mainly large arteries)**, leading to reduced resistance to ventricular emptying (afterload): this lowers blood pressure, decreases cardiac work and contributes to a reduced myocardial oxygen demand. Arterial dilation requires higher plasma nitrate concentrations; tolerance occurs less readily during long-term treatment.
- **Coronary arteries**: nitrates have little effect on total coronary blood flow in angina; indeed, flow may be reduced owing to a decrease in perfusion pressure. However, blood flow through collateral vessels may be improved, and nitrates also relieve coronary artery vasospasm. The net effect is increased blood supply to ischaemic areas of myocardium. Coronary artery dilation occurs at low plasma nitrate concentrations, and tolerance is slow to develop.

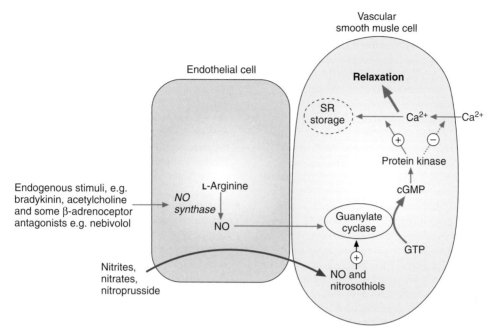

Fig. 5.2
Actions of endogenous and exogenous nitric oxide (NO). Endogenous NO from endothelial cells (EDRF) relaxes smooth muscle via generation of cGMP. Organic nitrates react with tissue thiols, generating NO or nitrosothiols, which then activate guanylate cyclase and increase cGMP. The steps involved in muscle relaxation are not yet certain but may include reduced Ca^{2+} influx, increased Ca^{2+} sequestering in sarcoplasmic reticulum (SR) and myosin light chain dephosphorylation (see also Fig. 6.5).

Pharmacokinetics

Glyceryl trinitrate is the most widely used organic nitrate. It is well absorbed from the gut but undergoes extensive first-pass metabolism in the liver to inactive metabolites. To increase its bioavailability, glyceryl trinitrate is given by one of four routes that avoid first-pass metabolism.

- **Sublingual**: the tablet is placed under the tongue and is absorbed rapidly across the buccal mucosa. The very short half-life of glyceryl trinitrate (less than 5 min) limits the duration of action to approximately 30 min. Tablets lose their potency with prolonged storage; a metered-dose aerosol spray is a more stable delivery mechanism.
- **Buccal**: a tablet containing glyceryl trinitrate in an inert polymer matrix is held between the upper lip and gum, which permits slow release of drug to prolong the duration of action.
- **Transdermal**: glyceryl trinitrate is absorbed well through the skin and can be delivered from an adhesive patch via a rate-limiting membrane or matrix. Steady release of the drug maintains a stable blood concentration for at least 24 h after application of the patch.
- **Intravenous**: the short duration of action of glyceryl trinitrate is an advantage for intravenous dose titration.

Isosorbide dinitrate is well absorbed orally but undergoes extensive first-pass metabolism, which produces both active and inactive metabolites. The majority of the sustained clinical effect results from the formation of isosorbide 5-mononitrate. Isosorbide dinitrate is longer acting than glyceryl trinitrate but still has a short half-life; therefore, sustained-release formulations are often used. It is also used as a chewable tablet for buccal absorption and a rapid onset of action, or by intravenous infusion.

Isosorbide 5-mononitrate is not subject to first-pass metabolism and can be used orally as an alternative to isosorbide dinitrate, when it gives a more predictable clinical response. Since the amount of isosorbide mononitrate absorbed is more than that generated during first-pass metabolism of the dinitrate, there is a greater antianginal action from an equal dose.

Unwanted effects

- Venodilation can produce postural hypotension, dizziness, syncope and reflex tachycardia.
- Arterial dilation causes throbbing headaches and flushing, but tolerance to these effects is common during treatment with long-acting nitrates.
- Tolerance to the therapeutic effects of nitrates develops rapidly if there is a sustained high plasma nitrate concentration. Contributory factors may include depletion of vascular thiol groups or activation of the sympathetic nervous system and

renin–angiotensin system in response to the low blood pressure; this leads to expansion of blood volume, which offsets the reduced preload. Recent evidence suggests, however, that tolerance is caused also by superoxide production within the target cells, leading to reduced generation of nitric oxide or to rapid degradation of the nitric oxide after it is produced by the drug. Tolerance can be avoided by a 'nitrate-low' period of several hours in each 24 h. This is preferable to a 'nitrate-free' period, which carries a risk of rebound angina. In practice, a nitrate-low period is achieved by asymmetric dosing with conventional formulations of isosorbide mononitrate or dinitrate (e.g., 8 a.m., 1 p.m.) or by using a once-daily formulation of isosorbide mononitrate that allows plasma nitrate concentrations to fall overnight. Transdermal nitrate patches have to be removed for part of each 24 h (e.g. overnight) to prevent tolerance, thereby creating a nitrate-free period. There is limited evidence that co-administration of an angiotensin-converting enzyme (ACE) inhibitor, angiotensin II receptor antagonist or hydralazine (Ch. 6) may reduce nitrate tolerance by impairing superoxide formation.

- Drug interactions are most troublesome with phosphodiesterase inhibitors, such as sildenafil, used in the treatment of erectile dysfunction (Ch. 16); co-administration can result in severe hypotension.

Beta-adrenoceptor antagonists (β-blockers)

Examples: atenolol, carvedilol, labetalol, propranolol, pindolol, nebivolol (information on individual β-adrenoceptor antagonists is given in the compendium to Chapter 8)

Mechanism of action and effects in angina

All β-adrenoceptor antagonists (often inadequately referred to as β-blockers) act as competitive antagonists of catecholamines at β-adrenoceptors. They achieve their therapeutic effect in angina by blockade at the cardiac β_1-adrenoceptor and thereby:

- decrease heart rate
- reduce the force of cardiac contraction
- lower blood pressure.

These effects are most marked during exercise, and reduce myocardial oxygen demand. The lengthening of diastole also gives more time for coronary perfusion and effectively improves oxygen supply.

Certain β-adrenoceptor antagonists have additional properties that may affect their pharmacological effects. These include the following.

- **Cardioselectivity**. Some β-adrenoceptor antagonists, for example atenolol, are relatively selective antagonists at the β_1-adrenoceptor, a property known as 'cardioselectivity' because of predominant effects on the heart. Other β-adrenoceptor antagonists, for example propranolol, have equal or greater antagonist activity at β_2-adrenoceptors; these drugs are referred to as 'non-selective' β-adrenoceptor antagonists. However, even cardioselective β-adrenoceptor antagonists produce β_2-adrenoceptor blockade at higher doses, so they are 'selective', rather than truly specific, for the β_1-adrenoceptor (Ch. 1).

- **Partial agonist activity**. Some β_1-adrenoceptor antagonists, such as pindolol, also possess partial agonist activity at the β_2-adrenoceptor (Chs 1 and 6). Such drugs weakly stimulate the β_2-adrenoceptor at rest. When the concentration of endogenous catecholamines rises, the drug becomes a competitive antagonist while retaining its mild stimulant activity. The rise in heart rate and force of cardiac contraction normally produced by catecholamines are, therefore, blunted to a lesser extent by a partial agonist than by a full antagonist, and myocardial oxygen demand remains higher. For this reason, β-adrenoceptor antagonists with partial agonist activity may be less effective than full antagonists in the treatment of severe angina, but partial agonists are less likely to cause a resting bradycardia. If the drug is a partial agonist at the β_2-adrenoceptor, it will produce vasodilation in some vascular beds (see Fig. 6.8).

- **Vasodilator activity**. Pure β_1-adrenoceptor antagonists do not cause vasodilation, and a consequence of β-adrenoceptor blockade is reflex vasoconstriction, which occurs in response to the fall in cardiac output. However, some β-adrenoceptor antagonists have additional properties that produce arterial vasodilation. This can be achieved by β_2-adrenoceptor partial agonist activity (e.g. pindolol), α-adrenoceptor blockade (e.g. labetalol), by increasing endothelial nitric oxide synthesis (nebivolol) or because of α_1-adrenoceptor blockade. Vasodilation does not have any proven advantage for the treatment of angina, but may be useful in the treatment of hypertension (Ch. 6). Of interest for future pharmacological developments is that nebivolol, like sotalol (Ch. 8) and propranolol, is a racemic mixture; the D-isomer is responsible for both β-adrenoceptor blockade and vasodilation, but the L-isomer has only vasodilator properties.

Pharmacokinetics

Lipophilic β-adrenoceptor antagonists, such as propranolol, are well absorbed from the gut but undergo extensive first-pass metabolism in the liver, with considerable variability between individuals. Reduction in exercise heart rate is closely related to the plasma concentration of β-adrenoceptor antagonist. Consequently, dose titration of lipophilic β-adrenoceptor antagonists is necessary to achieve the optimum clinical response in angina. Most lipophilic β-adrenoceptor antagonists have short half-lives.

Hydrophilic β-adrenoceptor antagonists, such as atenolol, are absorbed less completely from the gut and are eliminated unchanged by the kidney. The dose range to maintain effective plasma concentrations is narrower than for those drugs that undergo metabolism. The half-lives of hydrophilic drugs are usually intermediate.

Unwanted effects

- **Blockade of β_1-adrenoceptors**. Since β-adrenoceptor antagonists reduce cardiac output, they can precipitate heart failure if there is pre-existing poor left ventricular function, when high sympathetic nervous activity is necessary to maintain cardiac output. However, used with care, they can be given as part of the therapy of heart failure (Ch. 7). Reduction in cardiac output can also impair blood supply to peripheral tissues, which can increase symptoms of intermittent claudication when used together with vasodilators or can provoke Raynaud's phenomenon (Ch. 10). Excessive bradycardia occasionally occurs, and β-adrenoceptor antagonists should be used with caution or avoided in the presence of an atrioventricular conduction defect (heart block). Drugs with partial agonist activity are less likely to cause bradycardia or to reduce cardiac output.
- **Blockade of β_2-adrenoceptors**. Bronchospasm can be precipitated in asthmatics or those with chronic pulmonary disease, and even cardioselective drugs are not completely safe. Insulin-requiring diabetics may be prone to prolonged hypoglycaemic episodes while taking non-selective β-adrenoceptor antagonists. Gluconeogenesis, a component of the metabolic response to hypoglycaemia, is dependent on β_2-adrenoceptor stimulation in the liver. Beta-adrenoceptor antagonists also blunt the autonomic response that alerts the diabetic person to the onset of hypoglycaemia.
- **Effects on blood lipid levels**. Most β-adrenoceptor antagonists raise the plasma concentration of triglycerides and lower the concentration of high-density lipoprotein cholesterol (Ch. 48). These changes are modest, but are potentially atherogenic. They are most marked with non-selective β-adrenoceptor antagonists, and do not occur if the drug has partial agonist activity.
- **Central nervous system effects**. These include sleep disturbance, vivid dreams and hallucinations, and are more common with lipophilic drugs, which readily cross the blood–brain barrier. Fatigue and more subtle psychomotor effects, for example lack of concentration and sexual dysfunction, are less frequent.
- **Sudden withdrawal syndrome**. Upregulation of β-adrenoceptors (Ch. 1) during long-term treatment makes the heart more sensitive to catecholamines. Beta-adrenoceptor antagonists should be stopped gradually in people with ischaemic heart disease, to avoid precipitating unstable angina or myocardial infarction.
- **Drug interactions**. The calcium channel antagonists verapamil and, to a lesser extent, diltiazem (see below) have potentially hazardous additive effects with β-adrenoceptor antagonists, reducing the force of cardiac contraction and slowing heart rate.

Calcium channel antagonists (calcium antagonists)

>
> Examples: nifedipine, amlodipine, verapamil, diltiazem

Mechanism of action and effects

Calcium is essential for excitation–contraction coupling in muscle cells. Free Ca^{2+} must either enter the cell through transmembrane channels or be released from intracellular stores for contraction to occur. As myofilaments relax, Ca^{2+} is then either taken up by the sarcoplasmic reticulum or translocated out of the cell. In striated muscle, Ca^{2+} is almost entirely recycled intracellularly via the sarcoplasmic reticulum. However, in smooth muscle (such as that surrounding arteriolar resistance vessels) and, to a lesser extent, in cardiac muscle, intracellular Ca^{2+} recycling is poorly developed. Reduced Ca^{2+} entry into these cells will, therefore, inhibit muscle contraction.

There are at least five different types of Ca^{2+} channel, two of which are found in cardiovascular tissues. Calcium channel antagonists (often referred to inadequately as calcium antagonists) have widely different chemical structures, but act principally by reducing Ca^{2+} influx through voltage-operated L-type (long-acting) slow Ca^{2+} channels, which predominate in myocardial cells. Voltage-operated T-type (transient) channels are found at high concentrations in pacemaker cells of the sinoatrial and atrioventricular nodes, while both types are found in vascular smooth muscle. T-type channels are activated by lower voltages than L-type channels and produce more transient depolarisation. None of the currently available calcium channel antagonists affect T-type channels to any important extent, or influence receptor-mediated Ca^{2+} channels that are involved in neurotransmitter release and respond to endogenous agonists such as noradrenaline (Fig. 5.3).

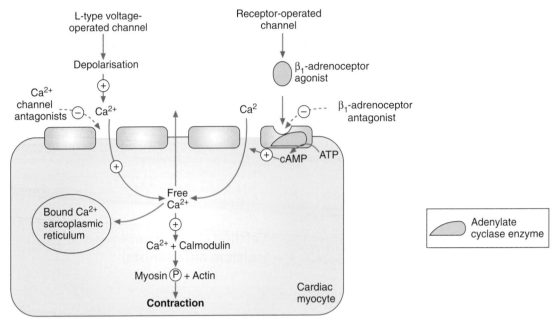

Fig. 5.3
Contraction of the cardiac myocyte by receptor and voltage-operated mechanisms. In the cardiac myocyte, depolarisation during the action potential activates the L-type voltage-operated channel. The influx of Ca^{2+} results in myosin phosphorylation and contraction. The Ca^{2+} influx is blocked by calcium channel antagonists. Adrenaline also causes contraction but acts via the β_1-adrenoreceptor to activate adenylate cyclase and increased intracellular cAMP. This results in phosphorylation of calcium channels, causing Ca^{2+} influx. The receptor-operated calcium channel is not blocked by calcium channel antagonists. +, stimulates activity; –, inhibits activity.

A number of effects of calcium channel antagonists may be important in angina.

- **Arteriolar dilation**. Dihydropyridine derivatives, such as nifedipine or amlodipine, are the most potent vasodilators. Arterial dilation reduces peripheral resistance and lowers the blood pressure, and therefore reduces the work of the left ventricle and, consequently, myocardial oxygen demand. Short-acting dihydropyridines produce a rapid drop in blood pressure, and reflex sympathetic nervous system activation leads to tachycardia (Fig. 5.4). Longer-acting compounds or modified-release formulations of short-acting drugs gradually reduce blood pressure and cause little reflex tachycardia.
- **Coronary artery dilation**. Prevention or relief of coronary vasospasm improves myocardial blood flow.
- **Negative chronotropic effect**. Verapamil and diltiazem (but not the dihydropyridines such as nifedipine or amlodipine) slow the rate of firing of the sinoatrial node and slow conduction of the impulse through the atrioventricular node. Thus, reflex tachycardia is not seen with these drugs and they slow the rate of rise in heart rate during exercise.
- **Reduced cardiac contractility**. Many calcium channel antagonists (particularly verapamil) have a negative inotropic effect. Amlodipine does not impair myocardial contractility.

There are clinically important differences among different calcium channel antagonists. They act on discrete receptors on the L-type Ca^{2+} channel; that for verapamil is intracellular, while diltiazem and the dihydropyridines (such as nifedipine) have extracellular binding sites, although the receptor domains for verapamil and diltiazem overlap. They also have different interaction kinetics with the receptor. Verapamil and diltiazem exhibit frequency-dependent interaction with their receptors, gaining access to the receptor when the channel is in the open state. By contrast, the dihydropyridines show voltage-dependent antagonism and bind to the channel in its inactivated state. The cardiac and vascular L-type Ca^{2+} channels also have differences in the structure of their subunits. These various factors are important in determining the antiarrhythmic properties of verapamil and diltiazem, and the vascular selectivity of the dihydropyridines. A comparison of the cardiovascular uses of the different calcium channel antagonists is shown in the drug compendium table at the end of this chapter.

Pharmacokinetics

Most calcium channel antagonists are lipophilic compounds with similar pharmacokinetic properties. They are almost completely absorbed from the gut lumen, undergo extensive and variable first-pass metabolism in the liver, and have short half-lives. Modified-release

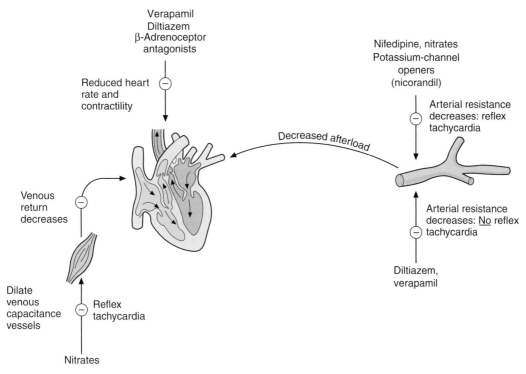

Fig. 5.4
The complementary major sites of action of some antianginal drugs and the reflex response of the heart to their actions. Reflex tachycardia results from the actions of nifedipine and potassium channel openers. This is not a problem with diltiazem and verapamil, which slow heart rate. Modified-release formulations of nifedipine or long-acting compounds such as amlodipine do not cause tachycardia.

formulations are widely used to prolong the duration of action. Nifedipine is also available in a liquid-containing capsule formulation; biting the capsule and swallowing the contents leads to a rapid onset of action.

Nifedipine is inactivated by metabolism, while verapamil and diltiazem have active, although less potent, metabolites. Verapamil can be given intravenously, a route that is usually reserved for the treatment of arrhythmias (Ch. 8).

Amlodipine differs from other calcium channel antagonists in that it is slowly, but more completely, absorbed and does not undergo first-pass metabolism. A high volume of distribution (Ch. 2), due to extensive membrane partitioning in cells, and slower metabolism by the liver give amlodipine a very long half-life of about 1–2 days.

Unwanted effects

- Arterial dilation: headache, flushing and dizziness may be troublesome, although tolerance often occurs with continued use. Ankle oedema, which is frequently resistant to diuretics, may be a consequence of increased transcapillary hydrostatic pressure. Tolerance to oedema does not occur. These unwanted effects are most common with the dihydropyridines.

- Reduced cardiac contractility can precipitate heart failure in susceptible people with pre-existing poor left ventricular function, particularly with verapamil. Amlodipine, a dihydropyridine, does not depress cardiac contractility.
- Tachycardia and palpitations with dihydropyridines.
- Bradycardia and heart block with verapamil or diltiazem. Both can slow the heart excessively, particularly if they are used in combination with other drugs that have similar effects on heart rate or atrioventricular nodal conduction, for example digoxin (Ch. 8) or β-adrenoceptor antagonists.
- Altered gut motility: constipation is most common with verapamil, less so with diltiazem. Nifedipine and related drugs can cause nausea and heartburn.
- Gum hyperplasia.

Potassium channel openers

Example: nicorandil

Mechanism of action
There are many different K^+ channels in cell membranes (Table 5.1). Nicorandil opens the adenosine triphosphate

Table 5.1
Selected examples of some K+ channels and associated currents

Voltage gated	Examples of distribution[a]	Comment
K_V channel family Delayed rectifying currents	Widely distributed including brain, heart, pancreas	Multiple subtypes of K+ channels are involved in delayed inward rectification and responsible for slow (I_{Ks}), rapid (I_{Kr}), ultra rapid (I_{Kur}) K+ currents involved in repolarisation in phases 2 and 3 the heart. (see Ch 8). Inhibited by quinidine and class III antiarrhythmics eg amiodarone and sotalol
Transient outward rectifying (I_{KTO}) current		A genetically distinct member of the K_V family of channels. Responsible for the I_{TO} transient current in phase 1. Activated by adenosine; inhibited by quinidine, amiodarone.
K_{ir} family Inward rectifying	Heart, muscle, brain, pancreas	Inward rectifying, rapidly inactivates cardiac Na+ channels; sets resting membrane potential (I_{K1}, I_{Kr}). Inhibited by amiodarone.
Ligand Gated Channels ATP sensitive channels (K_{ATP})	Heart, muscle, pancreas, mitochondria	Comprised of coexpressed K_{ir} channel and sulfonylurea. This provides a weak inward rectifying current; opened by ischaemia, inhibited by ATP, and sulfonylurea. Opened by minoxidil, nicorandil (Ch 6)
Acetylcholine sensitive channel (K_{ACh})	SA node, AV node and atria	This is G protein linked in SA node, atria and AV node and is a member of the K_{ir} family resulting in an inward rectifying (Kir) current. Opened by adenosine; inhibited by atropine and disopyramide.
Two pore channel (K_{2P})	Heart, brain pancreas	Opened by arachidonic acid; weak inward rectifying current; modulates resting membrane potential.
Calcium activated (K_{Ca} family) Large conductance channel (B_{Kca})	Heart, brain, pancreas	Members of K_{ir} family of channels. Being investigated for roles in neuroprotection, erectile dysfunction and other disorders.
Intermediate conductance channel (I_{Kca})	T lymphocytes, smooth muscle, brain, heart	Opened by hydralazine
Small conductance channel (S_{Kca})		

Potassium channels are diverse in structure and behaviour. Each channel consists of a variable number of membrane-spanning subunits. Each subunit consists of a variable number of linked membrane segments (maximum six) which make up the water filled pore. Some channels can be made up of just two subunits and some four. This diversity results in the possibility of dozens of genetically-determined different configurations of K+ channels many of which may have particular physiological roles. The genes encoding the channel proteins have in many cases been cloned. Channels with subunit variations are associated with different types of current which are involved in repolarization at different phases of the cardiac action potential. The channels can be open or closed depending upon the voltage across the cell or the presence of a selective ligand.
a: selected examples only are given

(ATP)-sensitive channel (a K_{ATP} channel with an ATP-sensitive K_{in} channel subunit) and hyperpolarises the cell membrane. When ATP binds to these channels, it inhibits K+ conductance; nicorandil opens the channels even in the presence of ATP. Hyperpolarisation of vascular smooth muscle cells inhibits opening of the L-type Ca^{2+} channels, which are voltage-dependent (Fig. 5.5). This produces vasodilation in systemic and coronary arteries.

Nicorandil also carries a nitrate moiety, and part of its vasodilator action is via generation of nitric oxide in vascular smooth muscle (see organic nitrates above). This may account for the venodilation produced by the drug.

Pharmacokinetics

Nicorandil is rapidly and almost completely absorbed from the gut. It is eliminated by hepatic metabolism and has a short half-life. However, the tissue effects correlate poorly with the plasma concentration, and the biological effect lasts up to 12 h.

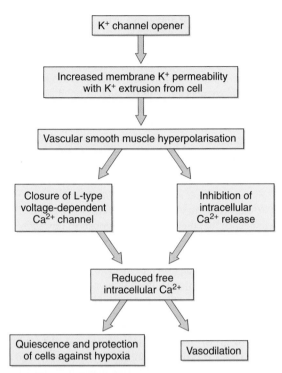

Fig. 5.5
The mechanism of action of potassium channel openers.

Unwanted effects

- arterial dilation causes headache in 25–50% of people, but tolerance usually occurs with continued use; palpitations (caused by reflex activation of the sympathetic nervous system) and flushing are less common
- dizziness
- nausea, vomiting.

Management of stable angina

The principal aims of treatment in stable angina are, firstly, to relieve symptoms and, secondly, to improve prognosis. There is no convincing evidence that the extent of suppression of the ischaemia will affect survival, or the risk of myocardial infarction. Angina has a circadian rhythm and occurs most frequently in the hours after waking, so a drug given for prophylaxis should ideally provide cover at this time.

There are several important principles of management.

- Lifestyle changes, such as stopping smoking, which substantially reduces the risk of developing an acute coronary syndrome by up to 50%, and weight loss, if obese, to reduce cardiac work should be implemented.
- Reduction of high blood pressure to reduce cardiac work and to reduce progression of atheroma, and control of diabetes to reduce progression of atheroma, are important.
- Provoking or exacerbating factors, such as anaemia, arrhythmias or thyrotoxicosis, should be controlled.
- Sublingual glyceryl trinitrate remains the treatment of choice for an acute anginal attack. It relieves symptoms within minutes, but gives only short-lived protection (20–30 min). Glyceryl trinitrate can also be taken for short-term prophylaxis before an activity that is likely to produce angina. For individuals who cannot tolerate a nitrate, a capsule of immediate-release nifedipine can be bitten and the contents swallowed to achieve a rapid effect.
- If anginal attacks are frequent, a longer-acting prophylactic antianginal drug should be used. A β-adrenoceptor antagonist – or, if this is contraindicated, a calcium channel antagonist – is the most effective treatment; nitrates are less suitable as first-line prophylactic agents because of the problems of tolerance. Since a rise in heart rate is one of the main precipitating factors for angina, a drug that lowers heart rate, such as a β-adrenoceptor antagonist, verapamil or diltiazem, may be most effective for first-line treatment. If symptoms are not controlled by optimal doses of a single drug, then a combination of a β-adrenoceptor antagonist with a calcium channel antagonist (not verapamil), or a β-adrenoceptor antagonist or calcium channel antagonist with a long-acting nitrate can be given. The role of nicorandil is less well established; it is generally used in combination therapy. 'Triple therapy' (e.g. β-adrenoceptor antagonist, calcium channel antagonist and a nitrate) has not been shown convincingly to be better than two agents, but may sometimes give further symptomatic benefit.
- Low-dose aspirin reduces the risk of subsequent myocardial infarction by about 35% (see Ch. 11).
- Treatment of a raised plasma cholesterol is desirable, initially by diet but by drugs (especially statins) if the response is inadequate (Ch. 48). Lowering the total plasma cholesterol to <4.0 mmol l^{-1} reduces the risk of subsequent non-fatal myocardial infarction, cardiac death and the need for surgical or percutaneous coronary artery revascularisation by an average of 30%.
- Coronary artery bypass grafting (CABG) improves long-term prognosis compared with medical treatment in subjects with left mainstem coronary artery stenosis, and in those with 'triple vessel disease' (significant left anterior descending, left circumflex and right coronary artery stenoses) who have impaired left ventricular function. In less severe disease, it is used for symptom relief.

- Percutaneous transluminal coronary angioplasty (PTCA) (often with insertion of a stent to maintain patency) is currently used for symptom relief only. Angioplasty alone is followed by a restenosis rate of about 40% at six months. This is reduced to about 20% by the use of a bare-metal stent, but with no difference in the risk of myocardial infarction or sudden death. Drug-eluting stents that are coated with a polymer matrix containing an antiproliferative drug such as sirolimus (Ch. 38) have further reduced the risk of restenosis at six months to about 6%. Insertion of a coronary artery stent is accompanied by intensive antiplatelet therapy to minimise early in-stent thrombosis. This usually comprises a combination of aspirin with clopidogrel for six weeks. The addition of a glycoprotein IIb/IIIa antagonist such as abciximab is common for high-risk procedures, especially in treatment of those with an acute coronary syndrome (Ch. 11).

Symptoms and response to treatment are a poor guide to the severity of coronary artery disease, and exercise stress testing is a more accurate predictor. A poor performance during such testing, as well as failure to respond to two prophylactic drugs in adequate dosages, should lead to consideration of coronary angiography, with a view to CABG or PTCA.

Management of acute coronary syndromes

Unstable angina usually presents with symptoms at rest, or a rapidly accelerating pattern of angina attacks that are produced by minimal exertion (*accelerated* or *crescendo angina*). It usually requires urgent treatment to reduce the 10% risk of subsequent myocardial infarction or death. When the blood concentration of a sensitive marker of myocardial damage, troponin I or T, is raised then a myocardial infarction has occurred. If this occurs without diagnostic changes of the ECG, it is termed a non-ST-elevation myocardial infarction.

- Low-dose aspirin should be given (Ch. 11), after a loading dose if aspirin was not previously taken. Full anticoagulation with intravenous heparin or subcutaneous low-molecular-weight heparin (Ch. 11) produces additive benefit; the risk of myocardial infarction or death within 14 days is reduced by about 60% after the onset of combined treatment with aspirin and heparin. The addition of the antiplatelet agent clopidogrel to aspirin for up to one year reduces the risk of myocardial infarction by a further 20% if the blood concentration of troponin I or T is raised.

- A β-adrenoceptor antagonist is the first-choice antianginal treatment, although a heart rate-limiting calcium channel antagonist, such as verapamil or diltiazem, can be used if a β-adrenoceptor antagonist is contraindicated or not tolerated. Dihydropyridine calcium channel antagonists, such as nifedipine, do not improve outcome when used alone, but they can be used with a β-adrenoceptor antagonist if the symptoms do not settle. These regimens reduce the risk of myocardial infarction by about 15% compared with no antianginal treatment.

- Nitrates are widely used, either sublingually or, for more prolonged effect, by the buccal or intravenous route. While they relieve symptoms, there is no evidence that they improve prognosis in unstable angina.

- Platelet inhibition with an intravenous glycoprotein IIb/IIIa antagonist such as tirofiban (Ch. 11) reduces the risk of myocardial infarction or death in those at high risk. These agents are most effective when there is a raised plasma concentration of troponin I or T.

- In the acute phase of an acute coronary syndrome, angiography – followed, when appropriate, by CABG or PTCA – is carried out for the 10% of people who are refractory to full medical treatment. If the unstable symptoms settle, then those who had evidence of myocardial damage during the acute episode (an increase in the plasma concentration of troponin I or T), or those who develop symptoms or ECG changes at an early stage during a standardised exercise test, should also be investigated by angiography.

- Cholesterol reduction to <4.0 mol l^{-1} should be initiated by diet, with addition of drugs (usually statins) at the time of the event (Ch. 48). This reduces the long-term risk of myocardial infarction or cardiac death by 25–30%.

Management of ST-elevation myocardial infarction

Acute management

Myocardial infarction is usually (but not invariably) associated with intense, prolonged chest pain and sympathetic nervous stimulation, which increases cardiac work. Drug therapy is directed initially towards two principal goals: pain relief and reperfusion of the occluded artery. For pain relief, an intravenous opioid analgesic, such as diamorphine (Ch. 19), is given, together with an antiemetic. Intramuscular injection should be avoided, since a low cardiac output and poor tissue perfusion often delay absorption. A nitrate (sublingual or intravenous) can also reduce pain by relief of coronary artery vasospasm at the site of the occlusion, with restoration of some blood flow. An intravenous β-adrenoceptor antagonist can be given to reduce cardiac work, especially if there is hypertension or tachycardia but no signs of heart failure.

Natural thrombolysis can be enhanced by intravenous thrombolytic therapy (Ch. 11) to limit the size of the infarct. Several agents are in wide clinical use, such as streptokinase and alteplase (rt-PA) or its rt-PA analogues. Alteplase produces more rapid reperfusion and opens a greater percentage of occluded vessels than streptokinase, but the extent of myocardial salvage and consequent reduction in mortality are similar for the two agents. Streptokinase is widely used but produces symptomatic hypotension during about 10% of administrations. Alteplase or related drugs are less likely to lower blood pressure and are given by choice if there is severe symptomatic hypotension prior to thrombolysis. They are also the treatment of choice if streptokinase has previously been used, since high titres of streptokinase-neutralising antibodies often persist for several years (Ch. 11). Alteplase and related compounds are usually followed by intravenous heparin for 48 h to reduce re-occlusion; this is unnecessary with streptokinase because of its longer duration of action.

Thrombolytic therapy significantly reduces mortality if given within 12 h of the onset of pain, but the survival advantage is greater the earlier treatment is given. Treatment within 6 h of the onset of pain saves 30 lives per 1000 people treated, whereas only 20 lives per 1000 are saved if treatment is delayed to 6–12 h after the onset of pain. Thrombolysis is used only if there are clear ECG changes of acute myocardial infarction (characteristic ST elevation in two or more leads) or left bundle branch block on the ECG and a good history of acute myocardial infarction. In the latter situation, an acute myocardial infarction cannot be easily diagnosed from the ECG but mortality is high. The greatest reduction in mortality is derived in those at highest risk (i.e anterior infarcts rather than inferior), the elderly (>65 years of age) and those with a presenting systolic blood pressure below 100 mmHg.

Other therapy

PTCA, usually with stenting, is helpful in the acute phase of myocardial infarction. It can be considered if access to a catheter laboratory is rapid, or if there are contraindications to thrombolysis; this is known as 'primary' PTCA. 'Rescue' PTCA can be considered if thrombolysis has failed to reperfuse the infarct-related vessel.

In addition to the management discussed above, complications of myocardial infarction may need specific treatment (Box 5.1).

Secondary prophylaxis after myocardial infarction

Secondary prophylaxis to reduce late mortality after myocardial infarction can be achieved with several approaches.

Box 5.1

Complications after myocardial infarction

Heart failure
Cardiogenic shock
Cardiac rupture
   Free wall rupture
   Ventricular septal defect
Arrhythmias
   Ventricular fibrillation
   Ventricular tachycardia
   Supraventricular tachycardias
   Sinus bradycardia and heart block
Pericarditis
Intracardiac thrombus

- Stopping smoking is of major benefit, since it reduces the mortality after a myocardial infarction by up to 50%. Rehabilitation programmes, which include exercise, also reduce mortality by up to 25% and improve psychological recovery.

- Low-dose aspirin (Ch. 11) reduces mortality in the first few weeks when started within 24 h of the onset of pain and reduces later mortality if continued long term (saving 20 lives per 1000 people treated). Initial benefits may result from reduced reocclusion of vessels that have undergone natural or therapeutic thrombolysis. A loading dose is required for a rapid onset of effect.

- Beta-adrenoceptor antagonists, started orally soon after the infarct, reduce later deaths and reinfarctions by about 25% each, although the mechanism is unknown. Greatest benefit is seen in those at highest risk, for example following anterior infarction and in those who have had serious postinfarct arrhythmias or postinfarct angina or heart failure. Heart failure must be controlled before a β-adrenoceptor antagonist is given (Ch. 7).

- An ACE inhibitor (Ch. 6) is of greater benefit if there is clinical or radiological evidence of heart failure after myocardial infarction, with a reduction in mortality of about 25% over the subsequent year. A lesser survival advantage is gained if there is significant left ventricular dysfunction after the infarction (an ejection fraction of 40% or less) but without clinical evidence of heart failure. In this group, a 20% reduction in mortality over 3–5 years after the event is accompanied by a significant reduction in non-fatal reinfarctions (although the mechanism of this effect is unknown). Most recently, a reduction in both non-fatal infarction and death has been shown when there is well-preserved left ventricular function. The benefits of an ACE inhibitor are additional to those of a β-adrenoceptor antagonist.

- Verapamil and diltiazem produce a small reduction in reinfarction, but do not reduce mortality. They may be detrimental if there have been symptoms or signs of heart failure. These drugs should be considered as an option only for those at high risk who cannot tolerate a β-adrenoceptor antagonist and who do not have significant left ventricular dysfunction. Nifedipine and similar calcium channel antagonists do not improve prognosis after myocardial infarction.

- Prophylactic anticoagulation with subcutaneous heparin (Ch. 11) can prevent deep vein thrombosis, but rapid mobilisation after a myocardial infarct minimises this risk. Long-term anticoagulation with warfarin (Ch. 11) reduces mortality and reinfarction

to a similar extent to low-dose aspirin. In combination with aspirin, warfarin produces a further reduction in both fatal and non-fatal events but with an increased risk of bleeding.

- Cholesterol reduction to <4.0 mmol l^{-1} should be attempted by diet and usually cholesterol-lowering drugs, especially the statins (Ch. 48). Statins reduce reinfarction and cardiac death by 25–30%. Fibrates are less effective, but may be useful if the total cholesterol is low but the high-density lipoprotein cholesterol is also low.

- A Mediterranean diet reduces mortality after myocardial infarction. A further reduction in mortality can be achieved with omega-3 fatty acids. An antiarryhthmic effect may be responsible for these benefits (Ch. 48).

FURTHER READING

Stable angina

Bales AC (2004) Medical management of chronic ischemic heart disease. Selecting specific drug therapies, modifying risk factors. *Postgrad Med* 115, 39–46

Fayers KE, Cummings MH, Shaw KM et al (2003) Nitrate tolerance and the links with endothelial dysfunction and oxidative stress. *Br J Clin Pharmacol* 56, 620–628

Feher MD (2003) Lipid lowering to delay the progression of coronary artery disease. *Heart* 89, 451–458

Fihn SD, Williams SV, Daley J et al (2001) Guidelines for the management of patients with chronic stable angina: treatment. *Ann Intern Med* 135, 616–632

Heidenreich PA, McDonald KM, Haslie T et al (1999) Meta-analysis of trials comparing β-blockers, calcium antagonists and nitrates for stable angina. *JAMA* 281, 1927–1936

Jain A, Wadehra V, Timmis AD (2003) Management of stable angina. *Postgrad Med J* 79, 332–336

Knight CJ (2003) Antiplatelet treatment in stable coronary artery disease. *Heart* 89, 1273–1278

Ko DT, Hebert PR, Coffey CS et al (2002) β-blocker therapy and symptoms of depression, fatigue, and sexual dysfunction. *JAMA* 288, 351–357

Levine GN, Kern MJ, Berger PB et al (2003) Management of patients undergoing percutaneous coronary revascularization. *Ann Intern Med* 139, 123–136

O'Toole, Grech ED (2003) Chronic stable angina: treatment options. *BMJ* 326, 1185–1188

Toda N (2003) Vasodilating β-adrenoceptor blockers as cardiovascular therapeutics. *Pharmacol Ther* 100, 215–234

Weisman SM, Graham DY (2002) Evaluation of the benefits and risks of low-dose aspirin in the secondary prevention of cardiovascular and cerebrovascular events. *Arch Intern Med* 162, 2197–2202

Acute coronary syndromes

Bavry AA, Kumbhani DJ, Quiroz R et al (2004) Invasive therapy along with glycoprotein IIb/IIIa inhibitors and

intracoronary stents improves survival in non-ST-segment elevation acute coronary syndromes: a meta-analysis and review of the literature. *Am J Cardiol* 93, 830–835

Braunwald E, Antman EM, Beasley JW et al (2002) ACC/AHA 2002 guideline update for the management of patients with unstable angina and non-ST-segment elevation myocardial infarction – summary article: a report of the American College of Cardiology/American Heart Association task force on practice guidelines (Committee on the Management of Patients With Unstable Angina). *J Am Coll Cardiol* 40, 1366–1374

Eikelboom JW, Anand SS, Malmberg K (2000) Unfractionated heparin and low molecular weight heparin in acute coronary syndrome without ST elevation: meta analysis. *Lancet* 355, 1936–1942

Fox KA (2004) Management of acute coronary syndromes: an update. *Heart* 90, 698–706

Jneid H, Bhatt DL, Corti R et al (2003) Aspirin and clopidogrel in acute coronary syndromes. Therapeutic insights from the CURE study. *Arch Intern Med* 163, 1145–1153

Kong DF, Hasselblad V, Harrington RA et al (2003) Meta-analysis of survival with platelet glycoprotein IIb/IIIa antagonists for percutaneous coronary interventions. *Am J Cardiol* 92, 651–655

Manhapra A, Borzak S (2000) Treatment possibilities for unstable angina. *BMJ* 321, 1269–1275

Task Force on the Management of Acute Coronary Syndromes of the European Society of Cardiology (2002) Management of acute coronary syndromes in patients presenting without persistent ST-segment elevation. *Eur Heart J* 23, 1809–1840

Timmis A (2003) Plaque stabilisation in acute coronary syndromes: clinical considerations. *Heart* 89, 1268–1272

Turpie AGG, Antman EM (2001) Low-molecular-weight heparins in the treatment of acute coronary syndromes. *Arch Intern Med* 161, 1484–1491

Myocardial infarction

American College of Cardiology/American Heart Association (1999) Update: ACC/AHA guidelines for the management of patients with acute myocardial infarction: executive summary and recommendations. *Circulation* 100, 1016–1030

Boersma E, Mercado N, Poldermans D et al (2003) Acute myocardial infarction. *Lancet* 361, 847–858

Brouwer MA, Clappers N, Verheugt FWA (2004) Adjunctive treatment in patients treated with thrombolytic therapy. *Heart* 90, 581–588

Dalal H, Evans PH, Campbell JL (2004) Recent developments in secondary prevention and cardiac rehabilitation after acute myocardial infarction. *BMJ* 328, 693–697

Keeley EC, Grines CL (2004) Primary coronary intervention for acute myocardial infarction. *JAMA* 291, 736–740

Klein L, Gheorghiade M (2004) Management of the patient with diabetes mellitus and myocardial infarction. *Am J Med* 116(5A), 47s–63s

Lee VC, Rhew DC, Dylan M et al (2004) Meta-analysis: angiotensin-receptor blockers in chronic heart failure and high-risk acute myocardial infarction. *Ann Intern Med* 41, 693–704

Ribichini F, Wijns W (2002) Acute myocardial infarction: reperfusion treatment. *Heart* 88, 298–305

Stenestrand U, Wallentin L (2003) Fibrinolytic therapy in patients 75 years and older with ST-segment-elevation myocardial infarction. *Arch Intern Med* 163, 965–971

Self-assessment

1. In the following questions, the first statement, in italics, is true. Is the accompanying statement also true?

   a. *The mechanism by which glyceryl trinitrate causes vasodilation is through its ability to release nitric oxide.* Nitric oxide causes vasodilation by increasing cyclic adenosine monophosphate (cAMP) synthesis in vascular smooth muscle cells.

   b. *Glyceryl trinitrate has a more rapid onset of action when given sublingually than when given by a transdermal patch.* Transdermal absorption of glyceryl trinitrate from a patch avoids first-pass metabolism.

   c. *The increased oxygen demand of a rise in workload in the heart is met by an elevation in coronary blood flow.* In angina, glyceryl trinitrate increases total coronary blood flow.

   d. *Glyceryl trinitrate can be safely administered with a β-adrenoceptor antagonist.* The benefit of glyceryl trinitrate in angina is only a result of its effect on coronary arteries.

   e. *Recombinant tissue-type plasminogen activator (rt-PA) is a genetically engineered copy of an endogenous fibrinolytic agent.* rt-PA inhibits the formation of plasmin.

2. From the following statements about angina and myocardial infarction, choose the one incorrect statement.

   a. Isosorbide-5 mononitrate is an active metabolite of isosorbide dinitrate and has the advantage that it does not undergo first-pass metabolism.

   b. Verapamil can reduce arterial blood pressure without causing reflex tachycardia.

   c. Platelet inhibitors such as the glycoprotein IIb/IIIa antagonist tirofiban can reduce the risk of myocardial infarction in high-risk individuals with unstable angina.

   d. Cholesterol reduction is of little benefit in reducing the risk of recurrence of myocardial infarction.

   e. Nifedipine does not improve prognosis after myocardial infarction.

3. Case history questions

   TK, a 45-year-old man who was a long-distance lorry driver, had been having episodes of chest pain that he likened to indigestion. They were brought on by moderately strenuous exercise and relieved by rest but were not relieved by antacids. They had been present for approximately 1 year, but recently the frequency and intensity of the pains had become worse and they were now occurring several times a week. He was hypertensive and his serum cholesterol level was 6.6 mmol l^{-1}. He smoked 40 cigarettes per day and was overweight. He drank about 10 units of alcohol a week. He performed well on an exercise test but his exercise ECG showed anterolateral ST-segment depression at peak exercise. There was no evidence of heart failure. A diagnosis of angina was made.

   a. How could his acute attacks of angina have been treated?

   b. The frequency of his attacks required prophylactic treatment. What options were available to reduce the frequency of anginal attacks?

   c. What other drugs could have been useful to improve his prognosis?

d. Would lifestyle changes help Mr TK?

e. If TK was an 80-year-old, what additional precautions should you have considered when prescribing his medication?

f. In unstable angina, which drug treatments would have been likely to reduce the progression of the episodes to myocardial infarction or sudden death?

> Despite continuing medication, 6 months later TK awoke with severe chest pains and dyspnoea that was not relieved by glyceryl trinitrate. Examination, biochemical tests and ECG recordings all led to the diagnosis of an acute myocardial infarction.

g. What was the likely cause of the myocardial infarction?

h. Why was it important to give thrombolytic therapy as quickly as possible?

i. TK was given the thrombolytic agent recombinant tissue-type plasminogen activator (rt-PA) because of fears that he would get an allergic response to streptokinase. Was this justified?

j. He was given 150 mg aspirin orally. Would this have any added benefit if thrombolytic therapy was also given?

k. The normal therapeutic dose of aspirin for headache is about 650 mg. Why was the dose given to TK so small?

l. Consideration was given to administering intravenous heparin to TK, but this was considered unnecessary because he had been given rt-PA. Was this decision correct?

m. Following his myocardial infarction, long-term prophylactic treatment of his condition was considered. Which of the following drugs would have been likely to be of benefit: low-dose aspirin, a β-adrenoceptor antagonist, an ACE inhibitor, verapamil, diltiazem or warfarin?

The answers are provided on pages 707–708.

Drugs used to treat ischaemic heart disease

Drug	Half-life (h)	Elimination	Comments
Beta-adrenoceptor antagonists			Acebutolol, atenolol, bisoprolol, carvedilol, metoprolol, nadolol, oxprenolol, pindolol, propranolol, and timolol are used for the treatment of angina – see Ch. 8 for details
Calcium channel antagonists			All are given orally unless stated otherwise; indications include angina, hypertension, Raynaud's phenomenon, arrhythmias and subarachnoid haemorrhage (see Chs 6 and 8–10)
Dihydropyridines			Metabolites are generally inactive; modified-release formulations are available for many of these drugs and are preferred for the treatment of angina and hypertension as they reduce fluctuations in blood pressure and reflex tachycardia
Amlodipine	30–60	Metabolism	Used for angina and hypertension; no detrimental effect in heart failure; given once daily; oral bioavailability is 60–80%; oxidised in liver
Felodipine	12–25	Metabolism	Used for angina and hypertension; no detrimental effect in heart failure; given once daily; oral bioavailability about 15% owing to first-pass metabolism; oxidised by CYP3A4
Isradipine	2–6	Metabolism	Used for hypertension only; oral bioavailability is 20% owing to first-pass metabolism
Lacidipine	7–8	Metabolism	Used for hypertension only; low and variable oral bioavailability (4–52%) (common to many dihydropyridines owing to variable intestinal and hepatic CYP3A4 activity)
Lercanidipine	3–5	Metabolism	Used for mild to moderate hypertension only; long duration of action (24 h) of undefined cause; oral bioavailability is 44% and increased by a fatty meal; eliminated by CYP3A4-mediated oxidation to inactive metabolites
Nicardipine	1–12	Metabolism	Used for angina and mild to moderate hypertension; bioavailability is dose-dependent owing to first-pass metabolism (5–10% at low doses and 30–45% at high doses); metabolised in liver
Nifedipine	2–4	Metabolism	Used for angina, hypertension and Raynaud's phenomenon; oral bioavailability is about 40% owing to first-pass metabolism by CYP3A4 in gut wall and liver
Nimodipine	8–9	Metabolism	Selective for cerebral arteries; use is confined to the prevention and treatment of ischaemic neurological deficits following aneurysmal subarachnoid haemorrhage; given orally or by intravenous infusion; oral bioavailability is 5–10%; eliminated by oxidation in the liver
Nisoldipine	2–4	Metabolism	Used for angina and mild to moderate hypertension; oral bioavailability is low (5–10%) and variable owing to intestinal and hepatic CYP3A4 metabolism; numerous metabolites
Non-dihydropyridines			Modified-release formulations are available for these drugs
Diltiazem	2–5	Metabolism	Used for angina and hypertension; reduces heart rate; some negative inotropic effect and should be avoided in heart failure; oral bioavailability is about 50% owing to first-pass metabolism; a number of metabolites, mostly inactive

continued

Drug compendium

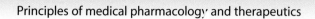

Drugs used to treat ischaemic heart disease *(continued)*

Drug	Half-life (h)	Elimination	Comments
Verapamil	2–5	Metabolism	Used for angina, hypertension and supraventricular arrhymias; reduces heart rate; marked negative inotropic effect and should be avoided in heart failure; given orally or by slow intravenous injection (over 2 min); oral bioavailability is about 20% owing to first-pass metabolism; oxidised by CYP3A4; metabolites retain activity but are rapidly eliminated by conjugation; half-life is longer after chronic dosing (5–12 h)
Nitrates			
Glyceryl trinitrate	1–3 min	Metabolism	Used for angina and left ventricular failure; given sublingually, bucally, topically or as an intravenous infusion; essentially complete first-pass metabolism if swallowed; the dinitrate metabolites have 10% of the activity but half-lives of about 40 min
Isosorbide dinitrate	0.5–2	Metabolism	Used for angina and left ventricular failure; given sublingually, orally (as normal or MR tablets), topically or by intravenous infusion; low bioavailability from sublingual (30–60%) and topical (10–30%); the active mononitrate metabolite inhibits clearance of the dinitrate during chronic treatment; high first-pass metabolism
Isosorbide mononitrate	3–7	Metabolism	Used for angina and as an adjunct in the treatment of congestive heart failure; given orally; bioavailability approaches 100%; metabolised by denitration and glucuronide conjugation; low first-pass metabolism
Potassium channel activators			
Nicorandil	1	Metabolism	Used for angina; given orally; essentially complete bioavailability; oxidised and denitrated in the liver; tolerance not a problem; biological effect much longer than predicted by half-life

Hypertension

Circulatory reflexes and the control of blood pressure

Systemic blood pressure is determined by the cardiac output and by peripheral resistance. It is maintained within fairly narrow limits by a series of physiological reflexes that respond to both acute and chronic changes in blood pressure. The two most important regulatory systems are:

- the sympathetic nervous system
- the renin–angiotensin–aldosterone system.

Any change in systemic blood pressure is detected by baroreceptors in the aorta and carotid arteries. Afferent impulses from these baroreceptors are integrated in the vasomotor centres in the medullary region of the brainstem (Fig. 6.1). A rise in blood pressure increases the input of impulses from the baroreceptors to the vasomotor centre, which inhibits the sympathetic nervous system output from the centre and accentuates the parasympathetic outflow. The sympathetic nervous system maintains arterial blood pressure by several mechanisms.

- On the heart, it acts mainly through β_1-adrenoceptors to increase myocardial contractility and heart rate, generating a greater cardiac output (Ch. 4).
- On arterial resistance vessels, it stimulates postsynaptic α_1-adrenoceptors, producing arteriolar vasoconstriction. This raises blood pressure and redistributes blood flow to specific vascular beds

to maintain perfusion of vital organs. This redistribution is helped by β_2-adrenoceptor-mediated vasodilation in selected vascular beds, such as skeletal muscle. Arterial vasoconstriction produces an increase in afterload on the heart, but in the healthy heart, cardiac output is maintained by an increase in cardiac contractility.

- On venous capacitance vessels, it stimulates postsynaptic α_1-adrenoceptors, producing venous constriction. This increases venous return to the heart (preload) and improves cardiac output (Fig. 6.2).

A slower compensatory mechanism to overcome reduction in blood pressure is initiated by release of renin from the juxtaglomerular apparatus of the kidney (Fig. 6.3). The major stimuli leading to renin release are reduced renal blood flow (often as a result of a decrease in blood pressure), decreased Na^+ in the distal renal tubule, and direct sympathetic stimulation via β_1-adrenoceptors at the juxtaglomerular apparatus.

Renin is a protease that acts on circulating renin substrate (angiotensinogen) to release the decapeptide

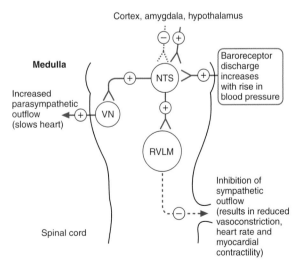

Fig. 6.1
The role of baroreceptors. Increased discharge from the baroreceptors results from stretch caused by increased blood pressure. This results in both a compensatory decrease in sympathetic outflow from the medulla and an increase in the vagal outflow. Both effects reduce peripheral resistance and are mimicked by centrally acting drugs that lower blood pressure (Fig. 6.9). NTS, nucleus of the tractus solitarius; VN, vagal nucleus (cardioinhibitory centre); RVLM, rostral ventrolateral medulla; +, stimulation; −, inhibition.

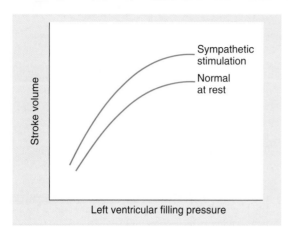

Fig. 6.2
The Frank–Starling phenomenon. The relationship between preload (left ventricular filling pressure) and stroke volume at different states of myocardial contractility.

angiotensin I. This in turn is cleaved by angiotensin-converting enzyme (ACE) to release the octapeptide angiotensin II. Angiotensin II is a potent vasoconstrictor that also enhances sympathetic nervous tone by an effect on presynaptic neurons. It has a number of additional properties, which can alter salt and water balance (Fig. 6.3). It also promotes the release of aldosterone from the adrenal cortex, which acts at the distal renal tubule to conserve salt and water at the expense of K^+ loss (Ch. 14). Thus, angiotensin II and aldosterone raise blood pressure by vasoconstriction and by increasing circulating blood volume.

The integration of the sympathetic nervous system and renin–angiotensin–aldosterone responses to a fall in blood pressure is shown in Figure 6.4. These mechanisms prevent hypotension due to peripheral pooling of blood on standing and during exercise.

Additional control mechanisms involved in the regulation of vascular tone and circulating blood volume include circulating or local hormones and metabolites such as atrial natriuretic peptide, prostaglandins, kinins, nitric oxide, endothelin and adenosine (Fig. 6.5). Their relative importance may differ in health and disease states.

Hypertension

Hypertension is a common condition, found in 20–30% of the population of the developed world. It is usually asymptomatic but produces progressive structural changes in the heart and circulation. These predispose to clinical complications that are often referred to as 'target organ damage'. The principal complications of hypertension are ischaemic heart disease (Ch. 5), which is twice as frequent as in normotensives, and cerebrovascular disease, which usually presents as thromboembolic stroke or, less commonly, as cerebral haemorrhage (Ch. 9). Such consequences are more common if hypertension is accompanied by hypercholesterolaemia and smoking. The underlying vascular lesions that occur in hypertension and their resulting complications, which together constitute target organ damage, are shown in Figure 6.6.

Sustained hypertension predisposes to left ventricular muscle hypertrophy (LVH). LVH is an independent risk factor for the complications of hypertension, particularly ischaemic heart disease (since the muscle outgrows its blood supply), diastolic heart failure (Ch. 7) and arrhythmias leading to sudden death (Ch. 8).

There is no absolute cut-off between normal and high blood pressure. Blood pressure in all populations is 'normally' distributed with a slight skew because of a small number of individuals with very high blood pressures. Defining a point at which blood pressure is 'high' is,

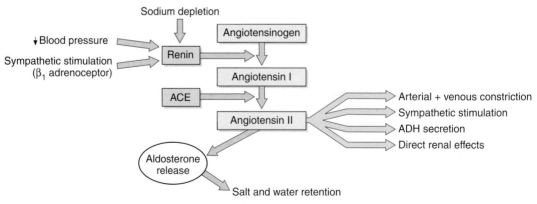

Fig. 6.3
Formation and actions of angiotensin II. ADH, antidiuretic hormone; ACE, angiotensin-converting enzyme.

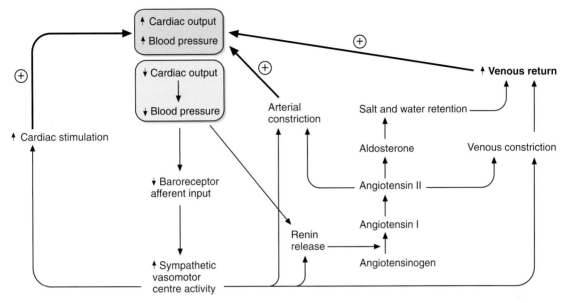

Fig. 6.4

The control of blood pressure via the sympathetic and angiotensin/aldosterone cascades. The integrated physiological compensatory mechanisms are shown in response to a fall in cardiac output or blood pressure (yellow box). The sympathetic-mediated responses on the left of the diagram are rapidly responding events, whereas the angiotensin/aldosterone events are more slowly responding. The final outcomes are increased venous return, increased arterial constriction and increased cardiac stimulation. Events that may be important at the level of the endothelium are shown in Fig. 6.5.

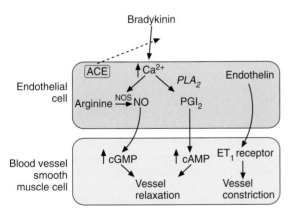

Fig. 6.5

The endothelial cell is an important site of production of vasoactive substances and enzymes that metabolise vasoactive substances. Both can be affected by many natural hormones and drugs, facilitating constriction or dilation. An example with potential clinical importance is bradykinin, which generates increased endothelial nitric oxide (NO) and the prostaglandin PGI$_2$ (prostacyclin). The endothelial cell also contains angiotensin-converting enzyme (ACE), which breaks down bradykinin to inactive peptides. This is reduced by ACE inhibitor drugs, amplifying the effects of bradykinin on the synthesis of endothelial vasodilators. Endothelin is a potent vasoconstrictor. Other substances such as adenosine also cause vasodilation. Atrial natriuretic peptide (ANP) is released from atrial cells and has effects to increase natriuresis and to increase cGMP, causing relaxation of blood vessels and a fall in blood pressure. ET$_1$, endothelin type 1 receptor; NOS, nitric oxide synthase; PLA$_2$, phospholipase A$_2$.

therefore, somewhat arbitrary. A widely accepted view is that hypertension exists if the blood pressure is maintained at a level above which treatment has been shown to reduce the risk of developing complications. Using this criterion, hypertension is present when the systolic pressure is sustained above 160 mmHg, or the diastolic blood pressure is sustained above 100 mmHg. However, once target organ damage is present, treatment at a lower level of blood pressure becomes desirable (i.e. at systolic pressure above 140 mmHg or a diastolic pressure above 90 mmHg).

The diagnosis of sustained hypertension requires at least three, and preferably more, blood pressure readings over several weeks, unless target organ damage gives a clear indication that earlier treatment is necessary. Sometimes, the blood pressure is raised only when the measurement is taken by a doctor or, to a lesser extent, by a nurse. This phenomenon is termed 'white coat' hypertension and appears to carry little risk of complications over the next few years. It can usually be detected either by repeated blood pressure readings that gradually approach the normal range, by measuring the blood pressure at home, or by use of an ambulatory 24-h blood pressure recorder. 'White coat' hypertension often persists despite drug treatment, which can result in quite troublesome hypotension away from the surgery or clinic.

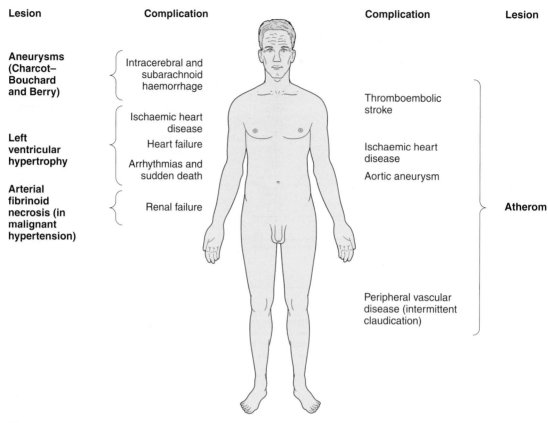

Lesion	Complication		Complication	Lesion

Aneurysms (Charcot–Bouchard and Berry) — Intracerebral and subarachnoid haemorrhage

Left ventricular hypertrophy — Ischaemic heart disease; Heart failure; Arrhythmias and sudden death

Arterial fibrinoid necrosis (in malignant hypertension) — Renal failure

Thromboembolic stroke

Ischaemic heart disease

Aortic aneurysm

Atherom

Peripheral vascular disease (intermittent claudication)

Fig. 6.6
Complications of hypertension. Hypertension causes vascular lesions and damage throughout the body.

Malignant or accelerated hypertension is an infrequently encountered condition, characterised by arterial fibrinoid necrosis. It is identified clinically by the presence of flame-shaped haemorrhages, hard exudates, and 'cotton wool' spots in the retina, which can lead to visual disturbance. Papilloedema can also occur. If untreated, it usually leads to death within 2 years from renal failure, heart failure or stroke.

Aetiology and pathogenesis of hypertension

Hypertension is usually associated with increased peripheral arterial resistance, which arises from arteriolar smooth muscle constriction and hypertrophy of the arteriolar wall. The cause of the inappropriately raised peripheral resistance is unknown in the majority of people with hypertension, who are said to have 'essential' hyperten-

sion. Essential hypertension probably has a polygenic inheritance, leading to several clinical subtypes with different underlying pathogenic mechanisms. Environmental influences and factors such as diet, level of exercise, obesity and alcohol intake all interact with the genetic programming to determine the final level of blood pressure. A secondary underlying cause of the high blood pressure, which is often renal or endocrinological, can be identified in about 5% of people with hypertension (Table 6.1).

Not surprisingly, since the cause of hypertension is unclear, treatment cannot be directed precisely at the underlying mechanism(s). Most antihypertensive drugs are vasodilators. They often modulate the natural hormonal or neuronal mechanisms responsible for blood pressure regulation. Less commonly, the hypotensive action is achieved by reducing cardiac output. The principal classes of antihypertensive drugs and their sites of action are shown in Table 6.2 and Figure 6.7.

Table 6.1
Principal causes of secondary hypertension

	Causes
Renal	Renal artery stenosis, glomerulonephritis, interstitial nephritis, arteritis, polycystic disease, chronic pyelonephritis
Endocrine	Conn's syndrome (aldosterone excess), Cushing's syndrome (glucocorticoid excess), phaeochromocytoma (catecholamine excess), acromegaly
Pregnancy	Pre-eclampsia and eclampsia
Drugs	Oestrogen, corticosteroids, non-steroidal anti-inflammatory drug (NSAIDs), ciclosporin

Antihypertensive drugs

Drugs acting on the sympathetic nervous system

Beta-adrenoceptor antagonists (β-blockers) (see the Compendium for Ch. 8 for individual drugs)

> Examples: atenolol, propranolol, pindolol

Mechanism of action in hypertension

The hypotensive action of the β-adrenoceptor antagonists is believed to have several components (Fig. 6.8). Selective β_1-adrenoceptor antagonists are as effective as non-selective drugs, indicating that β_2-adrenoceptor antagonism makes little contribution. The more important actions are probably:

- reduction of heart rate and myocardial contractility, which decrease cardiac output
- blockade of renal juxtaglomerular β_1-adrenoceptors, which reduces renin secretion
- peripheral vasodilation, but only with compounds that have a hybrid action, such as carvedilol, nebivolol or pindolol (Fig. 6.8c and Ch. 5)
- blockade of presynaptic β-adrenoceptors in sympathetic nerves supplying arteriolar resistance vessels – this may reduce the release of noradrenaline, but the clinical importance of this is uncertain.

For further details about β-adrenoceptor antagonists and their many uses, see Chapters 5 and 8, and Box 6.1.

Alpha-adrenoceptor antagonists (α-blockers)

> Examples: α_1-adrenoceptor selective antagonists: prazosin, doxazosin
> non-selective antagonists: phentolamine, phenoxybenzamin

Mechanisms of action

Blockade of postsynaptic α_1-adrenoceptors lowers blood pressure by:

Table 6.2
Principal classes of antihypertensive drugs and their sites of action

Sites of action	Drugs
Sympathetic nervous system	β-Adrenoceptor antagonists (β-blockers) α_1-Adrenoceptor antagonists (α_1-blockers) Selective imidazoline receptor agonists Centrally acting α_2-adrenoceptor agonists[a] Adrenergic neuron blockers[a] Ganglion blockers[a]
Hormonal control (renin–angiotensin system)	Angiotensin-converting enzyme (ACE) inhibitors Angiotensin II receptor antagonist
Vasodilation by other mechanisms	Diuretics Calcium channel antagonists Potassium channel activators Nitrovasodilators[a]

[a]Restricted use.

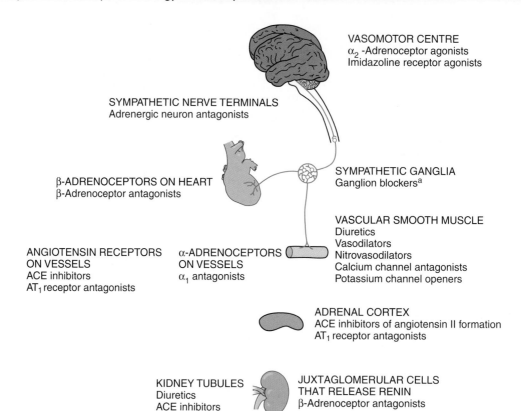

Fig. 6.7
The classes of antihypertensive drug and their sites of action. [a]Classes of drug that are rarely used now; ACE, angiotensin-converting enzyme.

- reducing tone in arteriolar resistance vessels
- dilating venous capacitance vessels, which reduces venous return and, therefore, cardiac output.

The fall in blood pressure is detected by arterial baroreceptors, which initiate a reflex increase in sympathetic discharge from the medulla (Fig. 6.1). The negative feedback produced by noradrenaline acting via inhibitory presynaptic α_2-adrenoceptors helps to blunt the expected reflex tachycardia (Fig. 6.8a). Selective α_1-adrenoceptor antagonists (they are often inadequately referred to as α-blockers) do not block the α_2-adrenoceptors on sympathetic nerve terminals, and, therefore, reflex tachycardia is unusual.

By contrast, non-selective α-adrenoceptor antagonists block both postsynaptic α_1-adrenoceptors and presynaptic α_2-adrenoceptors, and the latter blocks the negative feedback; in consequence, their use is accompanied by a marked reflex tachycardia. These agents now have little place in clinical practice except for the perioperative management of phaeochromocytoma. Phenoxybenzamine is an irreversible antagonist.

Alpha-adrenoceptor antagonists produce a potentially beneficial effect on plasma lipids; they increase high-density lipoprotein cholesterol and reduce triglycerides (Ch. 48). The relevance of this for the prevention of atheroma in hypertensive people is uncertain.

Pharmacokinetics

Selective α_1-adrenoceptor antagonists are well absorbed from the gut and undergo extensive first-pass metabolism and subsequent elimination in the liver. The compounds differ principally in their half-lives and, therefore, duration of action; for example, prazosin has a short half-life, while that of doxazosin is long.

Unwanted effects

- postural hypotension caused by venous pooling; this can be particularly troublesome after the first dose
- lethargy, headache, dizziness
- nausea, rhinitis
- urinary frequency or incontinence (see also Ch. 15)

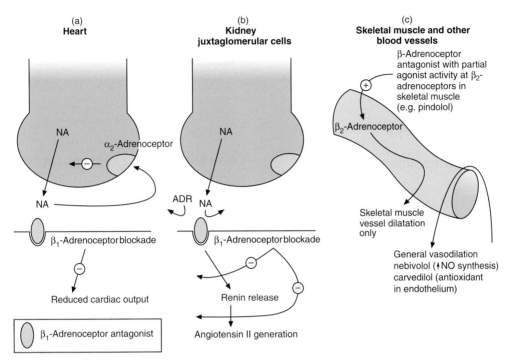

Fig. 6.8
Sites of action of the β-adrenoceptor antagonists relevant to their use as antihypertensive agents. (a) In the heart, the β_1-adrenoceptor antagonist drugs reduce noradrenaline- and adrenaline-induced stimulation of the β_1-adrenoceptors. The presynaptic stimulation of α_2-adrenoceptors, which inhibit noradrenaline release, still functions normally. (b) In the kidney, β_1-adrenoceptor blockade reduces the activity of the angiotensin II system. (c) Some β-adrenoceptor antagonists (e.g. pindolol) have partial agonist activity and stimulate the β_2-adrenoceptors in skeletal muscle blood vessels, which leads to vasodilation and a lowering of peripheral resistance. These drugs reduce heart rate and cardiac output less than those without partial agonist properties. Other β-adrenoceptor antagonists may dilate blood vessels more generally by actions on nitric oxide (NO) or free radicals. ADR, adrenaline; NA, noradrenaline.

- palpitations from reflex cardiac stimulation; these occur more commonly with non-selective drugs.

Ganglion blockers

Example: trimetaphan

Ganglion blockers are obsolete except for certain highly specialised indications such as during surgery.

Mechanism of action
Competitive blockade of nicotinic (N_1) receptors at autonomic ganglia reduces activity in both the sympathetic and parasympathetic nervous systems (Ch. 4 – see Table 4.4). Arterial and venous dilation both contribute to the hypotensive effects.

Pharmacokinetics
Trimetaphan is given by intravenous infusion or intermittent injection for controlled hypotension during surgery.

It is rapidly metabolised in the liver and has a duration of action of only a few minutes.

Unwanted effects
These are of little importance during brief intravenous administration:

> **Box 6.1**
>
> ### Clinical uses of β-adrenoceptor antagonists
>
> Treatment of hypertension (this chapter)
> Prophylaxis of angina (Ch. 5)
> Secondary prevention after myocardial infarction (Ch. 5)
> Prevention and treatment of arrhythmias (Ch. 8)
> Control of symptoms in thyrotoxicosis (Ch. 41)
> Alleviation of symptoms in anxiety (Ch. 20)
> Prophylaxis of migraine (Ch. 26)
> Topically for treatment of glaucoma (Ch. 50)

- blockade of parasympathetic outflow: constipation, urinary retention, blurred vision
- tachycardia
- respiratory depression.

Centrally acting antihypertensives

Selective imidazoline receptor agonists

Example: moxonidine

Mechanism of action

Imidazoline I_1 receptors are important for the regulation of sympathetic drive (Ch. 4, Fig. 4.7). They are concentrated in the rostral ventrolateral medulla, a part of the brainstem vasomotor centre. Increased neuronal activity in this area, either through baroreceptor stimulation or by direct stimulation of I_1 receptors, will decrease sympathetic outflow (Fig. 6.9). The result is a fall in blood pressure with no reflex tachycardia. Unlike other centrally acting drugs (clonidine and methyldopa), moxonidine has little affinity for α_2-adrenoceptors.

Pharmacokinetics

Moxonidine is well absorbed from the gut, and its principal route of elimination is the kidney. It has a short

half-life but a prolonged duration of action, which may reflect its high affinity for I_1 receptors.

Unwanted effects

- dry mouth
- nausea
- fatigue
- headache, dizziness.

Centrally acting α_2-adrenoceptor agonists

Examples: methyldopa, clonidine

Unwanted effects limit the use of the centrally acting α_2-adrenoceptor agonists, although methyldopa is a drug of choice in the treatment of hypertension in pregnancy (see below).

Mechanisms of action

The α_2-adrenoceptor agonists act at presynaptic autoreceptors in the central nervous system (CNS) to reduce central sympathetic nervous outflow and increase vagal outflow from the vasomotor centre (Fig. 6.9). This reduces both peripheral arterial and venous tone.

Methyldopa is a prodrug that is first metabolised in the nerve terminal as a 'false substrate' in the biosynthetic pathway for noradrenaline to produce α-methylnoradrenaline. This metabolite is a potent α_2-adrenoceptor agonist (Fig. 6.9). Clonidine is a direct-acting α_2-adrenoceptor agonist that is also an agonist at imidazoline I_1 receptors (see moxonidine). Clonidine has some peripheral postsynaptic α_1-adrenoceptor agonist activity, which produces direct peripheral vasoconstriction; this initially offsets some of the blood-pressure-lowering effect.

Pharmacokinetics

Methyldopa is incompletely absorbed from the gut and undergoes dose-dependent first-pass metabolism to an inactive sulphate conjugate. Its plasma half-life is short.

Clonidine is completely absorbed from the gut and is eliminated partly by the kidney and partly by liver metabolism. It has a long half-life.

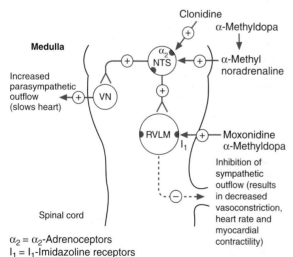

$\alpha_2 = \alpha_2$-Adrenoceptors
$I_1 = I_1$-Imidazoline receptors

Fig. 6.9
Mechanisms of centrally acting drugs in the control of blood pressure. Methyldopa and moxonidine mimic the responses of the medulla to raised blood pressure by stimulating α_2-adrenoceptors in the nucleus of the tractus solitarius (NTS) or imidazoline receptors (perhaps also a subtype of α-adrenoceptor) in the rostral ventrolateral medulla (RVLM). Methyldopa may also act through stimulating imidazoline receptors. VN, vagal nucleus (cardioinhibitory centre).

Unwanted effects

- sympathetic blockade: failure of ejaculation, and postural or exertional hypotension (unusual with clonidine, owing to its direct peripheral action)
- unopposed parasympathetic action: diarrhoea
- dry mouth
- CNS effects: sedation and drowsiness occur in up to 50% of those who take it; depression is occasionally seen

- fluid retention
- methyldopa induces a reversible positive Coombs' test in 20% of people, owing to production of IgG; however, haemolytic anaemia is rare
- sudden withdrawal of clonidine can produce severe rebound hypertension with tachycardia, sweating and anxiety.

Drugs affecting the renin–angiotensin system

Angiotensin-converting enzyme (ACE) inhibitors

Examples: captopril, lisinopril, ramipril

Mechanisms of action

The ACE inhibitors act by several mechanisms.

- Competitive inhibition of ACE reduces generation of angiotensin II and consequently reduces the release of aldosterone (Fig. 6.10). Inhibition of tissue ACE in the vascular wall (rather than plasma ACE) is most important for the hypotensive effect of these drugs (Fig. 6.10). Reduced tissue concentrations of angiotensin II lead to arterial and, to a lesser extent, venous dilation.
- There is no reflex tachycardia, probably because of stimulation of the vagus nerve and reduction in the potentiation of the sympathetic nervous system caused by angiotensin II (Fig. 6.3).
- Angiotensin II is also implicated in the development of arterial and left ventricular hypertrophy in hypertension. The importance of ACE inhibitors compared with other antihypertensives in limiting these effects is uncertain.
- ACE also degrades vasodilator kinins (Fig. 6.10). Increased kinins or vasodilator prostaglandins and nitric oxide in the vascular wall may contribute to the hypotensive actions of ACE inhibitors.

There are many clinical uses of these drugs apart from hypertension; these are listed in Box 6.2.

Pharmacokinetics

Most ACE inhibitors are given as prodrugs, because the active forms are water soluble and poorly absorbed from the gut. The prodrugs are converted in the liver to the active agent; for example, ramipril is converted to the active compound ramiprilat. In contrast, captopril and lisinopril are absorbed adequately as an active molecule. For most compounds, the active form is excreted unchanged by the kidney. The half-lives of captopril and ramiprilat

are short, whereas that of the active metabolite of enalapril (enalaprilat) is long.

Unwanted effects

- persistent dry cough that is not dose-related and may be caused by accumulation of kinins in the lung; it occurs in 10–30% of those who take the drug, is more common in women and can develop after many months of treatment
- postural hypotension, which is rare unless there is salt and water depletion, for example as a result of therapy with diuretics; in such people, profound hypotension can occur, particularly after the first dose; this is rarely a problem in the treatment of hypertension, but can be in the treatment of severe heart failure (Ch. 7)
- renal impairment, especially in people with severe bilateral renal artery stenosis who rely on angiotensin-mediated efferent glomerular arterial vasoconstriction to maintain glomerular perfusion pressure
- disturbance of taste, nausea, vomiting, dyspepsia or bowel disturbance
- rashes
- angioedema, more commonly in people of Afro-Caribbean origin.

Angiotensin II receptor antagonists

Examples: candesartan, losartan, valsartan

Mechanism of action

The angiotensin II receptor antagonists are selective for the AT_1 receptor subtype, which is found in the heart, blood vessels, kidney, adrenal cortex, lung and brain. Actions of angiotensin II via this receptor include vasoconstriction, cell growth and proliferation, aldosterone release, sympathetic stimulation, salt and water retention, and inhibition of renin release. They have less effect at the AT_2 receptor subtype, which inhibits vascular growth, vasodilates, and increases both renal Na^+ excretion and renin release. The overall effect of drugs like candesartan show similarities to those produced by ACE inhibitors, except that kinin degradation is unaffected and inhibition of the effects of angiotensin II on the AT_1 receptor is more complete (Fig. 6.10).

Pharmacokinetics

Losartan is well absorbed from the gut but has a low oral bioavailability because of first-pass metabolism. It is partially converted to an active metabolite, which is believed to be responsible for most of the pharmacological effects, and to several inactive metabolites. The metabolites are excreted by the kidney. The half-life of losartan

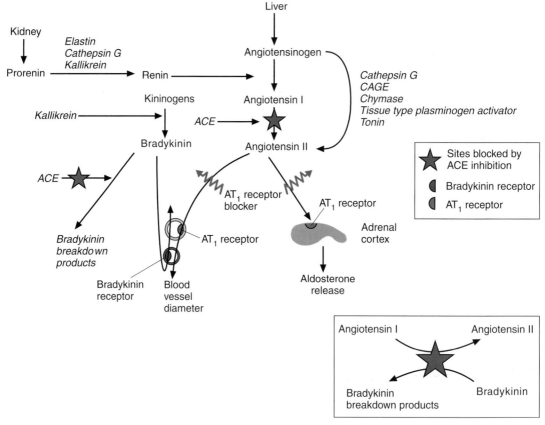

Fig. 6.10
The biological actions of bradykinin and angiotensin II and drugs that modify these actions. Bradykinin causes vasodilation by acting on vascular smooth muscle and on the endothelial cell (Fig. 6.5). Angiotensin II causes vasoconstriction by stimulating AT$_1$ receptors in the blood vessels and causes Na$^+$ retention by stimulating AT$_1$ receptors in the adrenal cortex, which results in aldosterone release. Angiotensin-converting enzyme (ACE) inhibitors block angiotensin II formation from angiotensin I, although an alternative pathway still remains that can result in some angiotensin II formation from angiotensinogen. Angiotensin II antagonists such as losartan act by inhibiting AT$_1$ receptors in blood vessels and on the adrenal cortex. CAGE, chymotrypsin-like angiotensin-II-generating enzyme.

is short, while that of the active metabolite is intermediate. Losartan is a competitive AT$_1$ receptor antagonist, but the active metabolite is a non-competitive antagonist.

Candesartan is given as a prodrug (candesartan cilextil); this is rapidly hydrolysed in the liver to the active candesartan, which has a long half-life. Valsartan is poorly absorbed from the gut. It is metabolised in the liver and has a short half-life.

Unwanted effects

Drugs in this class are usually well tolerated. Their major advantage over ACE inhibitors is the low incidence of cough. Angioedema is also rare. Unwanted effects include:

- headache
- dizzines
- arthralgia or myalgia
- fatigue.

Vasodilators

Diuretics

Three groups of diuretics are used to lower blood pressure: thiazide (and thiazide-like), loop and potassium-sparing diuretics.

Box 6.2

Clinical uses of ACE inhibitors

Treatment of hypertension (this chapter)
Treatment of heart failure (Ch. 7)
Secondary prevention after myocardial infarction (Ch. 5)
Diabetic nephropathy in insulin-dependent diabetes
    (Ch. 40 and this chapter)

Examples:
thiazide and thiazide-like diuretics:
  bendroflumethiazide, chlortalidone
loop diuretics: furosemide
potassium-sparing diuretics: spironolactone,
  amiloride, triamterene

Mechanism of action in hypertension
The sites and mechanisms of action of diuretics on the kidney and unwanted effects are considered in Chapter 14. There are several actions involved in lowering blood pressure.

- An initial hypotensive effect is produced by intravascular salt and water depletion. However, compensatory mechanisms such as activation of the renin–angiotensin–aldosterone system largely restore plasma and extracellular fluid volumes (see Fig. 6.4) (unless salt and water retention was a major component of the initial hypertension, e.g. in advanced renal failure or as a consequence of other antihypertensive treatment).
- Direct arterial dilation is responsible for the longer-term reduction in blood pressure. The mechanism of vasodilation is not well understood, but may result from reduced Ca^{2+} entry into the smooth muscle of the arteriolar resistance vessel walls (perhaps as a consequence of Na^+ depletion) and from synthesis of vasodilator prostaglandins.

Thiazide and thiazide-like diuretics. These produce their maximum blood-pressure-lowering effect at doses lower than those required for significant diuretic effects. This is an advantage, since most unwanted effects are dose related.

Loop diuretics. Unless used in a modified-release formulation, loop diuretics are usually less effective hypotensive agents than thiazides in the treatment of essential hypertension. Despite having a more powerful diuretic action, their duration of action is too short. However, hypertension with advanced renal impairment, or hypertension resistant to multiple drug treatment, is more likely to be associated with fluid retention and will respond better to a loop diuretic than to a thiazide.

Potassium-sparing diuretics. Spironolactone, a specific aldosterone antagonist, is most effective for hypertension caused by primary hyperaldosteronism (Conn's syndrome), but is increasingly used for resistant hypertension. Amiloride and triamterene are less effective than thiazides in essential hypertension.

Calcium channel antagonists (calcium antagonists)

Examples: amlodipine, nifedipine,
  verapamil, diltiazem (see Ch. 5 for
  individual drugs)

The calcium channel antagonists lower blood pressure principally by arterial vasodilation. For clinical uses, see Box 6.3. For further details, see Chapter 5.

Potassium channel openers

Example: minoxidil

Mechanism of action
Vascular smooth muscle possesses ubiquitous ATP-sensitive K^+ channels (K_{ATP}). Opening of a K_{ATP} channel occurs when minoxidil acts on an ATP-sensitive K_{ir} subunit causing inward rectification and an efflux of K^+; this results in hyperpolarisation and muscle relaxation (see also potassium channel openers, Ch. 5). Minoxidil is one of the most powerful peripheral arterial dilators.

Pharmacokinetics
Minoxidil is well absorbed from the gut, and mainly metabolised in the liver. It has a short half-life.

Unwanted effects

- arterial vasodilation produces flushing and headache
- the reflex sympathetic nervous system response to vasodilation causes tachycardia and palpitation (which can be blunted by concurrent use of a β-adrenoceptor antagonist, ACE inhibitor or angiotensin II receptor antagonist)
- increased transcapillary pressure can produce oedema, most marked in the ankles
- salt and water retention occur through stimulation of the renin–angiotensin–aldosterone system

---

Box 6.3

Clinical uses of calcium channel antagonists

Treatment of hypertension (this chapter)
Prophylaxis of angina (Ch. 5)
Treatment of Raynaud's phenomenon (Ch. 10)
Prevention and treatment of supraventricular arrhythmias (Ch. 8)
Subarachnoid haemorrhage (Ch. 9)

(Fig. 6.4); this can be reduced by the concurrent use of diuretics

- hirsutism; therefore rarely used for treatment of women.

Hydralazine

Mechanism of action

The mechanism of action of hydralazine is uncertain, but it may activate guanylate cyclase, leading to the intracellular production of cGMP. This will produce smooth muscle relaxation by a mechanism similar to that of organic nitrates (Fig. 6.5 and Ch. 5).

Pharmacokinetics

Hydralazine is well absorbed from the gut and then undergoes extensive first-pass metabolism in the gut wall and liver, principally by N-acetylation. Some individuals, who are genetically determined slow acetylators (Ch. 2), require lower doses of hydralazine and are more susceptible to some of the unwanted effects. The half-life of hydralazine is short.

Unwanted effects

- Arterial vasodilation with reflex sympathetic activation produces tachycardia, flushing, hypotension and fluid retention.
- Headache, dizziness.
- A systemic lupus erythematosus (SLE)-like syndrome, which usually occurs after several months of treatment, is dose-related and is more common in slow acetylators. It resembles the naturally occurring disease but does not produce renal or cerebral damage and is slowly reversed if treatment is stopped. A positive antinuclear antibody is found in many people who do not develop the syndrome.

Nitrovasodilators

Example: sodium nitroprusside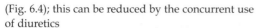

Mechanism of action

Nitroprusside is a nitrovasodilator with a mechanism of action similar to that of organic nitrates (Ch. 5). It produces dilation of arterioles and veins, reducing both peripheral resistance and venous return. Its use is limited to the emergency management of some hypertensive states.

Pharmacokinetics

Nitroprusside is given by intravenous infusion and has a duration of action of less than 5 min. Metabolism to cyanide within red blood cells (by electron transfer from haemoglobin iron) terminates its effect. The cyanide is partly bound in the erythrocyte and partly liberated, pro-

ducing inhibition of cellular cytochrome oxidase. Free cyanide is converted in the liver to less toxic thiocyanate. This accumulates with prolonged infusion; therefore, treatment is usually limited to a maximum of 3 days.

Unwanted effects

- headache, dizziness
- nausea, retching, abdominal pain
- thiocyanate accumulation causes tachycardia, sweating, hyperventilation, arrhythmias and metabolic acidosis from inhibition of aerobic metabolism in cells.

Treatment of hypertension

The morbidity and premature deaths associated with untreated hypertension are considerable, and increase with advancing age. Treatment of the older hypertensive, therefore, prevents more events in the short term than treating a similar number of younger people. However, early treatment will prevent vascular damage occurring in the younger hypertensive – an important consideration, since the vascular changes are not completely reversible once established.

The optimal target blood pressure is a systolic pressure below 140 mmHg and a diastolic pressure (phase V Korotkoff sound) below 85 mmHg in uncomplicated hypertension. When there is target organ damage or diabetes, then a lower target of 130/80 mmHg is recommended, to minimise the risk of progressive vascular disease. Even if the target pressures cannot be achieved, the progressively greater morbidity associated with higher blood pressures means that any blood pressure reduction in severe hypertension will be beneficial. Treating isolated systolic hypertension (systolic >160 mmHg, diastolic <90 mmHg) in the elderly gives similar benefits to the treatment of diastolic hypertension in this age group.

It is rarely possible to correct the underlying cause of hypertension. Lifestyle modifications, alone or combined with drug therapy, should be recommended initially, to reduce blood pressure, although their effectiveness in preventing complications is unknown. Weight loss, restriction of alcohol and excess salt intake, and increasing exercise may be enough to lower the blood pressure satisfactorily in some people with mild hypertension. In more severely hypertensive individuals, these measures can produce a substantial reduction in blood pressure but rarely restore it to normotensive values. It is important to advise all people with hypertension not to smoke, since smoking doubles the risk of cardiovascular and cerebrovascular events at any level of blood pressure.

The decision to treat a hypertensive person with drugs should be largely determined by an assessment of the overall risk of complications in that individual. Drug treatment is usually started if blood pressure remains above the levels discussed above despite non-pharmacological approaches.

Drug regimens in hypertension

Lowering blood pressure with drugs produces a substantial (≈40%) reduction in the risk of stroke, as well as reducing the risk of heart failure and renal failure. Drug treatment also reduces the risk of coronary artery disease in the elderly by about 25%; evidence for a similar reduction in the young is less convincing, which may reflect the short duration of the trials (up to 5 years). The target blood pressure in most people with hypertension is 140/85 mmHg or less. In people who also have diabetes, the risk of a cardiovascular event is further reduced if the blood pressure is lowered to 130/80 mmHg. There is no lower limit for blood pressure reduction, except in those with significant coronary artery disease. In this situation, lowering the diastolic blood pressure below 70 mmHg may reduce coronary artery perfusion and increase the risk of myocardial infarction.

Treatment regimens that are based on β-adrenoceptor antagonists, diuretics, calcium channel antagonists, ACE inhibitors or angiotensin II receptor antagonists have generally shown equal efficacy for reducing events, with the exception that β-adrenoceptor antagonists are less effective in the elderly. Treatment of hypertension should follow a 'stepped care' approach. A single drug will achieve good blood pressure control in about 35% of people with hypertension. If the initial choice of drug fails to produce an adequate reduction in blood pressure, then a change in therapy to an alternative first-line drug may be recommended. However, if the fall in blood pressure with the first drug is substantial but the target pressure is not reached, then the first drug should be continued and a second drug should be added.

The British Hypertension Society have endorsed the 'AB/CD' protocol for combining blood-pressure-lowering drugs that is based on their mode of action (Fig. 6.11). The underlying principle is that younger hypertensives are more likely to have high plasma renin concentrations, and therefore a drug that suppresses the production of renin, or reduces the generation or action of angiotensin II, is most likely to be effective. Conversely, elderly hypertensives are more likely to have 'low-renin' hypertension. Use of a drug that suppresses the renin–angiotensin system creates a low-renin state, while diuretics and calcium channel antagonists increase plasma renin. This provides the rationale for combination therapy with drugs from complementary classes in the algorithm. Both diuretics and β-adrenoceptor antagonists increase the risk of developing diabetes, and particularly when used together. This combination is not recommended in those who are at increased risk of glucose intolerance, such as obese people, those with a strong family history of type 2 diabetes, or people of South Asian or Afro-Caribbean origin.

If three drugs with complementary actions, taken in adequate dosage, are insufficient to control the blood pressure, then the person is said to have 'resistant' hypertension.

Resistant hypertension

There are several possible causes of apparently resistant hypertension. These include:

- poor adherence to prescribed therapy (see Ch. 55)
- 'white coat' hypertension, which responds poorly to drug treatment
- secondary hypertension, usually caused by renal artery stenosis or Conn's syndrome
- other, unidentified causes for poor response to drug treatments.

Some people with resistant hypertension benefit from treatment with a loop diuretic, which will help if expansion of the plasma volume is contributing to drug resistance. Spironolactone is an alternative if there is persisting evidence of hyperaldosteronism. In men, minoxidil can

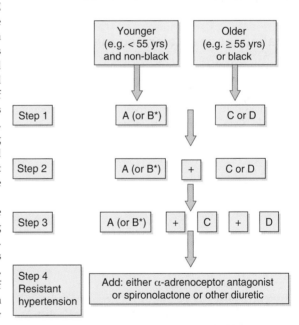

Fig. 6.11
The British Hypertension Society recommendations for combining blood-pressure-lowering drugs.
*Combination therapy involving B and D may induce more new-onset diabetes compared with other combination therapies.
From Williams et al (2004b) with permission.

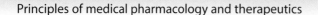
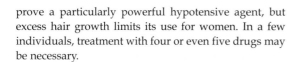

prove a particularly powerful hypotensive agent, but excess hair growth limits its use for women. In a few individuals, treatment with four or even five drugs may be necessary.

Additional treatment to reduce risk

The use of aspirin at low dosage reduces the risk of myocardial infarction in people with hypertension. It is recommended when the risk of coronary heart disease is greater than 15% in the subsequent 10 years. A statin is also recommended for primary prevention of cardiovascular disease in people with hypertension at a similar level of risk, or in those with diabetes (Ch. 48).

Hypertension in special groups

There are reasons for selecting particular classes of drugs under certain specific conditions or when concomitant illnesses are present (Table 6.3). Black people respond less well to β-adrenoceptor antagonists and ACE inhibitors than do Caucasians. Compared with younger people with hypertension, the elderly are less likely to achieve good blood pressure control with β-adrenoceptor antagonists.

Malignant or accelerated hypertension

Early treatment is important for hypertensives with retinal haemorrhages, exudates or papilloedema. Rapid blood pressure reduction is potentially dangerous, since it can lead to cerebral underperfusion and ischaemic damage. Oral atenolol or nifedipine are the most widely recommended treatments, which gradually reduce the blood pressure over 24 h or more.

Renal artery stenosis

ACE inhibitors or angiotensin II receptor antagonists usually produce an excellent reduction in blood pressure if hypertension is caused by renal artery stenosis, but they can lead to a deterioration in renal function, especially if there are bilateral stenoses. Renal artery angioplasty with stenting is usually recommended if there is associated renal impairment; however, while this may preserve renal function, it rarely results in a normalisation of blood pressure. Nevertheless, fewer drugs may subsequently be required to achieve target blood pressure levels.

Diabetic nephropathy

ACE inhibitors and angiotensin receptor blockers appear to protect the kidney more than other classes of antihypertensive drug in diabetic nephropathy. In particular, they reduce progression from microalbuminuria to overt nephropathy. The effect may be independent of blood pressure reduction and reflect a reduction in glomerular perfusion pressure. Other complications of hypertension in those with diabetes are prevented equally well by β-adrenoceptor antagonists, thiazide diuretics or calcium channel antagonists.

Phaeochromocytoma

Hypertension in this condition is caused by excessive release of catecholamines from a tumour that often arises

Table 6.3
Selection of antihypertensive drugs for patients with coexisting conditions

	Diuretic	β-Adrenoceptor antagonist	ACE inhibitor	Calcium antagonist	α₁-Adrenoceptor antagonist
Elderly	+	+/–	+/–	+	+/–
Black race	+	+/–	+/–	+	+
Angina	+/–	+	+/–	+	+/–
After myocardial infarction	+/–	+	+	–	+/–
Congestive heart failure	+	–	+	–	+/–
Diabetes mellitus (with or without nephropathy)	C	C	+	+/–	+/–
Raynaud's phenomenon	+/–	–	+	+	+
Gout	–	+/–	+/–	+/–	+/–
Prostatism	–	+/–	+/–	+/–	+
Supraventricular arrhythmias	+/–	+	+/–	+ᵃ	+/–
Dyslipidaemia	C	C	+/–	+/–	+/–
Migraine	+/–	+	+/–	+/–	+/–

ACE, angiotensin-converting enzyme. +, treatment of choice; +/–, no obvious advantage/not preferred; C, use with caution; –, usually contraindicated. ᵃDiltiazem or verapamil only.

in the adrenal glands. Noradrenaline-secreting tumours most often lead to sustained hypertension, through vasoconstriction mediated by α_1-adrenoceptor stimulation. Treatment is always started with an α-adrenoceptor antagonist to prevent the excessive vasoconstriction, followed by a β-adrenoceptor antagonist to block the arrhythmogenic effects of the catecholamines on the heart. Definitive treatment, whenever possible, is by surgical removal of the tumour.

Primary hyperaldosteronism (Conn's syndrome)

This can be caused by bilateral adrenal hyperplasia or, less commonly, by an adrenal tumour. The treatment of choice is spironolactone, to directly block the effects of aldosterone at its renal tubular receptor. If there is a tumour, then surgical excision should be considered.

Pregnancy

There are two issues peculiar to pregnancy.

Pre-existing chronic hypertension. The risk of hypertension to mother and fetus is probably not great until the systolic blood pressure reaches 150–160 mmHg, or the diastolic blood pressure reaches 100–110 mmHg. Treatment at lower levels carries a risk of impairment of fetal growth. Drugs given to the mother can carry a teratogenic risk for the fetus (Ch. 56). The drugs with the best safety record in this situation are methyldopa, nifedipine and labetalol. In the second trimester, although the risk of teratogenesis is past, diuretics and β-adrenoceptor antagonists are still contraindicated, since they may retard fetal growth, while ACE inhibitors or angiotensin II receptor antagonists may cause oligohydramnios, renal failure, hypotension and intrauterine death in the fetus.

Pre-eclampsia. This only occurs after 20 weeks of gestation. It presents as hypertension, with oedema and proteinuria or hyperuricaemia, in previously normotensive women. There is a risk to the mother of convulsions, cerebral haemorrhage, abruptio placentae, pulmonary oedema and renal failure if this condition is untreated. The fetal risk is of severe growth retardation or even death. Once the diagnosis is established, bed rest is supplemented by antihypertensive drugs as for pre-existing hypertension in pregnancy. Hydralazine, initially by intravenous bolus injection, is favoured in severe pre-eclampsia.

FURTHER READING

August P (2003) Initial treatment of hypertension. *N Engl J Med* 348, 610–617

Brown MA, Buddle ML, Martin A (2001) Is resistant hypertension really resistant? *Am J Hypertens* 14, 1263–1269

Brown MJ, Cruickshank JK, Dominiczak AF et al (2003) Better blood pressure control: how to combine drugs. *J Hum Hypertens* 17, 81–86

Ferrario C, Levy P (2002) Sexual dysfunction in patients with hypertension: implications for therapy. *J Clin Hypertens* 4, 424–432

Messerli FH, Grossman E, Goldbourt U (1998) Are β-blockers efficacious as a first-line therapy for hypertension in the elderly? A systematic review. *JAMA* 279, 1903–1909

Messerli FH, Grossman E, Lever A (2003) Do thiazides confer specific protection against strokes? *Arch Intern Med* 163, 2557–2560

Neal B, MacMahon S, Chapman et al (2000) Effects of ACE inhibitors, calcium antagonists, and other blood-pressure-lowering drugs: results of prospectively designed overviews of randomized trials. *Lancet* 355, 1955–1964

Oparil S, Zaman A, Calhoun DA (2003) Pathogenesis of hypertension. *Ann Intern Med* 139, 761–776

Psaty B, Lumley T, Furberg CD et al (2003) Health outcomes associated with various antihypertensive therapies used as first-line agents: A network meta-analysis. *JAMA* 289, 2534–2544

Safar ME, Smulyan H (2004) Hypertension in women. *Am J Hypertens* 17, 82–87

Snow V, Weiss KB, Mottur-Pilson C et al (2004) The evidence base for tight blood pressure control in the management of type 2 diabetic mellitus. *Ann Intern Med* 138, 587–592

Staessen JA, Wang J, Bianchi G et al (2003) Essential hypertension. *Lancet* 361, 1629–1641

Staessen JA, Wang J-G, Thijs L (2001) Cardiovascular protection and blood pressure reduction: a meta-analysis. *Lancet* 358, 1305–1315

Vijan S, Hayward RA (2003) Treatment of hypertension in type 2 diabetes mellitus: blood pressure goals, choice of agents, and setting priorities in diabetes. *Ann Intern Med* 138, 593–602

Williams B, Poulter NR, Brown MJ et al (2004a) British Hypertension Society guidelines for hypertension management 2004: summary. *BMJ* 328, 634–640

Williams B, Poulter NR, Brown MJ et al (2004b) Guidelines for management of hypertension: report of the fourth working party of the British Hypertension Society, 2004 – BHS IV. *J Hum Hypertens* 18, 139–185

Self-assessment

1. In the following questions, the first statement, in italics, is true. Is the accompanying statement also true?

   a. *Thiazide diuretics reduce sodium and water reabsorption in the distal convoluted tubule.* They are the drugs of choice for treating pregnancy-related hypertension.

   b. *Nifedipine shows selectivity for vasodilation over cardiac depression.* It does so principally by arterial vasodilation.

   c. *Moxonidine stimulates imidazoline receptors in the medulla.* This increases sympathetic outflow and decreases vagal tone, lowering blood pressure.

   d. *Propranolol lowers blood pressure.* It does so by (i) decreasing cardiac output, (ii) reducing renin secretion, and (iii) peripheral vasodilation.

   e. *Amiloride and spironolactone are potassium-sparing diuretics.* Their diuretic action is through different mechanisms in the distal tubule and early collecting duct.

   f. *Stretch of baroreceptors increases the afferent impulses to the vasomotor centre.* This results in enhanced sympathetic nervous outflow and a rise in blood pressure.

   g. *Stimulation of presynaptic α-adrenoceptors in arteriolar resistance vessels inhibits noradrenaline release.* α_1-Adrenoceptor blockade by prazosin increases noradrenaline release.

   h. *Thiazide diuretics initially lower blood pressure by depleting salt and water.* The long-term reduction in blood pressure by thiazide diuretics can be seen with doses that do not cause diuresis and natriuresis.

   i. *ACE inhibitors prevent the conversion of angiotensin I to the vasoconstrictor angiotensin II.* ACE inhibitors prevent the breakdown of the vasodilator bradykinin.

   j. *Minoxidil opens K^+ channels in smooth muscle membranes.* This K^+-channel opening destabilises the cell membrane, leading to vasoconstriction.

   k. *The antihypertensive effect of nitroprusside is limited to emergency management of some hypertensive states.* It can be administered for up to two months.

2. Choose the one incorrect statement from the following statements concerning drugs used in the treatment of hypertension.

   A. Thiazide diuretics lower blood pressure at doses lower than that are required for diuresis.

   B. ACE inhibitors cause cough by inhibiting the formation of bradykinin.

   C. Combinations of antihypertensive drugs are commonly used in the treatment of hypertension.

   D. Angiotensin receptor antagonists lower blood pressure by blocking the angiotensin type-1 receptor (AT_1).

   E. Nifedipine is more selective than verapamil for blockade of calcium channels in the arteries compared with calcium channels in the heart.

3. Case history questions

   > A 60-year-old man with non-insulin-dependent diabetes smoked 20 cigarettes a day. His plasma lipid levels were normal and there was no proteinuria. His height was 5'8" (1.70 m) and his weight 210 lb (95.5 kg). He had his blood pressure checked three times over a period of weeks and it was consistently 175/110 mmHg. He had no evidence of fluid retention or heart failure. His doctor prescribed propranolol, but the blood pressure was not fully controlled.

   a. Which of the following combinations would have been appropriate to prescribe to lower his blood pressure?

      A. Bendroflumethiazide plus propranolol
      B. Furosemide plus atenolol
      C. Amiloride plus ramipril
      D. Nifedipine plus atenolol.

   > Following several months of treatment with your chosen regimen, his blood pressure was still 165/100 mmHg and he then suffered a small myocardial infarction.

   b. What changes in his therapy would you consider?

   The answers are provided on pages 708–709.

Self-assessment questions

Drugs used in the control of hypertension

Drug	Half-life (h)	Elimination	Comments
β-Adrenoceptor antagonists			All β-adrenoceptor antagonists, except esmolol and sotalol, are used for hypertension (see Ch. 8)
Calcium channel antagonists			Isradipine, lacidipine, lercanidipine and nisoldipine are used only for the treatment of hypertension, while others have multiple uses (see Ch. 5)
Diuretics			Can be used to lower blood pressure; see Ch. 14 for individual drugs
α₁-Selective adrenoceptor antagonists			All drugs given orally
Doxazosin	9–12	Metabolism	Used for hypertension and benign prostatic hyperplasia; oral bioavailability is 65% owing to incomplete absorption; metabolised by oxidation
Indoramin	5	Metabolism	Used for hypertension and benign prostatic hyperplasia; oral bioavailability is 10–25%; eliminated by oxidation (CYP2D6) to an active hydroxyl metabolite
Prazosin	3	Metabolism	Used for hypertension, congestive heart failure, Raynaud's syndrome and benign prostatic hyperplasia; oral bioavailability is 60% owing to first-pass metabolism; high hepatic extraction and clearance by cytochrome P450
Terazosin	12	Metabolism	Used for mild to moderate hypertension and benign prostatic hyperplasia; high oral bioavailability (>90%); mostly eliminated by hepatic metabolism but some eliminated unchanged in urine (5%) and faeces (25%)
Non-selective adrenoceptor antagonists			Used in phaeochromocytoma only
Phenoxybenzamine	24	Metabolism	Used for hypertensive episodes associated with phaeochromocytoma; given orally or by intravenous infusion; low oral bioavailability (20–30%); metabolised in the liver
Phentolamine	1.5	Metabolism + renal	Used for hypertensive episodes in and diagnosis of phaeochromocytoma; given by intravenous injection; eliminated by poorly defined metabolism and unchanged via renal excretion (10%)
Angiotensin-converting enzyme inhibitors			All drugs given orally; many are prodrugs that undergo bioactivation by hepatic metabolism
Captopril	2	Renal + metabolism	Used for hypertension, congestive heart failure, post-myocardial infarction and diabetic nephropathy; good absorption (70–80%) with limited first-pass metabolism (10%); eliminated by renal filtration plus secretion, and formation of inactive metabolites

continued

Drug compendium

Drugs used in the control of hypertension *(continued)*

Drug	Half-life (h)	Elimination	Comments
Cilazapril	30 (cilazaprilat)[a]	Renal (cilazaprilat)	Used for hypertension and congestive heart failure; prodrug, which is well absorbed (60%);converted in liver to cilazaprilat, which shows biphasic elimination with half-lives of 1–2 and 30–50 h
Enalapril	35 (enalaprilat)[a]	Renal (enalaprilat)	Used for hypertension, congestive heart failure, and in subjects with left ventricular dysfunction; prodrug, which is well absorbed (60%); converted in liver to enalaprilat, both enalapril and enalaprilat are eliminated in the urine
Fosinopril	12 (fosinoprilat)[a]	Renal (fosinoprilat)	Used for hypertension and congestive heart failure; poorly absorbed prodrug of which about 30% is converted in the intestine and liver to fosinoprilat; fosinoprilat is eliminated unchanged in urine and faeces
Imidapril	8 (imidaprilat)[a]	Metabolism	Used for hypertension; prodrug, which is well absorbed and rapidly hydrolysed (half-life 2 h) to the active imidaprilat (the fate of which has not been published)
Lisinopril	12	Renal	Used for hypertension, congestive heart failure, post-myocardial infarction and diabetic nephropathy; incompletely absorbed from gut; excreted unchanged in urine (30%) and faeces (70%)
Moexipril	10 (moexiprilat)[a]	Renal (moexiprilat)	Used for hypertension; poorly absorbed prodrug; converted in liver to moexiprilat; significant amounts (50%) are excreted in faeces as moexiprilat (possibly formed in gut lumen from unabsorbed compound)
Perindopril	29 (perindoprilat)[a]	Renal (perindoprilat)	Used for hypertension and congestive heart failure; well-absorbed prodrug; about 20% is converted in liver to perindoprilat
Quinapril	2 (quinaprilat)[a]	Renal (quinaprilat)	Used for hypertension and congestive heart failure; well-absorbed prodrug; converted in liver to quinaprilat, which is eliminated rapidly by renal tubular secretion
Ramipril	1–5 (ramiprilat)[a]	Renal (ramiprilat)	Used for hypertension and congestive heart failure; well-absorbed prodrug; converted in liver to ramiprilat, which is excreted in urine
Trandolapril	16–24 (trandolaprilat)[a]	Metabolism + renal	Used for hypertension, post myocardial infarction and heart failure (unlicensed indication); well-absorbed prodrug; converted in liver to trandolaprilat and inactive metabolites; trandolaprilat is eliminated in urine and by metabolism and has a slow minor terminal half-life 50–100 h (which is not clinically significant)

continued

Drugs used in the control of hypertension (continued)

Drug	Half-life (h)	Elimination	Comments
Angiotension II receptor antagonists			All drugs given orally; all drugs used for hypertension
Candesartan	9–12	Renal + metabolism	Highly selective blockade of AT_1 receptors; given as the prodrug, candesartan cilexetil, which is rapidly hydrolysed during absorption to the active candesartan (15%); candesartan is eliminated by renal excretion (26%) and in faeces (possibly as metabolites)
Eprosartan	5–9	Renal + metabolism	Rapidly absorbed but with a low bioavailability (13%); eliminated largely unchanged in urine plus some conjugation with glucuronic acid
Irbesartan	11–15	Renal + metabolism	Also used for renal disease associated with type 2 diabetes mellitus; highly selective blockade at AT_1 receptors; oral bioavailability is 60–80%; metabolised by oxidation (CYP2C9) and conjugation; parent drug plus conjugates eliminated in urine and bile
Losartan	2	Metabolism	Also used for renal disease associated with type 2 diabetes mellitus; highly selective blockade at AT_1 receptors; extensive first-pass metabolism (50%) to inactive metabolites plus an active metabolite, which gives prolonged non-competitive selective blockade at AT_1 receptors
Olmesartan	13	Urine and bile	Given as medoxomil prodrug, which is rapidly and quantitatively converted to olmesartan in the gastrointestinal tract; olmesartan is eliminated unchanged
Telmisartan	16–23	Bile (+ metabolism)	Highly selective blockade at AT_1 receptors; good oral bioavailability (50%); eliminated unchanged in faeces, possibly after biliary excretion of the glucuronide conjugate, which is detected in blood
Valsartan	5–7	Metabolism	Highly selective blockade at AT_1 receptors; oral bioavailability is 25%; oxidised in liver to a hydroxy metabolite; duration of action is 24 h, allowing once-daily dosing
Vasodilator antihypertensive drugs			Drugs for hypertension and to control blood pressure under specified circumstances
Bosentan	5	Metabolism	Used for pulmonary arterial hypertension; endothelin-1- receptor anagonist; given orally; extensively metabolised by, and an inducer of, CYP2C9 and CYP3A4; blood levels change during the start of treatment due to autoinduction of metabolism; metabolites eliminated in bile
Diazoxide	28	Renal (+ metabolism)	For severe hypertension associated with renal disease; given in emergencies by intravenous bolus injection; eliminated largely by glomerular filtration; long half-life is a result of high protein binding

continued

Drug compendium

Drugs used in the control of hypertension (continued)

Drug	Half-life (h)	Elimination	Comments
Hydralazine	4	Metabolism	Used as an adjunct for treating moderate or severe hypertension, for heart failure and for hypertensive crisis; given orally, by slow intravenous injection or by intravenous infusion; undergoes first-pass metabolism by *N*-acetylation with a bioavailability of 10–15% in fast acetylators and 30–35% in slow acetylators; eliminated by acetylation and oxidation; slow acetylators have high circulating concentrations of hydralazine
Minoxidil	3–4	Metabolism + renal	Used for severe hypertension, in addition to a diuretic and β-adrenoceptor antagonist; given orally; complete oral bioavailability; mainly eliminated as a glucuronide conjugate
Sodium nitroprusside	Seconds	Decomposition + renal	Used for hypersensitive crisis, for controlled hypertension in anaesthesia and for acute or chronic heart failure; decomposes to NO and CN, which are eliminated largely in the urine as nitrite and thiocyanate ions; the clinical responses (owing to NO) are very rapid and short lived
Centrally acting antihypertensive drugs			Drugs for hypertension and to control blood pressure under specified circumstances
Clonidine	20–25	Renal + metabolism	Selective α_2-adrenoceptor agonist; used for hypertension, migraine and menopausal flushing; given orally or by slow intravenous injection; sudden withdrawal may give hypertensive crisis; good oral bioavailability (70%+); eliminated unchanged in urine (60%) and as hydroxyl metabolites
Methyldopa	1–2	Renal + metabolism	Selective α_2-adrenoceptor agonist; used for hypertension, particularly in pregnancy; given orally; oral bioavailability is 10–60% owing to conjugation with sulphate in the intestinal wall; eliminated by glomerular filtration and sulphate conjugation
Moxonidine	2–3	Renal + metabolism	Selective imidazoline I_1 receptor agonist; used for mild to moderate hypertension; given orally; bioavailability is about 90%; eliminated largely in the urine unchanged
Adrenergic neuron-blocking drugs			
Guanethidine	2 days	Renal	Used only for hypertensive crisis; given by intramuscular injection; eliminated by renal excretion and metabolism; very slow terminal phase (4–8 days) reported in some studies
Ganglion-blocking drugs			
Trimetaphan	–	–	Used for controlled hypotension during surgery; given by intravenous infusion; old drug with few data available

[a]The half-life and route of elimination relate to the active metabolite, which is named in parentheses.

7

Heart failure

The relationship between afterload and stroke volume is shown in Figure 7.2. Afterload is determined largely by peripheral resistance but also by the size of the ventricle. Enlargement of this chamber (e.g. as a result of increased venous return or preload) increases wall tension, and the heart must generate greater pressure both to initiate and to maintain contraction. Preload and afterload are therefore interrelated. In the healthy ventricle, a rise in afterload is met by an increase in myocardial contractility to maintain stroke volume. In the failing ventricle, inability to augment contraction as afterload rises leads to a progressive fall in stroke volume (Fig. 7.2).

Maintenance of cardiac output

There are four major determinants of cardiac output:

- preload: this is governed by the ventricular end-diastolic volume, which in turn is related to ventricular filling pressure and, therefore, to venous return
- heart rate
- myocardial contractility
- afterload: the systolic wall tension in the ventricle; this reflects the resistance to ventricular emptying.

These factors normally balance the output from both sides of the heart. In the healthy heart, changes in cardiac output are achieved mainly by changes in heart rate and preload.

The relationship between preload and stroke volume (the amount of blood ejected from the ventricle during systole) is shown in Figure 7.1. The degree of stretch of the ventricular muscle (preload) determines the force of cardiac contraction (the Frank–Starling phenomenon). The curve describing this relationship is governed by intrinsic myocardial contractility: thus, the curve is shifted downwards in the failing ventricle and upwards when contractility is augmented, for example by sympathetic nervous stimulation. The left ventricular filling pressure in a healthy heart with normal contractility falls on the steep part of the curve, making stroke volume sensitive to changes in preload. In the failing ventricle, the maximal achievable stroke volume is reduced. The Frank–Starling curve is also flatter, indicating that stroke volume is less dependent on changes in preload.

Pathophysiology of heart failure

There is no universally accepted definition, but heart failure is usually said to exist when the output of the heart is insufficient to meet the metabolic needs of the body. Heart failure is a syndrome with several underlying causes (Box 7.1). It can arise suddenly or develop gradually, depending on the cause.

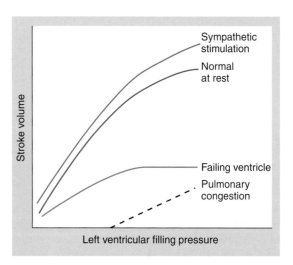

Fig. 7.1
The relationship between preload (left ventricular filling pressure) and stroke volume (the Frank–Starling phenomenon) in the healthy and failing heart. In the latter, if an increase in filling pressure and heart rate are insufficient to restore cardiac output, then pulmonary congestion will occur.

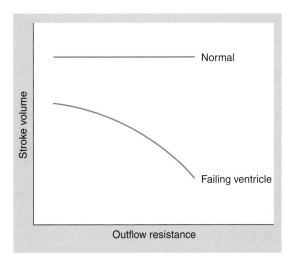

Fig. 7.2
The relationship between afterload (outflow resistance) and stroke volume in the presence of normal and reduced myocardial contractility.

Box 7.1

Causes of heart failure

Coronary artery disease
Hypertension
Myocardial disease; cardiomyopathies, myocarditis
Valvular heart disease
Constrictive pericarditis
Congenital: atrial septal defect, ventricular septal defect, aortic coarctation
Infiltrative: amyloid, sarcoid, iron
Iatrogenic: β-adrenoceptor antagonists, antiarrhythmics, calcium channel antagonists, cytotoxics, alcohol, irradiation
Arrhythmias, especially incessant tachyarrhythmias

Symptoms in heart failure are caused by a reduced cardiac output ('forward failure') or venous congestion ('backward failure'). The most common complaint is breathlessness, although fatigue is frequent, owing to reduced cardiac output and impaired muscle perfusion. Biochemical changes also occur in muscle, which are not immediately reversed when peripheral blood flow is improved. Other symptoms, such as the discomfort of peripheral oedema and anorexia due to bowel congestion, are attributable to a high systemic venous pressure.

The electrocardiograph (ECG) is almost always abnormal in heart failure (arrhythmias, ischaemic changes, previous myocardial infarction, etc.), and a chest X-ray examination may reveal cardiomegaly or pulmonary congestion. One of the most useful investigations is echocardiography. This may identify the cause of heart failure and establish the degree of left ventricular dysfunction, which is a guide to prognosis.

Although heart failure is often caused by reduced left ventricular systolic contractility (systolic heart failure), it can also arise from impaired diastolic relaxation (diastolic heart failure). If the left ventricle fails to relax adequately, it will not accommodate the venous return, leading to pulmonary venous congestion and a low cardiac output. Diastolic heart failure characteristically occurs in association with left ventricular hypertrophy, but it also occurs in ischaemic heart disease.

The syndrome of heart failure arises largely from neurohumoral counter-regulation in response to the low blood pressure and low renal perfusion pressure (Fig. 7.3). The consequences of these are vasoconstriction of both arteries and veins and excessive salt and water retention by the kidneys. These mechanisms are designed to increase the blood pressure, but in the setting of a failing heart can exacerbate the cardiac dysfunction. As a consequence the hydrostatic pressure in the veins rises, and when it exceeds the plasma colloid osmotic (oncotic) pressure that holds fluid in the blood vessel then tissue oedema occurs.

Acute left ventricular failure

Acute left ventricular failure usually results from a sudden inability of the heart to maintain an adequate output and blood pressure. This leads to reflex arterial and venous constriction (Fig. 7.3). There is a rapid rise in filling pressure of the left ventricle as a result of increased venous return. If the heart is unable to expel the extra blood, the hydrostatic pressure in the pulmonary veins rises until it exceeds the plasma oncotic pressure and produces pulmonary oedema. The principal symptom is breathlessness, occurring on exertion in the early stages, then at rest with orthopnoea. Left ventricular failure can follow acute myocardial infarction, acute mitral or aortic valvular regurgitation, or arise from brady- or tachyarrhythmias if there is pre-existing poor left ventricular function.

Cardiogenic shock

The syndrome of cardiogenic shock arises when the systolic function of the left ventricle is suddenly impaired to such a degree that there is insufficient blood flow to meet resting metabolic requirements of the tissues. This definition excludes shock caused by hypovolaemia. The clinical hallmarks are a low systolic blood pressure (usually <90 mmHg), with a reduced cardiac output and an elevated left ventricular filling pressure. Cardiogenic shock can follow acute myocardial infarction, and in this situa-

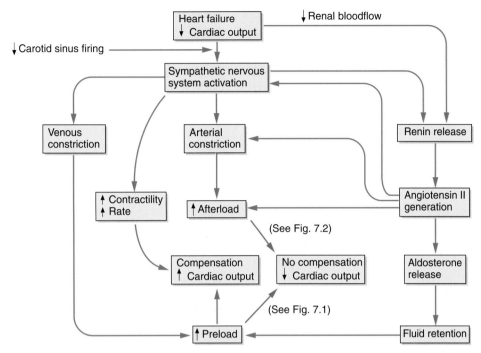

Fig. 7.3
Neurohumoral consequences of heart failure. The increase in preload can improve cardiac performance in the mildly impaired heart but will lead to oedema if cardiac function is significantly reduced, since the increased preload cannot restore a normal stroke volume (Fig. 7.1). The increased afterload will put additional strain on the failing heart and can further decrease cardiac output. These effects are compounded by downregulation of cardiac β_1-adrenoceptors.

tion, usually indicates loss of at least 40% of the left ventricular myocardium. Other mechanical disturbances, such as acute mitral regurgitation or ventricular septal rupture, can produce cardiogenic shock in association with a lesser degree of myocardial damage. Less commonly, the syndrome is associated with right ventricular infarction.

Chronic heart failure

Myocardial damage from ischaemic heart disease is the most common cause of chronic heart failure, but potentially correctable causes such as valvular lesions, as well as treatable exacerbating factors such as anaemia or arrhythmias, may be identified. In most people with heart failure, there are signs of both right and left ventricular failure (congestive heart failure). Chronic congestive heart failure is not a trivial complaint: even people with left ventricular systolic dysfunction who have symptoms only on exertion have a two-year mortality of about 20%, while if there are symptoms at rest, the one-year mortality is 80%. Death is either from progressive heart failure or from sudden arrhythmic death. The mortality in diastolic heart failure is about half that of systolic heart failure, but still four times that of the general population.

Positive inotropic drugs

Myocardial contractility can be improved by increasing the availability of free intracellular Ca^{2+} to interact with contractile proteins, or by increasing the sensitivity of the myofibrils to Ca^{2+}. Only drugs that increase myocardial intracellular Ca^{2+} are established in clinical use; they work by one of two distinct mechanisms:

- an action on the cell membrane Na^+/K^+-ATPase pump (e.g. digoxin)
- by increasing intracellular cyclic adenosine monophosphate (cAMP; e.g. phosphodiesterase inhibitors).

An additional advantage of the positive inotropic drugs that increase myocardial cAMP is their ability to enhance the reuptake of Ca^{2+} by the sarcoplasmic reticulum in diastole. This improves diastolic relaxation in addition to augmenting systolic contractility.

Digitalis glycosides

Example: digoxin

Mechanism of action and effects

Effect on myocardial contractility

Digitalis glycosides are compounds with a steroid nucleus that were originally isolated from a species of foxglove (*Digitalis purpura*). They bind to the energy-dependent Na^+ pump (Na^+/K^+-ATPase) in the myocyte membrane. This pump establishes and maintains the Na^+ and K^+ gradients across the cell (Fig. 7.4), producing low intracellular Na^+ and high intracellular K^+ concentrations. Partial inhibition of the pump by digitalis glycosides increases the intracellular Na^+ concentration and reduces the concentration gradient for Na^+ across the cell membrane. A separate passive transmembrane exchange of Na^+ and Ca^{2+} occurs down their concentration gradients. The activity of this ion-exchange mechanism is reduced by the increase in intracellular Na^+, and Ca^{2+} is therefore retained in the cell. The excess intracellular Ca^{2+} is stored in the sarcoplasmic reticulum during diastole and released during membrane excitation, leading to enhanced myocardial contraction.

Effects on cardiac action potential and conduction

Digoxin can have both arrhythmogenic and anti-arrhythmic actions. Direct actions of the drug can provoke arrhythmias by increasing myocardial excitability and automaticity (Ch. 8). The mechanisms for this are:

- a reduction of the resting membrane potential: the cell membrane Na^+/K^+- ATPase pump extrudes three Na^+ out of the cell for every two K^+ that enter, which increases the resting negative intracellular electrical potential and hyperpolarises the cell (see Ch. 8); inhibition of this membrane pump by digoxin, therefore, leads to the cell membrane potential becoming less negative and arrhythmias are more readily initiated

- triggering of spontaneous release of Ca^{2+} from the sarcoplasmic reticulum: this leads to transient depolarisation of the cell immediately following an action potential ('after potentials'), and is an important mechanism for initiating arrhythmias (Ch. 8).

Digitalis glycosides also have clinically useful indirect actions on the action potential via stimulation of the central vagal nucleus and enhanced cardiac sensitivity to acetylcholine. The vagal stimulation is antiarrhythmic (Ch. 8) through:

- decreased automaticity of the sinoatrial node, which slightly slows sinus rate
- an increased refractory period of the atrioventricular node, which results in a slower ventricular rate; this is useful in the management of certain arrhythmias, particularly atrial fibrillation (Ch. 8).

Digitalis glycosides produce distinctive changes on the ECG, which include non-specific T-wave changes and sagging of the S–T segment ('reverse tick') (Fig. 7.5). These effects can be mistaken for myocardial ischaemia.

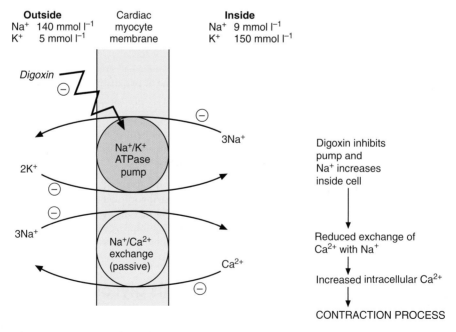

Fig. 7.4
The action of digoxin on the cardiac myocyte.

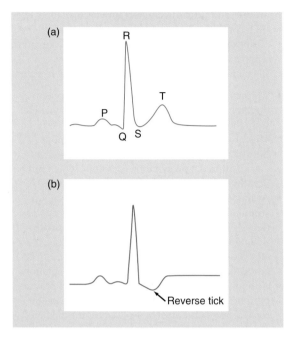

Fig. 7.5
The effect of digoxin on the S–T segment of an electrocardiograph (ECG). (a) Normal ECG trace. (b) Pronounced changes with digoxin include a sagging S–T segment and a flat T wave. Additionally, the resting membrane potential becomes less negative.

Pharmacokinetics

Digoxin is the most widely used of the digitalis glycosides in the UK. It is well absorbed from the gut; the kidney is the main route of elimination, partially by active tubular secretion. The half-life of digoxin is very long (about 1.5 days) and further lengthened when renal function is impaired. To achieve an early onset of action, initial loading doses should be given over 24–36 h (Ch. 2). If a rapid response is essential, digoxin can be given by slow intravenous injection.

Other digitalis glycosides are rarely used. Digitoxin is occasionally given in renal failure, since it is extensively metabolised and mainly excreted via the gut; however, it has the disadvantage of an even longer half-life (approximately 8 days).

Unwanted effects

Digitalis glycosides have a narrow therapeutic index. Toxicity is mostly dose related and includes:

- consequences of intracellular Ca^{2+} overload: increased automaticity of the atrioventricular node and Purkinje fibres produces junctional escape beats, junctional tachycardia, ventricular ectopic beats (including bigeminy or coupling of an ectopic after each normal beat) or (less commonly) ventricular tachycardia
- consequences of increased vagal activity: excessive atrioventricular nodal block can occur; when associated with increased atrial automaticity, this produces atrial tachycardia with 2:1 atrioventricular nodal block, a rhythm characteristic of digitalis toxicity
- gastrointestinal disturbances: anorexia, nausea and vomiting (largely a central effect at the chemoreceptor trigger zone; Ch. 32), and diarrhoea
- neurological disturbances: fatigue, malaise, confusion, vertigo, coloured vision (especially yellow halos around lights, possibly from inhibition of Na^+/K^+-ATPase in the cones of the retina)
- gynaecomastia or breast enlargement: the steroid structure allows digitalis glycosides to bind to oestrogen receptors.

Exacerbating factors for digitalis toxicity

- Hypokalaemia: a reduced extracellular K^+ concentration increases the effects of digitalis on the Na^+/K^+-ATPase pump. Care must be taken if potassium-losing diuretics, such as furosemide (Ch. 14), are used with digitalis glycosides.
- Renal impairment: this is not always obvious in the elderly, who may have a normal plasma creatinine concentration even when renal function is markedly reduced.
- Hypoxaemia: this sensitises the heart to digitalis-induced arrhythmias.
- Hypothyroidism: the renal elimination of digoxin is decreased because of a reduced glomerular filtration rate.
- Drugs that displace digoxin from tissue binding sites and interfere with its renal excretion: these include verapamil (Ch. 5) and quinidine (Ch. 8), which can double the plasma concentration of digoxin; amiodarone (Ch. 8) produces a less marked effect.

Treatment of digitalis toxicity

Digitalis toxicity can be treated by:

- withholding further drug
- using K^+ supplementation (Ch. 14) for hypokalaemia; this is usually given orally, but should be given by slow intravenous infusion if there are dangerous arrhythmias
- atropine (Ch. 8) for sinus bradycardia or atrioventricular block; temporary transvenous pacing is used for marked bradycardia unresponsive to atropine
- digoxin-specific antibody fragments for serious toxicity (Ch. 53).

Sympathomimetic inotropes

Examples:

non-selective β-adrenoceptor agonist: isoprenaline

selective β₁-adrenoceptor agonist: dobutamine

selective β₂-adrenoceptor agonist and dopaminergic agonist: dopexamine

mixed non-selective β-adrenoceptor, α-adrenoceptor and dopaminergic agonist: dopamine

Mechanisms of action and effects

The mechanisms of action of the sympathomimetic inotropes are also considered in Chapter 4.

Isoprenaline is a non-selective β-adrenoceptor agonist that increases both myocardial contractility (β_1-adrenoceptors) (Fig. 7.6) and heart rate (β_1- and β_2-adrenoceptors), and produces peripheral arterial vasodilation (β_2-adrenoceptors).

Dobutamine, a synthetic dopamine analogue, is a selective β_1-adrenoceptor agonist that produces a powerful inotropic response, with relatively less increase in heart rate and little direct effect on vascular tone, even at high concentrations.

Dopexamine acts on β_2-adrenoceptors and dopamine receptors, and does not cause vasoconstriction.

Dopamine has dose-related actions at several receptors.

- At low doses, it selectively stimulates peripheral dopamine receptors, which are structurally distinct from those in the central nervous system. This produces renal arterial vasodilation and diuresis (D_1 receptors) and peripheral arterial vasodilation (D_2 presynaptic receptors, which inhibit noradrenaline release from sympathetic nerves).
- At moderate doses, non-selective β-adrenoceptor stimulation produces a positive inotropic response (Fig. 7.6). Tachycardia is more marked than with dobutamine, because of stimulation of cardiac β_1- and β_2-adrenoceptors and the reflex response to β_2-adrenoceptor-mediated peripheral arterial dilation.
- At high doses, α_1-adrenoceptor stimulation produces peripheral vasoconstriction, which also affects the renal arteries and overcomes D_1-receptor-mediated renal vasodilation.

The doses that produce these different effects differ widely among individuals. There is no dose that can be relied upon to act selectively at dopamine receptors without stimulating adrenoceptors.

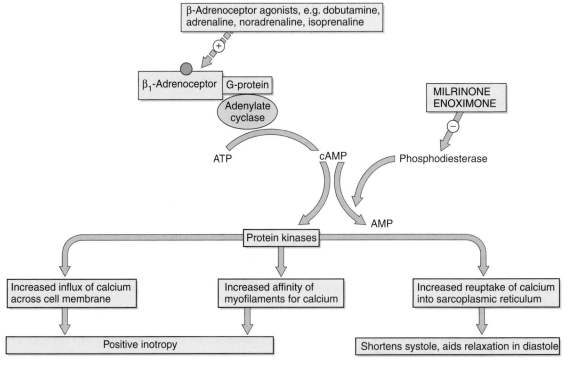

Fig. 7.6
Mechanisms by which sympathomimetics and phosphodiesterase inhibitors exert their positive inotropic effects.

Pharmacokinetics

Dobutamine, dopamine and isoprenaline are all administered by intravenous infusion because of their very short half-lives of about 2–10 min. Metabolic inactivation is by the same pathways as for noradrenaline (Ch. 4). Desensitisation and downregulation of β-adrenoceptors (Ch. 1) rapidly reduce the response to sustained infusions over 48–72 h. Owing to its vasoconstrictor actions, dopamine is usually given into a large central vein.

Unwanted effects

Unwanted effects can be predicted from agonist actions at adrenoceptors (Ch. 4) and mainly relate to excessive cardiac stimulation, with tachycardia, palpitations and arrhythmias.

Phosphodiesterase inhibitors

Examples: milrinone, enoximone

Mechanism of action and effects

Milrinone and enoximone are specific inhibitors of the isoenzyme of phosphodiesterase found in cardiac and smooth muscle (phosphodiesterase III). Their inotropic action on the heart results from an increase in intracellular cAMP with mobilisation of intracellular Ca^{2+} (Fig. 7.6). Unlike β-adrenoceptor agonists, the activity of phosphodiesterase inhibitors is not limited by desensitisation of cell surface receptors, because they act at a site beyond the receptor. Because of their complementary sites of action, phosphodiesterase inhibitors and β-adrenoceptor agonists will have additive effects on the heart. Phosphodiesterase inhibition in vascular smooth muscle produces peripheral arterial vasodilation.

Pharmacokinetics

Phosphodiesterase inhibitors are only given for short-term treatment by intravenous infusion. They are eliminated by the kidney (milrinone) or hepatic metabolism (enoximone), and have short half-lives.

Unwanted effects

The unwanted effects are mainly those produced by excessive cardiac stimulation, including:

- tachycardia
- palpitation
- potentially serious arrhythmias.

Large trials of oral formulations have indicated that phosphodiesterase inhibitors increase mortality during long-term use in heart failure.

Management of heart failure

Acute left ventricular failure

The immediate aim of treatment in acute left ventricular failure is to reduce the excessive venous return. Treatment includes:

- Intravenous injection of a loop diuretic such as furosemide (Ch. 14): this initially produces venous dilation, which increases peripheral venous pooling; symptoms, therefore, are improved even before the onset of a diuresis that reduces plasma volume and further decreases preload.
- Sublingual glyceryl trinitrate (Ch. 5): this dilates venous capacitance vessels and is a useful alternative or additional emergency treatment to diuretics.
- Intravenous opioid analgesic such as diamorphine (Ch. 19), often given to relieve distress and breathlessness.
- Oxygen in high concentration via a facemask.

Whenever possible, a precipitating or exacerbating cause should be treated – for example, arrhythmias, anaemia, thyrotoxicosis, acute mitral regurgitation or critical aortic stenosis. When this is not possible, maintenance treatment with an oral diuretic, and management as for chronic heart failure, is often required.

Cardiogenic shock

The mortality of cardiogenic shock, even with intensive treatment, is in excess of 70%. The immediate aim of treatment is resuscitation, while looking for a remediable cause. If appropriate, early coronary revascularisation is crucial to increase the probability of survival. Supportive measures include the following.

- Administer oxygen in high concentrations via a facemask.
- Correct any acid–base imbalance (especially acidosis) and electrolyte abnormalities (particularly hypokalaemia).
- Relieve pain, usually with an opioid analgesic such as diamorphine (Ch. 19).
- Correct any cardiac rhythm disturbance (Ch. 8).
- Ensure an adequate left ventricular filling pressure. This can be low after right ventricular infarction, despite a high central venous pressure

(right ventricular filling pressure). In this situation, monitoring of left heart function with a flow-guided balloon-tipped (Swan–Ganz) catheter is helpful to determine whether infusion of a colloid plasma expander is indicated.

- If intravenous volume is adequate but tissue perfusion remains impaired, dobutamine is the inotropic drug of choice. Dobutamine is often given in combination with low-dose dopamine, with the intention that the dopamine will improve renal perfusion; however, there is little evidence that the addition of dopamine is beneficial.
- Phosphodiesterase inhibitors are sometimes given to improve myocardial contractility and to produce peripheral vasodilation. They are usually reserved for those who fail to improve with maximum tolerated doses of dobutamine.
- When there is profound hypotension, noradrenaline (norepinephrine) (Ch. 4) can be infused intravenously to produce peripheral vasoconstriction and maintain vital organ perfusion.
- Vasodilators can be given to 'offload' the heart once an adequate blood pressure has been established. This strategy is particularly helpful if there is significant mitral regurgitation, since reduced resistance to left ventricular emptying will diminish the regurgitant volume; either glyceryl trinitrate (Ch. 5) or nitroprusside (Ch. 6) is used.
- Intra-aortic balloon pumping can temporarily maintain intra-aortic diastolic pressure and improve coronary perfusion. It is particularly useful prior to surgery, for example to repair an incompetent mitral valve or an acquired ventricular septal defect.

Chronic heart failure

Much of the treatment of chronic heart failure is directed towards counteracting the compensatory mechanisms for the reduced cardiac output and low blood pressure generated by a failing heart, i.e. arterial and venous vasoconstriction and fluid retention. A further desirable action is to reduce the shape change (remodelling) that occurs in the failing ventricle and makes contraction less efficient. Treatment has two main aims: symptom relief and improved prognosis.

Non-pharmacological treatment

A number of lifestyle changes can be helpful.

- Weight reduction should be encouraged for an obese person to improve exercise tolerance.
- Bed rest may be appropriate to rest the heart during acute episodes of fluid retention.
- Modest salt restriction is desirable (severe salt restriction is unpleasant and unnecessary).

- Fluid restriction is rarely required unless profound hyponatraemia accompanies severe oedema. In this situation, diuretics may be ineffective until the plasma Na^+ concentration is corrected.
- If possible, drugs that exacerbate heart failure by producing myocardial depression (e.g. high-dose β-adrenoceptor antagonists, most calcium channel antagonists) or by promoting fluid retention (e.g. non-steroidal anti-inflammatory drugs [NSAIDs]) should be withdrawn. Alcohol intake should be moderate at most, since alcohol depresses myocardial contractility and can be arrhythmogenic.
- A graded exercise programme for people with stable heart failure can improve symptoms.

Diuretics

Diuretics remain the mainstay of treatment for chronic heart failure (Ch. 14). They are usually taken once daily, in the morning. A thiazide diuretic, such as bendroflumethiazide, is only useful for mild symptoms, and a loop diuretic – usually furosemide – is used for moderate or severe fluid retention. Modest doses of furosemide are usually sufficient, unless renal function is impaired, when additional diuresis can be produced by much larger doses. Bumetanide has few advantages over furosemide, although its more predictable absorption is sometimes useful, for example in marked right-sided heart failure with gut congestion. Hypokalaemia is unusual when loop diuretics are used alone in chronic heart failure, but use of a potassium-sparing diuretic is advisable if the plasma K^+ falls below 3.5 mmol l^{-1} or if digoxin or antiarrhythmic therapy is given concurrently (because of an increased risk of generating rhythm disturbances). Potassium-sparing diuretics are a more effective and more palatable treatment for hypokalaemia than are K^+ supplements.

If fluid retention fails to respond to an oral loop diuretic, the addition of a distal tubular diuretic, such as bendroflumethiazide or metolazone, for a few days, often produces a profound natriuresis and diuresis. Care must be taken to avoid hyponatraemia, hypokalaemia, hypovolaemia and renal impairment with such combined diuretic regimens, and a potassium-sparing diuretic is almost always needed. Spironolactone is preferred in this situation since it improves symptoms and prognosis (at least in severe heart failure) if a low dose is added to maximal therapy with other drugs. For resistant fluid retention, an intravenous infusion of furosemide can initiate diuresis.

Angiotensin-converting enzyme inhibitors

An angiotensin-converting enzyme (ACE) inhibitor is now considered to be essential in the treatment of heart failure, and is usually started at the same time as a diuretic.

ACE inhibitors (Ch. 6) produce arterial and venous dilation, which improves peripheral haemodynamics and, therefore, cardiac function. Symptoms of breathlessness and fatigue are usually reduced, and exercise tolerance increases. The full symptomatic response is often delayed for 4 to 6 weeks after the start of treatment, despite early haemodynamic changes. A further benefit of ACE inhibitors is improved survival, which has been shown most clearly when there is severe left ventricular systolic dysfunction (a left ventricular ejection fraction below 40%). This may be due to a reduction in the harmful remodelling of the left ventricle. High doses of an ACE inhibitor are probably more effective than low doses, and reduce mortality by 20–25% in systolic heart failure.

There is a small risk of symptomatic hypotension after administration of the first dose of an ACE inhibitor; use of a small initial dose of ACE inhibitor reduces the duration of any hypotension. If the person has evidence of dehydration (e.g. a postural fall in blood pressure), diuretics should be omitted on at least the first day of ACE inhibitor treatment. Potassium-sparing diuretics are usually unnecessary when an ACE inhibitor is used, because ACE inhibitors promote K^+ retention by the kidney. However, the combination of an ACE inhibitor with spironolactone in severe heart failure is advantageous, although this carries a low risk of serious hyperkalaemia.

If an ACE inhibitor is not tolerated, usually because of a cough, an angiotensin II receptor antagonist (Ch. 6) can be substituted. These agents have similar efficacy to ACE inhibitors. ACE inhibitors or angiotensin II receptor antagonists improve symptoms in diastolic heart failure, but may not alter prognosis.

Beta-adrenoceptor antagonists

Contrary to traditional teaching, β-adrenoceptor antagonists (Ch. 5) are highly effective for treatment of heart failure that has been stabilised with an ACE inhibitor and diuretic. Because of their negative inotropic properties, these drugs were once considered to be contraindicated; however, if introduced very gradually in small doses, they improve both symptoms and survival. The survival advantage is additive to, and greater than, that produced by an ACE inhibitor, with a 30–35% reduction in mortality at all classes of severity of heart failure. Possible explanations for the benefit of β-adrenoceptor antagonists are numerous (Box 7.2). All patients with heart failure should now be treated with a β-adrenoceptor antagonist once stabilised on an ACE inhibitor or an angiotensin II receptor antagonist. The only compounds licensed for this use in the UK are bisoprolol and carvedilol, although there are also data to show the efficacy of a modified-release formulation of metoprolol.

Digoxin

Digitalis glycosides are widely used when heart failure is associated with atrial fibrillation and a rapid ventricular rate. The use of digoxin for heart failure associated with sinus rhythm has been more controversial, but there is now conclusive evidence that it is very effective as a supplement to diuretic and ACE inhibitor therapy when there is severe left ventricular systolic dysfunction. Symptoms are improved and the need for hospitalisation reduced, but survival is unaffected. In sinus rhythm, the effective dose of digoxin is smaller than that required for control of atrial fibrillation. Hypokalaemia should be avoided to minimise the risk of digoxin toxicity.

Other vasodilators

Treatment with a combination of hydralazine (Ch. 6) and isosorbide dinitrate (or mononitrate; (Ch. 5), in addition to a diuretic and digoxin, provides balanced arterial and venous dilation. This combination improves exercise tolerance in heart failure but only produces a modest reduction in mortality.

Box 7.2

Possible beneficial effects of β-adrenoceptor antagonists in heart failure

Reduced workload of the damaged myocardium
Suppression of the neurohumoral response to the low cardiac output
Antiarrhythmic effects
Inhibition of neutrophil-induced myocardial damage
Free radical scavenging in ischaemic myocardium

FURTHER READING

Amabile CM, Spencer AP (2004) Keeping your patient with heart failure safe. A review of potentially dangerous medications. *Arch Intern Med* 164, 709–720

Angeja BG, Grossman W (2003) Evaluation and management of diastolic heart failure. *Circulation* 107, 659–663

Cowie MR, Zaphiriou A (2002) Management of chronic heart failure. *BMJ* 325, 422–425

DiBianco R (2003) Update on therapy for heart failure. *Am J Med* 115, 480–488

Dimopoulos K, Salukhe TV, Coats AJS et al (2004) Meta-analyses of mortality and morbidity effects of an angiotensin receptor blocker in patients with chronic heart failure already receiving an ACE inhibitor (alone or with a β-adrenoceptor antagonist). *Int J Cardiol* 93, 105–111

Eichhorn EJ, Gheorghiade M (2002) Digoxin. *Prog Cardiovasc Dis* 44, 251–266

Farrell MH, Foody JM, Krumholz HM (2002) β-adrenoceptor antagonists in heart failure. Clinical applications *JAMA* 287, 890–897

Flather MD, Yuisuf S, Kober L et al (2000) Long-term ACE-inhibitor therapy in patients with heart failure or left ventricular dysfunction: a systematic overview of data from individual patients. *Lancet* 355, 1578–1581

Foody JM, Farrell MH, Krumholz HM (2002) β-adrenoceptor antagonist therapy in heart failure. Scientific review *JAMA* 287, 883–889

Goldstein S (2002) Benefits of β-blocker therapy for heart failure. *Arch Intern Med* 162, 641–648

Hollenberg SM (2001) Cardiogenic shock. *Crit Care Clin* 17, 391–410

Hunt SA, Baker DW, Chin MH et al (2001) ACC/AHA guidelines for the evaluation and management of chronic heart failure in the adult: executive summary: a report of the American College of Cardiology/American Heart Association Task Force on Practice Guidelines (Committee to revise the 1995 Guidelines for the Evaluation and Management of Heart Failure). *J Am Coll Cardiol* 38, 2101–2113

Koerner MM, Loebe M, Lisman KA et al (2001) New strategies for the management of acute decompensated heart failure. *Curr Opin Cardiol* 16, 164–173

McMurray J, Pfeffer MA (2002) New therapeutic options in congestive heart failure. *Circulation* 105, 2099–2106

Nohria A, Lewis E, Stevenson LW (2002) Medical management of advanced heart failure *JAMA* 287, 628–640

Ranvan SL, Ranvan MC, Deedwania PC et al (2002) Diuretic resistance and strategies to overcome resistance in patients with congestive heart failure. *Congest Heart Fail* 8, 80–85

Rathore SS, Curtis JP, Jeptha P et al (2003) Association of serum digoxin concentration and outcomes in patients with heart failure. *JAMA* 289, 871–878

Sowers JR (2004) Treatment of hypertension in patients with diabetes. *Arch Intern Med* 164, 1860–1857

Weber KT (1999) Aldosterone and spironolactone in heart failure. *N Engl J Med* 341, 753–754

Self-assessment

1. In the following questions, the first statement, in italics, is true. Is the accompanying statement also true?

   a. *One of the determinants of cardiac output is afterload.* In healthy hearts, myocardial contractility increases following a rise in afterload.

   b. *A major symptom of pulmonary oedema is breathlessness.* Oedema occurs when the pressure in the pulmonary veins is less than the plasma osmotic pressure.

   c. *Detrimental changes in body function in heart failure occur as a result of attempts by the body to compensate for the cardiac dysfunction.* In heart failure, sympathetic outflow increases because of an increase in the sensory input from the baroreceptors in the carotid sinus.

   d. *Treatment of chronic heart failure is directed towards the compensatory mechanisms, i.e. vasoconstriction and fluid retention.* Digoxin is the mainstay of treatment of the vasoconstriction and fluid retention.

   e. *The positive inotropic action of digoxin on the cardiac myocyte is a result of inhibition of the Na^+/K^+-ATPase pump on the myocyte membranes ultimately increasing intracellular Ca^{2+} concentrations.* Potassium ions and digoxin enhance the actions of each other at the Na^+/K^+-ATPase pump.

   f. *Digoxin has both direct and indirect effects on the electrical properties of the heart.* Digoxin inhibits the vagus, decreasing the refractory period of the atrioventricular node.

   g. *To improve tissue perfusion in cardiogenic shock, dobutamine or the phosphodiesterase inhibitor milrinone are given intravenously, as their half-lives are very short.* Desensitisation of the response to dobutamine but not to milrinone can occur with sustained infusion.

   h. *Dobutamine increases cardiac output and decreases ventricular filling pressure in heart failure.* Dobutamine produces peripheral vasodilation by its effect on $β_2$-adrenoceptors.

   i. *Digoxin has a half-life of about 1.5 days.* The toxicity of digoxin increases in renal failure.

   j. *In heart failure, drugs that do not have a direct action on the heart are very useful.* ACE inhibitors improve survival in chronic heart failure and have added benefit if given together with K$^+$-sparing diuretics such as spironolactone.

2. Case history questions.

DY was 78 years of age and had had a large anterior myocardial infarction 3 years ago. Echocardiography revealed marked left ventricular systolic dysfunction with reduced ejection fraction. He presented with several symptoms, including fatigue and decreased exercise ability, shortness of breath and peripheral oedema. Examination demonstrated cardiomegaly, a raised jugular venous pressure and crackles in the lungs. An ECG showed that he was in sinus rhythm.

---

a. Of the signs and symptoms stated, what was the main direct consequence of a reduced cardiac output?

b. Digoxin, a β-adrenoceptor antagonist and dobutamine were all considered as initial treatment for DY and were rejected. Would any of these treatments have been appropriate?

c. What were the choices of diuretic open to you in treating DY?

d. Potassium loss produced by diuretics may lead to hypokalaemia, which should be avoided in patients with heart failure, particularly those taking digoxin. What is an effective way of reducing urinary K$^+$ loss?

e. DY was then started on an ACE inhibitor. What are the precautionary measures that should be taken in starting this new medication and how would its effectiveness be assessed?

f. After 4 weeks of treatment with the ACE inhibitor and a diuretic, DY's symptoms of breathlessness, fatigue and exercise tolerance were much improved. However, he developed a cough while taking the ACE inhibitor, which became intolerable. What is thought to be the reason for the cough and what alternative therapy could be given to avoid this?

The answers are provided on pages 709–710.

Drugs used in heart failure

Drug compendium

Drug	Half-life	Elimination	Comments
Cardiac glycosides			Used in heart failure and for supraventricular arrhythmias (particularly atrial fibrillation)
Digitoxin	8 days (3–16 days)	Metabolism + renal + bile	Once-daily oral dosage, or even alternate-day dosage
Digoxin	40 h (20–50 h)	Renal	Given once daily as an oral dose; a loading dose may be given orally in divided dose over 24 h or by intravenous infusion in an emergency (see Ch. 2): eliminated by glomerular filtration
Phosphodiesterase inhibitors			
Enoximone	1.3 h	Metabolism	Used for congestive heart failure where cardiac output is reduced and filling pressure increased; given by intravenous infusion; half-life increased in chronic heart failure; metabolised to a sulphoxide which is eliminated in urine
Milrinone	0.8–0.9 h	Renal	Used for short-term treatment of severe congestive heart failure, and acute heart failure; given by intravenous injection followed by infusion (usually for up to 12 h); rapid elimination through renal tubular secretion, and low volume of distribution
Sympathomimetic inotropes			
Dobutamine	2 min	Metabolism	Used for inotropic effect after myocardial infarction, cardiac surgery, cardiomyopathies, septic shock and cardiogenic shock; acts on β_1-receptors in heart muscle to increase cardiac contractility with little effect on rate; given by intravenous infusion; at low doses, results in vasodilation
Dopamine	7–12 min	Metabolism	Used for cardiogenic shock in exacerbations of chronic heart failure and in heart failure associated with cardiac surgery; acts on β_1-receptors in heart muscle to increase cardiac contractility with little effect on rate; given by intravenous infusion; causes vasodilation
Dopexamine	7 min	Metabolism	Used for inotropic effect after myocardial infarction, cardiac surgery, cardiomyopathies, septic shock and cardiogenic shock; acts on β_2-receptors in heart muscle to increase cardiac contractility and on peripheral dopamine receptors to increase renal perfusion; given by intravenous infusion; allow at least 15 min prior to dose incrementation, causes vasodilation

Cardiac arrhythmias

Basic cardiac electrophysiology

Myocardial cells maintain transmembrane ion gradients by movement of the ions through membrane channels. Several specific channels exist for Na^+, Ca^{2+} and K^+. These channels cycle through three states: resting, open or closed (and therefore refractory) (Ch. 1). Whether the ion channels are open or closed is determined by the membrane potential across the cell; hence they are called voltage-gated ion channels. The direction in which ions move is dependent upon both the concentration gradient of the ions and on the transmembrane potential. The action potentials of sinoatrial (SA) and atrioventricular (AV) nodes, Purkinje fibres and ventricular cells vary in their characteristics (Fig. 8.1) as they have different membrane ion channels that are regulated at different membrane potentials.

The resting potential inside a cardiac cell is approximately −70 to −80 mV compared with the extracellular environment. Certain cells in the specialised conducting system of the heart are known as pacemaker cells; the primary example of this is the SA node, which controls the normal rhythm of the heart (sinus rhythm). Such cells are capable of spontaneous repetitive depolarisation, due to entry of positive ions into the resting cell. The intrinsic rate of firing of a pacemaker cell depends on three factors:

- the resting potential
- the threshold potential for initiating an impulse
- the rate of spontaneous depolarisation.

Spontaneous depolarisation in pacemaker cells is relatively slow and results from influx of Ca^{2+} into the cell, mainly through T-type Ca^{2+} channels and influx of Na^+ (Fig. 8.1). All pacemaker cells can therefore initiate a cardiac impulse, and their action potentials are propagated to and by other myocardial cells. The dominant pacemaker cells (i.e. those with the fastest intrinsic rate of depolarisation) are found in the SA node. Consequently, the normal cardiac impulse arises from the SA node, and the pacemakers elsewhere in the specialised electrical conducting tissue of the heart (e.g. Purkinje fibres) will only be utilised if there is a failure of pacemakers with a faster rate of spontaneous depolarisation.

Action potentials in the atria and the ventricles can visually be divided into four phases; these are most clearly seen in Purkinje fibres (Fig. 8.1). Phase 0 of the action potential is initiated by a rapid influx of Na^+ through specific voltage-gated ion channels. In most cardiac cells, phase 0 is triggered when sufficient Na^+ channels have been opened to allow the cell to reach the threshold potential. By contrast, in the AV node, phase 0 depolarisation arises from the slower influx of Ca^{2+} through L-type channels. This results in slower conduction of the impulse than in other parts of the heart and is responsible for the conduction delay in the AV node.

At the end of phase 0, the intracellular voltage potential briefly becomes positive, at which point a voltage-triggered 'gate' closes and inactivates the Na^+ or Ca^{2+} channels, preventing further inward ion flow and repetitive depolarisation. Although inactivation of these ion channels is triggered by the same depolarising impulse that opens the channels, closure of the channels occurs far more slowly. Recovery of the channels to the resting state, when they are closed but no longer refractory to further depolarisation, is dependent on repolarisation of the cell.

Repolarisation of the cell is achieved when depolarisation opens several types of outward-flowing K^+ channels. It begins when K^+ efflux from the cell exceeds Na^+ or Ca^+ influx (phase 1 of the action potential) due to I_{KTO} currents through K_v-type channels (Table 5.1). However, repolarisation is temporarily interrupted by a distinct period of influx of Ca^{2+} through L-type channels (plateau phase, or phase 2) which is balanced by K^+ efflux through K_v channels (I_{Ks}, I_{Kr} and I_{Kur} currents) which prolongs depolarisation. Repolarisation in phase 3 is achieved by increasing I_{Ks} and I_{Kr} currents but also through the inward-rectifying currents I_{K1} and I_{Kr} (K_{ir} channels, Table 5.1). The opening of most K^+ channels

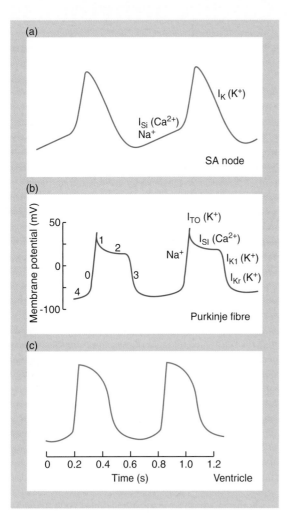

Fig. 8.1
Action potentials show patterns that vary with the region of the heart. The patterns are determined by the opening and closing of selective gates for Na^+, Ca^{2+} and K^+. The overall stability of the resting transmembrane ionic balance is maintained by active pumps such as the Na^+/K^+-ATPase pump (Fig 8.2). It is these pumps that maintain substantial concentration gradients of 140 mmol l^{-1} Na^+ outside and 10–15 mmol l^{-1} Na^+ inside the cell, and 140 mmol l^{-1} K^+ inside and 4 mmol l^{-1} K^+ outside the cell. This results in an electrical gradient at rest of approximately −70 to −80 mV inside the cell, relative to 0 mV outside the cell . Large ion fluxes at rest are prevented by specific pumps and closure of voltage-operated gates. The cardiac action potential is closely ordered. Action potentials in the atrioventricular node, bundle of His and ventricle are controlled by the sinoatrial (SA) node in the heart when it is in sinus rhythm. The rate of spontaneous depolarisation of the SA node determines its primary pacemaker status in the healthy heart.

Phase 0 (8.1b,c) occurs when the membrane potential reaches a defined threshold (threshold potential) and an 'all or none' influx of Na^+ through voltage-dependent channels occurs. This is transient and the gates close after a few milliseconds. Phase 0 is much slower in the SA node and depends mainly upon Ca^{2+} influx. This causes the conduction velocity in the SA node to be considerably less than that in the Purkinje fibres, and the refractory period is longer in proportion to the total duration of the action potential. Phase 1, called the early repolarisation and notch, results from K^+ efflux (the transient outward [TO] current) and reduced Na^+ influx. The phase 2 plateau is primarily a result of Ca^{2+} influx (slow inward, SI current) which is balanced by K^+ efflux over a slow time course. Phase 3 repolarisation results from inactivation of Ca^{2+} influx and increasing K^+ efflux via a number of currents (see text for explanation). Part of the overall importance of the K^+ currents is to maintain a stable resting membrane potential.

varies according to the membrane potential, giving rise to voltage-dependence of membrane resistance (rectification). The channels are therefore known as rectifiers. An inward rectification produces a larger current in response to a voltage driving a current into a cell than an identical voltage driving a current out of a cell.

In the resting phase between action potentials (phase 4), Na^+ and K^+ transmembrane concentration gradients are restored by a separate exchange pump (Na^+/K^+-ATPase) (Fig. 8.2). The negative internal resting membrane potential is maintained by high K^+ permeability of resting cell membranes through inward rectifying voltage and ligand-gated K_{ir} channels which close when the cell depolarises (see also Ch. 1).

During the period between phase 0 and the end of phase 2 of the action potential, the myocardial cell is refractory to further depolarisation (the absolute refractory period), because the depolarising channels are inactivated. During phase 3, a large depolarising stimulus can open sufficient Na^+ channels (many of which will have recovered to the resting state) to over-

come the K^+ efflux and initiate a further action potential. This part of the action potential is the relative refractory period.

The sum of the individual electrical currents that pass from one cell to another through the heart can be recorded on the surface electrocardiogram (ECG) (Fig. 8.3).

Mechanisms of arrhythmogenesis

Arrhythmias are disorders of rate and rhythm of the heart, which can arise as the result of either abnormal impulse generation or abnormal impulse conduction. There are three principal mechanisms of arrhythmogenesis.

Increased automaticity. Ectopic pacemakers (pacemakers other than the SA node) occur when pacemaker

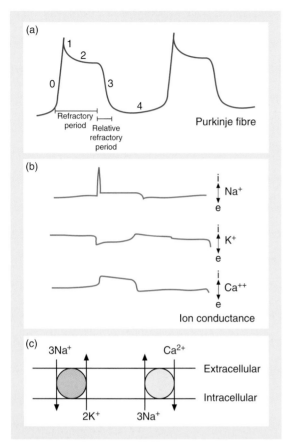

(a)

(b)

Na^+

K^+

Ca^{++}

Ion conductance

(c)

$3Na^+$

Ca^{2+}

Extracellular

Intracellular

$2K^+$ $3Na^+$

Fig. 8.2
A schematic representation of the influx and efflux of Na⁺, Ca²⁺ and K⁺ in Purkinje fibres. (a) The action potential pattern. (b) Overall conductance changes in relation to the action potential cycle. (c) The Na⁺/K⁺ and Na⁺/Ca²⁺ ion pumps and exchangers maintaining the membrane potential. The electrogenic Na⁺/K⁺ pump also contributes to the outward current in phase 4 of the action potential. In pacemaker cells, the upstroke is dependent on Ca²⁺ rather than Na⁺, and the clear Ca²⁺ influx maintaining the plateau phase is absent. i, intracellular; e, extracellular.

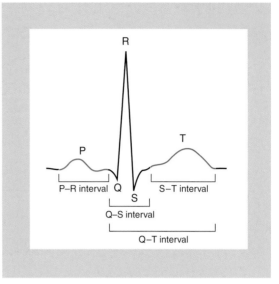

Fig. 8.3
The waveform for cardiac events seen on a surface electrocardiogram. The P wave represents the spread of depolarisation through the atria, and the QRS complex is the spread through the ventricles. The T wave represents repolarisation of the ventricle. The P–R interval is the time of conductance from atrium to ventricles, and the QRS time is the time the ventricles are activated. The duration of the ventricle action potential is given by the Q–T interval.

cells in the specialised conducting tissue develop a more rapid phase 4 depolarisation than the SA node. They can also arise when rapid spontaneous phase 4 depolarisation arises in myocardial cells that usually have a stable phase 4. Ischaemia, or other changes in the microcellular environment, can create conditions that allow a non-specialised myocardial cell to become a pacemaker.

Re-entry. This is the cause of most clinically important arrhythmias. If an impulse arrives at a part of the myocardium that is refractory to the stimulus because of abnormally slow repolarisation, the impulse will be conducted by an alternative route that bypasses the refractory tissue (Fig. 8.4b). If this impulse arrives at the 'blocked' tissue distally when it has had sufficient time to repolarise, it will then be conducted retrogradely (Fig. 8.4c).

If there has been sufficient time for the healthy myocardium proximal to the block to repolarise, a circuit of electrical activity will be initiated (a re-entry circuit). This circuit creates a self-perpetuating 'circus' of electrical activity that acts as a pacemaker. Such functional re-entry circuits can be localised within a small area of myocardium that has been damaged by scarring or ischaemia (micro-re-entry), and permits slow impulse conduction around the circuit. The slow conduction may be supported by L-type Ca²⁺ channels. In addition to functional re-entry circuits, the myocardium can also support large anatomical re-entry circuits. These can arise in congenital pathways that bypass the AV node, and conduct between the atria and ventricles. This will initiate a re-entry circuit that includes the AV node (such as occurs in the Wolff–Parkinson–White syndrome).

Triggered activity. A cell can develop transient depolarisations during, or following, repolarisation ('afterdepolarisations'), which will initiate an action potential if they reach the threshold potential. Afterdepolarisations are said to be 'early' if they occur during repolarisation (relative refractory period in Fig. 8.2a), or 'delayed' if they occur in phase 4. In many cases, conduction through L-type Ca²⁺ channels probably supports afterdepolarisation. Triggered rhythms are an uncommon mechanism of arrhythmogenesis but may be responsible for the proarrhythmic activity of class I and III antiarrhythmic agents and digitalis glycosides (see below).

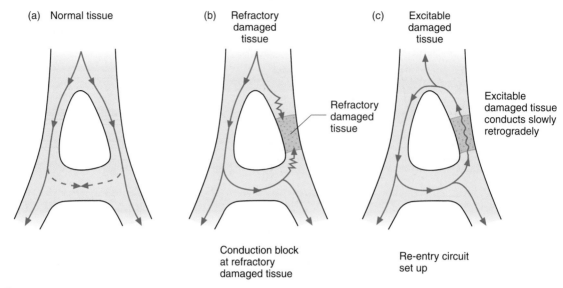

(a) Normal tissue

(b) Refractory damaged tissue

Refractory damaged tissue

(c) Excitable damaged tissue

Excitable damaged tissue conducts slowly retrogradely

Conduction block at refractory damaged tissue

Re-entry circuit set up

Fig. 8.4

Conduction in normal and damaged cardiac tissue. (a) In normal tissue, conduction is carefully ordered. When an impulse has passed, the tissue cannot be immediately reactivated because of refractoriness of the surrounding tissue. If conducted impulses meet, they die out. (b) If an area of damage is present, impulses are conducted abnormally. If an impulse arrives and the damaged tissue is refractory, the impulse is blocked. (c) If a distal impulse arrives when the damaged tissue is capable of being excited, it will be conducted retrogradely and could set up a perpetual re-entry circuit.

Classification of antiarrhythmic drugs

A widely used classification of antiarrhythmic drugs (the Vaughan Williams classification) is based on their effects on the action potential (Fig. 8.5) and explains the indications for use of each class of drug (Table 8.1). This classification has many flaws and does not take account of multiple actions possessed by some drugs, nor that the actions of drugs in diseased tissues may be different to those in healthy tissues.

An alternative method to predict antiarrhythmic drug efficacy is known as the Sicilian Gambit. This approach characterises drugs by their spectrum of activity on ion channels, receptors and pumps. It then attempts to identify the mechanism of the arrhythmia, and define the 'vulnerable parameter' of the arrhythmia. The drug most likely to affect this parameter is then selected. The Sicilian Gambit approach is hampered by its complexity and our lack of knowledge of the precise mechanisms of many arrhythmias.

The Vaughan Williams classification has four classes.

Class I

All class I drugs inhibit fast Na^+ channels and slow the rate of rise of phase 0. They are often called membrane

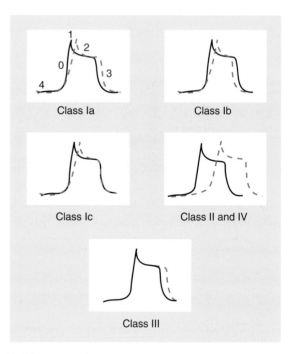

Class Ia

Class Ib

Class Ic

Class II and IV

Class III

Fig. 8.5

Effects of different classes of antiarrhythmic drug on the cardiac action potential. Class I block Na^+ channels and have variable effects on the effective refractory period. Class II decrease the phase 4 slope and automaticity. Class III prolong action potential duration and delay repolarisation by acting on K^+ currents. Class IV decrease the phase 4 slope and slow conduction in the sinoatrial and atrioventricular nodes.

Table 8.1
Principal indications for antiarrhythmic drugs

Class	Examples	Supraventricular arrhythmias	Ventricular arrhythmias
Ia	Disopyramide, procainamide, quinidine	+	+
Ib	Lidocaine, mexiletine, phenytoin	–	+ (especially after myocardial infarction)
Ic	Flecainide, propafenone	+	+
II	β-Adrenoceptor antagonists, sotalol	+	+ (especially after myocardial infarction)
III	Amiodarone, sotalol, bretylium[a]	+	+
IV	Calcium channel antagonists	+	–

[a]Used only is resuscitation and life-threatening arrhythmias.

stabilisers. They readily penetrate the phospholipid bilayers of the cell membrane, where they concentrate in the hydrophobic core and bind to hydrophobic amino acids in the channel. Class I drugs are subdivided according to their effects on the duration of the action potential.

- Class Ia, such as disopyramide, produce moderate Na^+ channel blockade and slow impulse conduction. In addition, there is blockade of some K^+ currents (Table 5.1, Fig. 8.1). These actions prolong repolarisation and the duration of the action potential.
- Class Ib, such as lidocaine, produce weak Na^+ channel blockade and slow impulse conduction, but only in abnormal tissue (such as ischaemic myocardium), with no effect in healthy tissue. They do not block K^+ channels and have no effect on repolarisation, or may shorten it.
- Class Ic, such as flecainide, produce marked Na^+ channel blockade and slow impulse conduction. There is weak blockade of some K^+ currents (Table 5.1), and they also block inward Ca^{2+} currents. There is only a slight effect on repolarisation.

The effects of the different class I subgroups result from their diverse binding characteristics to the ion channels. During the time course of the action potential, the access of the drug to its binding site is intermittent and dependent on the state of the channel. Class Ib drugs show marked use-dependency, i.e. the action increases with the frequency of opening of the channel. They associate more rapidly with Na^+ channels during depolarisation and they rapidly dissociate from the channel when it returns to the resting state. Therefore they are more effective when there are repetitive depolarisations, and they will block premature impulses. Class Ib drugs show relative selectivity for depolarised channels, such as are found in ischaemic tissue or digitalis toxicity. This explains their selectivity for ventricular arrhythmias in ischaemic heart disease (ischaemia mainly affects the ventricles). Class Ic drugs show use-dependent binding, but dissociate slowly from their binding sites in the Na^+ channel and therefore produce prolonged blockade of channels. This produces a widespread reduction in cellular excitability. Class Ia drugs have binding characteristics between those of the other two classes.

Class II

The class II drugs are the β-adrenoceptor antagonists which block the actions of catecholamines on the heart. They reduce the rate of spontaneous depolarisation of SA and AV nodal tissue and reduce conduction through the AV node. They also reduce spontaneous depolarisation in phase 4 of some ectopic foci by indirect blockade of adrenoceptor-activated Ca^{2+} channels.

Class III

Class III drugs prolong the duration of the action potential, thus increasing the absolute refractory period. This is achieved by inhibition of some K^+ channels involved in repolarisation (see Table 5.1). Drugs such as sotalol, that selectively block the I_{Kr} current (which is particularly involved in phase 2 and 3 repolarisation), show reverse use-dependency (higher receptor binding when the channel is closed) and are most effective at slow rates of cell depolarisation. Amiodarone, by contrast, blocks several K^+ channels and shows use-dependence.

Class IV

There are four types of calcium channel in the heart and the main one affected by current calcium channel blockers is the L type. The class IV drugs are predominantly L-type Ca^{2+} channel blockers (calcium antagonists). They stabilise phase 4 of the action potential, particularly in the AV node and slow the rate of depolarisation. The initiation of the pacemaker depolarisation in the SA node depends more on T-type Ca^{2+} channels and is relatively less affected by these drugs. The L-type Ca^{2+} channels are also responsible for maintaining the plateau phase 2 of the action potential in all myocardial cells.

Unclassified drugs

Four drugs used in the treatment of rhythm disturbances do not fit into the Vaughan Williams classification: digitalis glycosides, adenosine, magnesium sulfate and atropine.

Proarrhythmic activity of antiarrhythmic drugs

All antiarrhythmic drugs have the potential to precipitate serious arrhythmias, such as incessant ventricular tachycardia. Several of them (particularly class Ia agents and sotalol) prolong the Q–T interval on the ECG (Fig. 8.3). This predisposes to a polymorphic ventricular tachycardia known as *torsade de pointes*, which has a characteristic twisting QRS axis on the ECG and can degenerate into ventricular fibrillation. Drug-induced ventricular rhythm disturbances are particularly refractory to treatment. Many non-cardiac drugs, for example some antihistamines, that prolong the Q–T interval on the ECG have been withdrawn from clinical use because of their arrythmogenic potential.

The mechanisms of drug-induced arrhythmogenesis are probably multiple, and risk factors include:

- excessive slowing of cardiac impulse conduction, such as occurs with marked blockade of Na^+ channels
- excessive prolongation of the action potential, especially if due to blockade of the I_{Kr} current (Fig. 8.1), with generation of afterdepolarisations and triggered beats
- organic heart disease, especially ischaemic heart disease, with preferential slowing of conduction in diseased myocardium
- mutations in genes coding for channels that regulate Na^+, K^+ and Ca^{2+} transmembrane ion flows: these may exist in 5–10% of people who develop *torsade de pointes* when exposed to a drug that prolongs the Q–T interval, and probably represent subclinical variants of the congenital long Q–T syndrome.

Class Ia drugs

Disopyramide

Pharmacokinetics

Oral absorption of disopyramide is almost complete, but an intravenous formulation is available for rapid onset of action. Metabolism in the liver generates a compound with less antiarrhythmic activity but with greater antimuscarinic activity. About half the drug is eliminated unchanged in the urine. Disopyramide has an intermediate half-life.

Unwanted effects

- gastrointestinal disturbances
- powerful negative inotropic effect; disopyramide should be avoided in heart failure

- proarrhythmic effects
- antimuscarinic effects (see Ch. 4): especially urinary retention, dry mouth and blurred vision.

Procainamide

Pharmacokinetics

Procainamide is well absorbed from the gut but is also available for intravenous use. The majority of the drug is excreted unchanged by the kidney, but about 40% is acetylated in the liver. The rate of acetylation is subject to genetic polymorphism and is slow in some individuals (Ch. 2). The plasma half-life is short in fast acetylators but increased twofold in slow acetylators.

Unwanted effects

- gastrointestinal disturbances: nausea, vomiting, anorexia, diarrhoea
- negative inotropic effect, producing myocardial depression
- systemic lupus erythematosus-like syndrome with fever, arthralgia, rashes, pleurisy; the syndrome is more common in slow acetylators; it usually appears after at least 2 months of treatment and is common after 6 months; consequently, long-term treatment is usually avoided and this drug is no longer widely used in the UK
- proarrhythmic effects.

Quinidine

Pharmacokinetics

Oral absorption of quinidine is almost complete and about 30% undergoes first-pass metabolism. Metabolism in the liver is extensive and the drug has an intermediate half-life. Modified-release formulations are frequently used to reduce the peak plasma concentration and to minimise unwanted effects. Quinidine is little used in the UK.

Unwanted effects

- gastrointestinal disturbances: nausea, vomiting, abdominal pain, diarrhoea
- cinchonism: tinnitus, visual disturbance, flushing, abdominal pain, confusion, headache
- negative inotropic effect, producing myocardial depression
- proarrhythmic effects.

Class Ib drugs

Lidocaine

Pharmacokinetics

Extensive first-pass metabolism to a potentially toxic metabolite prevents oral administration of lidocaine. It is usually given intravenously, initially as a loading dose by bolus injection followed by an infusion. Lidocaine is extensively metabolised in the liver to compounds with little antiarrhythmic activity, but one can cause seizures. The half-life of lidocaine is short.

Unwanted effects

- nausea and vomiting
- central nervous system (CNS) toxicity: muscle twitching, convulsions, dizziness, drowsiness
- negative inotropic effect, producing myocardial depression
- bradycardia, proarrhythmic effects.

Mexiletine

Pharmacokinetics

Oral absorption is almost complete, but an intravenous formulation is also available for rapid onset of action. Metabolism in the liver is extensive and the half-life is long.

Unwanted effects

- nausea, vomiting, constipation
- CNS toxicity: drowsiness, tremor, confusion, ataxia, paraesthesiae, convulsions
- negative inotropic effect, producing myocardial depression
- bradycardia, proarrhythmic effects.

Class Ic drugs

Flecainide

Pharmacokinetics

Oral absorption of flecainide is complete. An intravenous formulation is also available for rapid onset of action. Flecainide is mainly eliminated by the kidneys and by hepatic metabolism, and has a long half-life.

Unwanted effects

- nausea, vomiting
- CNS toxicity: blurred vision, hallucinations, depression, convulsions, paraesthesiae, ataxia
- negative inotropic effect, producing myocardial depression
- may be particularly proarrhythmogenic after recent myocardial infarction, when it may increase mortality.

Propafenone

Propafenone has weak β-adrenoceptor antagonist activity in addition to its class Ic action.

Pharmacokinetics

Oral absorption of propafenone is almost complete, but dose-dependent first-pass metabolism can be extensive. Elimination is by hydroxylation, which is saturable and shows genetic polymorphism (Ch. 2). The half-life is therefore dose-dependent and much longer in slow metabolisers of CYP2D6 substrates.

Unwanted effects

- nausea, vomiting, diarrhoea, bitter taste
- CNS toxicity (as for flecainide)
- negative inotropic effect, producing hypotension
- weak β-adrenoceptor antagonist activity can cause bronchoconstriction in individuals with asthma
- antimuscarinic effects (see Ch. 4): especially urinary retention, dry mouth and blurred vision
- proarrhythmic effects.

Class II drugs

Beta-adrenoceptor antagonists (β-blockers)

The β_1-adrenoceptor antagonist activity is responsible for the therapeutic effects of this class. The most widely used agents are atenolol and propranolol; these are also discussed in Chapter 5.

Esmolol is an ultra-short-acting β_1-adrenoceptor-selective (cardioselective) agent that is used by bolus intravenous injection exclusively for the treatment of arrhythmias. It is most often used when arrhythmias arise during anaesthesia.

Pharmacokinetics

After bolus intravenous injection, the half-life of esmolol is very short (about 9 min). Its action is terminated by esterases after uptake by erythrocytes.

Class III drugs

Amiodarone

Amiodarone is actually a drug with non-specific antiarrhythmic actions. Although classified as a class III drug, it also has a class Ib-like action on Na^+ channels, as well as non-competitive β-adrenoceptor antagonist (class II) activity and calcium channel blocking (class IV) actions. The effects seen early after intravenous use are believed to be caused by β-adrenoceptor antagonist activity, while the class III effect is delayed.

Pharmacokinetics

Amiodarone is incompletely absorbed orally and has a large volume of distribution as a result of extensive tissue protein binding. Metabolism in the liver produces an active metabolite, and both amiodarone and its major metabolite have very long half-lives, averaging 50–60 days. An intravenous formulation is also available. Because of the long half-life, a prolonged loading dose regimen is used for both routes of administration.

Unwanted effects

- Gastrointestinal disturbances, for example constipation and nausea, most often occur during the loading period.
- Reversible corneal microdeposits are almost universal and can cause dazzling by lights when driving at night.
- Because of its iodine content, amiodarone produces thyrotoxicosis in up to one-third of those taking it. Inhibition of peripheral conversion of thyroxine to triiodothyronine (Ch. 41) produces hypothyroidism in a similar proportion of people. Thyrotoxicosis is often refractory to treatment, and at least temporary withdrawal of amiodarone may be necessary. Hypothyroidism can be treated by thyroxine replacement without stopping amiodarone (Ch. 41). Thyroid function should be checked every 6 months.
- Photosensitive skin rashes. Wide-spectrum sunscreen is recommended. Slate-grey skin discoloration can also occur.
- Peripheral neuropathy or myopathy.
- Hepatitis and cirrhosis occur rarely.
- Progressive pneumonitis or lung fibrosis are rare but serious effects of long-term treatment.
- Proarrhythmic effects.
- Drug interactions: the plasma concentrations of warfarin (Ch. 11) and digoxin (Ch. 7) are increased by amiodarone, with consequent potentiation of their effects. Amiodarone inhibits the metabolism of warfarin and both displace digoxin from tissue stores and inhibit the renal excretion of digoxin.

Unlike most antiarrhythmic drugs, amiodarone does not have negative inotropic effects and is safe to use in heart failure.

Bretylium tosilate

Bretylium is now used only during cardiac resuscitation for treatment of life-threatening ventricular arrhythmias when other agents have failed. In addition to its class III activity, bretylium concentrates in adrenergic nerve terminals, and produces myocardial adrenergic neuron blockade.

Pharmacokinetics

Oral absorption is poor and bretylium is only available for parenteral (usually intravenous) use. Selective concentration occurs in the myocardium. Bretylium is excreted unchanged by the kidney and has an intermediate half-life.

Unwanted effects

- hypotension
- nausea and vomiting after rapid intravenous injection.

Sotalol

Sotalol is a non-selective β-adrenoceptor antagonist (Ch. 5) with additional class III properties. As with many drugs, sotalol is a racemic mixture; both β-adrenoceptor-blocking and class III activity reside in the L-isomer, while the D-isomer only has class III activity. The class III activity gives sotalol a greater proarrhythmic potential than other β-adrenoceptor antagonists (see above). Sotalol is now reserved for treatment of significant rhythm disturbances and is not used for the other indications for β-adrenoceptor antagonists. Intracellular generation of cyclic adenosine monophosphate (cAMP) by sotalol, possibly related to its class III effect, counteracts the effect of β-blockade on myocardial contractility (see Ch. 5) and makes sotalol less negatively inotropic than most β-adrenoceptor antagonists.

Pharmacokinetics

Sotalol is almost completely absorbed from the gut and excreted unchanged in the urine. Its half-life is intermediate.

Unwanted effects

These are discussed in Chapter 5.

The additional proarrhythmic activity of sotalol is discussed above. It may be caused by the greater effect of sotalol on non-ischaemic ventricular cells, leading to differential rates of repolarisation that predisposes to re-entry circuits.

Class IV drugs

Calcium channel antagonists (calcium channel blockers)

Verapamil and diltiazem (Ch. 5), but not the dihydropyridine derivatives such as nifedipine, have antiarrhythmic activity. Verapamil can be given intravenously for a rapid effect, but this should not be given to someone taking a β-adrenoceptor antagonist, because of summation of myocardial depression and AV nodal conduction block. Details of calcium channel blockers are found in Chapter 5.

Other drugs for rhythm disturbances

Those drugs used for the management of rhythm disturbances that do not fit into the Vaughan Williams classification are considered here.

Digoxin

Digitalis glycosides (such as digoxin) are not strictly antiarrhythmic. They are, however, useful for controlling ventricular rate in atrial flutter and atrial fibrillation by reducing conduction through the AV node. Digitalis glycosides are discussed in Chapter 7.

Adenosine

Mechanism of action and effects

Adenosine is a purine nucleotide that has potent effects on the SA node, producing sinus bradycardia. It also slows impulse conduction through the AV node, but has no effect on conduction in the ventricles. Consequently, it is only useful for management of supraventricular arrhythmias, particularly those caused by AV nodal re-entry mechanisms. Its electrophysiological actions are mediated by the A_1 subtype of specific G-protein-coupled adenosine receptors, which activate inward rectifier KACh channels. This enhances the flow of K^+ out of myocardial cells and produces hyperpolarisation of the cell membrane (see Table 5.1). In addition, adenosine antagonises the stimulatory effects of noradrenaline on Ca^{2+} currents. These actions combine to stabilise the myocardial cell membrane.

The A_2 receptor subtype reduces Ca^{2+} uptake in vascular smooth muscle, and produces vasodilation. This receptor action enables adenosine to be used as a pharmacological stress to induce ischaemia in people with coronary artery disease. Preferential dilation of non-atheromatous arteries produces coronary blood flow 'steal' that reduces flow in other stenosed arteries. Myocardial ischaemia is then assessed by radionuclide scanning or echocardiography.

Pharmacokinetics

Adenosine is given by rapid bolus intravenous injection. The effect is terminated by uptake into erythrocytes and endothelial cells, followed by metabolism to inosine and hypoxanthine. Adenosine has a half-life of less than 10 s, and a duration of action of less than 1 min.

Unwanted effects

Unwanted effects are common, occurring in about 25% of those treated with adenosine; however, they are usually transient, lasting less than 1 min:

- bradycardia and AV block
- malaise, facial flushing, headache, chest pain or tightness, bronchospasm; adenosine should be avoided in people with asthma
- drug interactions: dipyridamole (Ch. 11) potentiates the effects of adenosine, while methylxanthines such as aminophylline (Ch. 12) inhibit its action.

Atropine

Atropine (see Ch. 4) is given by intravenous bolus injection and reduces the inhibitory effect of the vagus nerve on the heart. Blockage of muscarinic M_2 receptors increases the rate of firing of the SA node and increases conduction through the AV node. The second-messenger effects are mediated by activation of inward rectifying K_{ir} channels, which hyperpolarise the cell membrane. Atropine is used specifically for the treatment of sinus bradycardia and AV block. It is metabolised in the liver and has an intermediate half-life.

Magnesium sulphate

Intravenous magnesium sulphate is used to control the ventricular arrhythmia *torsade de pointes*, and digitalis-induced ventricular arrhythmias. The mechanism is not well understood, but may involve blockade of transmembrane Ca^{2+} currents. Flushing is the main unwanted effect.

Drug treatment of arrhythmias

Arrhythmias can be harmless, or they can produce a variety of symptoms that vary from mild to life-threatening. The probability of symptoms arising depends on several factors, the most important of which are the nature of the rhythm disturbance, the rate of an abnormal rhythm and the presence of underlying heart disease. The range of consequences of rhythm disturbances includes:

- awareness of palpitation
- dizziness
- syncope
- precipitation of angina or heart failure
- sudden death.

Treatment may not be necessary for benign or self-terminating arrhythmias; reassurance may be all that is required, but it is important to remove or treat any underlying cause. Vagotonic procedures such as the Valsalva manoeuvre or carotid sinus massage delay conduction through the AV node, and can terminate re-entrant tachycardias involving nodal tissue (but not atrial fibrillation or flutter).

The choice of treatment depends on the situation. With most tachyarrhythmias, sinus rhythm should, if possible, be restored. Direct current (DC) cardioversion is used to achieve this in severe, life-threatening or drug-resistant arrhythmias; drug therapy is used if there is less need for an immediate effect or to control the ventricular rate if the abnormal rhythm cannot be terminated. Radiofrequency ablation of an arrhythmogenic focus or pathway is increasingly used to prevent arrhythmia. This is carried out after intracardiac electrophysiological studies, using a cardiac catheter. Long-term drug treatment for bradyarrhythmias is rarely used, and an implanted pacemaker may be necessary. The principal indications for antiarrhythmic drugs are given in Table 8.1.

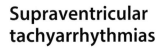

Supraventricular tachyarrhythmias

Atrial premature beats

Atrial premature beats are very common and usually benign. However, they can be produced by digoxin toxicity, and frequent multifocal atrial ectopics can result from organic heart disease. Other than treatment of an underlying cause, specific drug therapy is rarely needed. Some individuals are disturbed by a post-ectopic pause followed by a more forceful beat when sinus rhythm recommences. If treatment is required, then a β-adrenoceptor antagonist, or a calcium channel antagonist such as verapamil or diltiazem, can be used to suppress the ectopics.

Atrial tachycardia

Atrial tachycardia is an infrequent rhythm disturbance usually arising from an automatic focus, and it is often accompanied by AV conduction block. It is not usually associated with significant cardiac disease but can be a manifestation of digoxin toxicity. Treatment of the underlying disorder may be sufficient to restore sinus rhythm, but drug therapy may be necessary. An AV nodal blocking agent, such as a β-adrenoceptor antagonist or a calcium channel antagonist (verapamil or diltiazem), will sometimes control the ventricular rate but rarely restores sinus rhythm. This can be achieved with a class Ic antiarrhythmic agent such as flecainide, given with an AV nodal blocking drug (flecainide alone increases the risk of 1:1 AV nodal conduction if the atrial rate slows sufficiently, but sinus rhythm is not restored). Sotalol or amiodarone can also be used to suppress the rhythm disturbance. Ablation of the initiating focus may also be considered.

A less common form of atrial tachycardia is multifocal atrial tachycardia arising from several ectopic foci, usually in individuals with severe pulmonary disease. Calcium channel antagonists are usually used for ventricular rate control if treatment is needed.

Atrial flutter

In atrial flutter, the atrial rate is usually 250–350 beats min^{-1}, which is conducted to the ventricles with 2:1 or greater degrees of AV block. Flutter waves may be obvious on the ECG, or appear if the ventricular rate is slowed by vagal manoeuvres or the administration of adenosine. Atrial flutter usually arises from a macro re-entrant circuit in the right atrium. Underlying causes include cardiac surgery, *cor pulmonale* and congenital heart disease, but it can arise for no obvious reason. It may be paroxysmal, and it can degenerate into atrial fibrillation.

Drug therapy is relatively unsuccessful for restoring sinus rhythm, and DC cardioversion (synchronised to discharge on the R wave of the ECG) or rapid 'overdrive' electrical pacing to capture the ventricle, followed by a gradual reduction in the paced rate, may be required. Class Ia, Ic and III antiarrhythmic agents can prevent recurrence in paroxysmal atrial flutter. Disopyramide should be avoided as its antimuscarinic action can increase AV conduction and speed up the ventricular response. If a class Ic agent is used, then an AV nodal blocking drug should be given concurrently, since the flutter rate could slow and lead to normal 1:1 AV conduction, with an unacceptably high ventricular rate.

Control of the ventricular rate in atrial flutter can be achieved in a similar manner to that in chronic atrial fibrillation (see below), but treatment is often less successful. For this reason, radiofrequency ablation of the re-entrant pathway via a cardiac catheter is becoming increasingly popular. Prophylaxis against thromboembolism should be given, similar to that for atrial fibrillation.

Atrial fibrillation

Atrial fibrillation is the most common rhythm disturbance in clinical practice. It has a variety of underlying causes (Box 8.1), some of which may be treatable. In younger people, atrial fibrillation often occurs without any obvious underlying cause, when it is called 'lone' atrial fibrillation. The arrhythmia arises from multiple re-entry circuits in the atria. The ventricular rate will depend on AV nodal function, and when this is good, atrial fibrillation is accompanied by a rapid ventricular rate. Atrial fibrillation predisposes to atrial thrombus formation and subsequent systemic emboli, which commonly cause stroke. Clinically, three forms of atrial fibrillation are recognised: paroxysmal, persistent and permanent (the latter term is used after unsuccessful attempts to maintain sinus rhythm). Management has four underlying aims.

- **To identify and treat the underlying cause**.
- **To restore or maintain sinus rhythm in paroxysmal or persistent atrial fibrillation** (Box 8.2).

Box 8.1

Causes of atrial fibrillation

Structural heart disease
   Hypertension
   Coronary heart disease
   Valvular heart disease (especially mitral)
   Cardiomyopathies
   Cardiac surgery
   Congenital heart disease (especially atrial septal defect)

Other causes
   Major infections
   Throtoxicosis, myxoedema
   Alcohol intoxication
   Systemic illness (e.g. amyloid, sarcoidosis)

Box 8.2

Factors predicting a high probability of successful restoration of sinus rhythm in patients with atrial fibrillation

Short duration of atrial fibrillation (less than 1 year)
Younger age (<50 years)
Absence of underlying heart disease
Normal left ventricular function
Little or no enlargement of the left atrium
Withdrawal or treatment of a precipitating factor, e.g. thyrotoxicosis, alcohol

---

It is desirable to attempt to restore sinus rhythm in younger subjects or those who tolerate the rhythm disturbance poorly. In these individuals, symptoms and exercise tolerance are usually improved by restoring sinus rhythm, but the risk of stroke is not removed (see below). However, the case for restoring sinus rhythm is less clear-cut for older people who tolerate the rhythm well, because there is no reduction in the risk of thromboembolic events, and their quality of life may not improve. Restoration of sinus rhythm is usually possible in lone atrial fibrillation or when there is a treatable underlying cause. It can be achieved with drugs (pharmacological or chemical cardioversion), especially if the rhythm disturbance is of recent onset (40–80% success rate if the arrhythmia is of less than 7 days' duration), but often requires QRS-synchronised DC cardioversion. Pharmacological cardioversion is most rapidly achieved by using a single oral dose of a class Ic drug such as flecainide or propafenone. Intravenous amiodarone is also effective, but takes longer. Drugs are not usually recommended for routine use to maintain sinus rhythm after a first DC cardioversion, because of their proarrhythmic effects. However, if there is a high risk of recurrence, then sinus rhythm can be maintained with the same drugs used for chemical cardioversion, or with sotalol. Recurrence of atrial fibrillation is most frequent during the first 3–6 months after restoration of sinus rhythm. Amiodarone is most successful for long-term prevention of recurrence, but only maintains sinus rhythm in about 75% of people at 1 year. The addition of a second drug such as propafenone or verapamil to amiodarone, or the combination of propafenone and verapamil, can be more effective than amiodarone alone for reducing recurrence. Other drugs can be added to antiarrhythmic therapy to increase the probability of maintaining sinus rhythm. These include angiotensin-converting enzyme (ACE) inhibitors (Ch. 6) and angiotensin receptor blockers (Ch. 6), or β-adrenoceptor antagonists (see also Ch. 5) in people with ischaemic heart disease. The mechanisms of action, of these drugs, in atrial fibrillation are unknown. Antifibrillatory drugs are also useful for prophylaxis of paroxysmal atrial fibrillation. Digoxin is ineffective for restoring or maintaining sinus rhythm in paroxysmal atrial fibrillation and should be avoided. Radiofrequency isolation via a cardiac catheter of a trigger area in one of the pulmonary veins may prevent initiation of the re-entrant pathways. This is becoming increasingly used for younger individuals with paroxysmal atrial fibrillation.

- **To control a rapid ventricular response in persistent atrial fibrillation**. A β-adrenoceptor antagonist, or a ventricular-rate-controlling calcium channel antagonist such as verapamil or diltiazem, are the drugs of choice for rate control both at rest and on exercise. Rate control at rest can be achieved with digoxin, but a rapid heart rate often still occurs during exercise. A β-adrenoceptor antagonist, verapamil, diltiazem, flecainide or amiodarone can be used with digoxin if necessary. Sotalol has no particular value in sustained atrial fibrillation and should be avoided because of its greater proarrhythmic activity compared with that of other β-adrenoceptor antagonists. If drug combinations do not provide satisfactory rate control, then AV nodal ablation with insertion of a pacemaker can be considered

- **To reduce thromboembolism by long-term anticoagulation** (Ch. 11). Warfarin is the anticoagulant of choice in atrial fibrillation associated with rheumatic heart disease, thyrotoxicosis, and for one month before and at least one month after DC cardioversion. In non-rheumatic atrial fibrillation, the risk of emboli is greatest in the elderly (over 75 years of age) and if there is coexisting hypertension, diabetes mellitus or recent heart failure. Poor left ventricular systolic function or a very large left atrium on echocardiography also predicts increased risk (Table 8.2). Almost all people with atrial fibrillation, whether sustained or paroxysmal, should take either aspirin or warfarin. Warfarin (maintaining the international normalised ratio [INR] between 2 and 3; see Ch. 11) reduces the risk of thromboembolism by about two-thirds, and low-dose aspirin by one-third. Warfarin is therefore preferred for people at high risk of embolism, but has little advantage in those at low risk, when the increased risk of bleeding outweighs the benefit. Recent trial evidence suggests that continued use of warfarin by those at high risk of thromboembolic events will reduce the subsequent risk of stroke, even after restoration of sinus rhythm in paroxysmal

Table 8.2
Risk of stroke in 'non-rheumatic' atrial fibrillation

Patient group	Stroke risk without prophylaxis (% per year)	Anticoagulant of choice
High risk		
Previous ischaemic stroke or transient ischaemic attack	12	Warfarin
Age ≥75 years + one other risk factor[a]	8	Warfarin
Age 65–74 years + two or more other risk factors	8	Warfarin
Moderate risk		
Age <65 years + other risk factors	4	Aspirin
Age 65–74 years + one other risk factor	4	Aspirin
Low risk		
Age <65 years with no other risk factors	1	Aspirin

[a]Coexisting hypertension, diabetes mellitus, recent heart failure, poor left ventricular function on echocardiography (see text).

or persistent atrial fibrillation. This may reflect the high risk of recurrence of atrial fibrillation. The anticipated launch of the direct thrombin antagonist ximelagatran – currently delayed – may simplify the anticoagulation in atrial fibrillation (see Ch. 11).

Junctional (nodal) tachycardias

Junctional tachycardias usually arise from re-entry mechanisms, which can be within the AV node or involve an accessory AV pathway (e.g. in Wolff–Parkinson–White syndrome). Termination of an acute attack can often be achieved with vagotonic manoeuvres such as carotid sinus massage or by adenosine. Beta-adrenoceptor antagonists, diltiazem or verapamil can be used to treat acute episodes or for prophylaxis. Diltiazem, verapamil and digoxin should be avoided if there is an accessory AV pathway, because selective blockade of the AV node by these drugs can predispose to rapid conduction of atrial arrhythmias through the accessory pathway. Junctional tachycardias involving an accessory pathway often respond well to flecainide, sotalol or amiodarone. Radiofrequency ablation of the re-entry circuit, via a cardiac catheter, is being employed increasingly for troublesome junctional tachycardias.

Immediate management of narrow complex tachycardia of uncertain origin

If the rhythm is regular, then it is often not possible to determine from the ECG whether the arrhythmia has an atrial or nodal origin. If vagotonic manoeuvres are unsuccessful, and the person is haemodynamically stable, intravenous adenosine should be given. If there is a history of severe asthma, intravenous verapamil may be preferred.

Ventricular tachyarrhythmias

Ventricular ectopic beats

Ventricular ectopic beats can occur in healthy individuals or in association with a variety of cardiac disorders such as ischaemic heart disease and heart failure. Frequent ventricular ectopic beats after myocardial infarction predict a poorer long-term outcome; however, suppressing such ectopics with class I antiarrhythmic agents increases mortality, and should be avoided. Beta-adrenoceptor antagonists are useful after myocardial infarction and reduce the risk of sudden death (Ch. 5). A β-adrenoceptor antagonist can also suppress ventricular ectopic beats induced by stress or anxiety. In other situations, symptomatic ventricular ectopic beats can be suppressed by a class I drug such as mexiletine, flecainide or disopyramide.

Ventricular tachycardia

Ventricular tachycardia presents with broad QRS complexes on the ECG (*broad-complex tachycardia*). Although broad complexes can arise with supraventricular tachycardias (when there is bundle branch block), broad-complex tachycardia is usually treated on the assumption that it is ventricular tachycardia. Ventricular tachycardia is often associated with serious underlying heart disease, such as ischaemic heart disease or heart failure, and is more common following myocardial infarction. It can be either sustained or non-sustained. Sustained ventricular tachycardia can be associated with a minimal or absent cardiac output ('pulseless' ventricular tachycardia), when it is treated as ventricular fibrillation (see below). Polymorphic or incessant ventricular tachycardias can occur as a complication of antiarrhythmic drug therapy (see above) and with other drugs that prolong the Q–T interval on the ECG. For sustained ventricular tachycardias, drug options include class Ib antiarrhythmic agents such as lidocaine (especially after myocardial infarction), and amiodarone. Sustained ventricular tachycardia is often associated with a poor long-term outlook in ischaemic heart disease, and coronary revascularisation or an automatic implantable cardiac defibrillator may be beneficial. During and after the acute phase of myocardial infarction, a β-adrenoceptor antagonist is the treatment of choice for non-sustained ventricular tachycardias.

Polymorphic or incessant ventricular tachycardias do not respond well to conventional treatments. Withdrawal of a precipitant drug, correction of electrolyte imbalance and intravenous magnesium sulphate are the therapies of choice. Temporary transvenous overpacing at a rate of 90–110 beats min^{-1} may prevent recurrence. In the congenital form, a β-adrenoceptor antagonist is the mainstay of treatment.

Ventricular fibrillation

Ventricular fibrillation is a potentially lethal arrhythmia that constitutes one form of 'cardiac arrest'. An algorithm for the management of cardiac arrest is regularly updated by the European Resuscitation Working Party, and is shown in Figure 8.6. The important principles of resuscitation are maintenance of adequate cardiac output by external chest compression, and oxygenation by artificial inflation of the lungs while attempting to restore sinus rhythm. Ventricular fibrillation is the commonest arrhythmia in acute cardiac arrest and it should be assumed to be present; it should be treated with immediate DC cardioversion, if a good ECG monitor read-out is not available. Adrenaline (epinephrine; Ch. 4) may be given to vasoconstrict the peripheries and thus maintain pressure in the central arteries perfusing the heart and brain. For recurrent ventricular fibrillation, suppression is best achieved by long-term use of antiarrhythmic drugs such as sotalol or amiodarone (often combined with a β-adrenoceptor antagonist) or by an automatic implantable cardiac defibrillator.

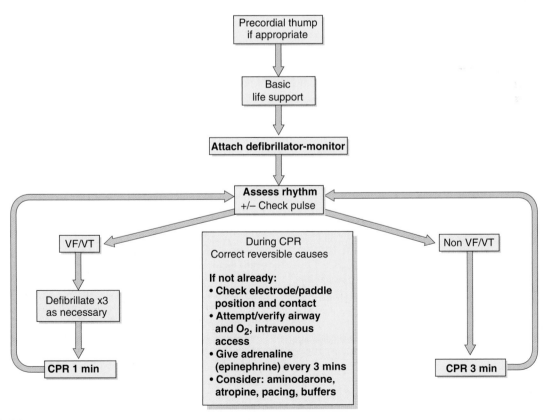

Fig. 8.6
An algorithm for the management of cardiac arrest. CPR, cardiopulmonary resuscitation; ETT, endotracheal tube; VF, ventricular fibrillation, VT, ventricular tachyarrhythmia.

Bradycardias

Sinus bradycardia

Treatment with atropine may be necessary if sinus bradycardia is causing symptoms (e.g. after myocardial infarction). Hypotension precipitated by drugs such as streptokinase (Ch. 11) or the first dose of an ACE inhibitor (Ch. 6) is often associated with vagally mediated bradycardia, which will respond to atropine.

Atrioventricular block ('heart block')

If AV block arises suddenly, then loss of consciousness (Stokes–Adams attack) or death can occur. An AV block can be congenital or accompany a variety of heart diseases.

If it occurs after myocardial infarction, it is usually temporary if the infarct is inferior but is often permanent after anterior infarction. First-degree heart block (prolongation of the P–R interval on the ECG) rarely requires treatment, but higher degrees of block (with non-conducted P waves) should be treated. If the onset is acute, atropine should be given intravenously to increase AV conduction, but external or temporary transvenous electrical cardiac pacing is usually required. The β-adrenoceptor agonist isoprenaline (Ch. 4) can be given by intravenous infusion if there is likely to be a delay in pacing; however, this usually produces excessive numbers of ectopic beats and rarely improves nodal conduction. If the AV block is permanent, the implantation of a permanent electrical cardiac pacemaker is usually necessary.

FURTHER READING

Blomström-Lundqvist C, Scheinman MM, Aliot EM et al (2003) ACC/AHA/ESC guidelines for the management of patients with supraventricular arrhythmias – executive summary. *Eur Heart J* 24, 1857–1897

Calò L, Sciarra L, Lamberti F et al (2003) Electropharmacological effects of antiarrhythmic drugs on atrial fibrillation termination. Part 1: molecular and ionic fundamentals of antiarrhythmic drug actions. *Ital Heart J* 4, 430–441

Crystal E, Connolly SJ (2004) Role of anticoagulation in management of atrial fibrillation. *Heart* 90, 813–817

De Latorre F, Nolan J, Robertson C et al (2000) European Resuscitation Council Guidelines 2000 for Adult Advanced Life Support. A statement from the Advanced Life Support Working Group and approved by the Executive Committee of the European Resuscitation Council. *Resuscitation* 48, 211–221

Goette A, Lendeckel U (2004) Nonchannel drug targets in atrial fibrillation. *Pharmacol Ther* 102, 17–36

Gowda RM, Khan IA, Wilbur SL et al (2004) Torsade de pointes: the clinical considerations. *Int J Cardiol* 96, 1–6

Grant AO (2001) Molecular biology of sodium channels and their role in cardiac arrhythmias. *Am J Med* 110, 296–305

Hancox JC, Patel KCR, Jones JV (2000) Antiarrhythmics – from cell to clinic: past, present, and future. *Heart* 84, 14–24

Iqbal MB, Taneja AK, Kip GYH et al (2005) Recent developments in atrial fibrillation. *BMJ* 330, 238–243

Katz AM (1998) Selectivity and toxicity of antiarrhythmic drugs: molecular interactions with ion channels. *Am J Med* 104, 179–195

Lau W, Newman D, Dorian P (2000) Can antiarrhythmic agents be selected based on mechanism of action? *Drugs* 60, 1315–1328

Markides V, Schilling RJ (2003) Atrial fibrillation: classification, pathophysiology, mechanisms and drug treatment. *Heart* 89, 939–943

McNamara RL, Tamariz LJ, Segal JB et al (2003) Management of atrial fibrillation: review of the evidence for the role of pharmacologic therapy, electrical cardioversion, and echocardiography. *Ann Intern Med* 139, 1018–1033

Page RL (2004) Newly diagnosed atrial fibrillation. *N Engl J Med* 351, 2408–2416

Reiffel JA, Reiter MJ, Blitzer M (1998) Antiarrhythmic drugs and devices for the management of ventricular tachyarrhythmias in ischemic heart disease. *Am J Cardiol* 82, 31I–40I

Reiter MJ, Reiffel JA (1998) Importance of beta blockade in the therapy of serious ventricular arrhythmias. *Am J Cardiol* 82, 9I–19I

Roden DM, Balser JR, George AL Jr, Anderson ME. (2002) Cardiac ion channels. *Annu Rev Physiol* 64, 431–475

Roden DM (2004) Drug-induced prolongation of the Q-T interval. *N Engl J Med* 350, 1013–1022

Shorofsky SR, Balke CW (2001) Calcium currents and arrhythmias: insights from molecular biology. *Am J Med* 110, 127–140

Snow V, Weiss KB, LeFevre M et al (2003) Management of newly detected atrial fibrillation: a clinical practice guideline from the American Academy of Family Physicians and the American College of Physicians. *Ann Intern Med* 139, 1009–1017

Tamargo J, Caballero, R, Gomez, R et al (2004) Pharmacology of cardiac potassium channels. *Cardiovascular Research* 62, 9–33

van Walraven C, Hart R, Singer D et al (2002) Oral anticoagulants vs aspirin in non-valvular atrial fibrillation: an individual patient meta-analysis. *JAMA* 288, 2441–2448

Self-assessment

1. In the following questions, the first statement, in italics, is true. Is the accompanying statement also true?

   a. *Pacemaker cells in the SA node initiate cardiac rhythm discharge at a higher frequency than those in other parts of the heart.* Spontaneous or pacemaker depolarisation occurring during diastole results from the fluxes of several anions.

   b. *The influx of Na^+ during phase 0 lasts only for milliseconds and the Na^+ channels for influx are closed during the plateau phase 2. Thus, cells are refractory to further action potentials during this period (refractory period).* The plateau phase (phase 2) results solely from the release of Ca^{2+} from the sarcoplasmic reticulum.

   c. *Reducing the rate of rise in the slope of phase 4 will slow the normal pacemaker rate.* β-Adrenoceptor stimulation, hypokalaemia and vagal stimulation reduce the slope of phase 4 depolarisation and, therefore, reduce pacemaker rate.

   d. *The SA node and the AV node have pacemaker activity.* Healthy non-pacemaker cells always remain quiescent if not excited by an impulse arising from other regions in the heart.

   e. *Antiarrhythmic drugs reduce the automaticity of ectopic pacemakers more than that of the SA node pacemaker.* The effect of the class I antiarrhythmic drugs is to block Na^+ channels, which prolongs the refractory period of the target cell.

   f. *Sympathetic AV stimulation increases pacemaker depolarisation rate and conduction through the AV node.* Beta-adrenoceptor antagonist drugs are useful in stress-induced tachycardias.

   g. *Verapamil has little benefit in ventricular arrhythmias.* Verapamil will affect both the plateau phase 2 and phase 4 of the action potential cycle.

   h. *Adenosine is currently the drug of choice for prompt conversion of AV-nodal re-entrant tachycardia to sinus rhythm.* Adenosine is effective in the treatment of ventricular arrhythmias.

2. Case history questions

> Mr GH, aged 48 years, consulted his GP complaining of palpitations and was found to have an irregular pulse with a ventricular rate of 120 beats min^{-1}. He had been suffering from shortness of breath and faintness for the previous 6 h. The symptoms had started after a drinking binge 36 h previously. Examination, blood tests (including thyroid function tests), ECG and chest radiograph revealed no coexisting heart disease, diabetes or hypertension. The ECG confirmed atrial fibrillation.

   a. What were the options available for treating this man?

> Before any treatment could be instituted, the patient spontaneously reverted to sinus rhythm. Mr GH was well for a year but then returned to his GP with a 3-day history of palpitations, breathlessness, chest pain and dizziness. Examination and an ECG again revealed atrial fibrillation. He was referred to a cardiologist and echocardiography showed no evidence of structural cardiac disease. Electrical DC cardioversion was carried out and the rhythm reverted to sinus rhythm.
>
> Over the next five years, episodes of atrial fibrillation occurred with increasing frequency and eventually sinus rhythm could not be restored with a variety of antiarrhythmic drugs or by DC conversion.

   b. What prophylactic treatment should be considered at the time of DC cardioversion? What drug treatments may be useful after DC cardioversion?

   The answers are provided on pages 710–711.

Drugs used in the treatment of arrhythmias

Drug	Half-life (h)	Elimination	Comments[a]
Class I drugs			
Disopyramide	4–10	Renal + metabolism	Used for SVT, VF, VT; given orally, or by slow intravenous injection (over at least 5 min) or intravenous infusion; oral bioavailability is 90%; main metabolite is less antiarrhythmic but more antimuscarinic
Flecainide	14	Renal + metabolism	Used for AF, N; treatment should be initiated in hospital; given orally, or by slow intravenous injection (over 10–30 min) or intravenous infusion (for ventricular tachyarrhythmias resistant to other treatments); oral bioavailability is >90%
Lidocaine	2	Metabolism	Used for VA (especially post-MI); given by intravenous injection or intravenous infusion; metabolites retain some activity
Mexiletine	13	Metabolism + renal	Used for VA (especially post-MI); given orally or by intravenous injection or intravenous infusion; inactive metabolites
Moracizine (moricizine)	3	Metabolism	Used for severe life-threatening VA on a named patient basis only; given orally; bioavailability is about 30–40% owing to first-pass metabolism; induces its own metabolism by cytochrome P450 (autoinduction)
Procainamide	3	Renal + metabolism	Used for AT, VA; given by slow intravenous injection or by intravenous infusion; metabolised by N-acetylation; N-acetyl metabolite is as active as the parent drug and has a longer half-life (6–9 h)
Propafenone	4	Metabolism	Used for SVT, N, VA; some β-adrenoceptor antagonist activity; given orally; low oral bioavailability (10%), which is increased at higher doses and by food; metabolised by oxidation by CYP2D6 + CYP3A4: longer half-life (17 h) in poor metabolisers of CYP2D6 substrates
Quinidine	7	Metabolism + renal	SVT, VA; specialist use; given orally; good oral bioavailability (70–80%); metabolised by oxidation; potent inhibitor of CYP2D6
Class II drugs: β-adrenoceptor antagonists			β-Adrenoceptor antagonists are used in a wide variety of indications; the list below first details those licensed for use in heart arrhythmias in the UK, and for completeness, then includes all other β-adrenoceptor antagonists irrespective of their value in arrhythmias
Antiarrhythmic β-adrenoceptor antagonists			Apart from esmolol, these drugs are also commonly used for angina, hypertension and other indications for β-adrenoceptor antagonists
Acebutolol	7	Metabolism + renal	Used for AF, SVT, VT; β$_1$-adrenoceptor selective; 10% β$_1$-adrenoceptor selective PAA; given orally; oral bioavailability is 50–70%; active acetylated metabolite; drug-induced lupus reported
Atenolol	7	Renal	Used for AF, SVT, VT; β$_1$-selective; given orally, or by injection or intravenous infusion; eliminated by glomerular filtration

continued

Drugs used in the treatment of arrhythmias *(continued)*

Drug	Half-life (h)	Elimination	Comments[a]
Esmolol	0.15	Metabolism	Used for SVT; β_1-adrenoceptor-selective; given by intravenous infusion; rapidly hydrolysed in erythrocytes
Metoprolol	3–10	Metabolism	Used for SVT, VT; β_1-adrenoceptor-selective (less than atenolol); given orally, or by injection or intravenous infusion; oral bioavailability is about 50%; wide variability in metabolism by CYP2D6
Nadolol	17–24	Renal + bile	Used for SVT, VT; β-adrenoceptor-non-selective; given orally but poor absorption (30%)
Oxpreonol	2	Metabolism	Used for SVT, VT; β-adrenoceptor-non-selective; 18% β-adrenoceptor-non-selective PAA; given orally; bioavailability is 20–80% owing to first-pass metabolism; hydroxy metabolite also active
Propranolol	4	Metabolism	Used for AF, SVT, VT; β-adrenoceptor-non-selective; given orally or by intravenous injection; oral bioavailability is 10–50% owing to first-pass metabolism; oxidised by P450 and conjugated with glucuronic acid (17%)
Sotalol			See under class III drugs; uses restricted to life-threatening arrhythmias
Beta-adrenoceptor antagonists not normally used as antiarrhythmics			Oral dosage unless otherwise indicated (typical uses shown)
Betaxolol	13–24	Metabolism + renal	Used for glaucoma, hypertension; β_1-adrenoceptor-selective; high oral bioavailability (80–90%); oxidised in liver and metabolites eliminated in urine
Bisoprolol	11	Renal + metabolism	Used for angina and hypertension; β_1-adrenoceptor-selective (less than atenolol); oral bioavailability is 90%; eliminated equally by glomerular filtration and secretion, and by metabolism in the liver
Carvedilol	6	Metabolism	Used for angina and hypertension; β-adrenoceptor-non-selective; vasodilator owing to α_1-adrenoceptor blockade; oral bioavailability is 20–30% owing to first-pass metabolism; metabolites eliminated in bile and urine
Celiprolol	5	Renal + some biliary	Used for mild to moderate hypertension; β_1-adrenoceptor-selective; vasodilator because of β_2 PAA; polar compound that has a bioavailability of 30–70% because of poor absorption
Labetalol	3	Metabolism	Used for hypertension; β_1-selective; vasodilator through α-adrenoceptor blockade; $\alpha{:}\beta$ selectivity is 1:2 orally and 1:7 intravenously; given orally, or by intravenous injection or intravenous infusion; oral bioavailability is variable (10–90%) owing to first-pass metabolism; metabolised by glucuronidation
Nebivolol	10	Metabolism	Used for hypertension; new β_1-adrenoceptor-selective drug; metabolised by oxidation. Produces NO and vasodilates
Pindolol	4	Metabolism + renal	Used for angina and hypertension; β-adrenoceptor-non-selective, vasodilator because of 35% β-adrenoceptor-non-selective PAA; high oral bioavailability (>90%); approximately equal elimination in urine and by metabolism

continued

Drugs used in the treatment of arrhythmias *(continued)*

Drug	Half-life (h)	Elimination	Comments[a]
Timolol	2–5	Metabolism + some renal	Used for angina, hypertension, post-MI; β-adrenoceptor-non-selective; oral bioavailability is 30–50%; eliminated by metabolism and renal excretion (20%)
Class III drugs			
Amiodarone	50–60 days	Metabolism	Used for all arrhythmias, with treatment usually initiated in hospital or under specialist supervision; given orally or by intravenous infusion; given by intravenous injection (over 3 min) for ventricular fibrillation; oral bioavailability is 20–100%; active metabolite, which also has a long half-life (50 days); accumulation occurs, with steady state reached after about 6 months of treatment
Bretylium	9	Renal	Used only in resuscitation for VA resistant to other treatments; given by slow intravenous injection, intramuscular injection, or intravenous infusion; can cause severe hypotension; clearance correlates with creatinine clearance
Sotalol	7–18	Renal	Also class II β-adrenoceptor antagonist; used for VT (life-threatening); β-adrenoceptor-non-selective; class III antiarrhythmic activity; greater proarrhythmic risk than other β-adrenoceptor antagonists; given orally or by intravenous injection (over 10 min); oral bioavailability is >90%; eliminated largely by glomerular filtration
Class IV drugs			Diltiazem (see Ch. 5) has antiarrhythmic properties but is not licensed in the UK for this indication
Verapamil	2–7	Metabolism	Used for SVT; given orally or by intravenous injection; low oral bioavailability (about 20%); S-isomer is more active form; metabolised by CYP3A4 or CYP1A2
Other drugs			
Adenosine	2 s	Metabolism (all cells)	Used as the treatment of choice for terminating paroxysmal SVT; given intravenously; cleared extremely rapidly by metabolism
Atropine	2–5	Metabolism + renal	Used for bradycardia, especially if complicated by hypotension; given intravenously
Digoxin	40 (20–50)	Renal	Used for AF; may need loading dose; oral or intravenous dosage (see Ch. 7)
(Phenytoin)	7–60	Metabolism	Has been used in the past for VA (especially that caused by cardiac glycosides); was given by slow intravenous infusion; now obsolete for arrhythmias (see Ch. 23)

[a]The types of arrhythmias commonly treated with different drugs are: AF, atrial fibrillation; AFL, atrial flutter; AT, atrial tachycardia;
SVT, supraventricular tachycardia; N, nodal; VF, ventricular fibrillation; VT, ventricular tachycardia; VA, ventricular arrhythmias.
Other abbreviations: MI, myocardial infarction, PAA, partial agonist activity. For other Ca^{2+} channel antagonists, see Chapter 5 compendium.

9

Cerebrovascular disease and dementia

Stroke

Aetiology

Strokes are a major cause of morbidity and mortality, particularly in older people. They present as a transient or permanent neurological disturbance caused by ischaemic infarction or haemorrhagic disruption of neuronal pathways in the brain. The extent and duration of the resulting functional deficit is very variable.

Ischaemic strokes account for about 85% of events. Transient cerebral ischaemic attacks (TIAs) arise from small cerebral arterial emboli which rapidly disperse. TIAs produce short-lived neurological signs and symptoms but leave no functional deficit 24 h later. However, there is a 30% risk of completed stroke within 5 years after a TIA. More severe cerebral ischaemia produces a cerebral infarction and the neurological disturbance persists for more than 24 h; frequently there is some permanent loss of function. Cerebral infarction can result from intracerebral arterial thrombosis or from cerebral arterial emboli (typically from the internal carotid arteries or from the heart).

Primary intracerebral haemorrhage is responsible for most of the remaining 15% of events. It often arises from rupture of small aneurysms on intracerebral arteries, usually in association with hypertension. Haemorrhagic strokes commonly leave a residual functional deficit.

Current treatments produce only a modest limitation of the neurological deficit in acute stroke; most management is directed to primary prevention of a first event, prevention of recurrence, or rehabilitation after the event. About one-third of strokes are recurrent. The recurrence rate for ischaemic stroke in people who are in sinus rhythm is about 3–7% per year; but higher, at about 12% per year, for those in atrial fibrillation.

Prevention and treatment

Primary prevention of ischaemic stroke

- Stopping smoking reduces the risk of stroke by up to 40% by 2–5 years after cessation.
- Hypertension is the single most powerful predictor of stroke. Pooled trial results indicate that a reduction in diastolic blood pressure by 5–6 mmHg reduces the risk of stroke by about 40% (Ch. 6). For isolated systolic hypertension, a similar reduction in risk has been shown after an average 11 mmHg reduction in systolic blood pressure (with a concurrent fall of 3–4 mmHg in diastolic blood pressure).
- Aspirin has not been shown to prevent a first stroke when taken by healthy individuals who are in sinus rhythm. By contrast, the antiplatelet action of aspirin (Ch. 11), in people with atrial fibrillation, can reduce the risk of a first event by almost one-third, although aspirin is less effective than warfarin (Ch. 8).
- Anticoagulation with warfarin in atrial fibrillation reduces the risk of a first stroke by 70–80%. Warfarin, at a dosage giving an INR (international normalised ratio) of 2–3, is superior to aspirin for stroke prevention, but at the expense of more major bleeds. If there are no other risk factors for cerebral embolic disease coexisting with atrial fibrillation, then the risk–benefit analysis may favour the use of aspirin (see Ch. 11). Warfarin reduces the risk of stroke following myocardial infarction if there is intracardiac clot associated with an akinetic area of the left ventricular wall.
- Reduction of a raised plasma cholesterol with a statin (Ch. 48) produces a 25% reduction in the risk of a first stroke, although much of this evidence derives from trials in people who have clinical evidence of vascular disease.
- Carotid endarterectomy is sometimes recommended for asymptomatic carotid artery disease. The annual risk of an ischaemic stroke is low in this situation, however, and there is little evidence to support this approach.

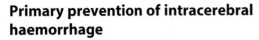

Primary prevention of intracerebral haemorrhage

Lowering blood pressure is the only means of preventing cerebral haemorrhage.

Treatment of acute stroke

Thrombolytic therapy with recombinant tissue plasminogen activator (rt-PA; Ch. 11) can be effective for ischaemic stroke. If treatment is started within 3 h of the onset of symptoms, thrombolysis reduces the risk of death or dependency at 3 months. There is an increased risk of intracerebral haemorrhage with thrombolysis, and if used after 3 h, there is an adverse effect on outcome because the risk of intracerebral haemorrhage outweighs the benefit from neuronal salvage.

Secondary prevention of recurrent stroke

Many treatments are similar to those used for primary prevention of ischaemic stroke (see above).

- Lowering blood pressure after a stroke will reduce the risk of recurrence by 30–40%. The reduction in risk is greatest following haemorrhagic stroke, when even lowering a 'normal' blood pressure may be effective. There is considerable reluctance to reduce blood pressure in the first few days after a stroke, because of concern that cerebral perfusion pressure may fall too much if the normal cerebral artery autoregulation has been disturbed by the stroke. However, there is some evidence that early treatment may not be detrimental.
- Aspirin at low dosage should be given to people who are in sinus rhythm following a TIA or a first ischaemic stroke. It reduces the risk of a further non-fatal stroke by about 20–30%. Dipyridamole or clopidogrel (Ch. 11) are alternatives if aspirin is not tolerated. Combining aspirin with dipyridamole may be more effective than low-dose aspirin given alone, but the evidence for this is not substantial and the outcome of ongoing trials is awaited. The combination is usually reserved for recurrence of stroke during treatment with low-dose aspirin alone. The combination of aspirin and clopidogrel is no more effective than aspirin alone. There is no added benefit from using warfarin for preventing recurrent stroke in people with sinus rhythm, owing to the greater risk of major bleeds.
- After a first stroke in people with atrial fibrillation, warfarin reduces the risk of a further stroke by two-thirds. By contrast, aspirin only has a modest protective effect in this situation (see Ch. 11).
- Cholesterol reduction with a statin is effective in secondary prevention of ischaemic stroke. However,

an important reason for cholesterol reduction in this situation is prevention of ischaemic cardiac events, since coronary artery disease often coexists with atheromatous cerebrovascular disease.

- Carotid endarterectomy reduces the risk of recurrent stroke if there have already been transient focal neurological symptoms in the cerebral territory served by a diseased carotid artery. If the stenosis is ≥70% of the vessel diameter (but without near occlusion), then endarterectomy reduces the risk of recurrent stroke by about 16% over the subsequent 5 years (despite a perioperative risk of stroke or death of 3–5%). There is no benefit if the occlusion is less than 50%, and only marginal benefit if the occlusion is between 50% and 69%.

Subarachnoid haemorrhage

Subarachnoid haemorrhage usually follows rupture of a Charcot–Bouchard aneurysm on a cerebral artery. These aneurysms are usually found in hypertensive subjects. Sudden onset of headache is the most common presenting feature, but focal neurological signs or progressive confusion and impaired consciousness can occur. Rebleeding is a major cause of disability and death, but with early surgical intervention in survivors of the initial bleed a more common cause of permanent neurological disability or death is cerebral ischaemia. This is produced by cerebral vasospasm, which develops in about 25% of cases, usually at least 3 days after the haemorrhage. The mechanism is poorly understood. Vasospasm leads to increased flow of Ca^{2+} into the cell and further ischaemic neuronal damage, which presents with confusion, decreased consciousness and new focal neurological deficit. The neuronal damage is fatal in 30% of those who develop vasospasm, and leaves a permanent neurological deficit in a further 50%.

Drugs for subarachnoid haemorrhage

Nimodipine

Nimodipine is a dihydropyridine calcium channel antagonist (for mechanism of action, see Ch. 5). It is a vasodilator with some selectivity for cerebral arteries, and reduces the risk of vasospasm following subarachnoid haemorrhage. However, it probably produces most of its benefits by protecting ischaemic neurons from Ca^{2+} overload. There is a theoretical risk that vasodilation may actually facilitate bleeding.

Pharmacokinetics

Nimodipine is well absorbed from the gut and undergoes extensive first-pass metabolism in the liver and gut wall. It has a short half-life and is metabolised in the liver. It is usually given intravenously immediately after the event, followed by oral dosing for a total of 5–10 days.

Unwanted effects

These are caused by arterial dilation:

- hypotension, which can have a detrimental effect on cerebral perfusion
- headaches, flushing.

Management of subarachnoid haemorrhage

The management of subarachnoid haemorrhage is mainly surgical, with clipping or endovascular coil occlusion of the aneurysm that produced the bleeding. Ischaemic cerebral damage can be reduced by using nimodipine in the first few days after the event. Although there is a lack of controlled clinical evidence, most neurosurgical units also use 'triple-H' therapy, a regimen of intravenous fluid replacement to create hypervolaemia, hypertension (or avoidance of hypotension) and haemodilution, to reduce ischaemic complications. This is achieved by a combination of intravenous crystalloid (typically isotonic saline) and colloid such as dextrans. The major risk of this approach is pulmonary oedema, which may be reduced by treatment with dexamethasone (Ch. 44). Optimal blood pressure in the early post-haemorrhage period is not known, but hypotension should be avoided and blood pressure lowered modestly in those who present with significant hypertension. In the last 20 years, early surgical intervention, combined with medical therapy, has reduced mortality from 20% to about 5–10%.

Dementia

Dementia usually begins with forgetfulness and is characterised by disorientation in unfamiliar surroundings, variable mood, restlessness and poor sleep. Deterioration in social behaviour with self-neglect often follows and may be accompanied by personality change, with loss of inhibition. Most dementia results from Alzheimer's disease or from cerebrovascular disease (multi-infarct dementia), but other causes may be identified (Box 9.1). Memory impairment in dementia tends to be associated with bilateral hippocampal damage.

Alzheimer's disease

Alzheimer's disease is the commonest cause of dementia in people over the age of 65 years. About 10% of people

---

Box 9.1

Causes of dementia

Treatable causes of dementia	Irreversible and partially treatable causes of dementia
Hypothyroidism	Vascular dementia
Neurosyphilis	Alzheimer's disease
Vitamin B_1 deficiency	Lewy body-type dementia
Normal pressure hydrocephalus	Parkinson's disease dementia
Frontal lobe tumours	Progressive supranuclear palsy
Cerebral vasculitis	Multisystem atrophy
Cerebral hypoperfusion	

---

over the age of 65 and nearly 50% of those over the age of 85 have some signs of Alzheimer's disease. The onset of symptoms is gradual, with progressive deterioration, unlike vascular dementia. There is a marked loss of cholinergic innervation to the cerebral cortex from the hippocampus. The initial defect may be in cholinergic signal transduction, followed by a progressive reduction in acetylcholine neurotransmitter synthesis in the cerebral cortex. Muscarinic receptor density appears normal but the number of nicotinic receptors is reduced. Depletion of other neurotransmitters is a late and inconsistent finding.

The cause of Alzheimer's disease is unknown, but there is a genetic predisposition, with the apolipoprotein E allele 4 (*apoE4*) conferring a higher risk. Beta-amyloid is deposited in the brain of those with Alzheimer's disease as senile plaques, which also contain typical neurofibrillary tangles. Activated microglia and reactive astrocytes surround the plaques, and there is local increase in proinflammatory mediators. Amyloid deposits may promote neuronal damage by increasing neuronal release of glutamate and thus promoting glutamate-induced excitotoxicity of cholinergic neurons. Hyperactivity of glutaminergic neurons is a common finding in Alzheimer's disease.

Drugs for Alzheimer's disease

Anticholinesterases

Examples: donepezil, galantamine, rivastigmine

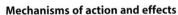

Mechanisms of action and effects

This class of drugs for the treatment of Alzheimer's disease acts by increasing cholinergic transmission in the brain via inhibition of cholinesterases.

- Donepezil is a reversible inhibitor of acetylcholinesterase with a high degree of selectivity for the central nervous system (CNS).
- Galantamine is a reversible competitive inhibitor of acetylcholinesterase that also has agonist activity at nicotinic receptors by allosterically enhancing the receptor response to acetylcholine.
- Rivastigmine is a slowly reversible, inhibitor of acetylcholinesterase with selectivity for the CNS; the duration of action is prolonged.

Pharmacokinetics

Donepezil, galantamine and rivastigmine are well absorbed from the gut; donepezil and galantamine are metabolised in the liver, whereas rivastigmine is rapidly inactivated by esterase-mediated hydrolysis. Donepezil and galantamine have long half-lives, while rivastigmine has a short half-life.

Unwanted effects

- anorexia, nausea, vomiting, diarrhoea, abdominal pain
- insomnia, confusion, agitation, headache.

NMDA receptor antagonists

> Example: memantine

Mechanism of action and effects

Memantine is a derivative of amantadine (Ch. 24), and is a non-competitive antagonist at glutamate NMDA (*N*-methyl-D-aspartate) receptors that demonstrates voltage-dependent activity and fast on/off receptor kinetics. This profile of receptor interaction may prevent glutamate-induced excitotoxicity (by limiting long-lasting influx of Ca^{2+} into neurons), but without interfering with the actions of glutamate that are involved in memory and learning. It can be administered together with anticholinesterases.

Pharmacokinetics

Memantine is well absorbed from the gut and is largely excreted unchanged by the kidney. It has a half-life of 60–80 h.

Unwanted effects

- diarrhoea
- insomnia, dizziness, headache, hallucinations.

Treatment of Alzheimer's disease

In the UK, it is recommended that drug treatment for Alzheimer's disease should be started only for people who have a Mini-Mental State Examination (MMSE) score of greater than 12 points (mid to moderate dementia). The diagnosis of Alzheimer's disease should be confirmed in a specialist clinic.

Cholinesterase inhibitors produce modest improvement, and a delay in the decline of cognitive function and memory, in up to 40% of sufferers and may be more effective in people who do not carry *apoE4*. Efficacy should be assessed after three months, and treatment stopped in non-responders. The decline in mental function is delayed by about 3–6 months but not arrested. Rapid progression resumes when the drugs are stopped, and there may be limited benefit from restarting treatment more than a month after withdrawal. Anticholinesterases produce some improvement in other functional measures and behaviour that also affect the quality of life.

Memantine produces moderate improvement in cognition and reduction in functional decline, and is usually well tolerated.

The National Institute for Clinical Excellence (NICE) advises that treatment should be started only in specialist units, should be reviewed every 6 months, and should be discontinued if the patient's MMSE score falls below 12 points and only continued if their 'global, functional and behavioural condition remains at a level where the drug is considered to be having a worthwhile effect'. A review of treatments for Alzheimer's disease is expected in mid 2005.

New treatment strategies are being developed that are directed either at enhancing the various neurotrophic proteins which protect neuronal systems, or at altering the production of amyloid protein or Tau protein found in neurofibrillary tangles. Such strategies may offer a more fundamental approach to retarding the progress of Alzheimer's disease. Early studies suggesting that treatment with non-steroidal anti-inflammatory drugs retards the progression of Alzheimer's disease have not been supported by recent evidence, but there is some suggestion that they may reduce the risk of developing the disease.

Vascular dementia

Cerebrovascular disease is a particularly common cause of dementia over the age of 85 years, and overall is the second most frequent cause of dementia. The deterioration in mental function is produced by multiple cerebral infarcts (multi-infarct dementia), particularly if they affect the white matter. The risk of dementia is increased ninefold in people with stroke. In some of these, dementia may be produced by specific strategically located infarcts, especially in the angular gyrus of the inferior parietal lobule. In contrast to Alzheimer's disease, the initial presentation is usually more acute, and cognitive decline has a stepwise course arising from recurrent cerebrovascular events.

Treatment

- Prophylaxis against cerebral emboli with aspirin or warfarin (see prevention of stroke, above).

The Cochrane database finds that there is no evidence, as yet, that aspirin is of benefit in vascular dementia.

- Control of hypertension (Ch. 6). Trials have shown that calcium channel antagonists are effective for reducing the risk of vascular dementia, but it is likely to be an effect related to blood pressure reduction rather than to a specific drug.
- Anticholinesterases or memantine may produce some improvement in vascular dementia.
- Immunosuppressive drugs (Ch. 39) in the rare cases caused by cerebral vasculitis.

FURTHER READING

The Cochrane database (**http://www.update-software.com/cochrane/**) analyses the trials that have been performed using aspirin, nimodipine and Ginkgo biloba in dementias and is worth referring to

Stroke

Amarenco P, Lavallee P, Touboul PJ (2004) Statins and stroke prevention. *Cerebrovasc Dis* 17(suppl 1), 81–88

Bedi A, Flaker GC (2002) How do HMG-CoA reductase inhibitors prevent stroke? *Am J Cardiovasc Drugs* 2, 7–14

Briel M, Studer M, Glass TR et al (2004) Effects of statins on stroke presentation in patients with and without coronary heart disease: a meta-analysis of randomized controlled trials. *Am J Med* 117, 596–606

Claiborne JS (2002) Transient ischemic attack. *N Engl J Med* 347, 1687–1692

De Schryver EL, Algra A, van Gijn J (2003) Cochrane review: dipyridamole for preventing major vascular events in patients with vascular disease. *Stroke* 34, 2072–2080

Fotherby MD, Panayiotou B (1999) Antihypertensive therapy in the prevention of stroke. *Drugs* 58, 663–674

Gubitz G, Sandercock P (2000) Acute ischaemic stroke. *BMJ* 320, 692–696

Koennecke HC (2004) Secondary prevention of stroke: a practical guide to drug treatment.

CNS Drugs 18, 221–241

Laws PE, Spark JI, Cowled PA, Fitridge RA (2004) The role of statins in vascular disease. *Eur J Vasc Endovasc Surg* 27, 6–16

Lindsberg PJ, Kaste M (2003) Thrombolysis for acute stroke. *Curr Opin Neurol* 16, 73–80

Powers WJ (2001) Oral anticoagulant therapy for the prevention of stroke. *N Engl J Med* 345, 1493–1495

Rashid P, Leonardi-Bee J, Bath P (2003) Blood pressure reduction and secondary prevention of stroke and other vascular events: a systematic review. *Stroke* 34, 2741–2748

Rothwell PM, Eliasziw M, Gutnikov SA et al (2003) Analysis of pooled data from the randomised controlled trials of endarterectomy for symptomatic carotid artery stenosis. *Lancet* 361, 107–116

Schellinger PD, Kaste M, Hacke W (2004) An update on thrombolytic therapy for acute stroke. *Curr Opin Neurol* 17, 69–77

Straus SE, Majumdar SR, McAlister FA (2002) New evidence for stroke prevention. Scientific review. *JAMA* 288, 1388–1395

Waldo AL (2003) Stroke prevention in atrial fibrillation. *JAMA* 290, 1093–1095

Subarachnoid haemorrhage

Sarkar PK, D'Souza C, Ballantyne S (2001) Treatment of aneurysmal subarachnoid haemorrhage in elderly patients. *J Clin Pharmacol Ther* 26, 247–256

Sen J, Belli A, Albon H et al (2003) Triple-H therapy in the management of aneurysmal subarachnoid haemorrhage. *Lancet Neurol* 2, 614–621

Dementia

Castro A, Conde S, Rodriguez-Franco MI, Martinez A (2002) Non-cholinergic pharmacotherapy approaches to the future treatment of Alzheimer's disease. *Mini Rev Med Chem* 2, 37–50

Clark RM, Karlawish JHT (2003) Alzheimer's disease: current concepts and emerging diagnostic and therapeutic strategies. *Ann Intern Med* 138, 400–411

Cummings JL (2004) Alzheimer's disease. *N Engl J Med* 351, 56–67

Doraiswamy PM (2002) Non-cholinergic strategies for treating and preventing Alzheimer's disease. *CNS Drugs* 16, 811–824

Doraiswamy PM (2003) Alzheimer's disease and the glutamate NMDA receptor. *Psychopharmacol Bull* 37, 41–49

Erkinjuntti T, Rockwood K (2003) Vascular dementia. *Semin Clin Neuropsychiatry* 8, 37–45

Forette F, Seux M-L, Staessen JA et al (2002) The prevention of dementia with antihypertensive treatment. New evidence from the Systolic Hypertension in Europe (Syst-Eur) study. *Arch Intern Med* 162, 2046–2052

Grutzendler J, Morris JC (2001) Cholinesterase inhibitors for Alzheimer's disease. *Drugs* 61, 41–52

Hermann N (2002) Pharmacotherapy for Alzheimer's disease and other dementias. *Curr Opin Psychiatry* 15, 403–409

Kawas CH (2003) Early Alzheimer's disease. *N Engl J Med* 349, 1056–1063

Muir KW (2004) Secondary prevention for stroke and transient ischaemic attacks. *BMJ* 328, 297–298

National Institute for Clinical Excellence (2001) Drugs for Alzheimer's disease – full guidance. **http://www.nice.org.uk/article.asp?a=14487** (accessed May 2004)

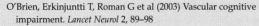

O'Brien, Erkinjuntti T, Roman G et al (2003) Vascular cognitive impairment. *Lancet Neurol* 2, 89–98

Ritchie K, Lovestone S (2002) The dementias. *Lancet* 360, 1759–1766

Scarpini E, Scheltens P, Feldman H (2003) Treatment of Alzheimer's disease: current status and new perspectives. *Lancet Neurol* 2, 539–547

Selkoe DJ, Schenk D (2003) Alzheimer's disease: molecular understanding predicts amyloid-based therapeutics. *Annu Rev Pharmacol Toxicol* 43, 545–584

Warlow C, Sudlow C, Dennis M et al (2003) Stroke. *Lancet* 362, 1211–1224

Self-assessment

1. In the following questions, the first statement, in italics, is true. Is the accompanying statement also true?

   a. *Aspirin has not been shown to prevent a first stroke when given to people in sinus rhythm.* Aspirin cannot prevent a first event in people with persistent atrial fibrillation.

   b. *Approximately 85% of all strokes have an ischaemic aetiology and the remaining 15% have a haemorrhagic basis.* If thrombolysis with tissue-type plasminogen activator (t-PA) is given in acute stroke, antiplatelet and anticoagulant therapies should not be given concurrently.

   c. *Glutamate receptor antagonists lower the neurotoxicity of the neuroexcitatory transmitter glutamate.* Cerebral ischaemia depolarises neurons and causes the release of large amounts of glutamate.

   d. *Cerebral emboli arising from the heart can be caused by atrial fibrillation, infected or damaged prosthetic valves or arise following damage to parts of the myocardium.* Anticoagulation with warfarin or antiplatelet therapy with aspirin are equally effective for secondary prevention of recurrent TIAs in the presence of sinus rhythm.

2. Choose the one correct statement from the following:

   A. Alzheimer's disease is associated with a relative lack of cholinergic and an excess of glutaminergic neurotransmission.

   B. It is recommended that rivastigmine is prescribed irrespective of the Mini-Mental State Examination (MMSE) score of the patient.

   C. Memantine acts by stimulation of glutamate receptors.

   D. Anticholinesterases should not be co-prescribed with memantine.

   E. Rivastigmine is metabolised by plasma cholinesterase.

3. Case history questions

   > A 70-year-old man had a blood pressure of 190/110 mmHg despite intensive antihypertensive drug treatment. He was admitted to hospital 6 h after the acute onset of unilateral weakness and sensory loss. At the time of admission to hospital, most of the neurological signs had resolved. He had no headache or vomiting and remained conscious. He was in sinus rhythm. Following clinical examination and a CT brain scan, this episode was diagnosed as a TIA.

   a. Should thrombolysis be given?

   b. What other therapies should be instituted immediately?

   c. What secondary prevention strategy should be employed?

   The answers are provided on pages 711–712.

Drugs used in cerebrovascular disease and dementia (given orally)[a]

Drug	Half-life (h)	Elimination	Comment
Clopidogrel	7	Metabolism	A prodrug which undergoes metabolism to both inactive and active species; slow elimination of major metabolites
Dipyridamole	12	Metabolism	Variable absorption (30–90%); metabolised by glucuronidation
Donepezil	70–80	Metabolism + renal	Used for mild to moderate dementia in Alzheimer's disease; oral bioavailability is high; metabolised by CYP2D6 (polymorphic) and CYP3A4 and excreted in urine as parent drug and metabolites; given once daily at night
Galantamine	5–7	Renal + some metabolism	Used for mild to moderate dementia in Alzheimer's disease; complete oral bioavailability (>90%); metabolised by CYP2D6 and CYP3A4 and excreted in urine as parent drug and metabolites
Memantine	60–80	Renal	Used for moderate to severe dementia in Alzheimer's disease; complete oral bioavailability (100%); renal excretion exceeds glomerular filtration rate (GFR) but is pH-dependent and markedly reduced at high urine pH
Nimodipine	8–9	Metabolism	Of benefit for preventing delayed ischaemic deficit after subarachnoid haemorrhage; given by intravenous infusion or orally (oral bioavailability is 10–20%); metabolised by hepatic cytochrome P450
Rivastigmine	1–2	Metabolism	Used for mild to moderate dementia in Alzheimer's disease; oral bioavailability is 30–70% (depending on dose); it is a carbamate inhibitor of choline esterases which is metabolised by hydrolysis; duration of effect is about 10 h

[a]Except nimodipine which can be given i.v.

Peripheral vascular disease

Atheromatous peripheral vascular disease

The risk factors for the development of atherosclerosis in peripheral arteries (principally the aorta, renal and lower limb arteries) are similar to those for coronary artery and cerebrovascular disease (Ch. 5 and Ch. 9). The strongest associations are with smoking and a raised systolic blood pressure, and, to a lesser extent, with diabetes mellitus, a raised plasma low-density lipoprotein (LDL) cholesterol and lack of exercise. Coexisting ischaemic heart and cerebrovascular disease are, not surprisingly, common in people with peripheral vascular disease and are responsible for most of their excess mortality. About 70% of deaths in people with peripheral vascular disease are due to coronary and cerebrovascular events, and only about 50% are alive at 10 years after diagnosis. This is three times the mortality of those without peripheral vascular disease.

Intermittent claudication

Intermittent claudication is a symptom produced by atherosclerosis of the lower limb arteries, when blood flow fails to increase to meet metabolic demand of the muscles on exercise. The limitation of blood flow leads to exercise-induced hypoxia of skeletal muscle, with pain in the limb which is precipitated by walking, especially up a slope, and relieved by rest. Depending on the site of vascular occlusion, pain can be experienced in the calf, thigh or buttock. Peripheral pulses may be absent if vessels are occluded or bruits heard over stenosed arteries. In three-quarters of those with peripheral vascular disease, the symptoms stabilise within a few months of presentation; the remainder have steady progression, but only 1% per year progress to critical ischaemia with pain at rest and distal gangrene (see below).

Drugs for peripheral vascular disease

Cilostazol

Mechanism of action
Cilostazol appears to have several actions. It is a reversible inhibitor of the enzyme phosphodiesterase type III, and therefore reduces breakdown of cyclic adenosine monophosphate (cAMP). Phosphodiesterase type III is present in vascular smooth muscle cells and platelets, and cilostazol causes vasodilation, inhibits platelet activation and aggregation, and prevents release of prothrombotic inflammatory and vasoactive substances. Cilostazol also inhibits adenosine reuptake and has favourable effects on atherogenic lipids in plasma by increasing plasma high-density lipoprotein (HDL) cholesterol. The vasodilatory actions of cilostazol are greater on femoral arteries than on vertebral, carotid or superior mesenteric arteries, and renal arteries do not dilate in response to cilostazol. This may reflect the differences in phosphodiesterase III abundance.

Pharmacokinetics
Cilostazol is well absorbed orally, and undergoes hepatic metabolism via cytochrome P450 to two metabolites with antiplatelet activity. Cilostazol has a long half-life.

Unwanted effects
- diarrhoea
- headache
- palpitation and tachycardia
- other phosphodiesterase inhibitors such as milrinone have been shown to decrease survival in people with heart failure (Ch. 7); cilostazol does not appear to increase the risk of life-threatening arrhythmias, but, at present, its use is contraindicated in heart failure and cardiac arrhythmias
- drug interactions: the pharmacokinetics of cilostazol will be altered by a long list of drugs that influence the liver cytochrome P450 CYP3A4 isoenzyme (Ch. 2).

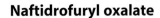

Naftidrofuryl oxalate

Mechanism of action and effects

Naftidrofuryl oxalate promotes the production of high-energy phosphates in ischaemic tissue by activating the enzyme succinic dehydrogenase. It also has 5-hydroxytryptamine type 2 ($5HT_2$) receptor-blocking activity, which leads to vasodilation and reduced platelet aggregation. These actions could improve blood flow and tissue nutrition, but the effect on walking distance is modest.

Pharmacokinetics

Naftidrofuryl is well absorbed from the gut and metabolised in the liver. It has a short half-life.

Unwanted effects

- nausea, epigastric pain
- rash
- hepatitis is a rare, but potentially serious, complication.

Management of intermittent claudication

Non-pharmacological treatment

- Stopping smoking slows the progression of peripheral atherosclerosis and may improve walking distance by improving blood oxygen transport.
- Regular exercise, up to the point of claudication, can improve walking distance.

Pharmacological treatment

- Low-dose aspirin inhibits platelet aggregation and reduces cardiac and cerebrovascular events (Chs 11 and 29).
- Intensive management of hypertension reduces progression of atheroma. Although β-adrenoceptor antagonists are often believed to exacerbate intermittent claudication by reducing cardiac output and impairing vasodilation of arteries supplying skeletal muscle (Ch. 5), there is little evidence that they are disadvantageous unless there is critical limb ischaemia.
- Lowering a raised serum cholesterol (Ch. 48) can stabilise or regress atherosclerotic plaques. This can improve walking distance, but whether it improves limb survival or reduces the need for subsequent surgery is not known. A greater benefit from cholesterol-lowering may be reduced morbidity and mortality from coexistent ischaemic heart disease (Ch. 5).
- Cilostazol can improve walking distance by more than 35%. The clinical significance of this is often

minimal, and the effect on long-term outcome or on the subsequent need for surgery is not known.
- Naftidrofuryl only has a modest effect on walking distance. It should not be used routinely, but a trial of treatment may be justified for those who remain restricted by the disease after 6–12 months of conservative treatment. Withdrawal is advised after 3–6 months of treatment, to see if spontaneous improvement has occurred.
- Pentoxifylline, nicotinic acid derivatives, and cinnarizine are licensed for treatment of peripheral vascular disease, but are relatively ineffective and are not recommended.

Surgical treatment

Surgical treatment is usually considered if quality of life is significantly impaired by claudication or if tissue integrity is at risk. The two options are percutaneous transluminal angioplasty, used particularly for stenoses above the inguinal ligament, often with insertion of a stent, and bypass surgery.

Acute and critical limb ischaemia

Acute or chronic limb ischaemia in peripheral vascular disease is usually caused by thrombosis superimposed on a pre-existing atheromatous plaque. Acute limb ischaemia is caused by an arterial embolus from an intracardiac or aortic thrombus, usually associated with atrial fibrillation (Ch. 8) or following a myocardial infarction (Ch. 5). Emboli can occlude previously healthy vessels. The clinical presentation is with acute onset of severe rest pain associated with signs of critically impaired tissue perfusion. Critical limb ischaemia results from chronic, severe, subtotal occlusion of an artery. The symptoms include rest pain, often worse at night and relieved by hanging the leg out of the bed.

Management

Unless treatment is rapid in acute or acute-on-chronic critical limb ischaemia, the person may be left with a chronically ischaemic limb or, occasionally, the limb may be lost through gangrene.

If the limb is still viable, then a peripheral arterial angiogram should be carried out. For acute embolic arterial occlusion, embolectomy is the treatment of choice. Intra-arterial thrombolysis (Ch. 11), either with streptokinase or tissue plasminogen activator (t-PA), is used for acute thrombosis occluding a previously diseased vessel. t-PA produces more rapid clot lysis, but there is no evidence that limb salvage is any better than with streptokinase. The thrombolytic agent can be either infused via a catheter for up to 24 h, given as a pulsed spray through a catheter with holes, or given as repeated boluses. Reperfusion takes several hours, and in about 25% of acute vascular occlusions lysis is not achieved. The risk of intracerebral haemorrhage is also a concern, and thrombolysis is often unsuccessful for embolic occlusion. A surgical bypass may be considered if there is no time for thrombolysis.

Secondary prevention measures to reduce other cardiovascular events (see above) should also be started.

Raynaud's phenomenon

Raynaud's phenomenon is a profound and exaggerated vasospastic response of blood vessels in the extremities on exposure to cold or during emotional upset. This leads to episodes of ischaemia, most commonly affecting the fingers (occasionally also occurs in the toes, ear lobes or the nipples), which can be provoked by even small degrees of temperature change. A typical attack initially produces pallor of the affected part, followed by cyanosis then redness as flow returns. About two-thirds of cases occur in women (typically presenting under the age of 40 years), in whom the overall prevalence is about 15%. Common symptoms include discomfort, numbness and tingling, with loss of function and pain if the condition is severe. Digital ulceration can occur rarely.

The majority of cases of Raynaud's phenomenon are idiopathic (primary Raynaud's phenomenon), when the cause of the excessive vascular reactivity is unknown. Vascular function in other tissues is often abnormal in primary Raynaud's phenomenon: for example, in the cerebral vessels (giving an association with migraine), the coronary circulation (producing variant angina) or, more rarely, in the pulmonary circulation (leading to pulmonary hypertension). In about 10% of cases, Raynaud's phenomenon is secondary to another disorder. This is most commonly scleroderma, but there are many other associations (Table 10.1). Structural damage to arteries is common in secondary Raynaud's phenomenon, and digital ulceration is much more common than in the primary type.

Other disorders of the peripheral circulation should be considered in the differential diagnosis of Raynaud's phenomenon.

- Acrocyanosis usually affects the hands and produces persistently cold, bluish fingers which are often sweaty or oedematous. The management of this condition is similar to that of Raynaud's phenomenon.
- Chilblains are an inflammatory disorder with erythematous lesions on the hands or feet that are precipitated by damp or cold. The lesions are often

Table 10.1
Conditions associated with Raynaud's phenomenon

Connective tissue disorders
  Systemic sclerosis
  Systemic lupus erythematosus
  Rheumatoid arthritis
  Dermatomyositis and polymyositis
Obstructive arterial disorders
  Carpal tunnel syndrome
  Thoracic outlet syndrome
  Atherosclerosis
  Thromboangitis obliterans
Drugs and chemicals
  Ergotamine
  Beta-adrenoceptor antagonists
  Bleomycin, vinblastine, cisplatin
  Oral contraceptives
  Vinyl chloride
Occupational
  Vibrating tools
  Cold environment
Blood disorders
  Polycythaemia
  Cold agglutinin disease
  Monoclonal gammopathies
Thrombocytosis

painful or itchy. Treatments used for Raynaud's phenomenon may help, with the addition of topical anti-inflammatory agents.
- Erythromelalgia is a painful, burning condition of the hands and feet that, unlike Raynaud's phenomenon, is usually provoked by heat. It sometimes responds to treatment with a β-adrenoceptor antagonist (Ch. 5).
- Vibration white finger is a patchy digital vasospasm associated with prolonged use of vibrating tools.

Management

Many people with Raynaud's phenomenon are only mildly inconvenienced by their symptoms and respond to simple measures. Drug treatment is usually reserved for those suffering from more intense vasospasm with pain, impairment of function or trophic changes. Responses to individual treatments are unpredictable, and are less satisfactory in secondary Raynaud's phenomenon because of the structural changes to the vessel wall.

Non-pharmacological treatment

- Often, minimising changes in ambient temperature with insulating clothing is enough to reduce the numbers of attacks, although electrically heated

gloves or socks may be useful for more severely affected people.
- Smoking should be strongly discouraged. Nicotine promotes vasospasm and may also reduce the threshold for other provoking factors.
- Aggravating factors should be withdrawn or corrected whenever possible (see Table 10.1). Beta-adrenoceptor antagonists (Ch. 5), in particular, produce peripheral circulatory problems sufficient to necessitate stopping treatment in about 3–5% of hypertensives.
- Surgical sympathectomy is occasionally used for advanced disease.

Pharmacological treatment

Arterial vasodilators

- Calcium channel antagonists (Ch. 5): modified-release nifedipine is the drug of first choice for Raynaud's phenomenon, and reduces the frequency, duration and intensity of vasospastic episodes. Several other dihydropyridines are probably equally effective, but diltiazem is less effective and verapamil ineffective in this condition.
- Naftidrofuryl may produce a modest reduction in the severity of attacks.
- Alpha-adrenoceptor antagonists (Ch. 6): moxisylyte may be effective and does not lower blood pressure, unlike other α-adrenoceptor antagonists. Prazosin has also been shown to be helpful.
- Angiotensin receptor blockers (Ch. 6): losartan has shown some benefit.

- Fluoxetine, a selective serotonin reuptake inhibitor (SSRI) antidepressant (Ch. 22), is effective in some people.
- Calcitonin gene-related peptide (CGRP) is effective for prolonged periods when given by intravenous infusion for 5 or more consecutive days. It is a neurotransmitter at vasodilator cutaneous sensorimotor nerves in the fingers and toes. CGRP is usually reserved for failure to respond to epoprostenol (see below).

Drugs acting primarily on blood components

- Prostaglandins: intravenous infusion of epoprostenol (prostacyclin, Ch. 11) over at least 5 consecutive days produces immediate and short-lived vasodilation, but long-term improvement in symptoms and healing of ulcers over a period of 10–16 weeks after a single prolonged infusion. These effects are believed to be caused by actions on the flow properties of blood, i.e. reduced platelet aggregation, increased red cell deformability and reduced neutrophil adhesiveness. Epoprostenol is rapidly inactivated in plasma by hydrolysis, and has a very short half-life of about 3 min. It is given by intravenous infusion. Unwanted effects are due to vasodilation, and include flushing, headache and hypotension.
- Inositol nicotinate (a nicotinic acid derivative) produces a gradual onset of clinical response and only modest improvement. Its action may result more from fibrinolysis (reducing plasma vicosity) and reduction in platelet aggregation than from vasodilation.

FURTHER READING

Bowling JCR, Dowd PM (2003) Raynaud's disease. *Lancet* 361, 2078–2080

Herrick AL (2003) Treatment of Raynaud's phenomenon: new insights and developments. *Curr Rheumatol Rep* 5, 168–174

Hiatt WR (2001) Drug therapy: medical treatment of peripheral arterial disease and claudication. *N Engl J Med* 344, 1608–1621

Hiatt WR (2002) Pharmacologic therapy for peripheral arterial disease and claudication. *J Vasc Surg* 36, 1283–1291

Hummers LK, Wigley FM (2003) Management of Raynaud's phenomenon and digital ischemic lesions in scleroderma. *Rheum Dis Clin North Am* 29, 293–313

Kim CK, Schmalfuss CM, Schofield RS et al (2003) Pharmacological treatment of patients with peripheral arterial disease. *Drugs* 63, 637–647

Ouriel K (2001) Peripheral arterial disease. *Lancet* 358, 1257–1264

Olin J (2003) Identifying and treating peripheral arterial disease. **http://www.medscape.com/viewarticle/459920_1**

Regensteiner JG, Hiatt WR (2002) Current medical therapies for patients with peripheral arterial disease: a critical review. *Am J Med* 112, 49–57

Tilley DG, Maurice DH (2002) Vascular smooth muscle cell phosphodiesterase (PDE) 3 and PDE4 activities and levels are regulated by cyclic AMP in vivo. *Mol Pharmacol* 63, 497–506

Wigley FM (2002) Raynaud's phenomenon. *N Engl J Med* 347, 1001–1008

Self-assessment

1. In the following questions, the first statement, in italics, is true. Is the accompanying statement also true?

    a. *There is an additive effect of diabetes mellitus, hypertension and smoking on the risk of developing peripheral vascular disease.* People with intermittent claudication do not have an increased risk of developing coronary disease.
    b. *'Statins' are indicated in people with symptomatic atherosclerotic peripheral vascular disease.* Simvastatin increases the expression of hepatic LDL receptors.
    c. *Drugs such as ergotamine, used in migraine treatment, can precipitate Raynaud's phenomenon.* Verapamil is the calcium channel antagonist of choice in the treatment of Raynaud's phenomenon.

2. Choose the one correct statement from the following:

    A. Cilostazol inhibits phosphodiesterase type III in vascular tissues.
    B. Cilostazol is useful in the treatment of congestive heart failure.
    C. Cilostazol is mainly excreted unchanged in the urine.
    D. Cilostazol has little effect on platelet aggregation.
    E. Cilostazol decreases plasma HDL cholesterol.

3. Case history questions

> Mr TH, aged 67 years, was an insulin-dependent diabetic and smoked 20 cigarettes a day. His plasma cholesterol level was raised at 7 mmol l^{-1} and his blood pressure was 160/110 mmHg. After walking 50 m, he developed pain in his left calf muscle, which was relieved by rest. He occasionally, but rarely, had rest pain at night. On examination, both popliteal and posterior tibial pulses were absent and femoropopliteal obstruction was diagnosed.

   a. Comment on the use of the following drugs to treat this patient:
      i.   Propranolol
      ii. Atenolol
      iii. Nifedipine
      iv. A statin
      v.   Low-dose aspirin
      vi. Cilostazol.
   b. What other therapy could be of benefit?
   c. Should the use of an electric blanket be discouraged?

The answers are provided on page 712.

Drug compendium

Drugs for peripheral vascular disease (all, except epoprostenol, given orally)

Drug	Half-life (h)	Elimination	Comment
Aspirin	15–20 min	Metabolism (hydrolysis)	Inhibitor of cyclo-oxygenase; half-life of active salicylic acid metabolite is 3–20 h
Cilostazol	12	Metabolism	Reversibly reduces platelet aggregation by inhibition of phosphodiesterase (PDE) type III; absorption increased by food; metabolised by CYP3A4 and CYP2C19 to active metabolites
Cinnarizine	24	Metabolism	Slow oral absorption; eliminated largely by CYP2D6 (polymorphic) metabolism
Epoprostenol	2 min	Metabolism	Given by intravenous infusion; eliminated as glucuronide
Inositol nicotinate	–	–	Few data available; probably eliminated by hydrolysis; also used for hyperlipidaemias
Moxisylyte	1 (DAM)	Metabolism	Good oral bioavailability; a prodrug which is rapidly deacetylated in plasma to an active metabolite (DAM)
Naftidrofuryl oxalate	3–4	Metabolism + some renal	Good oral bioavailability; metabolised by oxidation and hydrolysis
Pentoxifylline	1	Metabolism	Active after oral dosage; metabolised in liver and blood (clearance greatly exceeds liver blood flow)

11

Haemostasis

The descriptions of the processes of platelet aggregation and coagulation pathways in this chapter are restricted to essential knowledge required for understanding the actions of pharmacological agents.

Platelets and platelet aggregation

Platelets aggregate following adhesion to an injured blood vessel and subsequent activation. These functions are necessary occurrences in response to blood vessel damage, but, when abnormally evident, are risk factors for thrombotic disease. When the integrity of vascular endothelium is breached, subendothelial proteins are exposed to the blood. Proteins such as von Willebrand factor and collagen interact with a family of glycoprotein (GP) receptors (integrin receptors) on the surface of non-activated platelets; examples are GPIb/IX, GPIa/IIa, GPVI, which have different affinities for collagen, von Willebrand factor and other ligands (Fig. 11.1). These multiple actions lead to adhesion of the platelets at the site of injury, and formation of a platelet plug. Extension of the platelet plug results from exposure of platelet surface G-protein-linked receptors to soluble agonists such as thrombin, ADP, collagen and thromboxane A$_2$ (5-hydroxytryptamine [5HT], platelet activating factor

and vasopressin may also be involved). The processes of platelet activation involve an increase in intracellular Ca^{2+} and phosphorylation of myosin light chains in the platelet, and produce a rearrangement of the platelet cytoskeleton and a change in cell shape; there follows a critical upregulation and activation of GPIIb/IIIa receptors on platelets (Figs. 11.1, 2). At least 50000 of these receptors are found on each platelet. The increase in intracellular platelet Ca^{2+} also activates phospholipase A$_2$, which releases arachidonic acid, the precursor of the extremely pro-aggregating thromboxane A$_2$, in the platelet. Thromboxane A$_2$ further enhances expression of the GPIIb/IIIa surface receptors (Fig. 11.1).

Platelet aggregation occurs when upregulated GPIIb/IIIa receptors are cross-linked with fibrinogen. Platelet activation also enhances exocytosis of platelet storage granules, releasing substances such as platelet factor 4, β-thromboglobulin, ADP and 5HT, which initiate or enhance the coagulation cascade by causing:

- reduced prostacyclin (prostaglandin I$_2$) synthesis by vascular endothelium; prostacyclin is a vasodilator and a potent inhibitor of platelet aggregation
- inhibition of the action of heparin produced by the same cells; this enhances activity of the coagulation cascade
- induction of further platelet aggregation.

These processes lead to the deposition of fibrin thrombus and inhibition of fibrinolysis. In some circumstances, aggregates of platelets combined with fibrin thrombi can embolise and occlude more distal parts of the circulation. Platelets have a lifespan of 7–10 days in the circulation.

Both direct and thromboxane A$_2$-mediated expression of platelet GPIIb/IIIa surface receptors can be inhibited by increasing the concentration of cyclic adenosine monophosphate (cAMP) in the platelet. This is the mechanism by which prostacyclin released from vascular endothelium inhibits platelet aggregation. Polyunsaturated (omega-3) fatty acids in fish oils are precursors for thromboxane A$_3$, which causes less platelet aggregation than thromboxane A$_2$; they also increase production of a modified form of prostacyclin (PGI$_3$) by vascular endothelium which, however, has equal anti-aggregatory activity to PGI$_2$. A high intake of fish oils, therefore, creates a less pro-aggregatory state.

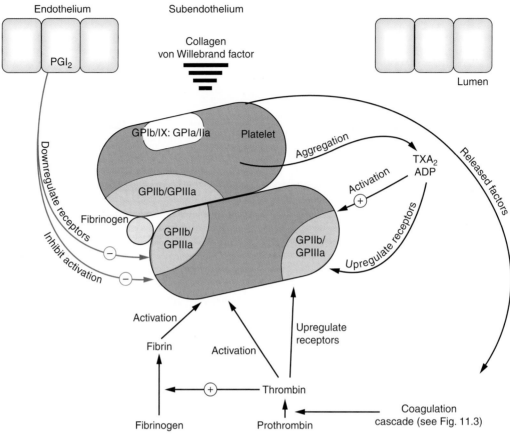

Fig. 11.1

Platelets and platelet aggregation. Subendothelial macromolecules such as collagen interact with glycoprotein receptors (GPIb/IX and GPIa/IIa) on platelets, causing activation of platelets and upregulation of GPIIb/IIIa receptors, which are cross-linked by fibrinogen during aggregation. Synthesis of the pro-aggregatory thromboxane A_2 (TXA_2) and release of ADP and 5-hydroxytryptamine occurs. TXA_2 and thrombin cause further platelet activation and release of pro-aggregatory platelet contents. This leads to further upregulation of GPIIb/IIIa receptors. Prostacyclin (PGI_2) from endothelial cells inhibits activation and upregulation of GPIIb/IIIa receptors. Thrombin is generated by the action of factor Xa on prothrombin (see Fig. 11.3).

Antiplatelet agents

Examples: aspirin, clopidogrel, dipyridamole

Aspirin

Mechanism of action on platelets

Irreversible inhibition of platelet cyclo-oxygenase type 1 (COX-1) by aspirin decreases platelet thromboxane A_2 synthesis. This reduces platelet aggregation, but does not eliminate it, because other pathways for platelet activation still function (Fig. 11.2). The antiplatelet action of aspirin occurs at very low doses that have little analgesic or anti-inflammatory actions. Details of the pharmacology of aspirin are found in Chapter 29.

Dipyridamole

Mechanisms of action

Dipyridamole inhibits the enzyme phosphodiesterase and this increases intracellular concentrations of cAMP. In the platelet, this reduces activation and expression of cell surface GPIIb/IIIa receptors (Fig. 11.2). Dipyridamole also blocks the cellular uptake of adenosine, but this is not relevant to its antiplatelet activity.

Pharmacokinetics

Dipyridamole is incompletely absorbed from the gut and is metabolised in the liver. It has an intermediate half-life. A modified-release formulation is better tolerated than the standard formulation.

Unwanted effects

- gastrointestinal effects
- myalgia

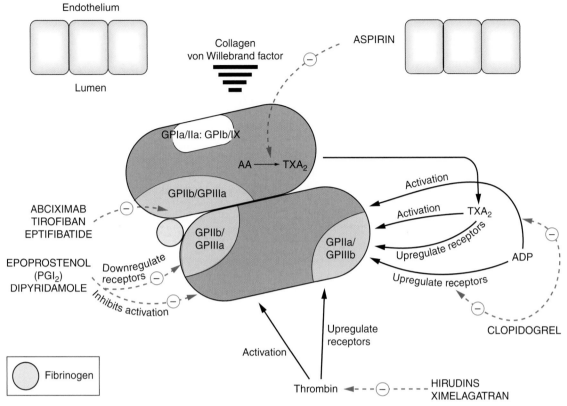

Fig. 11.2
Sites of action of major drugs used in haemostasis. Drugs act directly or indirectly to inhibit activation of platelets or to block or reduce upregulation of the glycoprotein GPIIb/IIIa receptors (integrin receptor family), which are necessary for aggregation of platelets. Abciximab is an antibody, tirofiban a non-peptide inhibitor, and eptifibatide a peptide inhibitor of these glycoprotein receptors. Epoprostenol and dipyridamole inhibit activation of platelets and downregulate the glycoprotein receptors. Clopidogrel prevents ADP-induced upregulation of the receptors and platelet aggregation. Hirudin prevents the effects of thrombin. Aspirin inhibits the generation of thromboxane A_2 (TXA_2), which causes activation of platelets and upregulation of GPIIb/IIIa receptors. AA, arachidonic acid. For effects of heparin, hirudins and ximelagatran on thrombin, see Fig. 11.3.

- dizziness, headache
- flushing, hypotension, tachycardia
- hypersensitivity reactions, including rash, urticaria, bronchospasm and angioedema.

Clopidogrel

Mechanisms of action
Clopidogrel inhibits platelet aggregation by irreversibly binding to the purinergic P_2 receptors for ADP on the platelet surface. This reduces the mobilisation of Ca^{2+} from intracellular platelet stores, and reduces expression of GPIIb/IIIa receptors.

Pharmacokinetics
Clopidogrel is a prodrug. It is well absorbed from the gut, and is activated by metabolism in the liver. It has an intermediate half-life and undergoes further metabolism to inactive derivatives in the liver.

Unwanted effects

- bleeding, although the risk is low
- gastrointestinal upset, especially with dyspepsia, abdominal pain and diarrhoea
- headache, dizziness, paraesthesia
- rashes.

Glycoprotein IIb/IIIa receptor antagonists

Examples: abciximab, tirofiban

Mechanism of action
Abciximab is a murine monoclonal antibody with the Fc fragment removed to prevent immunogenicity. The Fab fragment is then joined to a human Fc region to form a chimaeric molecule. Abciximab binds irreversibly to the

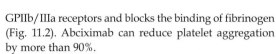
GPIIb/IIIa receptors and blocks the binding of fibrinogen (Fig. 11.2). Abciximab can reduce platelet aggregation by more than 90%.

Tirofiban is a non-peptide agent that binds reversibly to and blocks the GPIIb/IIIa receptor.

Pharmacokinetics

Abciximab must be given intravenously, usually as an initial bolus followed by continuous infusion. Platelet inhibition occurs rapidly with a bolus injection and largely recovers by 48 h after the infusion is stopped. However, small amounts of the antibody are still detected on platelets after one week or more.

Tirofiban also requires continuous infusion, has a shorter plasma and biological half-life than abciximab, and is eliminated by the kidney.

Unwanted effects

- bleeding, especially in the elderly and those of low bodyweight; the risk is reduced if the dose is adjusted for bodyweight
- thrombocytopenia
- abciximab can cause nausea, vomiting, hypotension, bradycardia, headache, and, occasionally, hypersensitivity reactions.

Epoprostenol

Mechanism of action

Epoprostenol (PGI$_2$) increases platelet cAMP, which at low concentrations inhibits platelet aggregation and at higher concentrations reduces adhesion. Epoprostenol also vasodilates peripheral arteries.

Pharmacokinetics

Epoprostenol is given by intravenous infusion. Unlike with most prostaglandins, lung metabolism is irrelevant, as it is rapidly metabolised by hydrolysis in plasma and peripheral tissues, giving a very short half-life.

Unwanted effects

These can be reduced by starting with a low dose and include:

- facial flushing
- headache
- hypotension
- gastrointestinal disturbances.

Clinical uses of antiplatelet agents

Dipyridamole, clopidogrel and aspirin show similar efficacy in many conditions that can be treated with oral antiplatelet agents. The more favourable unwanted-effect profile of low-dose aspirin, and the simple dosage regimen, make it the drug of choice for most indications.

- Prevention of embolic stroke and transient ischaemic attacks (aspirin; clopidogrel; dipyridamole). Dipyridamole combined with aspirin may have an additive effect in prevention of stroke (Ch. 9).
- Secondary prevention after myocardial infarction (aspirin; clopidogrel) (Ch. 5).
- Prevention of myocardial infarction in stable angina or peripheral vascular disease (aspirin; clopidogrel) (Chs 5 and 10). The evidence for the use of aspirin for primary prevention of myocardial infarction in healthy individuals who do not have evidence of established ischaemic heart disease is mainly inconclusive. However, it is recommended for people at high risk of developing ischaemic heart disease, particularly those with hypertension or diabetes.
- Treatment of acute coronary syndromes to reduce the risk of myocardial infarction or death (aspirin with the anticoagulant heparin) (Ch. 5). The GPIIb/IIIa inhibitor tirofiban further reduces events in non-ST-elevation myocardial infarction when added to aspirin and heparin.
- As an anticoagulant in extracorporeal circulations, for example cardiopulmonary bypass, and renal haemodialysis (epoprostenol).
- Symptom relief in Raynaud's phenomenon (epoprostenol) (Ch. 10).
- Abciximab is used to reduce ischaemic complications produced by sudden vessel closure following percutaneous transluminal angioplasty with stent insertion. These complications include myocardial infarction, the need for emergency revascularisation, and death.
- Dipyridamole is used as a pharmacological stress for the coronary circulation, in order to detect myocardial ischaemia in people who are unable to exercise. This is unrelated to its antiplatelet effect. Dipyridamole also blocks the cellular uptake of adenosine that is released by tissues when they become hypoxic. In the heart, the excess adenosine acts on specific receptors in the small resistance coronary arteries to produce vasodilation. Since these vessels are already maximally dilated in ischaemic tissue, the drug has no useful antianginal action. Indeed, dipyridamole can divert blood away from ischaemic tissue by dilating vascular beds in non-ischaemic myocardium (vascular steal). The heart is usually imaged at rest and again after stress by dipyridamole for radioisotope uptake (e.g. using technetium-labelled meta-iodobenzoyl isonitrile or thallium, which accumulate in aerobically metabolising myocardium) or by echocardiography to examine left ventricular wall motion.

Blood coagulation

There are two pathways for activation of the coagulation cascade, the extrinsic and intrinsic pathways. These amplify the coagulation response and work together to produce the thrombus. The extrinsic system is triggered by the release of thromboplastin from damaged tissue and is activated rapidly within minutes of endothelial disruption. The intrinsic system is triggered by contact of blood with a negatively charged surface such as subendothelial collagen and its activation is delayed by more than 10 min after tissue disruption. Both pathways respond much more slowly than platelet aggregation and vasoconstriction, the processes that initiate haemostasis.

Thrombin is responsible for activation of the final common step in the pathways of coagulation (Fig. 11.3). The action of thrombin is inhibited by circulating antithrombin. The coagulation cascade comprises a series of enzyme-mediated reactions involving activation of clotting factors, which leads to generation of thrombin. Each activated clotting factor is inactivated extremely rapidly so that the coagulation process remains localised at the site of the initiating event. Once sufficient thrombin has been produced to overcome the effect of circulating

antithrombin, the soluble protein fibrinogen is converted to a fibrin gel.

Anticoagulant agents

Anticoagulation can be achieved with either parenteral or oral drug therapy. A comparison of some of the properties of heparin, warfarin and ximelagatran are shown in Table 11.1.

Parenteral anticoagulants

Heparin

Mechanism of action and effects
Heparin is a highly sulphated acidic mucopolysaccharide (glycosaminoglycan) that has a variable molecular weight of 3000 to 30 000 Da. It forms a complex with the circulating protein antithrombin and induces a conformational change in antithrombin so that the activated heparin–antithrombin complex interacts with and neu-

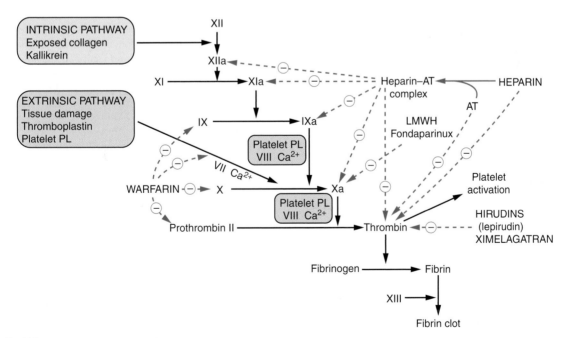

Fig. 11.3
The coagulation cascade and action of anticoagulants. The complex cascade of clotting factor synthesis is initiated extrinsically by tissue damage. Activation of the clotting factors after damage requires platelet factors and Ca^{2+}. The provision of platelet products is further enhanced by the formation of thrombin, which then activates further platelets as well as causing fibrin formation. Heparin acts at various sites in the cascade by activating the anticlotting factor antithrombin (AT) and inhibiting the activating protease clotting factors shown. Low-molecular-weight heparin (LMWH) acts on factor Xa. Hirudins and ximelagatran inhibit thrombin (IIa) action and formation. Warfarin inhibits the synthesis of the vitamin-K-dependent clotting factors VII, IX, X and II (prothrombin). Roman numerals indicate the individual clotting factors; PL, phospholipid.

Table 11.1
Comparison of some properties of heparin, warfarin and ximelagatran

	Heparin	Warfarin	Ximelagatran
Route of administration	Intravenous, subcutaneous	Oral	Oral
Onset	Immediate	1–3 days	<1 h
Site of action	Free thrombin, and clotting factors in blood	Clotting factors II, VII, IX, X in liver	Directly on free and fibrin-bound thrombin; inhibits thrombin formation
Duration of action	3–6 h	3–6 days	Hours
Antagonist	Protamine but this is less effective against LMWH	Vitamin K$_1$	No known antagonist
Monitoring	APTT	PT, INR	Does not affect APTT or PT; no INR monitoring required; liver function tests
Fate	Partially degraded in liver; does not cross the placenta	Inactivated in liver; crosses placenta; teratogenic	Metabolised to active melagatran
Variability in individual response	Little	Great, because of genetic diifferences	Little
Potential for drug interactions	Little	Many	Little

APTT, activated partial thromboplastin time; INR, international normalised ratio; LMWH, low-molecular-weight heparin; PT, prothrombin time.

tralises activated clotting factors (especially factors Xa, IXa and thrombin; Fig. 11.3). Heparin can also bind directly to, and inactivate, thrombin. Heparin is available as an unfractionated preparation, or as low-molecular-weight heparin (LMWH), which consists of the heparin subfraction that has a molecular weight less than 7000 Da. There are several major effects of heparin on haemostasis.

- Inhibition of the activated coagulation factors, especially Xa and thrombin. The higher-molecular-weight heparin–antithrombin complexes have greater affinity for thrombin than do LMWH–antithrombin complexes. However, heparin binds only to free circulating thrombin, since it binds to the substrate recognition site on thrombin. LMWH–antithrombin complexes mainly inactivate factor Xa; they are four times more active in this respect than unfractionated heparin.
- Release of tissue factor pathway inhibitor (TFPI) from the vascular wall contributes to the antithrombotic effects of heparin. TFPI inhibits formation of factor Xa.
- Inhibition of platelet aggregation through interaction with platelets and platelet factor 4.
- Activation of lipoprotein lipase, which in addition to promoting lipolysis also reduces platelet adhesiveness.

Danaparoid is a heparinoid related to heparin and derived from porcine gut mucosa. It contains heparan sulphate, dermatan sulphate and chondroitin sulphate. Its mechanism of action is similar to that of LMWH, and it can be used as an alternative to lepirudin (see below) when there is heparin-induced thrombocytopenia.

Pharmacokinetics

Heparins are inactive orally and are given intravenously or by subcutaneous injection. They have a rapid onset of action. Heparins do not cross the placenta or enter breast milk. Since the two principal forms of heparin have different structures, they also have different pharmacokinetic properties.

Unfractionated heparin. This is extracted from porcine intestinal mucosa or bovine lung, and consists of a mean of 45 polysaccharide units. Its kinetics are dose-dependent: the half-life is very short (about 30 min) at low doses, increasing some fivefold at higher doses. Most is metabolised in endothelial cells after binding to surface receptors. Some heparin is metabolised in the liver, with a small amount excreted unchanged by the kidney. Unfractionated heparin is given by repeated intravenous bolus injections or by continuous intravenous infusion for full anticoagulant effect. Low-dose subcutaneous injections are used for prophylaxis against thrombosis, although bioavailability by this route is only about 30%.

Low-molecular-weight heparin. LMWHs have a mean of 15 polysaccharide units. They have at least twice the duration of anticoagulant action and a more predictable anticoagulant effect compared with unfractionated heparin, because they have a low affinity for endothelial cell heparin receptors and plasma protein binding sites. LMWHs have two routes of elimination: a rapid, saturable liver uptake and slower renal excretion. They are almost completely absorbed after subcutaneous administration and only need to be given once or twice daily by subcutaneous injection for full anticoagulation. The various types of LMWH form complexes with antithrombin that differ in their affinity for factor Xa, but all have a lower affinity for thrombin than do the complexes formed by unfractionated heparin (see above).

Control of heparin therapy

The therapeutic index for heparin is low. The degree of anticoagulation with unfractionated heparin is usually monitored with the activated partial thromboplastin time (APTT, a global test of the intrinsic coagulation pathway), which should be prolonged by 1.5–2.0 times the control value for full anticoagulation. Monitoring is not required when low-dose subcutaneous unfractionated heparin is used (see below). The LMWHs can be monitored by factor Xa inhibition, but this is not carried out routinely, since their effect is much more predictable than that of unfractionated heparin.

Unwanted effects

- Haemorrhage is the most common problem. The risk is greater in the elderly, especially if there is a history of heavy alcohol intake. The effect of unfractionated heparin can be rapidly reversed by intravenous injection of protamine sulphate, a basic substance which binds strongly to the acidic heparin components. Protamine binds poorly to LMWHs and only partially reverses their action.
- Osteoporosis is a rare complication which can occur when heparin is given for several weeks. The risk is less with LMWH.
- Thrombocytopenia occurs due to the development of heparin-induced antiplatelet antibodies that cause platelet aggregation and arterial thrombosis. It rarely occurs until 7–10 days after starting intravenous heparin. Heparinoids (see above) or lepirudin (see below) are used if continued anticoagulation is necessary. LMWH has much less effect on platelet aggregation and its lower binding to endothelium also reduces interference with platelet–vessel wall interaction
- Hyperkalaemia by inhibition of aldosterone secretion. This is most likely to occur after 7 days of treatment.
- Hypersensitivity reactions.

Hirudins

Example: lepirudin

Mechanism of action and use

Lepirudin is a recombinant hirudin that binds directly to thrombin and inhibits its action. Lepirudin binds to both the substrate binding site and the catalytic site on the thrombin molecule and therefore inactivates both free and clot-bound thrombin. Its effect is monitored by measurement of the APTT. Lepirudin is used for anticoagulation in place of heparin when there has been heparin-induced thrombocytopenia.

Pharmacokinetics

Lepirudin is given intravenously, and is eliminated in urine and catabolised by hydrolysis; it has a short half-life.

Unwanted effects

- bleeding
- fever
- hypersensitivity reactions.

Fondaparinux

Mechanism of action and use

Fondaparinux is a synthetic pentasaccharide almost identical to the natural pentasaccharide sequence of heparin that binds to antithrombin. Like heparin, it enhances the innate ability of antithrombin to inhibit factor Xa. It is an alternative to heparin for the prophylaxis of deep vein thrombosis in orthopaedic surgery (Fig. 11.3).

Pharmacokinetics

Fondaparinux is given by subcutaneous injection. It is predictably absorbed from the injection site, eliminated unchanged by the kidney, and has a long half-life.

Unwanted effects

- haemorrhage
- thrombocytopenia
- oedema
- gastrointestinal upset.

Oral anticoagulants

Vitamin K antagonists

Example: warfarin

Mechanism of action

These drugs are antagonists of vitamin K and act by inhibiting the hepatic reductase enzyme that converts

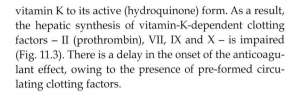
vitamin K to its active (hydroquinone) form. As a result, the hepatic synthesis of vitamin-K-dependent clotting factors – II (prothrombin), VII, IX and X – is impaired (Fig. 11.3). There is a delay in the onset of the anticoagulant effect, owing to the presence of pre-formed circulating clotting factors.

Pharmacokinetics

Warfarin is the most widely used oral anticoagulant. It is almost completely absorbed from the gut and is highly protein bound to albumin in plasma. It is eliminated by cytochrome P450-mediated hepatic metabolism and has a very long half-life of 1–1.5 days. The plasma concentration of warfarin does not correlate directly with the clinical effect of the drug, which is determined by the balance between the rates of synthesis and degradation of clotting factors. The maximum effect of an individual dose of warfarin is reflected in the blood coagulation time some 24–36 h later. On stopping treatment, the duration of anticoagulant action is determined largely by the time required to synthesise new clotting factors. Warfarin crosses the placenta and can adversely affect the fetus.

Control of oral anticoagulant therapy

Factor VII is the clotting factor that is most sensitive to vitamin K deficiency, since it has the shortest half-life of the vitamin-K-sensitive clotting factors; therefore, a test of the extrinsic coagulation pathway – the prothrombin time – is used as a measure of effectiveness. The degree of prolongation of the prothrombin time is standardised by comparison with a control plasma from a single source, and referred to as the INR (international normalised ratio). Therapeutic INR ranges differ according to the condition being treated:

- 2–2.5 for prophylaxis of deep vein thrombosis
- 2–3 for thromboprophylaxis in hip surgery and fractured femur operations, for treatment of deep vein thrombosis and pulmonary embolism, for treatment of transient ischaemic attacks and prevention of thromboembolism in atrial fibrillation
- 3–4.5 for prevention of recurrent deep vein thrombosis and for preventing thrombosis on mechanical prosthetic heart valves.

Unwanted effects

Warfarin is an important example of a drug that has a narrow therapeutic index.

- Haemorrhage. The most effective antidote to warfarin is phytomenadione (vitamin K_1). For major bleeding, this is given intravenously and controls bleeding within 6 h. An immediate coagulant effect is achieved by also giving an intravenous injection of prothrombin complex concentrate (vitamin K-dependent clotting factors) or an infusion of fresh frozen plasma. After giving a large dose of phytomenadione, it can be difficult to restore

therapeutic anticoagulation with warfarin for up to 3 weeks. If the INR is >8.0 but there is no bleeding or only minor bleeding, then a smaller dose of phytomenadione is given intravenously or orally.
- Warfarin has undesirable effects on the fetus. It is teratogenic and should be avoided in the first trimester of pregnancy, except when essential; furthermore, it should not be used in the last trimester, as it increases the risk of intracranial haemorrhage in the baby during delivery.
- Alopecia, skin necrosis and hypersensitivity reactions occur rarely.
- Drug interactions. These are particularly important. The anticoagulant effect of warfarin can be increased by broad-spectrum antibacterial agents which suppress the production of vitamin K by gut bacteria. Some non-steroidal anti-inflammatory drugs (Ch. 29) displace warfarin from its binding site on plasma proteins; this increases the plasma concentration of free (and therefore active) drug and briefly increases its effects. Amiodarone (Ch. 8) and the histamine H_2 receptor antagonist cimetidine (Ch. 33) inhibit the cytochrome P450-mediated metabolism of warfarin and enhance its effects. Drugs that induce hepatic microsomal drug-metabolising enzymes – for example, phenytoin, phenobarbital (Ch. 23) and alcohol (Ch. 54) – reduce the effect of warfarin by increasing its elimination.

Direct thrombin inhibitors

Example: ximelagatran

Ximelagatran is the first oral anticoagulant to reach phase III clinical trials in the past 50 years. Its role in venous thrombosis is still under investigation, and if the results of promising early studies are confirmed, then it will herald a significant advance in simplifying anticoagulation (Table 11.1).

Mechanism of action

Ximelagatran is converted to melagatran, a dipeptide which is a direct, competitive thrombin inhibitor that binds to free circulating and clot-bound thrombin. This is distinct from heparin, which only affects free thrombin, mainly via activation of antithrombin (see Table 11.1). At the time of writing, ximelagatran was not available in the UK.

Pharmacokinetics

Ximelagatran is a prodrug of melagatran that overcomes the poor oral absorption of the active compound. It is reliably and predictably absorbed, although bioavailability is still low. After absorption, it is converted to melagatran in the liver. Melagatran is excreted unchanged by the kidney, and has a short half-life. Because of the predictable pharmacokinetics, there is less risk of under- or over-anticoagulation, and monitoring is not required. There is no known antagonist.

Unwanted efffects

- bleeding, with a similar risk to warfarin; the coagulant effect cannot be reversed, and if there is bleeding, then maintaining a good urine flow rate, or haemodialysis to remove the drug, are the currently proposed strategies.
- elevation of liver enzymes. The long-term risk of liver damage is unknown.

Clinical uses of anticoagulants

Venous thromboembolism

Pulmonary embolism remains a major cause of morbidity and death and has been estimated to be responsible for 10% of all deaths in hospital. Most serious pulmonary emboli arise from lower limb deep vein thrombosis, particularly if this extends to the larger veins above the calf. Following a deep vein thrombosis, chronic post-phlebitic syndrome can develop, with pain, swelling and ulceration of the affected leg.

Predisposing factors to venous thromboembolism include use of the oral contraceptive pill in some women, particularly those who smoke (see Ch. 45), prolonged immobility and a variety of coexisting medical conditions such as cancer. Many episodes of deep vein thrombosis occur in hospital, particularly in those over 40 years of age following major illness, trauma or surgery. However, within this group, and in younger people, several additional factors predict the level of risk (Table 11.2).

Prevention of deep vein thrombosis

In hospitalised people, the methods used to prevent deep vein thrombosis vary according to the degree of risk.

Mechanical methods. These are used for people at moderate risk and include graduated elastic compression stockings and intermittent pneumatic compression devices to improve venous flow and limit stasis in venous valve pockets. They can also be used to supplement pharmacological prophylaxis in high-risk people.

Low-dose subcutaneous heparin. This is the treatment of choice in people at high-risk and in many people at moderate-risk. Heparin reduces both initiation and extension of fibrin-rich thrombi at doses which have little effect on measurements of blood coagulation. Therefore, laboratory monitoring is unnecessary, even with unfractionated heparin. Low-dose unfractionated heparin reduces deep venous thrombosis and fatal pulmonary emboli by about two-thirds, with minimal risk of serious bleeding, although minor bleeding is increased. For those at highest risk, particularly during orthopaedic surgery, LMWHs are more effective than unfractionated heparin. Prophylaxis should be started before surgery.

Low-dose aspirin and warfarin. Although a meta-analysis of several studies suggests that low-dose aspirin (see below) reduces deep venous thrombosis, it is less effective than heparin. Warfarin may be more effective than heparin for prophylaxis in people at highest risk.

Treatment of established venous thrombosis

The goals of treatment for deep vein thrombi are to prevent pulmonary emboli and to restore patency of the occluded vessel, with preservation of the function of venous valves.

Full anticoagulation. This is the treatment of choice for deep vein thrombosis and for most pulmonary emboli; it substantially reduces mortality. Heparin is given ini-

Table 11.2
Risk of thromboembolism in people admitted to hospital

Risk	Procedure
Low	Minor surgery, no other risk factor
	Major surgery, age <40 years, no other risk factors
	Minor trauma or illness
Moderate	Major surgery; age ≥40 years or other risk factor
	Heart failure, recent myocardial infarction, malignancy, inflammatory bowel disease
	Major trauma or burns
	Minor surgery, trauma or illness in patient with previous deep vein thrombosis or pulmonary embolism
High	Fracture or major orthopaedic surgery of pelvis, hips or lower limb
	Major pelvic or abdominal surgery for cancer
	Major surgery, trauma or illness in patient with previous deep vein thrombosis or pulmonary embolism
	Lower limb paralysis
	Major lower limb amputation

Table 11.3
Suggested duration of anticoagulant therapy for venous thromboembolism

Risk of recurrence	Patient type	Duration
Low	Temporary risk factors for thromboembolism	4–6 weeks
Intermediate	Continuing medical risk factors for thromboembolism	6 months
High	Recurrent thromboembolism, inherited thrombophilic tendency	Indefinite

tially for its rapid onset of effect. Unfractionated heparin by intravenous infusion (in preference to intermittent bolus injection, which carries a higher risk of serious bleeding) is now being replaced by LMWH given subcutaneously as a convenient and effective alternative. Heparin is usually given for 3–5 days, with concurrent initiation of treatment with warfarin. Once warfarin has produced adequate anticoagulation (i.e. the INR is within the therapeutic range; see above), heparin can be stopped. The optimal duration of anticoagulant therapy is not well defined, but suggested periods are shown in Table 11.3.

Surgical venous thrombectomy. This may be required for massive iliofemoral thrombosis if it threatens the viability of the limb. Pulmonary embolectomy is occasionally carried out for large pulmonary emboli.

Thrombolytic treatment with streptokinase. This treatment (see below) has no advantage over warfarin in uncomplicated deep venous thrombosis, but is sometimes used to disintegrate massive pulmonary emboli.

Other treatments. For pulmonary emboli that continue despite adequate anticoagulation, or if anticoagulation is contraindicated, inferior vena caval plication or insertion of a 'filter' device to trap emboli in the inferior vena cava can be considered.

Arterial thromboembolism

Warfarin is used long term for prevention of thrombosis on prosthetic heart valves. Atrial fibrillation (Ch. 8) and mural thrombus in the left ventricle following a myocardial infarction predispose to arterial embolism and are indications for anticoagulation with warfarin. Ximelagatran has shown equivalence to warfarin for stroke prevention in atrial fibrillation.

The fibrinolytic system

Fibrinolysis is the physiological mechanism for dissolving the fibrin meshwork in a thrombus. The process is initiated by activation of plasminogen, a circulating α_2-globulin (Fig. 11.4). Tissue plasminogen activator (t-PA), released from damaged vessels, can cleave plasminogen to the active enzyme plasmin. In the circulation, plasminogen activator inhibitors 1 and 2 rapidly clear tPA. However, t-PA binds locally at the site of release to fibrin, and converts fibrin-bound plasminogen to plasmin. Plasmin splits both fibrinogen and fibrin into degradation products; if this occurs at the site of a thrombus, it produces lysis of the clot matrix. Fibrinolytic therapy is given with a plasminogen activator in such large quantities that the inhibitory controls are overwhelmed.

Fibrinolytic (thrombolytic) agents

Examples: alteplase (recombinant tissue-type plasminogen activator, rt-PA), reteplase, streptokinase, tenecteplase

Mechanisms of action

All thrombolytic drugs activate plasminogen and enhance fibrinolysis. Alteplase is a genetically engineered copy of the naturally occurring t-PA which binds to fibrin. Reteplase is a recombinant deletion-modified form of t-PA with less fibrin binding but also less fibrinogen binding, similar sensitivity to plasminogen activator inhibitor, and a longer duration of action. Tenecteplase is a genetically engineered multiply-modified form of t-PA with increased fibrin specificity, less sensitivity to plasminogen activator inhibitor, and a longer duration of action than t-PA.

Streptokinase is obtained from haemolytic streptococci. Unlike alteplase and related compounds, streptokinase is inactive until it forms a complex with circulating plasminogen; the resultant streptokinase–plasminogen activator complex substitutes for t-PA in the fibrinolytic cascade, causing plasminogen activation.

The effectiveness of any thrombolytic agent depends on the age of the thrombus and the surface area of thrombus exposed to it.

Pharmacokinetics

All thrombolytic agents are given intravenously or intra-arterially. The streptokinase–plasminogen activator complex is degraded enzymatically in the circulation. Some streptokinase is cleared from the plasma before it

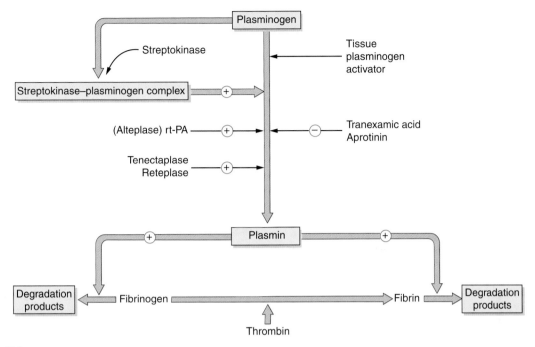

Fig. 11.4
The fibrinolytic system. The fibrinolytic system is linked intimately with the coagulation cascade and platelet function. When a clot is formed via the prothrombotic system, activation of plasminogen to the fibrinolytically active plasmin is initiated by several plasminogen activators, thus lysing the clot. The drugs promoting this act as plasminogen activators (rt-PA, urokinase) or bind to plasminogen (streptokinase), promoting plasmin activity. The antifibrinolytic drugs tranexamic acid and aprotinin inhibit plasminogen activation.

forms an active complex, by combining with circulating neutralising antibody formed during previous streptococcal infections. After the use of streptokinase, or following a streptococcal infection, neutralising antibodies can persist in high titre for several years and substantially reduce the effectiveness of subsequent therapy with streptokinase.

Alteplase and related compounds are metabolised in the liver.

Streptokinase has a slower onset of action than alteplase owing to slow combination with plasminogen. Consequently, the reperfusion of occluded vessels is slower. However, reocclusion is less common, because of the longer duration of action of streptokinase, with a half-life of about 23 min.

The half-life of streptokinase is longer than that of alteplase or reteplase, but similar to that of tenecteplase. Streptokinase is usually given as a short (1 h) infusion for the treatment of coronary artery occlusion, although longer infusions are usual for peripheral arterial occlusions or pulmonary embolism. Infusions of alteplase are given over longer periods, usually for between 3 and 24 h, depending on the condition being treated. Because of its short duration of action, when alteplase has been used to lyse coronary artery thrombus, subsequent anticoagulation with heparin for 48 h is necessary to reduce the reocclusion rate. Reteplase is given as two bolus injections separated by 90 min, and tenecteplase as a single

bolus. Although there are no clinical data, heparin is usually given after reteplase and tenecteplase.

Unwanted effects

- Haemorrhage is usually minor but can occasionally be serious – for example, intracerebral haemorrhage, which occurs in about 1% of those treated (and is slightly more frequent with alteplase and related drugs than with streptokinase). Bleeding can be stopped by antifibrinolytic drugs (see below) or by transfusion of fresh frozen plasma.
- Hypotension: this is dose related and more common with streptokinase. It may be caused by enzymatic release of the vasodilator bradykinin from its circulating precursor. If the infusion of the thrombolytic is stopped for a brief period, the blood pressure usually recovers rapidly and treatment can be continued.
- Allergic reactions: these are rare but can occur with streptokinase, as a consequence of its bacterial origin.

Clinical uses of fibrinolytic agents

Thrombolytic agents are used to treat the following:

- acute myocardial infarction (Ch. 5)
- pulmonary embolism or deep venous thrombosis, in a minority of cases (see above)

- peripheral arterial thromboembolism (Ch. 10)
- restoration of patency of intravenous catheters occluded by clot: this is particularly useful for 'long lines' inserted for intravenous nutrition or administration of cytotoxic drugs.

Antifibrinolytic and haemostatic agents

Antifibrinolytic agents

Examples: tranexamic acid, aprotinin

Mechanisms of action

Tranexamic acid binds to plasminogen, but does not prevent the binding of t-PA and conversion to plasmin. However, the plasmin–tranexamic acid complex cannot bind to fibrin, so fibrinolysis is inhibited.

Aprotinin is a broad-spectrum protease inhibitor. Effects include:

- inhibition of plasmin and therefore fibrinolysis
- inhibition of kallidinogenase (plasma kallikrein): this is involved in amplification of the coagulation cascade at the stage of activation of factor XII (Fig. 11.3); aprotinin therefore interferes with coagulation as well as having an antifibrinolytic effect
- inhibition of platelet activation by blocking the proteolytically activated thrombin receptor site: this confers an antithrombotic effect while still leaving the platelet responsive to formation of haemostatic plugs when exposed to collagen, ADP or adrenaline following endothelial disruption
- anti-inflammatory activity through inhibition of the production of inflammatory cytokines.

Pharmacokinetics

Tranexamic acid is a synthetic amino acid that is incompletely absorbed from the gut and can also be given intravenously. It is excreted unchanged by the kidney and has a short half-life. Aprotinin is a polypeptide that is not absorbed orally and must be given intravenously. It has an intermediate half-life and is filtered by the kidney, but most is then reabsorbed by the renal tubule and metabolised by lysosomal enzymes in the proximal renal tubule.

Unwanted effects

- hypersensitivity reactions occasionally occur with aprotinin
- nausea, vomiting or diarrhoea, and disturbances of colour vision can occur with tranexamic acid
- the theoretical risk of a thrombotic tendency does not appear to be a clinical problem.

Desmopressin

Desmopressin briefly increases the plasma concentration of clotting factor VIII and von Willebrand factor, an adhesion protein in blood vessel walls. Factor VIII accelerates the process of fibrin formation and von Willebrand factor enhances platelet adhesion to subendothelial tissue. Desmopressin is discussed in Chapter 43.

Clinical uses of antifibrinolytic and haemostatic agents

Haemostatic agents have a number of clinical uses:

- to prevent bleeding after surgery, especially of the prostate or after dental extraction in haemophilia
- desmopressin is used in mild congenital bleeding disorders such as haemophilia A or von Willebrand's disease; it is given to reduce spontaneous or traumatic bleeding, or as a prophylactic before surgery
- tranexamic acid is used for the treatment of menorrhagia, or bleeding following overdose of a thrombolytic drug
- aprotinin is mainly used prophylactically for reduction of bleeding during cardiovascular surgery with extracorporeal circulation
- tranexamic acid is used for treatment of hereditary angioedema.

FURTHER READING

Anticoagulants

Agnelli G, Becattini C, Kirschstein T (2002) Thrombolysis versus heparin in the treatment of pulmonary embolism. A clinical outcome-based meta-analysis. *Arch Intern Med* 162, 2537–2541

British Thoracic Society Standards of Care Committee Pulmonary Embolism Guideline Development Group (2003) British Thoracic Society guidelines for the management of suspected pulmonary embolism. *Thorax* 58, 470–483

Donnan GA, Dewey HM, Chambers BR (2004) Warfarin for atrial fibrillation: the end of an era? *Lancet Neurol* 3, 305–308

Geerts WH, Heit JA, Clagett GP et al (2000) Prevention of venous thromboembolism. *Chest* 119, 132s–175s

Ginsberg JS, Greer I, Hirsch J (2001) Use of antithrombotic agents during pregnancy. *Chest* 119, s122–s131

Goldhaber SZ (2004) Pulmonary embolism. *Lancet* 363, 1295–1305

Haemostasis and Thrombosis Task Force of the British Society For Haematology (1998) Guidelines on anticoagulation: third edition. *Br J Haematol* 101, 374–387

Hamm CW (2003) Anti-integrin therapy *Annu Rev Med* 54, 425–435

Hodl R, Klein W (2003) The role of low-molecular-weight heparins in cardiovascular medicine. *J Clin Pharm Ther* 28, 371–378

Hyers TM (2003) Management of venous thromboembolism. *Arch Intern Med* 163, 759–768

Nutescu EA, Wittkowsky AK (2004) Direct thrombin inhibitors for anticoagulation. *Ann Pharmacother* 38, 99–109

Schulman S (2003) Unresolved issues in anticoagulant therapy. *J Thromb Haemost* 1, 1464–1470

Tovey C, Wyatt S (2003) Diagnosis, investigation and management of deep vein thrombosis. *BMJ* 326, 1180–1184

Antiplatelet agents

Antiplatelet Trialist's Collaboration (2002) Collaborative meta-analysis of randomised trials of antiplatelet therapy for prevention of death, myocardial infarction and stroke in high risk patients. *BMJ* 324, 71–86

Behan MW, Storey RF (2004) Antiplatelet therapy in cardiovascular disease. *Postgrad Med J* 80, 155–164

Kong DF, Hasselblad V, Harrington RA et al (2003) Meta-analysis of survival with platelet glycoprotein IIb/IIIa antagonists for percutaneous coronary interventions. *Am J Cardiol* 92, 651–655

Micelli G, Cavallini A (2004) New therapeutic strategies with antiplatelet agents. *Neurol Sci* 25(suppl 1), s13–s15

Task force on the management of acute coronary syndromes of the European Society of Cardiology (2002) Management of acute coronary syndromes in patients presenting without persistent ST-segment elevation. *Eur Heart J* 23, 1809–1840

Vorchheimer DA, Badimon JJ, Fuster VV (1999) Platelet glycoprotein IIb/IIIa receptor antagonists in cardiovascular disease. *JAMA* 281, 1407–1414

Fibrinolytic drugs

Khan IJ, Gowda RM (2003) Clinical perspectives and therapeutics of thrombolysis. *Int J Cardiol* 91, 115–127

Nordt TK, Bode C (2003) Thrombolysis: newer thrombolytic agents and their role in clinical medicine. *Heart* 89, 1358–1362

Haemostatic drugs

Wellington K, Wagstaff AJ (2003) Tranexamic acid. A review of its use in the management of menorrhagia. *Drugs* 63, 1417–1433

Self-assessment

1. In the following questions, the first statement, in italics, is true. Is the accompanying statement also true?

   a. *Tenecteplase is a modified form of tissue-type plasminogen activator with a longer half-life.* Thrombolytic infusions of recombinant tissue-type plasminogen activator (rt-PA) for myocardial infarction are usually given for 1 h duration and streptokinase for 3–24 h.

   b. *Warfarin has a long half-life (36 h) in plasma.* Warfarin readily crosses the placenta.

   c. *Clopidogrel, dipyridamole and aspirin have similar clinical efficacies as antiplatelet agents.* Clopidogrel has its antithrombotic action by enhancing the action of ADP on platelets.

   d. *Abciximab in conjunction with heparin and aspirin is used before coronary angioplasty with stenting for high-risk procedures.* Abciximab is an antibody directed against the glycoprotein GPIIb/IIIa receptor on platelets.

   e. *Aspirin irreversibly inhibits cyclo-oxygenase enzymes.* Aspirin inhibits platelet aggregation at doses below those needed for an anti-inflammatory effect.

   f. *Warfarin inhibits the activation of clotting factors II, VII, IX and X, which depend upon vitamin K for their synthesis.* Anticoagulant activity of warfarin is inhibited by broad-spectrum antibacterial agents.

   g. *Tranexamic acid is an antifibrinolytic agent used in the treatment of menorrhagia.* Tranexamic acid enhances plasminogen activation.

   h. *LMWHs have longer half-lives than unfractionated heparin.* Once administered, the action of heparin cannot be reversed.

2. Comparing heparin, warfarin and ximelagatran, choose the one correct statement.

   A. Warfarin is a more predictable anticoagulant than ximelagatran.

   B. If a predictable oral anticoagulant is required before surgery, heparin is the drug of choice.

   C. Dosage adjustment of warfarin but not of ximelagatran would be required if a person subsequently started treatment with the proton pump inhibitor omeprazole.

   D. In overdose, the effects of ximelagatran but not of warfarin can be reversed with appropriate antagonists.

   E. During treatment with a broad-spectrum antimicrobial, the anticoagulant effects of warfarin and ximelagatran would be reduced.

3. Case history questions

   > A 51-year-old obese female was treated with oestrogen replacement therapy for 18 months because of perimenopausal symptoms. She was scheduled for a hip replacement.

   a. Was anticoagulant therapy necessary for this woman?

   b. Should thromboprophylaxis have been started before surgery?

c. Should heparin or warfarin have been chosen for prophylaxis and what routes of administration were appropriate?

The hip replacement was carried out successfully and the woman was discharged from hospital after 5 days, although heparin therapy was continued for a further 5 days.

d. Why was therapy continued for this extended period and what out-of-hospital therapeutic prophylaxis could be considered?

The answers are provided on pages 712–713.

Drugs used to affect haemostasis

Drug	Half-life (h)	Elimination	Comments
Antiplatelet drugs			
Abciximab	0.5	Metabolism?	Used as an adjunct to heparin and aspirin in high-risk subjects (specialist use only); antibody fragment to glycoprotein IIb/IIIa receptor on platelets; produces long-lasting blockade of receptors; given intravenously; mechanism of elimination not defined (probably tissue uptake and proteolysis)
Aspirin	0.25–0.35	Metabolism	Low dose used for the secondary prevention of thrombotic cerebrovascular or cardiovascular disease; given orally; half-life of active salicylic acid metabolite is 3–20 h
Clopidogrel	5–8 (inactive metabolite)	Metabolism	Used for the prevention of ischaemic events in subjects with a history of symptomatic ischaemic disease; given orally; prodrug requiring hepatic bioactivation by CYP1A; acts via an active metabolite which has not been identified; the half-life is for an inactive metabolite (and may not relate to the duration of clinical effect)
Dipyridamole	12	Metabolism	Used as an adjunct to oral anticoagulants in subjects with prosthetic heart valves and for the secondary prevention of ischaemic stroke; given orally or by intravenous injection (for diagnostic purposes); metabolised largely to glucuronic acid conjugates which are excreted in bile with some enterohepatic circulation
Epoprostenol	3 min	Metabolism	Used in combination with heparin during renal dialysis and in combination with oral anticoagulants for primary pulmonary hypertension resistant to other treatments; potent vasodilator; eliminated as glucuronide
Eptifibatide	1.5–2	Renal + metabolism	A cyclic hexapeptide used as an adjunct to heparin and aspirin in high-risk subjects with unstable angina (specialist use only); glycoprotein IIb/IIIa receptor inhibitor; given intravenously; eliminated unchanged and as a deaminated product
Tirofiban	2	Renal	A nonpeptide used as an adjunct to heparin and aspirin in high-risk subjects with unstable angina (specialist use only); glycoprotein IIb/IIIa receptor inhibitor; given intravenously; limited metabolism; eliminated in urine and bile
Anticoagulants (heparin-like)			All drugs are macromolecules and given by injection; they are eliminated by tissue uptake and degradation; LMWHs are as effective as unfractionated heparin and may be more effective in orthopaedic practice; the longer half-life allows treatment by once-daily subcutaneous injection
Bemiparin	4–5[a]	–	LMWH
Certoparin	–	–	LMWH; few data available
Dalteparin sodium	2–4[a]	Renal	LMWH; unlike heparin, elimination is not dose-dependent

continued

Drugs used to affect haemostasis (continued)

Drug	Half-life (h)	Elimination	Comments
Danaparoid sodium	17–28[a]	Renal?	LMWH; useful in prophylaxis of deep vein thrombosis on a named patient basis only; unlike heparin, elimination is not dose-dependent
Enoxaparin	3–6[a]	Metabolism + renal	LMWH; eliminated by hepatic degradation and limited renal excretion
Fondaparinux	18	Renal	Used for prophylaxis in subjects undergoing major orthopedic surgery of the legs; a synthetic pentasaccharide that inhibits factor X; excreted in the urine unchanged
Heparin (also known as unfractionated heparin)	0.4–2.5[a]	–	Used as the initial treatment for deep vein thrombosis and pulmonary embolism, as an intravenous loading dose followed by an intravenous infusion or intermittent subcutaneous injection; also given by subcutaneous injection for deep vein thrombosis and prophylaxis in general surgery; dose-dependent half-life
Lepirudin	1.5	Renal + metabolism?	Used for patients with heparin-associated thrombocytopenia type II who require parenteral anticoagulation; a recombinant hirudin (not related to heparins); acts directly on thrombin (independent of antithrombin III); given by slow intravenous injection or intravenous infusion; eliminated by glomerular filtration; very prolonged half-life in renal failure; possibly some metabolism
Reviparin	–	–	LMWH; few data available
Tinzaparin	3–4[a]	Metabolism + renal	LMWH; eliminated by hepatic degradation and renal excretion
Anticoagulants (oral)			Warfarin is the drug of choice and the others are seldom required (but see Table 11.1 for details of a new oral anticoagulant [ximelagatran] that is not yet available or licensed in the UK)
Acenocoumarol	7 (*R*) 1 (*S*)	Metabolism	Uses are as given for warfarin; *R*- and *S*-enantiomers show different kinetics
Phenindione	5–6	Metabolism + renal	Uses are as given for warfarin; urinary metabolites give a reddish colour to alkalinised urine
Warfarin	18–35 (*S*) 20–60 (*R*)	Metabolism	Used mainly for deep vein thrombosis; also used for pulmonary embolism, and for prophylaxis of embolism in rheumatic heart disease, atrial fibrillation and after insertion of prosthetic heart valves; activated by oxidation; *S*-enantiomer more active and oxidised by CYP2C9; *R*-enantiomer is reduced
Thrombolytic agents (also known as fibrinolytic agents)			Activate plasminogen to plasmin; used in the treatment of myocardial infarction; macromolecules that are given intravenously
Alteplase (rt-PA)	0.5	Hepatic uptake	Tissue-type plasmingen activator; given by intravenous injection (when the action may be limited by distribution, which has a half-life of only 3–11 min) or by intravenous infusion

continued

Drugs used to affect haemostasis *(continued)*

Drug	Half-life (h)	Elimination	Comments
(Anistreplase)	2	Deacylation	Prodrug that is no longer available in the UK; deacylation releases the active moiety over a prolonged period
Reteplase	0.4–0.5	Hepatic uptake	Given by intravenous injection over not more than 2 min; cleared by liver and kidney
Streptokinase	1	Binding to plasminogen	Also used for life-threatening venous thrombosis and pulmonary embolism; given by intravenous infusion; rapid initial decrease in concentrations when there is a high antibody titre
Tenecteplase	1.5–2	Metabolism	A modified tissue-type plasminogen activator produced by recombinant DNA technology; higher selectivity for fibrin than alteplase; given by intravenous injection over 10 s; eliminated by hepatic metabolism
Antifibrinolytic drugs and haemostatic agents			
Aprotinin	7	Metabolism in kidney	Used during and after major heart surgery to prevent blood loss and in subjects with hyperplasminaemia; an inhibitor that acts on plasmin and kallikrein; given by slow intravenous injection or infusion; rapid uptake by kidney (half-life 1 h), where it is degraded into oligopeptides; slower uptake and release from other tissues
Etamsylate	–	–	Reduces capillary bleeding, probably by affecting platelet adhesion; given orally; no published kinetic data available
Tranexamic acid	1.4	Renal	Used in hereditary angioedema, epistaxis and after excessive thrombolytic dosage; given orally or by slow intravenous injection; eliminated by glomerular filtration

[a]Value depends on the clotting factor measured to reflect drug presence and activity, rather than chemical analysis of the drug.
LMWH, low-molecular-weight heparin.

Drug compendium

The respiratory system

Asthma and chronic obstructive pulmonary disease

Asthma and chronic obstructive pulmonary disease (COPD) show several similarities in their clinical features, but are considered to be distinct entities with clinical overlap. Both are inflammatory disorders of the bronchi.

In asthma, the underlying problem is a persistent and excessive T-helper cell type 2 (Th2)-dominated immune response and resulting inflammation; this is accompanied by reduced Th1 involvement in the structural and defensive status of tissues (Ch. 38). The overall imbalance in T-helper cell types results in persistent inflammation, increased numbers of airways smooth muscle cells, proliferation of blood vessels, epithelial transformation into mucus-secreting cells and increased matrix deposition. Adequate suppression of the inflammation should be the basis of treatment, allowing resolution of the pathological changes. The predominant inflammatory cells are mast cells, eosinophils, and $CD4^+$ T-lymphoctes, with fewer macrophages. Important inflammatory mediators are leukotriene D_4 (LTD_4), histamine, a variety of cytokines including interleukin-4 (IL-4), IL-5, IL-9, IL-13, eotaxin, and RANTES (regulated on activation normal T-cell expressed and secreted), and there is relatively little evidence of oxidative stress. In asthma, all airways are involved in the inflammatory process, but the degree of fibrosis and mucus secretion are modest, with no parenchymal destruction.

By contrast, in COPD, the predominant infiltrating cells are neutrophils, macrophages and cytotoxic $CD8^+$ T-lymphocytes. The major inflammatory mediators are LTB_4, tumour necrosis factor alpha, IL-8 and growth-related oncogene alpha. There is increased oxidative stress due to reactive oxygen species, for example from cigarette smoke and released from neutrophils and inflammatory macrophages. The inflammatory process predominantly affects the peripheral airways, there is a marked fibrotic reaction, parenchymal destruction and excessive bronchial mucus secretion.

Asthma

Reversible airways obstruction is the characteristic feature of asthma, which is often associated with an atopic disposition. Exposure to allergens, or possibly other environmental determinants, may then result in expression of the condition. Despite the presence of atopy and eosinophilia, neither is absolutely required for asthma without other concurrent risk factors.

The most common symptoms of asthma are wheeze and breathlessness. In younger people, cough, especially at night, may be the only symptom.

The pathogenesis of asthma involves several processes (Figs 12.1 and 12.2). Chronic inflammation of the bronchial mucosa is prominent, with infiltration of activated T-lymphocytes and eosinophils. This leads to the release of several powerful chemical mediators that can damage the epithelial lining of the airways (see above). Many of these mediators are released following activation and degranulation of mast cells in the bronchial tree, which occurs in response to a variety of immunological or irritant insults to the airways. Some of the mediators act as chemotactic agents for other inflammatory cells. They also produce mucosal oedema, which narrows the airways and stimulates smooth muscle contraction, leading to bronchoconstriction (Table 12.1). Excessive production of mucus can cause further airways obstruction by plugging the bronchiolar lumen.

Viral upper respiratory tract infections exacerbate the mucosal inflammatory process, while exposure to allergens (such as pollen or the faeces of house-dust mite), irritants (such as dust or gases) or exercise can cause bronchoconstriction in sensitive airways. Attacks of asthma rapidly follow exposure to a provoking agent. Initial recovery may then be followed some 4–6 h later by a late-phase bronchoconstrictor response, which can leave the bronchi hyper-reactive to various irritants for several weeks.

Treatment of asthma has two aims:

- relief of symptoms
- reduction of airways inflammation.

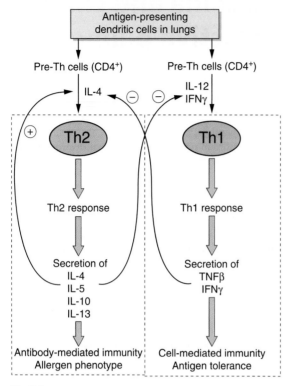

Fig. 12.1
Immune differentiation in response to antigens. In allergic asthma, the T-helper type 2 (Th2) response is amplified in preference to the type 1 (Th1) response. Th2-generated cytokines are responsible for developing and sustaining airway inflammation in asthma. IL-4 and IL-13 promote synthesis of IgE antibodies (Ch. 38), IL-5 and IL-9 attract and activate eosinophils, IL-10 inhibits IL-12 production. IFN, interferon; IL, interleukin; TNF, tumour necrosis factor.

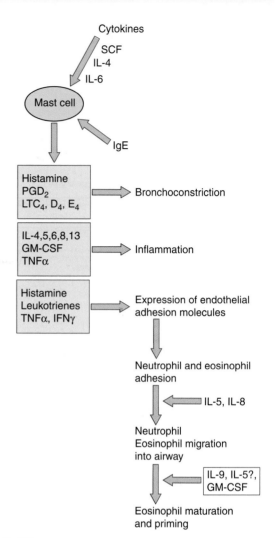

Fig. 12.2
Inflammatory mediators in asthma. Activation of mast cells results in secretion of several mediators that contribute to the pathogenesis of asthma. These mediators can directly produce bronchoconstriction and can both initiate the acute inflammatory response and attract and activate cells responsible for further inflammatory mediator production and maintaining chronic inflammation. GM-CSF, granulocyte and macrophage colony-stimulating factor; IFN, interferon; IL, interleukin; LT, leukotriene; PG, prostaglandin; SCF, stem cell factor TNF, tissue necrosis factor.

Chronic obstructive pulmonary disease

COPD is a symptom complex that is characterised by persistent airflow limitation which has a tendency to exacerbations triggered by respiratory infection. It is often accompanied by chronic bronchitis and emphysema. The airflow limitation is usually slowly progressive and largely irreversible. About 95% of people with COPD are, or have been, cigarette smokers. There is wide variability in the rate of decline in pulmonary function in smokers, with about 10–20% showing an accelerated decline, which may reflect a genetic susceptibility. The other causes are exposure to air pollution and inherited antiprotease deficiency. The airflow limitation results from a combination of decreased bronchial luminal diameter (produced by wall thickening, intraluminal mucus and changes in the fluid lining the small airways) and dynamic airways collapse due to emphysema. Corresponding histological changes include an

increase in goblet cells in the bronchial mucosa and an increase in muscle mass in the bronchial wall, with interstitial fibrosis. Airways wall inflammation, particularly with mononuclear cells, is common, especially in the early phases. Changes in small airways are most important in mild to moderate COPD.

Emphysema is largely a pathological description, and is defined as enlargement of airways distal to the terminal bronchioles owing to destructive changes that may involve the entire acinus (panacinar) or the central part of the acinus (centriacinar). Lung parenchymal destruction is largely mediated by tissue proteases such

Table 12.1
Mediators involved in the inflammatory process in asthma

	Bronchoconstriction	Mucosal oedema	Mucosal inflammation	Mucus secretion
Histamine	+	+		+
Leukotrienes C_4, D_4 and E_4	+	+		+
Prostaglandin D_2	+	+		+
Thromboxane A_2	+			+
Bradykinin	+	+	+	+
Platelet activating factor	+	+	+	+
Eosinophil chemotactic factors			+	
Neutrophil chemotactic factors			+	

as the matrix metalloproteinase gelatinase B (MMP-9) and cathepsins that are released by neutrophils and macrophages. Generation of excessive amounts of reactive oxygen species inhibits the antiproteases that normally protect the lung against such attack. Tissue destruction leads to a loss of lung recoil on expiration. Emphysema is probably the dominant factor in severe COPD.

The most frequent symptoms are gradually progressive breathlessness and cough. The cough is often productive and usually worse in the morning; its severity is unrelated to the degree of airflow limitation. Repeated respiratory infections are common. Unlike asthma, the airflow limitation is largely irreversible. However, about 10% of people with COPD show considerable reversibility of airflow limitation. These individuals have a mixed inflammatory pattern that probably represents an overlap between asthma and COPD (wheezy bronchitis).

Drugs for asthma and chronic obstructive pulmonary disease

Drug delivery to the lung

For the treatment of airways disease, direct delivery of drug to the lung by aerosol spray allows the use of smaller doses and therefore reduces the risk of unwanted effects (see Table 12.2). The size of the aerosol particle that is inhaled determines whether or not it will reach the airways and whereabouts in the airways it will be deposited. Particles larger than 5 µm will impact on the upper airways and will be swallowed. Particles smaller than 0.5 µm will not deposit in the lower respiratory tract and are exhaled. The optimal particle size for treatment is 1–3 µm. There are several methods for delivery of aerosols.

Pressurised metered-dose inhaler. This is the most common delivery device. Manually activated inhalers

are widely used since they are convenient and inexpensive, but they require coordination of inhalation and activation of the device. About one-third of users find this difficult, and even if coordination is optimal, about 70–90% of the aerosol is deposited in the oropharynx, then swallowed. Chlorofluorocarbon (CFC) propellants have been phased out and replaced by other propellants such as hydrofluorocarbons because of concerns over atmospheric ozone depletion. The inhaler should be shaken before use.

Large-volume spacers. Plastic reservoirs of about 750 ml volume can be attached to a metered-dose inhaler to remove the need to coordinate aerosol activation and breathing. The inhaler is activated into the spacer, and the person breathes through the mouthpiece, which is fitted with a valve to ensure the aerosol is inhaled. For young children, a small-volume (350 ml) spacer is used (attached to a facemask for very young children). The spacer also allows evaporation of propellant and thus may create more droplets of the correct size to deposit in the airways. Inhalation of the contents should be completed within 10 s. When the device is washed, it should not be wiped dry, since this creates an electrostatic charge which attracts particles and reduces drug delivery. Addition of a spacer makes a metered-dose inhaler system less portable. To overcome this, one manufacturer has incorporated a collapsible spacer into its inhaler device.

Breath-activated devices. There are several types, delivering either an aerosol or dry powder. The aerosol type is a modified metered-dose inhaler that is activated when air is drawn through the mouthpiece, provided airflow exceeds about 30 l min⁻¹. Dry-powder inhalers contain particles of drug of optimal size for deposition. Inspiration through the device generates turbulence, which disperses the particles in the inspired air. Breath-activated devices require a high airflow and are therefore less efficient than metered-dose inhalers, especially in those with severe airflow limitation.

Nebulisers. These are devices that are used with a facemask or mouthpiece to deliver drug from a reservoir solution. There are two types. Jet nebulisers use air or oxygen passing through a narrow orifice to suck drug solution from a reservoir into a feed tube with fine ligaments. The impact of the solution on these ligaments generates droplets (Venturi principle). Ultrasonic jet nebulisers use a piezoelectric crystal vibrating at high frequency. The vibrations are transmitted through a buffer to the drug solution and form a fountain of liquid in the nebulisation chamber. Ultrasonic nebulisers produce a more uniform particle size than do jet nebulisers. Up to ten times the amount of drug is required in a nebuliser to produce the same degree of bronchodilation achieved by a metered-dose inhaler. Delivery is more efficient via a mouthpiece than via a mask.

Symptom-relieving drugs or airflow obstruction

The β_2-adrenoceptor agonists

> Examples: salbutamol, terbutaline, salmeterol, formoterol

Mechanism of action and effects

The airways are rich in β_2-adrenoceptors, which are found on bronchial smooth muscle but also on several other cell types. Effects of receptor stimulation include:

- bronchodilation via generation of intracellular cyclic adenosine monophosphate (cAMP)
- inhibition of mediator release from mast cells
- enhanced mucociliary clearance.

Selectivity of an agonist for the β_2-adrenoceptor reduces systemic unwanted effects from stimulation of β_1-adrenoceptors.

Pharmacokinetics

The selectivity of β_2-adrenoceptor agonists is dose-dependent. Inhalation of drug aids selectivity since it delivers small but effective doses to the airways and minimises systemic exposure (Table 12.2). The dose–response relationship for bronchodilation is log-linear; therefore, a tenfold increase in dose is required to double the effect. A metered-dose aerosol inhaler is the most frequently used delivery mechanism, but breath-activated devices and nebuliser solutions are available.

After inhalation, the onset of drug action is rapid, often within 5 min. Agents such as salbutamol have an intermediate duration of action (producing bronchodilation for up to about 6 h), far longer than the natural adrenoceptor agonists. Their chemical structure prevents neuronal uptake and reduces their affinity for catechol-O-methyl transferase, which metabolises catecholamines (Ch. 4).

The long-acting agent salmeterol bronchodilates for up to 12 h by virtue of a long lipophilic side-chain on the molecule, which binds to an area adjacent to the active site of the receptor, producing prolonged receptor activation. Formoterol has a prolonged duration of action by entering the lipid bilayer of the cell membrane, from which it is gradually released to stimulate the receptor.

Salbutamol and terbutaline can also be given orally (as conventional or modified-release formulations), or by subcutaneous or intramuscular injections or intravenous infusion. However, larger doses are required to deliver an adequate amount to the lungs by any of these routes. This reduces the selectivity for β_2-adrenoceptors, and systemic unwanted effects can be troublesome.

Table 12.2
Comparison of aerosol and oral therapy for asthma

	Aerosol	Oral
Ideal pharmacokinetics	Slow absorption from the lung surface	Good oral absorption
	Rapid systemic clearance	Long systemic action
Dose	Low dose delivered direct to target	High systemic dose necessary to achieve an appropriate concentration in the lung
Systemic drug concentration	Low	High
Incidence of unwanted effects	Low	High
Distribution in the lung	Reduced in severe disease	Unaffected by disease
Compliance	Good with bronchodilators	Good
	Poor with anti-inflammatory	
Ease of administration	Difficult for small children and infirm people[a]	Good
Effectiveness	Good in mild to moderate disease	Good even in severe disease

[a]May be improved by breath-activated inhalers or spacing devices. Nebulisers can be used for severe exacerbations.

Tolerance to pharmacological bronchodilation can occur with β_2-adrenoceptor agonists but not with inhaled antimuscarinic drugs. The Committee on Safety of Medicines has advised that salmeterol and formoterol should not be used for relief of acute asthma and should only be used along with a concurrently administered corticosteroid.

Unwanted effects

- Fine skeletal muscle tremor from β_2-adrenoceptor stimulation.
- Tachycardia and arrhythmias result from both β_1- and β_2-adrenoceptor stimulation when high doses of inhaled drug are used, or after oral or parenteral administration.
- Acute metabolic responses to high-dose β_2-adrenoceptor stimulation include hypokalaemia, hypomagnesaemia and hyperglycaemia. They do not persist during long-term use.
- Paradoxical bronchospasm has been reported with inhalation, usually when given for the first time or with a new canister.
- Headache.

Concern has been expressed that regular use of high doses inhaled β_2-adrenoceptor agonists may be linked with asthma deaths by precipitation of serious arrhythmias. An alternative possibility is that high doses might allow people to tolerate initial exposure to larger doses of allergens or irritants, which then produce an enhanced late asthmatic response. However, it is more likely that the use of high doses is really a reflection of the severity of the underlying asthma.

Antimuscarinic agents

Examples: ipratropium, tiotropium

Mechanism of action and effects

There are three types of muscarinic receptors in the airways.

- M_1 receptors facilitate cholinergic neurotransmission at parasympathetic ganglia.
- M_2 receptors are presynaptic autoreceptors on cholinergic neurons and provide negative feedback that modulates acetylcholine release.
- M_3 receptors are postsynaptic and mediate bronchoconstriction and mucus secretion in response to parasympathetic stimulation, via generation of cyclic guanosine monophosphate (cGMP). Inhibition of M_3 receptors produces bronchodilation.

The antimuscarinic drugs used for bronchodilation are non-selective, and bind to all three types of muscarinic receptors in the lung. It remains uncertain whether they also have specific anti-inflammatory effects in addition to their actions on bronchial smooth muscle and mucus secretion. There is limited evidence that they may reduce pro-inflammatory mediator release from epithelial cells and reduce production of chemotaxins by alveolar macrophages. The clinical relevance of these effects is not known. Their main use is in COPD, where they are effective; they are of less value for bronchodilation in acute mild-to-moderate asthma, but may have a place when added to β_2-adrenoceptor agonists in severe exacerbations of asthma.

Pharmacokinetics

The antimuscarinic drugs used for bronchodilation are N-quaternary congeners of the tertiary-structured atropine; they are poorly absorbed orally and do not cross the blood–brain barrier. They are given exclusively by inhalation from a metered-dose aerosol or a nebuliser. They have a slower onset of action (30–60 min) than salbutamol (5–10 min), probably due to slow absorption from the surface of the airways. The duration of action is related to the rate of removal from the receptors in the airways, and not the half-life of elimination from the circulation. The duration of action of ipratropium is short, due to rapid dissociation from M_3 receptors, with a half-life at the receptor of 16 min. Tiotropium dissociates much more slowly from M_1 and M_3 receptors (its half-life at M_3 receptors is 35 h) than from M_2 receptors (half-life 3.5h), giving it a long duration of action.

Unwanted effects

Direct delivery of antimuscarinic drugs to the lung is the main reason for the relative lack of many of the systemic unwanted effects characteristically associated with atropine (Ch. 4).

- dry mouth is the most common effect
- nausea, constipation
- headache
- tiotropium can cause urinary retention in men with prostatism
- can contribute to angle-closure glaucoma (Ch. 50).

Methylxanthines

Examples: theophylline, aminophylline

Mechanism of action and effects

Methylxanthines are a group of naturally occurring substances found in coffee, tea, chocolate and related foodstuffs. Theophylline (1,3-dimethylxanthine), and its ester derivative aminophylline, are the only compounds in clinical use. They are chemically similar to caffeine.

Methylxanthines have vasodilator, anti-inflammatory and immunomodulatory actions. The mechanisms of action of methylxanthines are multiple, controversial and uncertain.

- Inhibition of the enzyme phosphodiesterase (PDE), which degrades cyclic nucleotide second messengers, has been suggested to explain methylxanthine actions. Theophylline preferentially inhibits PDE III and PDE IV isoenzymes – which are found in bronchial smooth muscle and several inflammatory cells, including mast cells – and increases intracellular cAMP. Theophylline also inhibits PDE V and reduces the breakdown of cGMP. The rise in intracellular cAMP and cGMP in bronchial smooth muscle leads to inhibition of large conductance voltage-gated Ca^{2+}-activated K^+ channels in the cell membrane. These channels are responsible for cell repolarisation. However, theophylline only produces bronchodilation at relatively high plasma concentrations (10–20 mg l^{-1}) and also drugs that have a greater effect as PDE inhibitors (such as dipyridamole) do not bronchodilate. PDE inhibition also stimulates ciliary beat frequency and water transport across the airway epithelium. These actions increase mucociliary clearance. By contrast, in cardiac muscle, theophylline increases the force and rate of contraction (Ch. 7).
- Increased diaphragmatic contractility has been reported at lower plasma theophylline concentrations than those required for bronchodilation. This may improve lung ventilation.
- Adenosine receptor antagonism may be relevant to some of the clinical effects of methylxanthines (see also adenosine; Ch. 8). Theophylline is a potent inhibitor of adenosine A_1- and A_2-receptors and may reduce bronchoconstriction by this mechanism. Adenosine releases histamine and leukotrienes from mast cells, which results in the constriction of hyper-responsive airways in people with asthma. (However, enprofylline, which is a much more potent bronchodilator than theophylline, does not inhibit adenosine, so this mechanism is equivocal.) Adenosine receptor antagonists also produce central nervous system (CNS) stimulation, which improves mental performance and alertness, and, in the kidney, reduces tubular Na^+ reabsorption and leads to natriuresis and diuresis.
- Activation of histone deacetylases. Acetylation of core histones activates pro-inflammatory transcription factors, such as nuclear factor-κB and activator protein-1. If the activity of histone deacetylases is increased, then the inflammatory genes will be suppressed. This anti-inflammatory effect of theophylline occurs at drug plasma concentrations of 5–10 mg l^{-1}, similar to those that produce clinical benefit. This action may only be relevant in potentiating the anti-inflammatory effects of corticosteroids (see Ch. 44), since histone deacetylases are only effective if recruited to the site of inflammation by activated glucocorticoid receptors.

Pharmacokinetics

The extent of theophylline absorption from the gut is unpredictable, with considerable inter-individual variation, and it is irritant to the stomach. This, and the short plasma half-life, has resulted in the widespread use of modified-release formulations. Theophylline has a narrow therapeutic index and since different formulations have dissimilar release characteristics, they are not readily interchangeable. Theophylline is metabolised in the liver by cytochrome P450 CYP1A2 isoenzyme and, to a lesser extent, by CYP3A4, giving the potential for drug interactions. Theophylline can also be given orally as a more soluble ester prodrug aminophylline, which is hydrolysed rapidly after absorption from the gut to theophylline and ethylenediamine. Aminophylline can also be given by intravenous infusion. Measurement of blood theophylline concentrations is valuable as a guide to effective dosing.

Unwanted effects

Most are dose-related and can arise within the accepted therapeutic plasma concentration range.

- Gastrointestinal upset, including nausea and vomiting (from PDE IV inhibition in the vomiting centre) and diarrhoea.
- CNS stimulation, including insomnia, irritability and, occasionally, seizures at high plasma concentrations (from adenosine receptor antagonism), and headache (from PDE inhibition).
- Hypotension from peripheral vasodilation. PDE III is present in the smooth muscle cells of many blood vessels. Unlike other peripheral vessels, cerebral arteries are constricted by methylxanthines; adenosine is a vasodilator of cranial blood vessels and methylxanthines may work in this vascular bed by inhibition of purinergic receptors.
- Cardiac stimulation produces various arrhythmias. Hypokalaemia can occur acutely, especially after intravenous injection, which also promotes cardiac arrhythmias.
- Tolerance to the beneficial effects of methylxanthines can occur.
- Drug interactions can be troublesome, due to the narrow therapeutic index of theophylline. Hepatic enzyme inhibitors such as ciprofloxacin, erythromycin, clarithromycin, fluconazole, ketoconazole (Ch. 51), and fluvoxamine (Ch. 22) can precipitate theophylline toxicity.

Anti-inflammatory drugs for airways obstruction

Corticosteroids

Examples: beclometasone dipropionate, budesonide, hydrocortisone, fluticasone propionate, mometasone, prednisolone

Mechanism of action and effects

Glucocorticoids are the most effective class of drug in the treatment of chronic asthma but are relatively ineffective in COPD. They are recommended as preventers when inhaled β_2-adrenoceptor agonists are used more than once daily. They act to suppress inflammation and the immune response. Powerful glucocorticoids, devoid of significant mineralocorticoid activity, are usually used.

Intracellular events involved in the anti-inflammatory action of corticosteroids are given in Chapter 44. A major effect in asthma is probably activation of glucocorticoid receptors that inhibit transcription of genes coding for the cytokines involved in inflammation. Glucocorticoid receptors recruit histone deacetylases to the transcription complex of activated inflammatory genes. The deacetylation of core histones at the transcription complex silences genes that have been activated by inflammatory stimuli. Used long-term, corticosteroids reduce airway responsiveness to several bronchoconstrictor mediators and block both the early and late reactions to allergen. Following a delay of 6–12 h, several anti-inflammatory actions occur which may be important in asthma.

Short-term anti-inflammatory effects include:

- reduced inflammatory cell activation (including macrophages, T-lymphocytes, eosinophils and airway epithelial cells)
- decreased IgE synthesis
- reduced mucosal oedema and decreased local generation of inflammatory prostaglandins and leukotrienes by inhibition of phospholipase A_2 (see also Ch. 29)
- β-adrenoceptor upregulation, which restores responsiveness to β_2-adrenoceptor agonists.

Long-term anti-inflammatory effects include:

- reduced T-cell cytokine production (Ch. 39) and reduced dendritic cell signalling to T-cells
- reduced eosinophil deposition in bronchial mucosa (by removing cytokine stimulation, reducing expression of epithelial adhesion molecules and enhancing apoptosis)
- reduced mast cell deposition in bronchial mucosa (although the release of mediators from these cells is unaffected)

- reversal of the excess epithelial cell shedding and goblet cell hyperplasia found in the bronchial epithelium in asthma.

Inhaled corticosteroids produce some improvement in asthmatic symptoms after 24 h and a maximum response after 1–2 weeks. Reduction in airway responsiveness to allergens and irritants occurs gradually over several months. Corticosteroids block the late-phase reaction to allergens in asthma. However, many of the chronic structural changes in the airways in asthma are unaffected by corticosteroids.

Pharmacokinetics

Corticosteroids can be used intravenously or orally in severe asthma. However, whenever possible, they are given by inhalation of an aerosol or dry powder to minimise systemic unwanted effects. Desirable properties of an inhaled corticosteroid include low rates of absorption across mucosal surfaces (such as the lung, but also including the gut for swallowed drug) and rapid inactivation once absorbed. Beclometasone dipropionate fulfils the former criterion, but it is only slowly inactivated once it reaches the systemic circulation. Budesonide (which is inactivated by extensive first-pass metabolism in the liver if systemically absorbed) and fluticasone (which is very poorly absorbed from the gut) are not given orally and may be preferred if high doses of inhaled drug are needed, or for the treatment of children.

Unwanted effects

The unwanted effects of oral and parenteral corticosteroids are described in Chapter 44. Inhaled corticosteroids only have systemic actions when given in high doses. The amount of swallowed drug can be minimised by using a large-volume spacer (see above); large aerosol particles, which would otherwise be deposited on the oropharyngeal mucosa, are trapped in the spacer and only the smaller particles are inhaled.

There are some specific problems with inhaled corticosteroids:

- dysphonia (hoarseness), caused by deposition on vocal cords and myopathy of laryngeal muscles, occurs in up to one-third of those using inhaled corticosteroids; this may be less troublesome with breath-activated delivery, since the method of inspiration leads to protection of the vocal cords by the false cords
- oral candidiasis can occur but can be prevented by using a spacer device or by gargling after use of the inhaler.

Cromones

Examples: sodium cromoglicate, nedocromil sodium

The cromones have no bronchodilator activity and are therefore of no use in acute attacks of asthma; rather, they are used as preventers. Prophylaxis with sodium cromoglicate is usually less effective than with inhaled corticosteroids. Currently, their major use is as a prophylactic agent in the treatment of mild to moderate antigen-, pollutant- and exercise-induced asthma. They are also used as a nasal inhalant to treat seasonal allergic rhinitis (Ch. 39) and as an ophthalmic solution to treat allergic conjunctivitis (Ch. 50).

Mechanisms of action and effects

- Mast cell stabilisation. Sodium cromoglicate was originally introduced as a mast cell stabiliser. It enhances phosphorylation of a protein that normally forms a substrate for the intracellular enzyme protein kinase C, and interferes with the signal transduction for inflammatory mediator release. This action may protect against immediate bronchoconstriction induced by allergen, exercise or cold air.
- Inhibition of sensory C-fibre neurons by antagonising the effects of the tachykinins, substance P and neurokinin B, which are involved in generation of sensory stimuli. This is probably responsible for protection against bronchoconstriction produced by irritants such as sulphur dioxide.
- Cromones inhibit accumulation of eosinophils in the lungs and reduce activation of eosinophils, neutrophils and macrophages in inflamed lung tissue. These actions may be important in preventing the 'late-phase' response to allergen and the development of bronchial hyperreactivity.
- Reduced IgE production. The inhibition of B-cell switching to IgE production probably also contributes to the long-term effects of these drugs.

A single dose of either nedocromil sodium or sodium cromoglicate will prevent the early-phase bronchoconstrictor response to allergen, but treatment for 1–2 months may be necessary to block the late-phase reaction. Only about one-third of people benefit from treatment with these agents, which are generally less effective than inhaled corticosteroids but produce few unwanted effects.

Pharmacokinetics

Both sodium cromoglicate and nedocromil sodium are highly ionised and poorly absorbed across biological membranes. They are therefore largely retained at the site of action on bronchial mucosa after inhalation as a powder or from a metered-dose aerosol inhaler. Swallowed drug is unabsorbed and voided in the faeces.

Unwanted effects

Cough, wheeze and throat irritation may be provoked transiently following inhalation.

Leukotriene receptor antagonists

Examples: montelukast, zafirlukast

These are oral agents for the prevention of chronic asthma and have an additive effect with corticosteroid treatment.

Mechanisms of action and effects

The leukotriene receptor antagonists are given orally and inhibit the bronchoconstriction induced by LTD_4, by blocking the receptor for the cysteinyl leukotrienes (LTC_4, LTD_4 and LTE_4). Cysteinyl leukotrienes are released from various cells, including activated mast cells and eosinophils. Their synthesis is increased in response to several challenges, including increased levels of cytokines. Cysteinyl leukotrienes can contribute to airway oedema, smooth muscle contraction and enhanced secretion of mucus.

The leukotriene receptor antagonists prevent both the early and late bronchoconstrictor responses to allergen. Leukotriene receptor antagonists may be most useful in mild and moderate asthma, exercise-induced asthma, and asthma provoked by non-steroidal anti-inflammatory drugs (NSAIDs; Ch. 29).

Unwanted effects

- headache, irritability
- gastrointestinal upset
- dry mouth, thirst
- oedema
- hypersensitivity reactions, including anaphylaxis, angioedema and skin rashes.

Magnesium sulphate

Mechanism of action and effects

The most recent British Thoracic Society guidelines for the treatment of severe asthma in adults in hospital advises that intravenous magnesium sulphate can be given if life-threatening features are present. Magnesium acts by reducing calcium influx by blocking calcium channels.

Pharmacokinetics

Magnesium sulphate is given intravenously and is widely distributed. It crosses the placenta and passes into breast milk.

Unwanted effects

- atrioventricular block
- enhancement of neuromuscular blockade by neuromuscular blocking agents
- potentiates the hypotensive effects of calcium channel antagonists.

Management of asthma

The acute attack

Mild infrequent attacks of asthma can often be controlled by occasional use of an inhaled β_2-adrenoceptor agonist. Antimuscarinic agents are most effective when asthma coexists with chronic obstructive airways disease. More severe attacks require intensive treatment with bronchodilators and systemic corticosteroids. The signs of severe and life-threatening asthma are shown in Table 12.3.

Treatment of severe asthma should include:

- ensuring adequate hydration
- 40–60% oxygen via a facemask
- nebulised β_2-adrenoceptor agonist such as salbutamol (preferably using oxygen)
- intravenous hydrocortisone and/or high-dose oral prednisolone.

If there are life-threatening features, additional treatment should be given:

- nebulised ipratropium
- intravenous aminophylline or β_2-adrenoceptor agonist such as salbutamol
- intravenous magnesium sulphate
- consider assisted ventilation if there is not rapid clinical improvement.

After recovery from a severe asthma attack, oral corticosteroids should be continued until there are no residual symptoms, especially at night, and the peak expiratory flow rate is at least 80% of the person's previous best. High doses of these drugs can be stopped abruptly if used for 3 weeks or less, or tapered off if they have been used for a longer period (Ch. 44).

Prophylaxis of recurrent attacks

An initial attempt should be made to identify and exclude precipitating factors – for example, allergens, occupational precipitants and β-adrenoceptor antagonists (includ-ing eye-drops). After initially gaining control of asthma symptoms, long-term treatment is guided by a stepwise treatment plan recommended by the British Thoracic Society/Scottish Intercollegiate Guidelines Network.

Step 1. Mild intermittent asthma. Inhaled short-acting β_2-adrenoceptor agonist, such as salbutamol, taken as required. For those who are intolerant to this treatment, inhaled ipratropium and oral theophylline are alternative options, but with a higher risk of unwanted effects with the latter.

Step 2. Regular preventer therapy. For adults, a corticosteroid such as beclometasone is most often used. In children and some adults, an initial trial of cromoglicate or nedocromil can be undertaken, but these agents are generally less effective than inhaled corticosteroid. A leukotriene receptor antagonist could also be tried at this stage.

Step 3. Add-on therapy. In people taking moderately high doses of inhaled corticosteroid, a suitable add-on therapy would be a long-acting β_2-adrenoceptor agonist such as salmeterol. If there is no beneficial response to the β_2-adrenoceptor agonist, it should be stopped and the corticosteroid further increased. If control still remains poor, the increased corticosteroid dose together with a long-acting β_2-adrenoceptor agonist should be given. For persistent poor control, sequential add-on therapy with either a leukotriene receptor antagonist, a modified-release theophylline formulation or a modified-release oral β_2-adrenoceptor agonist should be tried.

Step 4. Addition of fourth drug. High-dose inhaled corticosteroid with a short-acting β_2-adrenoceptor agonist as required, and usually an inhaled long-acting β_2-adrenoceptor agonist plus a sequential trial of one or more of the following:

- leukotriene receptor antagonist
- oral modified-release theophylline formulation
- oral modified-release β_2-adrenoceptor agonist.

Step 5. Continuous or frequent use of oral prednisolone. This is undertaken in addition to other measures outlined above.

Table 12.3
Signs of severe and life-threatening asthma

Severe	Life-threatening
Inability to complete a sentence	A silent chest
Pulse ≥110 beats min^{-1}	Bradycardia or hypotension
Peak expiratory flow rate ≤50% of predicted or previous best	Peak expiratory flow rate ≤33% of predicted or previous best
	Exhaustion, confusion or coma

Arterial blood gas markers of severe asthma
Normal (5–6 kPa) or high arterial carbon dioxide (Pa_{CO_2})
Severe hypoxaemia (Pa_{O_2} <8 kPa)
Low or high plasma pH

Aspirin-induced asthma

About 5% of individuals with asthma experience exacerbations when they take aspirin or other NSAIDs (Ch. 29). These people have an eosinophilic rhinosinusitis and nasal polyposis in addition to asthma. Symptoms begin within 3 h of ingesting aspirin, accompanied by profuse rhinorrhoea, conjunctival injection and, sometimes, flushing or urticaria. Airways inflammation can persist for many weeks after an aspirin challenge. The condition may be initiated by priming of the respiratory mucosa by an immune reaction to a viral infection or other insult. Upregulation of cysteinyl leukotriene receptors occurs, but lipoxygenase production is still under partial inhibitory control by PGE_2. Aspirin is a mixed cyclo-oxygenase type 1 (COX-1) and COX-2 inhibitor, and reduces PGE_2 synthesis and increases leukotriene synthesis, provoking bronchospasm. Only NSAIDs that inhibit COX-1 induce bronchoconstriction; the newer selective COX-2 inhibitors do not induce this unwanted effect. Leukotriene receptor antagonists produce symptom relief in some people with aspirin-induced asthma. Treatment of the asthmatic attack is the same as for any other episode. Sometimes, long-term use of an oral corticosteroid is the only way to control the persistent symptoms; then, desensitisation to aspirin should be attempted. Nasal polypectomy may be necessary to control rhinosinusitis.

Asthma resistant to treatment

For people with resistant disease, especially those requiring oral corticosteroids, the use of immunosuppressive drugs such as ciclosporin or methotrexate (Ch. 38) has been advocated.

Management of chronic obstructive pulmonary disease

There are several important aspects of treatment for COPD, which has two goals: to minimise symptoms and to preserve lung function.

- **Cessation of smoking**. Smoking (see Ch. 54) is the most important factor for altering the natural history of COPD. Cessation slows the rate of decline in lung function. Occupational exposure to inhaled pollutants should also be minimised.
- **Pneumococcal and influenza vaccination**. These can reduce infections in people with COPD.
- **Bronchodilators**. The principles are similar to those for asthma, although there is usually less marked benefit, except during an acute exacerbation of symptoms. Improvement in symptoms and functional capacity can occur without changes in lung function tests and the main benefit is improved lung emptying during expiration, with reduced hyperinflation at rest. Inhaled bronchodilators reduce the frequency of exacerbations of COPD. Either a β_2-adrenoceptor agonist or an antimuscarinic agent can be used, with theophylline as a second-line choice. Antimuscarinic drugs are often more effective for COPD than for asthma. Nebulised bronchodilators can be useful for severe exacerbations.
- **Corticosteroids**. Many of the inflammatory changes in COPD do not respond to corticosteroids, but an oral corticosteroid can be effective for short-term use over about two weeks when treating an exacerbation of symptoms. Long-term use of an inhaled corticosteroid may reduce the severity of future exacerbations, but responsiveness should be confirmed by spirometry after an initial 2–4-week treatment period. About 10% of people with COPD will have an improvement in their forced expiratory flow rate.
- **Antibacterial drugs**. One-third of infective exacerbations are due to viral infection, but antibacterial drugs (Ch. 51) produce earlier symptomatic improvement if there is moderate to severe acute exacerbation of symptoms with purulent sputum.
- **Mucolytic agents**. These are sometimes prescribed (Ch. 13) and may reduce the frequency of exacerbations.
- **Oxygen therapy**. This is extremely important during acute exacerbations. Care must be taken to raise the arterial oxygen saturation (if possible to ≥90%) without increasing the arterial carbon dioxide tension. Low-dose oxygen may be necessary (e.g. 24% by Venturi mask or 1–2 l min^{-1} by nasal cannulae) if there is a tendency to retain carbon dioxide (type 2 respiratory failure). Long-term domiciliary oxygen treatment, usually delivered via nasal cannulae, improves symptoms and survival in COPD with respiratory failure (with an arterial oxygen tension less than 7.3 kPa). It should not be used unless respiratory failure persists for 3–4 weeks despite optimal drug therapy and without a clinical exacerbation. It should not be used by smokers because of the fire risk. To improve survival, oxygen must be used for at least 15 h per day.
- **Ventilatory support**. This may be required during exacerbations. Intubation and mechanical ventilation may be necessary, but non-invasive assisted ventilation is preferable. Nasal intermittent positive pressure ventilation (NIPPV) is being increasingly used during exacerbations for people who fail to respond to maximal medical therapy. The respiratory stimulant doxapram (Ch. 13) may provide minor short-term improvement in blood gas tensions while awaiting initiation of non-invasive ventilation.
- **Pulmonary rehabilitation**. This improves exercise capacity, reduces the sensation of breathlessness, and can substantially improve morale.

FURTHER READING

Asthma

Barnes PJ (2000) Molecular basis for corticosteroid action in asthma. *Chem Immunol* 78, 72–80

Bloebaum RM, Grant JA, Sur S (2004) Immunomodulation: the future of allergy and asthma treatment. *Curr Opin Allergy Clin Immunol* 4, 63–67

British Thoracic Society, Scottish Intercollegiate Guidelines Network (SIGN) (2003) British guideline on the management of asthma. *Thorax* 58(suppl 1), i1–94, **http://www.brit-thoracic.org.uk/sign/** (accessed June 2004)

Corry DB (2002) Emerging immune targets for the therapy of allergic asthma. *Nat Rev Drug Discov* 1, 55–64

Davies DE, Holgate ST (2002) Asthma: the importance of epithelial mesenchymal communication in pathogenesis. Inflammation and the airway epithelium in asthma. *Int J Biochem Cell Biol* 34,1520–1526

Ducharme F, Schwartz Z, Hicks G, Kakuma R (2004) Addition of anti-leukotriene agents to inhaled corticosteroids for chronic asthma. *Cochrane Database Syst Rev* (2), CD003133

Foresi A, Paggiaro P (2003) Inhaled corticosteroids and leukotriene modifiers in the acute treatment of asthma exacerbations. *Curr Opin Pulm Med* 9, 52–56

Hamid Q, Tulic MK, Liu MC, Moqbel R (2003) Inflammatory cells in asthma: mechanisms and implications for therapy. *J Allergy Clin Immunol* 111(suppl), S5–S12; discussion S12–S17

Kaiser HB (2004) Risk factors in allergy/asthma. *Allergy Asthma Proc* 25, 7–10

Lin H, Casale TB (2002) Treatment of allergic asthma. *Am J Med* 113(9A), 8s–16s

Lipworth BJ, Jackson CM (2002) Second-line controller therapy for persistent asthma uncontrolled on inhaled corticosteroids. *Drugs* 62, 2315–2332

Livingston M, Heaney LG, Ennis M (2004) Adenosine, inflammation and asthma – a review. *Inflamm Res* 53, 171–178

Luft C, Hausding M, Finotto S (2004) Regulation of T cells in asthma: implications for genetic manipulation. *Curr Opin Allergy Clin Immunol* 4, 69–74

Naureckas ET, Solway J (2001) Mild asthma. *N Engl J Med* 345, 1257–1262

Nayak A (2004) A review of Montelukast in the treatment of asthma and allergic rhinitis. *Expert Opin Pharmacother* 3, 679–686

Ng D, Salvio F, Hicks G (2004) Anti-leukotriene agents compared to inhaled corticosteroids in the management of recurrent and/or chronic asthma in adults and children. *Cochrane Database Syst Rev* (2), CD002314

Rodrigo GJ (2003) Inhaled therapy for acute adult asthma. *Curr Opin Allergy Clin Immunol* 32, 169–175

Rodrigo GJ, Rodrigo C (2002) The role of anticholinergics in acute asthma treatment: an evidence-based evaluation. *Chest* 121, 1977–1988

Rowe BH, Bretzlaff JA, Bourdon C, Bota GW, Camargo CA Jr (2000) Intravenous magnesium sulfate treatment for acute asthma in the emergency department: a systematic review of the literature. *Ann Emerg Med* 3, 6181–6190

Salpeter SR, Ormiston TM, Salpeter EE (2004) Respiratory tolerance to regular β_2-agonist use in patients with asthma. *Ann Intern Med* 140, 802–814

Spina D (2003) Theophylline and PDE4 inhibitors in asthma. *Curr Opin Pulm Med* 9, 57–64

Szczeklik A, Stevenson DD (2003) Aspirin-induced asthma: advances in pathogenesis, diagnosis, and management. *J Allergy Clin Immunol* 111, 913–921

Szczeklik A, Sanak M, Nizankowska-Mogilnicka E, Kielbasa B (2004) Aspirin intolerance and the cyclooxygenase-leukotriene pathways. *Curr Opin Pulm Med* 10, 51–56

Vancheri C, Mastruzzo C, Sortino MA, Crimi N (2004) The lung as a privileged site for the beneficial actions of PGE2. *Trends Immunol* 25, 40–46

Vignola AM (2003) Effects of inhaled corticosteroids, leukotriene receptor antagonists, or both, plus long-acting beta2-agonists on asthma pathophysiology: a review of the evidence. *Drugs* 63(suppl 2), 35–51

Whittaker PA (2003) Genes for asthma: much ado about nothing? *Curr Opin Pharmacol* 3, 212–219

Chronic obstructive pulmonary disease

Altose MD (2003) Approaches to slowing the progression of COPD. *Curr Opin Pulm Med* 9, 125–130

Barnes PJ (2002) Theophylline. New perspectives for an old drug. *Am J Respir Crit Care Med* 167, 813–818

Barnes PJ, Ito K, Adcock IM (2004) Corticosteroid resistance in chronic obstructive pulmonary disease: inactivation of histone deacetylase. *Lancet* 363, 731–733

Calverly PMA, Walker P (2003) Chronic obstructive pulmonary disease. *Lancet* 362, 1053–1061

Chitkara RK, Sarinas PSA (2002) Recent advances in diagnosis and management of chronic bronchitis and emphysema. *Curr Opin Pulm Med* 8, 126–136

Disse B (2001) Antimuscarinic treatment for lung diseases. From research to clinical practice. *Life Sci* 68, 2557–2564

Knight DA, Holgate ST (2003) The airway epithelium: structural and functional properties in health and disease. *Respirology* 4, 432–446

Lipworth BJ (2005) Phosphodiesterase-4 inhibitors for asthma and chronic obstructive pulmonary disease. *Lancet*, 365, 167–175

MacNee W, Calverley PMA (2003) Chronic obstructive pulmonary disease 7: management of COPD. *Thorax* 58, 261–265

Man SPF, McAlister FA, Anthonisen NR et al (2003) Contemporary management of chronic obstructive pulmonary disease: clinical applications. *JAMA* 290, 2313–2316

Plant PK, Elliot MW (2003) Chronic obstructive pulmonary disease 9: management of ventilatory failure in COPD. *Thorax* 58, 537–542

Rennard SI (2002) New therapeutic drugs in the management of chronic obstructive pulmonary disease. *Curr Opin Pulm Med* 8, 106–111

Sin DD, McAlister FA, Man SPF et al (2003) Contemporary management of chronic obstructive pulmonary disease: scientific review. *JAMA* 290, 2301–2312

Singh JM, Palda VA, Stanbrook MB et al (2002) Corticosteroid therapy for patients with acute exacerbations of chronic obstructive pulmonary disease. *Arch Intern Med* 162, 2527–2536

Soto FJ, Varkey B (2003) Evidence-based approach to acute exacerbations of COPD. *Curr Opin Pulm Med* 9, 117–124

Stoller JK (2002) Acute exacerbations of chronic obstructive pulmonary disease. *N Engl J Med* 346, 988–994

Sutherland ER, Cherniak RM (2004) Management of chronic obstructive pulmonary disease. *N Engl J Med* 350, 2689–2697

Self-assessment

In the questions 1–8, the first statement, in italics, is correct. Are the accompanying statements also true?

1. *In asthmatics, an inherited tendency to develop allergy or airway hyper-responsiveness is exacerbated by allergens, irritants, infection and smoking.*

    a. An influx of Th2 lymphocytes occurs in the late phase of response following an asthmatic attack.
    b. Leukotriene C_4 is an important bronchodilator released from eosinophils.

2. *Exercise-induced asthma appears to involve only the immediate (early) phase response. The β_2-adrenoceptor agonists are effective in preventing exercise-induced asthma.*

3. *After recovery from the bronchospasm that follows an acute attack of asthma, increased hyperreactivity and inflammation can last for weeks. The late phase response is characterised by bronchial muscle hyperresponsiveness but a normal epithelial cell morphology.*

4. *In addition to their bronchodilator action, β_2-adrenoceptor agonists enhance mucus clearance by acting on cilia. Tolerance to β_2-adrenoceptor agonists can occur.*

5. *The mechanism of the bronchodilator action of the methylxanthines is unclear but may include inhibition of phosphodiesterases and antagonism at adenosine receptors.*

    a. The plasma concentration of theophylline is increased by simultaneous administration of erythromycin or ciprofloxacin.
    b. Methylxanthines cause drowsiness.
    c. An unwanted effect of theophylline is stimulation of the heart.

6. *The muscarinic receptor antagonist ipratropium can be given in combination with a β_2-adrenoceptor agonist and a corticosteroid.*

    a. Ipratropium is more effective than salbutamol for preventing brochospasm following challenge with an allergen.
    b. Ipratropium causes bradycardia.
    c. Ipratropium is poorly absorbed from the bronchi into the systemic circulation.

7. *Leukotriene C_4 may be important in the precipitation of asthma in subjects who are intolerant to aspirin.*

    a. Montelukast inhibits the lipoxygenase enzymes that convert arachidonic acid to leukotrienes.
    b. The leukotriene antagonists are only effective if given prophylactically.

8. *Glucocorticoids are ineffective in the treatment of the early-phase response in an asthmatic attack. Glucocorticoids reduce dendritic cell signalling to T cells, T-cell cytokine production and eosinophil deposition in bronchial mucosa.*

9. Extended-matching questions

Which is the most appropriate option A–H for add-on treatment to the current medication that is being prescribed in each case scenario (1–5).

    A. Ipratropium
    B. Ciprofloxacin
    C. Salmeterol
    D. A spacer
    E. Controlled-release theophylline
    F. Intravenous magnesium sulphate
    G. Oral prednisolone
    H. Controlled-release theophylline.

1. A 25-year-old woman was admitted to A&E with an acute exacerbation of her asthma. Her peak expiratory flow rate was 150 l min^{-1}. Her pulse rate was 145 beats min^{-1}, her respiratory rate was 30 min^{-1}, respiration was shallow and she was confused. She was treated with 60% oxygen, nebulised salbutamol, nebulised ipratropium, intravenous aminophylline and intravenous hydrocortisone. Blood gases on admission, breathing air, showed a P_{O_2} of 8.4 kPa, P_{CO_2} 7.2 kPa and pH 7.29. There was little clinical improvement and she was transferred to the intensive care unit.

2. A 64-year-old man had mild asthma that was well controlled taking salbutamol two to three times a week and inhaled beclometasone twice daily. He complained of soreness of the mouth and hoarseness and was advised about oral hygiene.

3. A 67-year-old man had COPD with a chronic cough producing clear sputum. The cough and sputum production had not recently changed. He had stopped smoking 3 months ago because of his dyspnoea. Prior to that time, he had smoked 20 cigarettes a day for 50 years. He denied alcohol use. He had no other significant medical illnesses. His FEV_1 was 1.34 (about 45% of that predicted). He was taking salbutamol four times daily. A trial of inhaled beclometasone 3 months previously had provided no benefit and had been stopped.

4. A 60-year-old woman attended the A&E department with increasing shortness of breath, increased production of green–yellow sputum and fever over the previous 4 days. She was known to have COPD. She was taking daily inhaled salbutamol and ipratropium.

5. A 30-year-old man had mild asthma and allergic rhinitis. He was taking inhaled salbutamol and beclometasone, both twice daily. Recently he had been waking most nights with a persistent cough. He was a non-smoker and had no other medical history.

10. Extended-matching questions

Which is the most appropriate option A–G that relates to the statements 1–5. The choice of options A–G must be used once only.

A. Theophylline
B. Celecoxib
C. Prostaglandin $F_{2\alpha}$
D. Salbutamol
E. Montelukast
F. Aspirin
G. Leukotriene B_4.

1. Increases the synthesis of cAMP.
2. Decreases the breakdown of cAMP.
3. Results in an increase in the synthesis of leukotriene C_4/D_4 in sensitive asthmatics.
4. Inhibits NSAID-induced bronchconstriction.
5. Causes bronchoconstriction.

The answers are provided on pages 713–714.

Drugs for use in asthma or chronic obstructive pulmonary disease (COPD)

Drug	Half-life (h)	Elimination	Comment
Beta-adrenoceptor agonists			
Bambuterol	8–22	Metabolism	Given orally; long-acting prodrug hydrolysed by plasma cholinesterase to terbutaline, which has a half-life of 14–18 h; not recommended for children
Fenoterol	6–7	Metabolism + renal	Given by inhalation in combination with ipratropium; eliminated by conjugation with sulphate
Formoterol	2–3	Metabolism	Given by dry-powder inhalation; duration of action in airways exceeds the elimination half-life; eliminated largely by glucuronidation
Orciprenaline	6	Metabolism	The 3,4-dihydroxy isomer of the old, non-selective drug isoprenaline; given orally but has a low bioavailability (about 10%); eliminated by conjugation with glucuronic acid
Salbutamol	4–6	Renal + metabolism	Given by inhalation, orally, intravenously or subcutaneously; conjugated with sulphate
Salmeterol	3–5	Metabolism	Given by inhalation; long acting; oxidised metabolite retains some activity; the half-life given is following oral dosage
Terbutaline	14–18	Renal + metabolism	Given by inhalation, orally, intravenously or subcutaneously; eliminated by glomerular filtration and by conjugation with sulphate
Ephedrine	6	Renal + metabolism	Direct + indirect acting sympathomimetic; given orally (high bioavailability); eliminated largely by renal excretion; metabolised to norephedrine, which has central stimulant effects
Methylxanthines			
Aminophylline	Minutes	Hydrolysis	Water-soluble mixture of theophylline and ethylenediamine; given orally or by injection; very rapidly broken down to constituents
Theophylline	1–13	Metabolism + some renal	Given orally; metabolised by CYP1A2, which is induced by smoking; half-life is shorter in children than in adults
Antimuscarinics			
Ipratropium	4	Renal + bile	Given by inhalation for short-term relief in asthma and for COPD; little drug enters the circulation after inhalation and most is swallowed and not absorbed from the gut
Tiotropium	5–6	Renal	Given by inhalation for COPD; the small amounts of drug that enter the circulation after inhalation are eliminated in the urine; not recommended for children
Corticosteroids			Given by inhalation (see Ch. 44 for corticosteroids such as prednisolone and hydrocortisone which are given orally or by intravenous injection in the treatment of asthma)

continued

Drugs for use in asthma or chronic obstructive pulmonary disease (COPD) *(continued)*

Drug compendium

Drug	Half-life (h)	Elimination	Comment
Beclometasone dipropionate	15	Metabolism	Hydrolysed rapidly by esterases to the 17-monopropionate, which is almost 30 times more potent, or 21-monopropionate, which is inactive
Budesonide	2	Metabolism	Metabolites are inactive; oral bioavailability is about 10%
Fluticasone propionate	3	Metabolism	Oxidised by liver to inactive acid metabolite, which is excreted in bile; any swallowed dose undergoes 100% first-pass inactivation
Mometasone furoate	?	Metabolism	Originally used as a topical corticosteroid in dermatology; eliminated by hydrolysis and conjugation with glucuronic acid; not recommended for children

Leukotriene activity modulators

Drug	Half-life (h)	Elimination	Comment
Montelukast	3–5	Metabolism	Given orally at bedtime; good bioavailability (about 70%); oxidised by hepatic CYP3A4 and CYP2C9
Zafirlukast	10	Metabolism	Given orally; not recommended for children under 12 years; believed to undergo extensive first-pass metabolism (but no intravenous formulation available for comparison); oxidised by hepatic CYP2C9

Cromones

Drug	Half-life (h)	Elimination	Comment
Nedocromil sodium	2	Renal	Similar to cromoglicate; high polarity gives slow absorption from lung; negligible absorption from gut, and oral half-life is 23 h because of absorption rate-limited kinetics
Sodium cromoglicate	1–1.5	Renal	Given by inhalation; high polarity gives slow absorption from lung; negligible absorption from gut

Other agents

Drug	Half-life (h)	Elimination	Comment
Ketotifen	22	Metabolism	An antihistamine with actions similar to cromoglicate, and which has proved to be of limited value in asthma; oral bioavailability is about 50%; eliminated by conjugation with glucuronic acid

Respiratory disorders: cough, respiratory stimulants, cystic fibrosis and neonatal respiratory distress syndrome

Cough

Cough is a protective mechanism for the airways that removes excessive mucus, abnormal substances such as oedema fluid or pus, or inhaled foreign material from the upper airways. Cough is under both voluntary and involuntary control.

The cough reflex is initiated by irritant receptors located at the epithelial surface of the airway mucosa that respond to either chemical or mechanical stimuli. These receptors have been identified at, and below, the oropharynx in the large airways, and are probably present in the external auditory canals and tympanic membrane in the ear as well as other sites such as the oesophagus and stomach that can initiate cough. Local production of neuropeptides such as tachykinins (including substance P) is important for sensitising the cough reflex. Afferent fibres travel in the vagus and superior laryngeal nerves to the medullary 'cough centre'. Efferent fibres from the medulla travel in somatic nerves to respiratory muscles. Projections from the cerebral cortex to the medulla can also initiate cough.

Several mediators are involved in the cough reflex in the medulla. One proposed model is that the afferent input to the cough centre is via glutamate neurons that stimulate NMDA (N-methyl-D-aspartate) receptors (Ch. 4). These neurons can be inhibited by presynaptic serotonergic nerve synapses via 5-hydroxytryptamine type 1 ($5HT_1$) receptors. Opioids facilitate the inhibitory action of these serotonergic neurons through further interneuronal connections. The complexity of cough is illustrated by the number of mediators and antagonists that can experimentally initiate and inhibit cough. Selective opioids such as κ- and δ-opioid receptor agonists, bradykinin receptor antagonists, vanilloid receptor VR_1 antagonists, and blockers of Na^+-dependent channels all have potential as future antitussives. Some studies also implicate thromboxanes and tachykinins as being associated with cough.

A cough is initiated by a rapid inspiration followed by brief closure of the glottis. Forced expiration against the closed glottis raises intrathoracic pressure, and sudden opening of the glottis expels air together with secretions and debris. Flow rates can approach the speed of sound, producing vibration of upper respiratory structures and the typical sound of cough.

Cough has several diverse causes (Box 13.1). There are two categories of cough: acute, lasting less than 3 weeks, and chronic. Acute cough is most often due to the common cold, while the most frequent causes of chronic non-productive cough in non-smokers are postnasal drip syndrome, asthma and gastro-oesophageal reflux disease. In some situations, a cough is unproductive and has no useful function. In others, a cough can be considered useful, clearing excess secretions or inhaled foreign matter. An effective cough depends on the ability to generate high airflow. An ineffective cough may result from respiratory muscle weakness, or when the mucus on the airway wall is thick and more adhesive.

Box 13.1

Common causes of cough

Acute respiratory infection
  Upper respiratory tract infection
  Pneumonia, including aspiration
Chronic respiratory infection
  Cystic fibrosis
  Bronchiectasis
  Postnasal drip
Airway disease
  Asthma
  Chronic obstructive pulmonary disease
Parenchymal lung disease
  Interstitial fibrosis
Irritant
  Cigarette smoke
  Inhaled foreign body
Bronchopulmonary malignancy
Drug-induced
  Angiotensin-converting enzyme inhibitors
  Inhaled drugs

Drugs for treatment of cough

Antitussives (cough suppressants)

Cough suppressants fall into three classes.

Centrally acting drugs (opioids). These increase the threshold for stimulation of neurons in the medullary cough centre. Weak opioid analgesics (Ch. 19) are most commonly used, especially codeine and pholcodine. They are less addictive than morphine, which should be reserved for terminal conditions. Dextromethorphan is structurally related to opioids but is an NMDA receptor antagonist; it has no analgesic or sedative activity but has antitussive properties.

Peripherally acting drugs. Local anaesthetics (Ch. 18) such as lidocaine are used as an oropharyngeal spray to reduce cough during bronchoscopy. Antihistamines (Ch. 39) reduce postnasal drip from allergic rhinitis, which can stimulate cough, but probably have little direct antitussive activity. Sedative antihistamines (Ch. 39), such as diphenhydramine, are commonly used in compound cough preparations on sale to the public.

Locally acting drugs. Demulcents line the surface of the airway above the larynx, reducing local irritation. The syrup in simple linctus acts by this mechanism.

Expectorants and mucolytics

Expectorants such as guaifenesin and squill are often included in compound cough preparations on sale to the public, with the intention of improving clearance of mucus from the airways. There is no evidence of clinical value.

Mucolytics such as mecysteine hydrochloride and carbocisteine can be given orally to reduce the viscosity of bronchial secretions by breaking disulphide cross-linking between molecules. Mucolytics are occasionally useful in chronic bronchitis (Ch. 12) or bronchiectasis.

Management of cough

Cough should be treated only if it is unproductive or excessive. A self-limiting non-productive acute cough, such as that caused by a viral illness, can be suppressed by simple linctus or a weak opioid. Any cough of unknown origin that is still present after 14 days should be investigated further, to identify an underlying cause.

For chronic cough, non-specific therapy has a limited role, since it should be possible to identify and treat the cause. Specific treatment for left ventricular failure, asthma, postnasal drip or gastro-oesophageal reflux disease should eliminate the cough associated with those conditions. Cough is a common unwanted effect of angiotensin-converting enzyme (ACE) inhibitors (Ch. 6) and occurs in up to 10% of those who take them. It sometimes appears soon after starting treatment, but

can arise after several months. The cough may improve with a reduction in drug dosage, but it is usually necessary to change to another class of drug to eliminate the cough.

When non-specific therapy is required for cough, there are few options. Opioids are most useful for chronic non-productive cough in terminal lung cancer. Mucolytics may make clearance of mucus easier, but are probably no more effective than hydration from inhaling steam or nebulised hypertonic saline. The value of mucolytics in chronic bronchitis is uncertain and they do not improve lung function in cystic fibrosis.

Respiratory stimulants (analeptic drugs)

Doxapram has a limited place in the short-term treatment of ventilatory failure, particularly in hypercapnoeic respiratory failure due to chronic obstructive pulmonary disease which is causing drowsiness. It increases respiratory drive and arousal, and improves both rate and depth of ventilation. When combined with physiotherapy, doxapram may encourage coughing and clearance of excessive secretions. Its use has largely been superseded by ventilatory support, such as with nasal intermittent positive pressure ventilation. There is also a minor role for doxapram to reverse postoperative respiratory depression. Doxapram stimulates the medullary respiratory centre both by a direct action and by peripheral stimulation of the carotid body. Given by intravenous injection, its action is very brief, owing to rapid metabolism by the liver, and a continuous infusion is often used. Restlessness, muscle twitching and vomiting are common unwanted effects, and convulsions can occur due to generalised stimulation of the central nervous system.

Acetazolamide (Ch. 14) stimulates the respiratory centre by creating a mild metabolic acidosis. This action may contribute to its ability to reduce the headache, nausea, vomiting and lethargy of acute mountain sickness by decreasing periodic nocturnal apnoea and maintaining arterial oxygen saturation. Use of acetazolamide is not a substitute for gradual acclimatisation to altitude.

Cystic fibrosis

Cystic fibrosis is an autosomal recessive disorder caused by a single gene mutation on the long arm of chromosome 7. This gene encodes the cystic fibrosis transmembrane conductance regulator (CFTR), which is a Cl^-

channel in epithelial cell membranes. If the *CFTR* gene is faulty, then Cl⁻ transport is defective in epithelial cells in many organs, including the respiratory, hepatobiliary, gastrointestinal and reproductive tracts and the pancreas. Impaired Cl⁻ transport leads to reduced Na⁺ and water transport. As a result, secretions become thicker, causing obstruction to, and destruction of, exocrine glandular ducts. There is a sustained and exaggerated inflammatory response to infection in the lung in cystic fibrosis, although the reasons are not fully understood. Over 1000 *CFTR* gene mutations have already been identified, but even a single type of mutation produces different severities of disease, suggesting involvement of other genes or environmental factors.

The most common clinical problems are lung disease (bronchiectasis and chronic airflow obstruction) and pancreatic exocrine insufficiency, which affect about 90% of those with cystic fibrosis. About 20% develop diabetes and a smaller number develop meconium ileus in infancy or obstructive biliary tract disease. Death in 90% of those with cystic fibrosis is due to progressive lung disease; however, owing to improved treatment, median survival is now over 30 years.

Drug treatment

Much of the treatment for cystic fibrosis is supportive, including intensive antibiotic therapy and physiotherapy for exacerbation of lung disease. One of the major problems is infection with *Pseudomonas aeruginosa*; *Staphylococcus aureus*, *Haemophilus influenzae* and *Stenotrophomas maltophilia* are also frequent pathogens. Prevention of infection, particularly during hospital admission, is important, and improved treatment of infection is the main reason for the prolongation of life expectancy in recent years. In the early years of life, anti-staphylococcal therapy is usually appropriate for exacerbations of lung disease (Ch. 51). By adolescence, *P. aeruginosa* becomes the predominant pathogen, and is treated with intravenous or nebulised antibiotics. Increasingly, nebulised tobramycin or colistimethate sodium, perhaps combined with oral ciprofloxacin, are preferred (Ch. 51). It is almost impossible to eradicate *P. aeruginosa* from sputum, but rapid, intensive treatment of clinical infection slows the decline in lung function.

Since inflammation is a major component of the airway disease, several anti-inflammatory therapies have been studied. Oral corticosteroids (Ch. 44) reduce the rate of decline in lung function and reduce the frequency of infections, but unwanted effects preclude their long-term use. Inhaled corticosteroid does not improve lung function, unless there is associated airway hyper-reactivity.

There are several pharmacological interventions under investigation for improving the conductance of the defective Cl⁻ channel in cystic fibrosis, but none has yet been shown to improve the long-term outcome of the lung disease. In addition to antimicrobial treatment of respiratory infection, current therapies for respiratory and gastrointestinal symptoms of cystic fibrosis include the following.

Dornase alfa (recombinant human deoxyribonuclease I; rhDNase I). This enzyme can digest extracellular DNA. DNA released from dying polymorphonuclear neutrophils in the airways contributes to the increased sputum viscosity in cystic fibrosis. Dornase alfa is given by inhalation using a jet nebuliser (see Ch. 12), and is probably most effective when given on alternate days. It reduces sputum viscoelasticity, improves lung function in the short term (although long-term benefits are much less certain), and results in fewer exacerbations of lung disease. Unwanted effects include transient pharyngitis and hoarseness. Currently, use of dornase alfa is usually confined to those with reduced lung function (but forced vital capacity preserved at greater than 40% of predicted) and chronic sputum production, who require regular courses of intravenous antibiotics for recurrent chest infections. Improved lung function should be measurable after 2 weeks in responders.

Pancreatic enzyme supplements (pancreatin). Pancreatin consists of protease, lipase and amylase, which are inactivated by gastric acid and by heat. Supplements, therefore, must be taken with food (but not mixed with very hot food), and either concurrently with gastric acid suppression therapy (e.g. with cimetidine; Ch. 33) or as enteric-coated formulations. Pancreatin preparations in clinical use are of porcine origin. Dosage is adjusted according to the size, number and consistency of stools. Unwanted effects include irritation of the mouth and perianal skin, nausea, vomiting and abdominal discomfort. Some higher-strength formulations should be avoided in children under 15 years of age with cystic fibrosis, since they have been associated with the formation of large-bowel strictures.

Ursodeoxycholic acid. This synthetic bile acid improves abnormal liver function tests in those with cystic fibrosis by improving bile acid flow, and by increasing the bicarbonate content of bile. It is not known whether this prevents progressive liver disease in the small group for whom this is a significant problem.

Neonatal respiratory distress syndrome

Pulmonary surfactant is responsible for reducing surface tension at the air–liquid interface in the alveoli, preventing lung collapse at resting lung pressures. Surfactant is a macromolecular complex largely composed of the phospholipids phosphatidylcholine and phosphatidylglycerol. These are stabilised during rapid compression and decompression as the lungs inflate and deflate, by the hydrophobic surfactant proteins B and C.

Surfactant is synthesised by epithelial cells lining the alveoli and is normally present in substantial amounts at full-term delivery. However, preterm infants may produce too little surfactant, leading to neonatal respiratory distress syndrome.

Mortality is high in neonatal respiratory distress syndrome, but it can be reduced by administration of surfactant via an endotracheal tube into the lung. There are two natural agents: beractant (bovine lung extract) and poractant alfa (porcine lung phospholipid fraction). A synthetic compound, colfosceril palmitate is also available. The natural agents have a more rapid onset of action, probably because of the presence of the surfactant proteins B and C. However, the natural agents appear to be slightly more effective than the synthetic compound.

The use of a surfactant in neonatal respiratory distress syndrome reduces the risk of death by 40%, whether the treatment is given prophylactically or as a rescue treatment. Surfactant is given as soon as possible after delivery to infants with neonatal respiratory distress syndrome, or to those considered to be at risk of developing it.

In women at risk of preterm delivery, corticosteroids such as dexamethasone will increase the production of surfactant in the fetal lung, which may prevent neonatal respiratory distress syndrome.

FURTHER READING

Cough

Cho YS, Park SY, Lee CK, Yoo B, Moon HB (2003) Elevated substance P levels in nasal lavage fluids from patients with chronic nonproductive cough and increased cough sensitivity to inhaled capsaicin. *J Allergy Clin Immunol* 112, 695–701

Chung KF (2003) Current and future prospects for drugs to suppress cough. *Drugs* 6, 781–786

Dicpinigaitis PV, Gayle YE (2003) Effect of guaifenesin on cough reflex sensitivity. *Chest* 124, 2178–2181

Fox AJ (1996) Modulation of cough and airway sensory fibres. *Pulm Pharmacol* 9, 335–342

Irwin RS, Boulet LP, Cloutier MM et al (1998) Managing cough as a defense mechanism and as a symptom. A consensus panel report of the American College of Chest Physicians *Chest* 114(suppl), 133S–181S

Irwin RS, Madison JM (2000) Primary care: the diagnosis and treatment of cough. *N Engl J Med* 343, 1715–1721

O'Connell F (2002) Central pathways for cough in man – unanswered questions. *Pulm Pharmacol Ther* 15, 295–301

Widdicombe JG (1999) Advances in understanding and treatment of cough. *Monaldi Arch Chest Dis* 54, 275–279

Cystic fibrosis

Lukacs GL, Durie PR (2003) Pharmacological approaches to correcting the basic defect in cystic fibrosis. *N Engl J Med* 349, 1401–1404

Ratjen F, Döring G (2003) Cystic fibrosis. *Lancet* 361, 681–689

Tonelli MR, Aitken LA (2001) New and emerging therapies for pulmonary complications of cystic fibrosis. *Drugs* 61, 1379–1385

Neonatal respiratory distress syndrome

Halliday HL (1996) Natural v. synthetic surfactants in neonatal respiratory distress syndrome. *Drugs* 51, 226–237

Whitsett JA, Weaver TE (2002) Mechanisms of disease: hydrophobic surfactant proteins in lung function and disease. *N Engl J Med* 347, 2142–2148

Self-assessment

In questions 1 and 2, the first statement, in italics, is correct. Are the accompanying statements also true?

1. *Postviral cough can last for 3–6 weeks. Treatment should include increased humidity of inspired air and cough suppressants. Other drugs are of little value.*

   a. Many compound cough preparations sold over the counter contain sedating antihistamines.
   b. Dextromethorphan is a synthetic opioid but has no analgesic action.

2. *There is little evidence that any preparation can specifically facilitate expectoration; they may serve a useful placebo function.*

   a. Pulmonary surfactant increases surface tension in the alveoli.

   b. Doxapram should not be used in postoperative respiratory failure.
   c. The mucolytic mecysteine acts by inhibiting the production of mucus.

3. Choose the one correct statement from the following statements concerning cough.

   A. Inhibitors of the angiotensin II receptor cause cough.
   B. Guaifenesin inhibits cough-reflex sensitivity.
   C. All opioids are equally effective as cough suppressants.
   D. Dextromethorphan has similar unwanted effects to the opioids.
   E. Antitussives are effective in the treatment of acute cough.

The answers are provided on page 714.

Drug compendium

Drugs for use in respiratory disorders

Drug	Half-life (h)	Elimination	Comment
Cough suppressants			
Codeine	3–4	Metabolism	Opioid given orally; see Ch. 19 for details
Dextromethorphan	3	Metabolism (+ renal)	Opioid given orally; extensive first-pass metabolism; metabolised by oxidation to dextrorphan, which is a non-opioid cough suppressant, and by glucuronidation
Methadone	6–8	Metabolism + renal	Opioid given orally; used in palliative care for the distressing cough of terminal lung cancer (used less than other opioids); see Ch. 19 for details
Morphine	1–5	Metabolism (+ renal)	Opioid given orally; used in palliative care for the distressing cough of terminal lung cancer; see Ch. 19 for details
Pholcodine	32–43	Metabolism + renal	Opioid given orally; slowly eliminated owing to very high apparent volume of distribution (50 l kg^{-1}) rather than low clearance, which is largely due to hepatic metabolism
Mucolytics			
Carbocisteine	–	Metabolism (+ renal)	Good oral absorption; eliminated unchanged and as metabolites in urine
Dornase alfa	–	–	Recombinant human DNAase preparation used for cystic fibrosis; given by inhalation of a nebulised solution; measurable concentrations have not been found in the blood after inhalation administration; activity in sputum is measurable for at least 6 h
Mecysteine	–	Metabolism (+ renal)	Given orally; few kinetic data available
Pulmonary surfactants			Used for respiratory distress in preterm infants
Beractant	–	–	Given by endotracheal tube; activity occurs at the alveolar surface without systemic absorption; respiratory distress syndrome may enhance permeability and uptake; the apparent half-life of the natural surfactant (phosphatidylglycerol) is about 30 h
Colfosceril palmitate	–	–	See beractant
Poractant alfa	–	–	See beractant
Pumactant	–	–	See beractant
Respiratory stimulants			Given only under expert supervision
Doxapram	2–4	Metabolism	Given by continuous intravenous infusion; metabolised by oxidation in the liver; the ketometabolite is less active than the parent drug but is eliminated more slowly

The renal system

14

Diuretics

Diuretics are drugs that act on the kidney to increase the tubular concentration of salt and/or water. An understanding of basic renal physiology is necessary to appreciate how they achieve their effects.

Functions of the kidney

The kidney has several important functions:

- regulation of plasma electrolyte concentrations
- regulation of acid–base balance
- elimination of waste products
- conservation of essential nutrients.

Maintenance of salt and water balance

Diuretics alter the body's electrolyte and fluid balance by increasing electrolyte (essentially salt) and water elimination. This can be useful in the management of a wide range of conditions that produce oedema (e.g. heart failure, cirrhosis of the liver and nephrotic syndrome) and for the treatment of hypertension. Basic knowledge of the mechanisms of electrolyte and fluid handling by the kidney is essential for understanding the use and the unwanted effects of diuretics.

A healthy adult will filter about 180 l of fluid and NaCl from plasma at the renal glomeruli each day. Since the urine output is only 1–2 l in 24 h, it is clear that the majority of filtered fluid and solutes is absorbed back from the tubule into the blood. Different regions of the tubule and collecting duct vary in their capacity to reabsorb solutes (Figs 14.1 and 14.2).

The proximal tubule. In the proximal tubule, about 60–70% of the filtered Na^+ is reabsorbed together with equivalent amounts of water. Therefore, on leaving the proximal tubule, the tubular fluid still has the same osmolarity as plasma. The proximal tubule has many transport mechanisms for the secretion of organic acids and bases and ammonia into the tubular lumen, and the reabsorption of water-soluble essential nutrients, such as glucose and amino acids, from the lumen. Reabsorption of ions from the proximal tubule through the renal tubular cells is both passive and active (Fig. 14.1; site 1). The activity of the Na^+/K^+-ATPase pump on the basolateral surface of the tubular cell (exchanging 3 Na^+ for 2 K^+) helps to establish the electrochemical gradient for passive Na^+ reabsorption from the tubular lumen into the tubule cell. The inward Na^+ gradient provides the energy to drive several other carriers, such as that for glucose. Bicarbonate is also reabsorbed from the proximal tubule by a mechanism dependent on the enzyme carbonic anhydrase (Fig. 14.1; site 2). Proximal tubular reabsorption of Na^+ and water is determined by two regulatory mechanisms: glomerulo-tubular feedback (enhanced tubular Na^+ reabsorption when the glomerular filtration rate rises), and various neural and hormonal influences such as the sympathetic nervous system, angiotensin II, endothelin, dopamine and parathyroid hormone.

The loop of Henle. The descending limb of the loop of Henle is permeable to water but not to Na^+. Water passes from the tubule into the interstitium of the renal medulla, where the fluid is hypertonic (see below). The thick ascending limb of the loop of Henle is impermeable to water but has an active $Na^+/K^+/2Cl^-$ cotransporter complex in the luminal (apical) membrane (Fig. 14.1; site 3). The gradient driving this cotransporter is the low intracellular Na^+, which is maintained by active extrusion of Na^+ by the Na^+/K^+-ATPase pump in the basolateral membrane. The ascending limb of the loop of Henle can reabsorb up to 30% of the Na^+ filtered at the glomerulus. K^+ that is carried into the cell by the cotransporter is then recycled back into the tubular lumen, which ensures that there is always enough tubular K^+ to continue to favour Na^+ reabsorption. K^+ recycling also creates a lumen-positive transepithelial voltage that drives a paracellular ionic current which carries half the total Na^+ reabsorbed by this region of the kidney, along with Ca^{2+} and Mg^{2+}. The reabsorption of Na^+ but not water by the thick ascending limb of the loop of Henle establishes the hypertonicity of the medullary interstitium. This, in turn, is responsible for the osmotic gradient across the collecting ducts that permits formation of hypertonic urine. Hormonal regulators of Na^+ reabsorption in the ascending limb of the loop of Henle include calcitonin, parathyroid hormone and prostaglandin E_2.

The proximal (cortical) diluting segment of the distal tubule. The filtrate leaving the loop of Henle is

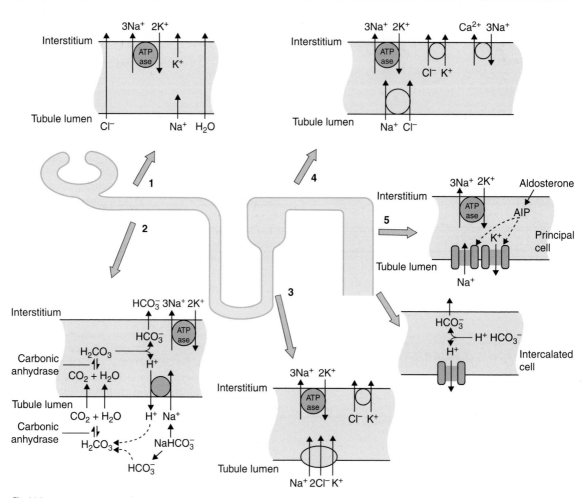

Fig. 14.1

Transport mechanisms for solutes in the kidney. In all segments of the renal tubule there is active transport of Na^+ out of and K^+ into the cell across the basolateral membrane using Na^+/K^+-ATPase. This sets up electrochemical gradients for the transport of other ions. In the proximal tubule *(sites 1 and 2)*, considerable amounts of Na^+ and glucose are taken up from the lumen along with water. Hydrogen ions are excreted in exchange for Na^+ uptake and this, in part, depends upon the activity of carbonic anhydrase. In the ascending limb of the loop of Henle *(site 3)*, the luminal membrane has a cotransport mechanism for $Na^+/Cl^-/K^+$ but is impermeable to water. In the proximal part of the distal tubule *(cortical diluting segment; site 4)*, Na^+ and Cl^- are co-absorbed but not water. Ca^{2+} also exchanges with 3 Na^+ at the basolateral border at this site. In the distal part of the distal tubule and collecting duct *(site 5)*, Na^+ is reabsorbed from the lumen in exchange for K^+ through selective channels. The channels transporting these ions are dependent upon aldosterone. Water is reabsorbed in the collecting duct under the influence of antidiuretic hormone (vasopressin) acting through receptors in the basolateral membrane. AIP, aldosterone-induced protein.

hypotonic and passes to the proximal part of the distal tubule (also known as the cortical diluting segment of the distal tubule). This part of the renal tubule is impermeable to water but has a luminal Na^+/Cl^- cotransporter (Fig 14.1; site 4). The driving force for this is again generated by the Na^+/K^+-ATPase pump in the basolateral membrane. About 5% of the filtered Na^+ load is reabsorbed at this site. The rich blood supply to this region allows rapid diffusion of the reabsorbed ions into the plasma and prevents the interstitium from becoming hypertonic. Reabsorption of Ca^{2+} is also regulated at this site, under the influence of parathyroid hormone and calcitriol (Ch. 42). The rate of Ca^{2+} transport is inversely related to that of Na^+ transport, because Na^+ inside the tubular cell either inhibits luminal voltage-gated Ca^{2+}

channels or reduces the activity of the basolateral Na^+/Ca^{2+} exchanger.

In this region of the kidney, the macula densa senses the luminal concentration of Na^+ or Cl^-, and if these rise, it initiates two responses that limit Na^+ loss. The first is tubulo-glomerular feedback that constricts the afferent glomerular arteriole to that nephron (possibly mediated by adenosine), and the second is secretion of renin. Renin, acting through the renin–angiotensin system, eventually increases the release of aldosterone from the adrenal cortex and increases Na^+ reabsorption at site 5 (Ch. 44 and below).

The distal part of the distal tubule and the collecting duct. The tubular fluid that has become yet more hypotonic in the cortical diluting segment of the distal

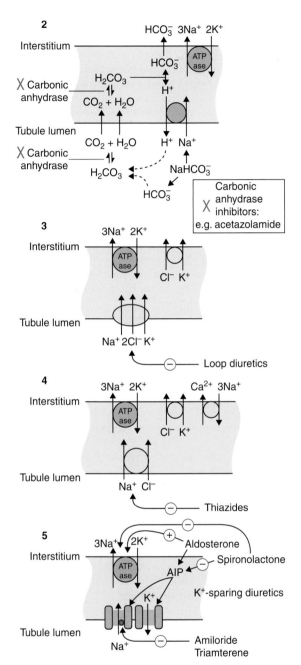

Fig. 14.2
Sites of action of diuretics. For location of these sites, see Fig. 14.1. Acetazolamide inhibits carbonic anhydrase and is a weak self-limiting diuretic, now largely used for other situations such as glaucoma. Osmotic diuretics increase osmotic pressure through the tubule, reducing electrolyte reabsorption across the luminal membrane. Loop diuretics can inhibit the cotransporter for $Na^+/Cl^-/K^+$ and inhibit up to 30% of filtered Na^+ reabsorption. Thiazide diuretics and K^+-sparing diuretics inhibit the reuptake of a maximum of about 5% of filtered Na^+. AIP, aldosterone-induced protein.

tubule, is delivered to the distal part of the distal tubule and then to the collecting duct. There are two cell types in this region. In the principal cell, Na^+ is reabsorbed through a highly specific amiloride-sensitive Na^+ channel (Fig. 14.2). This depolarises the luminal membrane, and activates inwardly rectifying K^+_{ATP} channels, which secrete K^+ into the tubule. Aldosterone enhances Na^+ reabsorption at this site by generating aldosterone-induced proteins (AIPs) that activate and increase the number of Na^+ channels. The driving force for the Na^+ reabsorption is again dependent upon the Na^+/K^+-ATPase in the basolateral membrane, the activity of which is also increased by aldosterone.

The principal cell is also the site of action of anti-diuretic hormone (ADH, vasopressin; Ch. 43). This hormone is secreted by the posterior pituitary gland and binds to receptors in the basolateral membrane, where it increases the permeability of the cell to water by upregulating aquaporin 2 channels. ADH increases water absorption and concentrates the urine as it passes through the collecting duct in the hypertonic medullary region. Other hormonal regulators of Na^+ reabsorption in the distal part of the distal tubule and the collecting duct include calcitonin, bradykinin and atrial natriuretic peptide.

The second cell type, intercalated cells, actively secrete H$^+$ into the lumen and conserve HCO$_3^-$. These cells are upregulated in acidosis.

Overall, only about 3–5% of filtered Na$^+$ is reabsorbed at the distal part of the distal tubule. The distal renal tubule is the primary site in the kidney responsible for maintenance of potassium homeostasis. Relatively small changes in extracellular K$^+$ concentration can affect cardiac muscle, skeletal muscle and brain function.

Diuretic drugs

Proximal tubular diuretics: carbonic anhydrase inhibitors

Example: acetazolamide

Mechanism of action

Acetazolamide interferes with the small proportion of Na$^+$ that is reabsorbed in the proximal tubule in exchange for H$^+$ (Fig. 14.2; site 2), a process dependent on the enzyme carbonic anhydrase. Acetazolamide inhibits carbonic anhydrase, and therefore increases HCO$_3^-$, Na$^+$ and K$^+$ secretion, causing alkaline urine. H$^+$ retention produces a mild acidosis in the blood, but the fall in plasma HCO$_3^-$ concentration stimulates carbonic anhydrase, which rapidly leads to tolerance to the diuretic action of acetazolamide. In consequence, acetazolamide does not have a useful diuretic action. Non-diuretic uses of acetazolamide are given at the end of this chapter.

Pharmacokinetics

Acetazolamide is well absorbed from the gut and is eliminated unchanged by the kidney. It is secreted into the proximal renal tubule via the organic acid transport mechanism, and works at the luminal surface of the proximal tubule. It has a long half-life.

Unwanted effects

- nausea and vomiting, anorexia
- paraesthesia, dizziness, fatigue
- hypokalaemia (see loop diuretics)
- drowsiness.

Osmotic diuretics

Example: mannitol

Mechanism of action

Mannitol is filtered at the glomerulus but not reabsorbed from the renal tubule. It exerts osmotic activity within the proximal renal tubule and particularly the descending limb of the loop of Henle, and limits passive tubular water reabsorption. Water reabsorption throughout the renal tubule is normally driven by the osmotic gradient across the tubular cells, which is created by active transport of Na$^+$ out of the cell across the basolateral membrane. Water loss produced by an osmotic diuretic is accompanied by a variable natriuresis (up to 25% of filtered Na$^+$). The initial expansion of plasma and extracellular fluid volume limits the clinical uses of osmotic diuretics.

Mannitol does not readily cross the blood–brain barrier. It is used to treat some forms of acute brain injury, when the main mechanism of action may be through haemodilution and reduced blood viscosity limiting the associated ischaemic damage, rather than a dehydrating action on cerebral tissues.

Pharmacokinetics

Mannitol is given by intravenous infusion and is excreted unchanged at the glomerulus. It has a short half-life, except in renal impairment.

Unwanted effects

- expansion of plasma volume can precipitate heart failure
- urinary K$^+$ loss can lead to hypokalaemia (see loop diuretics).

Loop diuretics

Examples: furosemide, bumetanide

Mechanism of action and effects

Loop diuretics act after they are secreted into the kidney tubule by the proximal tubule anion transport mechanism. Loop diuretics bind to the Na$^+$/K$^+$/2Cl$^-$ cotransporter complex at the luminal border of the thick ascending limb of the loop of Henle, and inhibit Cl$^-$ reabsorption. This reduces Na$^+$ reabsorption by diminishing the electrochemical gradient across the cell. Loop diuretics therefore reduce the generation of the medullary concentration gradient and prevent generation of concentrated urine in the collecting duct. Loop diuretics also prevent the tubulo-glomerular feedback mechanism and afferent artery vasoconstriction in response to the increased tubular Na$^+$ and Cl$^-$. They are powerful, 'high ceiling' diuretics which can inhibit reabsorption of up to 20–25% of the Na$^+$ that appears in the glomerular filtrate. The dose–response curve is steep, but the dose required to maximally inhibit Na$^+$ reabsorption shows wide interindividual variation. Their short duration of action can be followed by rebound Na^+ retention that offsets the effectiveness of the natriuresis. Loop diuretics remain effective even in advanced renal failure, but a larger dose is necessary to deliver enough drug to the renal tubule.

When injected intravenously, furosemide releases vasodilating prostaglandins, such as prostacyclin, from the kidney and produces a short-lived venodilation. Pooling of blood in the capacitance vessels reduces central blood volume, which can be useful in the treatment of acute left ventricular failure (Ch. 7). Loop diuretics also produce arterial vasodilation (see thiazide diuretics) but, because of their short duration of action, they are not widely used to treat hypertension.

Pharmacokinetics

Furosemide is incompletely and erratically absorbed from the gut, with considerable interindividual variation. Bumetanide is more completely absorbed and partially metabolised in the liver. Both drugs can be given intravenously by slow bolus injection or by infusion. In plasma, loop diuretics are highly protein bound and little drug is filtered at the glomerulus. The unmetabolised drug is actively secreted into the proximal tubular lumen via the proximal tubule anion transporter and the consequent rate of Na^+ excretion is directly related to the rate of urinary excretion of the diuretic. Renal failure impairs the delivery of drug to the tubular fluid through retention of organic anions that compete with the diuretic for tubular secretion. If renal function is normal, then the plasma half-lives of loop diuretics are short. Natriuresis and diuresis begin about 30 min after an oral dose and last up to 6 h, by which time the urinary concentration of drug has fallen below the diuretic threshold. Intravenous injection produces a more rapid effect, with an onset of diuresis within minutes, lasting about 2–3 h.

Unwanted effects

- Excessive salt and water depletion can cause intravascular volume depletion, hypotension and renal impairment.
- Dilutional hyponatraemia can arise from excessive Na^+ loss that exceeds water loss. Hyponatraemia is far more common with thiazide diuretics that block Na^+/K^+ cotransport in the distal tubule and impair free water clearance. It also arises from stimulation of ADH secretion, and consequent excessive water reabsorption in response to plasma volume contraction. Hyponatraemia can present with lethargy, impaired consciousness and, eventually, coma and seizures.
- Hypokalaemia can occur. This is dose related, and greater with longer-acting drugs. It arises from increased urinary K^+ loss from the distal renal tubule. Since diuretics increase the delivery of Na^+

to the distal tubule, there is enhanced Na^+ reabsorption at this site, which creates a negative luminal gradient favouring K^+ excretion. In addition, delivery of excess Na^+ to the lumen of the distal tubule stimulates renin release, causing secondary hyperaldosteronism. Aldosterone further enhances Na^+ reabsorption in the distal tubule at the expense of increased K^+ excretion. Obligatory urinary Cl^- loss with the cations creates a mild metabolic alkalosis in the plasma. To counteract the alkalosis, H^+ is shifted out of cells in exchange for intracellular accumulation of K^+, which exacerbates the hypokalaemia. Consequences and treatment of hypokalaemia are discussed below.

- Hypomagnesaemia may accompany hypokalaemia, which reduces tubular Mg^{2+} reabsorption. It also predisposes to arrhythmias and makes the correction of hypokalaemia more difficult. About 70% of filtered Mg^{2+} is reabsorbed by paracellular diffusion in the loop of Henle, and this is impaired by loop diuretics, contributing to hypomagnesaemia.
- Increased urinary Ca^{2+} excretion from inhibition of paracellular reabsorption of the ion at the loop of Henle can occur. This can be helpful in the management of hypercalcaemia if adequate hydration is maintained (Ch. 42).
- Hyperuricaemia arises from reduced glomerular filtration of uric acid following reduction of plasma volume. There may be an additional reduction of proximal tubular urate secretion as a result of competition between uric acid and the diuretic for the transporter. Clinical gout is unusual (Ch. 31), and less common with loop than with thiazide diuretics.
- Incontinence can result from the rapid increase in urine volume. In older males with prostatic hypertrophy, retention of urine can occur.
- Ototoxicity with deafness can result from cochlear damage, especially when renal failure reduces the rate of drug excretion or when very large doses of a loop diuretic are used. Vertigo may result from vestibular damage. Both are more common with furosemide and are usually reversible.

Thiazide and thiazide-like diuretics

Examples: bendroflumethiazide, chlortalidone, metolazone

Mechanisms of action and effects

The thiazides (or, more correctly, benzothiadiazines) are structurally related to sulphonamides. They act at the luminal surface of the cortical (proximal) diluting segment of the distal convoluted tubule and early collecting duct to inhibit the Na^+/Cl^- cotransporter. Although structurally different, several 'thiazide-like' drugs, such as chlortalidone and metolazone, share this site of action. Thiazides have a lower efficacy than loop diuretics, achieving a maximum natriuresis of about 5–8% of the filtered Na^+ load, and have a shallow dose–response curve. The onset of diuresis is slow, and they also have a longer duration of action than loop diuretics, although this varies among the drugs; for example, bendroflumethiazide produces a natriuresis over 6–12 h and chlortalidone over 48–72 h. Most thiazide diuretics are less effective in renal failure (especially when the glomerular filtration rate is below 20 ml min^{-1}). Metolazone differs from other thiazide diuretics in that it works in advanced renal failure.

Arterial vasodilation occurs during long-term use of thiazides, which produces a useful hypotensive effect (Ch. 6). This vascular action is maximal at lower dosages than are required for diuresis.

Pharmacokinetics

The thiazides and related drugs are fairly well absorbed from the gut and extensively metabolised in the liver. They are highly protein bound and little is filtered at the glomerulus. Thiazides act from the renal tubular lumen after secretion of the parent drug via the proximal tubule anion transport mechanism (see also loop diuretics).

Unwanted effects

- Hypokalaemia (see loop diuretics). The greatest reduction in plasma K^+ usually occurs within 2 weeks of starting treatment.
- Salt and water depletion. The combination of a thiazide with amiloride (see below) is particularly associated with dilutional hyponatraemia (see loop diuretics).
- Hyperuricaemia (see loop diuretics). Gout occurs infrequently and is less common in women.
- Decreased urinary Ca^{2+} excretion. This is in contrast to loop diuretics and the mechanism is not well understood. Hypercalcaemia is unusual unless there is another underlying disturbance of Ca^{2+} metabolism, such as hyperparathyroidism.
- Glucose intolerance, which is dose-related, with a progressive increase in plasma glucose over many months. The major cause is prolonged hypokalaemia; the consequent low intracellular K^+ concentration inhibits insulin release through altered secretion coupling, and impairs tissue uptake of glucose in response to insulin. The glucose intolerance usually reverses over several months if treatment is stopped.
- Hyperlipidaemia with a dose-related increase in low-density lipoprotein cholesterol and triglycerides. The long-term effects (>1 year) are small, but may increase atherogenic risk (Ch. 48).
- Impotence. This is reported by up to 10% of middle-aged hypertensive males treated with high doses of thiazides (Ch. 16).

- Nocturia and urinary frequency can result from prolonged diuresis.

Potassium-sparing diuretics

Examples: spironolactone, eplerenone, amiloride, triamterene

Mechanism of action and effects

These drugs act at the late distal convoluted tubule and cortical collecting duct. Aldosterone binds to a cytoplasmic mineralocorticoid receptor, a transcription factor that migrates to the nucleus and increases the synthesis of aldosterone-induced proteins (Fig. 14.2; site 5), such as serum- and glucocorticoid-inducible kinases (especially SGK 1); these phosphorylate and activate Na^+ channels. Spironolactone, its active metabolite canrenone, and eplerenone compete with aldosterone for its cytoplasmic receptors; receptors occupied by spironolactone do not attach to DNA. Spironolactone and eplerenone are the only diuretics that do not act at the luminal membrane of the tubular cells. They work in the presence of aldosterone and their effect is enhanced in hyperaldosteronism.

Amiloride and triamterene have a different mechanism of action, and block the Na^+ channel at the luminal surface of the renal tubule (Fig. 14.2). This action is independent of the presence of aldosterone.

The maximum natriuresis achieved by potassium-sparing diuretics is small (less than 2–3% of filtered Na^+) unless there is marked secondary hyperaldosteronism, when spironolactone is more effective. With this group of drugs, Na^+ and water loss is accompanied by preservation of plasma K^+, because of reduced Na^+/K^+ exchange. When used together with thiazide or loop diuretics, potassium-sparing diuretics reduce or eliminate the excess urinary K^+ loss.

Pharmacokinetics

All three drugs are given orally. Spironolactone is metabolised in the wall of the gut and the liver to canrenone, which is probably responsible for most of the diuretic effect. The half-life of spironolactone is short, but that of canrenone is long. The onset of action is slow, starting after one day and becoming maximal by 3–4 days; this slow effect is largely a consequence of its mechanism of action rather than its kinetics. Triamterene is extensively metabolised in the liver, and tubular secretion of the sulphate ester metabolite is responsible for the diuretic action. Triamterene has a short half-life. Amiloride is secreted unchanged into the proximal renal tubule and has a long half-life. The onset of action of amiloride and triamterene is rapid.

Unwanted effects

- Hyperkalaemia. This is more common in the presence of pre-existing renal disease, in the elderly and during combination treatment with angiotensin-converting enzyme (ACE) inhibitors (Ch. 6). Magnesium retention also occurs, in contrast to the situation with the thiazides and loop diuretics.
- Hyponatraemia. This is more common with thiazide–amiloride combinations.
- Spironolactone has a progestogenic and anti-androgenic effect, a consequence of its steroid structure and ability to bind to oestrogen receptors. This causes gynaecomastia and impotence in males, and menstrual irregularities in women. Eplerenone has greater steroid receptor specificity and does not cause these problems.
- Spironolactone is carcinogenic in rats but there is no evidence of a problem in humans.

Management of diuretic-induced hypokalaemia

A modest reduction in plasma K^+ concentration is common during treatment with loop or thiazide diuretics. Marked hypokalaemia (below 3.0 mmol l^{-1}) predisposes to cardiac rhythm disturbances, particularly in the presence of acute myocardial ischaemia, during treatment with digitalis glycosides (Ch. 7) or with antiarrhythmic agents that prolong the Q–T interval on the electrocardiogram (Ch. 8). It may also precipitate encephalopathy in people with liver failure. The risk of hypokalaemia is greatest with:

- thiazide rather than loop diuretics, because of their longer duration of action
- low oral intake of K^+
- high dosages of diuretic
- coexistent high aldosterone production, for example in hepatic cirrhosis and nephrotic syndrome.

Both treatment and prevention of diuretic-induced hypokalaemia can be achieved by using either KCl supplements or a potassium-sparing diuretic, but potassium supplements are less effective unless used in large quantities, which often cause gastric irritation. Modified-release tablets, effervescent formulations and intravenous solutions of K^+ are available. Supplements of greater than 30 mmol daily are usually needed, but many oral formulations of K^+ contain no more than 8 mmol in each tablet or sachet. Intravenous K^+ supplements are rarely needed unless there is severe K^+ depletion. Rapid intravenous injection can produce potentially lethal hyperkalaemia (provoking serious cardiac arrhythmias). A maximum infusion rate of 10 mmol h^{-1} is recommended, with hourly monitoring of the plasma K^+ concentration if such a high infusion rate is necessary.

It is unnecessary to routinely prescribe a potassium-sparing diuretic with a thiazide or loop diuretic, but they are widely used, often as fixed-dose combination tablets. A pragmatic approach would be to reserve their use for those at high risk from hypokalaemia, or those who develop significant hypokalaemia during regular diuretic treatment.

Major uses of diuretics

Diuretics can be used to control a number of conditions.

Oedema in heart failure (Ch. 7), nephrotic syndrome and hepatic cirrhosis. Mild oedema can sometimes be controlled by a thiazide diuretic. More marked oedema usually requires the use of a loop diuretic. Modest doses of a loop diuretic provide a near maximal response if renal function is normal, but large doses are sometimes necessary if there is renal failure (see above). The extent of diuresis is dependent on the rate of delivery of the drug to the renal tubule via proximal tubule secretory mechanisms. Once the optimal rate is exceeded, no further diuresis or natriuresis is achieved. Chronic use of a loop diuretic can occasionally produce tolerance, due to hypertrophy of epithelial cells of the cortical diluting segment of the distal convoluted tubule, with consequent increased Na^+ reabsorption at this site. If fluid retention is resistant to an oral loop diuretic, various strategies can be tried.

- Salt restriction, and avoidance of salt-retaining drugs, such as non-steroidal anti-inflammatory drugs (Ch. 29).
- Divided oral doses of a loop diuretic can be used to give more prolonged drug delivery to the kidney. This reduces post-diuretic rebound Na^+ retention.
- Oral bumetanide can be used rather than furosemide, because of its more consistent oral absorption.
- A loop diuretic can be given by intravenous infusion to prolong the duration of action. Slow intravenous infusion of higher drug doses will help to avoid ototoxicity.
- The addition of a thiazide diuretic or metolazone to a loop diuretic. Sequential inhibition of tubular Na^+ reabsorption can produce a dramatic diuresis and natriuresis; however, hyponatraemia, hypokalaemia, hypovolaemia and renal impairment can be troublesome with such combinations.
- If there is marked secondary hyperaldosteronism (e.g. in ascites associated with cirrhosis of the liver), spironolactone can be particularly useful. Eplerenone is currently reserved for people who are intolerant of spironolactone.

Hypertension (Ch. 6). Low doses of a thiazide diuretic are usually used. A loop diuretic or spironolactone are sometimes useful for resistant hypertension.

Acute renal failure. A loop or an osmotic diuretic may prevent incipient acute renal failure from becoming established. The mechanism of action in this situation is unknown.

Hypercalciuria with renal stone formation. Thiazides can be used to reduce urinary Ca^{2+} excretion.

Glaucoma. Acetazolamide can be used to reduce intraocular pressure (Ch. 50). Tolerance does not occur to this effect, unlike the diuretic action.

Mountain sickness. An unlicensed use for acetazolamide is the prevention and treatment of mountain sickness (Ch. 13). It should be taken for several days before ascending to altitude, and continued until descent. The mechanism is unknown.

Hypoventilation in chronic obstructive pulmonary disease. Acetazolamide creates a mild metabolic acidosis. This can stimulate respiration in the short term, and reduce carbon dioxide retention (Ch. 12).

Acute brain injury. Mannitol is occasionally useful, for example after neurosurgery or in acute traumatic brain injury, to reduce ischaemic cerebral damage. Fluid loss via the kidney should be replaced with intravenous crystalloid to avoid dehydration.

FURTHER READING

Brater DC (2000) Pharmacology of diuretics. *Am J Med Sci* 319, 38–50

De Bruyne LKM (2003) Mechanisms and management of diuretic resistance in congestive heart failure. *Postgrad Med J* 79, 268–271

Greenberg A (2000) Diuretic complications. *Am J Med Sci* 319, 10–24

Herbert SC (1999) Molecular mechanisms. *Semin Nephrol* 19, 504–523

Krämer BK, Schweda F, Riegger GAJ (1999) Diuretic treatment and diuretic resistance in heart failure. *Am J Med* 106, 90–96

Shankar SS, Brater DC (2003) Loop diuretics: from the Na-K-2Cl transporter to clinical use. *Am J Physiol Renal Physiol* 284, F11–F21

Self-assessment

In questions 1–11, the first statement, in italics, is correct. Are the accompanying statements also true?

1. *A fall in plasma K^+ concentration can affect cardiac muscle and brain function.* The main renal site of K^+ loss in the urine is from the proximal tubule.

2. *Electrogenic gradients are set up in many segments of the tubule by the Na^+/K^+-ATPase pump on the basolateral membrane.* The thick ascending limb of the loop of Henle is impermeable to water.

3. *Osmotic diuretics are poorly reabsorbed from the renal tubule.* Osmotic diuretics exert their activity on the proximal tubule, descending limb of the loop of Henle and the collecting ducts.

4. *Osmotic diuretics cause expansion of the extracellular fluid volume.* Osmotic diuretics should not be given in heart failure.

5. *The carbonic anhydrase inhibitor acetazolamide is used to inhibit the formation of aqueous humour in glaucoma.* Tolerance to the diuretic effect of acetazolamide develops.

6. *Approximately 20–30% of filtered Na^+ is reabsorbed in the thick ascending limb of the loop of Henle.* Loop diuretics increase the hypertonicity of the interstitium in the medullary region.

7. *In addition to its diuretic properties, furosemide has a venodilator action possibly as a result of the release of prostaglandins.*

   a. Loop diuretics are useful in the treatment of acute pulmonary oedema.
   b. Loop diuretics and thiazide diuretics should not be administered together.
   c. Loop diuretics do not produce hypokalaemia.
   d. There is no upper limit to the diuretic or natriuretic activity of a loop diuretic.
   e. Loop diuretics can produce ototoxicity.

8. *Unlike loop diuretics, which are short-acting, some thiazide diuretics such as chlortalidone can produce a diuresis over 48–72-h period.*

   a. Thiazide diuretics act by inhibiting the Na^+ and Cl^- cotransport in the basolateral membrane.
   b. Like the loop diuretics, the thiazides increase urinary Ca^{2+} excretion.
   c. The diuretic effect of metolazone is greater than that of other thiazide diuretics.
   d. Thiazide diuretics can produce glucose intolerance.

9. *Spironolactone and amiloride inhibit K$^+$ loss by reducing the uptake of Na$^+$ which exchange for K$^+$ in the late distal convoluted tubule and the cortical collecting duct.*

   a. Spironolactone and amiloride act by identical mechanisms to reduce K$^+$ loss.

   b. Potassium-sparing diuretics can cause a potentially harmful interaction if given with ACE inhibitors.

10. *Thiazide or loop diuretics are often given together with K$^+$-sparing diuretics.*

   a. The combination of amiloride and bendroflumethiazide produces no greater natriuresis than bendroflumethiazide given alone.

   b. Spironolactone is metabolised to the inactive metabolite canrenone.

11. *Non-steroidal anti-inflammatory drugs (NSAIDs) reduce the diuretic response to thiazide and loop diuretics.* Prostaglandins synthesised within the kidney increase renal blood flow and cause natriuresis.

12. Extended-matching questions
Choose the <u>most likely</u> option (A–G) that would relate to the case scenarios (1–4).

   A. Raised serum potassium levels
   B. Lowered serum potassium levels
   C. Reduced natriuresis
   D. Increased natriuresis

   E. Raised plasma glucose
   F. Lowered plasma glucose
   G. Lowered plasma calcium.

1. A 58-year-old woman was taken to the Accident and Emergency department with dyspnoea and bradycardia of 40 beats min^{-1}. She had previously had a myocardial infarction and coronary angioplasty. She was taking the ACE inhibitor lisinopril, and the diuretics bendroflumethiazide and amiloride, and had recently had the dose of lisinopril increased.

2. A 68-year-old woman with hypertension was taking bendroflumethiazide. Her blood pressure had been controlled at 136/88 mmHg. She had recently started taking naproxen for the aches and pains of osteoarthritis. Her blood pressure was found to be elevated (146/100 mmHg).

3. A 40-year-old man with type 1 diabetes and hypertension was being treated with insulin. He had started on chlortalidone two months previously for his hypertension and was seeking medical advice about his increased tiredness and lethargy.

4. A 55-year-old man with congestive heart failure was treated with digoxin and lisinopril. Furosemide was added because of oedema and he subsequently complained of palpitations. He was admitted to hospital and the electrocardiogram showed atrial tachycardia.

The answers are provided on pages 714–715.

Diuretic drugs (all given orally unless otherwise stated)

Drug	Half-life (h)	Elimination	Comment
Carbonic anhydrase inhibitors			
Acetazolamide	6–9	Renal	Of little clinical value as a diuretic, because of the rapid development of tolerance. Used in glaucoma (Ch. 50)
Osmotic diuretics			
Mannitol	2–36	Renal	Given by rapid intravenous infusion; used in cerebral oedema but not used in heart failure as it may expand plasma volume; half-life is 2 h in healthy subjects but very prolonged in cardiac or renal failure
Loop diuretics			Used for heart failure, oedema and oliguria due to renal failure
Bumetanide	1–2	Renal + metabolism	Given orally or by intravenous or intramuscular injection; well absorbed from the gut; about 50% is conjugated with glucuronic acid and excreted in urine and bile
Furosemide	1	Renal + metabolism	Given orally or by intravenous or intramuscular injection; incomplete and erratic absorption from gut; limited metabolism (15%) by glucuronidation
Torasemide	2–4	Metabolism + renal	Good oral absorption; about 25% cleared by kidney and remainder by metabolism; half-life unchanged in renal failure
Thiazide diuretics			Weak acids, therefore renal clearance affected by urine pH; used for heart failure, oedema and hypertension
Bendroflumethiazide	3–9	Metabolism + renal	Complete absorption from gut; 30% excreted in urine unchanged; metabolites not characterised
Chlorothiazide	15–27	Renal	Now little used in the UK
Chlortalidone	50–90	Renal	Incomplete oral absorption; long half-life because of its large volume of distribution and high plasma protein binding which reduces glomerular filtration
Cyclopenthiazide	–	Renal	Offers no advantages over other thiazides and is now little used in the UK
Hydrochlorothiazide	8–12	Renal	Offers no advantages over other thiazides and is now little used in the UK
Indapamide	10–22	Metabolism + renal	Rapidly and extensively absorbed from the gut; extensive hepatic metabolism; only 5% of dose is excreted unchanged
Metolazone	4–5	Renal	Good oral absorption; urine is main route of elimination (80% as the unchanged drug)
Polythiazide	25	Renal	Now little used in the UK
Xipamide	5	Renal + metabolism	Rapidly and extensively absorbed from the gut; about a half is excreted unchanged in the urine and a third as a glucuronide conjugate

continued

Drug compendium

Diuretic drugs (all given orally unless otherwise stated) *(continued)*

Drug	Half-life (h)	Elimination	Comment
Potassium-sparing diuretics			
Amiloride	6–9	Renal + faecal	Used in combination with thiazides and loop diuretics to conserve K^+; absorbed drug is excreted unchanged in urine
Eplerenone	4–6	Metabolism	Metabolised by CYP3A4. More selective for aldosterone receptor than spironolactone
Spironolactone	1	Metabolism	Variable absorption from gut, enhanced if taken with food; metabolised to an active metabolite (canrenone), which is eliminated in urine as an ester glucuronide and has a half-life of 17–22 h
Triamterene	2	Metabolism	Used in combination with thiazides and loop diuretics to conserve K^+; variable absorption owing to first-pass metabolism; metabolised by oxidation to a hydroxy metabolite and conjugated with sulphate; the conjugate retains activity

15

Disorders of micturition

Disorders of micturition

Disorders of micturition can arise from a disturbance of bladder function or from abnormalities affecting bladder outflow.

Detrusor instability

Detrusor instability produces uncontrolled bladder contractions during normal filling of the bladder. This results in urinary frequency, nocturia and urge incontinence. Most cases in women are idiopathic, but in men, bladder outflow obstruction is the commonest cause. Upper motor neuron lesions, such as those produced by stroke, spinal cord injuries or multiple sclerosis, also produce detrusor instability. Increased understanding of the neural pathways involved in initiating micturition is opening up new avenues for drug therapy to augment the relatively ineffective treatments currently available. Drugs used at present to treat detrusor instability act at peripheral muscarinic receptors to decrease bladder activity.

The urinary bladder is a smooth muscle organ composed chiefly of the detrusor muscle, which relaxes to allow bladder filling. A smaller muscle, the trigone, is found between the ureteric orifices and bladder neck. Internal and external distal sphincter mechanisms constrict to prevent bladder emptying and maintain continence (Fig. 15.1). Coordination of these components of the lower urinary tract is achieved by a complex neural control system. Sympathetic stimulation relaxes the bladder (via β-adrenoceptors in the detrusor and generation of intracellular cyclic adenosine monophosphate [cAMP]) to accommodate filling. At the same time, sympathetic stimulation to the internal sphincter (α_1-adrenoceptors) and somatic stimulation of the external sphincter maintains sphincter tone and continence. The signals for voiding can be initiated by myogenic stretch receptor activity produced by distention of the detrusor, or by signals from the urothelium. The sensory signal for voiding may be release of ATP from the urothelium, which stimulates subtypes of P2X receptors (the family of purinoreceptors) on the sensory afferent neurons. The sensitivity of this system is also modulated by other local factors and transmitters. The afferent nerves project to pontine areas of the brainstem that initiate activity in efferent pathways. Bladder contraction and initiation of voiding results from stimulation of parasympathetic muscarinic M_3 receptors in the detrusor muscle via generation of intracellular inositol 1,4,5-triphosphate (IP_3) and diacylglycerol (DAG) (Ch. 1). Stimulation of M_2 receptors inhibits intracellular cAMP production, and therefore opposes the effects of sympathetic activity. Non-cholinergic-mediated contraction becomes more prominent in unstable bladders, mediated by ATP acting via P2X receptors. Contraction of the detrusor is coordinated with inhibition of the tonic control of distal sphincter mechanisms and the bladder neck, and bladder emptying may be augmented by contraction of the diaphragm and abdominal muscles.

- Oxybutynin, tolterodine, trospium and propiverine all have antimuscarinic actions. Oxybutynin is selective for M_1 and M_3 receptors (with a higher affinity for M_3 receptors in the parotid than in the bladder) and has additional weak muscle relaxant properties through calcium channel antagonist actions and local anaesthetic activity. Oxybutinin is lipid-soluble, rapidly absorbed from the gut and readily crosses the blood–brain barrier. It is metabolised in the liver, and there is an active metabolite that may contribute to many of the unwanted effects of the drug. Oxybutinin has a short half-life. This results in large fluctuations in plasma drug concentrations, which increases the severity of unwanted effects; consequently, it is often given in a modified-release formulation. Tolterodine and trospium are non-selective muscarinic receptor blockers with no additional properties and less lipophilicity than oxybutynin. Tolterodine is well absorbed orally, metabolised in the liver and has a long half-life. It is better tolerated in a modified-release formulation. Trospium is poorly absorbed orally, and excreted by the kidney. It has a long half-life. Propiverine is also a non-selective muscarinic receptor blocker, with additional calcium channel

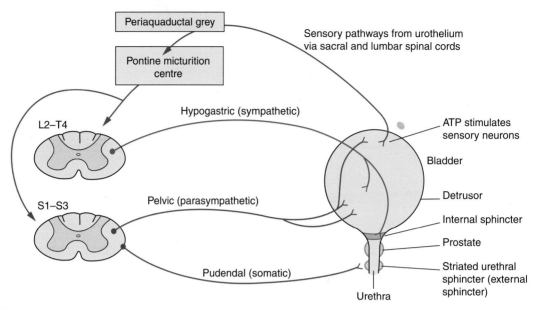

Fig. 15.1
Aspects of the bladder/prostate structures and the innervation involved in the micturition reflex. Other areas of the brain and peripheral control mechanisms are involved. For example, urine entry into the urethra stimulates afferents to the micturition centre. There are also gamma-aminobutyric acid (GABA) interneurons that inhibit bladder contraction. Sympathetic motor neurons operate through α_1-adrenoceptors, and the parasympathetic system through M_2 and M_3 muscarinic receptor subtypes. See text for further detail.

antagonist actions, which is well absorbed orally, metabolised in the liver and has a long half-life. Antimuscarinic unwanted effects (Ch. 4) are most troublesome with oxybutynin, particularly central nervous system effects (from M_1 receptor blockade) and dry mouth (from M_3 receptor blockade in salivary glands). The need for continued use of these drugs should be reviewed after 6 months.

- Tricyclic antidepressants, for example imipramine and amitriptyline (Ch. 22), have antimuscarinic actions but are now little used for detrusor instability, because of their troublesome unwanted effects.

Hypotonic bladder

Hypotonic bladder is often a result of lower motor neuron lesions, or can arise from bladder distension following chronic urinary retention. The condition leads to incomplete bladder emptying with urinary retention. Treatment depends on the cause.

- Chronic urinary retention is often caused by bladder outlet obstruction. If renal function is impaired, it should be managed by bladder catheterisation and correction of the underlying cause.
- Neurogenic problems can be helped by treatment with a muscarinic agonist (Ch. 4). The most frequently used drug is the anticholinesterase distigmine, which increases the force of detrusor contraction; it should not be used in the presence of

urinary outflow obstruction. The direct-acting agonist bethanechol is no longer recommended.

Urethral sphincter incompetence

Urethral sphincter incompetence produces stress incontinence in women or sphincter weakness incontinence in men. The most common cause in women is loss of collagenous support in the pelvic floor or perineum; it also arises from trauma to the membranous urethra (sphincter mechanism), such as may occur from pelvic trauma or following prostatectomy in males. Drug treatment is not appropriate, except for oestrogen replacement in postmenopausal women, either topically or as hormone replacement therapy (HRT) (Ch. 45), to reverse atrophic changes in the lower genital tract. Pelvic floor physiotherapy may be helpful, while minimal access surgical sling procedures to provide urethral support are gaining favour. Surgical intervention with colposuspension may be necessary.

Benign prostatic hypertrophy

Benign prostatic hypertrophy (BPH) produces symptoms in more than 25% of men above the age of 60 years, and up to 70% of men over the age of 70 years. The spectrum of symptoms is often called prostatism (Box 15.1). If left untreated, spontaneous improvement occurs or symptoms remain stable in up to half of all those with prostatism. Acute urinary retention occurs at a rate of 1–2% per year. Scoring systems can reliably quantify the extent to which symptoms affect the quality of life.

Medical management

Many symptomatic individuals do not require or want treatment, and a policy of 'watchful waiting' will be appropriate. The aim of drug treatment is either to reduce prostatic size or to relax the smooth muscle that restricts urine outflow. There is no evidence that medical treatment avoids the need for surgery in the long term. Current choices include:

- selective α_1-adrenoceptor antagonists
- 5α-reductase inhibitors
- plant extracts (a variety of 'nutraceuticals' are available via the web).

Alpha$_1$-adrenoceptor antagonists

Examples: prazosin, doxazosin, alfluzosin, tamsulosin

Selective α_1-adrenoceptor antagonists inhibit contraction in prostatic and bladder neck smooth muscle, without affecting the detrusor. Relaxation of these muscles improves urine flow rate and symptoms of BPH. Alfluzosin and tamsulosin are claimed to be more selective for the α_{1A}-adrenoceptor subtype in the urinary tract and may produce fewer vasodilatory unwanted effects than the other agents. However, the clinical advantages of these drugs are equivocal. Symptomatic improvement usually occurs within 1 month, and is seen in about two-thirds of those treated. Selective α_1-adrenoceptor antagonists are the first choice drugs for improving symptoms and urinary flow rates. More details of selective α_1-adrenoceptor antagonists can be found in Chapter 6.

5α-Reductase inhibitors

Examples: finasteride, dutasteride

Inhibition of the enzyme 5α-reductase does not affect circulating testosterone levels but reduces its conversion to dihydrotestosterone (DHT) within prostate cells. DHT is involved in prostate growth, and inhibition of

---

15.1

Symptoms of benign prostatic hypertrophy

Obstructive	*Irritative*
Hesitancy	Urgency
Poor stream	Frequency
Straining to pass urine	Nocturia
Prolonged micturition	Urge incontinence
Feeling of incomplete bladder emptying	
Urinary retention	

---

its production can reduce prostate volume by up to 30%. Finasteride only inhibits the type II isoenzyme of 5α-reductase, which is found in high concentration in the prostate; dutasteride inhibits both type I and II isoenzymes, but it is not yet known whether this will confer any clinical advantage. 5α-Reductase inhibitors usually take 3–6 months to improve symptoms, but the improvements are maintained. The drugs may be more effective with larger-volume prostates. The most recent trial evidence suggests that there can be additional symptomatic benefit from combining finasteride with an α_1-adrenoceptor antagonist.

Both finasteride and dutasteride are well absorbed after oral administration and eliminated by hepatic metabolism; the drugs differ in their half-lives (finasteride is short, whereas dutasteride is extremely long at about 4 weeks).

Unwanted effects occur in up to 10% of those taking the drugs, and include:

- reduced libido
- erectile impotence or decreased ejaculation.

Finasteride reduces the plasma concentration of prostate-specific antigen by an average of 50%, which should be considered when screening for prostate cancer.

Plant extracts

Examples: saw palmetto plant extracts, β-sitosterol plant extract

These products are available direct to consumers, but their composition varies between suppliers. Limited trial evidence suggests that they produce modest short-term improvements in symptoms of prostatism, and can be considered for those who have mild symptoms. The mechanism of action is uncertain, but these extracts may reduce the synthesis of testosterone, and inhibit the binding of DHT to prostatic receptors. They are well tolerated, with unwanted effects mainly confined to gastrointestinal upset.

Surgical treatment

Surgical treatment is usually required for severe symptoms or complications of BPH (Box 15.2). Transurethral resection of the prostate improves symptoms in 70–90% of those with prostatism. Long-term sequelae include impotence (5–10%), retrograde ejaculation (80–90%) and incontinence (<5%). Several less invasive procedures are now available, but they may be less successful for relieving symptoms, and do not reduce the risk of long-term consequences, although they produce fewer immediate postoperative complications.

Box 15.2

Indications for surgery in patients with benign prostatic hypertrophy (BPH)

Acute retention of urine
Chronic retention of urine
Recurrent urinary tract infection
Bladder stones
Renal insufficiency owing to BPH
Large bladder diverticula
Severe symptoms

FURTHER READING

Chapple RC, Yamanishi T, Chess-Williams R (2002) Muscarinic receptor subtypes and management of the overactive bladder. *Urology* 60(suppl 5A), 82–89

Foley CL, Kirby RS (2003) 5-alpha-reductase inhibitors: what's new? *Curr Opin Urol* 13, 31–37

Gerber GS (2002) Phytotherapy for benign prostatic hyperplasia. *Curr Urol Rep* 3, 285–291

Haeusler G, Leitich H, van Trotsenberg M et al (2002) Drug therapy of urinary urge incontinence: a systematic review. *Obstet Gynecol* 100, 1003–1016

Scientific Committee of the First International Consultation on Incontinence (2000) Assessment and treatment of urinary incontinence. *Lancet* 355, 2153–2158

Shefchyk SJ (2001) Sacral spinal interneurones and the control of urinary bladder and urethral striated sphincter muscle function. *J Physiol* 533, 57–63

Thakar R, Stanton S (2000) Management of urinary incontinence in women. *BMJ* 321, 1326–1331

Thorpe A, Neal D (2003) Benign prostatic hyperplasia. *Lancet* 361, 1359–1367

Wein AJ, Rovner ES (2002) Pharmacologic management of urinary incontinence in women. *Urol Clin North Am* 29, 537–550

Yoshimura N, Chancellor MB (2002) Current and future pharmacological treatment for overactive bladder. *J Urol* 168, 1897–1913

Self-assessment

1. In this question, the first statement, in italics, is correct. Are the accompanying statements also true? *Urinary bladder function is controlled by parasympathetic and sympathetic innervation of the detrusor and sphincter muscles.*

   a. Atropine causes urinary frequency and urge incontinence.
   b. The tricyclic antidepressant amitriptyline is effective in the management of the unstable bladder.
   c. The anticholinesterase distigmine can be safety given if there is urinary outflow obstruction.

2. Case history questions

   A 65-year-old man developed progressive urinary problems over a 5-year period. He had difficulty passing urine and was getting up three times in the night to pass urine. A rectal examination by his GP showed an enlarged prostate. Ultrasound, flow tests and prostate-specific antigen measurements suggested benign prostatic hypertrophy (BPH).

   a. What pharmacological approaches to the treatment of BPH could be considered?
   b. What are the unwanted effects of these treatments?

c. What are the possible outcomes of not treating?

3. Extended-matching questions
   Choose the <u>most appropriate</u> pharmacological option A–F to fit the case scenarios described in 1–3.

   A. Tamsulosin
   B. Finasteride
   C. Fluoxetine
   D. Amitryptiline
   E. Bethanecol
   F. Oxybutynin.

   1. A 50-year-old man with a 2-year history of difficulty in urinating and hesitancy was diagnosed with BPH. He was given a 1-month trial of an α-adrenoceptor antagonist, which did not improve his symptoms. He did not at this stage want to undergo surgery. What pharmacological treatment might be of benefit?

   2. A 30-year-old woman with normal bladder function complained of difficulty in urination after being prescribed new medication for her depression. She was found to have urinary retention. What agent could cause this effect?

   3. A 60-year-old woman had severe urge incontinence. She urinated 16–20 times a day and had leakage two to three times a day and at night. What treatment could she be given?

   The answers are provided on pages 715–716.

Drugs for use in disorders of micturition

Drug	Half-life (h)	Elimination	Comment
Drugs for urinary retention			All drugs taken orally
α₁-Adrenoceptor antagonists			
Alfuzosin	4–10	Metabolism (+ renal)	Reported to show selectivity for α_1-adrenoceptors in the genitourinary tract; oral bioavailability is about 50%; metabolised in the liver
Doxazosin	10–20	Metabolism (+ renal)	Oral bioavailability is 65%; longer half-lives (20 h) found after treatment to steady state; eliminated largely by oxidative metabolism to a number of products, one of which is a potent α_1-adrenoceptor antagonist
Indoramin	5 (2–10)	Metabolism (+ renal)	Undergoes extensive hepatic first-pass metabolism; oral bioavailability is about 10–20% (but 70% in patients with hepatic cirrhosis); longer half-life and much higher blood levels (five-fold) in the elderly
Prazosin	2–3	Metabolism (+ renal)	Oral bioavailability is about 60%; metabolised in the liver by dealkylation and conjugation
Tamsulosin	15	Metabolism (+ renal)	Selective for α_1-adrenoceptors in the genitourinary tract; normally taken with food (to reduce unwanted effects) but this reduces bioavailability to about 60%
Terazosin	12	Metabolism + renal	High oral bioavailability (90%); mainly eliminated via the bile and lost in the faeces as parent drug and metabolites
Parasympathomimetics			
Distigmine	70	Renal + hydrolysis	Given orally; very poor oral bioavailability (5%) especially if taken with food; hydrolysed by plasma esterases
5α-Reductase inhibitors			
Dutasteride	4–5 weeks	Metabolism	Given orally; bioavailability is about 60%; eliminated by CYP3A4 metabolism; the very long half-life results from low clearance (0.51 h⁻¹) and a large apparent volume of distribution (500 l); it takes about 6 months to reach steady state; safety profile similar to that of finasteride
Finasteride	6 (3–16)	Metabolism	Given orally; bioavailability is about 60–80%; eliminated as metabolites in faeces and in urine
Drugs for urinary frequency and incontinence			All drugs taken orally
Flavoxate	?	Renal + metabolism	Metabolised to a carboxylic acid derivative; few other kinetic data are available (high oral bioavailability in rats)
Oxybutynin	1–3	Metabolism	Very low oral bioavailability (6%) owing to extensive first-pass metabolism; cholinergic antagonism in vivo probably results from the desethyl metabolite, which is formed in the liver during first-pass metabolism and is as active as the parent compound
Propantheline	1–2	Metabolism	Oral bioavailability is about 5–10% (based on urinary excretion data); metabolites are inactive

continued

Drugs for use in disorders of micturition *(continued)*

Drug	Half-life (h)	Elimination	Comment
Propiverine	4	Metabolism	Oral bioavailability is about 50%; metabolised mainly by *N*-oxidation
Tolterodine	2 (EM) 10 (PM)	Metabolism	High oral bioavailability (about 75%); metabolised by CYP2D6 to an active metabolite responsible for part of the therapeutic effect; subjects with low CYP2D6 activity (poor metabolisers; PM) metabolise the drug by CYP3A4; PM have higher levels of parent drug and lower levels of the metabolite, but, as both compounds are active, they show similar responses to extensive metabolisers (EM); the drug shows dose-dependent kinetics in the therapeutic range
Trospium	1–2	Renal	A quarternary amino compound that has a very low oral bioavailability (3%); limited oxidative metabolism; about one half of that absorbed is excreted unchanged

Drug compendium

Erectile dysfunction

Physiology of erection

Achieving and maintaining an erection involves a complex series of interactions between the central nervous system, the autonomic nervous system and local mediators; both psychological and tactile stimuli are important. The primary erectile innervation is the parasympathetic nervous system. There are four phases of achieving an erection.

Phase 1. Parasympathetic stimulation leads to relaxation of arterial smooth muscle and the smooth muscle that forms bands (trabeculae) with connective tissue in the highly vascularised and neuronally innervated erectile tissues of the penis (corpus cavernosa and corpus spongiosum). This increases the influx of blood into the sinusoidal spaces of the corpus cavernosum, which engorges with blood (Fig. 16.1). Conversely, sympathetic stimulation inhibits erection by increasing vascular smooth muscle tone.

Phase 2. Intracavernous pressure rises and the sinusoids expand. The penis elongates and grows.

Phase 3. The rise in pressure in the sinusoids compresses the venous plexi and reduces venous outflow, thus maintaining the erection (the corporeal veno-occlusive mechanism).

Phase 4. The pudendal nerve (part of the parasympathetic innervation) stimulates the ischiocavernosal muscle. This squeezes the crura at the base of the penis and stops both arterial inflow and venous outflow, maintaining full erection. Skeletal muscle fatigue eventually allows return of perfusion.

Among the local mediators, nitric oxide synthesised by blood vessel endothelial cells and released from non-adrenergic non-cholinergic (NANC) nerves in the corpora appears to be crucial for cavernosal smooth muscle relaxation via generation of cyclic guanosine monophosphate (cGMP). In addition, vasoactive intestinal peptide (VIP), calcitonin gene-related peptide (CGRP), prostaglandin E_1 (via generation of cyclic adenosine monophosphate [cAMP]), and possibly other mediators all modulate penile vascular smooth muscle relaxation and blood flow.

Erectile dysfunction

Erectile dysfunction is defined as the consistent inability to achieve or sustain an erection of sufficient rigidity for sexual intercourse. It is a common problem, affecting up to 20% of adult men, with up to 10% over the age of 40 years having complete erectile dysfunction. Any disease process that affects penile neural supply, arterial inflow or venous outflow can produce erectile dysfunction. There is a physical cause in about 80% of cases (Box 16.1) but a psychological component often coexists. Psychogenic erectile dysfunction is more common in younger persons. Drugs are an important cause of erectile dysfunction, particularly antihypertensive, psychotropic and 'recreational' drugs, accounting for up to 25% of cases (Table 16.1).

Management of erectile dysfunction

A number of strategies can be used in the management of erectile dysfunction. Initially there should be an assessment and treatment of any underlying psychological cause or physical disease. Treatment options include:

- pharmacological agents described below
- mechanical aids, such as the vacuum constriction device; these are usually advised for older people who do not respond to pharmacological treatment and do not wish to have surgery
- penile implants using a malleable or inflatable prosthesis
- hypogonadism is an uncommon cause of impotence and responds to testosterone replacement therapy (Ch. 46)
- hyperprolactinaemia impairs erection; it is most commonly caused by drug therapy (e.g. with phenothiazines) and can be improved by oral bromocriptine (Ch. 43).

Oral phosphodiesterase inhibitors

Examples: sildenafil, tadalafil vardenafil

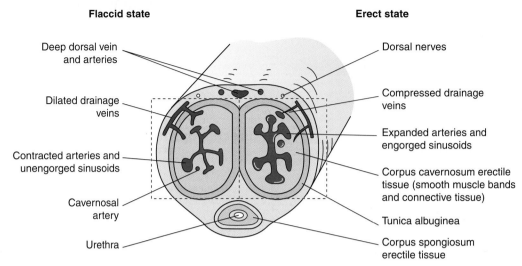

Fig. 16.1
Cross-section of the penis, showing structures involved in erection. This diagram shows only part of the rich nervous and vascular filling and drainage system in the penis. The left-hand area shows the situation in the flaccid penis and the right-hand area the erect penis. The rising pressure during erection limits the venous outflow, thus maintaining the erection. The penis contains three cylinders of erectile tissue: two corpora cavernosa and the corpus spongiosum. The corpus spongiosum contains the urethra. The cylinders of erectile tissue are divided into spaces known as sinusoids or lacunae, which are lined by vascular epithelium. The walls of these spaces are made up of thick bundles of smooth muscle cells within a framework of fibroblasts, collagen and elastin (trabeculae). The erectile tissues are supplied with blood from the cavernosal and helicine arteries, which drain into the sinusoidal spaces. Blood is drained from the sinusoidal spaces through emissary veins. The venules join together to form larger veins that drain into the deep dorsal vein or other veins at different parts of the penis. Arterial and sinusoid dilation is important for erection, while swelling is limited by the inelastic tunica albuginea.

These are analogues of cGMP and are orally active selective phosphodiesterase (type V) inhibitors that reduce the breakdown of cGMP and prolong the dilator effect of nitric oxide on penile vascular smooth muscle relaxation, resulting in erection. About 60% of men with erectile dysfunction will have improved erections sufficient to permit intercourse. Sexual stimulation is necessary for the drugs to work.

Box 16.1

Common causes of erectile dysfunction

Diabetes
Vascular disease
Surgery
Drugs, especially antihypertensives, antipsychotic drugs, antidepressants (Table 16.1)
Substance abuse, e.g. nicotine, alcohol, recreational drugs
Hormonal imbalance
Neurological disease, e.g. multiple sclerosis, Alzheimer's disease, epilepsy
Spinal cord injury
Psychological (20% as a primary cause, more commonly secondary to physical problems)

Pharmacokinetics

Sildenafil is relatively well absorbed orally, but vardenafil is less well absorbed, and there are no data for tadalafil. The absorption of sildenafil and vardenafil are delayed by a fatty meal, whereas the absorption of tadalafil is rapid and is unaffected by food. All are eliminated by hepatic metabolism. Sildenafil and vardenafil have moderate half-lives, and should be taken 30–60 min before sexual activity for maximum benefit. The half-life of tadalafil is long, with a duration of action ranging from 24 to 36 h; therefore, planning of sexual activity (and its timing in relation to drug dosage) is less relevant with this drug. Sildenafil and vardenafil both have active metabolites but tadalafil does not.

Unwanted effects

- Nausea, dyspepsia, vomiting.
- Slight hypotension, dizziness, flushing, headache and nasal congestion from vasodilation. Oral phosphodiesterase inhibitors are contraindicated in patients taking nitrates or nicorandil (see Ch. 5), because of a synergistic effect on vascular nitric oxide. The antiviral ritonavir (Ch. 51) has potentially hazardous interactions with oral phosphodiesterase inhibitors. Ritonavir inhibits the CYP3A isoenzyme that is the main metaboliser of sildenafil.

Table 16.1
Drugs that commonly cause male sexual dysfunction

	Ejaculatory dysfunction	Erectile dysfunction	Loss of libido
Antihypertensives			
β-Adrenoceptor antagonists		+	
α-Adrenoceptor antagonists	+		
Methyldopa	+	+	+
Thiazide diuretics		+	
Psychotropic drugs			
Phenothiazines	+	+	+
Benzodiazepines	+	+	+
Tricyclic antidepressants		+	+
Selective serotonin (5HT) reuptake inhibitors (SSRIs)		+	+
Other			
Spironolactone			+
Digoxin		+	
Cimetidine/ranitidine		+	+
Metoclopramide		+	+
Carbamazepine		+	+
Recreational drugs			
Alcohol	+	+	
Marijuana		+	
Cocaine		+	+
Amphetamines	+	+	+
Anabolic steroids		+	+

- Phosphodiesterase type VI is inhibited in the eye by high doses of sildenafil, but less so by tadalafil or vardenafil; they can cause visual disturbance (enhanced perception of bright lights, or a 'blue halo' effect) and raised intraocular pressure. Overall, the unwanted-effect profiles of tadalafil and vardenafil are similar to those of sildenafil.
- Additive orthostatic hypotension is seen if sildenafil is taken with an α_1-adrenoceptor antagonist.

Other vasodilators

Sublingual apomorphine. Apomorphine is a dopamine D_2-receptor agonist used in Parkinson's disease (Ch. 24); its mechanism of action in erectile dysfunction is uncertain and probably involves hypothalamic stimulation in the brain. Until recently it was available for treating erectile dysfunction only by subcutaneous administration, but is now given sublingually because the limited absorption through the buccal mucosa reduces the nausea and hypotension that were troublesome following subcutaneous injection. It is effective about 10–20 min after administration, and gives most benefit in psychogenic impotence.

Intracavernosal injection of vasodilators. These are more effective if arterial flow is normal, such as with neurogenic and psychogenic impotence. Bleeding ten-dencies preclude this form of treatment, as does poor manual dexterity or morbid obesity. The injection is made into the side of the penis directly into the corpus cavernosum.

Alprostadil. This is a synthetic prostaglandin E_1 analogue. It vasodilates by acting on smooth muscle cell surface receptors to increase intracellular cAMP, which in turn reduces the intracellular calcium concentration. Local pain after injection is a common unwanted effect, reported by one-third of users, and can be reduced by the addition of a local anaesthetic such as procaine (Ch. 18). Rapid local metabolism of alprostadil minimises systemic unwanted effects.

Phentolamine. This is a non-selective α-adrenoceptor antagonist (Ch. 6). It is relatively ineffective when used alone, because it does not reduce venous outflow, and is used in combination with papaverine.

Papaverine. This is a phosphodiesterase inhibitor that increases intracellular cAMP and cGMP, reduces intracellular calcium in smooth muscle and produces relaxation. Papaverine is not licensed in the UK. The success rate in impotence is about 50%, but there is a high incidence of prolonged erection (lasting more than 4 h) or priapism, so this drug is rarely used except in combination with alprostadil and phentolamine for non-responders to alprostadil given alone. Fibrosis within the penis can result from the acidity of the solution.

Intraurethral alprostadil. High doses of alprostadil can be given intraurethrally as a pellet using a plastic applicator, but are less effective than the injection. In responders, an erection develops within 15 min and lasts for 30–60 min. About 10% of administrations produce penile pain. Because of the uterine stimulant acitvity of alprostadil, a sheath is recommended if the partner is pregnant.

Many unapproved combinations of drugs, e.g. sildenafil and apomorphine, are being used where monotherapy fails.

FURTHER READING

Corbin JD, Francis SH (2002) Pharmacology of phosphodiesterase-5 inhibitors. *Int J Clin Pract* 56, 453–459

Fink HA, MacDonald R, Rutks I et al (2002) Sildenafil for male erectile dysfunction. *Arch Intern Med* 162, 1349–1360

Lue TF (2000) Erectile dysfunction. *N Engl J Med* 342, 1802–1813

Morgentaler A (1999) Male impotence. *Lancet* 354, 1713–1718

Park J-K, Moreland RB, Nehra A. The role of oxygen tension in penile erection and its relationship to erectile dysfunction. *Digital Urology Journal* **http://www.duj.com/Article/Nehra/Nehra.html (accessed October 2004)**

Self-assessment

1. Are the following statements true or false?

   a. Sildenafil should not be taken by men already taking nitrates.
   b. Sildenafil can cause an increase in blood pressure if taken with nitrates.
   c. Phosphodiesterase type V is only found in the vasculature in the penis.
   d. Increased parasympathetic outflow to the penis causes a failure of erection.
   e. Erections caused by injected drugs such as papaverine or alprostadil are not easy to control.
   f. Impotence caused by hypogonadism can be treated with oestrogen.
   g. Diabetes can cause impotence.
   h. The duration of biological actions of sildenafil and tadalafil are similar.
   i. Sildenafil inhibits the breakdown of cAMP.

2. Case history questions

> Mr JA, aged 56 years, presented with erectile dysfunction of gradual onset over the last 2–3 years. He was hypertensive, with a blood pressure of 160/96 mmHg, and was being treated with atenolol and bendroflumethiazide. There was a family history of coronary artery disease. He smokes 30 cigarettes a day and drinks 4 pints of beer a night. Examination revealed that he was hypercholesterolaemic and there were signs of coronary artery disease. Tests for liver function and testosterone were normal and no organic reason for the dysfunction was found. Mr JA also suffers from recurrent heartburn, for which he is taking cimetidine on most days.

> It was decided not to prescribe a pharmacological agent for his erectile dysfunction at this stage, but a number of suggestions and recommendations were made.

   a. Which of the above factors could contribute to his erectile dysfunction and what recommendations would you suggest?

> After 3 months, during which time Mr JA followed the advice he was given, his blood pressure was within normal limits and his cholesterol was lower. However, his erectile dysfunction persisted.
>
> Following discussions, it was decided that Mr JA should try sildenafil.

   b. From his history, what precautions should be taken in prescribing sildenafil and what advice should Mr JA be given?

The answers are provided on page 716.

Drugs used in erectile dysfunction (all should be used with caution in patients with cardiovascular disease)

Drug	Half-life	Elimination	Comments
Apomorphine	0.5 h	Metabolism	Taken sublingually 20 min before sexual activity
Alprostadil	30 s	Metabolism	Given by intracavernosal injection or urethral application; prostaglandin E_1 analogue; care if partner is pregnant; can cause priapism; can be given with papaverine (see below)
Papaverine	2 h	Metabolism	Smooth muscle relaxant given by intracavernosal injection; eliminated by oxidation in the liver; the 4-hydroxy metabolite is a phosphodiesterase inhibitor; not licensed in UK
Phentolamine	1.5 h	Metabolism + renal	Given by intracavernosal injection; eliminated in urine largely as oxidised metabolites plus some unchanged drug; not licensed in UK for this indication
Sildenafil	2 h	Metabolism	Given orally; incomplete oral bioavailability (about 40%) due to first-pass metabolism; usually taken 1 h before sexual activity, but absorption delayed by fatty food; eliminated by oxidation catalysed by CYP3A4 and CYP2C9; one metabolite retains some activity and contributes to the clinical effect; metabolites are eliminated mainly in the faeces (80%)
Tadalafil	17 h	Metabolism	Shows very high selectivity for phosphodiesterase type V; due to the long half-life and duration of action, it can be taken between 30 min and 12 h before sexual activity; bioavailability has not been defined, but absorption is not affected by food; eliminated by CYP3A4-catalysed oxidation in the liver
Vardenafil	4–5 h	Metabolism	Given orally; incomplete oral bioavailability (about 15%); usually taken 25–60 min before sexual activity, but absorption delayed by fatty food; eliminated by oxidation catalysed by CYP3A4; the major metabolite retains some activity; metabolites are eliminated mainly in the faeces (80%)

Drug compendium

The nervous system

17

General anaesthetics

General anaesthetics work in the brain to induce unconsciousness. This allows surgical or other painful procedures to be undertaken without the person being aware. General anaesthesia was introduced into clinical practice in the 19th century, with the inhalation of vapours such as diethyl ether and chloroform. Major drawbacks with such compounds included the time taken to cause loss of consciousness, slow recovery, unpleasant taste, irritant properties and their potential to explode. Cardiac and hepatic toxicity also limited the usefulness of chloroform. The perfect general anaesthetic would possess all the properties outlined in Box 17.1; however, since no single anaesthetic agent possesses all of these, it is now usual practice to use a combination of agents (balanced general anaesthesia). This utilises the advantages of each agent, and minimises the disadvantages. General anaesthesia for surgical procedures involves several steps:

- premedication
- induction
- muscle relaxation and intubation
- maintenance
- analgesia
- reversal.

Premedication in adults is usually with a benzodiazepine such as diazepam, temazepam or lorazepam (Ch. 20), to reduce anxiety and produce amnesia. In addition, an antiemetic such as metoclopramide (Ch. 32) may be given.

Anaesthesia was originally induced and maintained solely by inhalation of a volatile agent. If this method is used, several stages of general anaesthesia are passed through during induction and recovery. These are shown in Table 17.1. Some of these stages are undesirable. In adults, use of an inhalational anaesthetic for induction of anaesthesia is usually associated with troublesome excitation and struggling: this can be overcome by using a bolus of intravenous anaesthetic for induction, followed by an inhalational anaesthetic for maintenance. In children, this is less of a problem, and anaesthesia is often both induced and maintained with an inhalational anaesthetic agent. For some short surgical procedures in adults, total intravenous anaesthesia can be used.

For abdominal and thoracic surgery, and for long operations, adjunctive neuromuscular blocking drugs (Ch. 27) are used, in which case endotracheal intubation and mechanical ventilation are necessary. Analgesia can be provided by an intravenous opioid for systemic analgesia, or by a local anaesthetic (Ch. 18) to provide regional analgesia such as into the epidural space (epidural analgesia) or on peripheral nerves.

Resumption of consciousness (reversal of anaesthesia) occurs when intravenous anaesthetics are redistributed or metabolised, or when inhalational anaesthetics are redistributed or exhaled. Residual neuromuscular blockade may need reversal with neostigmine (Ch. 27). Attentiveness, and therefore the ability to drive safely, may be impaired for up to 24 h after general anaesthesia.

Mechanisms of action of general anaesthetics

General anaesthesia can be produced by compounds of widely differing chemical structure: from simple gases

---

Box 17.1

Properties of an ideal inhalational anaesthetic

Inherently stable

Non-flammable and non-explosive when mixed with air, oxygen or nitrous oxide

Potent, allowing the use of a high inspired oxygen concentration

Low blood solubility, allowing rapid induction (with minimal excitation stage); rapid emergence from anaesthesia, with no hangover; and rapid adjustment of the depth of anaesthesia

Non-irritant to the airways

Non-toxic

Lack of sensitisation of the heart to catecholamines

Analgesic

Easily reversible

Minimal interactions with other drugs

Inexpensive

Table 17.1
The stages of anaesthesia

Stage	Description	Effects produced
I	Analgesia	Analgesia without amnesia or loss of touch sensation; consciousness retained
II	Excitation	Excitation and delirium with struggling: respiration rapid and irregular; frequent eye movements with increased pupil diameter; amnesia
III	Surgical anaesthesia	Loss of consciousness; subdivided into four levels or planes of increasing depth; *plane I* shows a decrease in eye movements and some pupillary constriction; *plane II* shows loss of corneal reflex; *planes III and IV* show increasing loss of pharyngeal reflex, and a progressive decrease in thoracic breathing and general muscle tone
IV	Medullary depression	Loss of spontaneous respiration and progressive depression of cardiovascular reflexes: should be considered as an overdose requiring respiratory and circulatory support

such as nitrous oxide; volatile liquids such as isoflurane; and non-volatile solids such as propofol (Fig. 17.1). Anaesthetic potency is measured as the minimum alveolar concentration (MAC) of an agent necessary to immobilise 50% of subjects exposed to a noxious stimulus (which in humans is a surgical skin incision). Therefore, MAC is the equivalent of the ED_{50} (the 50% effective dose) for other drugs (Ch. 1). The MAC for inhaled anaesthetics correlates closely with their lipid solubility or oil:gas partition coefficient (see Table 17.2).

General anaesthetics act at cell membranes, and the relationship between lipid solubility and potency led to the hypothesis that their incorporation into lipids altered the cell membrane, perhaps resulting in the increased membrane fluidity and neural volume expansion. Although it is not known precisely how general anaesthetics work, there is increasing evidence that implicates actions at ligand-gated ion channels in the production of general anaesthesia. In particular, anaesthetic agents influence the function of the superfamilies of receptors for gamma-aminobutyric acid ($GABA_A$), glycine, acetylcholine (nicotinic) and 5-hydroxytryptamine ($5HT_3$), as well as the structurally unrelated NMDA (*N*-methyl-D-aspartate) receptor for glutamate. The actions of the first two (inhibitory) receptors are enhanced by general anaesthetics, whereas those of the latter three (excitatory) receptors are inhibited. The receptor binding sites for general anaesthetics have not yet been identified, but are probably on excitable membrane proteins. Binding of the drug to these proteins occurs preferentially when the ion channels are in their open state, and general anaesthetics may compete with endogenous ligands that are essential for the enzymatic function of these proteins.

The interaction of a general anaesthetic with the various ion channels alters postsynaptic receptor activity and inhibits both local and long-range (such as thalamocortical) cortical neural circuits. The amnesic and immobilising actions of an anaesthetic may result from effects on the hippocampus and spinal cord. The different receptor binding characteristics of the various inhaled anaesthetics may explain their distinct behavioural effects.

The different stages of anaesthesia (Table 17.1) probably arise from the different sizes of neurons and their accessibility to the anaesthetic agent. A rapid action on small neurons in the dorsal horn of the spinal cord (nociceptive impulses; Ch. 19) and inhibitory cells in the brain (cf. effects of alcohol; Ch. 54) explain the early analgesic and excitation phases. By contrast, neurons of the medullary centres are relatively insensitive and are affected last.

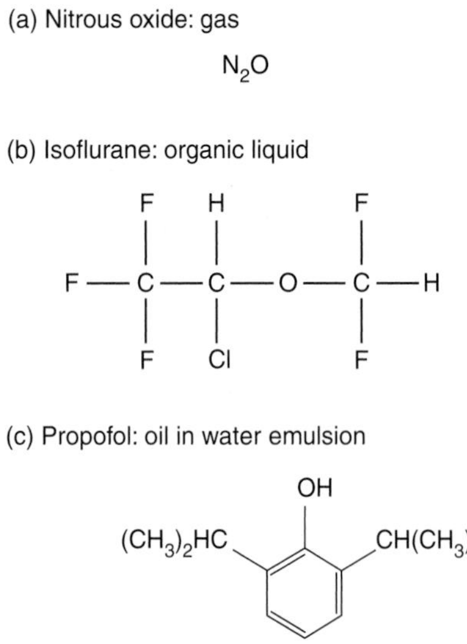

(a) Nitrous oxide: gas

N_2O

(b) Isoflurane: organic liquid

(c) Propofol: oil in water emulsion

Fig. 17.1
Examples of general anaesthetics of different chemical natures.

Drugs used in anaesthesia

General anaesthetics can be grouped according to their route of administration, which is either intravenous or inhalational.

Table 17.2
Inhalation anaesthetics[a]

Compound	Blood : gas partition coefficient	Oil : gas partition coefficient	Induction time (min)[b]	MAC (%)[c]	Metabolism (%)[d]
Nitrous oxide	0.5	1.4	2–3	>100[f]	0
Isoflurane	1.4	91	–	1.12	0.2
Enflurane	1.9	96	–	1.7	2.10
Halothane	2.3	224	4–5	0.8	15
Sevoflurane	0.6	53	–	2.1	approx 5
Diethyl ether[e]	12.1	65	10–20	2	5–10

[a]Most cause cardiac and respiratory depression and muscle relaxation. They have varying effects on cerebral blood flow.
[b]Time for induction if used as the sole anaesthetic; correlates with blood:gas coefficient
[c]Minimum alveolar concentration necessary for surgical anaesthesia (equivalent to potency); correlates inversely with oil:gas coefficient.
[d]Percentage eliminated as urinary metabolites; most of the remainder is eliminated in the expired air; influenced by volatility and blood:gas coefficient.
[e]No longer available for clinical use.
[f]Theoretical value.

Intravenous anaesthetics

Examples: propofol, thiopental, ketamine, etomidate

Intravenous anaesthetics are generally given for rapid induction of anaesthesia and are usually supplemented by inhalational anaesthetics. Propofol and ketamine can be given continuously without inhalational anaesthesia for short operations (total intravenous anaesthesia). Ketamine produces analgesia, unlike all other available intravenous anaesthetics, but it does not reliably suppress laryngeal reflexes, which can make intubation more difficult. Some properties of commonly used intravenous anaesthetics are shown in Table 17.3.

Pharmacokinetics

Thiobarbiturates, such as thiopental, have a very rapid onset of action (within 30 s) owing to their high lipid solu-

Table 17.3
Some properties of common intravenous anaesthetics

Drug	Type	Speed of induction	Recovery	Hangover effect	Analgesia	Comment
Thiopental	Barbiturate	Rapid	Slow owing to redistribution	Yes	No	Widely used; sloughing of tissue if extravascularisation occurs from the blood vessel or the site of injection; cannot be given by long-term continuous infusion; can cause bradycardia
Propofol	Phenol	Rapid	Rapid. Liver metabolism	Low	No	Does not accumulate during infusion; continuous infusion can be used in intensive care; occasional bradycardia
Etomidate	Imidazole	Rapid	Fairly rapid. Liver metabolism	Low	No	Not infused continuously; cardiac depressant; enhances GABA activity; repeated doses suppress adrenocortical function
Ketamine	Cyclohexanone	Slower	Slower	No	Yes	Hallucinations on recovery; cardiac stimulant, raises blood pressure; can be given continuously; analgesia that outlasts anaesthesia; bronchodilator

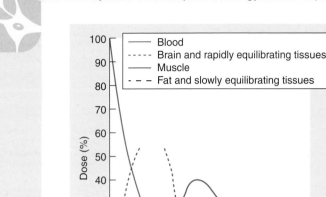

Fig. 17.2

The amounts of thiopental in blood, brain (and other rapidly equilibrating tissues), muscle, adipose tissue and other slowly equilibrating tissues after an intravenous infusion over 10 s.
NB: the time axis is not linear: the continued uptake into muscle between 1 and 30 min lowers the concentration in the blood and in all rapidly equilibrating tissues (including the brain); the terminal elimination slopes are parallel for all tissues; metabolism removes about 15% of the body load per hour.

bility and ease of passage across the blood–brain barrier. The delay in onset of action is largely a consequence of the circulation time between the site of injection in the arm and the brain. The duration of action after a bolus dose is very short (about 2–5 min) owing to redistribution from rapidly equilibrating tissues (including the brain) into more slowly equilibrating tissues such as muscle (Fig. 17.2; see also Ch. 2). With thiopental, total intravenous anaesthesia is not practicable, as the blood and slowly equilibrating tissues would reach equilibrium during anaesthesia; cessation of anaesthetic action would then depend on the elimination half-life (9–12 h for thiopental because of slow liver metabolism) not the distribution half-life (about 3 min). Therefore, following induction of anaesthesia with thiopental, an inhaled agent is used for maintenance of anaesthesia.

Propofol has a slightly slower onset of action (about 30 s) compared with thiopental; its duration of action is also limited by redistribution after a bolus dose. It can be given as an infusion for total intravenous anaesthesia (and for sedation in intensive care), when its duration of action is determined by a slower distribution phase (half-life 1–1.5 h) or, after prolonged use, by hepatic clearance (half-life about 6 h). Propofol is particularly useful for day surgery, because of its rapid elimination and absence of hangover effects. It also has an antiemetic action. Propofol can also be used by intravenous infusion for up to 3 days

for sedation in conscious patients requiring controlled ventilation in an intensive care unit.

Ketamine can be given by intramuscular injection or intravenously by bolus injection or infusion. The anaesthetic action is terminated by redistribution (half-life about 15 min), with some hepatic metabolism.

Etomidate has a rapid onset of action after intravenous injection, and its action is terminated by rapid metabolism in plasma and the liver, giving a duration of action of about 6–10 min, with minimal hangover.

Unwanted effects

- On the central nervous system (CNS): general depression of the CNS can also produce respiratory and cardiovascular depression. Slow release of thiopental distributed into tissues may result in some sedation for up to 24 h after use. Hallucinations and vivid dreams are common during recovery from ketamine (emergence reactions), but are less frequent in children.
- On muscles: extraneous muscle movement is common with etomidate, and can be reduced by a benzodiazepine or opioid analgesic given before induction. Ketamine increases muscle tone.
- On the heart: most intravenous anaesthetics depress the heart, producing bradycardia and reducing blood pressure. By contrast, ketamine produces tachycardia and an increase in blood pressure.
- Nausea and vomiting during recovery is experienced by up to 40% of people, but rarely persists for more than 24 h. Propofol has an antiemetic action.
- Convulsions have been reported after propofol. These can be delayed, indicating the need for special caution after day surgery.
- Pain on injection: propofol, being lipid soluble, is given in a complex vehicle, which may cause pain during intravenous injection. Thiopental is an alkaline solution that is irritant if injected outside the vein.

Intravenous opioids

Examples: alfentanil, fentanyl, remifentanil

Intravenous opioids are given at induction for intraoperative analgesia and to reduce the dose requirement of anaesthetic agents. In high doses, they stimulate the vagus and produce bradycardia; this can be helpful to reduce the tachycardia and hypertension produced by sympathetic nervous system activation during surgery. Attenuation of surgical stress can be particularly useful, for example during cardiac surgery. Details of the mechanism of action of opioids are found in Chapter 19.

Pharmacokinetics

After intravenous injection, fentanyl and remifentanil have a rapid onset of action, within 1–2 min. After a single dose, the action of fentanyl is short owing to rapid redistribution. The effect is maintained by repeated injections or infusion. With prolonged use, fentanyl has a long duration of action determined by its hepatic elimination (half-life 4 h), so that prolonged ventilatory support may be necessary after surgery. Alfentanil has a redistribution half-life of 5 min and an elimination half-life of 1.5 h.

Remifentanil is an opioid ester that has a very short half-life owing to metabolism by tissue and plasma esterases. After an initial bolus dose of remifentanil, continuous intravenous infusion is used to maintain its effects.

Unwanted effects

- muscle rigidity: this can be controlled during surgery with muscle relaxants, but after recovery, myoclonus and rigidity can persist, and require reversal with the opioid antagonist naloxone (Ch. 19)
- respiratory depression: this may be profound and means that assisted ventilation is usually necessary during surgery when large doses have been used.

Inhalational anaesthetics

Examples: halothane, isoflurane, nitrous oxide, sevoflurane

Inhaled anaesthetics are given with oxygen to avoid hypoxia during anaesthesia. Following induction with an intravenous anaesthetic, a single inhalational agent can be used to maintain anaesthesia. Nitrous oxide is not sufficiently potent to be used alone, but it has the advantage of producing analgesia (unlike the other inhalational anaesthetics) and is often used in combination with other anaesthetics, thus reducing the required dose of the other agent. Nitrous oxide can only be used as the sole inhalational agent when combined with an intravenous opioid and a neuromuscular junction blocking drug (Ch. 27), when there is a risk of awareness during surgery. Sevoflurane is widely used for children as it has a pleasant odour, an advantage when using it for induction; recovery is rapid, since it is eliminated more quickly than halothane or isoflurane, but, in consequence, early postoperative analgesia may be necessary.

Pharmacokinetics

The concentration of anaesthetic used in the inhaled gas (potency), and the duration of inhalation necessary to give sufficient concentration of drug in the CNS to produce general anaesthesia, depend on the relationships shown in Fig. 17.3 and Table 17.2. There are four factors that are important.

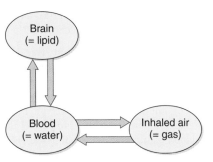

Fig. 17.3
Equilibration of inhaled general anaesthetics between air, blood and brain. The concentration ratio between blood and air at equilibrium is estimated from in vivo studies of the blood:gas partition coefficient (Table 17.2). The concentrations in brain and blood at equilibrium reflect the different affinities of the two media for general anaesthetics. The brain:blood ratio is 1–3:1 for all commonly used anaesthetics. The concentration in the inspired air required to give the necessary concentration in brain membranes (minimum alveolar concentration; MAC) is an indication of the potency of the compound.

1. The rate of absorption across the alveolar membranes. This depends on both the concentration of drug in the inspired air and the rate of drug delivery, i.e. the rate and depth of inspiration. These factors are important if an inhaled agent is used for induction, but less significant once an equilibrium has been established between the inhaled concentration and that in the brain. Lung conditions such as emphysema, which result in poor alveolar ventilation, will slow the induction of anaesthesia and also the recovery from agents eliminated by exhalation.
2. The rate at which the concentration of drug in the blood reaches equilibrium with that in the inspired air. An important factor in this context is the solubility of the anaesthetic in blood and rapidly equilibrating tissues such as the brain. A high solubility in blood will be associated with a slow attainment of equilibrium. Anaesthesia could be achieved more rapidly if the concentration inhaled during induction is higher than the maintenance concentration, since this would be equivalent to a loading dose (see Ch. 2).
3. The cardiac output, which will determine circulation time and drug delivery to the brain.
4. The relative concentrations of the drug in the brain and blood at equilibrium. The rate of entry of drug into the brain is not limiting because for lipid-soluble drugs, which are relatively insoluble in blood, the brain is part of the rapidly equilibrating central compartment. The rate-limiting step is the rate of delivery via the inhaled gas compared with the total amount in the body at equilibrium. The times to onset of anaesthesia (induction time) for a range of anaesthetic compounds are given in Table 17.2.

There are two physicochemical properties that affect the action of an inhaled anaesthetic agent.

- **The blood:gas partition coefficient.** This indicates the relative solubility of the drug in blood (or water) and air. A high solubility in water, and therefore in all rapidly equilibrating body tissues, means that a greater amount of the agent will need to be administered before the partial pressure of the agent in the blood equilibrates with that in the inspired air. Diethyl ether, although not used clinically, has been included in Table 17.2 since this illustrates well the relationship between a high blood:air partition coefficient and a long induction period.
  (Note: the data in Table 17.2 conform to the basic pharmacokinetic principle that compounds with a large apparent volume of distribution take longer to reach steady state during a constant rate of drug input.)
- **The oil:gas partition coefficient.** This reflects the ratio between the concentration in the lipid membranes of brain cells and the inhaled concentration. Since all anaesthetic agents must achieve approximately the same concentration in the membrane lipids of CNS neurons for effective anaesthesia, the higher the partition coefficient then the lower will be the inhaled concentration of gas required to maintain anaesthesia. This is well illustrated by the data in Table 17.2. Nitrous oxide has a low oil:gas partition coefficient, such that, if given alone, surgical anaesthesia could only be achieved with an inspired concentration of drug that would not allow an adequate inspired oxygen concentration.

The major route of elimination of inhaled anaesthetics is via the airways. Factors that influence the duration of the induction phase, such as ventilation rate and the blood:gas partition coefficient, will also affect the time taken to eliminate the anaesthetic and thus the recovery time. The recovery time may also depend on the duration of inhalation, which can affect the extent to which the drug has entered slowly equilibrating tissues. Elimination from these tissues is slow, which can maintain the plasma concentration of the drug and delay recovery. During recovery, the depth of anaesthesia reverses through the stages discussed above to consciousness; a rapid recovery which minimises stage II (Table 17.1) is beneficial. Comparing the data in Table 17.2, it is hardly surprising that diethyl ether is no longer used.

General anaesthetics are also partly eliminated by metabolism, the extent of which depends on the time that the agent is retained in the body and is available to the metabolising enzymes. Thus, exhalation and metabolism can be regarded as alternative pathways of elimination, the proportions of which are determined largely by the volatility of the agent and its blood:gas partition coefficient (see Table 17.2).

Unwanted effects

A number of unwanted effects are common to most clinically useful inhaled anaesthetics; however, each agent also has a unique profile of additional unwanted effects.

- **Cardiovascular system.** Most agents, and particularly halothane, depress myocardial contractility and produce bradycardia by interfering with transmembrane calcium flux. This decreases cardiac output and blood pressure. Halothane also sensitises the heart to catecholamines, which can lead to arrhythmias. Isoflurane is less cardiodepressant, but may reduce blood pressure by arterial vasodilation. Nitrous oxide also has less depressant effect on the heart and circulation and its use in combination with other agents may permit reduction in their dosage and, therefore, reduce their depressant effect on the heart. Inhaled anaesthetics often increase cerebral blood flow, which can exacerbate an elevated intracranial pressure.
- **Respiratory system.** All agents depress the response of the respiratory centre in the medulla to carbon dioxide and hypoxia. They also decrease tidal volume and increase respiratory rate. Some agents, e.g. isoflurane, are irritant and can cause coughing and laryngospasm if used for induction.
- **Liver.** Most agents decrease liver blood flow. Mild hepatic dysfunction because of specific hepatic toxicity is common after treatment with halothane. However, about 1 in 30 000 people will develop severe hepatic necrosis following the use of halothane, especially after repeat exposure within a short time interval. This is because of interaction of reactive metabolites with cellular proteins, which initiates an autoimmune reaction. Obesity, and hypoxia during anaesthesia appear to confer greater risk of this complication. Hepatotoxicity has resulted in the decreased use of halothane, and avoidance of repeat use within 3 months.
- **Kidney.** Both renal blood flow and renal vascular resistance decrease, resulting in a reduced glomerular filtration rate.
- **Uterus.** There is relaxation of the uterus, which may increase risk of haemorrhage if anaesthesia is used in labour. Nitrous oxide has less effect on uterine muscle compared with the other agents.
- **Skeletal muscle.** Most agents produce some muscle relaxation, which enhances the activity of neuromuscular blocking drugs (Ch. 27). With sevoflurane, this may be sufficient to enable tracheal intubation without the use of a neuromuscular blocker.
- **Chemoreceptor trigger zone.** Inhalational anaesthetics trigger postoperative nausea and vomiting. This may be most pronounced with nitrous oxide.

Table 17.4
The concept of 'balanced anaesthesia' – drugs are used in combination, each having more than one effect and having major or minor actions; overall contributing to a balanced effect

	Sedation	Analgesia	Muscle relaxation
Drugs exerting a major effect	Inhalational anaesthetics Propofol Premedicant benzodiazepines	Fentanyl Alfentanil Local anaesthetics	Neuromuscular blocking drugs (Ch. 27)
Drugs exerting a minor effect	Fentanyl, alfentanil Nitrous oxide	Nitrous oxide	Inhalational anaesthetics

- **Postoperative shivering.** This occurs in up to 65% of those recovering from general anaesthesia. The aetiology is unclear.
- **Malignant hyperthermia.** This is a rare but potentially fatal complication of inhalational anaesthesia. It is genetically determined, and results from a sudden increase in intracellular calcium in muscle cells. Tachycardia, unstable blood pressure, hypercapnoea, fever and hyperventilation occur, followed by hyperkalaemia and metabolic acidosis. Muscle rigidity may occur. Treatment is with dantrolene (Ch. 24).

The management of a person undergoing general anaesthesia requires the administration of several drugs having different desirable and unwanted effects. The appropriate combination of these agents produces a 'balanced anaesthesia' (Table 17.4).

FURTHER READING

Campagna JA, Miller KW, Forman SA (2003) Mechanisms of actions of inhaled anaesthetics. *N Engl J Med* 348, 2110–2124

Dodds C (1999) General anaesthesia: practical recommendations and recent advances. *Drugs* 58, 453–467

Fox AJ, Rowbottam DJ (1999) Anaesthesia. *BMJ* 319, 557–560

Millar KW (2002) The nature and sites of general anaesthetic action. *Br J Anaesth* 89, 17–31

Wiklund RA, Rosenbaum SH (1997) Anaesthesiology Parts I and II. *N Engl J Med* 337, 1132–1141, 1215–1219

Self-assessment

In questions 1–6, the initial statement, in italics, is true. Are the accompanying statements also true?

1. *The MAC of an inhalational anaesthetic required to produce surgical anaesthesia correlates with the oil:gas partition coefficient of drug.*

   a. Inhalational anaesthetics may have their effect by interacting with specific receptors.
   b. Inhalational anaesthetics are all gases.
   c. Most inhalational anaesthetics are sulphated compounds.

2. *Properties of an ideal inhalational anaesthetic are that it is stable, non-inflammable, potent, low lipid solubility, non-irritant, non-toxic, analgesic and does not sensitise the heart to catecholamines.*

   a. Halothane closely approaches the properties of an ideal inhalational anaesthetic.
   b. The risk of hangover effects with inhalational anaesthetics increases if the operation is long.

   c. Nitrous oxide, when administered alone, reaches the MAC necessary for surgical anaesthesia if its concentration in inspired air is 50%.
   d. Nitrous oxide is frequently given with oxygen and a fluorinated anaesthetic agent to produce effective surgical anaesthesia.

3. *Isoflurane is now the most widely used volatile anaesthetic.* Isoflurane is metabolised by the same pathway as halothane.

4. *The short duration of action of thiopental is due to its redistribution into richly perfused tissues such as muscles.*

   a. The elimination half-life of thiopental is similar to the distribution half-life.
   b. Propofol cannot be given as a continuous infusion for intravenous anaesthesia.
   c. Accidental injection of thiopental into an artery can have serious consequences.
   d. Ketamine is sedative but is without analgesic action.

5. *Fentanyl is a lipid-soluble opioid analgesic.* Fentanyl should not be administered concurrently with inhalational anaesthetics.

6. *Because of the rapid activity of modern anaesthetics, the individual well-defined stages of anaesthesia are not clearly seen.*

a. When administering an inhalational anaesthetic, the excitement stage of anaesthesia is prolonged if an intravenous anaesthetic is not given beforehand.

b. Most inhalational anaesthetics have a depressant effect on the cardiovascular system.

c. Inhalational anaesthetics reduce the sensitivity of the respiratory centre to carbon dioxide and hypoxia.

d. Sevoflurane has the advantage of a fast onset of action and eliminaton.

7. Considering the pharmacology of agents used in anaesthesia, choose the one <u>most appropriate</u> statement.

A. The minimum percentage concentration of nitrous oxide in alveolar air for surgical anaesthesia is 50%.

B. The major route of elimination of inhalational anaesthetics is via the liver.

C. Ketamine is an intravenous anaesthetic and also has analgesic properties.

D. The intravenous opioid fentanyl should not be administered together with sevoflurane.

E. Atropine is a commonly administered pre-operative agent.

8. Case history questions

> A 40-year-old lady is scheduled for a laparotomy because of an abdominal swelling. She has not had a previous operation and is otherwise healthy, with normal cardiovascular and respiratory function. She was premedicated with pethidine (meperidine) and atropine.

a. Why is atropine little used in adults as preanaesthetic medication nowadays?

b. Do the muscarinic antagonists atropine and hyoscine have the same properties?

> She was intubated after the administration of thiopental, fentanyl and suxamethonium (succinylcholine).

c. Why has the routine use of suxamethonium to facilitate endotracheal intubation been reduced?

> Following intubation, pancuronium and fentanyl were given and she was ventilated with nitrous oxide, enflurane and oxygen. An ovarian cyst was removed and the operation took 40 min.

d. Is pancuronium a suitable choice of muscle relaxant? What alternatives are available?

> After the operation, she did not breathe spontaneously, despite the administration of neostigmine and glycopyrronium.

e. What are the possible reasons for the apnoea and how could they be treated?

f. Would mivacurium (a short-duration muscle relaxant) have been a preferable muscle relaxant to use in this patient?

g. What is the reason for administering glycopyrronium with neostigmine at the end of the operation?

The answers are provided on pages 716–718.

General anaesthetics

Drug	Half-life (h)	Elimination	Comments
Intravenous anaesthetics			Following a bolus dose, the duration of action depends on the rate of redistribution and not the elimination half-life given below
Etomidate	2–11	Metabolism	Used for induction without hangover; suppresses adrenocortical function on continuous dosage and should not be used for maintenance anaesthesia; hydrolysed and oxidised in liver to inactive products
Ketamine	2–4	Metabolism	Can also be given by intramuscular injection for short procedures; redistribution half-life from well-perfused to poorly perfused tissues is about 15 min; hepatic metabolism produces numerous oxidation products
Propofol	3–12	Metabolism	Duration of action partly determined by redistribution, with a half-life of 0.5–1 h; rapid glucuronidation in the liver and other tissues contributes to recovery; drug that has entered poorly perfused tissues during prolonged administration is eliminated more slowly, with a half-life of about 3–12 h
Thiopental	4–12	Metabolism	Reconstituted solution is highly alkaline; duration of action determined by redistribution; slow oxidation to an inactive product; repeated doses have a cumulative and prolonged effect as the blood and poorly perfused tissues reach equilibrium
Intravenous opioids			Provide analgesia and enhance anaesthesia
Alfentanil	0.7–2	Metabolism	Used especially during short procedures and for outpatient surgery; respiratory depression may persist after the end of the procedure if repeated doses are given; oxidised in liver by CYP3A4, and conjugated with glucuronic acid
Fentanyl	1–6	Metabolism	Respiratory depression may persist after the end of the procedure if repeated doses are given; rapid initial uptake from the blood into lungs, followed by redistribution and elimination; high interindividual variability in kinetics; metabolised in the liver
Remifentanil	0.1	Metabolism	Given as an infusion; very rapid clearance by blood and tissue esterases (clearance is 3 l min^{-1}, which exceeds liver blood flow); metabolite inactive
Inhalational anaesthetics			
Desflurane	Various	Exhalation	Not recommended for induction in children because of cough, laryngospasm and increased secretions; <0.1% is metabolised by CYP2E1; brain:blood ratio is 1.3:1; rapid recovery (minutes) but present in exhaled air for days
Enflurane	Various	Exhalation + metabolism	Powerful cardiorespiratory depressant; about 8% is metabolised by CYP2E1; brain:blood ratio is 1.4:1; rapid recovery; multiple phases are present in the elimination curve, with half-lives ranging from 2 min to 34 h owing to uptake and release from tissues

continued

General anaesthetics *(continued)*

Drug	Half-life (h)	Elimination	Comments
Inhalational anaesthetics (continued)			
Halothane	Various	Exhalation + metabolism	Can be used for smooth induction of anaesthesia, because it is potent, non-irritant and does not produce cough; about 20% is metabolised; oxidation by CYP2E1 produces trifluoroacyl chloride, which may react with protein and trigger hepatotoxicity; brain:blood ratio is 2.9:1; half-lives similar to enflurane
Isoflurane	Various	Exhalation	An isomer of enflurane; <0.2% metabolism by CYP2E1; brain:blood ratio is 2.6:1; multiple half-lives reported, <1 min to 40 h, requires a five-compartmental mathematical model; rapid recovery during redistribution phases
Nitrous oxide	–	Exhalation	Low potency compared with other inhaled agents; rapid recovery owing to low potency and low tissue affinity; eliminated by exhalation, without metabolism; brain:blood ratio is 1.0:1; may reduce cerebrovascular effects of halothane when used in combination
Sevoflurane	–	Exhalation + metabolism	About 5% metabolism by CYP2E1; brain:blood ratio is 1.7:1; complex elimination kinetics; recovery may be particularly rapid after short procedures

18

Local anaesthetics

Local anaesthetics are drugs that reversibly block the transmission of pain stimuli locally at their site of administration.

Examples: lidocaine, cocaine, bupivacaine, benzocaine, ropivacaine, tetracaine, prilocaine

Mechanism of action

Local anaesthetics block the nerve transmission of pain by reducing the ion fluxes that are responsible for depolarisation of excitable cells. The neuronal cell membrane is freely permeable to K^+ at rest, but only semi-permeable to Na^+. The maintenance of a negative internal resting electrical potential is largely determined by K^+ alone. Conduction of a nerve action potential results from opening of Na^+ channels, and rapid influx of Na^+ to depolarise the cell (see Fig. 18.2). Local anaesthetics produce reversible conduction block by inactivating the Na^+ channel mainly when it is in its open state, although blockade is possible with some local anaesthetics even when it is in its inactivated state. There is considerable redundancy in the membrane Na^+ channels. Nerve conduction can continue even when up to 90% of the channels are blocked, and the peak membrane Na^+ current is about five times that required to initiate an action potential. Local anaesthetics progressively interrupt Na^+ channel excitability until conductance fails. Because local anaesthetics act by such a ubiquitous mechanism, they inhibit both afferent and efferent neural pathways as well as neuroeffector systems such as the neuromuscular junction.

The probability that propagation of a nerve impulse will fail at a particular segment of the nerve is related to the local concentration of the anaesthetic drug, the length of the nerve exposed to the drug, and to whether or not the nerve is myelinated. In myelinated nerves, the drug penetrates at the nodes of Ranvier and must block at least three consecutive nodes to produce conduction block. Unmyelinated nerves must be blocked over sufficient length, and around the full circumference of the nerve. The temporal onset of effect of a local anaesthetic is related to nerve fibre size, the spatial relationships within the nerve fibre and the concentration of the injected local anaesthetic. The most rapid and intense onset of anaesthesia is achieved in small diameter and/or myelinated fibres such as pain afferents, and these fibres also show the longest duration of effect. Therefore, pain pathways are considerably more sensitive to blockade by local anaesthetics than are the larger fibres involved in touch or pressure transmission (Table 18.1).

Structural requirements of local anaesthetics. Local anaesthetics act mainly by binding of the ionic form of the anaesthetic to the binding site on the inside of the

Table 18.1

Nerve fibres and their responsiveness to local anaesthetics

Fibre type	Site	Myelination	Diameter (μm)	Sensitivity to anaesthesia[a]
A				
Alpha	Motor	+	12–20	+
Beta	Touch, pressure	+	5-12	+
Gamma	Muscle spindle	+	3-6	++
Delta	Pain, temperature	+	2-5	+++
B	Preganglionic			
	Autonomic	(+)	1–3	+++
C	Dorsal horn	–	0.4–1.2	+++
	Postganglionic	–	0.3–1.3	+++

[a]Increasing number of + indicate increasing sensitivity to local anaesthesia.

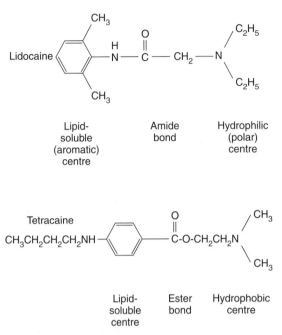

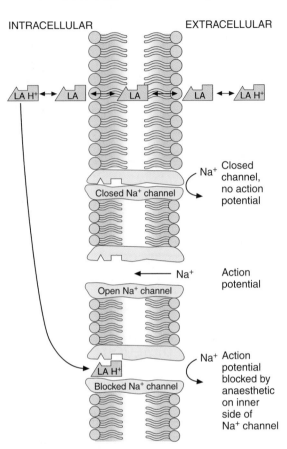

Fig. 18.1
General structure of local anaesthetics. Differences in structure alter the speed of onset, duration of action and the metabolism of the drugs (see the drug compendium table).

Fig. 18.2
Site and mechanism of action of local anaesthetics. Weakly basic local anaesthetics exist as an equilibrium between ionised (LA H$^+$) and un-ionised (LA) forms. The ionised form binds to the intracellular receptor, and the un-ionised form is lipid soluble and crosses the axonal membrane. Local anaesthesia may also result from incorporation of the compound into a ring of lipid around the Na$^+$ channel, which becomes rigid and cannot open.

channel. Membrane penetration, however, is better with the un-ionised form. The structural requirements for local anaesthetic activity appear to involve a minimum of a hydrophobic aromatic ring structure connected to a hydrophilic amine group by a short ester or amide linkage (Fig. 18.1). Clinically used potent local anaesthetics are secondary or tertiary amines with a central amide or ester structure. The lipophilic aromatic group enables the molecule to cross the nerve membrane, and the potency of the drug is directly related to its lipid solubility. The hydrophilic group binds to the sodium channel. Variation in the structures of the aromatic and hydrophilic groups alters the onset and duration of action of the drug. The length of the intermediate bonding chain is critical to local anaesthetic activity and is optimal between 3 and 7 carbon equivalents. Bupivacaine and ropivacaine have the same chemical structure but are different isomers (bupivacaine is the *R*-isomer and ropivacaine the *S*-isomer); levobupivacaine is the L-isomer of bupivacaine.

Specific intraneuronal binding. The protein binding of the drug within the Na$^+$ channel determines its duration of action. Those local anaesthetics with high protein-binding affinity reside at the site of action for longer: thus, procaine has low protein binding, a weak association with the nerve cell membrane and a short duration of action, while bupivacaine is highly protein bound and has a long duration of action.

The pKa of the drug (the pH at which 50% of the drug is in the base form and 50% in the cationic form) determines the extent of ionisation at physiological pH

and the speed of onset of the conduction block. All local anaesthetics are weak bases and will be relatively more ionised at a pH below the pKa, which for most local anaesthetics is between 7.7 and 9.1. Because the water solubility of a local anaesthetic is greatest in the ionised form, injectable preparations are prepared as the hydrochloride salts with a pH of 5.0–6.0. However, the base (un-ionised) form is more lipid soluble and more readily penetrates lipid membranes; therefore, after injection, the drug solution (pH 5.0–6.0) must be buffered to physiological pH (7.4) before a significant amount of base is available to penetrate the nerve and reach its site of action. The higher the pKa of the drug, the higher the percentage of the cationic form at physiological pH and the slower the speed of onset of anaesthesia. However, it is the ionised form of the drug that binds to an ionic structure within the axoplasmic opening of the Na$^+$ channel. The binding site is most accessible when the channel is in its open (activated) state (Fig. 18.2). Local anaesthetic effectiveness is also dependent on the frequency of firing of the neuron (use-dependency), and a faster onset of local anaesthesia occurs in rapidly firing neurons. Once the local anaesthetic has bound to the channel, the influx of Na^+ is blocked and the channel remains inactivated. It then slowly reverts to the resting state, with consequent loss of local anaesthetic binding.

Local anaesthetics also bind to other ion channels and cell receptors, including presynaptic Ca^{2+} channels, tachykinin type 1 receptors and acetylcholine receptors. The role of these interactions is unclear, but may be involved in the production of spinal anaesthesia (see below).

Pharmacokinetics

The onset of local anaesthetic action is largely determined by the physicochemical properties of the drug molecule. The duration of action of local anaesthetics is dependent on their rate of removal from the site of administration rather than their systemic elimination by metabolism. It is also affected by the extent of local vasodilation, and most local anaesthetics cause vasodilation at the site of injection. By contrast, cocaine, which blocks noradrenaline reuptake by noradrenergic neurons (uptake 1; Ch. 4), produces intense vasoconstriction and has a longer duration of action than would be expected given its polarity. This is one of the reasons that cocaine is never used by injection, and its medical use is restricted to topical anaesthesia in otolaryngology. The duration of action of any local anaesthetic can be extended considerably by co-administration with a vasoconstrictor such as an α_1-adrenoceptor agonist, for example adrenaline (epinephrine). However, the pH of the solution must be 2.0–3.0 to prevent decomposition of the adrenaline (epinephrine). There are several local anaesthetic preparations available which are combinations of a local anaesthetic and a vasoconstrictor.

Once the local anaesthetic has diffused away from the site of administration, it enters the general circulation and undergoes elimination from the body. Most local anaesthetics have a central amide bond, and are eliminated by hepatic hydrolysis of the amide bond. The half-life of amide local anaesthetics within the circulation is generally short (between 1 and 3 h). Ester bonds are very rapidly hydrolysed by plasma esterases; in consequence, the plasma half-lives of the ester drugs procaine and tetracaine are 3 min or less.

Unwanted effects

Local effects. These occur at the site of administration and include irritation and inflammation. Local ischaemia can occur if they are co-administered with a vasoconstrictor, therefore this should be avoided in the extremities such as the digits. Tissue damage/necrosis can follow inappropriate administration (e.g. accidental intra-arterial administration or spinal administration of an epidural dose).

Systemic effects. These are related to the local anaesthetic action, and usually result from excessive plasma concentrations that affect other excitable membranes such as the heart (see antiarrhythmic action of lidocaine; Ch. 8). After regional anaesthesia, the maximum plasma drug concentration occurs within 30 min.

- Excessive amounts (especially after accidental intravenous injection, or rapid absorption from inflamed tissues) can cause cardiovascular collapse owing to systemic vasodilation and a negative inotropic effect. Cardiotoxicity with serious arrhythmias is a particular problem with bupivacaine and is caused by its avid tissue binding in the heart. As a result of its high lipid solubility and high protein binding, it has a fast-in, slow-out kinetic pattern at the Na^+ channel. Bupivacaine blocks the normal cardiac conducting system and predisposes to ventricular re-entrant pathways and intractable ventricular arrhythmias. Bupivacaine is a racemic compound, and the optical isomer levobupivacaine has been introduced recently as a separate drug; it has about the same local anaesthetic potency but less potential to produce cardiac effects. Ropivacaine is a chemical analogue of bupivacaine with much less cardiotoxicity.
- In the central nervous system (CNS), local anaesthetics can produce light-headedness, then sedation and loss of consciousness. Severe reactions can be accompanied by convulsions. Metabolites of lidocaine can cause generalised excitation and convulsions.
- True allergy is rare, but can occur with ester agents, related to their metabolism to para-amino-benzoic acid.

For more details of individual local anaesthetics, see the drug compendium table at the end of this chapter.

Techniques of administration

The extent of local anaesthesia depends largely on the technique of administration.

Surface administration. High concentrations (up to 10%) of drug in an oily vehicle can slowly penetrate the skin or mucous membranes to give a small localised area of anaesthesia. Lidocaine can be applied as a cream to an area before a minor skin procedure or venepuncture. Benzocaine is a relatively non-polar weak non-amino local anaesthetic that is included in some throat pastilles to produce anaesthesia of mucous membranes. Cocaine is restricted to topical use in otolaryngeal procedures, to produce vasoconstriction and reduce mucosal bleeding.

Infiltration anaesthesia. A local injection of an aqueous solution of local anaesthetic, sometimes with a vasoconstrictor, produces a local field of anaesthesia. The anaesthetic effect produced is more efficient than surface anaesthesia, but requires a relatively large amount of drug. Smaller volumes can be used for field block anaesthesia, involving subcutaneous injection close to nerves around the area to be anaesthetised. This technique is extensively used in dentistry.

Peripheral nerve block anaesthesia. Injection of an aqueous solution around a nerve trunk produces a field of anaesthesia distal to the site of injection. This can be used for temporary sympathetic nerve block, such as the stellate ganglion, or for lumbar sympathectomy.

Epidural anaesthesia. Injection or slow infusion via a cannula of an aqueous solution adjacent to the spinal column, but outside the dura mater, produces anaesthesia both above and below the site of injection. The extent of anaesthesia depends on the volume of drug administered. This technique is used extensively in obstetrics and some other surgical procedures. The concentration of drug used is the same as that for spinal anaesthesia but the volume, and therefore the dose, is greater. For this reason, systemic unwanted effects are more frequent than with spinal anaesthesia. Sympathetic fibres are particularly sensitive to local anaesthetics; this can result in hypotension and may be particularly exaggerated during pregnancy (probably related to the concurrent effects of high progesterone concentrations). Backache is a frequent postoperative complication with epidural and spinal anaesthesia.

Spinal anaesthesia. This involves injection of an aqueous solution into the lumbar subarachnoid space, usually between the third and fourth lumbar vertebrae. The spread of anaesthetic within the subarachnoid space depends on the density of the solution (a solution in 10% glucose is more dense than cerebrospinal fluid) and the posture of the person during the first 10–15 min while the solution flows up or down the subarachnoid space. Spinal and epidural anaesthesia can be used together, often using an opioid (Ch. 17) alone or in combination with a local anaesthetic.

Intravenous regional anaesthesia. This involves injection of a dilute solution of local anaesthetic into a limb after application of a tourniquet (Bier's block). It is used for manipulation of fractures and minor surgical procedures. Arterial blood flow must be occluded for at least 20 min.

FURTHER READING

French RJ, Zamponi GW, Sierralta IE (1998) Molecular and kinetic determinants of local anaesthetic action on sodium channels. *Toxicol Lett* 100/101, 247–254

Tetzlaff JE (2000) The pharmacology of local anesthetics. *Anesth Clin North Am* 18, 217–233

Wiklund RA, Rosenbaum SH (1997) Anesthesiology. Part II. *N Engl J Med* 337, 1215–1219

Self-assessment

In questions 1 and 2, the first statement, in italics, is true. Are the accompanying statements true or false?

1. *Local anaesthetics exhibit use-dependence. The block is more rapid and complete when the nerve is actively firing. This is because local anaesthetics bind more readily to Na⁺ channels that are in the open state.*

   a. Local anaesthetics have no systemic unwanted effects.
   b. The main mechanism by which the effect of local anaesthesia wears off is through liver metabolism of the anaesthetic.
   c. Local anaesthetics block smaller myelinated axons more effectively than large myelinated axons.
   d. The α_1-adrenoceptor antagonist prazosin is added to local anaesthetics to extend their duration of activity.

2. *Local anaesthetics must be lipid soluble to penetrate the axon and reach the innerside of the Na⁺ channel before blocking it. It is the ionised component, however, which blocks the Na⁺ channel.*

   a. Ropivacaine is a long-acting local anaesthetic.
   b. Ropivacaine (also known as levobupivacaine) is the $S(-)$-bupivacaine enantioner of the racemate $R(+)$- and $S(-)$-bupivacaine. The $S(-)$-bupivacaine enantioner exhibits greater cardiotoxicity than the $R(+)$-bupivacaine enantiomer.

3. Choose the one <u>most appropriate</u> statement from the following options.

   A. Raising the pH of a local anaesthetic solution will increase its speed of onset.
   B. When locally administered, liver metabolism is the most important primary mechanism in terminating local anaesthetic action and reducing toxicity.
   C. The effectiveness of a local anaesthetic is not altered by local tissue pH.
   D. The direct effect on blood vessel diameter of most commonly used local anaesthetics prolongs their duration of action.

E. Adrenaline (epinephrine) is given with a local anaesthetic injection in digits and appendages to increase the duration of anaesthesia.

4. Extended-matching questions
   Choose the <u>most appropriate</u> option A–F that could be used in the situations 1–4 below.

   A. Cocaine
   B. Adrenaline (epinephrine)
   C. Salbutamol
   D. Tetracaine
   E. Lidocaine
   F. Benzocaine.

1. A child needed a minor surgical procedure on her nasopharynx and you chose to use a single agent that you could administer topically which would reduce mucous membrane bleeding.
2. An agent that would extend the duration and potency of a local anaesthetic.
3. An agent that could be applied topically to produce anaesthesia of the conjunctiva which would not cause vasoconstriction.
4. An agent that could be administered intravenously in the treatment of ventricular arrhythmias.

The answers are provided on page 718.

Drug compendium

Local anaesthetics (all given by injection, except for benzocaine)

Drug	Half-life[a]	Elimination	Comments
Articaine	1	Metabolism	Used in dentistry; concentrations in tooth alveolus are 100 times those in circulation; half-life data are from subjects treated to produce regional anaesthesia; hydrolysed to inactive articainic acid by serum esterases
Benzocaine	<1 min	Metabolism	Differs from other drugs by not having a secondary amino group; used in throat lozenges; minimal absorption; metabolised in liver
Bupivacaine	1–3 [2–4]	Metabolism	Bupivacaine is the R-isomer (with ropivacaine the S-isomer); used for local infiltration, peripheral nerve block, epidural block and sympathetic block; slow onset of action (30 min); metabolised mainly by N-dealkylation and hydroxylation; less than 10% is excreted in urine
Levobupivacaine	1.3	Metabolism	Newly introduced L-optical isomer of the drug bupivacaine; metabolised by hepatic CYP3A4; less cardiotoxicity than with bupivacaine
Lidocaine	1.5 [1–2]	Metabolism	Used for local infiltration, intravenous regional anaesthesia and nerve blocks and dental anaesthesia; also used topically; metabolised by dealkylation, catalysed by CYP3A4, followed by hydrolysis
Mepivacaine	2–3 [1–3]	Metabolism	Used in dentistry; metabolised in liver by N-dealkylation and hydroxylation
Prilocaine	1–2 [1.5]	Metabolism	Used for local infiltration anaesthesia, intravenous anaesthesia, nerve blocks and dental anaesthesia; may cause methaemoglobinaemia (especially in infants); metabolised mainly by amide hydrolysis in the liver
Procaine	Not relevant [0.5]	Metabolism	Seldom used now; local infiltration anaesthesia; very rapid ester hydrolysis at site of injection, any which escaped into the blood would be rapidly hydrolysed by plasma esterases, with a half-life of less than 1 min
Ropivacaine	2 [2–4]	Metabolism	Used for epidural, major nerve block and field block; oxidised by hepatic CYP1A2 and CYP3A4 isoenzymes; ropivacaine is the S-isomer form of bupivacaine (which is the R-isomer) and has less cardiotoxicity
Tetracaine	3 min [2–3]	Metabolism	Mostly used topically; poorly absorbed; hydrolysed by plasma pseudocholinesterase

[a]The effective duration of action is given in brackets

19

Opioid analgesics and the management of pain

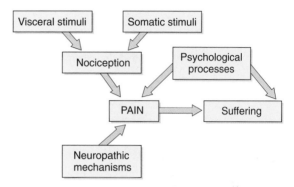

Fig. 19.1
The origin of pain and suffering.

Pain and pain perception

Pain is a complex phenomenon that involves both the generation of specific neuronal activity and the response of the patient to that activity. Pain is the subjective sensation that results from the perception of these impulses. Pain can last until the initiating trauma resolves (**nociceptive pain**), but can also become protracted, outlasting the original trauma, due to changes in the nociceptive neuronal pathways themselves (**neuropathic pain**).

Nociceptive pain can be an appropriate response to stimuli that activitate the peripheral mechanical, thermal or chemical nociceptor sensory units (units or receptors selectively sensitive to a noxious stimulus), initiating physiological protective responses in the nervous system. **Neuropathic pain** can be generated by damage, functional change or phenotypic change in the neural pathways. Chronic pain, which is usually recognised as persisting for longer than 3 months after the original pathology has resolved, may embrace the domain of neuropathic pain. Nociceptive pain is usually treatable by non-steroidal anti-inflammatory drugs (NSAIDs), opioids or neuronal blockade, but these are often less effective in treating chronic and neuropathic pain, which may require a variety of non-opioid or non-NSAID treatments. The response of the individual to the painful stimulus will be influenced by psychological factors; this will determine whether or not the pain produces or contributes to suffering or distress (Fig. 19.1).

Nociceptive pain can arise from somatic or visceral structures. Somatic pain is typically aching, stabbing, throbbing or pressure-like. Visceral pain is gnawing or cramp-like if it arises from a hollow viscus, or similar to somatic pain when arising from other structures. Sharp pain stimuli are transmitted to the central nervous system (CNS) by fast fibres in the neospinothalamic pathway; chronic visceral pain is transmitted by slow fibres in the paleospinothalamic pathway (Fig. 19.2).

NSAIDs (Ch. 29) and opioids are the major classes of pain-relieving (analgesic) drugs. They act at different levels in the pain-transmitting pathways to influence the production and recognition of pain as indicated in Figure 19.3.

Non-steroidal anti-inflammatory drugs. These act mainly by blocking the peripheral generation of the nociceptive impulses. They inhibit the production of prostaglandins by the cyclo-oxygenase type 1 and type 2 (COX-1, COX-2) isoenzymes and reduce the sensitivity of sensory nociceptive nerve endings to agents released by injured tissue that initiate pain, such as bradykinin, substance P, histamine and 5-hydroxytryptamine (5HT, serotonin). These drugs are considered fully in Chapter 29.

Opioids. These act on the spinal cord and limbic system, and stimulate the long descending inhibitory pathways from the midbrain to the dorsal horn. The contribution of peripheral actions is smaller. They produce their effects via specific receptors that are closely associated with the neuronal pathways which transmit pain from the periphery to the CNS.

Opioid analgesics

Examples: buprenorphine, codeine, diamorphine (heroin), dihydrocodeine, fentanyl, methadone, morphine, nalbuphine, pentazocine, pethidine (known as meperidine in the USA), tramadol

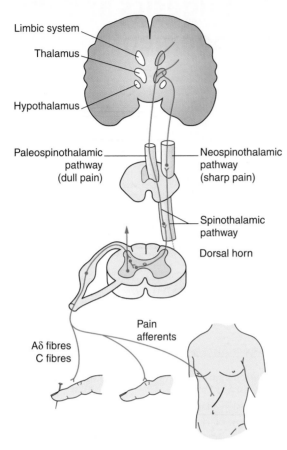

Fig. 19.2
Pathways of pain perception. Ascending pathways activated following stimulation of peripheral nociceptive nerve terminals. Many mediators are involved during afferent stimulation of the nociceptive pathway. Mediator release (bradykinin, 5-hydroxytryptamine, prostaglandins) stimulates the sensory nerve terminals of pain fibres. Onward afferent transmission of ascending nerve impulses at the synapses in the dorsal horn involves neuropeptides such as substance P, glutamate and nitric oxide. Hyperexcitability of pain fibres can also be promoted by other mediators. The ascending pathways innervate areas of the midbrain and thalamus.

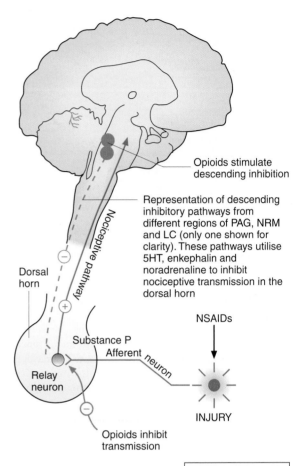

Opioid receptors ●

Fig. 19.3
Transmitters and receptors for pain perception and control. The afferent nociceptive pathways are subject to inhibitory control. Opioids act at opioid-receptor-rich sites in the periaqueductal grey matter (PAG), the nucleus raphe magnus (NRM) and other spinal sites to stimulate descending inhibitory fibres that inhibit nociceptive transmission in the dorsal horn. Descending pathways from the locus ceruleus (LC) that are noradrenergic are also involved. 5HT, 5-hydroxytryptamine; NSAIDs, non-steroidal anti-inflammatory drugs.

Opioid is a term used for both naturally occurring and synthetic molecules that produce their effects by an agonist action at opioid receptors. Use of the terms opiate analgesics (specifically, drugs derived from the juice of the opium poppy, *Papaver somniferum*) or narcotic analgesics (which literally means a 'stupor-inducing pain killer') is no longer preferred.

Mechanism of action

The brain produces several endogenous opioid peptides, which are neurotransmitters that act via specific opioid receptors. Among these are the two pentapeptide enkephalins: these each contain the amino acid sequence Tyr-Gly-Gly-Phe as the message domain, linked to either leucine or methionine, and are called leu-enkephalin and met-enkephalin. Other agonists incorporating the same amino acid sequence are dynorphin and the most potent β-endorphin, a 31-amino-acid peptide with met-enkephalin at its carboxyl end. More recently, two further peptides, endomorphins 1 and 2, have been identified that have a Tyr-Pro-Phe/Trp message domain sequence. All opioid peptides are derived from larger precursor molecules.

There is a distinctive regional distribution of opioid peptides in the CNS, with high concentrations in the limbic system and spinal cord, a distribution similar to that for opioid receptors. These regions also contain high concentrations of a neutral endopeptidase (enkephalinase), which rapidly hydrolyses the pentapeptides into fragments. Opioid receptors are found on the pre-synaptic membranes of neurons in the main pain

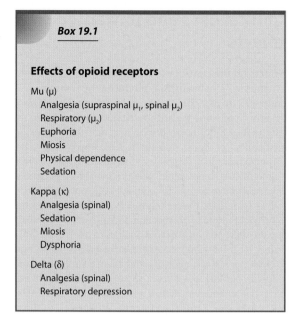

Box 19.1

Effects of opioid receptors

Mu (μ)
  Analgesia (supraspinal μ_1, spinal μ_2)
  Respiratory (μ_2)
  Euphoria
  Miosis
  Physical dependence
  Sedation

Kappa (κ)
  Analgesia (spinal)
  Sedation
  Miosis
  Dysphoria

Delta (δ)
  Analgesia (spinal)
  Respiratory depression

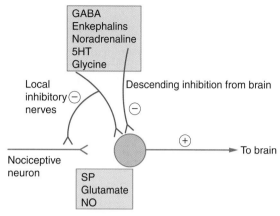

Fig. 19.4

Neurotransmitter substances involved in the genesis and modulation of neuropathic pain. Nociceptive pain resulting from an appropriate physiological response to stimulation of Aδ and C fibres is usually managed with opioids and/or non-steroidal anti-inflammatory drugs (NSAIDs; Ch. 29). However, neuropathic pain is far more complex and can result from neuronal damage and malfunction causing heightened responses to a normally painful stimulus (hyperalgesia) and painful responses to a stimulus that is not normally painful (allodynia); the latter may occur from phenotypic switching and sprouting of Aβ fibres that normally do not carry noxious sensations to become functionally like nociceptive fibres (Aδ and C fibres) and will carry ectopic noxious sensations. This can occur centrally and in the periphery. Following nerve injury, disinhibition of transmission at the dorsal horn can occur due to removal of inhibitory modulation by local and more distant neurons. Treatment of neuropathic pain can include non-standard treatments as well as opioids and NSAIDs acting at several sites where adequate inhibition can be regained (Table 19.1). Inhibitory transmitters are shown in a blue box and excitatory transmitters in a pink box. GABA, gamma-aminobutyric acid; SP, substance P; NO, nitric oxide.

pathways of the CNS, and have also been identified in the peripheral nervous system.

Morphine and related analgesics produce their effects largely by acting as agonists (see below) at specific opioid receptors in the CNS. Three major classes of opioid receptor have been identified, which mediate distinct effects (Box 19.1). The μ (mu), κ (kappa), and δ (delta) opioid receptors have been reclassified by an International Union of Pharmacology subcommittee as DOP (δ), KOP (κ), and MOP (μ), although this nomenclature has not been universally adopted. Each receptor has subtypes that have distinctive regional distributions. More recently, a distinct epsilon (ε)-receptor has been proposed, which is principally found in the medulla and facilitates descending enkephalinergic pathways in the spinal cord. All opioid receptors are coupled to inhibitory G-proteins, and receptor activation inhibits adenylate cyclase and the intracellular generation of cyclic adenosine monophosphate (cAMP). The G-proteins are also directly coupled to K^+ channels, and opioids increase K^+ conductance. Therefore, opioids hyperpolarise the target cells, making them less responsive to depolarising impulses, which in turn inhibits neuronal voltage-gated Ca^{2+} channels and reduces neurotransmitter release. The various endogenous opioid peptides show preferential receptor-binding affinities: β-endorphin binds equally to μ-, δ-, κ- and the putative ε-receptors; endomorphins bind mainly to μ-receptors; dynorphin binds mainly to κ-receptors; and the enkephalins bind mainly to δ-receptors. The different physiological effects produced by these receptors are due to their specific neuronal distributions.

The analgesic action of opioids is the end result of a complex series of neuronal interactions. In the nucleus raphe magnus of the brain, μ-receptor stimulation decreases activity in inhibitory gamma-aminobutyric acid (GABA) neurons that project to serotonergic neurons in the brainstem. Therefore, there is increased firing of these descending inhibitory serotonergic neurons that connect presynaptically with afferent nociceptive fibres in the dorsal horn of the spinal cord. Analgesia is produced by inhibition of the release of the pain pathway mediators, substance P, glutamate and nitric oxide, from the afferent nociceptive neurons (Fig. 19.4). Activation of κ-receptors antagonises the analgesia produced by μ-receptor stimulation, by inhibiting the descending serotonergic neurons in the pain pathway. Buprenorphine, which is a κ-receptor antagonist but a partial μ-receptor agonist, will therefore enhance its own analgesic action on the μ-receptors. Opioid receptors are also present on peripheral nerves in the pain pathways, and a μ-receptor agonist reduces the sensitivity of peripheral nociceptive neurons to pain stimuli, particularly in inflamed tissues. Non-neuronal κ-receptors are involved in the inflammatory response, and are found on endothelial cells, T-lymphocytes and macrophages; κ-receptor agonists are being developed to modulate the inflammatory response orchestrated by these cells.

Table 19.1
The mechanisms of action of some non-opioid analgesics

Drug	Mechanism (see Fig. 19.4)
Gabapentin	GABA concentrations increased
Baclofen	GABA$_B$ receptor antagonist
Clonidine	α_2-Adrenoceptor agonist
Tricyclic antidepressants	Increase noradrenaline availability
Ketamine, dextromethorphan	NMDA (glutamate) receptor antagonists
Local anaesthetics	Neuronal transmission (Na$^+$ channel block)
Anticonvulsants	(Na$^+$ channel block)
Capsaicin	SP depletion
Cannabinoids	Stimulation of cannabinoid receptors

GABA, γ-aminobutyric acid; SP, substance P.

Opioid drugs show receptor selectivity and can have agonist, partial agonist or antagonist properties at various receptor types. They are classified by their action at opioid receptors.

- Full agonists: these act principally at μ-receptors and include morphine, diamorphine, pethidine, codeine and dextropropoxyphene. They also have weak agonist activity at δ- and κ-receptors.
- Mixed agonist–antagonist: pentazocine has agonist effects at the κ-receptor (and, to a lesser extent, the δ-receptor) and is a weak μ-receptor antagonist; nalbuphine has similar actions but is a more potent μ-receptor antagonist.
- Mixed partial agonist–antagonist: buprenorphine is a potent partial agonist at the μ-receptor and has antagonist activity at κ-receptors.
- Opioids with additional properties: meptazinol is a μ-receptor agonist with muscarinic receptor agonist activity; tramadol and methadone are μ-receptor agonists that also inhibit noradrenaline and 5HT reuptake. This supplementary activity is of importance as enhanced amine-mediated neurotransmission potentiates descending inhibitory pain pathways (Table 19.1). Methadone is a potent opioid agonist and also an antagonist at glutamate NMDA (N-methyl-D-aspartate) receptors, and glutamate may be involved in pain transmission (Fig. 19.4).
- Opioid antagonists, such as naloxone, are without analgesic actions and are used in the treatment of opioid overdose (Ch. 53).

Clinical uses and unwanted effects

Effects on the central nervous system

Analgesia. The analgesia produced by morphine is most effective for chronic visceral pain, but the apparent resistance of some neuropathic pain is only relative. In addition to its antinociceptive effect, morphine alters the perception of pain, making it less unpleasant. This supraspinal effect, possibly at the limbic system, is less marked with some opioids such as pentazocine. Opioid analgesics have no anti-inflammatory effect and morphine can even release the inflammatory mediator histamine locally at the site of an injection. Full μ-receptor agonists are the most powerful opioid analgesics. However, some full μ-receptor agonists, e.g. dextropropoxyphene and codeine, are weak agonists and their ceiling analgesic effect in clinical use is low. There is growing evidence that the antagonist action of methadone at NMDA receptors can produce effective analgesia in those individuals who have become tolerant to high doses of morphine (see below).

The ceiling analgesic effect of a μ-receptor partial agonist is lower than that of an otherwise similar full agonist. If a person receiving high doses of a potent full μ-receptor antagonist is given a μ-receptor partial agonist (e.g. buprenorphine) or a μ-receptor antagonist (e.g. pentazocine), then some of the full-agonist molecules will be displaced from receptor sites by the less effective molecules. The degree of analgesia may then be reduced, and, in dependent individuals, withdrawal symptoms can be produced (see below and Table 19.2). Short-acting opioids such as alfentanil, fentanyl and remifentanil are used as analgesic supplements in anaesthesia. This use is considered in Chapter 17.

Euphoria. The use of morphine is often associated with an elevated sense of wellbeing (euphoria, mediated by μ-receptors), an action that contributes considerably to its analgesic efficacy. The opposite effect (dysphoria, mediated by κ-receptors) counteracts the euphoric action, and the degree of euphoria produced will depend on the receptor-binding characteristics of the drug.

Respiratory depression. The sensitivity of the respiratory centre to stimulation by carbon dioxide is reduced by morphine at doses that produce analgesia. Respiratory depression is a common cause of death in opioid overdose. Occasionally, the effect on respiratory rate can be of clinical benefit; for example, intravenous morphine relieves the dyspnoea associated with acute pulmonary oedema, and morphine is used orally, or diamorphine by subcutaneous infusion, for the treatment of breathlessness in palliative care. Meptazinol and tramadol are claimed to cause less respiratory depression than other opioids; for this reason, meptazinol is used for obstetric analgesia, to reduce the risk of respiratory depression in the neonate.

Table 19.2
Opioid analgesics

Compound	Analgesic potency	Tolerance and dependence	Clinical uses and comments
Alfentanil	+++	–	Used by injection for intraoperative analgesia; not used for management of chronic pain and therefore tolerance and dependence not relevant
Buprenorphine	++++	++	Used as an alternative to morphine for analgesia, but nausea may limit its tolerability; a partial agonist at μ opioid receptors
Codeine	+	+	See text; also used when the non-analgesic effects such as antitussive or antidiarrhoeal actions are needed; produces little respiratory depression
Dextropropoxyphene	(+)	+	Withdrawn in the UK, 2005. Reports of fatalities with overdose, especially when taken with alcohol
Diamorphine (heroin)	++++	++++	Clinical uses restricted because of high abuse potential; given orally or by infusion for the pain of terminal cancer; given for acute severe pain, e.g. myocardial infarction
Dihydrocodeine	+	+	Used largely as an alternative to codeine for moderate pain
Dipipanone	++	++	Less sedating than morphine, but the only available formulation in the UK contains cyclizine (an antiemetic), which makes it unsuitable for palliative care
Fentanyl	+++	+	Increasingly used by transdermal patch for intractable pain; intravenous adjunct in anaesthesia
Hydromorphone	+++	+++	Similar to morphine in most properties; shorter duration of action may limit usefulness in chronic pain compared with morphine
Meptazinol	+	–	Behaves as a mixed agonist/antagonist and lacks withdrawal and dependence symptoms
Methadone	+++	++	Major use is for withdrawal from morphine/heroin dependence
Morphine	+++	+++	See text
Nalbuphine	+++	+	Fewer side effects than morphine and a lower abuse potential; may produce opiate withdrawal if administered to opioid-dependent patients, due to its mixed opiate agonist and antagonist activity
Oxycodone	+++	++	Similar profile to morphine; used primarily to control pain in palliative care as an alternative in people who cannot tolerate morphine or hydromorphone.
Pentazocine	+++	++	See text; will provoke a withdrawal syndrome in a morphine-dependent subject because of weak antagonist or partial agonist action on μ-receptors (but not cross-tolerance to morphine)
Pethidine	++	+	Not useful for antitussive or antidiarrhoeal effects
Remifentanil	+++	–	Used by injection for intraoperative analgesia; not used for management of chronic pain and therefore tolerance and dependence not relevant
Tramadol	+	+	Obstetric analgesia; less potential for respiratory depression; WHO-classified step II agent; it is also a monoamine reuptake blocker

Suppression of the cough centre. Opioids possess an antitussive action. Compounds such as codeine and dextromethorphan are highly effective for cough suppression (Ch. 13), despite having relatively weak analgesic effects.

Vomiting. Opioids stimulate the chemoreceptor trigger zone, and cause vomiting in up to 30% of people. Tolerance to the nausea and vomiting can occur on repeated dosage. When used for acute pain, powerful opioids such as morphine are usually given with an antiemetic (Ch. 32).

Miosis. Stimulation of the third-nerve nucleus results in pupillary constriction. Pinpoint pupils, together with coma and slow respiration, are signs of opioid overdose (Ch. 53).

Endocrine effects. Opioids inhibit the hypothalamic–pituitary–adrenal axis, leading to a progressive decline in plasma cortisol levels (Ch. 44). They also increase prolactin and decrease luteinising hormone release, which leads to testosterone deficiency in men and a reduction in oestrogen in women (Chs 45 and 46). Men usually benefit from testosterone replacement during long-term opioid use (Ch. 46).

Peripheral effects

Gastrointestinal tract. There is a general increase in resting tone of the gut wall and sphincters. An increase in biliary pressure caused by opioid-induced spasm at the sphincter of Oddi can exacerbate biliary colic. In the stomach, a decrease in motility and pyloric tone can produce anorexia, nausea and vomiting. In the small and large intestines there is increased segmenting activity and decreased propulsive activity. Thus, opioid administration is associated with constipation, and up to 80% of those who take opioids long term will need a laxative. The effects of opioids on gastrointestinal motility make them useful in the treatment of diarrhoea (Ch. 35). These effects arise from stimulation of μ- and κ-receptors on neuronal plexuses in the gut wall. Pethidine and tramadol have less effect on the gastrointestinal tract than do equi-analgesic doses of morphine.

Cardiovascular system. Opioids have little effect on the heart or circulation except at high doses that can depress the medullary vasomotor centre. Hypotension can occur with parenteral use of morphine, possibly because of histamine release.

Other systems. Opioids have minor effects on other systems. For example, there is an increase in tone of the bladder wall and sphincter, which can lead to urinary retention. There is increasing evidence that chronic use of opioids suppresses immune function by inhibiting the development and differentiation of many types of immune cells. The clinical relevance of this is not known.

Tolerance and dependence

Tolerance and dependence result from changes in the functioning of opioid receptors during continuous opioid administration. In response to the inhibitory effects of morphine on intracellular cAMP generation, there is increased synthesis of stimulatory G-proteins and adenylate cyclase in an attempt to restore homeostasis. As a consequence of these adaptive changes, more drug is necessary to produce the same effect (tolerance) and withdrawal of the drug produces adverse physiological effects until the compensatory changes are reset (dependence).

Tolerance has two clinical types. Associative (learned) tolerance has a major psychological component. Non-associative (adaptive) tolerance involves downregulation or desensitisation of opioid receptors. This is associated with increased firing of neurons in the noradrenergic pathways of the locus ceruleus, which is rich in inhibitory opioid receptors, and activation of the reward pathway in the brain (see Ch. 54). It may also involve increased activity at NMDA receptors for excitatory glutamate-mediated neurotransmission in spinal and supraspinal circuits. Tolerance occurs rapidly during chronic opioid administration, despite constant plasma drug concentrations. Tolerance develops to analgesia, euphoria, respiratory depression and emesis, but much less to the constipatory effects or miosis. A high degree of cross-tolerance is shown by many opioids; consequently, individuals who develop tolerance to one opioid will usually be tolerant to another. However, not all opioids show cross-tolerance: the non-uniform nature of tolerance and cross-tolerance may be a result of splice variants of μ opioid receptors. Opioid rotation (alternating the opioid used during a period of long-term treatment) may overcome some problems with tolerance and limit the need for dose escalation.

Opioid-induced NMDA receptor activation can also produce abnormal pain sensitivity at spinal cord dorsal horn cells. This sensitisation process can be confused with tolerance and lead to opioid dose escalation. Methadone may be useful in this situation (see above).

Dependence manifests itself as a withdrawal syndrome, which can be precipitated when individuals who are abusing the drug have their intake stopped or are given an opioid antagonist or partial agonist. Dependence may be in part caused by effects on opioid neurons radiating from the locus ceruleus to the ventral tegmental area. The dopaminergic pathway projecting from the ventral tegmental area to the nucleus accumbens is believed to be involved in the euphoria of opioid administration. Details of the effects of dependence-inducing drugs on the reward pathways of the brain are found in Chapter 54.

During the first 12 h after opioid withdrawal, the effects, such as nervousness, sweating and craving, are largely psychological, because they can be alleviated by the administration of a placebo. Following this period, the effects of physiological dependence manifest themselves – for example, dilated pupils, anorexia, weakness, depression, insomnia, gastrointestinal and skeletal muscle cramps, increased respiratory rate, pyrexia, piloerection with goose-pimples, and diarrhoea. The time course for the development and loss of these symptoms varies among the opioids. In the case of morphine, the maximum withdrawal effects occur quickly (about 1–2 days) and subside rapidly (about 5–10 days), but the intensity of the symptoms may be intolerable. By contrast, withdrawal from methadone is a slow process because of its very long half-life, but the effects are far less intense (peak effect at almost 1 week and symptoms persist for about 3 weeks). Therefore, morphine- or heroin-dependent subjects are often transferred from their drug of abuse to methadone prior to withdrawal. Methadone also produces less euphoria than morphine or heroin. After a period of chronic treatment with methadone, the methadone dosage is gradually reduced and the person undergoes a more tolerable withdrawal.

More recently, buprenorphine has been used as an alternative to methadone, due to the low severity of withdrawal symptoms. It can be given for 6 days in a rapid detoxification programme. Long-term maintenance has also shown promise for reducing relapse, since the partial agonist activity of buprenorphine blocks the 'high' from illicit opioid use.

Rapid in-hospital tapering of opioids over 2 weeks has an 80% success rate; on an outpatient basis, slow tapering over 6 months is more successful, but still leads to only a 40% successful withdrawal rate. Long-term buprenorphine therapy, combined with high-intensity psychosocial group therapy treatment, has achieved up to 75% withdrawal rates after 1 year. Detoxification from opioids can also be helped by the presynaptic α_2-adrenoceptor agonists clonidine and lofexidine (a clonidine analogue with fewer unwanted effects). This inhibits the excessive sympathetic nervous system activity associated with opioid withdrawal, such as lacrimation, rhinorrhoea, muscle pain, joint pain and gastrointestinal symptoms. By contrast, lethargy, insomnia and restlessness persist.

Pharmacokinetics

The pharmacokinetic properties of individual opioid analgesics are summarised in the drug compendium at the end of this chapter. Most opioids are available for oral use. Buprenorphine is formulated for buccal absorption, and fentanyl is available as lozenges for rapid pain relief. Some opioids, such as morphine, buprenorphine, and diamorphine, can be given by intravenous, intramuscular or subcutaneous injection. Diamorphine is more soluble than morphine, and can be given by subcutaneous infusion since it is constituted in smaller volumes. Morphine can also be given as a suppository. Fentanyl, tramadol and buprenorphine can be delivered transdermally for prolonged analgesia.

Some opioids (e.g. morphine) have a low and variable absorption from the gut, so that a lower dose is necessary when they are given parenterally. Opioids are eliminated by hepatic metabolism, and some, such as dihydrocodeine, have a low oral bioavailability due to extensive first-pass metabolism. A major metabolite of morphine, morphine 6-glucuronide, has more analgesic activity than the parent compound and is excreted by the kidney. The dose of morphine must therefore be reduced in renal failure. Diamorphine is an acetylated morphine derivative that is converted to morphine by hydrolysis in plasma. Codeine is metabolised by CYP2D6, which shows genetic polymorphism, to several active metabolites, including morphine, that are responsible for much of the analgesic activity; in consequence, about 10% of people with low CYP2D6 have a reduced analgesic response to codeine.

Most opioid analgesics have short or intermediate half-lives. For long-term pain control, morphine is often given as a modified-release formulation to prolong the duration of action. Fentanyl has a short half-life, but pain relief takes 12–24 h after first applying a transdermal delivery patch, due to slow drug delivery (Ch. 2). In addition, the effects persist for several hours after removing the patch, owing to build-up of a subcutaneous drug reservoir. Care is necessary to maintain analgesia and avoid unwanted opioid effects if analgesia is changed between fentanyl patches and another opioid.

Unwanted effects

The unwanted effects of opioids (see above) are caused by their actions on those opioid receptors that are not the primary site for therapeutic benefit. For example, respiratory depression and constipation are unwanted effects when an opioid is used as an analgesic. Tolerance and dependence can also be regarded as unwanted problems associated with chronic use. However, concerns about tolerance and dependence should not inhibit the administration of adequate analgesia for patients with severe chronic pain, for example the pain experienced by terminally ill people with cancer.

Pain management

Appropriate management of pain depends on its origin and severity. The World Health Organization's (WHO) 'analgesic ladder' is useful for choosing drug therapy appropriate to the level of pain (Box 19.2).

Step 1 drugs. Paracetamol (Ch. 29) is a simple analgesic, suitable for mild pain. However, an NSAID (Ch. 29) may be more appropriate if there is local inflammation. The choice will be determined by the balance of benefits and risks of NSAIDs. Examples of pain that respond better to an NSAID are soft-tissue injury, tissue

---

Box 19.2

The 'analgesic ladder'

Step 1: simple analgesics, e.g. paracetamol, NSAIDs
Step 2: opioid suitable for moderate pain ± simple analgesics
Step 3: opioid suitable for severe pain ± simple analgesics

Adjuvant analgesics may be required at any step (see text).

compression, visceral pain caused by pleural or peritoneal irritation, and bone pain caused by metastatic deposits. Bone metastases cause local secretion of prostaglandins, and NSAIDs can be particularly effective. Individual responses to an NSAID vary; about 60% of people will respond to an alternative drug even if the first was ineffective.

Step 2 drugs. A weak opioid should be added for mild to moderate pain, or when the response to a stage 1 drug is inadequate. Opioids suitable for mild to moderate pain include codeine and dihydrocodeine. These are often used in combination with paracetamol, such as co-codamol (codeine and paracetamol), although the dose of opioid in some combinations is too low to produce additional analgesia. Tramadol has been advocated at this stage, but it is no more effective than co-codamol, and claims that it has less effect on respiration and gastrointestinal motility are of uncertain clinical importance.

Step 3 drugs. The drug of choice for moderate to severe pain is morphine. It is usually effective orally, using a rapid-onset formulation for initial pain control. Doctors are often unwilling to give adequate doses of strong opioid because of concern about addiction. In severe chronic pain with terminal illness, this is not an issue, and it should not be used as a reason for avoiding the use of morphine in non-cancer pain. Opioid addiction is not a problem when opioids are given appropriately for relief of pain.

Acute pain

Acute pain usually has an obvious cause and is accompanied by anxiety. For rapid pain relief in a self-limiting condition, for example migraine, a readily absorbed, short-acting drug will be appropriate. For more protracted conditions, for example sprains, a long-acting drug may be helpful to improve compliance by reducing the frequency of administration.

Minor pain can be effectively treated with a peripherally acting analgesic such as paracetamol or aspirin (Ch. 29). If there is an inflammatory component, for example soft-tissue injuries, then a drug with combined anti-inflammatory and analgesic properties from the NSAID class (Ch. 29) will be particularly useful. Very severe acute pain, for example with myocardial infarction, will require a powerful opioid such as morphine, given parenterally for rapid effect. Intramuscular injection should be avoided if possible, since severe pain is often accompanied by sympathetic nervous system stimulation, which produces peripheral vasoconstriction that delays drug absorption. Some acute severe pain, such as that arising postoperatively or from trauma, cholecystitis, pancreatitis or sickle cell crisis, should be treated initially with a powerful analgesic, then using less powerful analgesics as the condition resolves. This involves applying the principles of the WHO analgesic ladder in reverse.

Chronic pain

Chronic pain (usually defined as pain lasting for at least 3–6 months) can be a result of chronic nociceptive stimulation or can have a neuropathic origin. Drug therapy is not the only solution for chronic pain and, depending on the cause, non-pharmacological or local treatments are often appropriate. Examples include:

- surgery for neoplastic, structural or ischaemic disorders
- physical methods such as acupuncture, transcutaneous electrical nerve stimulation (TENS – which activates spinal inhibitory neurons by acting as a counter-irritant) and local anaesthetic nerve block (Ch. 18)
- behavioural modification, e.g. biofeedback, relaxation techniques, hypnosis
- corticosteroids for raised intracranial pressure or spinal cord compression, or to reduce inflammation which can be associated with cancer.

The principles of escalation of analgesia are described in the WHO analgesic ladder. For most severe chronic nociceptive pain, morphine is the treatment of choice. If pain remains severe with a low initial dosage of morphine, the dosage should be increased by 50–100% every 24 h; once the pain is moderate in intensity, increments of 25–50% daily are usually sufficient to achieve control without excessive unwanted effects. A modified-release formulation of morphine can be substituted once a stable dosage has been determined, although a rapid-acting formulation may still be required to treat breakthrough pain. Oral administration may not be possible if there is vomiting, dysphagia or intestinal obstruction. In these circumstances, rectal administration of morphine or subcutaneous infusion of diamorphine using a syringe driver can be used. Diamorphine can also be given by epidural or intrathecal injection for intractable pain. Transdermal delivery of an opioid such as fentanyl from an adhesive patch is an alternative to modified-release oral morphine. There is increasing evidence that intolerance to one opioid is often resolved by changing to an alternative opioid. The factors that predict intolerance to a particular agent are poorly understood, although it is now recognised that intolerance to morphine may be associated with a mutation in the multidrug resistance 1 transporter protein (Chs 2 and 52). Effective management of much chronic pain is facilitated by multidisciplinary pain teams.

Neuropathic pain

Neuropathic pain, such as trigeminal neuralgia, postherpetic neuralgia and phantom limb pain after an amputation, often responds poorly to conventional analgesia. Neuropathic pain can be spontaneous (stimulus-independent), when it is usually described by the sufferer as shooting or lancinating sensations, electric-shock-like pain or an abnormal unpleasant sensation (dysaesthesia). Alternatively, there may be stimulus-evoked pain such as an exaggerated response to a painful stimulus (hyperalgesia) or a painful response to a trivial stimulus (allodynia).

Mechanisms of neuropathic pain are now better understood, allowing a more rational approach to treatment. Stimulus-independent pain usually arises from spontaneous ectopic impulses arising in afferent nociceptive fibres. Stimulus-evoked pain can be due to this mechanism, especially following nerve injury, but is more likely to result from peripheral nociceptor sensitisation or loss of inhibitory controls at a spinal level (increased glutamate activity at excitatory NMDA receptors or decreased GABA-mediated inhibition). The afferent fibres involved in hyperalgesia are usually the lightly myelinated $A\delta$ fibres or unmyelinated C fibres (Ch. 18) that transmit nociceptive stimuli. By contrast, allodynia usually involves aberrant transmission in larger myelinated $A\beta$ fibres that normally transmit tactile stimuli.

Stimulus-independent symptoms respond best to membrane-stabilising agents, such as carbamazepine and phenytoin (Ch. 23). Burning pain can be treated with tricyclic antidepressants (Ch. 22) that increase synaptic noradrenaline and 5HT concentrations in the descending spinal inhibitory pathways (Fig. 19.4). The importance of noradrenaline is shown by the lack of efficacy of selective serotonin reuptake inhibitor (SSRI) antidepressants for neuropathic pain. Opioids are useful in some cases of stimulus-independent pain.

Of the stimulus-evoked pains, hyperalgesia may respond to topical treatment. Lidocaine cream may work, through its local anaesthetic actions (Ch. 18). Alternatively, capsaicin, a derivative of red chilli peppers that stimulates C fibres in the afferent nociceptive pathway, can be applied topically as a counter-irritant. This releases substance P and initially provokes hyperalgesia, but subsequent depletion of substance P then blocks nerve function. If local treatment is inappropriate or ineffective, a membrane-stabilising drug can be used. For allodynia, gabapentin (Ch. 23) is particularly effective for increasing inhibitory pathway activity. Alternatives include tricyclic antidepressants, the α_2-adrenoceptor agonist clonidine (Ch. 6), baclofen (Ch. 24) and the NMDA receptor antagonist ketamine (Ch. 17), all of which modulate spinal transmission of the pain signal. Opioids can be helpful in some cases of allodynia (Table 19.1).

The use of cannabinoids (the active components of cannabis; Ch. 54) for relief of hyperalgesia in conditions such as multiple sclerosis is receiving considerable attention. Stimulation of cannabinoid receptors produces an antinociceptive action and inhibits pain transmission in the spinal cord.

FURTHER READING

Ashburn MA, Staats PS (1999) Management of chronic pain. *Lancet* 353, 1865–1869

Ballantyne JC, Mao J (2003) Opioid therapy for chronic pain. *N Engl J Med* 349, 1943–1953

Berde CB, Sethna NF (2002) Analgesics for the treatment of pain in children. *N Engl J Med* 347, 1094–1103

Besson JM (1999) The neurobiology of pain. *Lancet* 353, 1610–1615

Carr DB, Goudas LC (1999) Acute pain. *Lancet* 353, 2051–2058

Croxford JL (2003) Therapeutic potential of cannabinoids in CNS disease. *CNS Drugs* 17, 179–202

Gonzalez G, Oliveto A, Kosten TR (2002) Treatment of heroin (diamorphine) addiction. *Drugs* 62, 1331–1343

Holdcroft A, Power I (2003) Management of pain. *BMJ* 326, 635–639

Jensen TS (2002) Anticonvulsants in neuropathic pain: rationale and clinical evidence. *Eur J Pain* 6(suppl A), 61–68

Johnson RW, Dworkin RH (2003) Treatment of herpes zoster and postherpetic neuralgia. *BMJ* 326, 748–750

McQuay H (1999) Opioids in pain management. *Lancet* 353, 2229–2232

Mendell JR, Sahenk Z (2003) Painful sensory neuropathy. *N Engl J Med* 348, 1243–1255

Ripamonti C, Dickerson ED (2001) Strategies for the treatment of cancer pain in the new millenium. *Drugs* 61, 955–977

Ward J, Hall W, Mattick RP (1999) Role of maintenance treatment in opioid dependence. *Lancet* 353, 221–226

Woolf CJ, Mannion RJ (1999) Neuropathic pain: aetiology, symptoms, mechanisms and management. *Lancet* 353, 1959–1964

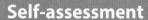

Self-assessment

In questions 1–4, the initial statement, in italics, is true. Are the accompanying statements also true?

1. *Opioids are analgesic by acting at the level of the dorsal horn to inhibit transmission in the ascending nociceptive pathway. They also act at the level of the periaqueductal grey matter to stimulate descending inhibitory pathways that further inhibit dorsal horn synaptic transmission.*

   a. Opioids can cause euphoria or dysphoria.
   b. Tolerance develops uniformly to all of the biological effects of the opioids.
   c. Methadone has a rapid onset of action and a short half-life.

2. *Concerns about dependence potential should not inhibit the administration of adequate doses of opioids to treat severe chronic pain.*

   a. Meptazinol is a pure μ-receptor stimulant.
   b. Naloxone is a short-acting opioid agonist.

3. *Opioids are less effective in treatment of neuropathic pain.*

   a. Drugs that inhibit the reuptake of noradrenaline can be effective analgesics in some cases of neuropathic pain.
   b. Anticonvulsants are ineffective in treatment of neuropathic pain.

4. *Pentazocine and buprenorphine are partial agonists at opioid receptors and have less abuse liability than morphine.* Pentazocine can precipitate withdrawal symptoms in morphine addicts.

5. Choose the <u>most appropriate</u> statement from the following options.

   A. In the elderly, tolerance rapidly develops to the constipatory effects of morphine.
   B. An opioid analgesic is the drug of choice for chronic limb pain following a below-knee amputation after a road traffic accident.
   C. Naloxone is an agonist at μ opioid receptors.
   D. Tolerance does not develop to the miotic effect of opioids.
   E. Fentanyl can be used for opioid withdrawal and maintenance of the chronically relapsing heroin addict.

6. Case history questions
   Pain control in terminal cancer. These case notes have been modified from original material written by Martin Church and Richard Hillier at the University of Southampton, and gratefully reproduced with their permission. The case notes highlight the

pharmacology of analgesic usage and concomitant drugs.

A 60-year-old man was admitted to a hospice. He had previously had a left nephrectomy because of renal cell carcinoma and now had intense metastatic bone pain in his ankles, right iliac crest and left upper arm. He was also having periods of dyspnoea. Prior to admission, his medication was the compound analgesic co-codamol and diclofenac (150 mg) at night. He was also taking cimetidine (400 mg) twice daily. His pain was not well controlled on admission. After a week of assessment and optimisation of drug therapy, his treatment comprised the following drugs:

morphine, slow release (MST)	260 mg	twice daily
morphine, oral solution	50 mg	when required
diclofenac, slow release	150 mg	at night
dexamethasone	2 mg	three times daily
metoclopramide (antiemetic)	10 mg	three times daily
cimetidine	400 mg	twice daily
docusate sodium (laxative)	100 mg	three times daily
temazepam	20 mg	at night

Morphine is the optimum drug of choice for pain control in the vast majority of patients with cancer.

a. How does morphine exert its pharmacological action as an analgesic?
b. Why was morphine oral solution (which is an immediate-release form) also made available in addition to the modified-release formulation?
c. Was the addictive potential of morphine likely to present a problem in this man?
d. What alternative opioids as an immediate replacement for morphine might you consider?
e. How does diclofenac control inflammation and inflammatory pain?
f. Why was diclofenac useful in this man?
g. What was the rationale for the use of dexamethasone in this man?
h. Metoclopramide is an antiemetic. Why do you think that this man was likely to suffer from nausea and possibly vomiting?
i. How does metoclopramide act to alleviate nausea?
j. What other drugs could be used to alleviate nausea?
k. Why might gastric or duodenal ulceration be a problem in this man?
l. How might cimetidine reduce the problem of gastric or duodenal ulceration?

m. Why was constipation likely to be a problem in this man?

n. What is the mechanism of action of docusate sodium?

o. What alternative laxative agents to docusate sodium could have been used?

p. Why was temazepam given?

The answers are provided on pages 718–720.

Drug compendium

Opioid analgesics

Drug	Half-life (h)	Elimination	Comments
Alfentanil	0.7–2	Metabolism	Used at surgery (Ch. 17); given by intravenous injection; respiratory depression may persist after the end of the procedure if repeated doses are given; oxidised in liver by CYP3A4, and conjugated with glucuronic acid
Buprenorphine	4–6	Metabolism	Has both agonist and antagonist properties and can precipitate withdrawal in individuals dependent on other opioids; bioavailability sublingual > oral; action only partly reversed by naloxone; metabolised by CYP3A4 to an active metabolite and by conjugation
Codeine	3–4	Metabolism (+ renal)	Given orally for mild to moderate pain, demethylated to morphine (5–15%) by the polymorphic enzyme CYP2D6; variability in response linked to CYP2D6 polymorphism
Diamorphine	2–5 min	Hydrolysis	Acetylated prodrug which is more lipid soluble and more potent than morphine; it readily crosses the blood-brain barrier and is rapidly hydrolysed to morphine
Dihydrocodeine	3–5	Metabolism	Similar potency to codeine; undergoes extensive first-pass metabolism; role of metabolites in activity is unknown
Diphenoxylate	2–3	Metabolism	Used in acute diarrhoea; may exert its effects locally on smooth muscle rather than via opioid receptors; low oral bioavailability owing to incomplete dissolution in gut; undergoes extensive hepatic metabolism to an active metabolite, diphenoxylic acid, which has a half-life of 3–14 h, and to inactive metabolites
Dipipanone	3–4	Metabolism	Clinical effects suggest good oral absorption but very few data are available
Fentanyl	1–6	Metabolism (+ renal)	Usually given by injection, or by transdermal or buccal routes; also used at surgery (Ch. 17); respiratory depression may persist after the end of the procedure if repeated doses are given; rapid initial uptake from the blood into lungs, followed by redistribution and elimination; high inter-individual variability in kinetics; metabolised in the liver
Hydromorphone	2–3	Metabolism	A potent μ-receptor agonist with a duration of action of about 3–4 h; given orally with a bioavailability of 60%; eliminated by conjugation with glucuronic acid and by reduction
Meptazinol	1–3	Metabolism (+ renal)	Less potent than morphine with possibly a reduced risk of respiratory depression; given orally or by injection; rapid absorption but low oral bioavailability (5–20%); eliminated by conjugation with sulphate and glucuronic acid
Methadone	6–8	Metabolism + renal	Potent μ-receptor agonist but less sedating than morphine; longer action with reduced excitation leads to its use in managing opioid withdrawal; good oral bioavailability (40–100%); substrate for P-glycoprotein, which may inhibit its absorption across the gut wall; eliminated by hepatic oxidation by a number of CYP isoenzymes which may undergo auto-induction on repeated dosage

continued

Opioid analgesics *(continued)*

Drug	Half-life (h)	Elimination	Comments
Morphine	1–5	Metabolism	Can be given orally, rectally as suppositories, or by subcutaneous, intramuscular or slow intravenous injection; oral bioavailability is low (10–50%); eliminated by conjugation with glucuronic acid to morphine-3-glucuronide (inactive major metabolite) and morphine-6-glucuronide (active minor metabolite, which crosses blood–brain barrier despite polarity)
Nalbuphine	2–4 (i.v.) 3–8 (oral)	Metabolism + renal	Similar potency and efficacy to morphine but with fewer adverse effects and a lower abuse potential; extensive first-pass metabolism (bioavailability 10–20%)
Naloxone	1–1.5	Metabolism	Opioid antagonist used to treat opioid overdose (Chs 53 and 54); administered by injection, giving a rapid onset of action (1–2 min); half-life is shorter than that of morphine and repeated doses may be necessary; eliminated by conjugation with glucuronic acid
Oxycodone	3–5	Metabolism (+ renal)	A potent μ-receptor agonist with similar efficacy and adverse effect profile to morphine; used largely in palliative care; given orally (normal or modified-release tablets) or rectally; bioavailability is about 50–90%; eliminated mostly by hepatic metabolism
Pentazocine	2–3	Metabolism (+ renal)	Is a racemate and the L-isomer has both agonist and antagonist properties; it can precipitate withdrawal in patients dependent on other opioids; oral bioavailability is 11–32%; eliminated by oxidation and conjugation
Pethidine	3–8	Metabolism + renal	Produces rapid but short-lasting analgesia; frequently used in labour; oral bioavailability about 50%; it is usually given by subcutaneous or intramuscular injection; metabolised by hydrolysis and demethylation to normeperidine (norpethidine), which is about 50% as potent as the parent compound but has a long half-life (15–30 h) and may accumulate on repeated dosage
Remifentanil	0.1	Metabolism	Used at surgery (Ch. 17); given as an infusion; very rapid clearance by blood and tissue esterases (clearance is 3 l min^{-1}, which exceeds liver blood flow); metabolite inactive
Tramadol	5–6	Metabolism (+ renal)	Acts as an opioid agonist and also produces analgesia via enhancement of 5HT and adrenaline pathways, with the different optical isomers of tramadol showing a different spectrum of affinities; oral bioavailability about 60–70%; undergoes CYP2D6-mediated *O*-demethylation to a metabolite which is a more potent agonist at μ-receptors and is responsible for most of the activity of the drug

Drug compendium

20

Anxiolytics, sedatives and hypnotics

> **Box 20.1**
>
> **Simplified classification of anxiety disorders**
>
> Phobic anxiety disorder
> Other anxiety disorder (including panic disorder and mixed anxiety and depressive disorder)
> Obsessive compulsive disorder
> Reaction to severe stress (including post-traumatic stress disorder)
> Conversion disorders
> Somatoform disorders
> Other neurotic disorders (including neurasthenia)

There is considerable overlap in the pharmacology of drugs that have anxiolytic (anxiety-relieving) and hypnotic (sleep-inducing) properties. Compounds with sedative properties (moderating excitement and calming) at low doses often have hypnotic effects at higher doses. In addition, sedative drugs may have anxiolytic properties when used at doses that are too low to produce sedation. More recently, compounds such as buspirone have been developed that have anxiolytic properties but do not sedate.

Biological basis of anxiety disorders

Anxiety disorders are among the most common psychiatric syndromes, and affect 15% of the general population during their lifetime. The clinical manifestations of anxiety are both psychological and physical. Anxiety is only pathological when it is inappropriate to the degree of stress to which the individual is exposed. A variety of anxiety disorders are recognised (Box 20.1). Of these, mixed anxiety and depressive disorder is the most common, followed by generalised anxiety disorder.

The symptoms vary among the disorders, but usually include apprehension, worry, fear and nervousness. Increased sympathetic nervous system activity frequently accompanies these feelings, causing sweating, tachycardia and epigastric discomfort. Sleep is often disturbed, with difficulty getting to sleep being a common feature. Many of the syndromes present early in life, and tend to become chronic if untreated. Anxiety syndromes are often associated with substance abuse.

Dysfunction of neurotransmission in the limbic region of the brain underlies the genesis of anxiety. The amygdala is a central part of the system that processes a fear stimulus and selects a response based on previous experience. Implementation of the response is through the locus ceruleus (autonomic and neuroendocrine responses) and nucleus paragigantocellularis (autonomic responses) in the brainstem, and the hypothalamus. There are many neurobiological theories that attempt to explain the origin of anxiety disorders. These try to integrate our understanding of the neurochemical disturbances with genetic predisposition and environmental triggers.

Excessive serotonergic and, to a lesser extent, noradrenergic excitatory neurotransmission in the limbic system has been implicated in many anxiety syndromes. In particular, overactivity at pre- and postsynaptic 5-hydroxytryptamine type 1A ($5HT_{1A}$) receptors, and postsynaptic $5HT_{2A}$ and $5HT_{1C}$ receptors may be important, associated with upregulation of presynaptic α_2-adrenoceptors. Deficient inhibition of limbic neurotransmission by gamma-aminobutyric acid (GABA) interneurons is found in many anxiety disorders, with subsensitivity of postsynaptic $GABA_A$ receptors. Excessive activity in excitatory glutamatergic neurons at NMDA (N-methyl-D-aspartate) receptors in the amygdala has also been implicated in anxiety disorders, and may be responsible for fear conditioning. Supersensitivity of receptors for peptide neurotransmitters such as cholecystokinin and neuropeptide Y may also be important.

In some anxiety syndromes, there is excess secretion of corticotrophin-releasing factor (CRF), but a low plasma cortisol concentration and upregulation of corticosteroid receptors. CRF is a neurotransmitter in the limbic system, and upregulation may occur from early adverse experiences conditioning those with a genetic predisposition to anxiety disorder in later life.

Drug therapy for anxiety

Drugs used to treat anxiety are called anxiolytics.

Benzodiazepines

Examples: chlordiazepoxide, diazepam, lorazepam, midazolam, temazepam

In addition to their anxiolytic effect, benzodiazepines have several other properties that are clinically useful. This section also considers drugs that are not primarily used for treatment of anxiety.

Mechanism of action and effects

Benzodiazepines act by potentiating the actions of GABA, the primary inhibitory neurotransmitter in the central nervous system (CNS). They act at a regulatory site closely linked to the $GABA_A$ receptor (Ch. 4) that mediates fast inhibitory synaptic neurotransmission. The $GABA_A$ receptor is also the binding site for volatile anaesthetics and alcohol, propofol, etomidate and barbiturates (Ch. 4). Binding of a benzodiazepine to subunits of the receptor induces a conformational change in the GABA receptor that enhances its affinity for the neurotransmitter (Fig. 20.1). GABA increases the influx of Cl^- into the neuron, hyperpolarises the cell membrane and decreases cell excitability. Benzodia-

zepines act only in the presence of GABA to enhance GABA-mediated opening of the ion channel; they have no direct action on the channel (Fig. 20.1). There are many subtypes of $GABA_A$ receptor, with specific regional distributions in the brain, and which differ in their sensitivity to benzodiazepines. The potential clinical relevance of this is not exploited by the currently available drugs. The increase in inhibitory neurotransmission produced by benzodiazepines has the following potentially useful effects:

- sedation from reduced sensory input to the reticular activating system
- sleep induction at high drug concentrations
- anterograde amnesia
- anxiolysis from actions on the limbic system and hypothalamus
- anticonvulsant activity (Ch. 23)
- reduction of muscle tone (Ch. 24).

Inhibitors of subunits of the GABA receptor result in improved memory in animal studies and are under investigation for the management of Alzheimer's disease.

Pharmacokinetics

Benzodiazepines are well absorbed from the gut, and their lipid solubility ensures ready penetration into the brain. Many, including diazepam, are subsequently metabolised in the liver to active compounds (see Fig 2.12) that contribute to a prolonged duration of action through relatively slow elimination from the body.

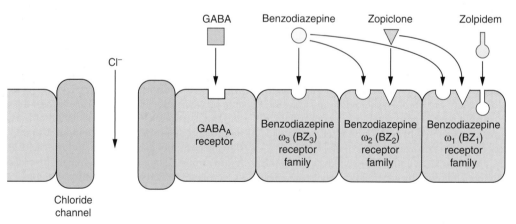

Fig. 20.1
Benzodiazepine receptor subtypes. Subtypes of receptors for benzodiazepine exist which in the literature are described using a variety of notations (see Barnard et al 1998; Mohler et al 2002). Previously, the three subtypes were called ω_{1-3} or BZ_{1-3}, respectively. This has now been reviewed in the light of cloning techniques that have identified a multitude of structurally diverse $GABA_A$ receptors with different subunits. There are α_{1-6}, β_{1-4}, γ_{1-3}, δ, ϵ, π and ρ_{1-3} subunit types. The benzodiazepine receptor ω_1 (BZ_1) is thus a family of receptors all containing the subunit α_1 and with a variable composition of other β and γ subunits, while the ω_2 (BZ_2) receptor family contains α_2 and α_3 or α_5 subunits and other subunits **excluding** α_1. The different receptors vary in abundance in different parts of the brain.

The ω_1 receptor subtype (α_1 subunit-containing) is thought to be associated with the sedative and amnesic actions of benzodiazepines. The ω_2 but not ω_3 receptor subtype is associated with anxiolysis. Muscle relaxation appears to be mediated by both α_1- and α_2-containing receptor subtypes, but generally higher doses of benzodiazepines are required for this action. Diazepam and lorazepam and other 'classic' benzodiazepines are non-selective, but compounds such as zolpidem have a higher affinity for the ω_1 receptor subtype (α_1 subunit-containing) than other subtypes. Benzodiazepines act allosterically to facilitate the actions of GABA on the $GABA_A$ receptor. Barbiturates have similar effects on the Cl^- channel but act by modulating the channel directly in high dose, although they may also have some allosteric influence on the $GABA_A$ receptor.

Metabolism of some benzodiazepines, for example temazepam (used as an hypnotic – see below), produces inactive derivatives. The pharmacokinetics of individual benzodiazepines determine their major clinical uses.

Benzodiazepines that are useful for inducing sleep are rapidly absorbed from the gut (e.g. temazepam). This produces a fast onset of sedation, then sleep. A brief duration of action is desirable to avoid hangover sedation in the morning; this is more likely if the drug is inactivated in the liver (e.g. temazepam). Repeated dosing, particularly with long-acting compounds such as diazepam, increases the risk of accumulation producing a prolonged sedative effect (see drug compendium at the end of this chapter).

The anxiolytic properties of benzodiazepines are best exploited by using a compound with a long duration of action. Smaller doses can then be used to minimise sedation, and the rebound in anxiety symptoms that can occur between doses of a short-acting drug is avoided.

Diazepam, lorazepam and midazolam can also be given by intravenous injection to provide rapid sedation pre-operatively or before procedures such as endoscopy. Intravenous lorazepam and diazepam can be useful for treatment of status epilepticus (Ch. 23). Long-acting benzodiazepines, such as clobazam, clonazepam and diazepam (rectally), are used in the treatment of epilepsy (see Ch. 23).

Unwanted effects

- drowsiness, which may cause problems with driving or operating machinery
- lightheadedness
- confusion, especially in the elderly
- paradoxical increase in aggression
- impaired memory
- ataxia
- muscle weakness
- potentiation of the sedative effects of other CNS depressant drugs, for example alcohol; in overdose, such combinations can lead to severe respiratory depression; flumazenil is a competitive antagonist of benzodiazepines and can be used in acute overdosage, particularly to reverse respiratory depression (Ch. 53)
- tolerance and dependence.

Tolerance. Tolerance to the therapeutic effects of benzodiazepines is common. Hypnotic effects are lost quite early, but the rebound insomnia on withdrawal can perpetuate benzodiazepine use.

Dependence. Dependence with physical and psychological withdrawal symptoms occurs during long-term treatment. The risk is highest in people with personality disorders, or a previous history of dependence on alcohol or drugs, and is more likely to occur if high doses of benzodiazepines are used. Restricting their use to a maximum of 4 weeks will minimise the risk of dependence. With long-acting drugs, withdrawal symptoms may be delayed by up to 3 weeks. Anxiety is the most frequent symptom, while insomnia, depression, and abnormalities of perception, such as altered sensitivity to noise, light or touch, also occur. More severe reactions such as psychosis or convulsions occasionally arise. Some withdrawal symptoms may resemble those for which the drug was originally prescribed, encouraging continued use. The symptoms may take several months to completely resolve. Gradual withdrawal of a benzodiazepine over 4–8 weeks is desirable after long-term use, although complete withdrawal may take up to a year. Lorazepam is a potent benzodiazepine with a relatively short action that proves particularly difficult to stop because of the intensity of withdrawal symptoms that begin a few hours after cessation of treatment. Substitution with the longer-acting drug diazepam may be helpful before withdrawal is attempted. There are no proven treatments for reducing symptoms associated with withdrawal. Beta-adrenoceptors antagonists (Ch. 5) are sometimes helpful, or an antidepressant (Ch. 22) if there are depressive symptoms or panic attacks.

Azapirones

Example: buspirone

Mechanism of action and effects

Buspirone is a partial agonist at presynaptic $5HT_{1A}$ receptors, producing negative feedback to inhibit 5HT release. It has no effect on GABA receptors. Initial exacerbation of anxiety may occur, possibly caused by postsynaptic $5HT_{1A}$ receptor stimulation. The onset of the anxiolytic action of buspirone is slow, over 1–2 weeks, reaching a maximum effect at approximately four weeks, so the mechanism of action may involve gradual changes in neural plasticity (enhancement of neural performance or changes in neural connections; Ch. 22). It has no sedative action, and is ineffective for panic attacks.

Pharmacokinetics

Buspirone is well absorbed from the gut and undergoes extensive first-pass metabolism in the liver. The half-life is short.

Unwanted effects

- nausea
- dizziness, lightheadedness and headache
- nervousness.

Neither tolerance nor dependence has been reported.

Management of anxiety

Symptoms of anxiety, if mild, may respond to counselling and psychotherapy, such as relaxation training. If they are more severe or persistent, benzodiazepines are the most effective drugs, with a rapid onset of action over a few minutes. Problems with dependence should limit their use to a maximum of 4 weeks, and the dose should be gradually reduced after the first 2 weeks. A minority of people may require long-term treatment, usually under specialist guidance. Buspirone has similar efficacy to benzodiazepines, but the slow onset of action (1–2 weeks) makes it less versatile for managing short-term anxiety. In addition, anxiety that responds well to benzodiazepines often responds less well to buspirone, possibly due to a relative lack of effect on somatic symptoms. Somatic symptoms of anxiety (e.g. tremor, palpitations) are often helped by a β-adrenceptor antagonist (Ch. 5). Novel approaches to the pharmacological management of anxiety are under investigation, including the use of tiagabine, an antiepileptic drug that modulates GABAergic neurotransmission (Ch. 23).

Anxiety frequently coexists with depression, and antidepressants (Ch. 22) provide a useful alternative treatment in this situation. Tricyclic antidepressants and selective serotonin reuptake inhibitors (SSRIs) appear to be equally effective. Antidepressants can initially exacerbate anxiety and a benzodiazepine may be necessary for the first week to prevent this. The optimal duration of antidepressant treatment in this situation is uncertain, but similar treatment periods as for depression (Ch. 22) are usually recommended.

Social anxiety disorder, in particular, responds to monoamine oxidase inhibitors (MAOIs) better than to most other agents (Ch. 22). Moclobemide is the treatment of choice, but phenelzine is also used.

Phobic disorders usually need a different approach. Behavioural techniques are often most effective in the long term.

Panic disorder is usually treated with tricyclic antidepressants or SSRIs; MAOIs are used for those who do not respond.

Table 20.1
Types of insomnia

Type of insomnia	Duration	Likely causes
Transient	2–3 days	Acute situational or environmental stress (e.g. jet lag, shift work)
Short term	<3 weeks	Ongoing personal stress
Long term	>3 weeks	Psychiatric illness, behavioural reasons, medical reasons

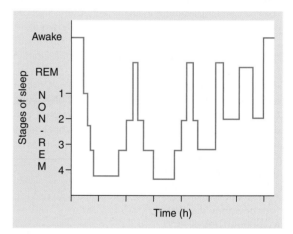

Fig. 20.2
Typical sleep pattern in a young adult. REM, rapid eye movement.

Insomnia

Defining insomnia is complicated by the considerable variability in the normal pattern of sleep. It is considered to be present if there is 'inability to initiate or maintain sleep'. There are three major categories of insomnia (Table 20.1).

The reticular formation in the midbrain, medulla and pons is responsible for maintaining wakefulness. This is dependent on sensory input via collateral connections from the main sensory pathways. Neurotransmitter systems involved in the regulation of sleep include noradrenergic pathways from the locus ceruleus and cholinergic ascending tracts, which are involved in cortical arousal. By contrast, GABA neurotransmission

inhibits these neurons, and release of 5HT from the rostral raphe nucleus also induces sleep.

Sleep patterns

The two main types of sleep pattern are non-rapid eye movement (non-REM) sleep and rapid eye movement (REM) sleep. These sleep patterns occur in cycles (Fig. 20.2), with non-REM sleep varying between light sleep (stages 1 and 2) and slow-wave sleep (stages 3 and 4). Two-thirds of sleep is usually spent in stages 2–4, characterised by continuous or intermittent delta waves (slow waves) on the electroencephalogram. These deeper stages of sleep are the recuperative phase, while most dreaming occurs during the REM-sleep periods. Increasing age is associated with more nocturnal awakening and longer periods of REM sleep.

Drug therapy for insomnia

Drugs used to treat insomnia are called hypnotics.

Benzodiazepines

Benzodiazepines have dose-related hypnotic effects. See above for details.

Non-benzodiazepine drugs that modulate the GABA/chloride channel

Examples: zopiclone, zolpidem

Mechanism of action and effects
Zopiclone and zolpidem (the 'Z' drugs) belong to different chemical classes, but interact in a similar manner with the postsynaptic $GABA_A$ receptor on neuronal membranes. They bind to modulatory sites on the receptor that are close to, but distinct from, the benzodiazepine binding site (Fig. 20.1) Like the benzodiazepines, they increase GABA-mediated Cl^- influx into the cell, which inhibits neurotransmission. Zolpidem shows selectivity for the receptor subtype ω_1. Zopiclone acts at the ω_2 receptor subtype and produces a marked hypnotic effect, but although it possesses anxiolytic and anticonvulsant activity, its short duration of action makes it unsuitable for these indications.

Pharmacokinetics
These drugs show rapid absorption and short half-lives, which makes them well suited to their use as hypnotics. Metabolism in the liver is responsible for elimination.

Unwanted effects
- bitter metallic taste (zopiclone)
- gastrointestinal disturbances, including nausea and vomiting
- drowsiness, dizziness, headache and fatigue
- depression, confusion
- there is only anecdotal evidence for tolerance, but dependence with withdrawal symptoms has been reported.

Clomethiazole

Mechanism of action, effects and clinical uses
Clomethiazole is structurally similar to thiamine (vitamin B_1). It probably enhances GABA receptor activity by interaction with a site similar to that of the barbiturates (Fig. 20.1 and Ch. 23). Clomethiazole has sedative, hypnotic and anticonvulsant properties, but is now rarely used as a hypnotic. Clinical uses are limited, but it is sometimes used in the management of alcohol withdrawal (Ch. 54), status epilepticus (Ch. 23) and control of agitation in the elderly.

Pharmacokinetics
Clomethiazole is readily absorbed from the gut but undergoes extensive first-pass metabolism in the liver. The half-life is short.

Unwanted effects
- nasal congestion and conjunctival irritation early in use
- headache
- hangover effects
- respiratory depression in overdose, especially if taken with alcohol
- dependence is common, which restricts the drug's usefulness; to reduce the risk of dependence, clomethiazole should not be given for more than 9 days.

Chloral derivatives

Examples: chloral hydrate, triclofos sodium

Mechanism of action and effects
The alcohol metabolite trichloroethanol is mainly responsible for the hypnotic effects of chloral derivatives. It may act in part by modulating GABAergic inhibitory neurotransmission, although it has effects on several other receptors and ligand-activated ion channels. Chloral derivatives have a narrow therapeutic index and therefore are not ideal hypnotic drugs. They are considered less suitable than other hypnotics and are only for short-term use.

Pharmacokinetics
Chloral is a prodrug that is well absorbed from the gut, then rapidly metabolised to trichloroethanol by alcohol dehydrogenase. The drug competes with ethanol for metabolism.

Unwanted effects
- unpleasant taste and gastric irritation
- ataxia and nightmares
- hangover effects
- tolerance and dependence are frequent, as with benzodiazepines
- respiratory and myocardial depression can occur in overdose.

Management of insomnia

Drugs play only a small part in the treatment of insomnia. Explanation of the normal variations in sleep patterns and avoidance of diuretics or of drinks containing caffeine or alcohol in the hours before retiring can help. Eliminating excessive noise or heat in the bedroom, encouraging regular exercise in the day and minimising daytime napping may also be useful.

Hypnotic drugs are reserved for when abnormal sleep markedly affects quality of life. The ideal hypnotic will induce good-quality prolonged sleep without disturbance of the normal sleep pattern. It should have a rapid onset of action, with no 'hangover' sedation in the morning and should not produce tolerance or dependence. Few drugs come close to this ideal profile. Benzodiazepines reduce sleep latency (the time between settling down and falling asleep) and prolong sleep duration. However, they reduce the time spent in REM sleep, with more time spent in stage 2 sleep. Of the other hypnotic drugs, zopiclone and zolpidem produce less disturbance of sleep 'architecture', having less effect on the amount of REM sleep while increasing the duration of slow-wave sleep.

Hypnotic drugs should be used only for short periods and intermittently if possible; tolerance to hypnotics frequently occurs after 2 weeks. If a benzodiazepine is used continuously for 4–6 weeks, rebound insomnia is common when the drug is stopped, caused by mild dependence. However, benzodiazepines are still widely used since they are safe in overdose. Short-acting benzodiazepines may produce wakefulness early in the morning but longer-acting drugs carry the risk of hangover effects the following day. Zopiclone and zolpidem are equally as effective as a benzodiazepine and carry a similar risk of dependence.

Of the other hypnotics, chloral derivatives and clomethiazole should usually be avoided. Compounds with sedative actions as a part of their therapeutic profile can be useful to aid sleep – for example, a sedative antihistamine such as promazine (Ch. 39) for children suffering from somnambulism (sleep walking) or night terrors. Sedative antidepressants (Ch. 22) – for example, a tricyclic antidepressant such as amitriptyline – should be considered if there is an underlying depressive illness. If less-sedative antidepressants are used, short-term concurrent use of a benzodiazepine may be necessary while awaiting the onset of the antidepressant effect.

FURTHER READING

Aranda M, Hanson CW (2000) Anesthetics, sedatives and paralytics. Understanding their use in the intensive care unit. *Surg Clin North Am* 80, 933–947

Barnard EA, Slolnick P, Olsen RW et al (1998) International Union of Pharmacology. XV. Subtypes of gamma-aminobutyric acid$_A$ receptors: classification on the basis of subunit structure and receptor function *Pharmacol Rev* 50, 292–310

Blanco C, Antia SX, Liebowitz MR (2002) Pharmacotherapy of social anxiety disorder. *Biol Psychiatry* 51, 109–120

Doble A (1999) New insights into the mechanism of action of hypnotics. *J Psychopharmacol* 13, S11–S20

Estivill E, Bov A, Garca-Borreguero D et al (2003) Consensus on drug treatment, definition and diagnosis for insomnia. **http://www.medscape.com/viewarticle/456734?src=search** (accessed May 2004)

Fricehione G (2004) Generalized anxiety disorder. *N Engl J Med* 351, 675–682

Gale C, Oakley-Browne M (2000) Anxiety disorder. *BMJ* 321, 1204–1211

Gottesmann C (2002) GABA mechanisms and sleep. *Neuroscience* 111, 231–239

Lader MH (1999) Limitations on the use of benzodiazepines in anxiety and insomnia: are they justified? *Eur Neuropsychopharmacol* 9(suppl 6), S399–S405

Lerch C, Park GR (1999) Sedation and analgesia. *Br Med Bull* 55, 76–95

Longo LP, Johnson B (2000) Addiction: Part I. Benzodiazepines – side effects, abuse risk and alternatives. *Am Fam Physician* 61, 2121–2128

Lydiard RB (2003) The role of GABA in anxiety. *J Clin Psychiatry* 64(suppl 3), 21–27

Mohler H, Fritschy JM, Rudolph U (2002) A new benzodiazepine pharmacology. *J Pharmacol Exp Ther* 300, 2–8

National Institute for Clinical Excellence Guidelines (2004) Newer hypnotic drugs for insomnia **http://www.nice.org.uk/cat.asp?c=113330** (accessed May 2004)

Schenk CH, Mahowald MW, Sack RL (2003) Assessment and management of insomnia. *JAMA* 289, 2475–2479

Sramek JJ, Zarotsky V, Cutler NR (2002) Generalised anxiety disorder. *Drugs* 62, 1635–1648

Tancer ME, Uhde TW (1995) Social phobia: a review of pharmacological treatment. *CNS Drugs* 3, 267–278

Whiting PJ (2003) GABA receptor subtypes in the brain: a paradigm for CNS drug discovery *Drug Discovery Today* 8, 445–450

Young C, Knudsen N, Hilton A, Reves JG (2000) Sedation in the intensive care unit. *Crit Care Med* 28, 853–866

Self-assessment

In questions 1–3, the first statement, in italics, is true. Are the accompanying statements also true?

1. *Benzodiazepines with a medium to long duration of action are useful for treating anxiety states.*

   a. Long-term use of benzodiazepines is recommended in anxiety states.
   b. Potentiation of CNS effects occurs with concurrent alcohol administration.

2. *CNS depressant effects of benzodiazepines can be reversed with the antagonist flumazenil.*

   a. Lower doses of benzodiazepines should be used in the elderly.
   b. Buspirone is more sedative than temazepam.

3. *Benzodiazepines used to treat anxiety should be administered for as short a time as possible and in the lowest dose possible.* Benzodiazepines have no effect on sleep patterns as measured by the duration of REM sleep.

4. You are considering options for the treatment of a patient with insomnia and anxiety who has been taking diazepam for several months without clear benefit. Choose the one <u>most appropriate</u> statement from the following.

   A. If there is no response to one hypnotic, it is advisable to switch to another.
   B. Withdrawal symptoms abate within 3 weeks of abruptly stopping diazepam.
   C. Barbiturates are the drugs of choice in patients with insomnia and anxiety.
   D. Buspirone decreases anxiety by acting at the GABA receptor site.
   E. Benzodiazepines act to potentiate the inhibitory actions of GABA at its receptor.

5. Case history questions

   > Mrs FL was a 46-year-old mother of three who was finding it very hard to cope following the sudden death of her husband 5 weeks previously. She had returned to work from bereavement leave but did not sleep properly, experienced occasional periods of anxiety during the day and felt that she was at risk of losing her job because tiredness and anxiety about her financial difficulties prevented her concentrating on her work.

   a. What drug might you prescribe to help Mrs FL's insomnia? What factors may determine your choice of this drug?
   b. How does your chosen drug work to reduce insomnia and anxiety? What potential unwanted effects and drug interactions should you warn Mrs FL about?
   c. Mrs FL returned 2 weeks later, saying that she regularly woke at 4 a.m. and could not get back to sleep. Consider the 'pros' and 'cons' of changing her to a longer-acting drug or to another 'newer' hypnotic.
   d. What are the problems associated with long-term use of benzodiazepines? What other options should be considered to help to manage Mrs FL's problems in the long term?

6. Extended-matching questions

   Choose the <u>most appropriate</u> statement A–E that fits the case scenarios described in 1 and 2. These are not 'complete' case studies. Only the pharmacological aspects of cases are dealt with; the equally important roles of psychological and psychiatric help must always be considered.

   A. Gradual tapering of the medication over many months.
   B. Gradual tapering of the medication over several days.
   C. Switch to another type of benzodiazepine.
   D. Prescribe another course of the same benzodiazepine.
   E. Consider giving paroxetine.

   1. A 54-year-old woman had a history of anxiety. Seven years earlier, she had received a prescription of lorazepam, the first of a series of prescriptions. For the last 3 years, her doctor had been refilling prescription requests without reassessing the clinical need. The woman now wishes to stop her medication.

   2. You have been treating a woman aged 25 for a year. She has been having up to ten intense panic attacks a month. At any time of day, she suddenly developed a peculiar and very strong feeling of being lightheaded, jumpy and being smothered. Her heart rate increased dramatically. It came on so quickly and was so severe that she felt she might be dying. Then she felt very shaky, sweaty, and unsteady. This whole experience reached peak intensity within 2 min but she was often unable to continue work and needed to go home. She had been treated with intermittent courses of diazepam for a year without improvement.

   The answers are provided on pages 720–721.

Drug compendium

Anxiolytics, sedatives and hypnotics (all given orally unless otherwise stated)

Drug	Half-life (h)	Elimination	Comments
Anxiolytics			
Alprazolam	6–16	Metabolism	Almost complete oral bioavailability; eliminated largely by oxidation by CYP3A4 to inactive metabolites which are conjugated with glucuronic acid
Buspirone	2–4	Metabolism	Rapid absorption but extensive first-pass metabolism, so that the bioavailability is only about 4%, but increased if taken with food; metabolised by CYP3A4-mediated oxidative dealkylation and hydroxylation
Chlordiazepoxide	5–30	Metabolism	Complete oral bioavailability; slowly eliminated by hepatic metabolism; a number of the metabolites retain activity, have very long half-lives (15–100 h) and contribute significantly to the effect
Clorazepate	30–200 (metabolite)	Metabolism	A prodrug that undergoes pH-dependent decarboxylation in the gut to *N*-desmethyldiazepam, which is then absorbed into systemic circulation and has a half-life of 30–200 h
Diazepam	20–100	Metabolism	May be given orally, rectally or by intramuscular or slow intravenous injection; complete oral bioavailability; metabolised to *N*-desmethyl metabolite, which has a longer half-life (30–200h), and to temazepam; *N*-desmethyldiazepam is oxidised to oxazepam
Lorazepam	4–25	Metabolism	May be given orally or by intramuscular or slow intravenous dosage; high bioavailability; eliminated mainly as the glucuronic acid conjugate
Meprobamate	8–11	Metabolism (+ renal)	Good oral absorption; eliminated by hepatic metabolism to inactive metabolites and some renal excretion of the parent drug
Oxazepam	4–25	Metabolism	High bioavailability; eliminated mainly as the glucuronic acid conjugate
Sedative and hypnotics			
Clomethiazole	4–6	Metabolism	Used only in the elderly (with little hangover); may be given orally (or by intravenous infusion for acute alcohol withdrawal); rapid absorption but extensive (40–95%) first-pass metabolism; metabolised by dechlorination and oxidation
Chloral hydrate	0.1	Metabolism	Limited current use; not recommended; extensive first pass metabolism; rapidly reduced to trichloroethanol (TCE) (half-life 8–12 h) and oxidised to trichloroacetic acid (half-life 60–70 h), the hypnotic effect is believed to be caused by TCE
Flunitrazepam	23	Metabolism	Good oral bioavailability; a large number of metabolites, some of which retain pharmacological activity

continued

Anxiolytics, sedatives and hypnotics (all given orally unless otherwise stated) *(continued)*

Drug	Half-life (h)	Elimination	Comments
Sedative and hypnotics (continued)			
Flurazepam	2–3		Good oral absorption; oxidised in the liver to active metabolites which have half-lives of 30–100 and 2–4 h
Loprazolam	7	Metabolism (+ biliary)	Good oral absorption; metabolised by formation of a more polar *N*-oxide; metabolite and parent drug are eliminated in bile
Lormetazepam	8–10	Metabolism	Unlike many benzodiazepines, it is not extensively oxidised but is eliminated as the glucuronic acid conjugate of the parent drug; limited oxidation (about 10%) to lorazepam (the *N*-desmethyl analogue)
Nitrazepam	20–48	Metabolism	Rapid absorption but variable bioavailability (50–90%); metabolism is mainly by nitro-reduction, followed by N-acetylation of the resultant amino group; only the parent drug is active
Promethazine	7–14	Metabolism	Sedative and hypnotic antihistamine that has a prolonged effect; incomplete oral bioavailability (about 20%); metabolised by *S*-oxidation and *N*-dealkylation in the liver; the *S*-oxide (which is the main metabolite) is inactive
Temazepam	5–12	Metabolism	High oral bioavailability, oxidised by *N*-demethylation to oxazepam and by conjugation with glucuronic acid; most activity is probably due to the parent compound
Triclofos	–	Metabolism	Similar to chloral hydrate (see above); few published data available; phosphate ester of trichloroethanol that is hydrolysed in vivo; causes fewer gastrointestinal effects than chloral hydrate
Zaleplon	1	Metabolism	Binds to ω_1 benzodiazepine receptor on the GABA channel; rapid absorption with a bioavailability of 30%; metabolised by aldehyde oxidase and CYP3A4 to inactive products
Zolpidem	2–4	Metabolism	Binds to ω_1 benzodiazepine receptor on the GABA channel; good oral bioavailability (about 70%); metabolised largely by CYP3A4 to inactive metabolites
Zopiclone	4–6	Metabolism	Binds to ω_2 benzodiazepine receptor on the GABA channel; rapid absorption and a high bioavailability (about 80%); metabolised by *N*-dealkylation, *N*-oxidation and decarboxylation, the metabolites and about 5% of unchanged parent drug are eliminated in the urine

21

The major psychotic disorders: schizophrenia and mania

Psychotic disorders

The term psychosis indicates that the person affected has lost contact with reality. This is usually experienced as hallucination, delusion or a disruption in thought processes. The two most profound functional psychotic conditions are schizophrenia and mania. These disorders probably form extremes of a continuum that embraces the so-called schizoaffective disorders (Box 21.1). Organic disease caused by metabolic disturbance, toxic substances or psychoactive drugs can also cause psychosis.

Schizophrenia

Schizophrenia is more common in males and usually presents relatively early in life. The onset is usually gradual but can be abrupt. Once established, it can have a relapsing or persistent course. Clinical features are categorised as positive or negative (Table 21.1), although none are pathognomonic of the disorder. The positive features are disordered versions of thinking, perception, formation of ideas, or sense of self. They include hallucinations (false sensory perceptions) and delusions (false beliefs held with absolute certainty and un-explained by the person's socioeconomic background). The negative features are often the most debilitating in the long term.

Box 21.1

Classification of major psychotic disorders

Schizophrenia

Persistent delusional disorders (includes paranoid psychosis, paraphrenia)

Acute and transient psychotic disorders

Schizoaffective disorders

Manic episode

Bipolar affective disorder

Table 21.1
Clinical features of schizophrenia

Features	Characteristics
Positive features	
Hallucinations	Third-person auditory hallucinations (voices talking about the person as 'he' or 'she') Second-person commands Olfactory, tactile or visual hallucinations
Delusions	Thought withdrawal (thoughts being taken from your mind) Thought insertion (alien thoughts inserted in your mind) Though broadcast (thoughts are known to others) Actions are caused or controlled from outside Bodily sensations are imposed from outside Delusional perception (a sudden, fully formed delusion, in the wake of a normal perception)
Negative features	Loss of interest in others, initiative or sense of enjoyment Blunted emotions Limited speech

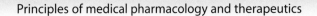

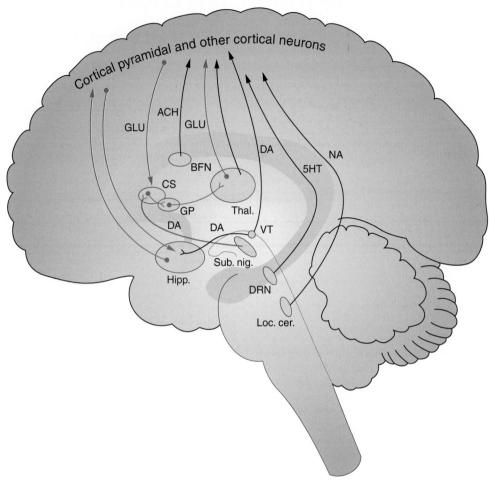

Fig. 21.1
Pathways in the central nervous system that appear to be involved in schizophrenia. This cartoon shows only representative pathways relating to schizophrenia, without the myriad of connecting interneurons. Neurons that are information repositories and processors such as pyramidal neurons in the cortex are said to be excessively responsive in psychoses. These neurons are normally under the appropriate control of many other interneurons that are themselves controlled by dopaminergic (DA), serotoninergic (5HT), noradrenergic (NA) and cholinergic (ACH) neurons which feed into the cortex. The interneurons utilise other transmitters such as GABA. Some pathways also facilitate glutamate (GLU) release, e.g. 5HT. BFN, basal forebrain nucleus; CS, corpus striatum; DRN, dorsal raphe nucleus; GP, globus pallidus; Hipp., hippocampus; Loc. cer., locus ceruleus; Sub. nig., substantia nigra; Thal., thalamus; VT, ventral tegmentum.

Biological basis of schizophrenia

The neurobiology of schizophrenia is poorly understood; it is believed to involve abnormal function in dopaminergic circuits in the central nervous system (CNS), and yet blockade of dopamine receptors does not completely remove symptoms. It is possible that psychosis results from an excessive response of cortical processing neurons (pyramidal neurons) to sensory information relayed by excitatory glutamatergic projections from the thalamic nuclei and other afferent inputs. The response to glutamate in the cortex is facilitated by dopaminergic, serotonergic, noradrenergic and cholinergic afferent projections from the mesolimbic system (Fig. 21.1). Treatment is based on modulation of these afferent inputs to the cortex.

There is a strong genetic component to schizophrenia, with environmental influences only affecting those with a genetic predisposition. Many neurobiological abnormalities have been described in schizophrenia, including disturbances in neuronal numbers and synaptic connections in the cortical, thalamic, and hippocampal areas. These disturbances become more marked as the illness progresses.

The dopaminergic systems in the CNS arise from the substantia nigra and ventral tegmental area in the midbrain (Fig. 21.1). Within the basal ganglia, dopaminergic neurons from the substantia nigra project to gamma-aminobutyric acid (GABA)-ergic inhibitory interneurons in the corpus striatum and globus pallidus via the nigrostriatal pathways (Ch. 24) and modulate motor and behavioural function via ongoing projections to the thalamus and cortex. The striatum receives input from the cortex, and projects back to the cortex via the globus pallidus and thalamus. Neurons from the ventral tegmental area connect via the mesolimbic projections to the limbic region (especially the hippocampus) and via the mesocortical projections to the prefrontal cortex. The limbic region also receives cortical afferents. The limbic region and prefrontal cortex are involved in cognition, emotional memory and the initiation of behaviour. Two neuronal circuits are believed to be of particular importance in the genesis of schizophrenia: the reciprocal connection between the hippocampus and cortex, and the striatal-pallidal-thalamic-cortical loop.

Several receptors for the neurotransmitter dopamine are found in the brain (Ch. 4). CNS dopamine receptors belong to two families, D_1 (which includes subtypes D_1 and D_5) and D_2 (which includes subtypes D_2, D_3 and D_4). Both D_1 and D_2 subtypes are found in the striatum, limbic system, thalamus and hypothalamus. These are all areas that receive dopaminergic innervation. D_2 receptors are also present in the pituitary. Presynaptic D_3 receptors on the dopaminergic neuronal terminals in the striatum and limbic system inhibit dopamine release in these areas. D_4 receptors are present in the limbic system and frontal cortex.

The positive symptoms of schizophrenia are believed to result from dopaminergic overactivity in the mesolimbic system (and thus the hippocampus) of the dominant hemisphere. This overactivity may be attributable to a primary dysfunction in NMDA (*N*-methyl-D-aspartate) receptor-mediated glutamatergic neuronal projections from the prefrontal cortex to dopaminergic neurons in the limbic system. Consistent with this hypothesis, the general anaesthetic ketamine (Ch. 17), which is a non-competitive antagonist at NMDA receptors, can produce many symptoms similar to those of schizophrenia. The response to glutamate at the other glutamate receptors in the cortex (AMPA and kainite receptors) may be excessive in schizophrenia. These receptors can mediate 'glutamate excitotoxicity', leading to oligodendrocyte cell death, loss of white matter and reduced synaptic connections of cortical neurons.

By contrast, the negative symptoms of schizophrenia may be determined by underactive tonic dopaminergic neurotransmission in the mesocortical system. Abnormalities of other neurotransmitter systems may also be important in schizophrenia. Inhibitory noradrenergic activity from the locus ceruleus nucleus to inhibitory GABA interneurons in the cortex may be enhanced, and neuropeptides such as neurotensin, cholecystokinin and somatostatin may also be be involved.

Mania and bipolar disorder

Mania is a disorder of elevated mood that can occur alone or be interspersed with episodes of depression (bipolar affective disorder or manic-depressive illness); unipolar mania is uncommon. Mild mania is termed hypomania. Sometimes, the fluctuations of mood are less marked, and the disorder is termed cyclothymia.

Mania can occur gradually or suddenly and varies in severity from mild elation, increased drive and sociability, to grandiose ideas, marked overactivity, overspending and socially embarrassing behaviour. Onset is usually early in adult life and both mania and bipolar disorder have (and share) a stronger genetic component than any other major psychiatric disorder.

Biological basis of mania

The biological basis for mania is not well understood, but probably involves altered neurotransmission in the prefrontal cortex, limbic and subcortical circuitry. Increased CNS monoamine neurotransmitter activity (noradrenaline, dopamine and possibly 5-hydroxytryptamine [5HT]), reduced acetylcholine and GABA neurotransmission, and disruption of the hypothalamic–pituitary–adrenal axis may all be important in orchestrating the changes in neuronal function. However, these are in turn probably triggered by altered expression of critical neuronal proteins, determined by the genetic predisposition.

Increased G_s protein activity in the target cells, and therefore increased levels of the intracellular second messenger cyclic adenosine monophosphate (cAMP), has been implicated in the pathogenesis of bipolar disorder. cAMP increases protein kinase A activity and leads to gene expression mediated by cAMP-responsive element-binding protein (CREB). These changes are the opposite of those described in unipolar depression (Ch. 22). Excessive phosphoinositide pathway signalling has also been found in bipolar disorder, with increased levels of inositol triphosphate (IP_3) and diacylglycerol (DAG). IP_3 enhances intracellular calcium signalling. DAG activates protein kinase C, which phosphorylates a number of substrates, the most prominent of which in the brain is myristoylated alanine-rich C-kinase substrate (MARCKS). MARCKS activates nuclear transcription regulatory factors and therefore modulates genes that increase synthesis of neuromodulatory peptide hormones, stimulate neuroplastic processes and alter cell signalling. These effects may contribute to the changes in neurotransmitter synthesis and neuronal excitability, neuroplastic changes (especially synaptic plasticity) and neuronal cell loss that are features of mania and bipolar disorder.

Antipsychotic drugs

Classification

Antipsychotic drugs (also known as neuroleptics or major tranquillisers) belong to various chemical classes

Table 21.2
Consequences of different receptor antagonist activities among antipsychotic drugs

Drug type	Example	Sedative	Anticholinergic	Extrapyramidal	Hypotension
Phenothiazines					
Group 1 (aliphatic)					
	Chlorpromazine	+++	++	++	+++
	Levomepromazine	+++	++	++	+++
	Promazine	+++	++	++	+++
Group 2 (piperidine)					
	Pericyazine	++	+++	+	++
	Pipotiazine	+	++	++	++
	Thioridazine	++	+++	+	++
Group 3 (piperazine)					
	Fluphenazine	++	+	+++	+
	Perphenazine	++	++	+++	++
	Prochlorperazine	++	++	+++	++
	Trifluoperazine	++	++	+++	+
Thioxanthenes					
	Flupentixol	+	+	+++	+
	Zuclopenthixol	+	+	+++	+
Butyrophenones					
	Benperidol	+	+	+++	+
	Haloperidol	+	+	+++	++
Diphenylbutylpiperidines					
	Pimozide	0	+	+++	+
Substituted benzamides					
	Sulpiride	+	+	+	0
Atypical antipsychotics					
	Amisulpride	+	+	0	+
	Clozapine	++	+	0	+
	Olanzapine	++	+	0	+
	Quetiapine	++	0	0	+
	Risperidone	+	0	+	+
	Sertindole	+	0	0	++
	Zotepine	++	0	0	+

Key +++, high risk; ++, moderate risk; +, low risk; 0, minimal risk.

that vary in their sedative, antimuscarinic and extrapyramidal effects (Table 21.2).

Mechanism of action and effects

The antipsychotic action involves blockade of CNS dopamine receptors in mesolimbic pathways. High affinity for the D_2 receptors is common to all conventional antipsychotics, and the affinity for these receptors correlates well with the effective dose of the drugs. Conventional antipsychotics bind to D_2 receptors more than does dopamine, with slow dissociation from the receptor. At least 65% D_2 receptor occupancy is required for clinical benefit during long-term treatment. However, 80% or more D_2 receptor blockade in the striatum will produce extrapyramidal unwanted effects (see below). Many conventional antipsychotics also block serotonin $5HT_{2A}$ and $5HT_{2C}$ receptors, an action that may contribute to their clinical effects. Antagonist activity at other receptors, including α_2-adrenoceptors and histamine H_1 receptors (in which respect they resemble tricyclic antidepressants), does not influence their efficacy in psychotic illness but can produce unwanted effects. The severity of which varies considerably among the different drugs.

Compared with conventional drugs, the 'atypical' antipsychotic drugs (e.g. clozapine, olanzapine and risperidone) have different receptor affinities. In particular, their affinity for D_2 receptors is much lower than that of conventional antipsychotics, and less than that of dopamine, with much more transient receptor occupancy. This may underlie their lower propensity for producing movement disorders (Ch. 24). Clozapine is a relatively weak D_2 receptor antagonist with selective cortical receptor occupancy, and shows greater blockade at D_1 and D_4 receptors. It has a much higher affinity for blockade of $5HT_{2A}$ and $5HT_{2C}$ receptors, and also blocks α-adrenoceptors and muscarinic receptors. Olanzapine has a similar profile to clozapine, with additional antagonist activity at some other 5HT receptors and histamine H_1 receptors. Risperidone has higher affinity binding to D_2 receptors, with dose-dependent limbic selectivity. It also binds to $5HT_{2A}$ receptors, and to $α_1$- and $α_2$-adrenoceptors, but not to muscarinic or histamine receptors. Indeed, the atypical antipsychotic drugs increase the release of acetylcholine from neurons. Since 'atypical' antipsychotics cause markedly fewer extrapyramidal effects than do conventional drugs, this improves compliance and may explain their apparently greater efficacy when compared with conventional drugs. Clozapine uniquely is clearly superior to all other drugs for refractory schizophrenia.

Despite immediate production of dopamine receptor blockade, clinical improvement after initiation of treatment with antipsychotic drugs is delayed. There is increasing evidence that these drugs affect neuroplasticity, leading to changes in synaptic connections in areas of the brain known to be involved in psychotic illness. This may be achieved through D_2 receptor activation, phosphorylation of transcription factors in the nuclei of target neurons and expression of genes under the control of calcium and cAMP second messenger pathways.

Clinically useful effects produced by antipsychotic drugs include:

- a depressant action on conditioned responses and emotional responsiveness; in psychoses, this is particularly helpful for management of thought disorders, abnormalities of perception and delusional beliefs
- a sedative action, which is useful for treatment of restlessness and confusion; sensory input into the reticular activating system is reduced by blockade of collateral fibres from the lemniscal pathways, but spontaneous activity is preserved; arousal stimuli therefore produce less response
- an antiemetic effect through dopamine receptor blockade at the chemoreceptor trigger zone (CTZ),

which is useful to treat vomiting, such as that associated with drugs (e.g. cytotoxics, opioid analgesics) and uraemia; some antipsychotic drugs are also effective in motion sickness, through muscarinic receptor blockade (Ch. 32)
- antihistaminic activity produced by histamine H_1 receptor blockade can be used for treatment of allergic reactions (Ch. 39).

Pharmacokinetics

Antipsychotics are rapidly absorbed from the gut but most undergo extensive first-pass metabolism. For some drugs, the plasma concentrations of active drug (including metabolites) can vary up to tenfold between individuals, but there is not a close relationship between plasma drug concentration and clinical response. Elimination is by metabolism in the liver. Several antipsychotic drugs, such as chlorpromazine, haloperidol, perphenazine, risperidone, sertindole, thioridazine and zuclopenthixol, are metabolised predominantly by the polymorphic enzyme CYP2D6: significant relationships have been reported between the steady-state plasma concentrations (see Ch. 2) and the CYP2D6 genotype; however, there are not clear relationships between CYP2D6 activity and clinical response to the drug. Sulpiride and amisulpride do not undergo first-pass metabolism and are largely eliminated unchanged by the kidney. The half-lives of the antipsychotics vary widely; for example, that of sulpiride is intermediate, while that of pimozide is very long at two days. Many antipsychotics can be given by intramuscular injection for more rapid onset of action in disturbed people. Since adherence to treatment is often poor in psychotic disorders, depot formulations of many antipsychotics have been developed. They are given by intramuscular injection as a prodrug – which is the active compound esterified to a long-chain fatty acid and dissolved in a vegetable oil – that slowly releases the drug for between 1 and 12 weeks (depending on the formulation). When given as a depot preparation or by intramuscular injection, the doses used are smaller than those for oral treatment, because of the lack of first-pass metabolism. The half-lives given in the drug table do not reflect the slow absorption rate-limited half-life of the depot form (see Ch. 2).

Unwanted effects

The antipsychotic drugs differ mainly in the degree of associated or unwanted effects (Table 21.2).

- Extrapyramidal effects such as akathisia (restlessness), acute dystonias (tongue protrusion, torticollis, oculogyric crisis) or parkinsonism arise from D_2 receptor blockade in the nigrostriatal pathways. Extrapyramidal effects (Ch. 24) occur in more than half of those being treated with conventional antipsychotics, but are usually reversible if the drug is stopped. With prolonged use, tardive dyskinesias or dystonias can develop. These consist of choreo-athetoid and repetitive orofacial movements that arise after months or years of continued treatment and often do not resolve when the drug is withdrawn. Their aetiology is uncertain: upregulation of D_2 receptors may contribute, but damage to inhibitory GABAergic neurons and/or dysfunction in other neurotransmitter pathways probably participate. Atypical antipsychotics have a much lower risk of extrapyramidal effects, and they do not occur with clozapine.

- Drowsiness and cognitive impairment can occur as a result of histamine and dopamine receptor blockade. Risperidone, by contrast, causes insomnia and agitation.
- Galactorrhoea, with gynaecomastia, amenorrhoea, and impotence. Greater than 70% D_2 receptor blockade in hypothalamic pathways produces hyperprolactinaemia and reduced gonadotrophin secretion. It may be less common with atypical antipsychotics.
- Antimuscarinic effects, such as dry mouth, constipation, micturition difficulties and blurred vision (Ch. 4). In addition to peripheral antimuscarinic actions, CNS muscarinic receptor blockade predisposes to acute confusional states.
- Postural hypotension, nasal stuffiness and impaired ejaculation, due to α_1-adrenoceptor blockade.
- Hypothermia as a consequence of depressed hypothalamic function. Altered 5HT neuronal activity may be responsible.
- Increased risk of seizures, especially in those with a history of epilepsy.
- Hypersensitivity reactions include cholestatic jaundice, skin reactions and bone marrow depression.
- Photosensitivity and skin discoloration (especially with chlorpromazine).
- Agranulocytosis is a particular problem with clozapine (1–2% risk) and regular blood tests are mandatory during treatment with this drug.
- Cognitive impairment, which is less marked with atypical antipsychotics.
- Weight gain with atypical antipsychotics, with an increased risk of insulin resistance and glucose intolerance.
- Prolongation of the Q–T interval on the electrocardiogram, a particular problem with pimozide, predisposes to ventricular arrhythmias (Ch. 8).
- Neuroleptic malignant syndrome is a rare genetically determined disorder caused by a polymorphism in the D_2 receptor and consequent abnormal dopamine receptor blockade in the corpus striatum and hypothalamus. In those with a receptor abnormality, antipsychotic drugs produce high fever, muscle rigidity, autonomic instability with hypertension, urinary incontinence and sweating, and altered consciousness. Immediate withdrawal of the antipsychotic and treatment with dantrolene or a dopamine agonist (Ch. 24) may be life-saving. Symptoms can take 2 weeks to subside, or longer after a depot preparation. Cautious reintroduction of an antipsychotic may be possible without recurrence, but at least 2 weeks should be allowed after symptoms of the syndrome have resolved.
- Sudden withdrawal after long-term use can produce symptoms of nausea, vomiting, anorexia, diarrhoea, sweating, myalgias, paraesthesiae, insomnia and agitation. These usually subside within 2 weeks.

Mood-stabilising drugs

Lithium

Mechanism of action
The mechanism of action of lithium is not well understood, but it has multiple effects in the CNS.

- Lithium has complex effects on intracellular generation of cAMP in cortical neuronal pathways. It attenuates the function of G_s-proteins coupled to adenylate cyclase but increases basal adenylate cyclase activity. Lithium also inhibits intracellular inositol monophosphatase, which interferes with substrate generation for second messengers for phosphoinositide pathway signalling. This will affect several aminergic and cholinergic systems in the CNS. The overall action of lithium may be to stabilise intracellular signalling by enhancing basal activity but decreasing maximum activity.
- Suppression of the expression of pro-apoptotic genes and increased expression of anti-apoptotic genes, with consequent neuroprotection, occurs. Lithium inhibits the multifunctional protein kinase glucose synthase kinase-3 (GSK-3), a regulator of many signal transduction pathways that are involved in neuronal apoptosis. Inhibition of the activity of the pro-apoptotic enzyme caspase-3 by lithium also confers neuroprotection.
- Increased neurogenesis has been found in the hippocampus after lithium treatment, which may be one consequence of these complex changes in intracellular signalling.

Pharmacokinetics
Lithium is given as a salt (e.g. carbonate, citrate), which is rapidly absorbed from the gut. To avoid high peak plasma concentrations (which are associated with

unwanted effects), modified-release formulations are normally used. Lithium is widely distributed in the body but enters the brain slowly. It is selectively concentrated in bone and the thyroid gland. Excretion is by glomerular filtration, with 80% reabsorbed in the proximal tubule by the same mechanism as Na^+. Unlike Na^+, lithium is not reabsorbed from more distal parts of the kidney. When the body is depleted of salt and water, for example by vomiting or diarrhoea, then enhanced reabsorption of Na^+ in the proximal tubule is accompanied by enhanced lithium reabsorption, which can produce acute toxicity. Lithium has a long half-life of about 1 day and has a narrow therapeutic index. Regular monitoring of plasma concentrations (which should be measured 12 h after dosing so that the absorption and distribution phases are completed) is mandatory at least every 3 months during long-term treatment.

Unwanted effects

- Nausea and diarrhoea can occur at low plasma concentrations.
- CNS effects, including tremor, giddiness, ataxia and dysarthria, occur commonly with moderate intoxication.
- Severe intoxication produces coma, convulsions, and profound hypotension with oliguria.
- Hypothyroidism can be caused by interference with thyroxine synthesis during long-term treatment.
- The distal renal tubule becomes less responsive to antidiuretic hormone (ADH, vasopressin). This occasionally produces a reversible nephrogenic diabetes insipidus with polyuria.

Drug interactions

Diuretics can reduce lithium excretion by producing dehydration (see above). This is most marked with thiazides (Ch. 14) because of their prolonged action. Angiotensin-converting enzyme inhibitors (Ch. 6) and some non-steroidal anti-inflammatory drugs (Ch. 29) also reduce the excretion of lithium. When lithium is prescribed concurrently with antipsychotic drugs, the risk of extrapyramidal effects may be increased.

Anticonvulsants used in mania

Mechanism of action in mania

The mode of action of the anticonvulsants carbamazepine and sodium valproate (Ch. 23) in mania may be related to facilitation of GABAergic inhibitory neurotransmission, and consequent modulation of excitatory glutamatergic neurons. Like lithium, anticonvulsants modulate cAMP-mediated intracellular events, produce inositol depletion in the phosphoinositide signalling pathway and activate neuroprotective anti-apoptotic genes. They also stimulate hippocampal neurogenesis. Antiepileptic drugs are discussed in Chapter 23.

Management of psychotic disorders

Management of schizophrenia

Acute psychotic symptoms such as hallucinations and delusions can be controlled relatively rapidly with an antipsychotic drug such as haloperidol or chlorpromazine. The initial sedative actions of these drugs can be particularly helpful. However, reductions in thought disturbance, withdrawal and apathy are delayed. Therefore, the clinical improvement is gradual over several weeks of treatment. For newly diagnosed schizophrenia, or for those in whom there is concern about extrapyramidal effects, an atypical antipsychotic is increasingly preferred for maintenance treatment.

Treatment for schizophrenia is not curative, and long-term maintenance therapy is usually required to prevent relapse. The duration of this treatment is determined by the number of acute episodes, and is usually at least 2–5 years. Intermittent treatment that is introduced only for relapses is associated with a higher overall relapse rate (50–80%, compared with 25–40% in those taking prophylactic therapy). The relapse rate is lowest with use of atypical antipsychotics. Adherence to maintenance treatment is often poor in schizophrenia, and can be improved by depot injections given every 1–4 weeks. Continuous antipsychotic treatment provides relief of symptoms for more than 70% of schizophrenic persons. Resistance to conventional antipsychotics is often found, particularly if negative symptoms predominate.

Atypical antipsychotics should be considered:

- when choosing first-line treatment for newly diagnosed schizophrenia
- if there are unacceptable unwanted effects with a conventional drug
- if there is an acute schizophrenic episode when discussion with the person is not possible.

Atypical antipsychotic drugs and amisulpride produce greater relief of negative symptoms than the conventional antipsychotic drugs, although this may be due to better adherence to treatment. There is limited evidence to support the concurrent use of a selective serotonin reuptake inhibitor (SSRI; Ch. 22) with an atypical antipsychotic drug for those whose negative symptoms do not respond to monotherapy. Clozapine is the only drug shown to be effective in treatment resistance (incomplete recovery), but the risk of agranulocytosis has limited its use. It should always be tried if symptoms have failed to respond to two antipsychotic drugs, one of which should be an atypical drug, each given for 6–8 weeks. Between 30% and 50% of those who are resistant to other treatments will respond to clozapine.

Various psychological treatments to improve social skills are important as an adjunct to drug treatment and should be provided along with social support.

Management of mania and bipolar disorder

When symptoms of acute mania are mild or moderate, they can usually be controlled by lithium, although the therapeutic effect may be delayed for at least a week. A benzodiazepine (Ch. 20) is usually given as well for the first 7 days. The anticonvulsants carbamazepine or sodium valproate (Ch. 23) are effective alternatives to lithium. Carbamazepine has a delayed onset of action, and is also used initially with a benzodiazepine. The sedative action of sodium valproate produces a response in 1–4 days when used alone.

If manic symptoms are more severe, it is usually necessary to give an antipsychotic drug in combination with lithium, carbamazepine or sodium valproate. Conventional antipsychotic drugs are only recommended for short-term use, because of their extrapyramidal unwanted effects, but combination therapy, and perhaps use of a benzodiazepine, can reduce the dose of antipsychotic drug needed to control symptoms. The atypical antipsychotic drugs such as olanzapine have antimanic activity, with a lower risk of extrapyramidal unwanted effects.

If a person with bipolar disorder has had at least two episodes of either mania or depression in 5 years, then prophylactic therapy is recommended. Lithium is the conventional treatment of choice for prophylaxis, but carbamazepine is equally effective. There is less evidence to support the use of sodium valproate, which is usually reserved for those who do not tolerate first-line treatments, or for when these are ineffective. Other anticonvulsant drugs, including lamotrigine, gabapentin and topiramate, may be useful as alternatives to carbamazepine for prophylaxis, but the evidence is limited at present. The optimal duration of prophylactic therapy is unknown, but if a decision is made to discontinue treatment, then gradual withdrawal is recommended, to reduce the risk of rebound recurrence, especially of mania.

Treatment of depression in bipolar disorder usually requires a combination of lithium and an antidepressant. However, the response to antidepressant therapy is less than with unipolar depression, and there is a risk of provoking a manic 'switch'. There is limited evidence that mania is less likely to be provoked by an SSRI than by a tricyclic antidepressant (Ch. 22). As an alternative, lamotrigine has been reported to be effective as sole therapy for bipolar depression.

Electroconvulsive therapy is used for refractory episodes of both mania and depression, and has a much more rapid action than drug therapy. As for schizophrenia, psychological treatments are an important adjunct to drug therapy in bipolar disorder.

FURTHER READING

Altamura AC, Sassella F, Santini A et al (2003) Intramuscular preparations of antipsychotics. *Drugs* 63, 493–512

Belmaker RH (2004) Bipolar disorder. *N Engl J Med* 351, 476–486

Freedman R (2003) Schizophrenia. *N Engl J Med* 349, 1738–1749

Geddes J, Freemantle N, Harrison P, Bebbington P (2000) Atypical antipsychotics in the treatment of schizophrenia: systematic overview and meta-regression analysis. *BMJ* 321, 1371–1376

Harwood AJ, Agam G (2003) Search for a common mechanism of action of mood stabilizers. *Biochem Pharmacol* 66, 179–189

McGrath J, Emmerson WB (1999) Treatment of schizophrenia. *BMJ* 319, 1045–1048

Miyamoto S, Duncan GE, Marx CE et al (2005) Treatments for schizophrenia: a critical review of pharmacology and mechanisms of action of antipsychotic Drugs. *Molecular Psychiatry* 10, 79–104

Möller H-J (2003) Management of the negative symptoms of schizophrenia. *CNS Drugs* 17, 793–823

Mueser KT, McGurk SR (2004) Schizophrenia. *Lancet* 363, 2063–2072

Müller-Oerlinghausen B, Berghöfer A, Bauer M (2002) Bipolar disorder. *Lancet* 359, 241–247

National Institute for Clinical Excellence. Core interventions in the treatment and management of schizophrenia in primary and secondary care. **http://www.nice.org.uk** (accessed May 2004)

Seeman P (2002) Atypical antipsychotics: mechanism of action. *Can J Psychiatry* 47, 27–38

Xiaohua L, Ketter TA, Frye MA (2002) Synaptic, intracellular, and neuroprotective mechanisms of anticonvulsants: are they relevant for the treatment and course of bipolar disorders? *J Affective Dis* 69, 1–14

Self-assessment

In questions 1–3, the first statement, in italics, is true. Are the accompanying statements also true?

1. *Some antipsychotic drugs such as clozapine have relatively few effects on the extrapyramidal system and have low affinity for the dopamine receptors in the substantia nigra.*

    a. The phenothiazine fluphenazine has greater antimuscarinic activity than chlorpromazine.
    b. Clozapine causes agranulocytosis.
    c. Chlorpromazine given as decanoates in a depot preparation has to be injected weekly.

2. *The beneficial effects of antipsychotics take several weeks for full effect to be seen.*

    a. The 'positive' symptoms of schizophrenia (e.g. delusions) are more readily controlled than negative (withdrawal) symptoms.
    b. There is a close correlation between plasma levels of chlorpromazine and its antipsychotic effect.

3. *Antipsychotics are effective in treating only about 70% of schizophrenics.* Clozapine and thioridazine cause relatively few extrapyramidal symptoms.

4. From the following statements regarding properties of antipsychotics, choose the one <u>most appropriate</u> option.

    A. Clozapine is associated with a high incidence of extrapyramidal side-effects.
    B. Regular blood tests are required in people taking clozapine.
    C. Thioridazine causes little hypotension.
    D. Haloperidol causes nausea.
    E. Lithium is reabsorbed through the distal convoluted tubule in the kidney.

5. You wish to compare the beneficial- and unwanted-effect profile of a new antipsychotic. Which one of the following is likely to contribute to its antipsychotic rather than unwanted-effect potential?

    A. Its potential to block dopamine receptor blocking activity in the substantia nigra.
    B. Its potential to block muscarinic receptors.
    C. Its potential to block α_1-adrenoceptors.
    D. Its potential to block serotonin (5HT) receptors.
    E. Its potential to block histamine receptors.

6. Case history questions

    > A 25-year-old man (Mr PS) with schizophrenia had been treated with high-dose oral chlorpromazine for 2 years. His main symptoms of auditory hallucinations and delusional thoughts (*'The people in the flat above are broadcasting my thoughts on their radio'*) had improved, but he remained socially withdrawn and apathetic and described a number of new problems, including feeling very tired, faintness on standing up, dry mouth, sexual problems, blurred and darkened vision, occasional difficulty with fine control of movement (writing/typing) and weight gain.

    a. Which neural pathways are thought to be dysfunctional in schizophrenia and what is the evidence for this? How does chlorpromazine exert its antipsychotic action?
    b. Which adverse effect(s) reported by Mr PS are likely to be caused by chlorpromazine acting at dopamine receptors? Why are movement disorders caused by chlorpromazine less than those associated with some other antipsychotic drugs?
    c. Which unwanted effects reported by Mr PS are likely to be caused by blockade of histamine receptors, muscarinic receptors and α-adrenoceptors?
    d. Mr PS has had two severe relapses requiring hospitalisation within the last 18 months and is vague on whether he always takes his medication as directed. How might you improve adherence to treatment?
    e. Consider alternative antipsychotic drugs that might help Mr PS. What special care is required with the drug(s) you suggest?

    The answers are provided on pages 721–722.

Antipsychotic drugs

Drug compendium

Drug	Half-life (h)	Elimination	Comments
Amisulpride[a]	12	Renal	Oral dosage; D_2/D_3 antagonistic with presynaptic and limbic system selectivity; oral bioavailability is about 50%; eliminated largely by the kidneys
Benperidol	5–7	Metabolism	Oral dosage; incomplete oral bioavailability (about 40–50%); metabolites are inactive
Chlorpromazine	8–35	Metabolism	Oral, suppository and injection formulations available; incomplete oral bioavailability (10–33%); numerous pathways of metabolism, with some metabolites detectable months after cessation of treatment
Clozapine[a]	12 (6–33)	Metabolism	High affinity for D_1 and D_4 receptors; oral dosage with good bioavailability (30–50%); metabolised by hepatic oxidation (CYP1A2, CYP2D6 and CYP3A4); the desmethyl metabolite is pharmacologically active and its formation may be related to the negative effects on neutrophil counts
Flupentixol	35	Metabolism	Given orally (as hydrochloride) or by depot injection (as the decanoate ester prodrug); oral bioavailability is about 40%; the half-life for release from the depot injection is about 17 days; parent drug undergoes enterohepatic circulation following biliary excretion as a glucuronide
Fluphenazine	16	Metabolism	Given orally (as hydrochloride) or by depot injection (as the decanoate ester prodrug); oral bioavailability is about 50%; the half-life for release from the depot injection is about 26 days; metabolites of fluphenazine retain activity and may be responsible for about 50% of the total activity
Haloperidol	20 (9–67)	Metabolism	Given orally and by injection, or by depot injection (as the decanoate prodrug); oral bioavailability is about 60%; the half-life for release from the depot injection is about 21 days; reduced to an active metabolite in liver and extrahepatic tissues; undergoes enterohepatic circulation
Levomepromazine	15–70	Metabolism	Given orally or by injection (i.m. or i.v.); oral bioavailability is about 50%; numerous metabolites and wide interindividual variation in kinetics
Lithium	8–45	Renal	Complete oral absorption; filtered at the glomerular and reabsorbed (about 80%) in the proximal, but not distal, parts of the renal tubule
Olanzapine[a]	30 (21–54)	Metabolism	Given orally; antagonist at D_1, D_2, D_4 and $5HT_2$ receptors; oral bioavailability is 60%; metabolised by CYP1A2 and CYP2D6 to inactive products
Pericyazine	–	Metabolism (?)	Given orally, early drug, and few published data available
Perphenazine	9	Metabolism	Given orally; low and high variable oral bioavailability CYP2D6; metabolites eliminated over many weeks after cessation of treatment
Pimozide	55	Metabolism	Given orally; oral bioavailability is about 60–80%; metabolised to inactive products by CYP3A4
Pipotiazine palmitate	15–16 days	Metabolism	Depot injection formulation; long half-life results from slow release from depot injection; the active drug (pipotiazide) has an elimination half-life of a few hours only
Prochlorperazine	6–7	Metabolism	Given orally, rectally or by deep i.m. injection; variable absorption of oral doses; undergoes extensive hepatic metabolism
Promazine	–	Metabolism	Given orally or by i.m. injection; it is a low-potency metabolite of chlorpromazine; metabolised in the liver by N-demethylation and S-oxidation
Quetiapine[a]	6	Metabolism	Given orally; antagonist at $5HT_2$ and D_2 receptors; metabolised by hepatic CYP3A4

continued

Drug compendium

Antipsychotic drugs (continued)

Drug	Half-life (h)	Elimination	Comments
Risperidone[a]	2–4 (EM) 17–22 (PM)	Metabolism (+ renal in PM)	Given orally or by deep i.m. injection; oral bioavailability is about 70%; antagonist at $5HT_2$ and D_2 receptors; metabolised by hepatic CYP2D6 with extensive metabolisers (EM) eliminating the drug 5–10 times more rapidly than poor metabolisers (PM), who excrete about 30% unchanged in urine
Sertindole[a]	60–90	Metabolism	Given orally; selective antagonist at $5HT_2$ receptors; metabolised by CYP2D6 and CYP3A4; poor metabolisers of CYP2D6 substrates show lower clearance
Sulpiride	6–8	Urine	Given orally; incomplete oral bioavailability (about 30–40%) owing to poor absorption; water-soluble compound eliminated largely unchanged in urine and faeces; clearance approximates to glomerular filtration rate
Thioridazine	10	Metabolism	Given orally; oral bioavailability is about 60%; metabolised in liver to a number of S-oxidised products of which the simple sulphoxide (SO) and sulphone (SO_2) analogues retain activity
Trifluoperazine	14 (7–18)	Metabolism	Given orally; oral bioavailability has not been defined (because of the absence of i.v. reference data); numerous metabolites formed
Zotepine[a]	12–24	Metabolism	Given orally; low oral bioavailability (7–13%); antagonist at $5HT_2$ and D_2 receptors; numerous metabolites formed
Zuclopenthixol	20 (13–23)	Metabolism	Given orally (as the dihydrochloride) or as deep i.m. depot injection (as the acetate or decanoate ester); oral bioavailability (of zuclopenthixol dihydrochloride) is about 60%; the half-lives of the depot forms (acetate and decanoate) are about 19 days; zuclopenthixol is converted into numerous inactive metabolites

i.m., intramuscular; i.v., intravenous.
[a]Atypical antipsychotic.

Depression

Clinical depression is characterised by diverse psychological symptoms such as low mood, loss of interest and enjoyment of activities, and reduced energy. It is often accompanied by a sense of guilt and worthlessness, as well as physical symptoms including sleep disturbance, reduced appetite and loss of libido. If severe, there may be marked suicidal tendencies and psychotic symptoms (hallucinations and delusions). Depression can present with physical rather than psychological symptoms. The existence of mixed anxiety–depression disorder is now also well accepted.

Biological basis of depression

The cause of depression is unknown, but the most widely accepted hypothesis proposes that there is a fundamental abnormality in central nervous system (CNS) monoaminergic neurotransmission. Simplistically, it has been hypothesised that the following occur (Fig. 22.1):

- low levels of monoamine transmitters
- upregulation of postsynaptic monoamine receptors
- upregulation of the presynaptic and somatodendritic autoreceptors that control monoamine release.

Some evidence indicates that disordered serotonin (5-hydroxytryptamine, 5HT) and noradrenaline neurotransmission is involved in the genesis of depression, the apocryphal 'amine hypothesis'. Most of the current clinically used antidepressants target the mechanisms involved in the control of neurotransmitter monoamine turnover or monoamine receptor function. Although there are differences in unwanted effects, there seems to be little difference in efficacy between drugs that act predominantly on serotonergic or on noradrenergic mechanisms. A schematic of these mechanisms and the ways that major antidepressants work to modify monoamine turnover and function is shown in Figure 22.1.

Serotonergic and noradrenergic mechanisms

Most serotonergic neurons are found in the raphe area of the midbrain, from where they project to the hippocampus in the limbic system and the cerebral cortex. $5HT_{1B/1D}$ autoreceptors are present presynaptically on neuronal terminals, where they tonically inhibit 5HT release. Somatodendritic $5HT_{1A}$ α_1- and β-adrenergic autoreceptors on the neuronal cell bodies of the raphe nuclei also regulate firing in serotonergic neurons. Postsynaptic $5HT_{2A}$ and $5HT_{2C}$ receptors are found widely in the cerebral cortex, especially the prefrontal cortex (Fig. 22.1).

Most noradrenergic neurons, on the other hand, arise in the locus ceruleus and the lateral tegmental areas of the brainstem. The locus ceruleus and the raphe region in particular have reciprocal neural projections. Adrenergic neurotransmission stimulates serotonergic neurons by activating somatodendritic α_1-adrenoceptors. However, noradrenaline also inhibits 5HT synthesis and release through presynaptic α_2-adrenoceptors.

Overall support for the monoamine theory as a molecular basis for depression in man is patchy; it is suggested that there are increased $5HT_2$ receptor numbers in the frontal cortex of depressed suicide victims, while other studies have indicated that 5HT concentrations in the brain may be reduced in depression. Altered neurotransmission in pathways dependent on glutamate, gamma-aminobutyric acid (GABA) or substance P may also modulate monoaminergic neurotransmission in depressive illness.

Extending the monoamine theory of depression

Although the mechanisms of many current pharmacological treatments for depression would support the monoamine theory, it has long been recognised that this explanation of depression is far from complete. In particular, the clinical benefit of antidepressant therapy is delayed, despite rapid increases in CNS monoamine concentrations or rapid blockade of monoamine receptors, and only a limited number of patients benefit from antidepressant treatment. There is upregulation of β-adrenoceptors in depression, but β-adrenoceptor antagonists do not have antidepressant activity. It is therefore likely that the benefit of rapidly altering the monoamine turnover or receptor function proceeds to much more gradual adaptive changes which may only in part depend upon elevating monoamine activity. These pharmacologically induced adaptive changes are relatively poorly understood but may lead to a normalisation of the fundamental dysfunctions in intra-

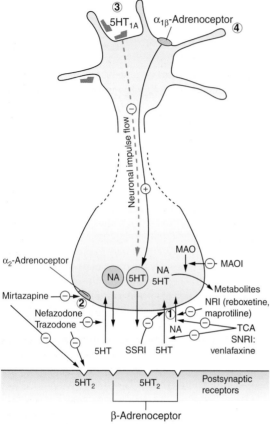

Fig. 22.1
The effect of drugs used in the treatment of depression on CNS serotonergic and adrenergic functioning. Some of the bewildering array of adrenergic and 5-hydroxytryptamine (5HT, serotonin) receptor subtypes are omitted for clarity. In depression it is hypothesised that there is a reduction in monoamine neurotransmission, resulting in upregulation of some postsynaptic *and* somatodendritic receptors; these changes are associated with a myriad of complex cellular and signal transduction dysfunctions that underlie depression. Using 5HT as an example, it is considered that the lack of 5HT results in an upregulation of postsynaptic $5HT_2$ receptors and presynaptic (somatodendritic) $5HT_{1A}$ receptors, and an uncoupling of these receptors from their G-proteins. The primary actions of many drugs in current clinical use is to enhance serotonin and noradrenaline availability, therefore inducing a downregulation of elevated receptors, or to functionally reduce receptor numbers by using selective antagonists. The majority of released 5HT and noradrenaline is rapidly removed from the synapse by reuptake into the neuron (**site 1**). Stimulation of presynaptic α_2-adrenoceptors (**site 2**) or similarly sited $5HT_{1B/D}$ receptors (not shown) acts to reduce monoamine release. Stimulation of the somatodendritic $5HT_{1A}$ autoreceptors (**site 3**) inhibits the neuronal impulse flow in the axon and reduces 5HT release, whereas stimulation of α_{1B}-adrenoceptors (**site 4**) enhances 5HT release. There is now a range of antidepressants having a variety of different actions on serotoninergic and noradrenergic neurotransmission, via actions on single or multiple receptor subtypes (see Fig 22.1 and text below). Similar actions may occur at somatodendritic receptor sites. It is not clear whether the different types of antidepressants have advantages in terms of their antidepressant activity, but they differ markedly in their side-effect profiles. TCA, 'classic' tricyclic antidepressants; SSRI, selective serotonin reuptake inhibitors; SNRI, serotonin *and* noradrenaline reuptake inhibitors; NRI, (selective) noradrenaline reuptake inhibitor; MAO, monoamine oxidase; NA, noradrenaline. Other drugs act by significantly blocking pre- and postsynaptic receptors.

cellular signalling pathways and transduction mechanisms that have been described in depression. The myriad of molecular events that follows from antidepressant treatment is now being investigated to try and complement and complete the jigsaw of the monoamine theory.

In depression, there may be uncoupling of receptor actions from G-proteins. There is reduced generation of intracellular cyclic adenosine monophosphate (cAMP). As a result, synthesis of the cAMP-responsive element-binding protein (CREB) is reduced, and this impairs gene regulation for the production of brain-derived neurotrophic factor (BDNF), which promotes neuroprotection and neuronal survival, both of which may be compromised in depression. There is also hypersecretion of the 'stressor' hormone corticotrophin-releasing factor (CRF) (Ch. 43), which has detrimental effects on neural synaptic plasticity, neurogenesis and neurotoxicity, and depresses serotonergic neurotransmission. CRF orchestrates the CNS control of behavioural, endocrine, autonomic and immunological responses. In individuals genetically predisposed to depression, stress can initiate remodelling and elimination of hippocampal circuits involved in regulation of mood, cognition and behaviour. Many of these circuits involve glutamatergic neurotransmission via the excitatory NMDA (*N*-methyl-D-aspartate) receptor. Cortisol also reduces the expression of BDNF in the hippocampus. Cortisol also produces hyperactivity in dopaminergic neurons, and excessive production may contribute to the genesis of psychotic depression.

Finally, a cautionary note: a unifying hypothesis for the genesis of depression still escapes us, and the illuminating 'new' theories of the molecular basis for depression have resulted mainly from animal work and have yet to result in novel treatments.

Antidepressant drug action

Increasingly, it is recognised that long-term treatment with antidepressants has important effects through promoting both the structural and functional integrity of the neural circuits that regulate mood. The mechanisms of action are complex.

- **Enhanced CNS monoamine levels.** The initial action of drugs used in the treatment of depression is to increase CNS monoaminergic neurotransmission, and particularly serotonergic neurotransmission. However, although they rapidly enhance synaptic monoamine levels, clinical improvement is delayed. In part, this delay may be due to slow adaptational changes in the inhibitory somatodendritic $5HT_{1A}$ and terminal $5HT_{1B/1D}$ autoreceptors. Desensitisation and downregulation of these receptors gradually regulates activity in serotonergic pathways. Increased noradrenergic activity enhances serotonergic neurotransmission by stimulating somatodendritic α_1-adrenoceptors on serotonergic neurons.

- **Effects on intracellular signal transduction**. With all antidepressants, a long-term (but not acute) effect is increased responsiveness to 5HT in the prefrontal cortex. There is considerable evidence that antidepressants reverse the changes in intracellular signalling that are found in depression. Antidepressants downregulate $5HT_2$ receptors, but enhance G_s coupling to adenylate cyclase. The ultimate intracellular response is increased expression of BDNF and its receptor, leading to differentiation of progenitor cells into neurons and increased neuronal survival.
- **Regulation of CRF production**. During long-term antidepressant use, there is normalisation of CRF secretion. This may be related to upregulation of CNS glucocorticoid receptors, with feedback inhibition of CRF.
- **Antagonism of NMDA receptor action**. Antidepressant drugs bind to a site in NMDA receptor-associated ion channels in the hippocampus and cerebral cortex. Receptor-related function in the hippocampus is not impaired, but antidepressants may protect against stress-induced 'glutamate excitotoxicity'.

Antidepressant drugs

Tricyclic antidepressant drugs and related compounds

> Examples:
> tricyclic compounds: amitriptyline, imipramine, lofepramine
> non-tricyclic compounds: maprotiline, amoxapine

Mechanism of action

The first-generation compounds in this class have a triple carbon ring structure (tricyclic antidepressants; TCAs). Many of the newer drugs are structurally unrelated to tricyclic compounds despite having a similar mechanism of action. These include bicyclic, tetracyclic and non-cyclic structures.

TCAs and related drugs inhibit the reuptake of monoamine neurotransmitters into the presynaptic neuron by competitive inhibition of the ATPase in the membrane monoamine pump (Fig. 22.1). Some drugs show little monoamine selectivity, while other compounds are more selective for one monoamine (Table 22.1). However, monoamine selectivity has not been shown to influence efficacy.

A major contribution to the unwanted effects of these drugs is their ability to block other postsynaptic receptors (e.g. muscarinic and histamine H_1 receptors and α_1-adrenoceptors) to varying degrees (Table 22.1). This probably does not influence their antidepressant action, but contributes to the profile of unwanted effects.

Pharmacokinetics

All TCAs and related drugs are well absorbed from the gut and highly protein bound in plasma. Those with a tertiary amine structure, such as imipramine and amitriptyline, undergo extensive first-pass metabolism by demethylation in the liver. Active metabolites (for example, desipramine from imipramine and lofepramine, and nortriptyline from amitriptyline) are formed and are partially responsible for the long duration of action of these drugs.

There is no clear dose relationship for therapeutic effects, although unwanted effects are dose related. This may reflect the considerable interindividual variability in the first-pass metabolism of most TCAs (leading to up to 40-fold differences in the plasma concentrations of the parent drug), and the difficulty in quantifying the contribution of both parent drug and active metabolites to the clinical response. Dose titration is usually necessary to optimise the therapeutic response; this should be gradual over 1–2 weeks to minimise unwanted effects.

Unwanted effects

The incidence and nature of unwanted effects vary widely among the different drugs. In general, tertiary amine TCAs have greater α_1-adrenoceptor, histamine H_1 and muscarinic receptor blocking activity. TCAs tend to be cardiotoxic, especially in overdose, although lofepramine is less cardiotoxic than other TCAs. These differences are outlined in Table 22.1, which compares the profiles for selected compounds.

- Sedation. This is a result of histamine H_1 and α-adrenoceptor blockade (Ch. 39). Some compounds are highly sedative, for example amitriptyline, and others less so, for example amoxapine. Sedation can be useful to help restore sleep patterns in depression (using a larger dose of a sedative drug at night) but can be troublesome or dangerous during the day.
- Antimuscarinic effects (see Ch. 4). These are common with tricyclic drugs and include, in particular, dry mouth, and, less commonly, constipation, urinary retention, impotence and visual disturbance. Tolerance can occur and gradual increases in dose may reduce these problems.
- Excessive sweating and tremor. The mechanisms behind these effects are uncertain.

Table 22.1
Comparative properties of some commonly used antidepressant drugs[a]

	Uptake inhibition	Muscarinic receptor block	Alpha₁-adrenoceptor block	Histamine H₁ receptor block	P-450 related metabolism[b]	Sedative
TCA						
Amitriptyline	5HT=NA	+++	+++	+++++	Inhibition	+++
Imipramine	5HT=NA	++	++	+++	Inhibition	++
Amoxapine	5HT=NA	+	+++	+++	+	+
Clomipramine	5HT>NA	+++	+++	+++	Inhibition	++
Doxepine	5HT>NA	++	+++	+++++	?	++
Dosulepin	5HT=NA	++	+	++	–	++
Lofepramine	NA>>5HT	+	+	+	?	+/–
SSRI						
Citalopram	5HT>>NA	0	+	+	Weak inhibition	0
Fluoxetine	5HT>>NA	0	0	0	Inhibition	0
Fluvoxamine	5HT>>NA	0	0	0	Inhibition	0
Paroxetine	5HT>NA	++	+	+	Inhibition	0
Sertraline	5HT>>NA	0	++	0	Weak inhibition	0
Other drugs						
Mirtazapine*	–	+	+	+++++	Weak inhibition	+
Nefazodone	5HT>>NA	0	+++	+++	Inhibition	0
Reboxetine	NA>>5HT	Low	Low	Low	–	0
Venlafaxine	Weak NA=5HT	0	0	0	Weak inhibition	0
Maprotiline	NA>>5HT	+	0	++	+	+
Mianserin*	–	+	Low	+++++	+	+
Trazodone*	Weak 5HT	Low	+	+	+	+

[a]The table is constructed for approximate comparison only and is derived from a number of sources where data are available but mainly from Anderson et al (2000) and Richelson (2002). The drugs are listed under their major actions or conventional groupings but many of them have mixed actions or their mechanism is uncertain.
[b]Many antidepressants utilise particular isoforms of P450 enzymes for metabolism and thus can result in drug interactions. Many are inhibitors of discrete CYP isoforms and this is particularly true for some SSRIs. Other antidepressants can be weaker inhibitors of some CYP isoforms. Several are substrates for the CYP2D6 isoform and are subject to polymorphic metabolism.
TCA, tricyclic antidepressants; SSRI, selective serotonin reuptake inhibitors; SNRI, serotonin and noradrenaline reuptake inhibitors; 5HT, 5-hydroxytryptamine; NA, noradrenaline.
*Variable 5HT and NA receptor blockade.

- Postural hypotension produced by peripheral α_1-adrenoceptor blockade (Ch. 4), which can be particularly troublesome in the elderly, although tolerance can occur.
- Epileptogenic effects. Fits can be provoked, even when there is no previous clinical history.
- Cardiotoxicity in overdosage. Most tricyclic drugs depress myocardial contractility or produce tachycardia and severe arrhythmias when taken in overdose. Antimuscarinic effects and excessive noradrenergic stimulation both contribute to the genesis of arrhythmias. Lofepramine appears to be the safest drug in this group in overdose.
- Weight gain. Appetite stimulation is common with tricyclic drugs, probably due to histamine H₁ receptor blockade.

- Hyponatraemia from inappropriate antidiuretic hormone (ADH) secretion, leading to drowsiness, confusion and convulsions.
- Sudden withdrawal syndrome. During long-term treatment, doses should be gradually reduced over four weeks to avoid agitation, headache, malaise, sweating and gastrointestinal upset, which can accompany sudden withdrawal. This may be a result of excessive cholinergic activity following prolonged muscarinic receptor blockade.

Drug interactions

Several important drug interactions are recognised. TCAs potentiate the central depressant activity of many drugs, including alcohol. A dangerous interaction can result from giving a monoamine oxidase (MAO) inhibitor (MAOI) (see below) and a TCA together. Potentiation arises from the prolonged action of excess 5HT released from the neuron and can lead to hyperpyrexia, convulsions and coma. The long duration of MAO inhibition means that the interaction can occur up to 2 weeks after stopping an MAOI.

The risk of serious arrhythmias is increased when TCAs are taken with drugs that prolong the Q–T interval on the electrocardiogram (Ch. 8). Such drugs include the class III antiarrhythmic sotalol, and all class I antiarrhythmics.

Selective serotonin reuptake inhibitors and related antidepressants

Examples: fluoxetine, paroxetine, sertraline, citalopram

Mechanism of action

Unlike the TCAs, the selective serotonin reuptake inhibitors (SSRIs) reduce the neuronal reuptake of serotonin but have no or much reduced effect on noradrenaline reuptake (Table 22.1). They have a generally more favourable profile of unwanted effects because of low affinity for muscarinic, histaminergic and adrenergic receptors. Paroxetine is unusual in having affinity for muscarinic M_3 receptors, found in the brain, salivary glands and smooth muscle. The hypothetical mechanism of action of SSRIs is as follows.

- An initial increase in 5HT concentration in the somatodendritic and axon terminal presynaptic areas produces downregulation of $5HT_{1A}$ and $5HT_{1B/1D}$ inhibitory autoreceptors.
- As a consequence of reduced inhibitory autoreceptor activity, there is increased 5HT release at the axon terminal. The prolonged increase in synaptic 5HT concentration results in downregulation of postsynaptic $5HT_2$ receptors and subsequent alterations in cellular function as described for TCAs.

Pharmacokinetics

SSRIs are well absorbed from the gut and metabolised in the liver. Paroxetine has a long half-life. Citalopram, fluoxetine and sertraline all have half-lives in excess of 24 h. Norfluoxetine, the active metabolite of fluoxetine, has a half-life of seven days, and the resulting very long duration of action can be a disadvantage if an MAOI (see below) is used subsequently.

Unwanted effects

In contrast to the TCAs, SSRIs (apart from paroxetine) have few antimuscarinic effects, cause little sedation or weight gain, and are not cardiotoxic in overdose. However, they may cause:

- nausea (can be frequent), abdominal pain or diarrhoea (less frequent)
- insomnia, anxiety and agitation
- anorexia with weight loss
- decreased libido
- dry mouth and constipation with paroxetine
- sudden withdrawal syndrome after long-term use, which may be most troublesome with paroxetine; it presents in a similar manner to the syndrome after withdrawal of TCAs.

Drug interactions

The most serious interaction is with MAOIs (see TCAs above). An interval of 5 weeks is recommended after stopping fluoxetine, or 2 weeks after paroxetine or sertraline, before an MAOI (including selegeline, Ch. 24) is prescribed. Fluoxetine inhibits hepatic CYP2D6, and this can give elevated plasma concentrations of co-prescribed CYP2D6 substrate.

Serotonin and noradrenaline reuptake inhibitors

Example: venlafaxine

Mechanism of action

Venlafaxine is classed as a serotonin and noradrenaline reuptake inhibitor (SNRI) although it has a greater effect on serotonin reuptake at lower doses (Table 22.1). It has properties that place it between the tricyclic and SSRI antidepressants. Like the TCAs, it inhibits neuronal reuptake of both serotonin and noradrenaline, but it shares with SSRIs a low affinity for muscarinic, histaminergic and adrenergic receptors. Its unwanted effect profile is therefore closer to that of the SSRIs than the TCAs.

There is limited evidence that clinical improvement with venlafaxine may begin earlier than with other antidepressant drugs.

Pharmacokinetics

Venlafaxine is rapidly absorbed from the gut and undergoes extensive first-pass metabolism in the liver. The active metabolites have long half-lives.

Unwanted effects

- somnolence
- dry mouth, nausea, constipation
- dizziness, confusion.

Selective noradrenaline reuptake inhibitors

Example: reboxetine

Mechanism of action

Reboxetine is related to fluoxetine but selectively inhibits noradrenaline reuptake. Increased noradrenergic activity at somatodendritic α_2-adrenoceptors enhances serotonergic neurotransmission. Reboxetine, in common with the SSRIs, has little or no activity at histamine H_1, muscarinic and adrenergic receptors. It has fewer cardiovascular unwanted effects than TCAs.

Pharmacokinetics

Reboxetine is rapidly absorbed orally. It is eliminated by hepatic metabolism and has a long half-life.

Unwanted effects

- insomnia
- sweating
- postural hypotension
- dizziness, paraesthesia.

Presynaptic α_2-adrenoceptor blockers

Example: mirtazapine

Mechanism of action

Mirtazapine is a tetracyclic drug unrelated structurally to the TCAs. In addition to potent $5HT_{2A}$ receptor-blocking activity in the cortex, mirtazapine blocks presynaptic α_2-adrenoceptors (Fig. 22.1) and reduces negative feedback control on 5HT release from raphe nucleus neurons in their terminal projections to regions such as the cortex and hippocampus. Mirtazapine blocks histamine H_1 receptors but has a low affinity for muscarinic receptors and postsynaptic α_1-adrenoceptors. It has minimal effects on monoamine reuptake.

Pharmacokinetics

Mirtazapine is well absorbed from the gut. It is metabolised in the liver and has a very long half-life.

Unwanted effects

- drowsiness and sedation, especially at lower doses, due to histamine H_1 receptor blockade; at higher doses, increased noradrenergic neurotransmission offsets some of the sedative effects
- increased appetite and weight gain.

Serotonin receptor blockers

Example: trazodone

Mechanism of action

Trazodone is structurally unrelated to TCAs. A significant action is blockade of postsynaptic $5HT_{2C}$ receptors in addition to weak inhibition of presynaptic 5HT reuptake, which may also contribute to its antidepressant activity; it does not inhibit noradrenaline reuptake. Trazodone also blocks α_1-adrenoceptors and weakly blocks muscarinic and histamine H_1 receptors.

Pharmacokinetics

Trazodone is well absorbed orally, and metabolised in the liver. The half-life is intermediate.

Unwanted effects

- sedation
- hypotension and reflex tachycardia as a result of α_1-adrenoceptor blockade
- nausea.

Classic (non-selective) monoamine oxidase inhibitors

Examples: phenelzine, tranylcypromine

Mechanism of action

The mechanism of action of classic (non-selective) MAOIs is complex, but their primary action is to inhibit intracellular MAO, which is the enzyme responsible for degrading free monoamines. The accumulation of monoamine neurotransmitters in the presynaptic neuron leads to increased release when the nerve is stimulated (Fig. 22.1). Two MAO isoenzymes have been identified (Fig. 22.2). MAO-B is the predominant enzyme in many parts of the brain, but MAO-A is present in noradrenergic and serotonergic neurons, especially in the locus ceruleus and other cells of the brainstem, as well as being the main enzyme in peripheral tissues. Inhibition of MAO-A in the brain produces the therapeutic effects of these drugs, but classic inhibitors (MAOIs) are not selective for this isoenzyme. MAO-A inhibition in the gut wall

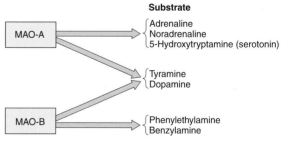

Fig. 22.2
Actions of monoamine oxidase. The relative selectivity of the substrates for MAO is shown. MAO-A is the target for drugs useful in treating depression. Non-selective inhibition of both MAO-A and MAO-B blocks the metabolism of tyramine, which is responsible for the food reaction that occurs with these drugs. Reversible inhibition of MAOA (RIMA) blocks only type MAO-A. Therefore tyramine is still metabolised by type B and the food reaction is reduced.

and liver also has important consequences (see below). MAOIs also inhibit various drug-metabolising enzymes in the liver; this predisposes to drug interactions but does not contribute to clinical efficacy.

Pharmacokinetics

All drugs in this class are well absorbed from the gut. Structurally, they are either derivatives of hydrazine (e.g. phenelzine) or similar to amfetamine (e.g. tranylcypromine). They are irreversible enzyme inhibitors and therefore their prolonged duration of action is unrelated to the half-life of the drug. Drug withdrawal is followed by gradual restoration of normal MAO activity over about 2 weeks as new enzyme is synthesised.

Unwanted effects

- Compared with the TCAs, antimuscarinic effects are unusual and there is no predisposition to fits.
- Dose-related postural hypotension can occur. Unlike with the tricyclic compounds, tolerance does not arise. The mechanism may involve conversion of tyramine (normally degraded by MAO) to octopamine, a false neurotransmitter which competes with noradrenaline at sympathetic nerve terminals.
- CNS stimulation with tranylcypromine leads to irritability and insomnia. These are amfetamine-like actions (Ch. 54) and doses should be given early in the day to avoid disturbing sleep.
- Hepatitis is a rare idiosyncratic reaction to the hydrazine derivative phenelzine.
- Acute overdose produces delayed toxic effects after some 12 h. Excessive adrenergic stimulation leads to chest pain, headache and hyperactivity, progressing to confusion and severe hypertension, with eventually profound hypotension and fits.
- Food interactions can occur because MAO in the gut wall and liver usually prevents the absorption of natural amines, particularly tyramine, which is an indirect-acting sympathomimetic (Ch. 4). If food containing tyramine, for example cheese, yeast extracts (such as Bovril®, Oxo® or Marmite®), pickled herrings, chianti or caviar, or broad bean pods (which contain L-dopa), is eaten, the increased release of noradrenaline produces vasoconstriction and severe hypertension. The first indication of this is a throbbing headache. A warning card should be supplied to people who are prescribed MAOIs.

Drug interactions

A number of drug interactions can occur. Indirect-acting sympathomimetics (Ch. 4) in cold remedies (e.g. ephedrine, phenylpropanolamine), and levodopa (given for treatment of Parkinson's disease, Ch. 24) will be more active, with a risk of hypotensive crisis. The toxicity of the triptans (5HT$_1$ receptor agonists used for treatment of migraine, Ch. 26) and sibutramine (given for treatment of obesity, Ch. 37) will be potentiated. All these drugs

should be avoided for 2 weeks after stopping an MAOI. The combination of MAOIs with TCAs or SSRIs (see above) can be dangerous. Other important interactions occur because MAOIs can impair the hepatic metabolism of certain drugs, especially opioid analgesics.

Reversible inhibitors of monoamine oxidase A

Example: moclobemide

Mechanism of action and effects

Moclobemide is a selective reversible inhibitor of MAO-A (RIMA). This isoenzyme is the target for the antidepressant action of classic MAOIs. If tyramine is absorbed from the gut, MAO-B is able to degrade it, and the food reaction described above for classic MAOIs is very unlikely to occur. Also, since the action of moclobemide on MAO-A is reversible, high concentrations of tyramine will displace the drug from the enzyme, further facilitating degradation of tyramine. If moclobemide is taken after meals, then inhibition of MAO-A in the gut during absorption of tyramine will be minimised, providing further protection. Enzyme inhibition by moclobemide lasts less than 24 h after a single dose.

Pharmacokinetics

Oral absorption is good but there is substantial first-pass metabolism, partially to an active metabolite. Extensive hepatic metabolism gives moclobemide a short half-life.

Unwanted effects

- CNS stimulation can produce sleep disturbance or agitation
- nausea
- dizziness, headache.

Drug interactions

Inhibition of cytochrome P450 activity in the liver by cimetidine (Ch. 33) substantially reduces the metabolism of moclobemide, and smaller starting doses are recommended in this situation. Moclobemide should not be given with other antidepressants, and the recommendations for stopping these drugs before prescribing moclobemide are the same as for classic MAOIs.

Management of depression

Drugs form only part of the management of depression but are usually necessary for moderate, severe or protracted symptoms. However, in mild to moderate depression, cognitive therapy is as effective as drug treatment. The herbal remedy *Hypericum perforatum* (St John's Wort) is an effective alternative to drug treatment for mild depression, and does not often cause unwanted effects. The concentrations of the active constituents vary between different preparations, and St John's Wort can induce drug-metabolising enzymes. St John's Wort should not be taken with a prescribed antidepressant. All antidepressant drugs have a delayed onset of action, and persons who are severely ill should be considered for electroconvulsive therapy (ECT), which gives a more rapid response.

The TCAs or related compounds are still considered by some psychiatrists to be the drugs of choice for initial management in carefully defined subsets of depressed people, although other drugs such as the SSRIs are in general being prescribed more frequently. TCAs have serious cardiotoxic effects when taken in overdose and should usually be avoided when treating those who are at high risk of attempting suicide. The newer drugs, for example SSRIs and some drugs related to the TCAs, are no more effective than TCAs (and some analyses suggest that they are rather less effective) and do not work any faster, but they are slightly better tolerated. They are certainly safer than TCAs when there is a high risk of suicide.

Encouraging adherence to treatment with TCAs may initially be difficult, since antimuscarinic unwanted effects can be troublesome before any benefit is perceived. Starting with a small dose with gradual dose titration is desirable. There is now evidence that large doses of a TCA do not necessarily enhance the treatment response but do increase unwanted effects. The use of low dosages may therefore be preferred.

Up to 70% of depressed individuals will respond to drug therapy if the dosage is adequate, compared with about 30% taking placebo. However, only 50% will respond to an individual drug, and up to a further 20% of depressives will respond if the drug is changed after failure of the initial treatment. Responders show an initial improvement in sleep pattern within a few days. Psychomotor retardation responds more gradually over several days, leading to greater involvement with everyday activities and to enjoyment of life. Improvement in the depressed mood is delayed, beginning up to two or more weeks after treatment with adequate dosages. The response of most symptoms tends to be erratic, with good and bad days.

Initial treatment with an antidepressant should be for 6 weeks. If there is no response after this time, and if it is believed that there is not a problem with adherence to treatment, then either the dose should be increased further if unwanted effects permit, or an alternative drug can be substituted. If there is a good response then, the dosage can usually be reduced, but maintenance treatment should be continued for at least 4–6 months after the first episode of depression, to minimise the risk of relapse. A longer period of maintenance treatment to prevent recurrence (at least 1 year) is often recommended for the elderly, for others who are at high risk of recurrence, and for those who have experienced two or more depressive episodes. About half of all those who experience depression only have a single episode. In recurrent illness, relapse occurs in up to 65% of those who stop treatment within a year, but only in 15% of people who continue treatment.

Classic MAOIs are usually reserved for atypical depression with hypochondriacal and phobic symptoms, or when TCAs have failed. The therapeutic place of the newer antidepressants such as SNRIs and RIMAs has yet to be fully established. Small doses of a phenothiazine such as flupentixol (Ch. 21) are sometimes recommended for the depressed elderly person; evidence for a true antidepressant effect is slight, but some symptoms undoubtedly do improve.

Treatment is most difficult in severe depression, especially if there are psychotic features, or where depression forms part of a bipolar affective disorder (Ch. 21). ECT is used for treatment-resistant depression, and in the elderly who are particularly likely to show a response. Overall, ECT is probably more effective than drug therapy but does produce some lasting cognitive impairment, especially if given bilaterally rather than unilaterally, given frequently or with high currents. ECT should be combined with prolonged antidepressant drug treatment. Lithium (Ch. 21) is used for those with severe recurrent depressive episodes and for prophylaxis of bipolar affective disorder. The effect of lithium can take several months to become fully established. The treatment of depression in bipolar disorder is discussed in Chapter 21.

FURTHER READING

Anderson IM, Nutt DJ, Deakin JFW (2000) Evidence-based guidelines for treating depressive disorders with antidepressants: a revision of the 1993 British Association for Psychopharmacology guidelines. *J Psychopharmacol* 14, 3–20

Cryan JF, Leonard BE (2000) 5HT$_{1A}$ and beyond: the role of serotonin and its receptors in depression and the antidepressant response. *Hum Psychopharmacol Clin Exp* 15, 113–135

Donati RJ, Rasenick MM (2003) G-protein signaling and the molecular basis of antidepressant action. *Life Sci* 73, 1–17

Duman RS (2004) Role of neurotrophic factors in the etiology and treatment of mood disorders. *Neuromolecular Med* 5, 11–25

Edwards JG, Anderson I (1999) Systematic review and guide to selection of selective serotonin reuptake inhibitors. *Drugs* 57, 507–533

Furukawa TA, McGuire H, Barbui C (2002) Meta-analysis of effects and side effects of low dosage tricyclic antidepressants in depression: systematic review. *BMJ* 325, 991–995

Geddes JR, Carney SM, Davies C et al (2003) Relapse prevention with antidepressant drug treatment in depressive disorders: a systematic review. *Lancet* 361, 653–661

Kent JM (2000) SNaRIs, NaSSAs, and NaRIs: new agents for the treatment of depression. *Lancet* 355, 911–918

Leonard BE (2001) The immune system, depression and the action of antidepressants. *Prog Neuropsychopharmacol Biol Psychiatry* 25, 767–780

Leonard BE, Richelson E (2000) Synaptic effects of antidepressants: relationship to their therapeutic and adverse effects. In: Buckley P, Waddington J (eds) Schizophrenia and Mood Disorders. The New Drug Therapies in Clinical Practice. Oxford: Butterworth Heinemann; pp 67–84

Manji HK, Drevets WC, Charney DS (2001) The cellular neurobiology of depression. *Nat Med* 7, 541–547

Pacher P, Kecskemeti V (2004) Trends in the development of new antidepressants. Is there a light at the end of the tunnel? *Curr Med Chem* 11, 925–943

Richelson E (2002) The clinical relevance of antidepressant interaction with neurotransmitter transporters and receptors. *Psychopharmacol Bull* 36, 133–150

Skolnick P (2002) Beyond monoamine-based therapies: clues to new approaches. *J Clin Psychiatry*. 63 Suppl 2, 19–23

Spollen JJ, Gutman DG (2003) Recent findings in depression. http://www.medscape.com/viewprogram/2104

Stone EA, Lin Y, Rosengarten H, Kramer HK, Quartermain D (2003) Emerging evidence for central epinephrine-innervated alpha adrenergic system that regulates behavioral activation and is impaired in depression. *Neuropsychopharmacology* 28, 1387–1399

Whooley MA, Simon GE (2000) Primary care: managing depression in medical outpatients. *N Engl J Med* 343, 1942–1950

Young LT, Bakish D, Beaulieu S (2002) The neurobiology of treatment response to antidepressants and mood stabilizing medications. *J Psychiatry Neurosci* 27, 260–265

Self-assessment

In questions 1–4, the first statement, in italics, is true. Are the accompanying statements also true?

1. *Despite the fact that the monoamine hypothesis does not adequately explain all the processes of depression, alteration of monoamine transmission remains the mainstay of successful drug treatment.*

   a. Downregulation of $5HT_2$ receptors occurs during antidepressant treatment.
   b. Most TCAs inhibit the reuptake of noradrenaline and 5HT equally.
   c. TCAs have a less satisfactory therapeutic ratio than SSRIs.

2. *Although there are variations in responses of individuals, inhibitors of noradrenaline or 5HT reuptake are equally effective as antidepressants.*

   a. Lofepramine is more cardiotoxic than amitriptyline.
   b. Co-administration of an SSRI and an MAOI can cause cardiovascular collapse.

3. *Atypical antidepressants include compounds such as trazodone, which have a different mechanism of action to the TCAs.*

   a. Trazodone is an antidepressant that is only a weak inhibitor of monoamine reuptake.
   b. Venlafaxine has marked sedative and antimuscarinic actions.

   c. Venlafaxine requires longer than most antidepressants to produce clinical improvement.

4. *During antidepressant treatment, only 30–40% of people with depression improve as a result of the drug.*

   a. TCAs potentiate the central depressant effects of alcohol.
   b. The half-life of lithium is about 30 min.
   c. Lithium is only used for treatment of bipolar affective disorder.

5. Which one of the following statements concerning antidepressant drugs is the <u>most appropriate</u>?

   A. A TCA would be more suitable than an SSRI for a patient with urinary outflow problems due to benign prostate hypertrophy.
   B. A drug that blocks muscarinic receptors would be a more effective antidepressant than one that blocks serotonin receptors.
   C. A person on moclobemide is likely to get an adverse reaction if he or she ingests cheese.
   D. An SSRI would be more suitable than a TCA to treat a person with serious depression and suicidal tendencies.
   E. Increase in brain monoamine levels occurs only after 4–5 weeks treatment with a TCA.

6. Which is the one <u>most appropriate</u> statement concerning the antidepressant venlafaxine?

   A. It is a $5HT_2$ receptor antagonist.
   B. It inhibits the neuronal reuptake of noradrenaline and 5HT.

C. It has potent antimuscarinic activity.

D. It does not exhibit drug interactions with MAOIs.

E. It is slower in onset of action than TCAs.

7. Case history questions

DW, a 30-year-old female financier, was a former Olympic athlete. In 1994 she was appointed manager of the Emerging Countries Fund of a large Unit Trust Company. In early 1996 the company was taken over and DW had a new boss and was moved to assistant manager of the Fund. From 1994 to 1996 she had put on 10 kg in weight, and in January 1996 started a strict diet and worked out at a gym four times a week. In June 1996 she visited her GP with a 6-month history of increasing insomnia, lack of concentration, irritability and anxiety. She had begun to withdraw from a busy social calendar and was becoming indecisive. This was now affecting her work. For the previous 4 weeks she had had recurrent thoughts of suicide. She had also lost 4 kg in weight during that period. The GP diagnosed that she was depressed, arranged a psychiatric consultation for her and started her on a TCA.

a. What are the causes of depression?

b. What are the risk factors for depression? Was DW at risk prior to the diagnosis?

c. What neurochemical and receptor changes are associated with depressive illness?

d. Are TCAs an appropriate first choice of drug for this patient?

e. What are the unwanted effects of TCAs?

f. How successful is antidepressant treatment? After therapy for 3 months and some improvement, DW decided that the side-effects of the TCAs were unacceptable. What alternative antidepressant therapies could be given and what are the unwanted effects?

The answers are provided on pages 722–723.

Antidepressant drugs[a]

Drug	Half-life (h)	Elimination	Comments
Tricyclic antidepressants (TCAs) and related compounds			Most show high apparent volumes of distribution (Ch. 2) (10–50 l kg^{-1} bodyweight), which explains the combination of high first-pass metabolism and high clearance but a long elimination half-life
Amitriptyline	10–28	Metabolism	Particularly useful when sedation is required and for nocturnal enuresis in children; bioavailability is 30–60%; oxidised by hepatic CYP3A4-mediated demethylation to nortriptyline (see below) which has a slightly longer half-life
Amoxapine	8–14	Metabolism	Bioavailability is 18–54%; metabolised to hydroxy compounds which are eliminated as conjugates; 8-hydroxy-amoxapine is active and has a longer half-life (30 h) and is present at two-fold greater concentrations than amoxapine during repeated dosage
Clomipramine	12–36	Metabolism	Also useful for phobic and obsessive states; oral bioavailability is about 50%; oxidised by demethylation followed by hydroxylation and conjugation; selective and potent inhibitor of 5HT uptake
Dosulepin	11–40	Metabolism	Particularly useful when sedation is required; absolute bioavailability has not been defined; oxidised by demethylation and *S*-oxidation
Doxepin	8–25	Metabolism	Particularly useful when sedation is required; bioavailability is about 30%; extensive demethylation in the liver by the polymorphic CYP2D6 to the active desmethyl metabolite, which has a half-life of 30–50 h; subjects who are poor metabolisers are at increased risk of unwanted effects
Imipramine	8–20	Metabolism	Also useful for nocturnal enuresis in children; bioavailability is about 50%; metabolised by demethylation to an active metabolite (desipramine) and by hydroxylation; desipramine is metabolised by CYP2D6
Lofepramine	5	Metabolism	Undergoes extensive first-pass metabolism but absolute bioavailability is not known; metabolised to desipramine, which is probably responsible for much of the activity
Maprotiline	30–60	Metabolism	Particularly useful when sedation is required; tetracyclic compound; oral bioavailability is 40–70%; extensively metabolised, with metabolites eliminated in urine and bile; the desmethyl metabolite retains activity
Mianserin	10–20	Metabolism	Particularly useful when sedation is required; tetracyclic compound; oral bioavailability is 20–30%; major metabolite is desmethyl compound (demethylation product) which has weak α_2-adrenoceptor agonist properties
Nortriptyline	18–90	Metabolism	Also useful for nocturnal enuresis in children; bioavailability is 50–60%; oxidised by CYP2D6 to a 10-hydroxy metabolite (which retains some activity) that is conjugated and excreted; CYP2D6 poor metabolisers have higher plasma concentrations of the parent drug but do not show an increased incidence of unwanted effects
Trazodone	7–13	Metabolism	Particularly useful when sedation is required; tetracyclic compound; complete oral bioavailability (100%); rapidly metabolised by CYP3A4 oxidation to an active metabolite (that has higher plasma concentrations than the parent compound)

continued

Drug compendium

Antidepressant drugs[a] *(continued)*

Drug	Half-life (h)	Elimination	Comments
Tricyclic antidepressants (TCAs) and related compounds (continued)			
Trimipramine	20–26	Metabolism	Particularly useful when sedation is required; bioavailability is 40%; metabolised by demethylation and hydroxylation catalysed by multiple P450 isoenzymes; the desmethyl metabolite is active but is present only at low concentrations
Selective serotonin (5HT) reuptake inhibitors (SSRIs)			
Citalopram	23–75	Metabolism (+ renal)	Also useful for panic disorder; oral bioavailability is 80%; oxidised in liver by CYP3A4 and CYP2C19 to a range of metabolites, some of which retain weak activity; weak inhibitor of, but not a substrate for, CYP2D6; about 20% cleared by the kidneys
Escitalopram	27–32	Metabolism (+ renal)	Also useful for panic disorder; an isomer of citalopram; oxidised in liver mostly by CYP3A4 and CYP2C19; about 8% cleared by the kidneys
Fluoxetine	48–72	Metabolism	Also useful for bulimia nervosa and obsessive–compulsive disorder; essentially complete bioavailability; metabolised by CYP2D6; poor metabolisers have a two-fold longer half-life and excrete more of the parent compound in the urine; the major desmethyl metabolite (norfluoxetine) is as active as the parent drug and has a longer half-life (6 days); both parent drug and metabolite are potent inhibitors of CYP2D6 (which metabolises desipramine)
Fluvoxamine	7–70	Metabolism	Also useful for obsessive–compulsive disorder; high oral bioavailability (absolute bioavailability is not known); extensively metabolised by oxidation (not by CYP2D6)
Paroxetine	10–20 (EM) 30–50 (PM)	Metabolism	Also useful for obsessive–compulsive disorder, panic disorder, social phobia, post-traumatic stress disorder and general anxiety disorder; good but variable absorption; eliminated by CYP2D6-catalysed oxidation; the half-life in poor metabolisers (PM) is longer than in extensive metabolisers (EM); the metabolites are inactive; during repeated dosage the steady-state plasma concentrations are similar in EM and PM subjects because CYP2D6 is saturated in both groups, and other non-saturated enzymes (e.g. CYP3A4) determine the clearance
Sertraline	26	Metabolism	Also useful for obsessive–compulsive disorder and post-traumatic stress disorder; oral bioavailability is low and increased if given with food (absolute bioavailability is not known); undergoes hepatic demethylation and oxidation to largely inactive metabolites

continued

Antidepressant drugs[a] (continued)

Drug	Half-life (h)	Elimination	Comments
Serotonin and noradrenaline reuptake inhibitors (SNRIs)			
Venlafaxine	5	Metabolism	Also useful for general anxiety disorder; high oral bioavailability (>90%); oxidised by hepatic CYP2D6 to the active *O*-desmethyl metabolite which is responsible for much of the therapeutic activity and has a longer half-life (11 h); other minor metabolites, such as the *N*-desmethyl metabolite, are inactive
Classic (non-selective) monoamine oxidase inhibitors (MAOIs)			
Isocarboxazid	2–3	Metabolism	Essentially complete bioavailability; rapidly hydrolysed by esterases; duration of action is measured in days; slow onset of clinical action (weeks)
Phenelzine	1	Metabolism	Extensively absorbed; rapidly metabolised by *N*-acetylation; produces profound and prolonged inhibition of MAO with a slow onset of clinical action (weeks)
Tranylcypromine	2–3	Metabolism	Extensively absorbed; metabolised by oxidation, *N*-acetylation and *N*-glucuronidation (a rare metabolic reaction); onset of action is more rapid than for the other drugs in this group
Reversible inhibitors of monoamine oxidase A (RIMAs)			
Moclobemide	1–2	Metabolism	Also useful for social phobia; bioavailability is about 50%; numerous metabolites formed; metabolised by polymorphic CYP2C19 (CYP2C19 metabolises mephenytoin); poor metabolisers of mephenytoin (low CYP2C19) have a half-life of moclobemide which is 4 h, compared with 2 h in extensive metabolisers of mephenytoin (high CYP2C19)
Other antidepressant drugs			
Flupentixol	35	Metabolism	Particularly useful for associated psychoses; bioavailability is about 40%; parent drug undergoes enterohepatic circulation following biliary excretion as a glucuronide
Lithium	8–45	Renal	Used for severe recurrent depressive episodes and for prophylaxis of bipolar affective disorder; complete oral absorption; filtered at the glomerular and reabsorbed (about 80%) in the proximal, but not distal, parts of the renal tubule
Mirtazapine	20–40	Metabolism	Principal action is inhibition of central presynaptic α_2-adrenoceptors and blocking of postsynaptic $5HT_2$ receptors; bioavailability is about 50%; metabolised by oxidation followed by glucuronidation; metabolised by CYP2D6 and CYP3A4

continued

Drug compendium

Antidepressant drugs[a] *(continued)*

Drug	Half-life (h)	Elimination	Comments
Other antidepressant drugs (continued)			
Reboxetine	15	Metabolism (+ renal)	Selective inhibitor of noradrenaline uptake; complete oral bioavailability; oxidised by hepatic CYP3A4 plus some renal clearance (10%)
Tryptophan	2	Metabolism	Very restricted hospital use as an adjunct to conventional treatments; actively absorbed from the intestinal tract and transported across the blood–brain barrier (in competition with other amino acids); undergoes decarboxylation and deamination

[a]All drugs given orally unless otherwise stated; they are all lipid soluble and well absorbed but many undergo extensive first-pass metabolism, which limits their bioavailability.

23

Epilepsy

Pathological basis of epilepsy

Epilepsy affects 0.1% of the population and is charac-terised by recurrent epileptic seizures without any immediate provoking cause. Epileptic seizures are sudden and transient episodes of motor, sensory, autonomic or psychic disturbance triggered by abnormal neuronal discharges in the brain. The clinical manifestations depend on the site of the discharge. In partial (localisation-related) epilepsy, the discharge starts in a localised area of the brain and may remain localised or spread to affect the whole brain (secondary generalisation). In generalised epilepsy, the abnormal discharge affects the whole of the brain from the onset (Table 23.1). Identification of the type of seizure is useful as a guide to treatment.

The origin of epilepsy is complex. Structural damage in the brain, such as that resulting from trauma, tumours, cerebrovascular disease or haemorrhage, may provide the initial focus of abnormal neuronal activity. Acute symptomatic seizures may be caused by metabolic disturbance, such as hypoglycaemia or alcohol abuse. However, in most people with epilepsy, there is probably a genetic component.

Neurotransmitters and epilepsy

Coordinated activity among neurons depends on a controlled balance between excitatory and inhibitory influences on the electrical activity across the cell membrane. The development and evolution of an epileptic seizure probably arises from a local imbalance between excitatory neurotransmission, principally mediated by glutamate, and inhibitory neurotransmission, mediated by gamma-aminobutyric acid (GABA), which leads to a focus of neuronal instability. Generalised epilepsy involves abnormally synchronised activity in large-scale neuronal networks, in particular involving interaction between cortical and subcortical structures such as the thalamus.

In healthy neuronal circuits, depolarising inward Na^+ and Ca^{2+} ionic currents (activated by glutamate receptors) are balanced by repolarising outward K^+ currents (via $GABA_B$ receptors). Influx of Cl^- ions into the cell, produced by $GABA_A$ receptor activation, hyper-polarises the neuron, with inhibition of impulse generation. Any defect in these pumps that results in incomplete repolarisation of the cell will leave the

Table 23.1
Simplified classification of epileptic seizures

Seizures type	Characteristics
Partial (focal) seizures	
Simple partial seizures	Motor, somatosensory or psychic symptoms; consciousness is not impaired
Complex partial seizures	Temporal lobe, psychomotor; consciousness is impaired
Secondary generalised seizures	These begin as partial seizures
Generalised seizures	Affect whole brain with loss of consciousness
Clonic, tonic, or tonic–clonic	Initial rigid extensor spasm, respiration stops, defecation, micturition and salivation occur (tonic phase, ~1 min); violent synchronous jerks (clonic phase, 2–4 min)
Myoclonic	Seizures of a muscle or group of muscles
Absence	Abrupt loss of awareness of surroundings, little motor disturbance (occur in children)
Atonic	Loss of muscle tone/strength

Unclassified seizures

neuron closer to its threshold potential for firing, and create a hyperexcitable state. This instability could initiate the burst of firing that produces epileptiform activity. Once an electrical discharge is triggered, spontaneous repetitive firing of the focus is maintained by a feedback mechanism known as post-tetanic potentiation (see Ch. 27 for a description of post-tetanic potentiation in relation to the neuromuscular junction). Several inherited epilepsy syndromes have now been characterised at a cellular level, and arise from mutations of proteins involved in ion channel function. Reduction in the activity of membrane-bound ATPases linked to neuronal transmembrane ion pumps has also been found in the brains of people with epilepsy. Ion channel dysfunction may therefore provide the substrate for the genesis of many types of generalised seizures.

The genesis of partial seizures is less well understood. These arise from focal lesions in the brain that promote formation of abnormal hyperexcitable circuits. These circuits may be enhanced by disruption of glial cell function and changes in the neuronal microenvironment.

Most antiepileptic drugs act either by blockade of depolarising ion channels, or by enhancing the inhibitory actions of GABA.

Antiepileptic drugs

Carbamazepine and oxcarbazepine

Mechanism of action and uses

Carbamazepine and oxcarbazepine are used in most types of epilepsy, except myoclonic epilepsy or absences, which they can exacerbate. Their mechanisms of action are incompletely understood, and may include:

- inhibition of repetitive neuronal firing by use-dependent blockade of Na^+ channels; this is probably the principle mechanism
- attenuation of the action of glutamate at NMDA (N-methyl-D-aspartate) receptors, and reduced glutamate release.

Carbamazepine is also used in the management of neuropathic pain (Ch. 19) (oxcarbazepine is also effective), and in the management of bipolar disorder (Ch. 21).

Pharmacokinetics

Absorption of carbamazepine is slow and incomplete after oral administration. It is metabolised in the liver. Its major epoxide metabolite is also active but is present in lower concentrations than the parent drug. The half-life of carbamazepine is initially very long at about 1.5 days but decreases by two-thirds over the first 2 to 3 weeks of treatment because of 'autoinduction' of its own metabolism in the liver. Seizure control may then require an increase in dose. The plasma or salivary

concentration of carbamazepine correlates well with its clinical efficacy, but the substantial fluctuations in plasma concentration between doses make interpretation of a single value difficult. Transient unwanted neurological effects can occur in association with the peak plasma drug concentration when using the conventional formulation of carbamazepine, and these can be minimised by use of a modified-release formulation.

Oxcarbazepine is well absorbed orally and is rapidly and extensively converted in the liver to an active metabolite with an intermediate half-life.

Unwanted effects

The unwanted effects with oxcarbazepine are less severe than with carbamazepine.

- Nausea and vomiting, especially early in treatment. Constipation, diarrhoea and anorexia also happen.
- Skin rashes, especially transient generalised erythema, but more severe reactions also occur. If a rash is produced by carbamazepine, oxcarbazepine can often be given without recurrence.
- Central nervous system (CNS) toxicity leads to double vision, dizziness, drowsiness or confusion. Ataxia can occur at high doses.
- Transient leucopenia is common, especially early in treatment, but severe bone marrow depression is rare.
- Hyponatraemia, caused by potentiation of the action of antidiuretic hormone, can lead to confusion and decreased control of seizures. This may be more pronounced with oxcarbazepine.
- Teratogenicity is common, especially with carbamazepine (see below).
- Induction of hepatic drug-metabolising enzymes (Ch. 2) with carbamazepine. The most common interaction is with the oral contraceptive pill (Ch. 45), and the dose of oestrogen should be increased to avoid failure of contraception. The metabolism of warfarin (Ch. 11) and ciclosporin (Ch. 38) are also accelerated. Interactions of carbamazepine with other antiepileptic drugs are discussed below. Oxcarbazepine has little effect on cytochrome P450 and therefore has few drug interactions.

Phenytoin and fosphenytoin

Mechanism of action and effects

Phenytoin and its prodrug fosphenytoin have a broad spectrum of activity and are effective against all forms of epilepsy, except absences. They have several actions that may contribute to the anticonvulsant activity:

- use-dependent blockade of Na^+ channels, which reduces cell excitability, is the main mechanism of action
- blockade of voltage-activated L-type Ca^{2+} channels
- potentiation of the action of GABA at $GABA_A$ receptors.

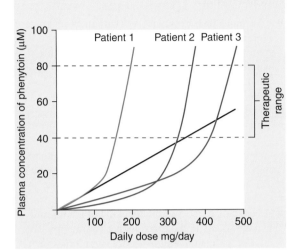

Fig. 23.1
Increasing the daily dose of phenytoin results in marked interindividual variation in plasma concentrations of phenytoin at steady state. The figure illustrates the types of relationships between dose and plasma concentration that can be seen in three patients. The non-linear relationship within the desired therapeutic range leads to difficulties in dosage adjustment. The straight line illustrates the increase in plasma concentrations of phenytoin in subject 1 that would occur if the metabolism were not saturated (i.e. first-order kinetics).

Phenytoin is sometimes used in the management of neuropathic pain (Ch. 19) and for cardiac arrhythmias (Ch. 5).

Pharmacokinetics

Phenytoin is well, but slowly, absorbed from the gut. Slow intravenous injection can be used if a rapid onset of action is needed. Intramuscular injection of phenytoin should be avoided since absorption by this route is erratic and unpredictable, and muscle damage can occur. Phenytoin is eliminated by hepatic metabolism, but the enzyme is saturated within the therapeutic dose range, and at saturating doses the elimination changes from first-order (linear) kinetics to zero-order (non-linear) kinetics (Ch. 2; Fig. 23.1). This occurs in some individuals at plasma drug concentrations near the lower end of the therapeutic range. Once the enzyme is saturated, a small change in dose produces a large change in the plasma concentration at steady state (Ch. 2), and the elimination half-life is increased fourfold to almost 2 days. Plasma phenytoin concentrations are closely related to the clinical effect, and their measurement is useful as a guide to dosing. Phenytoin is highly protein bound (about 90%) and can be displaced from its binding sites by sodium valproate and salicylates, which enhance the clinical effect of phenytoin to an unpredictable extent. The concentration of phenytoin in saliva reflects the free or unbound drug concentration in plasma, and measurement of the salivary concentration can be useful if protein binding is altered, for example in pregnancy or renal failure. Collection of saliva is non-invasive, and salivary measurements are useful for monitoring the treatment of children.

Fosphenytoin is only available for parenteral use, and can be given by intramuscular injection (absorption from this route is good, unlike that of phenytoin) or by intravenous infusion. It is completely metabolised to phenytoin.

Unwanted effects

Most unwanted effects of these drugs are dose-related:

- nausea or vomiting
- impaired brainstem and cerebellar function, producing confusion, dizziness, tremor, nervousness or insomnia; nystagmus, blurred vision, ataxia, and dysarthria are signs of overdosage
- chronic connective tissue effects: gum hyperplasia, coarsening of facial features, hirsutism and acne (for this reason, it is usual to avoid phenytoin in young women or adolescents)
- skin rashes
- folic acid deficiency producing megaloblastic haemopoeisis, although anaemia with a macrocytic blood picture is rare; folic acid metabolism is increased by phenytoin
- vitamin D deficiency as a result of increased vitamin D metabolism; in rare cases, this can produce osteomalacia
- teratogenic effects, including facial and digital malformations; these occur in up to 10% of pregnancies
- induction of hepatic drug-metabolising enzymes (Ch. 2) predisposes to several drug interactions; in particular, the metabolism of warfarin and ciclosporin is increased; interactions with other anticonvulsants are discussed below.

Lamotrigine

Mechanism of action and uses

Lamotrigine has a wide spectrum of efficacy for partial and generalised seizures. It produces use-dependent inhibition of neuronal Na^+ channels, but, unlike carbamazepine and phenytoin, it selectively targets neurons that synthesise glutamate and aspartate. Lamotrigine also reduces glutamate release, possibly through inhibition of voltage-sensitive Ca^{2+} channels.

Pharmacokinetics

Lamotrigine is well absorbed orally and extensively metabolised in the liver. The half-life is long.

Unwanted effects

- fever, malaise, influenza-like symptoms
- skin rashes: some disappear despite continued treatment; occasionally, severe skin reactions arise, particularly with rapid dose escalation

- gastrointestinal disturbances, including vomiting
- CNS effects: drowsiness, headache, dizziness, double vision and ataxia; tremor can be troublesome at high dosages.

Sodium valproate

Mechanism of action and uses

Valproate has a wide spectrum of antiepileptic activity, and suppresses the initial seizure discharge as well as the spread of seizure activity. It is effective for all forms of epilepsy. Valproate has multiple actions, but their contributions to the clinical effects are incompletely understood. The actions of valproate include:

- use-dependent blockade of transmembrane Na^+ channels, thus stabilising neuronal membranes; this is probably not the most important action of the drug
- potentiation of the effect of the inhibitory amino acid GABA, possibly by enhanced synthesis and release, and reduced degradation
- attenuation of the excitatory action of glutamate at NMDA receptors
- inhibition of T-type Ca^{2+} channels
- activation of neuroprotective/neurotrophic intracellular proteins (see also Ch. 21).

The immediate effects may be due to extracellular actions on neuronal ion channels, while slow diffusion into neurons produces delayed intracellular effects. The full benefit of treatment may be delayed by several weeks. Sodium valproate is also used for the management of bipolar disorder and mania (Ch. 21), prophylaxis of migraine (Ch. 26) and in the management of neuropathic pain (Ch. 19).

Pharmacokinetics

Sodium valproate is well absorbed from the gut. To reduce gastric upset, conventional-formulation tablets should be taken with food. Plasma protein binding of valproate is high (90–95% at low to moderate plasma concentrations), but the proportion of free (and therefore active) drug rises with increasing blood concentration of the drug. Although valproate is highly ionised at physiological pH, it is rapidly transported across the blood–brain barrier via an anion exchange transporter, then passively and slowly diffuses into neurons. Slow diffusion into and out of neurons may in part explain why the drug concentration in plasma does not correlate well with its therapeutic effect. Monitoring of blood concentrations is only useful to assess compliance. Valproate is extensively metabolised in the liver and the half-life is long. Sodium valproate is also available in a modified-release formulation (as sodium valproate with valproic acid), and there is an intravenous preparation for rapid seizure control.

Valproate is also available as a formulation containing only valproic acid, rather than the sodium salt.

Unwanted effects

- Gastrointestinal upset: nausea, vomiting, anorexia, abdominal pain and bowel disturbance. These can be minimised by gradual dosage titration. Sodium valproate can cause pancreatitis, and a serum amylase should be measured if symptoms such as abdominal pain or nausea and vomiting arise.
- Weight gain caused by appetite stimulation.
- Transient hair loss, with regrowth of curly hair.
- Ataxia, tremor, confusion and, rarely, encephalopathy and coma. These can be minimised by slow dosage titration.
- Thrombocytopenia or impaired platelet activity.
- Oedema.
- Severe hepatotoxicity can develop but is rare, and usually occurs in the first 6 months of therapy. This is most frequent in children under age 3 years or those with organic brain disorders, who are receiving multiple drug therapy for seizures. Raised liver enzymes without severe liver disturbance is not uncommon during therapy with sodium valproate.
- Teratogenicity (see below).
- Inhibition of hepatic drug-metabolising enzymes, leading to interactions with other antiepileptic drugs (see below).

Phenobarbital and primidone

Mechanism of action and effects

These drugs have a wide spectrum of activity and are effective in most forms of epilepsy, but unwanted effects limit their use. Phenobarbital is a barbiturate, and the major mechanism of action is activation of postsynaptic neuronal $GABA_A$ receptors (Ch. 20). This increases the duration of opening of the transmembrane Cl^- channel associated with the receptor, and the neuronal membrane is therefore hyperpolarised and less likely to fire. This effect is independent of the presence of the inhibitory amino acid GABA, but phenobarbital will also potentiate the effect of GABA (Ch. 20). The action of primidone is in part due to its conversion to phenobarbital. Primidone has no advantage over phenobarbital and is generally less well tolerated. People with epilepsy who do not respond to, or tolerate, phenobarbital are unlikely to benefit from primidone.

Pharmacokinetics

Oral absorption of phenobarbital is almost complete. Elimination is by hepatic metabolism and renal excretion, with about 25% excreted unchanged in the urine. The half-life is very long at about four days, but with considerable interindividual variation.

Primidone is well absorbed orally and converted in the liver to two active metabolites.

The plasma concentrations of phenobarbital and primidone relate poorly to control of seizures; they are only useful as a guide to adherence to treatment. Control of seizures or unwanted effects should determine dosages.

Unwanted effects

- CNS effects: sedation and fatigue are common in adults; paradoxical excitement, confusion and restlessness can occur in the elderly, and hyperactivity in children. Depression has also been reported.
- Folate deficiency and, rarely, megaloblastic anaemia can occur (cf. phenytoin).
- Tolerance to both unwanted and therapeutic effects tends to occur during long-term administration.
- Dependence with a physical withdrawal reaction is seen after long-term treatment.
- Teratogenicity (see below).
- Induction of hepatic drug-metabolising enzymes (Ch. 2) leads to increased metabolism of phenobarbital itself and warfarin, ciclosporin and oestrogen (reducing the effectiveness of oral contraception). Interactions with other antiepileptic drugs are considered below.

Gabapentin

Mechanism of action and uses

The major use of gabapentin is in partial seizures, with or without secondary generalisation. Although designed as a structural analogue of GABA, gabapentin does not mimic GABA in the brain. Possible mechanisms of action include:

- increased synthesis and release of GABA, and reduced breakdown
- inhibition of L-type voltage-gated Ca^{2+} channels
- interaction with the L-amino acid transport system.

Gabapentin is also used in neuropathic pain (Ch. 19).

Pharmacokinetics

Gabapentin is incompletely absorbed from the gut, via a saturable transport mechanism, and is excreted unchanged by the kidney. It has a short half-life.

Unwanted effects

- CNS effects, including drowsiness, dizziness, ataxia, fatigue, headache, tremor and double vision
- rhinitis
- nausea and vomiting.

Topiramate

Mechanism of action and uses

Topiramate is used as an add-on treatment for drug-resistant partial or generalised seizures. The mechanisms of action are not fully understood, but may include:

- use-dependent blockade of neuronal Na^+ channels
- inhibition of L-type voltage-gated Ca^{2+} channels

- enhancement of the action of GABA at $GABA_A$ receptors, although the mechanism of this interaction is unknown
- antagonist activity at the AMPA/kainite subtype of receptor for the excitatory amino acid glutamate.

Pharmacokinetics

Topiramate is rapidly absorbed orally and up to 50% is metabolised in the liver; the rest is eliminated unchanged by the kidney. The half-life is long.

Unwanted effects

- CNS effects, including impaired concentration, cognitive impairment, confusion, dizziness, ataxia, and headache
- agitation, emotional lability or depression
- gastrointestinal upset, with abdominal pain, nausea, anorexia and weight loss
- acute angle-closure glaucoma, especially within 1 month of starting treatment.

Tiagabine

Mechanism of action and uses

Tiagabine is used as an adjunctive therapy for partial seizures, with or without secondary generalisation. It is a potent inhibitor of GABA transporter 1 (GAT-1) and decreases glial and, to a lesser extent, neuronal uptake of the inhibitory amino acid GABA. This is the mechanism that normally limits the duration of action of GABA in the brain. The action is relatively selective for the hippocampus and thalamus.

Pharmacokinetics

Tiagabine is well absorbed from the gut. It is metabolised in the liver and has an intermediate half-life.

Unwanted effects

- CNS effects: dizziness, lethargy, nervousness, impaired concentration, tremor
- nausea, diarrhoea.

Vigabatrin

Mechanism of action and uses

Vigabatrin is only used in combination with other drugs to treat epilepsy that is resistant to other drug combinations, or when they are poorly tolerated. It is effective in partial epilepsy, with or without secondary generalisation, but its use is now restricted because of the unacceptably high risk of visual field defects (see below). It is, however, still useful for infantile spasms. Vigabatrin has a unique mechanism of action. It is a structural analogue of GABA and produces irreversible inhibition of GABA transaminase (GABA-T), the enzyme that inactivates GABA. The generalised increase in CNS concentrations of GABA inhibits the spread of epileptic discharges.

Pharmacokinetics

Vigabatrin is rapidly absorbed from the gut and excreted unchanged by the kidney. The half-life is intermediate. Irreversible drug binding to the target enzyme means that the half-life of the enzyme, which is much longer than that of the drug, determines the duration of action. GABA-T activity recovers to about 60% of baseline after 5 days. The efficacy of vigabatrin, therefore, is unrelated to the plasma drug concentration, and blood concentration monitoring is of no value.

Unwanted effects

- CNS effects: sedation and fatigue, dizziness, nervousness, irritability, depression, impaired concentration, ataxia, nystagmus and tremor
- psychotic reactions, especially if there is a history of psychiatric disorder
- severe peripheral visual field defects during prolonged use; they can arise from 1 month to several years after starting use, and are usually irreversible; regular monitoring at 6-month intervals is recommended
- weight gain and oedema.

Levetiracetam

Mechanism of action and uses

Levetiracetam is used for adjunctive treatment of partial seizures, with or without secondary generalisation. Its mechanisms of action remain uncertain. Levetiracetam binds to an unidentified site on the neuronal synaptic plasma membrane, and may modulate activity at $GABA_B$ receptors or suppress NMDA receptor firing in response to glutamate. The end result is selective inhibition of synchronised epileptiform burst firing and propagation of seizure activity in the hippocampus, without affecting neuronal excitability.

Pharmacokinetics

Levetiracetam is rapidly absorbed after oral administration, and largely eliminated unchanged by the kidney. Up to one-third undergoes hepatic metabolism. Levetiracetam has an intermediate half-life.

Unwanted effects

- drowsiness, lethargy, dizziness
- anorexia, nausea, dyspepsia, diarrhoea.

Benzodiazepines

Examples: clonazepam, clobazam, diazepam, lorazepam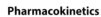

Mechanism of action and uses

These drugs enhance the action of the inhibitory neurotransmitter GABA (Ch. 20). Clonazepam and clobazam are used orally for prophylaxis, usually as an adjunct to other drugs. Lorazepam, diazepam or clonazepam can be used intravenously to treat individual fits; if intravenous access is not available, then rectal diazepam or buccal or intranasal midazolam can be used. Intravenous diazepam is formulated as an emulsion to reduce the incidence of thrombophlebitis.

Pharmacokinetics

These are long-acting benzodiazepines. Their pharmacokinetics are described in Chapter 20.

Unwanted effects

These are discussed in Chapter 20. Partial or complete tolerance to the antiepileptic action of benzodiazepines often occurs after about 4–6 months of continuous treatment.

Ethosuximide

Mechanism of action and uses

Ethosuximide is a drug of choice in absence seizures, and may be effective for myoclonic seizures, and tonic or atonic seizures. It is ineffective in other types of epilepsy. In absence seizures, T-type Ca^{2+} channels are believed to generate excessive activity in thalamocortical relay neurons. Ethosuximide inhibits these channels and prevents synchronised neuronal firing.

Pharmacokinetics

Absorption of ethosuximide from the gut is almost complete. Metabolism in the liver is extensive and the half-life is very long, at 2–3 days, although it is shorter in children. Plasma and salivary drug concentrations correlate well with control of seizures and can be used to monitor treatment.

Unwanted effects

- nausea, vomiting, anorexia (less frequent if the drug is taken with food and if the dose is gradually increased)
- drowsiness, dizziness, ataxia, dyskinesia, photophobia, headache and depression
- skin rashes
- agranulocytosis and aplastic anaemia are rare complications
- teratogenicity.

Drug interactions among anticonvulsants

Many antiepileptics affect hepatic drug-metabolising enzymes such as the cytochrome P450 isoenzymes; therefore, drug interactions are frequent. Interactions when two or more antiepileptics are used together can have major clinical implications for seizure control or toxicity. Plasma drug concentration monitoring is often advisable when more than one drug is used. Common interactions are listed below.

Carbamazepine. This is an enzyme inducer that can lower the plasma concentrations of clobazam, clonazepam, lamotrigine, tiagabine, topiramate, sodium valproate and an active metabolite of oxcarbazepine.

Phenobarbital and primidone. These are enzyme inducers that lower the plasma concentrations of carbamazepine, clonazepam, lamotrigine, tiagabine, phenytoin, sodium valproate and an active metabolite of oxcarbazepine.

Phenytoin. This is an enzyme inducer and it often lowers the plasma concentrations of carbamazepine, clonazepam, lamotrigine, tiagabine, topiramate, sodium valproate and an active metabolite of oxcarbazepine.

Valproate. Inhibition of hepatic drug metabolism by valproate often increases the plasma concentrations of phenobarbital and lamotrigine, as well as those of an active metabolite of carbamazepine. Sodium valproate can displace phenytoin from plasma protein binding sites but also inhibits the metabolism of phenytoin, and the net result is an increase in the active free component.

Vigabatrin. This drug often reduces plasma phenytoin concentration by an unknown mechanism.

Management of epilepsy

Treatment of individual seizures

The initial management of a seizure involves positioning the person to avoid injury. Particular attention must also be given to maintaining the airways and ensuring adequate oxygenation. A correctable cause such as hypoglycaemia should be sought and treated, and intravenous thiamine given if alcohol abuse is suspected.

Prolonged or repetitive seizures (status epilepticus) usually require urgent parenteral drug treatment. Intravenous lorazepam is the drug of choice; diazepam can be used but has a shorter duration of action owing to more rapid redistribution. If intravenous access is not available, then midazolam can be given by the buccal or intranasal route. Diazepam is available as a rectal solution, and may be particularly useful for children or initial treatment out of hospital. Close observation for signs of drug-induced respiratory depression should be maintained after giving a benzodiazepine.

If there is no response after 30 min, or seizures recur, then a slow intravenous injection of phenytoin, or a more rapid injection of fosphenytoin or phenobarbital, should be given. If seizures are still not controlled with these measures, then full anaesthesia using thiopental or propofol (Ch. 17) with assisted respiration in an intensive care unit will be necessary.

Prophylaxis for seizures

A diagnosis of epilepsy requires two or more spontaneous seizures. After a single event, up to 80% of people will have a second fit within 3 years. If a predisposing cause cannot be identified and avoided (e.g. alcohol withdrawal, photosensitive epilepsy precipitated by viewing a television from too close a distance), drug treatment will usually be recommended after a second seizure, unless the seizures were separated by very long intervals or were mild.

Treatment should begin with a single drug, the choice depending on the type of epilepsy and relative toxicity of the drugs (Table 23.2). If the type of epilepsy is uncertain, then sodium valproate is often recommended, since it has the broadest spectrum of activity. If seizures are not controlled with the first-choice drug, it becomes more important to accurately identify the type of seizure. A second single drug should then be tried while the first is gradually withdrawn (Table 23.2). A single drug will usually control seizures in up to 90% of people with epilepsy, although this may not be achieved with the first drug chosen. However, if the first drug does not control the seizures, then the chance of a second single drug being successful is 13%, and with a third, only 4%.

Refractory epilepsy can indicate poor adherence to treatment, inappropriate drug choice or dosage, or that the seizures are 'pseudo seizures' rather than true epilepsy. Multiple drug treatment (e.g. with two first-line drugs, or a first- and a second-line drug) should be reserved for seizures that have not been resolved by treatment with two or three drugs given alone. Drugs like vigabatrin, gabapentin and topiramate are only used in combination with other agents. Sometimes, despite good adherence to treatment recommendations, combination therapy at maximally tolerated doses does not control the seizures. This is more frequent if their onset was at an early age, if there are generalised, atonic or absence seizures, or if there is structural brain damage. Some recent evidence suggests that the origin of some of this resistance may lie in overexpression of proteins that help to maintain the blood–brain barrier, such as P-glycoprotein or members of the multidrug resistance-associated protein family of transporters that transport drugs out of the CNS. For temporal lobe epilepsy, there is now good evidence that if more than two consecutive anticonvulsants fail to control the seizures, then surgical treatment should be considered.

It is not usually necessary to monitor plasma drug concentrations to determine whether they are within the 'therapeutic range' unless seizure control is poor, or if poor adherence or drug toxicity are suspected. Good seizure control will often be achieved at plasma drug concentrations that are below the accepted 'therapeutic range', and, under such circumstances, an increase in dosage would not be necessary. Conversely, those who continue to have seizures may need plasma drug con-

Table 23.2
Drug choice in the treatment of epilepsy

Type of seizure	First-line drugs	Second-line drugs
Partial seizures	Carbamazepine, or phenytoin, or valproate[a], or Lamotrigine[b]	Phenobarbital/primidone[b] Clonazepam/clobazam[b] Gabapentin[b] (as adjunct) Vigabatrin[b] (as adjunct) Topiramate[b] (as adjunct)
Generalised seizures Tonic–clonic (grand mal)	Valproate, or carbamazepine, or phenytoin[a], or Lamotrigine[b]	Phenobarbital/primidone[b] Vigabatrin[b] (as adjunct)
Myoclonic	Valproate[a]	Clonazepam[b] Ethosuximide[c]
Absence	Ethosuximide[c] or valproate	Clonazepam[b] Lamotrigine[b]
Atonic	Valproate[a]	Phenytoin[a] Lamotrigine[b] Clonazepam[b] Ethosuximide[c] Phenobarbital[b]

Valproate, sodium valproate.
[a]Blocks Na^+ channels.
[b]Enhances gamma-aminobutyric acid activity.
[c]Inhibits T-type Ca^{2+} channels.

centrations above the standard therapeutic range to achieve control, provided there is no evidence of toxic effects. The only drug for which monitoring is of proven benefit for dosage adjustment is phenytoin, primarily because metabolism may be saturated at therapeutic doses and the kinetics become non-linear (Fig. 23.1). Adjustment of the dosages of carbamazepine or ethosuximide may be easier if the plasma concentration is known; however, for other drugs, monitoring is only of value to confirm that the drug is being taken.

In the UK, a driving licence is revoked until the individual has been seizure-free for one year, or has only suffered nocturnal seizures for three years. Driving is not advised during withdrawal of antiepileptic drugs, or for six months afterwards.

Once started, treatment should usually be continued for at least 2–3 years after the last seizure. If there is a continuing predisposing condition or the person wishes to drive, treatment should probably be lifelong. If withdrawal is undertaken, then it should be gradual, in order to minimise the risk of rebound seizures; when several drugs are used, one should be withdrawn at a time.

Prophylaxis for seizures is often given for up to three months following neurosurgical procedures or head injury, particularly if there was a depressed skull fracture or an associated intracranial haematoma. Evidence that such routine use is beneficial is not secure.

Febrile convulsions occur commonly in infancy and usually do not lead to epilepsy or produce CNS damage. About 4% of children have them and they recur in about one-third. Measures to reduce pyrexia during febrile episodes, such as removal of clothes and use of paracetamol (Ch. 29), are essential. Routine prophylaxis with antiepileptic drugs is not recommended, but rectal diazepam is sometimes given when a child who has previously had a febrile convulsion becomes pyrexial.

Anticonvulsants in pregnancy

No anticonvulsant has a proven safety record in pregnancy and many carry a high risk of teratogenesis if the fetus is exposed in the first trimester. Fetal abnormalities are most frequent if more than one drug is used. Neural tube defects are particularly common with carbamazepine and sodium valproate (1–2% of pregnancies), and other developmental abnormalities occur with phenytoin. Women taking antiepileptic drugs who wish to become pregnant should be counselled about the risk and offered antenatal screening during pregnancy, with α-fetoprotein measurement (to detect neural tube defects) and second-trimester ultrasound scanning. Folic acid supplements may reduce the risk of neural tube defects and should be advised before and during pregnancy. Of all the anticonvulsant drugs, cautious optimism has been expressed for the lack of teratogenicity with lamotrigine. It is important to advise a potential mother with epilepsy that the risks of uncontrolled seizures during pregnancy, both to her and to the fetus, may be greater than the risk associated with drug therapy.

When the mother is taking carbamazepine, phenobarbital or phenytoin, there is an increased risk of neonatal bleeding. Prophylactic vitamin K_1 should be given to the mother before delivery at 36 weeks' gestation, and to the neonate.

FURTHER READING

Ängehangen M, Ben-Menachem E, Rönnbäck L et al (2003) Novel mechanisms of action of three antiepileptic drugs, vigabatrin, tiagabine, and topiramate *Neurochem Res* 28, 333–340

Anon (1998) Consensus statements: medical management of epilepsy. *Neurology* 51(suppl 4), S39–S43

Brodie MJ, French JA (2000) Management of epilepsy in adolescents and adults. *Lancet* 356, 323–329

Eadie MJ (1997) The single seizure. To treat or not to treat? *Drugs* 54, 651–656

Lowenstein DH, Alldredge BK (1998) Status epilepticus. *N Engl J Med* 338, 970–976

Morrell MJ (2002) Antiepileptic medications for the treatment of epilepsy. *Semin Neurol* 22, 247–258

Neville BRG (1997) Epilepsy in childhood. *BMJ* 315, 924–930

Nulman I, Laslo D, Koren G (1999) Treatment of epilepsy in pregnancy. *Drugs* 59, 525–533

Rosenow F, Arzimanoglou A, Baulac M (2002) Recent developments in treatment of status epilepticus: a review. *Epileptic Disord* 4(suppl 2), S41–S51

Sills GJ, Brodie MJ (2001) Update on the mechanisms of action of antiepileptic drugs. *Epileptic Disord* 3, 165–172

Tatum WO IV, Liporace J, Benbadia SR et al (2004) Updates on the treatment of epilepsy in women. *Arch Intern Med* 164, 137–146

Self-assessment

In questions 1–6, the first statement, in italics, is true. Are the accompanying statements also true?

1. *Generalised seizures involving the whole brain include tonic–clonic seizures (grand mal) and absences (petit mal).* Absences occur mainly in adults.

2. *Partial (or focal) seizures are localised and can involve motor, sensory or psychic symptoms without loss of consciousness.* In partial seizures, generalised muscle contractions do not occur.

3. *The excitatory amino acid glutamate acting on NMDA receptors is increased in some seizures and can lead to excitotoxic damage to cells.*

   a. Control of glutamate transmission is an important approach to current drug therapy.
   b. Enhanced neurotransmission by GABA is useful for treating epilepsy by decreasing Na^+ influx.

4. *The two main mechanisms by which drugs act as anticonvulsants is to inhibit Na^+ channel actions and enhance the activity of GABA.* The effect of phenytoin diminishes with long-term use.

5. *Phenytoin is highly protein bound.*

   a. Salicylates and sodium valproate reduce the effectiveness of phenytoin.
   b. The plasma concentration of phenytoin varies in a linear manner with the dose administered over the whole therapeutic dose range.

6. *The abrupt withdrawal of antiepileptics should be avoided.* Vigabatrin is a first-line drug for the treatment of all types of epilepsy.

7. A 10-year old boy was diagnosed with absence seizures, and the drugs that might be used and their unwanted effects were assessed. Which one of the following statements is <u>most likely</u> to apply in this boy?

   A. Phenytoin would be a suitable drug to use first.
   B. Ethosuxamide would be a suitable drug to use first.
   C. Valproate may reduce the effectiveness of ethosuximide.
   D. Ethosuximide probably acts principally to block Na^+ channels.
   E. The full benefit of sodium valproate is seen within 2 h of administration.

8. Regarding the effects of drugs used in the treatment of epilepsy, choose the one <u>most appropriate</u> statement.

   A. The risk of fetal abnormalities is similar with the use of either one or two antiepileptic drugs to control epilepsy in the pregnant woman.
   B. The effectiveness of phenobarbital diminishes with time.

Self-assessment questions

C. Plasma concentrations of phenytoin relate linearly to the dose given over a wide dose range.

D. The effect of phenytoin is reduced by aspirin.

E. Diazepam is used orally as a sole treatment for long-term prophylaxis in tonic–clonic seizures.

9. Case history 1 questions

> A 7-year-old boy was described as dreamy by his mother. He was making slow progress at school and his mother and teachers both commented that he could not concentrate and had frequent episodes of staring vacantly for a few seconds and then carrying on as normal. Following an electroencephalogram (EEG), a synchronous discharge characteristic of petit mal or absence form of epilepsy was demonstrated.

a. Which of the following drugs would you prescribe: phenytoin, phenobarbital, sodium valproate, ethosuximide?

b. What are the major relevant unwanted effects of those drugs you could have prescribed in this child?

c. If control of absence seizures is inadequate with your chosen antiepileptic, can combination therapy be given?

10. Case history 2 questions

> A 19-year-old woman had a long-term history of epilepsy of the complex partial seizure type, which often gravitated to generalised seizures. For several years her epilepsy had been well controlled with a stable drug regimen. She sought advice on contraception.

a. What antiepileptic drugs might be effective in the type of epilepsy this woman has?

b. What suitable options are available for contraception?

c. What potential problems can arise if the woman takes the oral combined contraceptive?

d. Would an injected progestogen contraceptive be worth considering?

e. If the oral combined contraceptive were the chosen method, what strategies should be adopted to ensure its efficacy?

f. Would the progestogen-only pill be a suitable method of contraception?

The answers are provided on pages 723–724.

Drugs used for epilepsy and status epilepticus

Drug	Half-life (h)	Elimination	Comments
Drugs used for epilepsy			Drugs given orally, usually once or twice daily, to encourage better compliance
Acetazolamide	6–15	Renal	Low efficacy and used as a second-line drug for partial and tonic–clonic seizures; negligible metabolism
Carbamazepine	25–65 (initial) 12–17 (chronic)	Metabolism	Used for partial and secondary generalised tonic–clonic seizures, some primary generalised seizures; also used for trigeminal neuralgia and for bipolar disorder unresponsive to lithium (Ch. 21); given orally or rectally; good oral bioavailability; epoxide metabolite has anticonvulsant actions; induction of CYP3A4 leads to drug interactions; wide intersubject variation in the extent of enzyme induction; autoinduction of its metabolism results in a shorter half-life after repeated dosage
Clobazam	10–50	Metabolism	Used as adjunctive therapy in epilepsy; also used short term for anxiety; high oral bioavailability; oxidised in the liver to numerous metabolites; the *N*-desmethyl metabolite is active and plasma concentrations are 5–10 times those of the parent drug
Clonazepam	18–45	Metabolism	Used in all forms of epilepsy; also used in myoclonus; oral bioavailability about 80%; metabolites formed by nitro-reduction in the liver have negligible activity
Ethosuximide	50–60	Metabolism + renal	Used for absence seizures, myoclonic seizures and some atypical seizures; about 80% is metabolised by CYP3A4-mediated hydroxylation and then conjugation; half-life is shorter in children (30 h)
Gabapentin	5–7	Renal	Used as adjunctive treatment in partial epilepsy with or without secondary generalised tonic–clonic seizures; also used for neuropathic pain; absorption from gut is rapid but dose dependent (possibly because of saturation of active amino acid transporter); oral bioavailability (60%) decreases at high doses; clearance approximates to glomerular filtration rate
Lamotrigine	15–60	Metabolism + renal	Used for partial and primary and secondary generalised tonic–clonic seizures; rapid and complete absorption; metabolised to various products, including a *N*-glucuronide (unusual reaction)
Levetiracetam	–	Renal + metabolism	Used as adjunctive treatment in partial epilepsy with or without secondary generalised tonic–clonic seizures; rapid absorption and 100% bioavailability; eliminated largely by glomerular filtration and some hydrolysis to an inactive carboxyclic acid (25%)
Oxcarbazepine	2	Renal	Used for partial seizures with or without secondary generalised tonic–clonic seizures; oxcarbazepine is the keto analogue of carbamazepine; rapid and complete absorption; reduced in the liver to the active metabolite (10-hydroxy oxcarbazepine), which has a longer half-life (9 h) and is responsible for most of the anti-seizure activity

continued

Drugs used for epilepsy and status epilepticus *(continued)*

Drug	Half-life (h)	Elimination	Comments
Drugs used for epilepsy *(continued)*			
Phenobarbital	50–150	Metabolism + renal	Used for all forms of epilepsy except absence seizures; oral bioavailability >90%; mostly eliminated by hepatic CYP2C9-mediated oxidation; potent inducer of cytochrome P450 isoenzymes, which leads to numerous drug interactions; about 25% is excreted unchanged in urine and renal clearance is increased by alkalinisation of the urine
Phenytoin	7–60	Metabolism + renal	Used for all forms of epilepsy except absence seizures; complete oral bioavailability; dose-dependent elimination because of saturation of metabolism; there is wide inter-subject variation in the concentration at which metabolism is saturated; renal elimination is 7% of dose at low doses; potent inducer of cytochrome P450 isoenzymes, which leads to numerous drug interactions
Primidone	4–22	Metabolism	Used for all forms of epilepsy except absence seizures; also used for essential tremor; active metabolites (phenobarbital and phenylethyl malonamide) have longer half-lives than primidone and accumulate; the metabolites account for most activity during chronic treatment; potent inducer of cytochrome P450 isoenzymes, leading to numerous drug interactions
Tiagabine	5–8	Metabolism	Used as adjunctive treatment in partial epilepsy with or without secondary generalised tonic–clonic seizures; rapidly and completely absorbed; oxidised by hepatic CYP3A4; does not induce cytochrome P450; elimination is increased by drugs which induce cytochrome P450
Topiramate	20–30	Renal + metabolism	Used as monotherapy or adjunctive treatment in generalised tonic–clonic seizures and in partial epilepsy with or without secondary generalisation; absorbed rapidly with a high bioavailability; about 70% is eliminated unchanged, but there is extensive reabsorption in the renal tubule; there is some metabolism, and elimination is enhanced by cytochrome P450 inducers
Valproate sodium	9–21	Metabolism	Used in all forms of epilepsy; oral bioavailability is >95%; metabolised by oxidation (CYP2C19 and CYP2C9) and by glucuronidation; some metabolites have activity but their importance is not known; interactions with other substrates of CYP2C19 and CYP2C9 have been reported
Vigabatrin	7–8	Renal	Used under specialised supervision as adjunctive treatment in partial epilepsy with or without secondary generalised tonic–clonic seizures; clearance is similar to, and correlates with, glomerular filtration rate; the duration of the effect greatly exceeds the drug half-life
Drugs used for status epilepticus			
Clonazepam	See above	See above	Given by intravenous injection or infusion; see above for other information
Diazepam	–	Metabolism	Given rectally or by intravenous injection; see Ch. 20 for other details

continued

Drugs used for epilepsy and status epilepticus *(continued)*

Drug	Half-life (h)	Elimination	Comments
Drugs used for status epilepticus (continued)			
Fosphenytoin sodium	0.15–0.25	Hydrolysis	Given by intravenous injection or infusion; ester prodrug for phenytoin
Lorazepam	8–25	Metabolism	Given by intravenous injection; see Ch. 20
Paraldehyde	10 (neonates)	Metabolism	Given rectally using a glass syringe (it dissolves plastic!)
Phenytoin sodium	See above	See above	Given by intravenous injection or infusion; the solution for injection is highly alkaline and venous irritation is reduced by injecting physiological saline before and after drug administration; see above for other information

24

Extrapyramidal movement disorders and spasticity

The neuronal connections of the area of the brain known as the basal ganglia are intimately involved in the co-ordination of motor function in conjunction with the motor cortex, cerebellum and spinal cord. Several neurotransmitters are involved in regulating the function of the basal ganglia (Fig. 24.1). Degeneration of vital neurons in these pathways produces disordered regulation of neuronal activity and dysfunctional motor activity. Treatment for these disorders is directed at restoring the balance among the neurotransmitters.

Parkinson's disease and parkinsonism

Parkinson's disease is a disorder characterised by a triad of:

- resting tremor
- skeletal muscle rigidity
- bradykinesia (poverty of movement).

The underlying pathology involves loss of neurons in the substantia nigra pars compacta and deposition of intracytoplasmic Lewy bodies. Lewy bodies are complex structures that produce functional changes in dopaminergic neurons of the nigrostriatal pathway, possibly involving impaired handling of free radicals generated during dopamine metabolism. This ultimately leads to neuronal death and degeneration of the nigrostriatal pathway (Fig. 24.1). The trigger for the condition is unknown, but genetic susceptibility and environmental toxins have been implicated. More than 50% of substantia nigra pars compacta neurons have degenerated before symptoms are apparent.

Two clinical subtypes of Parkinson's disease are recognised that have different morphological patterns. The *akinetic-rigid form* of the syndrome is associated with greatest cell loss in the ventrolateral part of the substantia nigra pars compacta, with dopaminergic denervation of the striatum. The motor symptoms are due to over-activity of the gamma-aminobutyric acid (GABA)-ergic motor loop, with a decrease in the glutamatergic thalamocortical pathway leading to reduced cortical activation. The *tremor-dominant type* has more severe cell loss in the medial substantia nigra pars compacta that projects to the dorsolateral striatum and thalamus.

The symptoms of Parkinson's disease correlate poorly with the extent of loss of dopaminergic activity in the substantia nigra and probably arise from overactivity of thalamocortical and cerebellar projections. The proposed changes in some transmitter substances in the basal ganglia that may contribute to the disordered motor function are shown in Figure 24.1. Several non-dopaminergic neural systems outside the basal ganglia are variably involved in contributing to Parkinson's disease, including cholinergic, serotonergic and noradrenergic pathways.

In some conditions that have clinical similarities to Parkinson's disease, for example the Steele–Richardson–Olszewski (progressive supranuclear palsy) and Shy–Drager syndromes, the GABA neurons also degenerate, which explains the poor response of these conditions to treatment with dopamine replacement therapy. Drugs that block striatal dopamine receptors, such as antipsychotic drugs (Ch. 21, Fig. 21.1), can produce a parkinsonian syndrome which also responds poorly to dopamine replacement therapy.

Drugs for Parkinson's disease

Treatment of Parkinson's disease is directed at enhancing dopaminergic activity (Fig. 24.2) or inhibiting cholinergic activity.

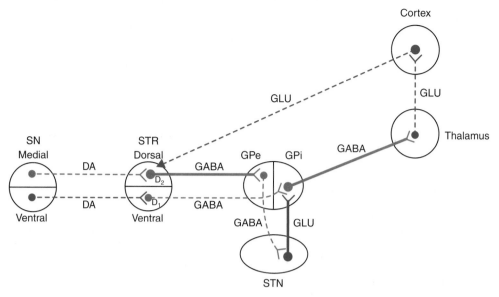

Fig. 24.1

A simplified model of events occurring in the basal ganglion that help to explain the disordered motor control in Parkinson's disease.
For the purposes of clarity, only selected interconnections and anatomical areas are shown. Many other complex excitatory and inhibitory interconnections exist. The figure shows two different neuronal circuitry loops where the degeneration of dopaminergic neurons results in dysfunctional motor control. It is suggested that if *akinetic-rigid* symptoms predominate, then this is associated with greater cell loss in the ventral part of the substantia nigra (SN) relative to the medial part (*the ventral nigral-striatal-pallidus interna-thalamic-cortex loop*), and if there are *tremor-dominant* symptoms, there is less SN cell loss overall, but that the medial SN shows relatively greater cell loss (*the medial nigral-striatal-pallidus externa-subthalamic nuclei-thalamic-cortex loop*). The basal ganglia contains the SN, the striatum (STR), the globus pallidus externa (GPe) and interna (GPi) segments, and the subthalamic nucleus (STN). The green interconnections mark excitatory neurotransmitter connections, and the red, inhibitory connections. The neurotransmitter utilised in each interconnecting pathway is also shown. The dotted lines in the interconnecting pathways between structures indicate *relative* underactivity, and the thicker solid lines, *relative* overactivity of the pathway compared with normal function. In parkinsonism, reduced activation of the D_2 receptors in the striatum by nerves from the <u>medial</u> SN leads to increased gamma-aminobutyric acid (GABA)-mediated inhibition of the GPe neurons. This, in turn, leads to increased firing rates of excitatory glutamatergic (GLU) neurons from the subthalamic nucleus to the GPi, leading to greater GABA-mediated inhibitory control in the motor thalamus and diminished glutamatergic input, particularly to the frontal cortex. The <u>ventral</u> nigrostriatal dopaminergic pathway utilises predominantly D_1 receptors in the striatum to enhance GABAergic input into the GPi. Reduction of this also results in enhanced GABAergic feed into the thalamus. Oscillatory bursts of the neuronal activity from the subthalamic nucleus and GPi are seen in parkinsonism and may contribute to the excessive thalamic and brainstem locomotor area inhibition. (For more detail, see Lang and Lozano (1998) and Jellinger (2002), from whom this figure was adapted.)

Dopaminergic drugs

Levodopa

Mechanism of action

Dopamine cannot be given to replace the deficiency in the basal ganglia because it does not cross the blood–brain barrier. However, the large neutral amino acid levodopa can be transported into the brain, where it is taken up into dopaminergic neurons and converted to dopamine by L-aromatic amino acid decarboxylase (Ch. 4).

Pharmacokinetics

Levodopa is absorbed from the small intestine by an active transport mechanism for large neutral amino acids. A similar transport system is used to transfer levodopa across the blood–brain barrier. Decarboxylation of levodopa to dopamine occurs extensively in peripheral tissues such as the gut wall, liver and kidney. This reduces the amount of levodopa that reaches the brain

(to about 1% of an oral dose) and generates substantial amounts of extracerebral dopamine that produce unwanted effects. Therefore, levodopa is given in combination with a peripheral dopa decarboxylase inhibitor (with carbidopa as co-careldopa or with benserazide as co-beneldopa) that does not cross the blood–brain barrier and only inhibits peripheral decarboxylation. About 80% of the peripheral metabolism of levodopa can be inhibited by this means, thereby increasing the amount of levodopa that crosses the blood–brain barrier to 5–10% of the oral dose.

The half-life of levodopa is short. In the early stages of the disease, storage of dopamine in striatal neurons can ensure a stable response despite infrequent doses of levodopa. Modified-release formulations of levodopa are also available to provide a more continuous supply of drug to the neurons. These formulations are often preferred by people with mild to moderate symptoms who do not experience levodopa-related dyskinesias (see below). Transition from conventional levodopa to a

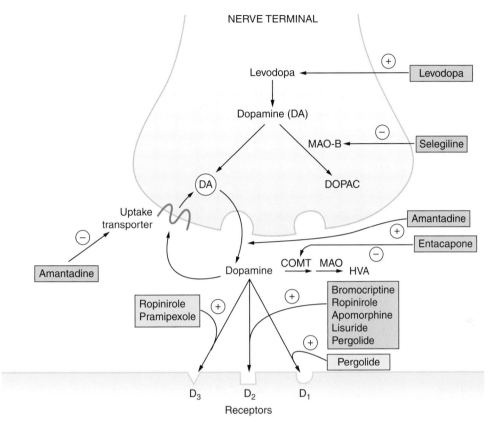

NERVE TERMINAL

Fig. 24.2
The major effects of drugs on the dopaminergic nerve terminal. Drugs act a number of different sites to amplify dopaminergic signalling. COMT, catechol-O-methyltransferase; DA, dopamine; DOPAC, 3,4-dihydroxyphenylacetic acid; HVA, homovanillic acid; MAO-B, monoamine oxidase B; +, stimulation; −, inhibition.

modified-release formulation requires care, because the latter has a lower bioavailability, which makes estimations of dosage equivalence difficult.

Unwanted effects
Unwanted effects fall broadly into two categories.

- Effects arising mainly from peripheral dopamine generation. These are reduced by use of a peripheral decarboxylase inhibitor. They include nausea and vomiting, caused by stimulation of the chemoreceptor trigger zone (CTZ) of the medullary vomiting centre, which lies outside the blood–brain barrier (Ch. 32), and postural hypotension caused by vasodilation.
- Effects arising from excessive central nervous system (CNS) dopamine generation. These include dyskinetic involuntary movements, especially of the face and neck, or akathisia (restlessness). Psychological disturbance can also occur, including hallucinations and confusion.

Dopamine receptor agonists

Examples: apomorphine, bromocriptine, pergolide, ropinirole

Mechanism of action
In contrast to levodopa, these drugs are direct agonists at central dopaminergic receptors. They have a longer duration of action than levodopa. The orally active drugs act on the inhibitory dopamine D_2-type receptor family (mainly D_2 and D_3), showing less activity at excitatory D_1 receptors (see Ch. 4). Bromocriptine and pergolide are structurally related to ergot alkaloids (Ch. 26), and bromocriptine has weak α-adrenoceptor agonist properties.

Pharmacokinetics
Bromocriptine is incompletely absorbed from the gut and undergoes extensive first-pass metabolism in the

liver. Pergolide and ropinirole have higher bioavailability, but are also eliminated by hepatic metabolism. The half-lives vary from short to very long.

Apomorphine is given parenterally by subcutaneous injection or continuous infusion, giving a very rapid onset of action. It has a short duration of action because of rapid hepatic metabolism.

Unwanted effects

Gradual dosage titration over several months may limit unwanted effects:

- nausea and vomiting (particularly with apomorphine)
- dyskinesias
- neuropsychiatric effects with hallucinations and confusion
- peripheral vasospasm with bromocriptine, especially in those with Raynaud's phenomenon
- postural hypotension (especially with bromocriptine)
- retroperitoneal fibrosis with bromocriptine or pergolide
- respiratory depression with high dosages of apomorphine (an opioid derivative), which is antagonised by naloxone (Ch. 19).

Amantadine

Mechanism of action

Amantadine was introduced originally as an antiviral drug. It is believed to act in Parkinson's disease by stimulating release of dopamine stored in nerve terminals and by reducing reuptake of released dopamine by the presynaptic neuron (Fig. 24.2). Its usefulness tends to be short-lived, because of the development of tolerance. It can be useful in treatment of levodopa-induced dyskinesias.

Pharmacokinetics

Amantadine is well absorbed from the gut and has a long half-life. It is excreted unchanged by the kidney.

Unwanted effects

Most are mild and dose-related. They include:

- ankle oedema
- postural hypotension
- nervousness, insomnia or hallucinations with high doses
- livedo reticularis (skin vasoconstriction caused by local catecholamine release).

Selective monoamine oxidase B inhibitors

Example: selegiline

Mechanism of action and effects

Selegiline inhibits the enzyme monoamine oxidase (MAO), which is responsible for the intraneuronal degradation of monoamine neurotransmitters (Ch. 4). It is selective at low doses for the isoenzyme (MAO-B) found in the striatum. This isoenzyme is distinct from MAO-A, which is also present in the CNS, as well as in the gut wall and other peripheral tissues; consequently, the interactions with drugs and foods containing tyramine, which is a problem with conventional non-selective MAO inhibitor (MAOI) antidepressants (Ch. 22), do not occur. Selegiline prolongs the duration of action of levodopa and reduces the levodopa dosage requirement by about one-third. It produces a small degree of clinical benefit when used alone.

Pharmacokinetics

Selegiline is completely absorbed from the gut and has a short half-life. It is extensively metabolised in the liver at first pass, in part to the L isomers of amfetamine and metamfetamine, which have long half-lives.

Unwanted effects

- nausea, vomiting, constipation or diarrhoea
- dry mouth, sore throat
- transient dizziness or lightheadedness is common
- insomnia, agitation, confusion, hallucinations caused by production of active amfetamine metabolites (Ch. 54).

Catechol-O-methyltransferase inhibitors

Example: entacapone

Mechanism of action and effects

Catechol-O-methyltransferase (COMT) is responsible for breakdown of between 10% and 30% of levodopa both peripherally and in the CNS (Ch. 4). In the presence of a peripheral dopa decarboxylase inhibitor, COMT is responsible for most of the peripheral metabolism of levodopa. Inhibition of COMT in conjunction with a dopa decarboxylase inhibitor doubles the half-life of levodopa and produces a 50% increase in the motor response to each dose of levodopa. The dose of levodopa may therefore need to be reduced when entacapone is started. Entacapone does not cross the blood–brain barrier.

Pharmacokinetics

Entacapone is variably absorbed from the gut. It undergoes extensive first-pass metabolism in the liver and has a short half-life.

Unwanted effects

- dyskinesias, hallucinations
- nausea, vomiting, abdominal pain, diarrhoea.

Antimuscarinic drugs

Examples: trihexyphenidyl hydrochloride, benzatropine, orphenadrine, procyclidine

Mechanism of action and effects
Drugs that block central muscarinic receptors (Ch. 4) restore the balance between cholinergic and dopaminergic activity. They have little effect on bradykinesia, and are less effective than levodopa for treating tremor and rigidity.

Pharmacokinetics
Most antimuscarinic drugs are fairly well absorbed from the gut, and undergo extensive hepatic metabolism with intermediate to long half-lives. High lipid solubility ensures transfer across the blood–brain barrier.

Unwanted effects
These are predictable and a result of blockade of peripheral muscarinic receptors (Ch. 4). Reduced saliva production can be helpful in some parkinsonian patients, in whom sialorrhoea is a problem. Blockade of CNS muscarinic receptors can produce confusion in the elderly.

Management of Parkinson's disease and parkinsonian syndromes

Treatment is usually witheld in Parkinson's disease until symptoms become troublesome. Levodopa (with a peripheral decarboxylase inhibitor) is still widely used for treatment of idiopathic Parkinson's disease, and is particularly useful for reducing bradykinesia. A useful clinical response is achieved in about 70% of those with idiopathic Parkinson's disease, whereas, in contrast, drug-induced parkinsonism responds poorly. Frequent doses of levodopa may be needed, especially in advanced disease, to prevent the response 'wearing off'. There is increasing reluctance to use levodopa in the early stages of Parkinson's disease. It is possible that pulsatile dopaminergic stimulation produced by oral doses of levodopa, with its short half-life, may increase the risk of dykinesias developing later in treatment. For this reason, early disease is often treated with amantadine or selegiline, changing to a dopamine receptor agonist when the symptoms become more severe. There is significantly less risk of response fluctuation to levodopa or of dyskinesias later in therapy when a dopamine receptor agonist is used in preference to levodopa as initial treatment.

Levodopa is still preferred to a dopamine receptor agonist for older people with Parkinson's disease (over 65 years) or those with cognitive impairment, because of its lower propensity to cause confusion. Combinations of drugs are often necessary in advanced disease, but unwanted effects can be troublesome.

Motor complications with levodopa can occur immediately on starting treatment, but become progressively more likely with prolonged use. They can be extremely disabling, and involve a change from a long-duration response to levodopa to a short-duration response. The duration of symptomatic benefit after each dose may be reduced ('wearing off'), the dose may take longer to work ('delayed on') or it may sometimes fail to produce any improvement ('no on'). Treatment strategies aim to provide more stable plasma concentrations of levodopa, and include combining levodopa with an MAO-B inhibitor such as selegiline, or with a COMT inhibitor such as entacapone. Alternatively, a dopaminergic receptor agonist could be added. Poor responses to individual doses of levodopa may be due to interference with absorption by a high protein meal or by delayed gastric emptying, and can be improved by taking the drug before meals. The rapid action of subcutaneous apomorphine can be invaluable to abort the 'off' state, but it is highly emetogenic; this can be prevented by domperidone, a dopamine receptor blocker that does not cross the blood–brain barrier (Ch. 32). Domperidone should be taken 30 min before apomorphine, but it is often necessary to 'load' with domperidone for 24 h before starting apomorphine. The 'on–off' phenomenon with rapid swings between severe bradykinesia and toxic dyskinesias should be treated by a reduction in total levodopa dosage as well as using the above strategies. Amantidine can be helpful to reduce levodopa-associated dyskinesias. High-frequency bilateral stimulation of the subthalamic nuclei is effective for those who respond to levodopa but continue to have marked motor complications despite optimising therapy. It is used as an alternative to ablation therapy since it allows the clinician to vary the site and area of the stimulation with time.

Antimuscarinic agents are rarely used, but may be given for tremor that responds inadequately to levodopa. They can also be helpful in reducing excessive salivation.

Symptomatic treatment for a variety of associated symptoms may be necessary in Parkinson's disease. These include treatment of autonomic symptoms such as postural hypotension, vomiting, constipation, urinary frequency and impotence. Parkinsonian psychosis should be treated with an atypical antipsychotic drug (Ch. 21).

Drugs improve symptoms and quality of life in idiopathic Parkinson's disease, but there is little evidence that they alter the underlying rate of neuronal degeneration. Levodopa therapy increases life expectancy, probably by reducing complications. Several studies are underway to look at a potential neuroprotective effect of dopamine receptor agonists. Other neuroprotective strategies, such as with antioxidants or glutamate receptor blocking agents, have so far proved disappointing.

In advanced Parkinson's disease, surgical treatment is sometimes advocated. Severe tremor may respond to stereotactic thalamotomy or pallidotomy. Pallidotomy can also be helpful for severe dyskinesias.

Parkinsonism resulting from antipsychotic drug therapy responds best to drug withdrawal. If this is not possible, then an atypical antipsychotic drug should be used and an antimuscarinic drug given for residual symptoms.

Other involuntary movement disorders (dyskinesias)

Dyskinesias are abnormal involuntary movement disorders that can present in several ways.

- Tremor is a rhythmic sinusoidal movement caused by repetitive muscle contractions. It may be an exaggeration of the normal physiological tremor, or an abnormal movement such as seen in Parkinson's disease.
- Akathisia is a compulsive need to move, often in stereotyped patterns.
- Chorea is irregular, unpredictable, jerky and non-stereotyped movement that involves several different parts of the body.
- Myoclonus is rapid shock-like movements that are often repetitive.
- Tics are rapid repetitive movements that can sometimes be voluntarily controlled with difficulty for short periods.
- Dystonias are sustained spasms of muscle contraction that distort a part of the body into a dystonic posture. The dystonia is often exaggerated by voluntary movement. Examples include spasmodic torticollis (twisted neck) and oculogyric crisis.

Movement disorders have numerous causes, and can be precipitated by drug therapy. For example, a tremor can be caused by lithium, sodium valproate, tricyclic antidepressants, and sympathomimetics. Antipsychotic drugs (Ch. 21) are associated with a wide variety of movement disorders, ranging from acute dystonia to akathisia, and tardive dyskinesias (involving choreodystonic movements often of the face and mouth).

Some movement disorders have a genetic origin. One such is Huntington's chorea, an autosomal dominant hereditary disease that presents in adult life with progressive impairment of motor coordination, bizarre limb movements and dementia. The pathology is a loss of GABA inhibitory neurons within the neostriatum,

which connect with the substantia nigra. There is a consequent reduction of inhibitory activity on dopaminergic cells in the substantia nigra and cells in the globus pallidus. Therefore, these cells generate uncoordinated discharges that produce bursts of excess motor activity.

Drug treatment

Tetrabenazine

Mechanism of action
Tetrabenazine produces selective monoamine depletion from neurons in the CNS. Storage vesicles become leaky and the released contents are degraded by MAO.

Pharmacokinetics
Tetrabenazine has a low oral bioavailability. It is extensively metabolised by first-pass metabolism in the liver to an active derivative. The half-life is intermediate.

Unwanted effects
- drowsiness
- postural hypotension
- depression
- dysphagia, which may be caused by extrapyramidal dysfunction.

Management of dyskinesias

Treatment options depend on the cause. Some common strategies are listed below.

- Cessation of the provoking drug. Symptoms may initially be exacerbated but usually settle. Withdrawal dyskinesias usually respond to gradual drug discontinuation. Tardive dyskinesias associated with antipsychotic treatment may become worse on drug withdrawal, then slowly improve over many months.
- Exaggerated physiological tremor (e.g. anxiety tremor or tremor of thyrotoxicosis) may respond to a non-selective β-adrenoceptor antagonist such as propranolol (Ch. 8). Benign essential tremor is an action tremor that may benefit from a β-adrenoceptor antagonist or from primidone (Ch. 23). Gabapentin is an alternative second-line treatment (Ch. 23).
- Tetrabenazine is sometimes effective for treatment of choreiform movements.
- Many acute dystonias will respond to an antimuscarinic drug such as trihexyphenidyl given orally, or benzatropine given by intramuscular or intravenous injection for more severe symptoms.

- Enhanced inhibitory GABA neurotransmitter activity with baclofen (see below), sodium valproate or clonazepam (Ch. 23) may help some dystonias.
- Botulinum toxin (Ch. 27), which impairs acetylcholine release from nerve endings in the neuromuscular junction, can be injected into dystonic muscles to provide temporary relief. Spread of the paralytic effect to adjacent muscles can cause problems; for example, dysphagia after injection of neck muscles for torticollis. There are two types of botulinum toxin; some people who are refractory to type A may respond to type B.

Spasticity

Spasticity is a state of sustained muscle tone or tension which is often associated with an increase in stretch reflexes. The increase in muscle tone can arise from continued spinal reflex activity in the absence of inhibitory input from the motor cortex, such as can result from a stroke or in multiple sclerosis. Spasticity in skeletal muscles is often associated with partial or complete loss of voluntary movement and can produce painful and deforming contractures. Skeletal muscle relaxants are sometimes used for treatment of spasticity. The primary sites of action of these agents are the spinal reflexes or the release of Ca^{2+} in the muscle fibre, rather than the neuromuscular junction. Drugs that block the neuromuscular junction (Ch. 27) are not used to treat spasticity, because their main effect would probably be a further loss of voluntary movement.

Drugs for spasticity

Diazepam

Diazepam (and other benzodiazepines) enhance spinal inhibitory pathways by facilitating GABA-mediated opening of Cl^- channels (Ch. 20). The main disadvantage is sedation, as a result of inhibitory activity in higher centres at the doses necessary for a spasmolytic action.

Baclofen

Mechanism of action

Baclofen is an analogue of GABA that inhibits excitatory activity at mono- and polysynaptic reflexes at the spinal level. It binds stereoselectively to, and is an agonist at, $GABA_B$ receptors. This is believed to increase presynaptic inhibition of reflex pathways by reducing presynaptic Ca^{2+} influx and thus reducing excitatory neurotransmitter release. Baclofen also has an analgesic action, probably by inhibition of the release of substance P.

Pharmacokinetics

Baclofen is absorbed rapidly from the gastrointestinal tract. It has a short half-life and is eliminated largely unchanged in the urine. It can be given by intrathecal infusion using an implantable pump if severe spasticity is resistant to oral therapy.

Unwanted effects

- sedation and drowsiness
- muscle hypotonia
- nausea
- various CNS effects (e.g. lightheadedness, confusion, dizziness, ataxia and headache)
- hallucinations or other psychiatric disturbance
- hyperactivity, autonomic dysfunction and convulsions can be precipitated by sudden withdrawal.

Tizanidine

Mechanisms of action

Tizanidine is an α_2-adrenoceptor agonist that increases presynaptic inhibition of motor neurons in the spinal cord via descending noradrenergic pathways. Inhibition is greatest in polysynaptic rather than monosynaptic pathways. Tizanidine has only 10% of the antihypertensive activity of the α_2-adrenoceptor agonist clonidine.

Pharmacokinetics

Tizanidine is well absorbed from the gut but undergoes extensive first-pass metabolism in the liver. Its elimination half-life is short.

Unwanted effects

These are mainly dose-related, and can be minimised by slow dose titration.

- dry mouth
- drowsiness and fatigue
- dizziness
- gastrointestinal disturbances
- increased liver enzymes and, occasionally, acute hepatitis.

Dantrolene

Mechanism of action and uses

Dantrolene inhibits the release of Ca^{2+} from the sarcoplasmic reticulum of skeletal muscles, and uncouples muscle excitation from activation of the contractile apparatus. Dantrolene is also used for the treatment of malignant hyperthermia (Ch. 17) and as an adjunctive treatment in neuroleptic malignant syndrome (Ch. 21).

Pharmacokinetics

Dantrolene is slowly absorbed from the gut and can also be given by intramuscular or slow intravenous injection.

It is metabolised in the liver and has a variable and unpredictable half-life, which is short in some individuals and long in others.

Unwanted effects

- drowsiness, dizziness, weakness and malaise (usually transient)
- anorexia, nausea or diarrhoea
- headache
- dose-related risk of hepatitis.

Management of spasticity

Muscle hypotonia is a common problem in the drug therapy of spasticity. Mild spasticity may be useful, since the increased tone provides support for a weak limb, and should not be treated with drugs. Excessive spasticity following a stroke is most effectively prevented by adequate physiotherapy. Drug therapy can be useful for deforming or painful spasticity, particularly if the person is not ambulant. In severe spasticity, intramuscular injection of botulinum toxin (see above, and Ch. 27) can be helpful for up to 3 months.

FURTHER READING

Parkinson's disease

Djaldetti R, Melamed E (2002) New drugs in the future treatment of Parkinson's disease. *J Neurol* 249(suppl 2), 30–35

Jellinger KA (2002) Recent developments in the pathology of Parkinson's disease. *J Neural Transm Suppl* 62, 347–376

Korczyn AD, Nussbaum M (2002) Emerging therapies in the pharmacological treatment of Parkinson's disease *Drugs* 62, 775–786

Lang AE, Lozano AM (1998) Parkinson's disease. Part 1 and Part 2. *N Engl J Med* 339, 1130–1143

Samil A, Nutt JG, Ransom BR (2004) Parkinson's disease. *Lancet* 363, 1783–1793

Schapira AHV, Olanow CW (2004) Neuroprotection in Parkinson disease: mysteries, myths and misconceptions. *JAMA* 291, 358–364

Siderowf A, Stern M (2003) Update on Parkinson disease. *Ann Intern Med* 138, 651–658

Tanner CM (2000) Dopamine agonists in early therapy for Parkinson disease. *JAMA* 284, 1971–1973

Tintner R, Jankovic J (2002) Treatment options for Parkinson's disease. *Curr Opin Neurol* 15, 467–476

Dyskinesias and dystonias

Blanchet PJ (2003) Antipsychotic drug-induced movement disorders. *Can J Neurol Sci* 30(suppl 1), S101–S107

Klein C, Ozelius LJ (2002) Dystonia: clinical features, genetics, and treatment. *Curr Opin Neurol* 15, 491–497

Louis ED (2001) Essential tremor. *N Engl J Med* 345, 887–891

Shale H, Tanner C (1996) Pharmacological options for the management of dyskinesias. *Drugs* 52, 849–860

van Harten PN, Hoek HW, Kahn RS (1999) Acute dystonia induced by drug treatment. *BMJ* 319, 623–626

Self-assessment

In questions 1–4, the first statement, in italics, is true. Are the accompanying statements also true?

1. *In Parkinson's disease, there is abnormally reduced dopaminergic transmission which results in overexpression of GABAergic, glutamatergic and cholinergic transmission.*

   a. Symptoms of Parkinson's disease only become apparent when approximately 25% of dopaminergic neurons have been lost.
   b. Glutamate receptor antagonists are being investigated for use in Parkinson's disease.
   c. Levodopa has a long half-life.

2. *In people with young-onset disease (below 40 years of age), treatment with levodopa will usually lead to complications such as dyskinesias and on/off fluctuations after about 5 years.*

   a. In very early Parkinson's disease, ropinirole is as effective as levodopa.
   b. Antimuscarinic drugs such as trihexyphenidyl have a low incidence of unwanted effects.

3. *The motor complications associated with long-term use of levodopa may be helped by reducing the dosage and increasing the frequency of administration.*

   a. Bromocriptine is a potent agonist at dopamine (D_2) receptors.
   b. Some of the movement disorder in Parkinson's disease arises from abnormalities in non-dopaminergic innervated areas of the brain.
   c. The chemoreceptor trigger zone (CTZ) is stimulated by peripheral dopamine, as the CTZ lies outside the blood–brain barrier.
   d. The monoamine oxidase inhibitor (MAOI) selegiline causes the 'cheese' reaction with ingestion of tyramine-containing foods.
   e. Entacapone is a direct-acting dopamine receptor agonist.

4. *Dantrolene is useful in spasticity as it reduces the Ca^{2+} release that contributes to contraction of skeletal muscle.*

   a. Baclofen enhances muscle spasticity.
   b. Botulinum toxin has a duration of action of up to 3 months.

5. A number of drugs are used for the treatment of Parkinson's disease. Which one of the following is a true statement about the properties of these drugs?

   A. Dysfunction in both dopaminergic and cholinergic transmission occurs in Parkinson's disease.
   B. Selegiline is a selective MAO-A inhibitor used for Parkinson's disease.
   C. More than 50% of administered levodopa enters the brain unaltered.
   D. Currently used drugs for parkinsonism are mainly potent stimulators of D_1 receptors.
   E. Systemically absorbed carbidopa is an effective CNS dopamine decarboxylase inhibitor.

6. Case history 1 questions

A 75-year-old woman had been suffering from progressive symptoms of Parkinson's disease for 5 years. From the outset she had been treated continuously with levodopa, but problems had developed in controlling the symptoms with this drug.
---

   a. What is the cause of Parkinson's disease?
   b. What symptoms is this woman likely to have?
   c. Levodopa was given as co-beneldopa. What are the benefits of this formulation compared with levodopa alone?
   d. What difficulties can arise in controlling symptoms with levodopa in the early stages and later stages of treatment, and what changes in therapy could then be considered?
   e. What precautions need to be followed if this woman started to take vitamin supplements?
   f. Could a β-adrenoceptor antagonist be of use as part of this woman's treatment?
   g. Can any treatment protect against progressive deterioration in Parkinson's disease?

7. Case history 2 questions

A married man aged 40 years was newly diagnosed as suffering from Parkinson's disease. His symptoms were tremor, bradykinesia, hypokinesia and rigidity, which were sufficiently mild that he was still able to carry out his work and pursue his hobbies. He was a security guard and had previously fought as a relatively unsuccessful professional boxer for 10 years, before retiring from the ring at the age of 35.

Suggest possible treatment regimens for this man, with reasons for your suggestions.

The answers are provided on pages 724–726.

Drug compendium

Drugs used for extrapyramidal movement disorders and spasticity

Drug	Half-life (h)	Elimination	Comments
Drugs used for Parkinson's disease			Given orally unless otherwise stated
Dopaminergic drugs			
Amantadine	10–15	Renal	Complete oral bioavailability: renal clearance (400 ml min^{-1}) indicates extensive tubular secretion; half-life increases in elderly in relation to changes in renal function
Apomorphine	0.5–1	Metabolism	D_2 agonist; given by subcutaneous injection; not effective orally, probably as a result of presystemic metabolism; undergoes hepatic N-demethylation and also sulphate conjugation to inactive metabolites
Benserazide	No data	Metabolism	Peripheral decarboxylase inhibitor used in combination with levodopa (co-beneldopa); incomplete absorption; metabolised by hydrolysis
Bromocriptine	3	Metabolism	D_2 agonist; low oral bioavailability (about 10%) as a result of poor absorption and first-pass metabolism; extensively metabolised by hydrolysis to inactive products
Cabergoline	60–90	Metabolism (+ renal)	D_2 agonist; used as an adjunct to levodopa; hydrolysed to metabolites that are excreted in bile and urine
Carbidopa	1–3	Renal + metabolism	Peripheral decarboxylase inhibitor used in combination with levodopa (co-careldopa); variable oral bioavailability (40–90%); limited metabolism
Entacapone	2–3	Metabolism	Catechol-O-methyltransferase inhibitor; oral bioavailability is about 30–50%; metabolised by glucuronidation
Levodopa	1.3	Metabolism	Precursor of dopamine; normally given with carbidopa or benserazide to reduce first-pass metabolism and increase duration of action; metabolised by dopa decarboxylase to dopamine and by O-methylation
Lisuride	2–3	Metabolism	D_2 agonist; low oral bioavailability (about 10%) with large inter-patient variability because of first-pass metabolism; metabolised to inactive products
Pergolide	27	Metabolism	Agonist at both D_2 and D_1 receptors; rapid absorption but high first-pass metabolism; converted to numerous metabolites, some of which retain activity
Pramipexole	8–12	Renal	Selective for D_3 receptors; high oral bioavailability; eliminated by renal tubular secretion and filtration
Ropinirole	6	Metabolism (+ renal)	Agonist at D_3 and D_2 receptors; bioavailability is about 50%; main metabolic pathway is oxidation by CYP1A2 in the liver
Selegiline	1–2	Metabolism	An irreversible inhibitor of monoamine oxidase type B; high bioavailability; metabolised in the liver to an active desmethyl metabolite and amfetamine analogues

continued

Drugs used for extrapyramidal movement disorders and spasticity *(continued)*

Drug	Half-life (h)	Elimination	Comments
Antimuscarinic drugs			
Benzatropine	No data	Metabolism	Given orally, or by intramuscular or intravenous injection; few data available; numerous metabolites found in rat studies
Orphenadrine	14–16	Metabolism (+ renal)	Given orally; bioavailability is about 70%; eliminated by P450-mediated oxidation
Procyclidine	13	Metabolism	Given orally, or by intramuscular or intravenous injection; about 75% oral bioavailability; eliminated by oxidation and conjugation
Trihexyphenidyl hydrochloride	3–7	Metabolism + renal	High bioavailability; 56% recovered as hydroxy metabolites within 3 days
Drugs used for essential tremor, chorea, tics and related disorders			Given orally unless otherwise indicated
Chlorpromazine	–	–	See Ch. 21
Clonidine	–	–	See Ch. 6
Haloperidol	–	–	See Ch. 21
Pimozide	–	–	See Ch. 21
Piracetam	4	Renal	Mostly eliminated by glomerular filtration; non-renal elimination (route undefined) accounts for about 30% of elimination
Primidone	–	–	See Ch. 23
Propranolol	–	–	See Ch. 8
Riluzole	12	Metabolism	Used only in motor neuron disease; modulates the release of glutamate; bioavailability is 60%; oxidised by CYP1A2 with wide intersubject variations
Sulpiride	–	–	See Ch. 21
Tetrabenazine	7	Metabolism	Low oral bioavailability (5%); response is probably caused by a metabolite, dihydrotetrabenazine, which is as active as the parent drug and has a longer half-life (12 h)
Trihexyphenidyl	–	–	See above
Drugs used for spasticity			Given orally except where indicated
Baclofen	3–4	Renal + metabolism	Good oral bioavailability (95%); good oral absorption; about 15% undergoes deamination in the liver and the remainder is eliminated by the kidneys
Dantrolene	4–24	Metabolism	Good oral bioavailability (40–80%); metabolites are largely inactive and eliminated in urine and bile

continued

Drug compendium

Drugs used for extrapyramidal movement disorders and spasticity *(continued)*

Drug	Half-life (h)	Elimination	Comments
Drugs used for spasticity *(continued)*			Given orally except where indicated
Diazepam	–	–	See Ch. 20
Tizanidine	2–4	Metabolism	α_2-Adrenoceptor agonist; oral bioavailability is about 20–40% because of first-pass metabolism; metabolites are inactive
Other muscle relaxants			
Botulinum A toxin	–	–	Specialist use; given by local intramuscular injection; onset and duration of action depend on the clinical use of the drug
Botulinum B toxin	–	–	Specialist use; given by local intramuscular injection; onset and duration of action depend on the clinical use of the drug
Carisoprodol	6–8	Metabolism	Active orally; rapid absorption; numerous metabolites, including meprobamate, formed by polymorphic CYP2C19
Methocarbamol	1–2	Metabolism	Active orally; rapid and complete absorption; extensively metabolised in the liver (more published data for race horses than for humans!)

25 Other neurological disorders: multiple sclerosis, motor neuron disease and Guillain–Barré syndrome

Multiple sclerosis

Multiple sclerosis is characterised by an immunologically mediated inflammatory demyelination of the central nervous system (CNS). The blood–brain barrier is breached by T- and B-lymphocytes and macrophages. T-cells secrete inflammatory cytokines, such as interleukin-4 (IL-4) and interferon-γ, and release chemokines and matrix metalloproteinases. These cytokines activate macrophages that selectively attack myelin antigens and destroy the myelin sheath around nerves. The destruction is enhanced by B-cell-derived autoantibodies. The immunological damage also affects oligodendrocytes, the cells that produce the myelin. The end result is generation of demyelinated plaques that disturb normal conduction of electrical impulses in the CNS. The long-term disability is mainly due to axonal damage, which occurs most extensively in the first year after disease onset. Demyelination may predispose axons to cytotoxicity from upregulation of Ca^{2+} channels, or to secondary injury from cytotoxic T-lymphocytes. Axon degeneration may also be enhanced by oligodendrocyte dysfunction and failure to remyelinate the nerves. Some T-lymphocytes found in the inflammatory lesions have neuroprotective or neurotrophic properties, but it is not yet possible to selectively encourage the action of these potentially restorative cell populations.

The cause of multiple sclerosis is unknown, but it may result from exposure of genetically susceptible individuals to a virus with an antigenic structure similar to myelin basic protein (molecular mimicry). Multiple sclerosis usually begins in the second or third decades of life and in 80% of cases presents with relapsing and remitting symptoms and signs of multifocal CNS dysfunction. Such episodes must be separated in both time and place (more than one episode in more than one area of the brain) to secure the diagnosis. The usual clinical course is initially one of stepwise, eventually progressive deterioration. The areas of the CNS most often involved are the optic nerves, spinal cord, brainstem and cerebellum. Common presentations are optic neuritis, spasticity, weakness, and bladder and bowel involvement.

Drug treatment

There is no proven cure for multiple sclerosis, but drugs can be used to reduce the symptoms. There is increasing evidence that modulating the immune response as early as possible in the disease process may reduce disability.

- Corticosteroids (Ch. 44) are often used to treat an acute relapse (e.g. intravenous methylprednisolone for 3 days or oral prednisolone for 3 weeks). They probably shorten the duration of an attack but have no effect on long-term outcome.
- Interferon-β can reduce the inflammatory response in an acute attack and reduce the frequency of relapses. Proposed mechanisms include downregulation of the production of inflammatory interferon-γ, and enhanced activity of suppressor T-cells. It is given by intramuscular or subcutaneous injection. About 50% of people who have a single demyelinating episode will develop multiple sclerosis. The use of interferon-β at this first episode significantly reduces the risk of developing multiple sclerosis at 2 years after treatment. Otherwise, the use of interferon-β is reserved for ambulant individuals who have had at least two attacks of relapsing and remitting disease over the previous 2 or 3 years. However, although the drug may reduce relapses, it does not prevent ultimate disability, and although it is licensed for ambulatory people with relapsing–remitting disease who have had at least two clinical relapses in the previous 2–3 years, it is not recommended by the National Institute for Clinical Excellence (NICE). (NICE guidelines issued in 2002 were on balance of cost and effectiveness, and were unable to recommend the use of either interferon-β or glatiramer acetate.) The most frequent unwanted effects are influenza-like symptoms, which occur commonly and may persist for several months, and pain or ulceration at the injection site.

- Glatiramer acetate is a synthetic polypeptide immunomodulator that has some structural similarities to myelin basic protein. It may produce immunological tolerance and is used for reducing relapses. Like interferon-β, it does not alter long-term disability and, although it is licensed for ambulatory individuals with relapsing–remitting disease who have had at least one clinical relapse in the previous 2 years, it is not recommended by NICE (see above). Unwanted effects include flushing, chest pain, palpitation and dyspnoea immediately after injection, and reactions at the injection site.
- Mitoxantrone, a cytotoxic antibiotic (Ch. 52), has shown encouraging results in reducing disability when given at 3-monthly intervals. These results require confirmation.
- Natalizumab is a monoclonal antibody that is a selective adhesion molecule inhibitor. In inhibits alpha-4 integrin and prevents T-cells from crossing the blood–brain barrier. It reduces relapse rate in relapsing multiple sclerosis.
- Symptomatic treatment of spasticity may be necessary, for example with baclofen (Ch. 24).

Motor neuron disease

Motor neuron disease is an uncommon, rapidly progressive disorder of motor neurons that occurs most often in middle-aged males. It leads to both upper motor neuron signs (hypertonia, impaired fine movement and hyperreflexia) and lower motor neuron signs (fasciculations, muscle cramps, weakness and muscle atrophy). Death from respiratory failure usually occurs 3–5 years from the onset of symptoms. The pathophysiology involves neuronal loss but the cause is unknown; an autoimmune origin is unlikely, since treatment with immunosuppressive drugs is ineffective. There is evidence of excessive activation of excitatory glutamate receptors in the CNS. Consequent prolonged depolarisation of motor neurons may lead to intracellular Ca^{2+} overload, mitochondrial damage and cell death (excitotoxicity). Oxidative stress from excessive free radical generation may be important. Mutations in the genes coding for superoxide dismutase, the cytosolic enzyme that protects against oxidative damage, have been described in motor neuron disease. A third mechanism of neuronal death, accelerated apoptosis, may also be involved.

Drug treatment

Riluzole is the only available agent that alters the course of the disease. This crosses the blood–brain barrier and may block the release of glutamate, and is also an indirect antagonist at glutamate NMDA (*N*-methyl-D-aspartate) receptors; thus, it may inhibit glutamate-induced excitotoxicity. Treatment does not arrest the disease but may slow its progression to a modest extent, improving survival by an average of 3 months after 18 months of treatment. Unwanted effects of riluzole include lethargy, nausea and dizziness.

Physiotherapists can help with advice on posture and exercise early in the disease, and later with passive movement to reduce musculoskeletal pain. Symptomatic treatment is often necessary for pain, breathlessness or dysphagia.

Guillain–Barré syndrome

Guillain–Barré syndrome is an autoimmune demyelinating disorder, probably triggered by a bacterial or viral infection. It only affects the peripheral nervous system and it produces rapid onset of limb weakness with loss of tendon reflexes, few sensory signs, and autonomic dysfunction. About 10% of those affected die in the acute illness and a further 10% are left with severe long-term disability.

The pathological process involves acute lymphocytic infiltration into peripheral nerves and spinal roots, with both T-lymphocytes and autoantibodies contributing to demyelination. In those with long-term disability, macrophages invade the nerve in the spinal root and cause axonal degeneration.

Management

There are several aspects to the management of Guillain–Barré syndrome.

- Supportive treatment may be life-saving, and is the cornerstone of management. For example, ventilatory support is necessary for respiratory muscle weakness or paralysis. Haemodynamic disturbance, including significant bradycardia and asystole, can result from autonomic involvement and may require cardiovascular support. Prophylaxis for deep venous thrombosis with subcutaneous heparin (Ch. 11) should be used. Pain may require analgesia and can be reduced by passive limb movement.
- Plasma exchange, when used within 2 weeks of the onset of symptoms, improves the long-term outcome. The benefit is probably due to removal of autoantibodies.
- High-dose intravenous immunoglobulin (IgG) is equally effective as plasma exchange, and is now the preferred treatment. Unwanted effects include malaise, chills and fever.
- Corticosteroids are of no benefit, either alone or in combination with immunoglobulin.

FURTHER READING

Dib M (2003) Amyotrophic lateral sclerosis. Progress and prospects for treatment. *Drugs* 63, 289–310

Howard RS, Orrell RW (2002) Management of motor neurone disease. *Postgrad Med J* 78, 736–741

Kieseier BC, Hartung H-P (2003) Multiple paradigm shifts in multiple sclerosis. *Curr Opin Neurol* 16, 247–252

National Institute for Clinical Excellence. Full guidance on the use of beta interferon and glatiramer acetate in multiple sclerosis. http://www.nice.org.uk/page.aspx?o=27635 (Issue reviewed 2004)

Noseworthy JH (2003) Management of multiple sclerosis: current trials and future options. *Curr Opin Neurol* 16, 289–297

Noseworthy JH, Lucchinetti C, Rodriguez M, Weinshenker BG (2000) Multiple sclerosis. *N Engl J Med* 343, 938–952

Shaw PJ (1999) Motor neuron disease. *BMJ* 318, 1118–1121

Tselis AC, Lisak RP (1999) Multiple sclerosis. A therapeutic update. *Arch Neurol* 56, 277–280

Winer JB (2002) Treatment of Guillain–Barré syndrome. *Q J Med* 95, 717–721

Self-assessment

1. Are the following statements true or false?

   a. Treatment with interferon-γ is of benefit in reducing relapses in multiple sclerosis.
   b. Multiple sclerosis is characterised in the early years by a steady progressive worsening of symptoms in the majority of people.
   c. Glutamate can cause neuronal damage.
   d. Riluzole is of benefit in motor neuron disease by blocking the release of gamma-aminobutyric acid (GABA).
   e. In multiple sclerosis, prednisolone does not shorten the duration of relapses.

2. The following statements relate to the treatment of multiple sclerosis. Choose the one <u>most appropriate</u> statement.

   A. Beta-interferon causes influenza-like symptoms in a small percentage of those who receive it.
   B. Expert opinion does not recommend glatiramer acetate as a first-line drug for use in all people with multiple sclerosis.
   C. Glatiramer acetate causes no unwanted effects following injection.
   D. Corticosteroid treatment is of benefit in reducing the progression of multiple sclerosis.
   E. Neuronal conduction is unimpaired in multiple sclerosis.

The answers are provided on page 726.

Self-assessment questions

Drug compendium

Drugs used in multiple sclerosis, motor neuron disease and Guillain–Barré syndrome

Drug	Half-life (h)	Elimination	Comments
Baclofen	3–4	Renal + metabolism	May be of benefit for spasticity in people with multiple sclerosis (Ch. 24)
Corticosteroids	–	–	Corticosteroids such as methylprednisolone or prednisolone may be of benefit for acute relapse in people with multiple sclerosis – see Ch. 44
Glatiramer acetate	?	Metabolism	Given by subcutaneous injection to patients with multiple sclerosis; not recommended by NICE[a]; hydrolysed locally at the site of injection and absorbed parent compound and fragments enter the blood and lymphatic system; metabolised by proteolysis
Interferon beta	2–4	Metabolism	Given by subcutaneous or intramuscular injection to people with multiple sclerosis; rapid elimination is because of tissue uptake and catabolism (especially in the liver); not recommended by NICE[a]; metabolised by proteolysis
Mitoxantrone	4–220	Renal + metabolism	A cytotoxic antibiotic given by intravenous infusion for the treatment of cancer (Ch. 52); not currently licensed for multiple sclerosis
Riluzole	12	Metabolism	A glutamate antagonist used for motor neuron disease; given orally; high oral bioavailability (90%); eliminated by hepatic CYP1A2-mediated oxidation

[a]The National Institute for Clinical Excellence guidelines issued in 2002 did not recommend its use on balance of cost and effectiveness.

26

Migraine

Headache has many causes (Box 26.1). Tension is by far the most common primary cause, accounting for about two-thirds of cases, and migraine is the second most frequent cause. When headache is prolonged or recurrent, secondary causes may need to be excluded by a full history and examination for associated neurological symptoms and signs.

Migraine is an episodic headache typically lasting 4–72 h. Diagnostic features are listed in Box 26.2. These are the only symptoms in the majority of migraineurs. However, in up to one-third, the headache is preceded or accompanied by focal neurological symptoms (migraine with aura), which often consist of visual disturbances but occasionally comprise more severe focal neurological episodes.

Pathogenesis of migraine

The pathogenesis of migraine, and other related types of headache, is as yet imperfectly understood but involves neuronal and vascular dysfunction (Fig. 26.1). The intracranial structures that can produce pain are the blood vessels and the dura mater, and pain can also arise from extracranial blood vessels such as the frontal branch of the superficial temporal artery. Intracranial blood vessels are innervated by the ophthalmic division of the trigeminal nerve. Efferent innervation includes vasoconstrictor sympathetic nerves, mediated by co-transmission of noradrenergic, peptidergic (neuropeptide Y) and purinergic (adenosine triphosphate [ATP]) neuro-transmission. Vasodilator parasympathetic innervation is mediated by vasoactive intestinal peptide, other neuropeptides and possibly nitric oxide. Other neuronal pathways utilising 5-hydroxytryptamine (5HT, serotonin) produce vasoconstriction by stimulation of $5HT_{1B}$ receptors and vasodilation by stimulating $5HT_2$ receptors.

The aura of migraine is caused by a slowly propagated wave of cortical depolarisation that transiently depresses spontaneous and evoked neuronal activity (cortical spreading depression). This wave is preceded by intense but brief neuronal excitation producing cortical hyperaemia, which may be responsible for the visual aura of flashing or jagged lights. The depressant wave is associated with vasoconstriction, which can produce focal neurological symptoms and signs. The generation of the aura and headache are probably parallel, independent processes activated by the migraine trigger.

Box 26.1

Causes of headache

Primary headache
   Tension-type headache
   Migraine
   Idiopathic stabbing headache
   Exertional headache
   Cluster headache

Secondary headache
   Systemic infection
   Head injury
   Drug-induced headache
   Vascular disorders
   Brain tumor

Box 26.2

Diagnostic features of migraine

Two or more of the following features:

● Unilateral pain
● Throbbing
● Aggravation on movement
● Pain of moderate or severe intensity

and one of the following:

● Nausea or vomiting
● Light or noise sensitivity (photophobia or phonophobia)

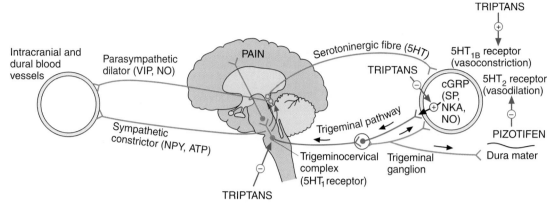

Fig. 26.1

Some factors associated with the genesis of migraine and putative sites of action of antimigraine drugs. The sequence and nature of neurogenic and vascular involvement in migraine are vigorously debated and may vary in different kinds of migraine-type headache. The trigeminal system (red) is activated by calcitonin gene-related peptide (cGRP). This transmitter is elevated in migraine in association with the pronounced blood vessel dilation. Antidromic stimulation (green) via the trigeminal ganglion, which has cGRP receptors, causes dilation and inflammation of blood vessels and dura mater. Bipolar activation of the trigeminal ganglion also stimulates the trigeminocervical complex (the trigeminal nucleus and C1, C2) and activates fibres responsible for pain, nausea and vomiting. The trigeminocervical complex is rich in $5HT_{1B/1D}$ receptors and their stimulation inhibits neurotransmission. 5-Hydroxytryptamine (5HT), substance P (SP), neurokinin A (NKA) and nitric oxide (NO) also play a role in these vascular and neurological phenomena. Parasympathetic outflow may also be stimulated. Triptans ($5HT_{1B/1D/1F}$ agonists) are thought to relieve the symptoms of migraine activity at presynaptic receptors, to inhibit cGRP release ($5HT_{1D}$ agonist) and inhibit vasodilation ($5HT_{1B}$ agonist). Serotoninergic fibres to blood vessels can also cause vasodilation by stimulating $5HT_2$ subtype receptors; this may explain the benefit of pizotifen, which blocks $5HT_2$ receptors. Some triptans (e.g. naratriptan) act on the trigeminocervical complex. ATP, adenosine triphosphate; NPY, neuropeptide Y; VIP, vasoactive intestinal peptide.

The primary defect in migraine is believed to be dysfunction of ion channels in aminergic pathways of the brainstem (the migraine generator). These pathways are responsible for sensory (mainly nociceptive) modulation of afferent nerves to cranial blood vessels and may initiate neurogenic vasodilation in the dural and extracranial vessels. Vasodilation in the dural meninges activates the trigeminal ganglion via the first (ophthalmic) division of the trigeminal nerve (the trigeminovascular pathway). The impulses are then relayed through the trigeminocervical complex (the trigeminal nucleus caudalis and the dorsal horns of C1 and C2 in the spinal cord to the brainstem), from where they are transmitted to the thalamus. Thalamic stimulation produces pain, nausea and vomiting. Pontine neurons in the brainstem link this pathway via a reflex parasympathetic vaso-dilator connection back to the dural vessels (Fig. 26.1).

When a migraine attack begins, activation of the trigeminovascular pathway and trigeminal nucleus results in antidromic release ('feed-forward' stimulation) of the vasodilator substance calcitonin gene-related peptide and substance P (and possibly neurokinin A and nitric oxide) from sensory C-fibre terminals. This results in dilation of dural blood vessels and neurogenic in-flammation. Neural activity in the brainstem potentiates the vasodilation by activating the parasympathetic vasodilator pathways to the meningeal vessels. The trigeminocervical complex is rich in $5HT_{1B/1D/1F}$ receptors and their stimulation (particularly $5HT_{1B}$ receptors) inhibits neurotransmission.

Drugs for migraine

Specific drugs for the acute migraine attack

Triptans

Examples: sumatriptan, naratriptan, zolmitriptan

Mechanisms of action and effects

The triptans are $5HT_{1B/1D}$ receptor agonists, with additional activity at $5HT_{1F}$ receptors that may contribute to their actions. Possible mechanisms of action are illustrated in Figure 26.1 and include:

- cranial vasoconstriction ($5HT_{1B}$)
- peripheral neuronal inhibition ($5HT_{1D}$)
- inhibition of the trigeminocervical complex ($5HT_{1B/1D/?1F}$).

Sumatriptan does not cross the blood–brain barrier. Naratriptan, zolmitriptan and other 'second-generation' triptans penetrate the blood–brain barrier and can directly inhibit excitability of the trigeminocervical complex in the brainstem. Triptans relieve both the pain and the nausea associated with migraine.

Pharmacokinetics

Absorption of sumatriptan from the gut is rapid but erratic, whereas second-generation triptans such as naratriptan and zolmitriptan have better absorption. Effective plasma concentrations are usually reached within 30 min. Sumatriptan is also available for subcutaneous injection or administration by nasal spray. Some triptans undergo first-pass metabolism by monoamine oxidase A (MAO-A); bioavailability varies from 15% for sumatriptan to 70% for naratriptan (which is not a substrate for MAO-A). Elimination is by hepatic metabolism via MAO-A and cytochrome P450, although 50% of naratriptan is excreted unchanged by the kidney. Sumatriptan and zolmitriptan have short half-lives; that of naratriptan is intermediate. Most migraineurs prefer oral treatment, but nasal or subcutaneous (sumatriptan only) administration relieves symptoms within 15 min. This can be more effective if there is nausea, since gastric stasis often delays oral drug absorption during a migraine attack.

Unwanted effects

The frequency and intensity of unwanted effects is highest after subcutaneous use of sumatriptan:

- tingling, paraesthesiae or sensation of warmth in the head, neck, chest and limbs
- dizziness or vertigo
- nausea or vomiting
- chest discomfort or pressure in up to 40% of users, which is probably not caused by myocardial ischaemia
- angina caused by coronary artery vasoconstriction ($5HT_{1B}$ receptors) if there is pre-existing coronary artery disease; such individuals should not take a triptan
- pain or irritation at the injection site, or in the nose after local use.

Ergotamine

Mechanism of action

Ergotamine probably has an antimigraine action similar to the triptans, stimulating $5HT_{1D}$ receptors. Unwanted effects arise from agonist activity at several other receptors, including α_1-adrenoceptors, and dopamine D_2 receptors in the chemoreceptor trigger zone (CTZ).

Pharmacokinetics

Oral administration is often accompanied by nausea, and it is better tolerated as a rectal suppository. Absorption is poor, erratic and delayed whichever route is chosen. Ergotamine undergoes extensive metabolism in the liver and has a short half-life. However, tight receptor binding produces a long duration of action.

Unwanted effects

- Nausea and vomiting are caused by dopaminergic stimulation at the CTZ (Ch. 32).
- Abdominal cramps and diarrhoea.
- Muscle cramps.
- Severe vasoconstriction is a result of α_1-adrenoceptor stimulation and can lead to peripheral gangrene (acute ergotism). Ergotamine should be avoided in known vascular disease (including ischaemic heart disease).
- Chronic intoxication with dependence can occur after prolonged use. Withdrawal then produces nausea and headache similar to an acute migraine attack. For this reason, ergotamine treatment should not be repeated at intervals of less than 4 days and should not be used more than twice a month.

Prophylactic drugs

Beta-adrenoceptor antagonists

Examples: propranolol, atenolol

Mechanism of action in migraine

Full details of the β-adrenoceptor antagonists are found in Chapter 5. In migraine, drugs with partial agonist activity that cause vasodilation (e.g. pindolol) are ineffective, suggesting that it is vasoconstriction that contributes to anti-migraine action.

Antiepileptic drugs

The mechanism of action of sodium valproate, gabapentin and topiramate in migraine is not well understood, and some other antiepileptics that have been studied are ineffective. It is possible that there are multiple mechanisms, one of which may be gamma-aminobutyric acid (GABA)-mediated suppression of neurotransmission through the trigeminocervical complex in the brainstem. Full details of these drugs are found in Chapter 23.

Amitriptiline

The mechanism of action in migraine is unknown. Several other antidepressants have been studied, but, with the possible exception of fluoxetine, are ineffective. Full details of amitriptiline are found in Chapter 22.

Pizotifen

Mechanism of action

Pizotifen is an antagonist at $5HT_2$ receptors, producing vasoconstriction of cranial arteries.

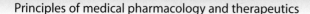

Pharmacokinetics

Oral absorption is almost complete and extensive metabolism occurs in the liver. The half-life of pizotifen is 26 h.

Unwanted effects

- appetite stimulation with weight gain (may be caused by enhanced insulin release)
- drowsiness.

Methysergide

Mechanism of action

Methysergide is similar to pizotifen, having $5HT_2$ antagonist activity and some additional partial agonist activity at $5HT_{1B/1D}$ receptors.

Pharmacokinetics

Oral absorption is complete, and methysergide undergoes extensive first-pass metabolism in the liver. It has an intermediate half-life.

Unwanted effects

- restless or painful legs
- retroperitoneal fibrosis with long-term use, producing ureteric compression, hydronephrosis and renal failure; this is reversible, but methysergide should be given for a maximum of 6 months, followed by a 1-month drug-free interval to avoid this complication.

Management of migraine

The acute attack

Withdrawal of possible triggers such as cheese, chocolate, citrus fruits or alcoholic drinks may reduce the frequency of attacks by up to 50%. The combined oral contraceptive pill is a potential exacerbating factor, but, by contrast, can be helpful for menstrual-related migraine.

For relief of a mild acute attack, simple analgesia – for example, with aspirin, paracetamol or a non-steroidal anti-inflammatory drug (NSAID) (Ch. 29) – may be sufficient. Nausea delays gastric emptying and frequently accompanies a migraine attack; absorption of the analgesic will be more rapid if an antiemetic such as metoclopramide or domperidone (Ch. 32) is given. If vomiting is prominent, rectal or intramuscular analgesia, for example with the NSAIDs diclofenac or naproxen, can be given. Analgesics are usually more effective when given early after the onset of pain. Opioid analgesics are not recommended as they are short-acting, produce dependence and frequent use can also promote 'analgesic headaches' (pain which appears as the effect of the drug wanes). Analgesic headaches are also more common with compound analgesics, especially those that contain caffeine.

If attacks are poorly controlled by standard therapies or are moderate to severe in intensity, a triptan is usually highly effective. It can relieve pain even if taken more than 4 h after the onset of an attack, but is less effective in those migraineurs who have developed cutaneous allodynia (Ch. 19) in the trigeminal nerve distribution in association with the headache. Subcutaneous sumatriptan is useful if a rapid response is required or if nausea precludes oral therapy. Headache recurs in more than 25% of those who take a triptan, and the risk of recurrence may be related to the half-life of the drug. Naratriptan has a longer half-life, and may have a lower recurrence rate than the other agents. Ergotamine can be used to treat acute attacks, and also has a place for treating relapse after use of a triptan. The risk of vasospasm and habituation means that ergotamine should be avoided in older persons (who may have cardiovascular disease) and in those with frequent attacks. For these reasons, and because of the frequency of other unwanted effects, ergotamine is now infrequently used.

Prophylaxis

Prophylaxis is usually recommended for people experiencing at least two attacks of migraine each month. Beta-adrenoceptor antagonists are widely held to be the best choice if there are no contraindications. The antiepileptic drugs sodium valproate and topiramate are effective alternatives. There is less consistent evidence for the use of gabapentin. The major disadvantage of these agents is the risk of teratogenicity in women of childbearing age. The acceptability of pizotifen is limited, especially in young women, by weight gain. Amitryptyline can be helpful for migraine as well as tension headache, but other antidepressants that have been studied are ineffective. Methysergide can be given provided there are brief drug-free periods. Less well-evaluated preventive treatments include the angiotensin receptor antagonist candesartan (Ch. 6), and botulinum toxin type A (Ch. 24) by injection into glabellar, frontalis and temporalis muscles, which produces benefit for up to 4 months.

The efficacy of all current prophylactic treatments is limited. Although the response to an individual drug class is unpredictable, only about half of all migraineurs can expect to have a 50% reduction in the frequency of attacks

FURTHER READING

Agostoni E, Frigerio R, Santoro P (2003) Antiepileptic drugs in the treatment of chronic headaches. *Neurol Sci* 249suppl 2), S128–S131

Ashkenazi A, Silberstein SD (2003) The evolving management of migraine. *Curr Opin Neurol* 16, 341–345

Cutrer FM (2001) Antiepileptic drugs: how they work in headache. *Headache* 41(suppl 1), S3–S10

Dahlöf C (2002) Integrating the triptans into clinical practice. *Curr Opin Neurol* 15, 317–322

Krymchantowski AV, Bigal ME, Moreira PF (2002) New and emerging prophylactic agents for migraine. *CNS Drugs* 16, 611–634

Montagna P (2004) The physiopathology of migraine: the contribution of genetics. *Neurol Sci.* 25 Suppl 3:S93–6

Rapoport AM, Bigal ME (2004) Preventive migraine therapy: what is new? *Neurol Sci.* Suppl 3:S177–85. Review

Silberstein SD (2004) Migraine. *Lancet* 363, 381–391

Snow V, Weiss K, Wall EM et al (2002) Pharmacologic management of acute attacks of migraine and prevention of migraine headache. *Ann Intern Med* 137, 840–849

Self-assessment

In the following questions, the first statement, in italics, is true. Are the accompanying statements also true?

1. *Both antagonists at $5HT_2$ receptors and agonists at $5HT_{1D}$ receptors are used for the treatment of migraine.*

   a. Ergotamine is used prophylactically for migraine.
   b. Sumatriptan is not of use for acute attacks of migraine as it is slow-acting.

2. *The contraceptive pill can enhance the frequency of migraine attacks in some women.* There is a large release of 5HT (possibly from platelets) in a migraine attack.

3. *Headache in migraine is thought to be caused by stimulation of sensory nerve endings in arteries.*

   a. Pizotifen is used prophylactically and inhibits $5HT_2$ receptors.
   b. Ergotamine is safe to use in ischaemic heart disease.
   c. Sumatriptan causes chest discomfort in 40% of people as a result of coronary vasoconstriction.
   d. Prophylactic treatment for migraine is highly effective.

4. *A variety of drugs such as tricyclic antidepressants, β-adrenoceptor antagonists and pizotifen may be useful in prophylaxis of migraine.* Where migraine is associated with vomiting, metoclopramide and paracetamol given together is a useful combination.

5. *Beta-adrenoceptor antagonists are widely used in the prophylaxis of migraine.* Dietary or stress factors play little part in the precipitation of migraine attacks.

The answers are provided on pages 726–727.

Drugs used in migraine

Drug	Half-life (h)	Elimination	Comments
Almotriptan	3–4	Metabolism + renal	5HT$_1$ agonist used in acute attacks; given orally; high oral bioavailability (70%); eliminated by oxidation via monoamine oxidase and P450 and also by renal tubular secretion
Amitriptiline	10–28	Metabolism	Used for prophylaxis; see Ch. 22
Antiepileptic drugs	–	–	Some antiepileptic drugs are used for prophylaxis; see Ch. 23
Beta-adrenoceptor antagonists	–	–	Some β-adrenoceptor antagonists are used for prophylaxis; see Ch. 8
Clonidine	20–25	Renal + metabolism	Used orally for prophylaxis but is not recommended; see Ch. 6
Dihydroergotamine	1–2	Metabolism	Very low oral bioavailability (1%); there is a terminal half-life of about 18 h, but this contributes minimally to elimination
Eletriptan	4–5	Metabolism + some renal	5HT$_1$ agonist used in acute attacks; given orally; good oral bioavailability (50%); metabolised by CYP3A4; a demethylated metabolite retains the activity and has a longer half-life (13 h) but contributes little to the overall response
Ergotamine	2	Metabolism	Given orally or as suppositories; very low oral bioavailability (2%); pathways of metabolism not defined
Frovatriptan	26	Metabolism	5HT$_1$ agonist used in acute attacks; given orally; fair oral bioavailability (20–30%); metabolised by CYP1A2
Isometheptene	?	Metabolism	Used orally for acute attacks; metabolised in animals but kinetic data are not available for humans
Methysergide	10	(Renal + metabolism)?	Used orally for prophylaxis but should only be administered under hospital supervision; rapid and complete absorption; extent and route of metabolism are poorly defined
Naratriptan	6	Metabolism + renal	5HT$_1$ agonist used in acute attacks; inhibits trigeminocervical complex (unlike sumatriptan); given orally with a high bioavailability (70%); inactive metabolites; 50% excreted unchanged
Non-steroidal anti-inflammatory drugs	–	–	Most migraine headaches respond to analgesics, but reduced gastric emptying and peristalsis may reduce the rate of oral absorption; tolfenamic acid is licensed specifically for oral treatment of acute attacks; see Ch. 29
Pizotifen	26	Metabolism	Used for prophylaxis; good oral bioavailability (80%); metabolised to a polar quaternary N-glucuronide (very unusual reaction – see Ch. 2)

continued

Drugs used in migraine (continued)

Drug	Half-life (h)	Elimination	Comments
Rizatriptan	2–3	Metabolism + renal	$5HT_1$ agonist used in acute attacks; given orally; more rapid absorption than sumatriptan; good oral bioavailability (45%); oxidised by monoamine oxidase to inactive metabolites; administration by subcutaneous injection is the treatment of choice for cluster headaches
Sumatriptan	2	Metabolism + renal	$5HT_1$ agonist used in acute attacks; given orally, intranasally or by subcutaneous injection; low oral bioavailability (15%) but essentially complete availability after subcutaneous injection; eliminated equally by metabolism to inactive products and by renal excretion of the parent drug
Zolmitriptan	3	Metabolism + renal	$5HT_1$ agonist used in acute attacks; given orally or intranasally; oral bioavailability about 40%; one of the three main metabolites (the N-desmethyl metabolite) is a $5HT_{1D}$ agonist and probably contributes significantly to the activity in vivo; also eliminated by renal excretion of the parent drug

The musculoskeletal system

The neuromuscular junction and neuromuscular blockade

Neuromuscular transmission

The neuromuscular junction represents a specialised part of the sarcolemma of skeletal muscle, the motor endplate (Fig. 27.1a). In mammals, depolarisation of the postsynaptic membrane at the motor endplate causes contraction of the muscle fibre in an all-or-none response. For stronger contractions, more motor units are recruited.

The neurotransmitter at the neuromuscular junction is acetylcholine (ACh), acting at nicotinic N_2 receptors. The processes of synthesis and release of ACh have been described briefly in Chapter 4, in relation to the general properties of neurotransmitters in the nervous system. The presynaptic nerve terminal at the neuromuscular junction contains 300 000 or more vesicles, each of which may contain up to 5000 molecules of ACh (known as a quantum). In response to an action potential, up to 500 vesicles are discharged over a very short period (0.5 ms). Each N_2 receptor is capable of binding two molecules of ACh. When both binding sites are occupied, the Na^+ channel in the centre of the receptor opens (Ch. 1), allowing an influx of Na^+ into the muscle cell and depolarisation of the motor endplate. If this depolarisation reaches the firing threshold, then voltage-gated Na^+ channels open, full depolarisation of the muscle cell is triggered and an action potential is generated. Therefore, muscle contraction will depend on sufficient ACh release and binding to nicotinic N_2 receptors (Fig. 27.1b). The action potential opens voltage-gated Ca^{2+} channels in the muscle cell membrane, and also passes along the sarcolemma into the T tubules, where Ca^{2+} is released from the sarcoplasmic reticulum. The increased availability of intracellular Ca^{2+} brings about the processes that produce muscle contraction. Contraction of a muscle fibre usually requires the release of 50–200 quanta of ACh, which will activate 10–15% of motor endplate N_2 receptors.

The action of ACh on N_2 receptors is very short lived (about 0.5 ms) because both the junctional cleft and the motor endplate contain large amounts of acetylcholin-

(a)

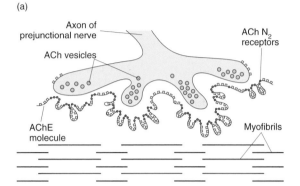

(b)

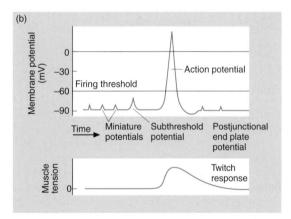

Fig. 27.1
Acetylcholine (ACh) at the neuromuscular junction. (a) Released ACh acts upon a postsynaptic nicotinic (N_2) receptor on the motor endplate, opening a cation channel, and an influx of Na^+ occurs, resulting in depolarisation. (b) At rest, insignificant amounts of ACh are released, and miniature endplate potentials generated are insufficient to reach the threshold potential to cause a propagated action potential. If sufficient ACh is released, an action potential is propagated, causing muscle contraction. Non-depolarising muscle relaxants prevent the generation of the action potential by blocking N_2 receptors.

esterase (AChE). Plasma cholinesterase (pseudocholinesterase) hydrolyses ACh more slowly than does AChE. However the plasma enzyme is important pharmacologically because of its ability to metabolise several drugs with ester bonds. Tissue esterases that break down ACh are also present in many cells, notably in the liver.

Although ACh is the neurotransmitter that causes contraction of both skeletal muscle and most smooth muscles, the basic organisation and functioning of these neuroeffector systems are very different, as shown in Table 27.1.

Table 27.1
Comparison of skeletal and smooth muscle innervation

Property	Skeletal muscle fibre	Smooth muscle fibre
Nerves supplying fibre	Single	Multiple
Junction	Highly organised motor endplate	Simple
Neurotransmitter	Ach	Ach
Receptor subtype	Nicotinic N_2	Muscarinic (mainly M_3)
Receptor distribution	Only at motor endplate, only one motor endplate per muscle fibre	Widely on the muscle surface
Effects of stimulation	Single nerve contracts the whole muscle fibre (all-or-none response)	Each nerve contracts part of muscle fibre (graded response)
Overdose by inhibition of AChE	Flaccid paralysis	Spasticity

Ach, acetylcholine; AchE, acetylcholinesterase.

Drugs acting at the neuromuscular junction

Acetylcholinesterase inhibitors

Further details of this class of drug are given in Chapter 28.

AChE inhibitors block the breakdown of ACh following its release in neuronal synapses and at neuroeffector junctions. The mechanisms of action of different types of AChE inhibitor have been described in Chapter 4, but it is important to remember that they are non-selective and affect the actions of ACh at all its receptors (nicotinic N_1 and N_2 and muscarinic). An important clinical use for these drugs is in the treatment of myasthenia gravis (Ch. 28).

Inhibitors of release of acetylcholine

Botulinum toxin A from the anaerobic bacillus *Clostridium botulinum* decreases the release of ACh from vesicles. It binds selectively to cholinergic nerve terminals, and after internalisation into the terminal via a cell membrane vesicle, it is released into the cytoplasm. The toxin cleaves a cytoplasmic protein on the cell membrane that is required for neurotransmitter release. This chemical denervation stimulates collateral axon growth and eventual formation of a new neuromuscular junction. Botulinum toxin is extremely dangerous, as evidenced by the consequences of botulinum poisoning, but it also has a clinical role. Injection into muscles produces local muscle paralysis that is employed to treat involuntary movements such as blepharospasm (spasm of the eyelids) or torticollis (wry-neck) and to relieve spasticity

(Ch. 24). It is given by injection as botulinum A toxin–haemagglutinin complex into the affected muscles, after which it can be effective for many weeks. It is also used by local injection to reduce excessive sweating, because of its action in inhibiting ACh at sweat glands, and it is being used increasingly for cosmetic reasons to temporarily remove frown lines and wrinkles.

Antagonists/blockers at the neuromuscular junction

Relaxation of skeletal muscles is an essential prerequisite for many surgical operations (see also Ch. 17). It is also required to relax the vocal cords prior to passage of an endotracheal tube ('intubation'). To reduce the concentrations of general anaesthetic needed for deep anaesthesia, muscle relaxation is achieved by drugs that specifically block the neuromuscular junction without affecting autonomic function (that is, the actions of ACh on muscarinic and nicotinic N_1 receptors). Drugs that block the neuromuscular junction almost all resemble ACh in that they have a quaternary amino group that binds strongly to the anionic site of the nicotinic N_2 receptor (Fig. 27.2).

A neuromuscular blocker must occupy more than 75% of the postsynaptic N_2 receptors to produce neuromuscular blockade. Therefore, the number of molecules of drug that must enter the junctional cleft is similar for all drugs, regardless of potency. The potency of a neuromuscular blocker is measured by the ED_{95}, which is the dose required to produce 95% depression of muscular twitch (Table 27.2). About twice this dose is required for adequate muscle relaxation to permit tracheal intubation. The laryngeal muscles are more rapidly paralysed than other muscle groups, but the effect is often of shorter

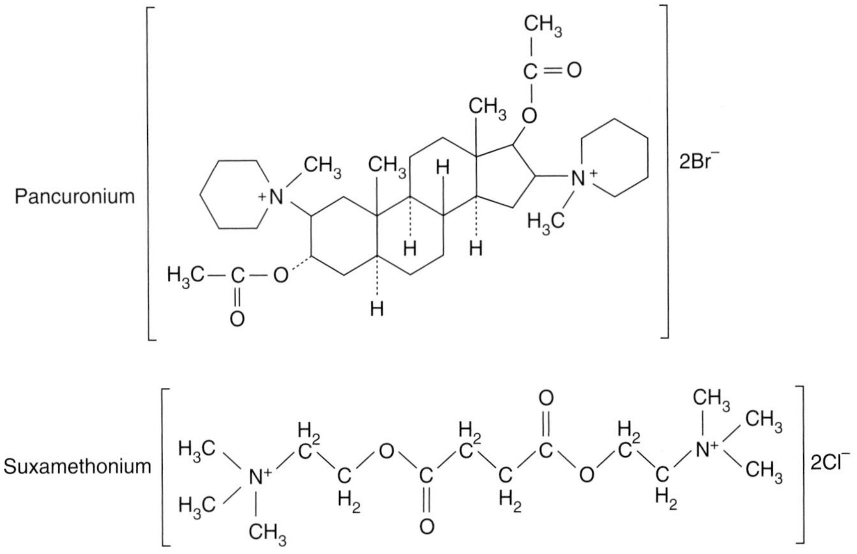

Pancuronium

Suxamethonium

Fig. 27.2
The structures of pancuronium, a non-depolarising blocking drug, and suxamethonium, a depolarising blocker.

Table 27.2
Properties of some non-depolarising skeletal muscle relaxants

Muscle relaxant	ED_{95} mg/kg[a]	Time to max block (min)[b]	Duration (min)[c]	Comment
Pancuronium	0.06	4–5	90	Tachycardia, increase in cardiac output
Vecuronium	0.05	3–4	45	
Atracurium	0.25	3–4	40	Histamine release; increase in heart rate and decrease in SVR
Cisatracurium	0.05	4.5–5.5	30–40	
Rocuronium	0.4	2–3	30	Increase in heart rate
Mivacurium	0.08	2–3	15–20	Histamine release; increase in heart rate and decrease in SVR

[a]ED95 is the dose required to suppress the twitch by 95%.
[b]Time to maximum block following administration of the dose used for intubation (2× the ED_{95}).
[c]Time taken to recover to 25% of the original twitch height after an intubation dose (2× the ED_{95}).
SVR, systemic vascular resistance.

duration. This may reflect either the higher blood flow to this muscle, or the greater density of N_2 receptors. A rapid loss of activity depends on the rate of clearance of the drug from the plasma. For many neuromuscular blockers, after a bolus dose this is more a result of redistribution to tissues than metabolism. Redistribution lowers the plasma concentration (see Ch. 2) and, there-fore, the concentration at the motor endplate. For those drugs which undergo rapid redistribution, the duration of neuromuscular blockade will be more prolonged after repeated boluses or infusions that allow equilibrium between plasma and tissue concentrations. The duration

of effect then becomes dependent on the elimination half-life.

Competitive (non-depolarising) antagonists

Examples: pancuronium, rocuronium, vecuronium, atracurium, cisatracurium, mivacurium

Mechanism of action and effects

The competitive neuromuscular blockers bind to the nicotinic N_2 receptor without causing depolarisation of the postsynaptic membrane. This blocks the depolarising effect of ACh. Inhibition of ACh breakdown by an AChE inhibitor (usually neostigmine, see Ch. 28) will prolong the action of ACh and reverse the blockade. Competitive blockade can be characterised by post-tetanic potentiation. A period of continuous nerve stimulation (tetanic stimulation) decreases neuronal ACh stores and increases ACh synthesis. If tetanic stimulation occurs during partial blockade of the N_2 receptor, the release of ACh decreases, the extent of blockade increases, and the tetanic contraction fades. However, after cessation of tetanic stimulation, there is an enhanced response to a subsequent single stimulation (due to the increased ACh synthesis), which is known as post-tetanic potentiation.

Pharmacokinetics

Because of their high polarity, conferred by the quaternary N atom (Fig. 27.2), these drugs are not absorbed from the gastrointestinal tract (hence the successful use of curare as an arrow-tip poison in hunting) and they are given by intravenous injection. They have a low apparent volume of distribution and do not cross the blood–brain barrier. Vecuronium is partially metabolised in the liver and partially excreted unchanged in the bile. Pancuronium and rocuronium are mainly excreted unchanged by the kidney. Atracurium (a mixture of 10 isomers) and cisatracurium (a single isomer of atracurium) undergo non-enzymatic spontaneous degradation as well as hydrolysis by non-specific esterases in the plasma. Only 10% of a dose is excreted unchanged by the kidney which is an advantage in hepatic or renal impairment. Mivacurium, like suxamethonium (see below), is metabolised by plasma cholinesterase.

The speed of onset of action and duration of action of competitive blockers differ (Table 27.2). Rocuronium has the fastest onset of action, within 2 min, which may facilitate intubation. With the exception of atracurium and cisatracurium, the duration of action of competitive antagonists at the neuromuscular junction (from about 30 min for vecuronium up to 75 min for pancuronium) is determined by redistribution of the drug into the body tissues. This leads to prolonged action with repeated doses (see above). The duration of effect of atracurium and cisatracurium is about 40 min. This is longer than predicted from their plasma half-lives and may be a consequence of high-affinity binding sites close to the ACh receptor acting as a reservoir for the drug. The lack of accumulation with repeated doses may make them more suitable for long-term muscle relaxation.

Unwanted effects

- pancuronium blocks cardiac muscarinic receptors and has a sympathomimetic effect, which leads to tachycardia and hypertension

- atracurium and mivacurium can cause the release of histamine from mast cells, producing flushing, hypotension, tachycardia and bronchospasm
- mivacurium can cause prolonged muscle paralysis in people with plasma cholinesterase deficiency (see suxamethonium below)
- the other agents have few unwanted effects at clinically used doses, although allergic reactions have been reported.

Depolarising blockers

Example: suxamethonium (succinylcholine)

Mechanism of action and effects

Suxamethonium is succinic acid with a choline molecule attached at each carboxylic acid group, and resembles two ACh molecules joined back to back. When two molecules of suxamethonium bind to the nicotinic N_2 receptor, it acts as an agonist and depolarises the motor endplate. Suxamethonium is not hydrolysed by AChE and, therefore, produces more prolonged depolarisation than ACh. This leads to a conformational change in the receptor that allows the Na^+ channel to close despite the continued presence of an agonist. As a result, the muscle repolarises and, although it can respond to direct electrical stimulation, it can no longer be stimulated via the neuronal release of ACh. Indeed, if the amount of available synaptic ACh is enhanced (such as occurs with the use of an AChE inhibitor), it will add to a partial depolarising blockade and not reverse it. After about 20 min of depolarising blockade, suxamethonium produces a 'dual block' with the onset of non-depolarising competitive blockade. At this stage, tetanic stimulation no longer produces a sustained contraction and is accompanied by post-tetanic potentiation; in addition, the blockade can now be partially reversed by an AChE inhibitor.

Pharmacokinetics

Suxamethonium is highly polar, is not absorbed orally and must be given intravenously. It has a low volume of distribution and does not cross the blood–brain barrier. Thus, suxamethonium has an onset of action within 1 min. It is rapidly hydrolysed by plasma cholinesterase and this results in a very short duration of action (about 3–12 min); therefore, an infusion is necessary to give a prolonged effect. A very prolonged paralysis occurs in about 1 in 2000–3000 individuals, who have a genetically determined deficiency of plasma cholinesterase. In this population, the action of suxamethonium is terminated after some 2–3 h by renal excretion.

Unwanted effects

- There is an initial depolarisation of the motor endplates prior to blockade; this results in muscle fasciculation and postoperative muscle pain.
- Prolonged apnoea occurs if there is a low circulating concentration of plasma cholinesterase, through either a genetic deficiency or a decreased synthesis of the enzyme in severe liver disease.
- The use of suxamethonium during anaesthesia has been linked with the development of a rare but potentially fatal disorder of muscles known as malignant hyperthermia, with a rapid rise in temperature, muscle rigidity, tachycardia and acidosis. Predisposition to this condition has an autosomal dominant inheritance, producing a defect in Ca^{2+} flux across the cell membrane.
- Stimulation of ACh receptors at autonomic ganglia (nicotinic N_1) and muscarinic receptors produce bradycardia, especially with repeated doses.
- Hyperkalaemia occurs especially in the presence of major tissue trauma and severe burns.

Indications for neuromuscular-blocking drugs

The neuromuscular-blocking drugs are used in both surgical procedures and intensive care.

Tracheal intubation. Relaxation of the vocal cords allows easy passage of an endotracheal tube. A rapid onset of action is essential to minimise the risk of aspiration of gastric contents. This is the only current major use for suxamethonium. Because of frequent unwanted effects, suxamethonium is being superseded by rapidly acting non-depolarising blockers such as rocuronium.

During surgical procedures. Neuromuscular blockade produces muscle relaxation for procedures such as abdominal incisions. It can be achieved either by single injection or by intravenous infusion for more prolonged surgery. At the end of the operation, the effect of a non-depolarising blocker can be reversed within 1 min by intravenous injection of neostigmine. Glycopyrrolate or atropine (Ch.4) is given before neostigmine to prevent bradycardia or excessive salivation produced by stimulation of muscarinic receptors.

In intensive care. Neuromuscular blockade is used in addition to analgesia and sedation during mechanical ventilation, particularly if respiratory drive is suppressed (e.g. in adult respiratory distress syndrome), in status asthmaticus, for status epilepticus or tetanus, and for those with elevated intracranial pressure.

FURTHER READING

Denborough M (1998) Malignant hyperthermia. *Lancet* 352, 1131–1136

Miinchau A, Bhatia KP (2000) Uses of botulinum toxin injection in medicine today. *BMJ* 320, 161–165

Moore EW, Hunter JM (2001) The new neuromuscular blocking agents: do they offer any advantages? *Br J Anaesth* 87, 912–925

Wiklund RA, Rosenbaum SH (1997) Anesthesiology Part 1. *N Engl J Med* 337, 7132–7141

Self-assessment

In questions 1–4, the initial statement, in italics, is true. Are the accompanying statements also true?

1. *Vecuronium, unlike atracurium, has no haemodynamic effects as it does not cause histamine release.*

   a. Suxamethonium blockade is antagonised by lowered body temperature.
   b. All non-depolarising muscle relaxants cause similar amounts of histamine release.

2. *Malignant hyperthermia is a rare genetically determined disorder that causes hyperthermia and muscle spasms in response to suxamethonium, halothane and other drugs.*

   a. Dantrolene is used to treat malignant hyperthermia.
   b. A skeletal muscle fibre is innervated by one motor endplate.
   c. The nicotinic receptor on skeletal muscle is identical to the nicotinic receptor in autonomic ganglia.

3. *Except for mivacurium and atracurium, the action of competitive neuromuscular junction-blocking drugs is mainly limited by redistribution of the drug.*

   a. Suxamethonium is the only muscle relaxant used for tracheal intubation.
   b. Competitive neuromuscular-blocking drugs such as vecuronium are relatively well absorbed orally.

4. *Botulinum toxin poisoning results from long-lasting blockade of parasympathetic and motor function.*

   a. Botulinum toxin acts postsynaptically to block ACh-induced depolarisation.
   b. Botulinum toxin is administered only by discrete local injection.
   c. Botulinum toxin inhibits pathological excessive sweating as sweat glands are innervated by sympathetic cholinergic nerve fibres.

5. You are evaluating the properties of different neuromuscular-blocking drugs. Choose the <u>most appropriate</u> statement from the following options.

   A. Rocuronium will have direct central nervous system effects as it crosses the blood–brain barrier.
   B. Pancuronium is the neuromuscular-blocking drug of choice for a surgical procedure that will take less than 30 min.
   C. Suxamethonium is the only muscle relaxant that can be used for electroconvulsive therapy.
   D. To produce complete block of an evoked twitch, about 50% of nicotinic receptors need to be occupied by a non-depolarising neuromuscular-blocking drug.
   E. Atracurium causes the release of histamine.

6. Case history – see the case history for Chapter 17, page 246.

The answers are provided on page 727.

Drugs acting at the neuromuscular junction

Drug	Half-life (h)	Elimination	Comments
Acetylcholine esterase inhibitors			
Distigmine	? (long)	Renal + hydrolysis	Used for myasthenia gravis (but rarely) and urinary retention; see Ch. 28
Edrophonium	1.8	Renal + metabolism	Given by i.v. or intramuscular injection in the diagnosis and management of myasthenia gravis and to reverse the effects of a non-depolarising blocker; very short duration of action; given i.v. over 30 s; see Ch. 28
Neostigmine	0.4–1.7 (i.v.)	Hydrolysis + renal	Given i.v. to reverse the effects of a non-depolarising blocker (with atropine to minimise effects of acetylcholine on the parasympathetic system); given orally or by subcutaneous or intramuscular injection for treatment of myasthenia gravis; see Ch. 28.
Pyridostigmine	0.4–1.9 (i.v.)	Renal + hydrolysis	Given orally for treatment of myasthenia gravis; see Ch. 28
Non-depolarising blockers			All are used for muscle relaxation for surgery; all show negligible oral absorption and are given by i.v. injection or infusion
Atracurium	0.3	Spontaneous hydrolysis	Also used for muscle relaxation during intensive care; a complex mixture of 10 isomers; very rapidly breaks down within blood; unaffected by hepatic or renal failure; cardiovascular effects due to histamine release
Cisatracurium	0.5	Spontaneous	Also used for muscle relaxation during intensive care; a single isomer of atracurium; spontaneous degradation; does not cause histamine release
Gallamine	2–2.5	Renal	Rarely used, because of sympathomimetic effects on heart rate and blood pressure; increased half-life in elderly
Mivacurium	2 min (trans–trans); 50–60 min (cis–cis)	Plasma hydrolysis	Consists of three isomers; the cis–trans and trans–trans have similar half-lives, are 10 times more potent than the cis–cis isomer, and are responsible for the clinical response; hydrolysed by plasma cholinesterase and shows prolonged effect in the rare individuals with a genetic deficiency of this enzyme
Pancuronium	0.5	Renal + biliary + metabolism	Often used for long-term muscle relaxation during mechanical ventilation in intensive care; hydrolysis product (3-hydroxy metabolite) retains activity; sympathomimetic effects on heart rate and blood pressure can cause tachycardia and hypertension
Rocuronium	1.2	Renal + metabolism	Also used for muscle relaxation during intensive care; most rapid onset of action of drugs in this class; minimal cardiovascular effects

continued

Drug compendium

Drugs acting at the neuromuscular junction (continued)

Drug	Half-life (h)	Elimination	Comments
Non-depolarising blockers (continued)			
Vecuronium	1.0	Bile + metabolism	Bile is major route of elimination (note molecular weight – 638 D – exceeds the threshold for biliary excretion); lacks cardiovascular effects
Depolarising blockers			
Suxamethonium (succinylcholine)	2–5 min	Plasma hydrolysis	Rapid onset but short duration of action; paralysis is preceded by painful fasciculations; prolonged paralysis can cause a so-called dual block in which a non-depolarising block follows the initial depolarising block (edrophonium – see above – can be used to determine the nature of the block); hydrolysed by plasma cholinesterase and shows prolonged effect in those with a genetic deficiency of this enzyme; half-life shorter in infants and children

i.v., intravenous

28

Myasthenia gravis

Myasthenia gravis is a comparatively rare autoimmune disease in which there is an autoantibody to the acetylcholine nicotinic N_2 receptor system that impairs the responsiveness of the neuromuscular junction (Ch. 27). The antibody in myasthenia gravis reduces the number of functional N_2 receptors on the motor endplate by three distinct mechanisms:

- increased receptor destruction by complement binding
- cross-linking of receptors, which causes increased receptor internalisation
- receptor blockade by steric hindrance.

Therefore, fewer functional receptors are available to acetylcholine to reach the firing potential in the muscle cell. As a result, in myasthenia gravis, there is voluntary muscle weakness. Repetitive nerve impulses result in a progressive decrement in the availability of sensitive receptors. This is without physiological consequences in a healthy neuromuscular junction, but in myasthenia, the smaller receptor pool leads to a more rapid reduction in receptor availability with repetitive stimulation, and increasing numbers of muscle fibres fail to fire. This produces the characteristic rapid muscle fatigue on exertion. The earliest symptoms of myasthenia gravis are often diplopia or ptosis, arising from weakness of the extraocular muscles. In 85% of cases, the symptoms progress to involve many other muscle groups, particularly bulbar, facial and proximal limb weakness.

The thymus gland plays a part in the genesis of the immune response in myasthenia gravis, although the precise role is as yet uncertain. There are associated abnormalities of the thymus in 80% of people with myasthenia gravis, usually lymphoreticular hyperplasia if the onset of the condition is at an early age or thymoma if the onset is over the age of 40 years.

Drug treatment of myasthenia gravis is based on prolongation of the action of acetylcholine by inhibiting its hydrolysis. The type of interaction between the antibody and the receptor probably determines the effectiveness of treatment in an individual. In myasthenia gravis, there is altered sensitivity to muscle relaxant drugs: there is increased sensitivity to competitive (non-depolarising) neuromuscular blockers but resistance to depolarising neuromuscular blockers (Ch. 27).

Acetylcholinesterase inhibitors

Examples: neostigmine, pyridostigmine, edrophonium

Mechanism of action and effects

Acetylcholinesterase (AChE) inhibitors block the breakdown of acetylcholine released from presynaptic neurons, and details of their mechanisms of action are found in Chapter 4. They are non-selective and have actions at all synaptic connections that use acetylcholine as a neurotransmitter. AChE inhibitors produce beneficial effects in myasthenia gravis through their action at nicotinic N_2 receptors (Ch. 4); unwanted effects arise from the excessive actions of acetylcholine at nicotinic N_1 and muscarinic receptors.

Pharmacokinetics and clinical uses

Neostigmine and pyridostigmine are quaternary amines that are slowly and incompletely absorbed from the gut; as a result, oral doses need to be approximately 10 times greater than parenteral doses to be effective. They have short elimination half-lives, due to a combination of renal tubular secretion and some hepatic metabolism; the plasma half-life after oral dosage is probable longer, due to absorption-rate-limited kinetics (Ch. 2). They do not readily cross the blood–brain barrier (see Ch. 9 for anticholinesterases that cross the blood–brain barrier and are used in Alzheimer's disease). Both neostigmine and pyridostigmine can be used to treat myasthenia gravis, but pyridostigmine is the preferred choice, due to a longer duration of action. Neostigmine has a faster onset of action, and is used by intravenous injection to reverse the effect of competitive neuromuscular blockers (Ch. 27).

Edrophonium is given as an intravenous bolus to test the therapeutic response to AChE inhibitors in myasthenia gravis (see below); it has a very short duration of action (2–5 min), largely owing to tissue redistribution, and is of no value in treatment.

Unwanted effects

Unwanted effects arise from the non-specific inhibition of AChE, and are experienced by up to one-third of those treated. They are more troublesome with neostigmine than with pyridostigmine. Peripheral muscarinic receptor agonist effects, which can be blocked by administration of the muscarinic receptor blocking drug propantheline, include:

- diarrhoea, abdominal cramps, excessive salivation
- bradycardia, hypotension (uncommon)
- miosis and lacrimation
- bronchoconstriction (see Ch. 12)
- nausea.

Excessive dosage will lead to a depolarising neuro-muscular blockade by acetylcholine. Initially, there may be muscle twitching and cramps, followed by weakness through the build-up of excess acetylcholine (see below).

Management of myasthenia gravis

Diagnosis

When the diagnosis of myasthenia is suspected, useful information can be obtained rapidly by pharmacological testing. An intravenous injection of the short-acting AChE inhibitor edrophonium will produce clinical improvement within 1 min, lasting about 5 min. Detection of circulating N_2 receptor antibodies, and electromyographical tests that demonstrate abnormal fatiguability in multiple muscle fibres, are used to confirm the diagnosis.

Treatment

Symptomatic treatment of myasthenia gravis is with an AChE inhibitor, which reduces the normal rapid breakdown of acetylcholine and thereby enhances the activity of acetylcholine released by nerve stimulation. Pyridostigmine is commonly used since its action is more consistent than that of neostigmine, the dosing frequency is less, and there are fewer muscarinic unwanted effects. The onset of action is after about 30–45 min, lasting for 3–6 h. An antimuscarinic agent (such as propantheline; Ch. 4) may be necessary to block any parasympathomimetic actions of pyridostigmine, especially if large doses are given. Some individuals do not respond well to AChE inhibitors, while in others, unwanted effects preclude the use of adequate doses.

Excessive dosage of an AChE inhibitor can lead to prolonged stimulation of the N_2 receptors by acetylcholine, resulting in a depolarising blockade of the neuromuscular junction similar to that produced by suxamethonium (succinylcholine; Ch. 27). Therefore, muscle weakness in myasthenia gravis can be the result of either inadequate dosage ('myasthenic crisis') or excessive dosage ('cholinergic crisis') of an AChE inhibitor. The safest way to distinguish these problems is to use assisted ventilation and temporarily withdraw the AChE inhibitor. Muscle groups do not all respond equally well to AChE inhibitors; ptosis and diplopia appear to be the most resistant.

Generalised myasthenia is now usually treated by immunosuppression with a corticosteroid, such as prednisolone (Ch. 44). Corticosteroids are also used for initial immunosuppression in those who are severely ill. They probably act by suppressing T-cell proliferation and reducing antibody synthesis. Initial high-dose corticosteroid therapy can make the weakness worse, particularly in the first few hours, possibly due to a direct effect on neuromuscular transmission. A clinical response is usually apparent after 1 month, but maximum benefit is delayed for up to 9 months. Azathioprine (Ch. 38) produces a clinical response over 2–4 months, but with maximum benefit delayed for 6–24 months. For this reason, it is usually used in combination with a corticosteroid, and often permits a reduction in the long-term dosage of corticosteroid. Mycophenolate mofetil or ciclosporin (Ch. 38) are used if there is a poor response to other immunosuppressive therapy or for intolerance to azathioprine, but the dosage of ciclosporin is usually limited by significant nephrotoxicity. Long-term immunosuppression is usually necessary, since relapse frequently occurs on withdrawal of therapy.

Plasma exchange to remove circulating acetylcholine receptor antibodies can produce a short-term response in severe disease. With repeated exchanges, improvement is seen after 1 day, with a maximum response after 1–2 weeks that is sustained for 2–8 weeks. An alternative is the use of intravenous immunoglobulin, of which IgG is the active component. It produces improvement after about 4 days, and an optimal response after 1–2 weeks that is sustained for 6–15 weeks. Immunoglobulin treatment is usually better tolerated than plasma exchange.

Thymectomy can induce remission, although this can be delayed for up to 5 years. Thymectomy is usually used for early-onset disease with positive receptor antibodies, when it produces complete remission within 5 years in about 40% and significant improvement in a further 35%. It is also used to remove a thymoma, although the clinical benefit is often less clear-cut.

Some drugs can interfere wth neuromuscular transmission and worsen the symptoms of myasthenia gravis. Those most often implicated include aminoglycoside antibiotics (Ch. 51), β-adrenoceptor antagonists (Ch.5), phenytoin (Ch. 23), chloroquine and penicillamine (Ch. 30).

FURTHER READING

Lindstrom JM (2000) Acetylcholine receptors and myasthenia. *Muscle Nerve* 23, 453–477

Newsom-Davis J (2003) Therapy in myasthenia gravis and Lambert-Eaton myasthenic syndrome. *Semin Neurol* 23, 191–197

Nicolle MW (2002) Myasthenia gravis. *The Neurologist* 8, 2–21

Self-assessment

In questions 1 and 2, the first statement, in italics, is true. Are the accompanying statements also true?

1. *Caution is required when administering pyridostigmine to people with asthma.*

   a. Overdosage causing respiratory depression can be treated with atropine.
   b. In severe myasthenia gravis, the response to an anticholinesterase may be poor because of increased breakdown of the drug.

2. *Pyridostigmine produces less muscarinic receptor activity than neostigmine.*

   a. An AChE inhibitor should not be given with depolarising muscle relaxants such as suxamethonium.
   b. A cholinergic crisis should be confirmed by administering pyridostigmine.

3. Regarding a person who has been diagnosed with myasthenia gravis, choose the <u>most appropriate</u> statement from the following options.

   A. All people diagnosed with myasthenia gravis have a thymoma.
   B. In order to be effective, anticholinesterases used in treating myasthenia gravis should be able to cross the blood–brain barrier.
   C. Glucocorticoids which can be of benefit in some people with myasthenia gravis are effective because of their anti-inflammatory actions.
   D. Many of the unwanted effects that physostigmine has on the autonomic nervous system can be reduced with a muscarinic receptor blocking drug.
   E. The aim of plasmapheresis is to reduce the plasma (pseudo) cholinesterase which breaks down acetylcholine.

4. Case history questions

   A 35-year-old woman with no previous illness noticed that she had ptosis and occasional diplopia. Over a period of time she became aware that on exertion she suffered from leg weakness although her coordination was normal. Following a sustained upward gaze for a minute, ptosis and diplopia could be elicited. Myasthenia gravis was suspected.

   a. What tests should be performed to verify the diagnosis?
   b. What is the pathogenesis of myasthenia gravis?
   c. Why is edrophonium injection used as a test for myasthenia gravis?

   Treatment was commenced following diagnosis.

   d. What principles should treatment follow?

   The answers are provided on pages 727–728.

Acetylcholinesterase inhibitors for the treatment of myasthenia gravis

Drug	Half-life (h)	Elimination	Comments
Distigmine	? (long)	Renal + hydrolysis	Rarely used; also used for urinary retention (Ch 15); given orally; very poor oral bioavailability (1–2%), especially if taken with food; hydrolysed by plasma esterases
Edrophonium	1.8	Renal + metabolism	Very short duration of action and mainly used for diagnosis; given i.v. over 30 s; not given orally; pathways of elimination not defined but severe renal impairment reduces total clearance by more than 50%
Neostigmine	0.4–1.7 (i.v.)	Renal and hydrolysis	Given orally or by subcutaneous or i.v. injection; very low oral bioavailability (1–2%); food delays absorption but does not affect AUC (of absorbed drug); elimination after oral dosage is probably longer than after i.v. dosage (absorption rate-limited); metabolised by plasma and hepatic esterases
Pyridostigmine	0.4–1.9 (i.v.)	Renal + hydrolysis	Given orally; low oral bioavailability (10–20%); food delays absorption but does not alter bioavailability; most of the absorbed fraction is excreted in the urine unchanged; terminal half-life after oral dosage is probably longer than after i.v. dosage (absorption rate-limited); longer acting than neostigmine

AUC, area under the plasma concentration versus time curve; i.v., intravenous.

29

Non-steroidal anti-inflammatory drugs

The role of cyclo-oxygenase enzymes in the actions of non-steroidal anti-inflammatory drugs

The major therapeutic and unwanted actions of non-steroidal anti-inflammatory drugs (NSAIDs) are achieved because they inhibit in various ways the cyclo-oxygenases (COX). These enzymes are essential in the production of the ubiquitous local hormones prostanoids (prostaglandins and thromboxanes) which are members of the family of eicosanoids.

Eicosanoids (molecules that comprise 20 carbon atoms and have two double bonds) are members of a family of related polyunsaturated fatty acids that includes the prostanoids and leukotrienes. These are local hormones, which are generally synthesised and catabolised close to their site of action, and have numerous physiological and pathological actions. The immediate fatty acid precursor of most eicosanoids in individuals on a standard mixed diet is arachidonic acid; this is formed from dietary linoleic acid found in quantities in vegetable oils such as sunflower oil. Linoleic acid is converted in the liver in several steps to the eicosanoid precursor arachidonic acid, which is then incorporated into glycerophospholipids in cells; arachidonic acid is released under the influence of lipases like phospholipase A_2 and can then be converted to eicosanoids (Fig. 29.1).

Arachidonate (which has four double bonds) is converted to prostanoids containing two double bonds (e.g. prostaglandin E_2 [PGE_2]). Prostanoids having three double bonds (e.g. thromboxane A_3 [TXA_3]) can be produced from another fatty acid precursor, eicosapentaenoic acid (EPA), which is found in oily fish. Consumption of fish can enrich EPA in glycerophospholipids and increase the formation of prostanoids of the 3 series. TXA_3 is less pro-aggregatory for platelets than TXA_2 produced from arachidonic acid, and fish-oil intake may be of benefit in cardiovascular diseases (Ch. 48).

Prostanoids are synthesised by oxygenation and ring closure of arachidonic acid, controlled by the rate-limiting enzyme COX. The initial products of the action of COX on arachidonic acid are unstable intermediates known as cyclic endoperoxides. Specific synthases, the occurrence and abundance of which differs from cell to cell, then convert the endoperoxide PGH_2 to various prostanoids (Fig. 29.1). The products of the COX pathways therefore differ among various tissues, reflecting the diverse nature of their multitude of actions and the individual requirements of each cell type. Most cell types form different prostanoids simultaneously, but the pattern and abundance of formation depends upon the type of COX enzymes and synthases present, which themselves depend upon the presence of many disparate hormones and other controlling factors.

COX occurs as a least three isoenzymes, COX-1, COX-2 and COX-3, and other variant enzymes also exist. Until relatively recently it was considered that the different forms of COX had clearly distinct functions. COX-1 was thought to be mainly a constitutive 'housekeeping' enzyme localised to the endoplasmic reticulum. It can be produced in the resting state by many cells and contributes to the regulation of several homeostatic processes such as renal and gastric blood flow, gastric cytoprotection and platelet aggregation (Table 29.1). COX-2 was thought to be mainly an inducible enzyme, present in the nuclear envelope in greater concentrations than in the endoplasmic reticulum. COX-2 was originally found to be present in cells in only low amounts; however, it is expressed in many cells such as endothelial cells, macrophages, synovial fibroblasts, mast cells, chondrocytes and osteoblasts in response to elevated inflammatory cytokine concentrations. COX-2 was thought to be the enzyme mainly responsible for generation of prostaglandins involved in inflammation, pain and fever. COX-3 is an enzyme variant of COX-1 that retains all the COX-1 transcript, with an additional conserved intron sequence. It is mainly expressed in the brain and spinal cord and to a lesser extent in the heart, endothelial cells and monocytes. COX-3 may have a role in central nervous system (CNS) pain perception, but its precise functions are as yet uncertain. Recent studies have shown that in many biological systems there is no clear separation between the functions of 'physiological, constitutive, housekeeping' COX-1 and the 'inflammatory, inducible, pathological' COX-2, and these descriptions are probably misleading. This applies particularly to the kidney, CNS, cardiovascular and reproductive systems.

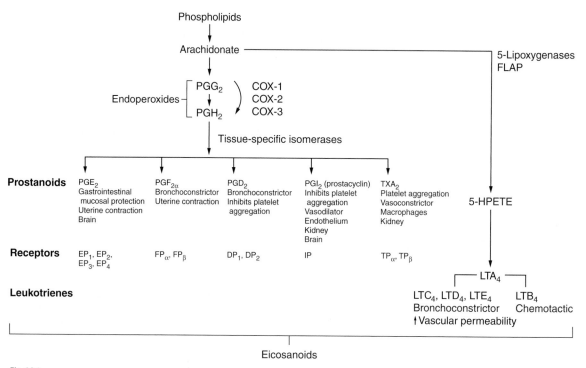

Fig. 29.1

The arachidonic acid cascade. Arachidonic acid can be utilised by cyclo-oxygenases (COX) 1, 2 or 3 to form prostanoids (prostaglandins and thromboxanes) having two double bonds in their side chains. They have a multitude of actions and stabilities depending upon the prostanoid, the site of formation and the amount formed. The receptors they act on are G-protein coupled. Other properties are shown in Table 29.2 and in the text. PG, prostaglandin; TX thromboxane; HPETE, hydroperoxyeicosatetraenoic acid; LT, leukotriene; FLAP, five (5) lipoxygenase activating protein.

Either isoform may be involved in the production of 'physiological' or 'pathological' prostanoids. Table 29.1 shows that there are roles for constitutive COX-2 in homeostasis in many cell types and that COX-1 isoenzymes may be involved in some pathological events.

The actions of prostaglandins and thromboxanes depend upon the circumstances and site of their formation, and whether they are formed in excessive amounts. For example, PGE_2 is generated in low physiological amounts by COX-1 in gastric mucosa and is important for maintaining mucosal integrity by a variety of mechanisms, including increased bicarbonate production, increased blood flow and a cytoprotective role of uncertain mechanism. During tissue damage, there is increased prostaglandin synthesis via elevated COX-2 expression, and this contributes to inflammation and pain. In particular, production of PGE_2 induces vasodilation, increased vascular permeability and sensitises pain fibre nerve endings to the nociceptive action of bradykinin and 5-hydroxytryptamine (5HT) and other mediators (Ch. 19). However, in the later stages of repair following tissue damage, COX-2-derived prostanoids may contribute to the processes of wound healing. TXA_2 is generated by COX-1 in platelets and promotes appropriate platelet aggregation to prevent blood loss from damaged vessels (Ch. 11). However, inappropriate

platelet aggregation induced by TXA_2 can also contribute to thrombus formation in ischaemic heart disease.

Prostanoids act via five main classes of G-protein-coupled receptors on cell surfaces. Some of the many actions of prostaglandins are shown in Table 29.2.

The second route for arachidonic acid metabolism is via the lipoxygenase pathway, to produce leukotrienes (Fig. 29.1). These are also involved in the inflammatory process by enhancing vascular permeability (leukotrienes [LT] C_4, D_4 and E_4) and through chemotactic attraction of leucocytes (particularly LTB_4; see also Ch. 12).

Non-steroidal anti-inflammatory drugs

Mechanisms of action

The NSAIDs share a common mode of action – that is, inhibition of the COX isoenzymes (Table 29.3). Different NSAIDs do not inhibit the two main isozymes (COX-1 and COX-2) to the same extent either in blood or in the gastric mucosa, and this partly explains the variations in their therapeutic and unwanted-effect profiles. Inhibition

Table 29.1
Some biological roles of cyclo-oxygenase enzymes COX-1 and COX-2[a]

COX-1 'Homeostasis–physiological–housekeeping' roles – constitutive	COX-2 'Homeostasis–physiological–housekeeping' roles – constitutive
Gastrointestinal protection	Renal function
Platelet aggregation	CNS function
Blood flow regulation	Tissue repair and healing (including gastrointestinal)
CNS function	Reproduction
	Uterine contraction
	Blood vessel dilation
	Pancreas
	Inhibition of platelet aggregation
	Airways
COX-1 'Pathological'	**COX-2 'Pathological'**
(Possible involvement in inflammation)	Inflammation
Raised blood pressure	Pain
Pain	Fever
	Blood vessel permeability
	Reproduction
	Alzheimer's
	Promotion angiogenesis, inhibition apoptosis

[a]The separation of the roles of COX-1- and COX-2-derived prostanoids into 'physiological' and 'pathological' is increasingly indistinct. The actions of the prostanoids may be permissive in allowing and enhancing the actions of other agents while not having marked direct effects themselves.

of COX reduces the generation of prostanoids but does not directly affect the production of leukotrienes, which may, as a consequence, exert unopposed actions. Leukotriene production may even increase as a result of diversion (shunting) of arachidonic acid into the lipoxygenase pathway. In aspirin-induced asthma, the COX-1-generated PGE_2 that normally applies a 'brake' to leukotriene synthesis is diminished and leukotrienes are increased.

The responses observed with individual NSAIDs will reflect the ability of the drug to inhibit the different COX isoenzymes involved in the biological actions shown in Table 29.1 and Table 29.2. The extent of selectivity will depend not only on the type of NSAID but also on the dosage used. In some situations, the clinical implications of inhibition of different COX isoenzymes has not yet been fully worked out.

The main clinically important therapeutic and unwanted effects of COX inhibition and the predominant COX involved are shown in Table 29.4. Selective COX-2 inhibitors seem to be weaker analgesics than non-selective COX-1 and COX-2 inhibitors.

NSAIDs have even more complex anti-inflammatory effects than can be explained by inhibition of COX. They also have agonist activity at peroxisome proliferator-activated receptors (PPARs). PPARs have a key role in modulation of immune responses by suppressing pro-inflammatory gene expression (for production of tumour necrosis factor alpha, interleukin-1 and inducible nitric oxide synthase) in macrophages. This action occurs at higher drug concentrations than are required to produce analgesia. NSAIDs also have complex effects on lymphocytes, including inhibition of T-cell activation and increased T-cell apoptosis, some of which may reflect PPAR-mediated actions.

Classification of NSAIDs

Table 29.5 shows the principal chemical types of NSAIDs.

Most NSAIDs bind reversibly to the channel in COX that accepts arachidonic acid, but the irreversible inactivation produced by aspirin involves acetylation of a serine residue in the enzyme. Many conventional NSAIDs produce greater inhibition of COX-1 than of COX-2. Other drugs show greater selectivity for COX-2 (Table 29.3).

Actions and effects of non-selective NSAIDs

A comparison of some of the properties and actions of a few of the commonly used analgesic drugs are compared in Table 29.6.

Analgesia. This is in part a peripheral action at the site of pain and is most effective when the pain has an

Table 29.2
Some of the myriad effects of the prostanoids[a]

Tissue	Effect	Eicosanoid
Platelets	↑ Aggregation	TXA_2
	↓ Aggregation	PGI_2, PGD_2
Vascular smooth muscle	Vasodilation	PGI_2, PGE_2, PGD_2
	Vasoconstriction	TXA_2
Other smooth muscle	Bronchodilation	PGE_2
	Bronchoconstriction	PGD_2, PGF_2, TXA_2, LTC_4, LTD_4, LTE_4
	GI tract (contraction/relaxation, depends on muscle orientation)	PGF_2, PGE_2, PGI_2, PGD_2
	Uterine contraction	PGE_2, PGF_2
Vascular endothelium	Increased permeability	LTC_4, LTB_4
	Potentiates histamine/bradykinin	PGE_2, PGI_2
Neutrophils/macrophages	Chemotaxis	LTB_4
Gastrointestinal mucosa	Reduced acid secretion	PGE_2, PGI_2
	Increased mucus secretion	PGE_2
	Increased blood flow	PGE_2, PGI_2
Nervous system	Inhibition of noradrenaline release	PGD_2, PGE_2, PGI_2
	Endogenous pyrogen in hypothalamus	PGE_2
	Sedation, sleep	PGD_2
Endocrine/metabolic	Secretion of ACTH, GH, prolactin, gonadotrophins	PGE_2
	Inhibition of lipolysis	PGE_2
Kidney	Increased renal blood flow	PGE_2, PGI_2
	Antagonism of ADH	PGE_2
	Renin release	PGI_2, PGE_2, PGD_2
Pain	Potentiates pain through bradykinin, 5HT	PGE_2, PGD_2
Temperature	Pyretic in hypothalamus	PGE_2

[a]Only the main prostanoids involved are shown. The prostanoids involved can also vary depending upon the influence of other hormones and mediators.

ACTH, adrenocorticotrophic hormone. ADH antidiuretic hormone; GH, growth hormone; 5HT, 5-hydroxytryptamine; LT, leukotriene; PG, prostaglandin; TX, thromboxane.

inflammatory origin (see also Ch. 19). It appears to be achieved predominantly through inhibition of COX-2-derived prostaglandins in inflamed or injured tissues. A component of the analgesic action of NSAIDs is also due to inhibition of COX-1, COX-2 and COX-3, with reduction of prostaglandin production in the pain pathways of the CNS. Some evidence suggests that selective inhibition of COX-1 may potentiate the analgesic actions of opioids; COX-2 inhibition decreases PGE_2 production in the spinal cord and reduces the excitability of second-order neurons in the pain relay pathway. The analgesic action of NSAIDs is apparent after the first dose, but does not reach a maximal effect until about 1 week.

Anti-inflammatory effect. This is partly related to reduced peripheral COX-2-generated prostaglandin synthesis. NSAIDs also affect several other inflammatory processes unrelated to their effects on prostaglandins. For example, they probably reduce harmful superoxide free radical generation by neutrophils. They may also uncouple G-protein-regulated processes in the cell membrane of inflammatory cells. This would reduce cell responsiveness to a variety of agonists released by damaged tissues. The anti-inflammatory effects of NSAIDs develop gradually over about 3 weeks.

Antipyretic effect. Fever is reduced through hypothalamic COX-2-generated prostaglandin inhibition. Circulating pyrogens enhance PGE_2 production in the hypothalamus, which depresses the response of temperature-sensitive neurons. NSAIDs do not affect normal body temperature.

Reduction of platelet aggregation. This action is mediated by reduced platelet COX-1- generated TXA_2 synthesis. The effect is marked for aspirin, because it has an irreversible action on COX and platelets are unable to synthesise more enzyme. The reversible action of most other NSAIDs (with the exception of naproxen) produces

Table 29.3
The relative abilities of a selection of non-steroidal anti-inflammatory drugs to inhibit cyclo-oxygenase 1 (COX-1) and COX-2 isoenzymes

Ratio COX-1/COX-2 inhibition in blood assays[a]		COX-1 inhibition in human gastric mucosa (IC$_{50}$ μM)[b]	
1 : 5–10	Flubiprofen Ketoprofen Fenoprofen	0.1–0.4	Flurbiprofen Ketoprofen Indometacin Diclofenac Ketorolac
1 : 2–5	Aspirin	1.0–5.9	Piroxicam Fenoprofen Aspirin Ibuprofen
1 : 1–2	Indometacin Ibuprofen	10–32	Etodolac Naproxen
1 : 0.5–1	Naproxen Piroxicam Ketorolac Nabumetone Sulindac	32–60	Nabumetone Sulindac Paracetamol
1 : 0.1–0.5	Etolodac Paracetamol Celecoxib	>60	Celecoxib Valdecoxib Etoricoxib Dexamethasone
1 : 0.09	Meloxicam		
1 : 0.05	Diclofenac		
1 : 0.02	Rofecoxib		
1 : 0.01	Etoricoxib		
1 : 0.002	Dexamethasone		

[a]Values in blood are ratios of serum assays of COX-1 (thromboxane A$_2$ generation following clotting) and COX-2 (lipopolysaccharide-stimulated prostaglandin E$_2$ synthesis). The lower ratios indicate increased selectivity for COX-2 inhibition.
[b]Values in human gastric tissue are the concentrations of non-steroidal anti-inflammatory drug required to inhibit synthesis of prostaglandin E$_2$ following ex vivo incubation (only the COX-1 isoform is present). The relative abilities to cause gastric damage relate approximately to inhibition of COX-1 in gastric mucosa. Therefore, much higher concentrations of celecoxib are required to cause gastric damage than aspirin.
These data are modified from reviewed data (Cryer and Feldman 1998; Del Tacca et al 2002; Stichtenoth and Frolich 2003).

relatively weaker platelet inhibition, and the COX-2-selective 'coxibs' are without effect (Table 29.3).

Other actions. Considerable work is being carried out in other areas of medicine to examine the place of the NSAIDs. Amongst these are the treatment of colonic cancer and Alzheimer's disease.

Pharmacokinetics

Most NSAIDs are weak acids that undergo some gastric absorption by pH partitioning (Ch. 2). This explains the relatively high drug concentration in cells of the gastric mucosa. However, most absorption occurs from the larger surface area of the small bowel. Enteric-coated formulations can be used to reduce release of drug in the stomach and limit direct exposure of the gastric mucosa. Some compounds, such as nabumetone, are inactive prodrugs (Ch. 2), which limits direct exposure of the gastric mucosa to the active form of the drug. These are converted (usually in the liver after absorption) to an active metabolite.

Absorption of NSAIDs from the gut is usually fairly rapid from conventional formulations. Some NSAIDs can be given by intramuscular injection for rapid onset of analgesia, or rectally to achieve a prolonged action and to reduce gastric irritation. Transcutaneous delivery was introduced with the intention of providing high local drug concentrations while attempting to minimise systemic unwanted effects. However, once the drug has penetrated the skin, it is widely distributed, and this route has little advantage for reducing systemic toxicity.

Many NSAIDs undergo hepatic metabolism to inactive compounds. The compounds differ widely in their elimination half-lives (see drug table). Short-acting drugs require frequent dosing to maintain continuous therapeutic effect, although synovial fluid concentrations in joint disease fluctuate less than the plasma concentrations. Modified-release formulations are widely used to reduce dosing frequency during long-term treatment. Piroxicam undergoes enterohepatic cycling, which contributes to its long half-life.

Aspirin (acetylsalicylic acid) is initially converted to an active metabolite, salicylic acid, and finally inactivated by conjugation with glycine and, to some extent, glucuronic acid (Ch. 2). Conjugation with glycine is saturable at higher doses and the metabolism of salicylate then changes from first-order to zero-order elimination kinetics (Ch. 2). This has important implications for aspirin overdose (Ch. 53).

Unwanted effects

Most unwanted effects arise from the inhibition of prostaglandin synthesis throughout the body. They are usually dose related.

Gastrointestinal effects

- Nausea, dyspepsia, gastric irritation and gastric ulceration are the most frequent unwanted effects. They are thought to occur principally as a result of inhibition of mucosal production of COX-1-generated PGE_2 and PGI_2, although inhibition of COX-2 may interfere with some aspects of tissue healing. The 'coxibs' cause a lower incidence of gastrointestinal disturbance. The propensity of the NSAID to produce gastrointestinal irritation more closely relates to the inhibition of COX-1 than the ratio of inhibition of COX-1:COX-2. PGE_2 has several actions that confer

Table 29.4
The predominant cyclo-oxygenase (COX) enzyme inhibited by non-steroidal anti-inflammatory drugs resulting in therapeutic and unwanted events

Predominant COX enzyme involved	
Therapeutic effect	
Analgesia	COX-2 and COX-1
Anti-inflammatory	COX-2 > COX-1
Antipyretic	COX-2 > COX-1
Antiplatelet	COX-1
Unwanted effect	
Gastrointestinal toxicity	COX-1 > COX-2
Sodium and water retention	COX-1 > COX-2
Decreased endothelial prostacyclin	COX-1
Bronchoconstriction	COX-2

Table 29.5
Classification of non-steroidal anti-inflammatory drugs, with major drug examples

Chemical type	Major examples
Salicylates	Aspirin Benorilate
Fenamates	Mefenamic acid
Propionic acid derivatives	Ibuprofen Naproxen Fenbufen Flurbiprofen Ketoprofen
Indoles	Indometacin Sulindac
Phenyl acetic acids	Diclofenac
Pyrazole derivatives	Phenylbutazone
Oxicams	Piroxicam Meloxicam
Selective COX-2 inhibitors ('coxibs')	Celecoxib[a] Etoricoxib Valdecoxib[a]

[a]Sulphonamides.
COX-2, cyclo-oxygenase 2.

Table 29.6
Properties of some commonly used analgesic drugs

	Aspirin (moderate doses)	Paracetamol	Indometacin	Ibuprofen	Celecoxib
Analgesic	++	++	++	+	+
Anti-inflammatory	+	–	+++	+	+
Antipyretic	+	+	+	+	+
Gastrointestinal bleeding	+	–	+	low	low

cytoprotection in the stomach (Ch. 33). The acidic nature of NSAIDs and their local concentration in gastric mucosal cells results in a decrease of the surface hydrophobicity of the mucus gel layer, reducing its barrier effect. Uncoupling of cellular oxidative phosphorylation by the drugs increases mucosal permeability, with consequent back-diffusion of H^+, which is trapped in the mucosal epithelium and leads to cytotoxicity. Inhibition of prostaglandin generation reduces mucosal blood flow, which probably enhances cytotoxicity by producing tissue hypoxia and local free radical generation. Mucus secretion and bicarbonate secretion are also reduced and acid secretion increased. Increased local production of leukotrienes may also be involved in the development of gastric toxicity. NSAIDs accumulate within gastric mucosal cells by direct absorption of the drug from the gastric lumen and also by systemic delivery of the drug to the mucosa. Consequently, rectal administration or the use of a prodrug may reduce, but will not eliminate, the risk of gastric damage. Occult blood loss from the bowel is increased during regular treatment with NSAIDs and the risk of overt gastrointestinal bleeding is greater. Not all NSAIDs carry the same risk of serious upper gastrointestinal unwanted effects and this is loosely related to their ability to inhibit COX-1. Management of NSAID-induced gastric damage is considered in Chapter 33.

- Rectal administration of NSAIDs can result in local irritation and bleeding.
- Exacerbation of inflammatory bowel disease (Ch. 34).
- Lower gastrointestinal bleeding or perforation.

Renal effects

- Prostaglandins (PGE_2, PGI_2) generated by both COX-1 and COX-2 are involved in the maintenance of renal blood flow and have additional effects on the renal tubule that promote natriuresis (Ch. 14). NSAIDs can produce a reversible decline in renal function, with a rise in serum creatinine. The problem is more common if renal function is already impaired (as is often the case in the elderly), or in the presence of heart failure or cirrhosis. These conditions are associated with reduced effective circulating blood volume, when prostaglandins play a greater role in maintenace of renal blood flow.
- Salt and water retention can occur even without renal insufficiency. Reduced prostaglandin synthesis in the ascending limb of the loop of Henle decreases expression of the $Na^+/K^+/2Cl^-$ cotransporter complex, and prostaglandins antagonise the action of vasopressin (Ch. 14). Water retention may exceed that of Na^+, resulting in dilutional hyponatraemia. Suppression of prostaglandin-mediated renin secretion can lead to hypoaldosteronism and

hyperkalaemia. Salt and water retention produced by NSAIDs can exacerbate heart failure and raise blood pressure by an average of 3–5 mmHg. In addition, the efficacy of drug treatments for these conditions (e.g. diuretics, angiotensin-converting enzyme inhibitors, β-adrenoceptor antagonists) is blunted by NSAIDs (Ch. 14).

Hypersensitivity

Hypersensitivity reactions occasionally produce asthma, urticaria, angioedema and rhinitis. People with nasal polyps and known allergic disorders appear to be most susceptible. Aspirin can precipitate 'pseudo-allergic' asthma in a subgroup of sensitive asthmatics, through inhibition of COX-1-generated PGE_2 production in the lung. It is suggested that as many as one in five asthmatics may be affected. Reduction of PGE_2 lowers its partial inhibitory effect on leukotrienes and mast cell degranulation, and is accompanied by increased synthesis of cysteinyl leukotrienes (particularly LTE_4) (Ch. 12). COX-2-selective NSAIDs do not cause this phenomenon.

Other unwanted effects

Other unwanted effects are unrelated to prostaglandin inhibition and are sometimes specific for individual compounds.

- CNS unwanted effects such as headache, dizziness, drowsiness, insomnia and confusion can occur, particularly in the elderly.
- Skin reactions can occasionally be severe, especially with fenbufen.
- Aspirin produces tinnitus in toxic doses; overdose of aspirin can be particularly hazardous (Ch. 53).
- Aspirin is associated with Reye's syndrome in children, a rare condition producing acute encephalopathy and fatty degeneration of the liver. The use of aspirin should be avoided in children under the age of 12 years.
- Phenylbutazone can produce bone marrow aplasia; its use is now restricted to ankylosing spondylitis, for which it is particularly effective.

COX-2-selective inhibitors

Examples: celecoxib, etoricoxib, valdecoxib, meloxicam

Mechanism of action

Selective COX-2 inhibitors have much less inhibitory action on COX-1, but the degree of selectivity for COX-2 varies among the drugs in this class. Etoricoxib has the greatest selectivity in whole blood tests (Table 29.3). Although diclofenac is selective for COX-2 inhibition, it is a potent COX-1 inhibitor in the human gastrointestinal tract and this is reflected in its ability to cause gastro-intestinal damage. They have anti-inflammatory actions similar to conventional non-selective NSAIDs, but there is some evidence that they may be less effective analgesics. This may be due to less inhibition of COX-3 in the brain and spinal cord. Selective COX-2 inhibitors have little direct effect on platelet TXA_2 production; how-ever, they can suppress the production of the anti-aggregating and vasodilating PGI_2 by blood vessels, which may allow thromboxanes to exert greater un-wanted cardiovascular effects. COX-2-selective drugs also interact with PPARs and impair macrophage activity and T-cell-mediated immune responses (see above).

Pharmacokinetics

Celecoxib, etoricoxib and valdecoxib are all well absorbed from the gut. They are eliminated by hepatic metabolism. The half-lives of celecoxib and valdecoxib are inter-mediate, while that of etoricoxib is long.

Unwanted effects

- COX-2-selective inhibitors have fewer upper gastrointestinal unwanted effects than NSAIDs, and reduce the risk of ulcers and ulcer complications by up to 50% compared with conventional NSAIDs. However, there is increasing evidence that the risk of ulceration increases with duration of therapy. Furthermore, if low-dose aspirin is concurrently being taken for its antiplatelet benefit, this negates the gastrointestinal-sparing benefits of COX-2-selective inhibitors. The strategy of reducing the upper gastrointestinal toxicity of COX inhibition by greater isozyme selectivity, therefore, has limited effectiveness. New molecules that are under investigation look likely to have even better gastroduodenal tolerability by combining COX inhibition with the protective effects of either lipoxygenase inhibition (COX-LOX inhibitors) or nitric oxide generation (nitric oxide-donating NSAIDs).
- Exacerbation of inflammatory bowel disease (Ch. 34).
- Stomatitis or mouth ulcers.
- Palpitation.
- Selective COX-2 inhibitors are much less likely to induce asthmatic attacks in NSAID-sensitive individuals.
- Overall risks of cardiovascular complications, stroke and raised blood pressure associated with COX-2 inhibitors are still being assessed. Celecoxib, etoricoxib and valdecoxib are contraindicated in severe congestive heart failure and caution should be exercised if there is a history of cardiac failure, left ventricular dysfunction, hypertension, or oedema for any other reason. Rofecoxib has recently been withdrawn from the market because of an increased incidence of cardiovascular complications when taken for more than 18 months. Further investigation into the effects of all selective COX-2 inhibitors on the occurrence of unwanted cardiovascular events is being undertaken.

Paracetamol

Mechanism of action

Paracetamol (acetaminophen in the USA) is a simple analgesic without anti-inflammatory activity. It has very little inhibitory effect on COX-1 or COX-2 in peripheral tissues, but inhibits COX-3 in the CNS. This inhibition is weak, however, and cannot explain all of the properties of paracetamol. Hydroperoxides are generated from the metabolism of arachidonic acid by COX and exert a positive feedback to stimulate COX activity. This feed-back is probably blocked by paracetamol. Several additional biochemical effects may contribute to the analgesic action, including modulation of serotonergic neurotransmission and inhibition of nuclear transcription of specific CNS proteins.

Pharmacokinetics

Paracetamol is rapidly absorbed from the gut. It is meta-bolised mainly by conjugation, but a minor hydroxylated metabolite is produced by cytochrome P450 in the liver and kidneys. This is detoxified by the limited supply of glutathione in these organs. In overdose, failure to con-jugate this metabolite can lead to liver and renal damage (Ch. 53).

Unwanted effects

- Paracetamol is usually well tolerated, and because it does not inhibit peripheral prostaglandin synthesis, it does not cause problems with homeostatic functions of prostanoids, for example gastrointestinal disturbances.
- Hepatic damage and renal failure in overdose (Ch. 53).

Indications for NSAIDs

NSAIDs are indicated for pain relief, particularly for:

- inflammatory conditions affecting joints, soft tissues, etc.
- postoperative pain
- renal colic
- headache
- dysmenorrhoea.

About 60% of people will respond to any one NSAID, but those who fail to respond to one may derive benefit from another. Adequate time must be allowed for the full analgesic or anti-inflammatory effect to develop (see above). The choice of NSAID is mainly determined by their unwanted effects, particularly on the stomach.

Other indications

NSAIDs are also used:

- as an antipyretic in febrile conditions
- to achieve closure of a patent ductus arteriosus in a neonate where patency may be inappropriately maintained by prostaglandin production; NSAIDs should not be given to a pregnant mother in the third trimester to avoid premature closure of the ductus
- for primary dysmenorrhoea; stimulation of the uterus by prostaglandins can be responsible for the pain in this condition
- for modest reduction of menstrual blood loss in menorrhagia (excessive blood loss at menstruation)
- for prevention of vascular occlusion by inhibition of platelet aggregation (especially low-dose aspirin [Ch. 11])

- for reduction in colonic polyps and prevention of colonic cancer
- NSAIDs may reduce the risk of developing Alzheimer's disease (Ch. 9).

In 2001, the National Institute for Clinical Excellence (NICE) advised that "Cox II selective inhibitors are not recommended for routine use in rheumatoid arthritis (RA) or osteoarthritis (OA). They should be used, in preference to standard NSAIDs, when clearly indicated as part of the management of RA or OA only in people who may be at 'high risk' of developing serious gastro-intestinal adverse effects." The drugs available for consideration at that time were celecoxib, rofecoxib, etodolac and meloxicam.

FURTHER READING

Bleumink GS, Feenstra J, Sturkenboom CJM et al (2003) Nonsteroidal anti-inflammatory drugs and heart failure. *Drugs* 63, 525–534

Camu F, Shi L, Vanlersberghe C (2003) The role of COX-2 inhibitors in pain modulation. *Drugs* 63, 1–7

Cryer B, Feldman M (1998) Cyclo-oxygenase-1 and cyclo-oxygenase-2 selectivity of widely used nonsteroidal anti-inflammatory drugs. *Am J Med* 104, 413–421

Del Tacca M, Colucci R, Fornai M, Blandizzi C (2002) Efficacy and tolerability of meloxicam, a COX-2 preferential nonsteroidal anti-inflammatory drug. *Clin Drug Invest* 22, 799–818

Epstein M (2002) Non-steroidal anti-inflammatory drugs and the continuum of renal dysfunction. *J Hypertens* 20(suppl 6), S17–S23

Garner S, Fidan D, Frankish R et al (2004) Celecoxib for rheumatoid arthritis (Cochrane Review). In: The Cochrane Library, Issue 2. Chichester, UK: John Wiley

James MW, Hawkey CJ (2003) Assessment of non-steroidal anti-inflammatory drug (NSAID) damage in the human gastrointestinal tract. *Br J Clin Pharmacol* 56, 146–155

Jones C. Practical COX-1 and COX-2 pharmacology: what's it all about? http://www.vetmedpub.com/cp/pdf/symposium/nov 1.pdf (accessed May 2004)

Kismet K, Akay MT, Abbasogulu O, Ercan A (2004) Celecoxib: a potent cyclo-oxygenase-2 inhibitor in cancer prevention. *Cancer Detect Prev* 28, 127–142

Lichtenstein DR, Wolfe M (2000) COX-2-selective NSAIDs. *JAMA* 284, 1297–1299

Micklewright R, Linley SLW, McQuade C et al (2003) NSAIDs, gastroprotection and cyclo-oxygenase-II-selective inhibitors. *Aliment Pharmacol Ther* 17, 321–332

National Institute for Clinical Excellence (2001) Guidance on the use of cyclo-oxygenase (Cox) II selective inhibitors, celecoxib, rofecoxib, meloxicam and etodolac for osteoarthritis and rheumatoid arthritis. http://www.nice.org.uk/Docref.asp?d=18034 (accessed May 5, 2004)

Paccani SR, Boncristiano M, Baldari CT (2003) Molecular mechanisms underlying suppression of lymphocyte responses by nonsteroidal antiinflammatory drugs. *Cell Mol Life Sci* 60, 1071–1083

Parente L, Perretti M (2003) Advances in the pathophysiology of constitutive and inducible cyclooxygenases: two enzymes in the spotlight. *Biochem Pharmacol* 65, 153–159

Stichtenoth DO, Frolich JC (2003) The second generation of COX-2 inhibitors – what advantages do the newest offer? *Drugs* 63, 33–45

Szczeklik A, Stevenson DD (2003) Aspirin-induced asthma: advances in pathogenesis, diagnosis, and management. *J Allergy Clin Immunol* 111, 913–921

Self-assessment

In questions 1–4, the first statement, in italics, is true. Are the accompanying statements also true?

1. *At least three isoenzymes, COX-1, COX-2 and COX-3, are involved in the synthesis of prostaglandins and thromboxanes.*

   a. COX-2 is not found constitutively in cells.
   b. PGE$_2$ does not cause pain itself but enhances the activity of algesic substances such as bradykinin.
   c. All NSAIDs inhibit COX-1 and COX-2 isoenzymes with equal potency.
   d. Paracetamol is a potent analgesic and anti-inflammatory agent.

2. *Gastrointestinal complications are the most common unwanted effects of NSAIDs.*

   a. NSAIDs reduce gastric blood flow.
   b. Aspirin and warfarin can be safely administered concurrently.
   c. Celecoxib causes a greater incidence of gastrointestinal symptoms than naproxen.

3. *The PGE$_1$ analogue misoprostol, if administered with NSAIDs, reduces their potential to cause gastric damage.*

   a. Small daily doses of aspirin (75 mg) can compromise renal function.
   b. The elderly have a greater risk of gastrointestinal adverse events when given NSAIDs.
   c. Ibuprofen is an effective first-choice NSAID in severe rheumatoid arthritis.

   d. Aspirin is a good choice of analgesic therapy for people with asthma.

4. *Celecoxib causes fewer gastrointestinal symptoms because it is a highly selective COX-2 inhibitor.*

   a. Celecoxib is useful for the inhibition of platelet aggregation in patients with myocardial infarction.
   b. Celecoxib is an antipyretic.

5. Extended-matching questions
   Choose the one <u>most appropriate</u> NSAID A–E that you would initially give in each case scenario 1–3.

   A. Aspirin
   B. Celecoxib
   C. Diclofenac plus misoprostol
   D. Paracetamol
   E. Indometacin.

   1. An elderly man with a long history of hypertension, congestive heart failure with oedema and chronic gastritis has chronic mild knee pain due to osteoarthritic changes which is interrupting his sleep.
   2. A 32-year-old severely asthmatic woman with a diagnosis of rheumatoid arthritis and recurrent dyspepsia and no other relevant history.
   3. A 45-year-old man who recently had a myocardial infarction. He was prescribed an angiotensin-converting enzyme inhibitor and simvastatin.

   The answers are provided on page 728.

Non-steroidal anti-inflammatory drugs (NSAIDs) and related drugs

Drug	Half-life (h)	Elimination	Comments
NSAIDs			All drugs have broad indications for pain relief (unless the use is indicated below); all are given orally (unless otherwise stated); many of the drugs are carboxylic acid derivatives which are eliminated as acyl glucuronides
Aceclofenac	–	Metabolism	Oxidation in liver by CYP2C9 is the major pathway; a minor hydrolytic pathway results in bioactivation by forming diclofenac
Acemetacin	1	Metabolism	Prodrug of indometacin, with high bioavailability and quantitative conversion to indometacin
Aspirin	0.25	Rapid hydrolysis	Salicylic acid is an active metabolite (half-life 3–20 h)
Azapropazone	13–17	Renal (?)	Use restricted to rheumatoid arthritis, ankylosing spondylitis and acute gout when other NSAIDs have been tried and failed; high oral bioavailability; clearance correlates with creatinine clearance
Celecoxib	11	Metabolism	Used for pain and inflammation in osteoarthritis and rheumatoid arthritis; good oral absorption; metabolised by polymorphic CYP2C9 to inactive products
Dexketoprofen	1–3	Metabolism	Used for short-term treatment of mild to moderate pain; optical isomer of ketoprofen (see below)
Diclofenac	1–2	Metabolism	Given orally, rectally, by deep intramuscular injection or intravenous infusion; oral bioavailability is about 60%; eliminated by a combination of CYP2C9- and CYP3A4-mediated oxidation and by conjugation
Diflunisal	8–12	Metabolism	Good oral absorption; major route of elimination is conjugation with glucuronic acid
Etodolac	6–7	Metabolism	Used for pain and inflammation in osteoarthritis and rheumatoid arthritis, good oral bioavailability (80%); eliminated by both oxidation and conjugation with glucuronic acid
Etoricoxib	25	Metabolism	Used for pain and inflammation in osteoarthritis, rheumatoid arthritis and in acute gout; good oral bioavailability (90%); eliminated largely by CYP3A4-mediated oxidation
Fenbufen	10–17	Metabolism	Prodrug which is oxidised to active metabolites
Fenoprofen	2–3	Metabolism	Rapidly and completely absorbed; eliminated by both oxidation and conjugation with glucuronic acid
Flurbiprofen	3–9	Metabolism + renal	Given orally or rectally; rapidly and completely absorbed, metabolised by polymorphic CYP2C9 and also by direct conjugation; about 25% is eliminated unchanged by the kidneys
Ibuprofen	2–4	Metabolism + renal	Good oral bioavailability (80%); about 10% is eliminated unchanged by the kidneys and the remainder via metabolism by polymorphic CYP2C9
Indometacin	3–5	Metabolism + renal	Given orally or rectally; rapidly and completely absorbed; eliminated by oxidation and conjugation while the remainder is excreted unchanged by the kidneys
Ketoprofen	1–3	Metabolism	Given orally, rectally or by deep intramuscular injection; high oral bioavailability (90%); glucuronidation is the major route of elimination but the conjugate can be hydrolysed back to the parent drug if elimination is impaired, for example in renal failure

continued

Non-steroidal anti-inflammatory drugs (NSAIDs) and related drugs (continued)

Drug	Half-life (h)	Elimination	Comments
NSAIDs (continued)			
Ketorolac	3–9	Renal + metabolism	Used in short-term management of postoperative pain; given orally or by intramuscular or slow intravenous injection; renal excretion is major route (60% of dose) of elimination; metabolism is by both oxidation and conjugation
Mefenamic acid	3–4	Metabolism	Rapidly and completely absorbed; absorption reduced if taken with food; metabolised by polymorphic CYP2C9 and also by direct conjugation; metabolites are known to be inactive
Meloxicam	12–20	Metabolism	Used for pain and inflammation in rheumatoid arthritis, osteoarthritis (short-term) and in ankylosing spondylitis; given orally or rectally; absorption is slow but essentially complete; metabolised by polymorphic CYP2C9 to inactive metabolites
Nabumetone	16–27	Metabolism	Used for pain and inflammation in osteoarthritis and rheumatoid arthritis; undergoes complete first-pass metabolism by hydrolysis of methyl ester group to yield an active naphthylacetic acid derivative
Naproxen	12–15	Metabolism	Given orally or rectally; rapidly and completely absorbed; metabolised by oxidation and conjugation to inactive products
Parecoxib	5–9	Metabolism	Used in short-term management of postoperative pain; give by deep intramuscular or intravenous injection; metabolised to a range of products, including valdecoxib
Piroxicam	30–60	Metabolism + renal	Given orally, rectally or by deep intramuscular injection; rapid absorption; metabolised in the liver to inactive products; renal excretion accounts for about 10% of dose (99% protein binding minimises glomerular filtration of the drug)
Sulindac	7–8	Metabolism + renal	Prodrug for active thioether metabolite, which is formed by reduction in the liver and lower bowel
Tenoxicam	44–100	Metabolism	Given orally or by intramuscular or intravenous injection; metabolites are known to be inactive
Tiaprofenic acid	2–4	Metabolism	Oxidised by P450 (little other information available)
Tolfenamic acid	2	Metabolism	Licensed for the treatment of migraine – see Ch. 26; metabolites are eliminated in bile
Valdecoxib	8–11	Metabolism	Used for pain and inflammation in osteoarthritis and rheumatoid arthritis and for dysmenorrhoea; high oral bioavailability (83%); eliminated by oxidation via CYP3A4 and CYP2C9 and also by formation of an *N*-glucuronide
Related drugs			All drugs given orally (unless otherwise stated)
Benorylate	<0.1	Hydrolysis	Ester of paracetamol and acetylsalicylic acid; absorbed intact and hydrolysed rapidly in blood and liver
Paracetamol (acetaminophen)	3–4	Metabolism	Rapidly and completely absorbed; most is metabolised by conjugation with glucuronic acid and sulphate; a minor oxidation pathway leads to hepatotoxicity – see Ch. 53

30

Rheumatoid arthritis, other inflammatory arthritides and osteoarthritis

Rheumatoid arthritis is a chronic inflammatory condition of unknown cause. Autoimmune processes contribute to the maintenance of the condition, but it is uncertain whether it is initiated by an autoimmune reaction or an exogenous antigen. The primary process is lymphoid cell infiltration of the synovium around the joint, formation of new blood vessels and a proliferation of the synovial membrane. The synovium subsequently becomes locally invasive (pannus) and osteoclasts destroy joint cartilage and bone. Apart from psoriatic arthritis, other forms of inflammatory arthritis do not produce erosive changes in periarticular bone or marked joint destruction to the same degree.

The chronic inflammatory process is initiated by T-lymphocytes; then, cellular infiltration with T-cells, B-cells, macrophages and plasma cells and subsequent cytokine and cytokine receptor production sustain the condition (Fig. 30.1). Macrophages and fibroblasts produce cytokines, and of these, interleukins IL-1 and IL-6, and tumour necrosis factor alpha (TNFα) are prominent. This pattern differs from most other immune-mediated diseases. TNFα and IL-1 orchestrate the recruitment of inflammatory cells such as leucocytes by increasing the expression of adhesion molecules (integrins) on vascular endothelial cells. They also stimulate synovial fibroblasts, osteoclasts and chondrocytes to release tissue-destroying matrix metalloproteinases (MMPs) and chemokine receptors. The ubiquitous gene transcription factor nuclear factor kappa B (NF-κB) is also thought to be involved in the destructive cycle of events. Activated macrophages, lymphocytes and fibroblasts stimulate angiogenesis in the synovium. Antibodies are produced to the collagen exposed in the damaged cartilage. Complexes of collagen antibody with IgM rheumatoid factor (autoantibodies reactive with IgG) in the cartilage activate the complement path-way, although the contribution of this to joint damage is not known. The activated T-cells stimulate osteoclastogenesis that increases bone resorption. The end result of this complex inflammatory process is irreversible destruction of cartilage and erosion of periarticular bone.

The symptoms of rheumatoid arthritis usually appear gradually and most often involve the proximal interphalangeal joints of the fingers, metacarpophalangeal joints and wrists. Other joints such as the ankles and hips may be involved later. The affected joints are warm, swollen and painful. Stiffness is troublesome, particularly in the morning, as a result of an increase in extracellular fluid in and around the joint. Systemic disturbance is common, including general fatigue and malaise, while extra-articular manifestations such as vasculitis and neuropathy can occur.

Disease-modifying antirheumatic drugs or second-line drugs for rheumatoid arthritis

Non-steroidal anti-inflammatory drugs (NSAIDs – Ch. 29) provide symptomatic relief but do not alter the long-term progression of joint destruction in rheumatoid arthritis. A diverse group of compounds can reduce the rate of progression of joint erosion and destruction, leading to improvement both in symptoms and in the clinical and serological markers of rheumatoid arthritis activity. These drugs produce long-term depression of the inflammatory response even though they have little direct anti-inflammatory effect. They all have a slow onset of action, with many producing little improvement until about 3 months after starting treatment. Such drugs are grouped together and known as second-line drugs or disease-modifying antirheumatic drugs (DMARDs).

Sulfasalazine

The action of sulfasalazine in arthritis is poorly understood. It is hydrolysed in the colon to 5-aminosalicylic acid (which is believed to contribute little to the antirheumatic action) and to sulfapyridine. The latter moiety may reduce absorption of antigens from the colon that promote joint inflammation. However, sulfasalazine and sulfapyridine are both absorbed and are found at similar concentrations in synovial fluid. Sulfasalazine can influence several signal transduction pathways involved in the synthesis of pro-inflammatory cytokines, such as gene transcription mediated by NF-κB.

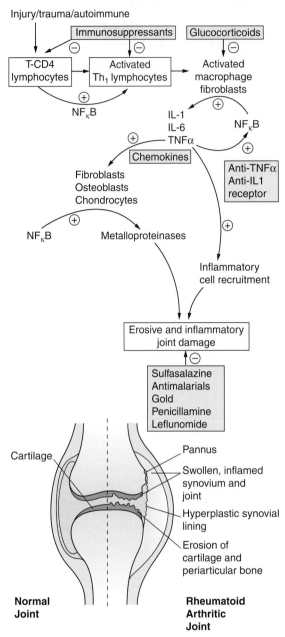

Fig. 30.1
The sites of drug action in rheumatoid arthritis. The affected synovial joint is characterised by inflamed and swollen synovium with increased presence of fibroblasts, osteoclasts, plasma cells, mast cells, B cells and angiogenesis. The synovial fluid contains increased numbers of polymorphonuclear neutrophil leucocytes. There is erosion of cartilage and adjacent bone. The cascade of self-perpetuating inflammatory events involves many factors, including upregulation of the ubiquitous gene transcription superfamily nuclear factor kappa B (NF-κB) which not only can induce gene transcription for many inflammatory, proliferative and remodelling factors but also can be a target for their actions. Many of the drugs shown act at multiple sites. IL, interleukin; TNFα, tumour necrosis factor alpha.

High doses of sulfasalazine are required for the treatment of rheumatoid arthritis and these often produce gastrointestinal upset. This can be minimised by increasing the dose slowly and by using an enteric-coated formulation. Other problems include reversible oligospermia (therefore sulfasalazine should be avoided in males who wish to have a family) and blood dyscrasias. Sulfasalazine is discussed more fully in Chapter 34.

Antimalarials

Examples: chloroquine, hydroxychloroquine

The antimalarial drugs are believed to reduce T-lymphocyte transformation and chemotaxis. Their weakly basic nature permits their uptake and concentration in tissues in a non-ionised form. Having entered the lysosomes inside the cell, the acidic environment traps and concentrates the drug in its ionised state. Macrophages depend on acid proteases in their lysosomes for digestion of phagocytosed protein. Antimalarial drugs slightly increase the pH inside the macrophage lysosomes, which alters the processing of peptide antigens and their subsequent presentation on the cell surface. Thus, the interaction between T helper cells and antigen-presenting macrophages responsible for joint inflammation is reduced, with a reduction in the inflammatory response. Recent evidence also suggests that these drugs reduce the production of several inflammatory cytokines.

The major toxic effect of antimalarial drugs is on the retina, although at the low doses that are now recommended they are relatively safe. Hydroxychloroquine is better tolerated than chloroquine and is now the preferred agent. Specialist assessment of the eyes is recommended during treatment with hydroxychloroquine if there is a change in visual acuity or blurring of vision, or if treatment continues for more than 5 years. The pharmacokinetics and unwanted effects of these drugs can be found in Chapter 51.

Leflunomide

Mechanism of action and uses

Leflunomide is an isoxazole derivative that binds to dehydroorotate dehydrogenase, which is a key mitochondrial enzyme in the de novo synthesis of the pyrimidine ribonucleotide uridine monophosphate (UMP). Activated lymphocytes require an eightfold increase in their pyrimidine pool to proliferate. Inadequate provision by de novo synthesis increases expression of the tumour-suppressor p53 that translocates to the cell nucleus and arrests the cell cycle in the G_1 phase. This reduces the expansion of the activated and autoimmune T- and B-lymphocyte pool. The result is suppression of immunoglobulin production and cellular immune processes. Other dividing cells can obtain adequate pyrimidines from a separate salvage pathway. Other potential contributory mechanisms of immunomodulation, such as inhibition of tyrosine kinases and reduced production of transcription factors that regulate inflammatory cytokines, are probably of lesser importance.

Pharmacokinetics

Leflunomide is a prodrug. It is well absorbed from the gut and converted non-enzymatically in the intestinal mucosa and plasma, and, to a lesser extent, by first-pass metabolism in the liver to its active metabolite. The metabolite has a very long half-life of 15 days and is excreted via the bile and kidney. Enterohepatic circulation contributes to the long plasma half-life.

Unwanted effects

- gastrointestinal upset, especially diarrhoea
- increase in blood pressure
- headache, dizziness, lethargy
- leucopenia
- skin rash
- alopecia
- reversible abnormalities of liver function
- teratogenicity: it is advised that conception should be avoided for 2 years after stopping treatment in women and 3 months in men.

Prevention and management of unwanted effects

Monitoring of full blood count (especially white cell count) and liver function should be carried out regularly during treatment. If serious unwanted effects occur, elimination of the drug can be increased by the use of colestyramine (Ch. 48) to bind the active metabolite present in the gut after biliary excretion.

Immunosuppressive drugs

Several drugs with immunosuppressive actions have been shown to be effective in rheumatoid arthritis. These include:

- antimetabolites: methotrexate, azathioprine (Ch. 52)
- calcineurin inhibitors: ciclosporin (Ch. 38).

Tacrolimus (Ch. 38) and mycophenolate mofetil (Ch. 38) may also be useful in rheumatoid arthritis but are not licensed for this indication in the UK.

Methotrexate is one of the most effective antirheumatic drugs. Although its primary mechanism of action is by folate antagonism, co-administration of folic acid supplements prevents much of the mucosal and gastrointestinal toxicity of the drug but does not reduce its immunomodulatory effect. A possible additional mechanism of action to explain the effect in arthritis is accumulation of adenosine, an intermediate in purine biosynthesis. Adenosine is a potent anti-inflammatory

mediator through its effects on neutrophil adhesion and cytokine production, macrophage function and endothelial adhesion molecules. For the treatment of inflammatory arthritis, methotrexate is usually given orally once a week. However, if it produces intractable gastrointestinal symptoms, then it can be given intramuscularly.

Gold

Examples: sodium aurothiomalate, auranofin

Mechanism of action

The precise mechanism by which gold acts is unknown. A popular concept is that gold is taken up by mononuclear cells and inhibits their phagocytic function. This will reduce the release of inflammatory mediators and inhibit inflammatory cell proliferation. Production of inflammatory cytokines such as IL-1 and IL-6 and TNFα is inhibited, and superoxide production by neutrophils is reduced. There is also evidence for inhibition of other cell-signalling pathways involved in inflammation, including NF-κB.

Oral gold (auranofin) has a rather slower onset of action than intramuscular gold and is less efficacious, but is much better tolerated. The advent of more effective drugs has reduced the use of gold salts in current clinical practice.

Pharmacokinetics

The parenteral form of gold (sodium aurothiomalate) is given by deep intramuscular injection. An initial test dose is given to screen for acute toxicity (see below), followed by injections at weekly intervals to gradually achieve a therapeutic concentration in the tissues. Subsequently, a smaller dose is used to maintain remission. Oral gold is taken daily. Gold binds readily to albumin and several tissue proteins and accumulates in many tissues such as the liver, kidney, bone marrow, lymph nodes and spleen. Accumulation also occurs in the synovium of inflamed joints. Elimination is largely by the kidney, and to a lesser extent by biliary excretion. Gold has a half-life of several weeks, probably as a result of its extensive tissue binding.

Unwanted effects

The unwanted effects can be serious and all but the most minor effects should lead to immediate cessation of treatment:

- oral ulceration
- proteinuria from membranous glomerulonephritis: proteinuria can develop after several weeks of treatment, sometimes progressing to nephrotic syndrome; recovery can take up to two years following drug withdrawal

- blood disorders, especially thrombocytopenia but also agranulocytosis and aplastic anaemia
- skin rashes
- pulmonary fibrosis
- diarrhoea: common with oral gold.

Prevention and management of unwanted effects

Urine should be checked for protein and a blood count obtained before each injection of gold, and regularly during oral therapy. Major complications may require chelation of gold with dimercaprol or penicillamine (Ch. 53) to increase its elimination. Corticosteroids can be helpful to treat blood dyscrasias. Gold should not be used if there is a history of renal or hepatic disease, blood dyscrasias or severe skin rashes. If stomatitis, a pruritic rash, neutropenia, thrombocytopenia or significant proteinuria (>1 g in 24 h) develop, gold should be stopped.

Penicillamine

Mechanism of action and uses

The details of its mechanism of action are uncertain. Modulation of the immune system is believed to underlie the action of penicillamine, but it is not classified with other drugs affecting the immune response in the British National Formulary. Actions are thought to include reduced production of immunoglobulins, reduction in the number of activated lymphocytes, and stabilisation of lysosomal membranes in inflammatory cells. Penicillamine has not been shown to slow the progression of joint erosions.

Penicillamine is a thiol compound that can chelate many metals. This is probably of little relevance to its use in arthritis but has given the drug a role in the management of poisonings (Ch. 53) and in Wilson's disease, a genetically determined illness that is associated with copper overload.

Pharmacokinetics

Penicillamine is well absorbed from the gut, although oral iron supplements substantially reduce its absorption. The half-life is short, but penicillamine binds tightly via disulphide bonds to plasma and tissue proteins. Penicillamine is partially metabolised in the liver, but is also excreted unchanged in the urine.

Unwanted effects

Unwanted effects occur frequently and are responsible for about 30% of people stopping treatment. They can be reduced by slow increases in dose. Many unwanted effects resemble those of gold:

- nausea, vomiting, abdominal discomfort and rashes (often with fever), especially early in treatment
- loss of taste is common, but may resolve despite continued treatment

- oral ulceration
- proteinuria, which is caused by immune-complex glomerulonephritis and is dose related; nephrotic syndrome can occur
- blood disorders, especially thrombocytopenia but also neutropenia and, rarely, aplastic anaemia.

Regular monitoring of urine protein and blood counts should be carried out during treatment.

Antibodies against tumour necrosis factor alpha

Examples: adalimumab, etanercept, infliximab

Mechanism of action

TNFα stimulates several inflammatory processes:

- release of pro-inflammatory cytokines such as IL-1, IL-6 and IL-8
- increased expression of adhesion molecules by fibroblasts, with increased leucocyte migration into inflamed tissues
- release of MMPs from synovial fibroblasts, osteoclasts and chondrocytes, contributing to cartilage degradation
- stimulation of osteoclasts, causing bone resorption
- stimulation of angiogenesis, contributing to pannus formation in the synovium.

TNFα acts by binding to one of two cell surface receptors, p55 and p75, that are found in several tissues.

Adalimumab is a monoclonal antibody specific for TNFα.

Etanercept is a fusion protein consisting of two recombinant soluble extracellular portions of the human TNF p75 receptor, fused to the constant (Fc) domain of human immunoglobulin (IgG$_1$). It binds to TNFα and the cytokine lymphotoxin α (also known as TNFβ). Etanercept reduces the pro-inflammatory activity of TNFα, but it is not known whether the effect on lymphotoxin is of clinical importance.

Infliximab is a chimeric monoclonal antibody, with the variable region of a murine antibody that neutralises TNFα combined with the constant region of a human antibody. It does not neutralise TNFβ.

Pharmacokinetics

Adalimumab is given by subcutaneous injection. The long half-life allows the drug to be given once every two weeks. The mechanism of elimination has not been defined.

Etanercept is given by twice-weekly subcutaneous injection. It is slowly absorbed from the injection site, and has a very long half-life of about 5 days. It is believed to be metabolised by proteolytic processes.

Infliximab is given by intravenous infusion, initially at 2- and 4-week intervals, then every 2 months. It has a very long half-life of 9 days, and its route of elimination is not well understood.

Unwanted effects

- Adalimumab appears to be well tolerated when used in conjunction with other DMARDs, but comparative data with etanercept or infliximab are not available.
- Etanercept produces mild injection site reactions and upper respiratory tract symptoms, e.g. rhinitis.
- Infliximab produces fever, chills, pruritis or urticaria after infusion in about 15% of people. It less commonly causes dyspnoea or headache.
- There are reports of an increased risk of serious infection, but the causal relationship is uncertain. An increased risk of tuberculosis does appear to be causally related, and screening for evidence of tuberculosis is recommended before initiation of therapy.

Interleukin-1 receptor antagonists

Example: anakinra

Mechanism of action

Anakinra is a recombinant human IL-1 receptor antagonist. IL-1 is a pro-inflammatory cytokine released by macrophages and fibroblasts in inflamed synovium, and by neutrophils in synovial fluid. IL-1 is actually a family of three cytokines, comprising two agonists (IL-1α and IL-1β) and the IL-1 receptor antagonist. The theoretical basis for the use of anakinra is that joint destruction arises from an imbalance between the agonists and the antagonist. The IL-1 family peptides compete for occupancy of the IL-1 receptor on the outer membrane of synovial cells; as little as 2–3% occupancy by the agonists produces maximal pro-inflammatory cell activation.

Pharmacokinetics

Anakinra is given by daily subcutaneous injection. Elimination is via the kidneys, and anakinra has a short half-life.

Unwanted effects

- injection site reactions
- increased risk of serious infections, particularly in people with asthma
- neutropenia.

Management of rheumatoid arthritis and other inflammatory arthritides

NSAIDs (Ch. 29) are the mainstay of symptomatic drug treatment for all types of inflammatory arthritis. Physical aids such as splinting and bed rest are important for acute episodes. The choice of NSAID is arbitrary, with considerable variation in individual responses to different drugs. Propionic acid derivatives are often used first; they have a weaker anti-inflammatory activity than other classes of NSAID, but generally have fewer unwanted effects. More powerful drugs such as diclofenac can be used when others fail to control symptoms, although the increased risk of unwanted gastrointestinal effects may limit their use, especially in the elderly. About 60% of people can be expected to respond to the first-choice agent, and most derive some benefit from taking one of the NSAIDs. Predicting which drug will be most effective in an individual is currently impossible. Morning stiffness is often disabling in inflammatory arthritis: this is helped by giving a late evening dose of an NSAID with a long half-life, a modified-release formulation of a compound with a short half-life, or an NSAID suppository. Topical NSAIDs applied over the affected joint(s) are not usually recommended. Cyclo-oxygenase 2 (COX-2)-selective drugs are usually reserved for those who are intolerant of NSAIDs, or who have a higher risk of serious gastrointestinal complications with an NSAID (Ch. 29).

Inflammatory arthritides other than rheumatoid arthritis (the seronegative spondylarthritides) do not usually progress to extensive erosive arthritis with joint destruction. By contrast, progressive joint damage is common in rheumatoid arthritis, and, to a lesser extent, in psoriatic arthritis. There is now a sustantial body of evidence that early use of second-line drugs (DMARDs) leads to a better long-term outcome, and this has led to a more intensive approach to the treatment of rheumatoid arthritis with earlier use of DMARDs. Indications for DMARDs include:

- the prevention of erosive damage
- the suppression of persistent inflammation that fails to respond to three months of treatment with NSAIDs
- intolerance to NSAIDs
- a high titre of rheumatoid factor or extra-articular manifestations of rheumatoid disease.

DMARDs are almost always used in combination with NSAIDs, particularly in the first few weeks of treatment, since they do not have significant anti-inflammatory action and require 2–3 months before an effect is established. Sulfasalazine is often given initially for its perceived low toxicity; however, methotrexate is probably the most effective agent and is now the first-choice DMARD for most rheumatologists. Used correctly, it also is well tolerated. Hydroxychloroquine can be an effective alternative, but is seldom used as monotherapy, while leflunomide is often reserved for people who are intolerant of methotrexate. Gold and penicillamine are now less widely used, due to toxicity and limited efficacy, while immunomodulators other than methotrexate are generally reserved as third-line agents. Cytotoxic drugs, especially cyclophosphamide, are particularly useful for the management of extra-articular manifestations of rheumatoid disease, such as vasculitis, pericarditis or pleurisy.

Increasingly, combinations of DMARDs are being used as standard therapy. If a single second-line drug is insufficient to suppress disease activity and methotrexate has not been used, then methotrexate should be tried. Combination therapy is used for failure to respond to methotrexate within 3 months. If methotrexate has been well tolerated, then another second-line drug such as hydroxychloroquine, sulfasalazine or ciclosporin is usually added. Leflunomide is of comparable efficacy to methotrexate, and is used for those who are intolerant of methotrexate. Drug combinations are more effective than single agents, and triple therapy may have advantages over two drugs. Anti-TNFα agents and anakinra are reserved for those who fail to respond to more-conventional therapies or are intolerant of several drugs. Criteria for the use of anti-TNFα agents have been produced in the UK and specify that previous DMARD therapy should have been tried, and the level of clinical activity of the disease assessed by a composite scoring system. The National Institute for Clinical Excellence (NICE) guidelines should be referred to for details.

The role of corticosteroids in rheumatoid arthritis has been controversial. Intra-articular injections are used for individual inflamed joints (especially knee and shoulder). In active disease, short courses of oral prednisolone or pulse therapy with intravenous methylprednisolone (Ch. 44) can produce a rapid relief of symptoms before DMARDs work. In early rheumatoid disease, a small dose of oral prednisolone given for 6 months in combination with sulfasalazine or methotrexate retards bone damage and slows disease progression. Pulsed intramuscular corticosteroid therapy is also given for disease flares, or to ameliorate symptoms in the first few weeks after initiating DMARD therapy (because of the slow reponse).

Although most evidence for the use of DMARDs has been obtained in the treatment of rheumatoid arthritis, there is increasing evidence for their efficacy in the seronegative spondylarthritides. Sulfasalazine and methotrexate may be effective for peripheral joint disease. Anti-TNFα agents are used in the short-term treatment of ankylosing spondylitis and psoriatic arthritis, but it is not known whether they will slow ankylosis.

Clinical trials are taking place with drugs that block chemokines and their receptors. Initial clinical data show some benefit.

Osteoarthritis

Osteoarthritis is the clinical manifestation of joint degeneration that results from loss of articular cartilage and becomes more common with increasing age. Most osteoarthritis is idiopathic (when it can be localised or generalised) but a small proportion is secondary to other conditions such as joint injury or chondrocalcinosis. It is not known whether the initiating factors originate in the articular cartilage or subchondral bone.

The integrity of articular cartilage depends on the balance of synthetic and catabolic activity of the chondrocytes embedded in the cartilage matrix. Mechanical compression of cartilage produces many physical and biochemical stimuli that influence chondrocyte metabolism. Mechanical overload, the principal cause of secondary osteoarthritis, produces changes that promote matrix destruction and apoptotic chondrocyte death. It remains uncertain whether most osteoarthritis is caused primarily by increased degradation or decreased synthesis of cartilage.

Synthesis of cartilage is promoted by the expression of growth factors by chondrocytes, especially insulin-like growth factor 1 and transforming growth factor beta. Degradation of cartilage proteins is carried out by MMPs, particularly stromelysin 1 (MMP-3) in early osteoarthritis and gelatinase A (MMP-2) and MMP-13 in late disease. MMPs are synthesised by chondrocytes in response to stimulation by the pro-inflammatory cytokines IL-1β and TNFα. Synovial inflammation often occurs adjacent to the damaged cartilage. Chondrocytes produce a chemokine, RANTES (regulated upon activation normal T cell expressed and secreted), and synovial cells produce chemokine receptors CXCR4 (chemokine receptor type 4) which is on the surface of white blood cells and has a role in the trafficking of cells in the immune response. Some but not all chemokines are upregulated in osteoarthritis and may contribute to disease progression.

Loss of matrix leads to disruption of the cartilage, with swelling and fissuring of the surface. Subchondral bone becomes increasingly vascular and new bone is laid down. There is recent evidence that stiffening of subchondral bone, with less effective shock absorption, may be the initiating factor for cartilage loss.

The cardinal symptom of osteoarthritis is pain during physical activity, which is most pronounced with use of the affected joint, and relieved by rest. Pain also occurs at rest with advanced disease. Stiffness may be troublesome for short periods after rest. Various joints can be involved, particularly the distal interphalangeal joints of the fingers and the carpometacarpal joint of the thumb. Large joints such as the knee, hip, elbow and shoulder are often asymmetrically affected.

Management of osteoarthritis

Treatment currently remains symptomatic. Non-pharmacological therapy such as weight loss, exercise and physical therapy is often useful. If pain is troublesome, simple analgesics should usually be considered as first-line treatment. NSAIDs may be helpful for inflammatory episodes or if paracetamol is ineffective. In vitro studies suggest that some NSAIDs may accelerate the loss of articular cartilage in osteoarthritis; clinical studies are inconclusive, but avoidance of powerful NSAIDs is probably desirable. Intra-articular or peri-articular injection of a corticosteroid (Ch. 44) can provide short-term symptomatic relief in osteoarthritis, even if there is little clinical evidence of joint inflammation. Corticosteroids inhibit pro-inflammatory mediators in synovial tissue, such as IL-1 and TNFα.

Oral glucosamine (an over-the-counter preparation in the UK) can produce symptomatic relief in osteoarthritis, and may have a chondroprotective effect. Joint injection with hyaluronic acid remains a controversial treatment, with conflicting evidence of efficacy from clinical trials. Long-term management of osteoarthritis may eventually require surgical joint replacement. Compounds under development, particularly metalloproteinase inhibitors and IL-1 receptor antagonists, may in future offer the possibility of prevention of cartilage degeneration or even promote regeneration.

FURTHER READING

Rheumatoid arthritis and other inflammatory arthritides

Braun J, Brandt J, Listing J et al (2003) Biologic therapies in the spondyloarthritis: new opportunities, new challenges. *Curr Opin Rheumatol* 15, 394–407

Brockbank J, Gladman D (2002) Diagnosis and management of psoriatic arthritis. *Drugs* 62, 2447–2457

Canella AC, O'Dell JR (2003) Is there still a role for traditional disease-modifying antirheumatic drugs (DMARDs) in rheumatoid arthritis? *Curr Opin Rheumatol* 15, 185–192

Conn DL, Lim SS (2003) New role for an old friend: prednisone is a disease-modifying agent in early rheumatoid arthritis. *Curr Opin Rheumatol* 15, 193–196

Drosos AA (2002) Newer immunosuppressive drugs. Their potential role in rheumatoid arthritis *Drugs* 62, 891–907

Haringman JJ, Ludikhuize J, Tak PP (2004) Chemokines in joint disease: the key to inflammation? *Ann Rheum Dis* 63, 1186–1194

Katz WA (2002) Use of nonopioid analgesics and adjunctive agents in the management of pain in rheumatic diseases. *Curr Opin Rheumatol* 14, 63–71

Kremer JM (2001) Rational use of new and existing disease-modifying agents in rheumatoid arthritis. *Ann Intern Med* 134, 695–706

Lee DM, Weinblatt ME (2001) Rheumatoid arthritis. *Lancet* 358, 903–911

Makarov SS (2001) NFκB in rheumatoid arthritis: a pivotal regulator of inflammation, hyperplasia, and tissue destruction. **http://arthritis-research.com/content/3/4/200** (accessed July 2004)

National Institute for Clinical Excellence (2001) Full guidance on Cox II selective inhibitors. **http://www.nice.org.uk/page.aspx?o=18034** (accessed July 2004). (Update expected 2005)

O'Dell JR (2004) Therapeutic strategies for rheumatoid arthritis. *N Engl J Med* 350, 2591–2602

Olsen NJ, Stein CM (2004) New drugs for rheumatoid arthritis. *N Engl J Med* 350, 2167–2179

Shanahan JC, Moreland LW, Carter RH (2003) Upcoming biologic agents for the treatment of rheumatic diseases. *Curr Opin Rheumatol* 15, 226–236

Smith JM (2001) Anti-TNF agents for rheumatoid arthritis. *Br J Pharmacol* 51, 201–208

Smolen JS, Steiner G (2003) Therapeutic strategies for rheumatoid arthritis *Nat Rev Drug Discov* 2, 473–488

Osteoarthritis

Chard J, Dieppe P (2002) Update: treatment of osteoarthritis. *Arthritis Rheum* 47, 686–690

Dieppe P, Brandt KD (2003) What is important in treating osteoarthritis? Whom should we treat and how should we treat them? *Rheum Dis Clin North Am* 29, 687–716

Haq I, Murphy E, Dacre J (2003) Osteoarthritis. *Postgrad Med J* 79, 377–383

Jubb RW (2002) Oral and intra-articular remedies: review of papers published from March 2001 to February 2002. *Curr Opin Rheumatol* 14, 597–602

Sharma S (2002) Nonpharmacological management of osteoarthritis. *Curr Opin Rheumatol* 14, 603–607

Self-assessment

In questions 1–6, the first statement, in italics, is true. Are the following statements also true?

1. *Disease-modifying antirheumatic drugs (DMARDs) are commonly also called second-line antirheumatic drugs.*

   a. NSAIDs reduce the symptoms of rheumatoid disease and retard the progress of the disease.
   b. If penicillamine does not lead to clinical benefit within 6 months, it should be stopped.

2. *When tolerated, intramuscular gold is an effective drug for achieving remission in rheumatoid arthritis but unwanted effects limit tolerability.*

   a. Gold can be given by intramuscular or oral routes.
   b. Intramuscular gold can cause proteinuria.

3. *Methotrexate or sulfasalazine are often chosen as initial second-line therapy for rheumatoid arthritis partly because of their rapid onset of action (4–6 weeks methotrexate, 8–12 weeks sulfasalazine).*

   a. During methotrexate therapy, folic acid is contraindicated.
   b. The combination of sulfapyridine and 5-amino salicylic acid (sulfasalazine) is more effective than either component alone.
   c. Methotrexate has relatively fewer unwanted effects compared with most other DMARDs for rheumatoid arthritis.

4. *Sulfasalazine can scavenge toxic oxygen metabolites produced by neutrophils, and this may contribute to its effect in rheumatoid arthritis.* Combination therapy with DMARDs should not be used in rheumatoid arthritis.

5. *A major role of corticosteroids is to bridge the gap between starting treatment and the onset of action of the second-line treatments for rheumatoid arthritis.*

   a. Intra-articular injections of corticosteroids slow progression of erosions.
   b. Prolonged treatment with high doses of corticosteroids can cause adrenal atrophy.

6. *Ciclosporin is valuable when used in combination with methotrexate in very active early rheumatoid disease.* The antimalarials chloroquine and hydroxychloroquine are of little benefit in the treatment of rheumatoid arthritis.

7. Extended-matching questions

   For each of the scenarios 1–3, choose the best option A–H in answer to the question.

   A. An NSAID such as ibuprofen
   B. Indometacin
   C. Methotrexate
   D. Methotrexate plus ibuprofen
   E. Infliximab
   F. Hydroxychloroquine
   G. A disease-modifying antirheumatic drug
   H. Sulfasalazine.

   1. 30-year-old woman had gradually developed painful wrists over 4 weeks; she had not experienced similar episodes of pain before. On examination, both wrists and the metacarpophalangeal joints of both hands were tender but not deformed. What treatment would you choose?
   2. There was some initial symptomatic improvement, but subsequently the pain, stiffness and swelling of the hands persisted and 8 weeks later both knees became similarly affected. She saw a rheumatologist who altered her treatment. What drug might she be given?
   3. She was commenced on treatment that required the supplement folic acid to counteract folate depletion. What drug treatment had been started?

   The answers are provided on pages 728–729.

Second-line drugs[a] used to suppress the rheumatic disease process

Drug	Half-life (h)	Elimination	Comments
Auranofin	17–25 days	Metabolism	Used for active progressive rheumatoid arthritis; given orally; the available kinetic data are for gold (not the drug form); 13–33% absorbed; the molecule is metabolised rapidly; the products are eliminated equally in urine and faeces
Aurothiomalate (sodium salt)	250 days	Metabolism	Used for active progressive rheumatoid arthritis and juvenile arthritis; given by deep intramuscular injection; the available kinetic data are for gold (not the drug form); the drug is probably metabolised and the products eliminated in urine and faeces
Chloroquine	30–60 days	Metabolism	Used for moderate active rheumatoid arthritis and juvenile arthritis; given orally; see Ch. 51 for other details
Hydroxychloroquine	18 days	Renal + metabolism	Used for moderate active rheumatoid arthritis and juvenile arthritis; given orally; extensive oral absorption; metabolised by dealkylation and side-chain oxidation
Penicillamine	1–6 h	Metabolism + faecal + renal	Used for active progressive rheumatoid arthritis; given orally; incomplete oral absorption; the thiol group forms mixed disulphides with cysteine and other thio-compounds
Sulfasalazine	Parent drug (3–11 h) Sulfapyridine (6–17 h) 5-Aminosalicylate (4–10 h)	Parent drug undergoes reductive metabolism	Used to suppress the inflammatory activity of rheumatoid arthritis; also used for ulcerative colitis; see Ch. 34 for details
Drugs affecting the immune response			
Azathioprine	3–5 h	Metabolism	Used for moderate to severe rheumatoid arthritis in people who have not responded to other DMARDs; more toxic than methotrexate and used for patients who have not responded to methotrexate; given orally; see Ch. 38 for other details
Ciclosporin	27 h	Metabolism	Used for severe active rheumatoid arthritis when conventional second-line therapy is inappropriate or ineffective; see Ch. 38 for other details
Cyclophosphamide	4–10 h	metabolism + renal	Used for rheumatoid arthritis with severe systemic manifestations when response to other DMARDs has been inadequate; given orally; see Ch. 52 for other details

continued

Drug compendium

Drug compendium

Second-line drugs[a] used to suppress the rheumatic disease process (continued)

Drug	Half-life (h)	Elimination	Comments
Drugs affecting the immune response (continued)			
Leflunomide	2 weeks (the active metabolite)	Metabolism	Used for moderate to severe rheumatoid arthritis; more toxic than methotrexate and used for people who have not responded to methotrexate; given orally; parent drug not detected in plasma; 90% is converted to an active metabolite which is eliminated by biliary excretion and further metabolism; the metabolite has a very long but highly variable half-life
Methotrexate	8–10 h	Metabolism	Used for moderate to severe rheumatoid arthritis; see Ch. 52 for other details
Cytokine inhibitors			Should be used under specialised supervision – recombinant human proteins
Adalimumab	12 days	Protein clearance	Monoclonal antibody; used in combination with methotrexate for moderate to severe active rheumatoid arthritis when response to other DMARDs has been inadequate; given by subcutaneous injection
Anakinra	4–6 h	Renal	Interleukin-1 receptor antagonist; licensed for use in the UK in combination with methotrexate for rheumatoid arthritis in people who have not responded to methotrexate alone[b]; given by subcutaneous injection
Etanercept	5 days	Protein clearance	Monoclonal antibody against TNFα; used for severe, active and progressive rheumatoid arthritis in people who have failed to respond to at least two standard DMARDs; given by subcutaneous injection
Infliximab	8–10 days	Protein clearance	Monoclonal antibody against TNFα; used for severe, active and progressive rheumatoid arthritis in people who have failed to respond to at least two standard DMARDs; given by intravenous infusion

[a]These drugs affect the disease process and are also known as **disease-modifying antirheumatic drugs.** Unlike non-steroidal anti-inflammatory drugs, they do not produce a rapid response and may require 4–6 months for a full response.
[b]The National Institute for Clinical Excellence guidelines issued in 2003 did not recommend the use of anakinra for the treatment of rheumatoid arthritis, except in the context of a controlled, long-term clinical study.
DMARD, disease-modifying antirheumatic drug; TNFα, tumour necrosis factor alpha.

31 Hyperuricaemia and gout

The pathophysiology of gout

Uric acid is a relatively insoluble product of catabolism of the nucleic acid purine bases guanine and adenine (Fig. 31.1). Its immediate precursors, xanthine and hypoxanthine, are more water-soluble. Uric acid is normally eliminated by the kidney. It is filtered at the glomerulus and then reabsorbed from the proximal tubule. Subsequently, there is net secretion into the late proximal tubule.

Hyperuricaemia results from:

- overproduction of uric acid: from excessive cell destruction (e.g. lymphoproliferative or myeloproliferative disorders, especially during their treatment; Ch. 52), inherited defects that increase purine synthesis, high alcohol intake
- reduced renal excretion of uric acid: the majority of uric acid (>90%) is reabsorbed in the early proximal tubule, but 6–10% is secreted by an active process in the second part of the proximal tubule and this is the main component of urinary uric acid; renal failure and drugs (e.g. most diuretics, low-dose aspirin and lactate formed from alcohol) can reduce the tubular secretion of uric acid; reduced excretion accounts for at least 80% of cases of gout.

A high plasma concentration of uric acid is often asymptomatic, but when the plasma concentration exceeds $0.42\,mmol\,l^{-1}$ (normal about $0.25\,mmol\,l^{-1}$) monosodium urate crystals can be deposited in tissues, forming a tophus (a deposit of urate crystals). When monosodium urate crystals are shed from a tophus in the synovial membrane or cartilage of a joint, they produce an extremely painful acute arthritis that presents with the clinical syndrome of gout. In brief, the crystals interact with phagocytic synoviocytes (phagocytic cells within the synovium) that release mediators such as cytokines, prostaglandins and leukotrienes. The synoviocytes also trigger mast cells and activate endothelial cells, leading to release of other inflammatory mediators such as histamine, tumour necrosis factor alpha (TNFα)

and various chemokines (Ch. 30). The activated endothelial cells attract further phagocytic cells, principally neutrophil leucocytes and monocytes. These cells internalise the crystals, and release proteolytic and lysosomal enzymes that enhance tissue inflammation and destroy cartilage, damaging the joint. Attacks of gout are self-limiting, probably in part due to coating of the crystals with protein, which reduces their irritant properties.

Gout in younger people is usually a recurrent condition affecting a single joint, with repeated acute attacks if the underlying cause is not treated. In the elderly, a chronic arthritis affecting multiple joints can occur. The diagnosis of gout is confirmed by the finding of monosodium urate crystals in the affected joint. With persistent hyperuricaemia, chronic urate deposits are sometimes found in tendon sheaths and soft tissues. Excess uric acid can be deposited in the interstitium of the kidney or form stones in the renal calyces. Both mechanisms will produce progressive renal damage.

There are two reasons to consider drug treatment:

- treatment of an acute attack of gout
- reduction of plasma uric acid concentration for prophylaxis against recurrent attacks of gout or to prevent kidney damage.

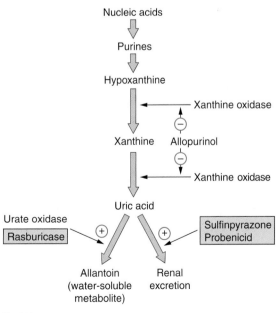

Fig. 31.1
The pathway for production of uric acid and the sites of action of drugs used in treatment.

379

Drugs for the treatment of gout and prevention of hyperuricaemia

Colchicine

Mechanism of action

Colchicine interferes with several steps in the inflammatory cascade. It reduces the production of TNFα by macrophages and downregulates its receptors on macrophages and endothelial cells. This may inhibit priming of leucocytes before they are activated by monosodium urate crystals. Colchicine inhibits production of chemotaxins such as leukotriene B_4 and interleukin-8 that attract leucocytes into inflamed tissue. Colchicine also disrupts self-assembly of microtubules in neutrophil leucocytes, by forming a complex with tubulin in the cell. This interferes with the process of adhesion of neutrophils to endothelial cells, which reduces their recruitment into the joint, and also impairs phagocytosis of crystals once the neutrophil has reached the joint. In addition, once crystals are phagocytosed into the neutrophil, colchicine inhibits the subsequent release of enzymes and free radicals that damage the joint. All these actions give colchicine a specific anti-inflammatory effect in the gouty joint; it is ineffective in other forms of inflammatory arthritis.

Pharmacokinetics

Colchicine is poorly absorbed from the gut and is partially eliminated by hepatic metabolism. It is also partially excreted unchanged in the urine and bile. The initial half-life of colchicine is very short, but enterohepatic circulation prolongs its action. It is usually given every 2 h until symptomatic relief is achieved or unwanted effects occur. Pain relief usually begins after about 18 h and is maximal by 48 h.

Unwanted effects

Colchicine has a low therapeutic index.

- gut toxicity caused by inhibition of mucosal cell division produces abdominal pain, nausea, vomiting and diarrhoea; these effects are common and are often dose-limiting
- bone marrow toxicity with long-term use
- myopathy with proximal weakness if used in renal impairment.

Allopurinol

Mechanism of action

Allopurinol is an analogue of hypoxanthine and competitively inhibits the enzyme xanthine oxidase, thereby reducing uric acid formation (Fig. 31.1). Although plasma xanthine and hypoxanthine concentrations increase, they do not crystallise, because of their greater water solubility; concentrations remain well below saturation levels even if uric acid is reduced to 0.1 mmol l^{-1}. Xanthine and hypoxanthine are reincorporated into the purine metabolic cycle, and by a feedback mechanism this decreases de novo purine formation.

Pharmacokinetics

Allopurinol is well absorbed from the gut and converted in the liver to a long-acting active metabolite, oxipurinol (alloxanthine). Both compounds are excreted by the kidney. The half-life of oxipurinol is long, due to tubular reabsorption in the kidney.

Unwanted effects

- there is an increased risk of acute gout during the first few weeks of treatment; this may be caused by fluctuations in plasma uric acid, perhaps through release from tissue deposits
- allergic reactions, especially rashes; these can be particularly serious in those with renal impairment
- hepatotoxicity
- drug interactions: allopurinol inhibits the metabolism of the cytotoxic drugs mercaptopurine and azathioprine (Ch. 52), which are metabolised by xanthine oxidase.

Rasburicase

Mechanism of action

Rasburicase is a recombinant version of the enzyme urate oxidase which catalyses the oxidation of uric acid to a soluble metabolite, allantoin. This enzyme is present in mammals other than humans; the recombinant version is produced by a genetically modified fungal strain. Rasburicase is used for prophylaxis of hyperuricaemia during treatment of malignancies with chemotherapy.

Pharmacokinetics

Rasburicase is given intravenously. It is metabolised by peptide hydrolysis in plasma, and has a long half-life.

Unwanted effects

- fever
- vomiting
- anaphylaxis; rasburicase induces antibody responses in about 10% of those treated, although allergic reactions are rare
- rashes
- haemolysis from production of hydrogen peroxide as a by-product of the formation of allantoin.

Uricosuric agents

Examples: probenecid, sulfinpyrazone

Mechanism of action

The uricosuric drugs compete with uric acid for both secretion and reabsorption at the renal tubule. Low doses preferentially inhibit tubular secretion of uric acid, which can raise plasma uric acid levels. There is a risk of precipitation of uric acid crystals in the kidney, particularly during the early stages of treatment, which can be prevented by maintaining a high fluid intake and an alkaline urine (using potassium citrate or sodium bicarbonate). Aspirin and other salicylates should not be given with uricosurics, because small doses of these drugs inhibit tubular uric acid secretion.

Pharmacokinetics

Both probenecid and sulfinpyrazone are well absorbed from the gut. Probenecid is metabolised in the liver, and has an intermediate half-life. Sulfinpyrazone is eliminated partly by metabolism and partly by renal excretion, and has a short half-life.

Unwanted effects

- gastrointestinal upset
- renal uric acid deposition; deterioration of renal function can occur if there is pre-existing impairment
- allergic rashes
- urinary frequency, headache, flushing, dizziness with probenecid
- probenecid reduces urinary elimination of several drugs, for example penicillins, cephalosporins (Ch. 51), non-steroidal anti-inflammatory drugs (NSAIDs; Ch. 29) and sulphonylureas (Ch. 40).

Treatment of gout

Acute gout

Efforts should always be made to identify and remove precipitating causes, particularly enquiring about alcohol intake and reviewing concurrent drug therapy. For acute attacks, NSAIDs (Ch. 29) are the treatment of choice, especially indometacin. Aspirin should be avoided because at some doses it can inhibit renal excretion of uric acid and increase plasma urate concentration. Recent studies have shown that cyclo-oxygenase 2 (COX-2)-selective anti-inflammatory drugs are as effective as classic NSAIDs. Colchicine is usually reserved for those who are intolerant of NSAIDs. Intra-articular injection of corticosteroid can be very effective if other treatments are contraindicated. Oral corticosteroids, for example prednisolone (Ch. 44), are reserved for resistant episodes of gout, and should be reduced gradually over 8 days to minimise the risk of a rebound flare of symptoms.

Prevention of gout attacks

Allopurinol is given for prophylaxis against recurrent attacks of acute gout, for chronic tophus formation in the tissues, or for uric acid-induced renal damage. It is also given prophylactically before cytotoxic chemotherapy, when tissue breakdown generates large amounts of uric acid. To prevent gout, the serum uric acid concentration should be reduced to less than 0.36 mmol l^{-1}, although it may be necessary to go below 0.30 mmol l^{-1} to reabsorb gouty tophi. Allopurinol should not be used during an acute attack of gout since it can prolong the attack. To reduce the risk of provoking an attack when allopurinol is started in someone with hyperuricaemia, cover with a low dosage of an NSAID or a low dosage of colchicine should be given during the first 3 months of treatment (or for 1 month after correction of the plasma uric acid concentration). Uricosuric drugs are reserved for those who do not tolerate allopurinol, or are used in combination with allopurinol for resistant cases. They should be avoided if there is renal impairment.

Prophylactic treatment should usually be life-long, since recurrence of gout or tophi frequently occurs if treatment is stopped.

Short-term prophylaxis is possible when allopurinol is used during cytotoxic chemotherapy. Rasburicase is used when intravenous prophylaxis is required for chemotherapy.

FURTHER READING

Lioté F (2003) Hyperuricaemia and gout. *Curr Rheumatol Rep* 5, 227–234

Molad Y (2002) Update on colchicine and its mechanism of action. *Curr Rheumatol Rep* 4, 252–256

Rott KT, Agudelo CA (2003) Gout. *JAMA* 289, 2857–2860

Wortmann RL (2002) Gout and hyperuricaemia. *Curr Opin Rheumatol* 14, 281–286

Self-assessment

1. You are investigating the pathophysiology of gout and drugs used in its treatment. Choose the one <u>most appropriate</u> statement from the choices A–E.

    A. Sodium urate is more water-soluble than its precursor hypoxanthine.
    B. The cause of joint pain in gout is the high plasma level of urate.
    C. Allopurinol enhances the renal secretion of uric acid.
    D. Colchicine is an anti-inflammatory agent that inhibits the release of proteinases from neutrophils that cause joint damage.
    E. Aspirin is safe to use in acute attacks of gout to reduce the pain and inflammation.

2. Case history questions

    > A 56-year-old man awoke in the night with sudden severe pain in his first metatarsophalangeal joint which lasted for a week. Over the next few months, he had similar acute episodes of pain in his ankles and knees, as well as his big toe. He had hypertension but no other vascular disease. The GP suspected gout and referred him to a specialist.

    a. What treatment should the GP institute for the acute attacks, prior to the specialist diagnosis?
    b. What test could the rheumatologist do to confirm the suspected diagnosis?

    > The diagnosis of gout was confirmed.

    c. What was the cause of his gout?
    d. Which drugs would you prescribe and what are the mechanisms by which the drugs act for acute attacks?
    e. What would you prescribe for prophylaxis to reduce recurrent attacks and how does this agent act?
    f. The chosen treatment was only partially effective; what additional treatment could you prescribe?
    g. What might be the consequences of inadequate treatment of this patient?

    The answers are provided on page 729.

Drugs used for gout and hyperuricaemia

Drug	Half-life (h)	Elimination	Comments
Allopurinol	0.5–2	Metabolism + renal	Used for prophylaxis of gout and of hyperuricaemia associated with cancer chemotherapy; given orally; high oral bioavailability; eliminated by metabolism to oxipurinol and unchanged in urine (about 10%); oxipurinol is biologically active and, although less potent than allopurinol, it has a longer half-life (10–40 h) and accumulates on repeated dosage.
Colchicine	0.2–1 (?)	Renal + metabolism	Used for acute gout and short-term prophylaxis during initial therapy with other drugs; given orally; good oral absorption; rapid eliminated from plasma but the reported half-life may reflect the distribution phase, because the half-life in leucocytes is about 60 h
Probenecid	4–17	Metabolism + renal	Used for nephrotoxicity associated with the use of the antiretroviral drug cidofovir; given orally; complete oral bioavailability; eliminated by hepatic oxidation, glucuronic acid conjugation and by renal excretion (5–10%); the oxidised metabolites are uricosuric
Rasburicase	22 (data for children)	Metabolism	Used for the hyperuricaemia arising during the initial chemotherapy of haematological malignancy; a recombinant form of fungal urate oxidase which converts urate to allantoin, which is inactive and soluble; given intravenously; no evidence of accumulation on repeated dosage
Sulfinpyrazone	4–5	Metabolism	Used for gout prophylaxis and hyperuricaemia; given orally; good oral absorption; metabolised at the SO group to an inactive sulphone (SO_2) and a sulphide (S) analogue (which inhibits platelet aggregation); also metabolised by oxidation and formation of a C-glucuronide (a rare reaction)

The gastrointestinal system

32

Nausea and vomiting

Nausea and vomiting

Nausea, retching and vomiting are part of the body's defence against ingested toxins. Vomiting is a reflex that is integrated by the 'vomiting centre' in the medulla oblongata of the brainstem. The exact location of the vomiting centre is unclear. It is composed of a series of nuclei in the nucleus tractus solitarius and the dorsal motor nucleus of the vagus. Efferent connections from the vomiting centre include the vagus and phrenic nerves; when stimulated, the fundus and body of the stomach and the lower oesophageal sphincter relax, and retrograde giant contractions occur in the small intestine. Diaphragmatic and abdominal muscle contractions compress the stomach, and together these factors produce vomiting.

The afferent input to the vomiting centre comes from several sources (Fig. 32.1):

- abdominal and cardiac vagal afferents, activated by mechano- or chemosensory receptors; some drugs induce vomiting by an effect on gastric chemosensory receptors
- the area postrema on the floor of the 4th ventricle; this is often referred to as the chemoreceptor trigger zone (CTZ), and lies outside the blood–brain barrier; the CTZ has many receptors for both neurotransmitters and hormones and has many afferent and efferent connections with the underlying nucleus tractus solitarius; many drugs produce vomiting by an action on the CTZ, which responds to both endogenous and exogenous influences (Box 32.1)
- the vestibular system, which is involved in the emetic response to motion
- other brainstem structures, such as the amygdala.

Several neurotransmitter receptors are involved in activation of the vomiting centre and CTZ, including those for dopamine (D_2), 5-hydroxytryptamine ($5HT_3$ and $5HT_4$), acetylcholine (muscarinic), histamine (H_1), glutamate (*N*-methyl-D-aspartate [NMDA]) and substance P (neurokinin 1 [NK_1]) (Fig. 32.1). How these multiple neurons and receptors are involved in nausea and vomiting is as yet not clear. For example, $5HT_3$ receptor antagonists will provide protection against nausea and vomiting induced by cytotoxic drugs and radiation but not by motion or apomorphine.

Vomiting can result from the summation of several subemetic stimuli, for example in the genesis of post-operative nausea and vomiting. This frequently occurs in the first 24 h after anaesthesia and surgery; it is provoked by inhalational rather than intravenous anaesthesia, more often by abdominal, ophthalmic or ear, nose and throat procedures, by the use of opioid analgesics and by postoperative pain, hypotension and gastric stasis.

Antiemetic agents

Antihistamines

Examples: cyclizine, promethazine

Mechanism of action and clinical use
Antihistamines used for treatment of vomiting block histamine H_1 receptors (Ch. 39), and many also have antimuscarinic effects. Promethazine also blocks some 5HT receptors. They are effective against most causes of vomiting, but, apart from the use of cyclizine for drug-induced vomiting, they are rarely treatments of choice. Promethazine is used to treat vomiting in pregnancy since it appears to be free from teratogenic effects.

Pharmacokinetics
These drugs are well absorbed orally; promethazine and cyclizine can also be given by intramuscular and, in the case of cyclizine, intravenous injection. After oral dosing, promethazine undergoes extensive first-pass metabolism. They are eliminated by hepatic metabolism; the half-life of promethazine is intermediate, while that of cyclizine is long.

Unwanted effects
- sedation, particularly with promethazine
- antimuscarinic effects (Ch. 4), especially dry mouth and blurred vision.

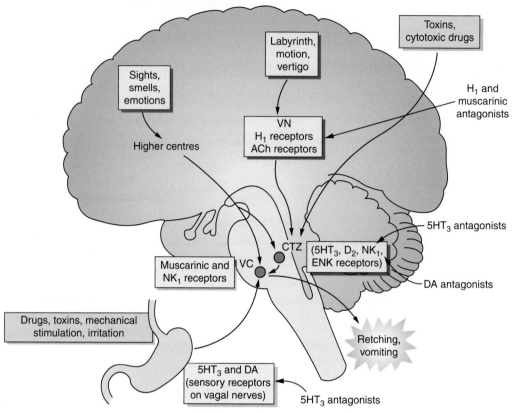

Fig. 32.1
Some of the neuronal pathways and receptors involved in the control of nausea and vomiting. The pathways and neurotransmitter receptors utilised underpin the mechanisms of action of the antiemetic drugs. The chemoreceptor trigger zone (CTZ) has neuronal connections to the vomiting centre (VC) which is a collection of nuclei including the dorsal motor nucleus of the vagus and the nucleus tractus solitarius. $5HT_3$, 5-hydroxytryptamine type 3 receptor; ACh, muscarinic receptor; DA, dopamine receptor; ENK, enkephalin receptor; H_1, histamine type 1 receptor; NK_1, neurokinin 1 receptor; VN, vestibular nuclei. $5HT_4$ receptors may also be involved in the gut and CNS.

Box 32.1

Drugs that produce a high incidence of nausea and vomiting

Allopurinol
Antimicrobials (oral use)
Bromocriptine
Cytotoxic agents (especially cisplatin, cyclophosphamide, doxorubicin, nitrosoureas)
Digoxin
Gold
Iron (oral use)
Levodopa
Non-steroidal anti-inflammatory drugs
Oestrogens (oral use)
Opioid analgesics
Penicillamine
Sulfasalazine
Theophylline

Antimuscarinic agents

Example: hyoscine

Mechanism of action and clinical use

Muscarinic receptors are involved in the visceral afferent input from the gut to the vomiting centre and in the tract that the VIII cranial nerve takes from the labyrinth to the CTZ via the vestibular nucleus. Hyoscine (known as scopolamine in the USA) is used for the treatment of motion sickness and postoperative vomiting. Some antihistamines such as promethazine and cyclizine (see above), and dopamine receptor antagonists, for example prochlorperazine (see below), also have antimuscarinic activity.

Pharmacokinetics

Hyoscine is available for oral, parenteral or transdermal use. Oral absorption is good, but hyoscine is also available in an adhesive patch that can be placed behind the ear and delivers a therapeutic dose for 72 h. Hyoscine is metabolised in the liver and has an intermediate half-life.

Unwanted effects

- typical antimuscarinic actions (Ch. 4)
- sedation.

Dopamine receptor antagonists

Examples: metoclopramide, domperidone, prochlorperazine

Mechanism of action and clinical use

Domperidone, metoclopramide and the antipsychotic drugs block dopamine D_2 receptors and inhibit dopaminergic stimulation of the CTZ (Fig. 32.1).

The pharmacology of the antipsychotic drugs is discussed in Chapter 21; their ability to block dopamine and also muscarinic receptors contributes to their antiemetic effects. Antiemetic doses of antipsychotic drugs are generally less than one-third of those used to treat psychoses.

Domperidone acts solely by dopamine receptor blockade. Metoclopramide, too, acts as a dopamine antagonist at usual oral doses, but it also acts as a $5HT_3$ receptor antagonist at higher doses. This enhanced efficacy is utilised by intravenous administration of metoclopramide to treat the vomiting induced by cytotoxic agents such as cisplatin.

Metoclopramide also has additional antiemetic actions on the gut, increasing the tone of the gastrooesophageal sphincter and enhancing both gastric emptying and small intestinal motility (prokinetic properties). These effects may be a result of indirect cholinergic stimulation following agonist activity at the $5HT_4$ receptor subtype in the enteric nervous system.

Dopamine receptor antagonists are mainly used to reduce vomiting induced by drugs and surgery. Antipsychotic drugs, such as prochlorperazine, can also be used to treat vestibular disorders and motion sickness, probably as a result of their antimuscarinic activity. Pure dopamine receptor antagonists are ineffective in motion sickness.

Pharmacokinetics

Metoclopramide and domperidone are well absorbed orally, and undergo extensive first-pass metabolism in the liver. Metoclopramide is also available for intravenous or intramuscular use, while domperidone can also be given rectally by suppository. They are eliminated mainly by metabolism in the liver; metoclopramide has a short half-life and domperidone has an intermediate half-life. Unlike metoclopramide, domperidone only crosses the blood–brain barrier to a limited extent.

Unwanted effects

Central nervous system (CNS) unwanted effects are produced by metoclopramide and the antipsychotics, but to a lesser extent by domperidone (as a result of lower CNS penetration).

- Acute and chronic extrapyramidal effects from dopamine receptor blockade in the basal ganglia can lead to acute dystonias (especially in children and young adults), akathisia and a parkinsonian-like syndrome. Tardive dyskinesias can be a problem with prolonged use (see also Ch. 24).
- Galactorrhoea and amenorrhoea caused by hyperprolactinaemia can result from pituitary dopamine receptor blockade.
- Drowsiness can occur with metoclopramide.

$5HT_3$ receptor antagonists

Examples: ondansetron, tropisetron

Mechanism of action and clinical use

The $5HT_3$ receptor antagonists block the $5HT_3$ receptors in the CTZ and in the gut (Fig. 32.1). They are particularly effective against the acute vomiting induced by highly emetogenic chemotherapeutic agents used for treating malignancy (e.g. cisplatin; Ch. 52) and postoperative vomiting that is resistant to other agents. They are also used when the consequences of vomiting could be particularly deleterious, for example after eye surgery.

Pharmacokinetics

Oral absorption of ondansetron is rapid, and it can also be given by intravenous or intramuscular injection or by rectal suppository. It undergoes first-pass metabolism, and is eliminated by metabolism in the liver. The half-life of ondansetron is short. Other drugs show similar profiles, except for dolasetron, which has a very short half-life but is converted to an active metabolite with an intermediate half-life.

Unwanted effects

- headache is common
- constipation can occur, probably caused by $5HT_3$ receptor blockade in the gut
- flushing
- hiccups.

Neurokinin receptor antagonists

Example: aprepitant

Mechanism of action

Aprepitant blocks CNS NK_1 receptors. It augments the efficacy of $5HT_3$ receptor antagonists and corticosteroids in preventing the acute and delayed emetic response to the cancer chemotherapeutic agent cisplatin. Aprepitant is not currently licensed in the UK.

Pharmacokinetics

Aprepitant is well absorbed from the gut, and is extensively metabolised in the liver by CYP3A4 isoenzyme. It has a long half-life. Aprepitant is an inhibitor of CYP3A4, and an inducer of CYP2C9.

Unwanted effects

- fatigue, dizziness
- abdominal pain, diarrhoea
- drug interactions: the effect of warfarin may be decreased by aprepitant.

Cannabinoids

Example: nabilone

Mechanism of action and clinical use

Nabilone, a synthetic derivative of tetrahydrocannabinol (an active substance in cannabis; Ch. 54), is effective in combating sickness induced by cytotoxic drugs, providing it is given before chemotherapy is started. The mechanism is uncertain, but it may involve inhibition of cortical activity and anxiolysis; cannabinoid receptors are found in several areas of the CNS.

Pharmacokinetics

Nabilone is absorbed from the gut. It is extensively metabolised in the liver and has a short half-life. However, some of its metabolites may be active, and have long half-lives.

Unwanted effects

- sedation, dry mouth and dizziness are common
- dysphoric reactions with hallucinations and disorientation are most disturbing to older persons; these may be reduced by concurrent use of prochlorperazine (see dopamine receptor antagonists).

Corticosteroids

Dexamethasone and methylprednisolone are weak antiemetics. However, they produce additive effects when given with high-dose metoclopramide or with a $5HT_3$ receptor antagonist such as ondansetron. High doses of dexamethasone can be given intravenously before chemotherapy, with subsequent oral doses to prevent delayed emesis. The mechanism of action is unknown but may involve reduction of prostaglandin synthesis.

Table 32.1
Common indications for various antiemetic agents

Cause of vomiting	Treatment
Motion sickness	Hyoscine, cyclizine, promethazine
Postoperative vomiting	Hyoscine, metoclopramide, domperidone, prochlorperazine ondansetron (reserved for resistant vomiting)
Drug-induced vomiting	Prochlorperazine, metoclopramide, cyclizine (particularly for opioid-induced vomiting)
Cytotoxic drug-induced vomiting	Prochlorperazine, metoclopramide (especially high doses), nabilone, ondansetron Adjunctive treatment, e.g. corticosteroids, benzodiazepines
Pregnancy-induced vomiting	Promethazine, metoclopramide, pyridoxine

The pharmacology of corticosteroids is discussed in Chapter 44.

Benzodiazepines

Benzodiazepines have no intrinsic antiemetic activity. They are given orally or intravenously to sedate and produce amnesia before cancer chemotherapy. They are especially useful if there has previously been vomiting with a cytotoxic treatment, since anticipatory nausea and vomiting are then common with subsequent courses. Benzodiazepines are discussed in Chapter 20.

Management of nausea and vomiting

Antiemetics are used in a number of situations where nausea and vomiting can be problematic. Some specific clinical uses are considered in more detail (Table 32.1).

Drug-induced vomiting

It is sometimes necessary to use drugs that carry a high risk of inducing nausea and vomiting (Box 32.1). Cyclizine, prochlorperazine or metoclopramide are often effective for prevention of opioid-induced vomiting.

More problematic are the highly emetogenic agents used for cancer treatment. Cancer chemotherapy is accompanied by an increase in 5HT release in the gut and the brainstem. 5HT in the gut probably stimulates vomiting via vagal afferent nerve fibres. For low-risk treatments, routine prophylaxis is not needed. For moderately emetogenic treatments, a corticosteroid such as dexamethasone, or metoclopramide is usually recommended. For highly emetogenic chemotherapy, a $5HT_3$ receptor antagonist such as ondansetron combined with dexamethasone can achieve control in up to 80% of cases. When there is intolerance of $5HT_3$ receptor antagonists or corticosteroids, then prochlorperazine, domperidone or nabilone have been used.

Delayed emesis, arising at least 16 h after the chemotherapy, may be mediated by CNS $5HT_4$ and NK_1 receptors. Dexamethasone combined with metoclopramide is recommended for control of delayed emesis, with a $5HT_3$ receptor antagonist substituted for metoclopramide for resistant symptoms. Aprepitant has been used in clinical trials for resistant vomiting with cisplatin, in combination with a $5HT_3$ receptor antagonist and dexamethasone for 3 days, starting immediately before the chemotherapy.

Anticipatory vomiting prior to cycles of chemotherapy usually occurs if previous cycles have been accompanied by nausea and vomiting. It is most effectively prevented by including a benzodiazepine with the chemotherapy regimen from the start of treatment, to produce amnesia.

Postoperative vomiting

Postoperative nausea and vomiting is more common in females, in non-smokers, after a previous episode of postoperative nausea and vomiting, and with the use of opioid analgesics. Dexamethasone, prochlorperazine, hyoscine (using a transdermal patch), promethazine and haloperidol are all effective for preventing postoperative vomiting. By contrast, metoclopramide and nabilone appear to be ineffective. If vomiting is severe, or if it carries high risk for the patient (e.g. after eye surgery), then a $5HT_3$ receptor antagonist such as ondansetron is particularly effective.

Motion sickness

Hyoscine and cyclizine are often used to treat motion sickness, with promethazine as an alternative. Antimuscarinic unwanted effects or drowsiness may be troublesome with all these agents.

Vomiting in pregnancy

Vomiting in pregnancy can be troublesome and there is a natural desire to avoid drugs whenever possible. Some clinicians advocate a trial of pyridoxine (vitamin B_6) or of ground ginger in this situation. Psychotherapeutic counselling or hypnotism may also be considered, since psychological abnormalities are a frequent trigger. If drugs are necessary, promethazine is

---

Box 32.2

Causes of vertigo

Ménière's disease
Benign positional vertigo
Migraine
Vestibular neuronitis
Multiple sclerosis
Brainstem ischaemia
Temporal lobe epilepsy
Cerebellopontine angle tumours

---

the treatment of choice, with metoclopramide as an alternative.

Vertigo

Vertigo is a hallucination of motion, usually perceived as spinning, which is generated in the vestibular system of the inner ear. There are several causes of vertigo (Box 32.2). The mechanisms of vertigo are poorly understood. Treatment is empirical and involves modulation of neurotransmitters and receptors involved in the vestibular sensory pathway to the oculomotor nucleus. The neurochemistry of vertigo overlaps with that of emesis and motion sickness, and involves:

- glutamate, excitatory, acting through NMDA receptors at both peripheral and central neurons
- acetylcholine, excitatory, acting through muscarinic M_2 receptors in peripheral and central neurons
- gamma-aminobutyric acid (GABA), inhibitory, acting through $GABA_A$ and $GABA_B$ receptors in central neurons
- histamine, excitatory, acting through H_1 and H_2 receptors in central neurons
- noradrenaline, involved in central modulation of vestibular sensory transmission
- dopamine, excitatory at central neurons.

Ménière's disease is one of the causes of vertigo for which the pathogenesis is better understood. It usually presents with episodic vertigo and associated signs of vagal disturbance such as pallor, sweating, nausea and vomiting. Tinnitus and, later, sensorineural deafness can be troublesome. The basic defect is an excess of endolymph in the membranous labyrinth of the middle ear. There may be a genetic predisposition, while anatomical abnormalities in the middle ear and various immunological, vascular or viral precipitating insults may be involved.

Drugs for treatment of vertigo

Antihistamines (histamine H_1 receptor blockers). These are the most widely used drugs for vertigo, for example cyclizine and promethazine (Ch. 39).

Antimuscarinic agents. Vestibular suppression can be achieved with hyoscine, and the mechanism of action may be similar to that involved in the treatment of motion sickness.

Benzodiazepines. The use of these agents for short periods may help for severe attacks of vertigo.

Cimetidine. This drug probably produces symptom relief by blockade of histamine H_2 receptors in the CNS (Ch. 33).

Histamine receptor agonists. The use of betahistine to treat Ménière's disease illustrates a paradox that both histaminergic and antihistaminic drugs can be effective in this condition. Betahistine is an analogue of L-histidine, the metabolic precursor of histamine. It is a partial agonist at postsynaptic histamine H_1 receptors and an antagonist at presynaptic H_3 receptors, an action that facilitates central histaminergic neurotransmission. Betahistine also increases blood flow to the inner ear. It is metabolised to an active derivative in the liver, which has a long half-life. The main unwanted effects are headache and nausea.

Dopamine receptor antagonists. Several antipsychotic drugs such as prochlorperazine are used in vertigo, mainly to treat the associated nausea. Their use for treatment of dizziness in the elderly is not recommended, because of the risk of extrapyramidal effects.

Management of vertigo

Many forms of vertigo are brief and self-limiting. Acute vertigo, such as that caused by vestibular neuronitis, is often treated with antiemetic agents until vestibular compensation occurs, which is usually encouraged by maintaining activity. The drug should usually be withdrawn as soon as the acute symptoms subside.

Benign paroxysmal positional vertigo responds poorly to drugs and is most effectively treated by vestibular exercises. Drug therapy should be avoided if possible, since it can blunt the effectiveness of the exercises.

Ménière's disease is often treated initially with sedative drugs such as promethazine, cinnarizine or pro-chlorperazine. Modification of the endolymph production in the inner ear with diuretics such as furosemide or hydrochlorothiazide (Ch. 14) is often attempted for chronic symptoms, although clear evidence of efficacy is lacking. Betahistine is often co-prescribed with a diuretic. For persistent symptoms, the vestibular apparatus can be ablated, for example using local delivery of gentamicin (Ch. 51), which is toxic to the inner ear. Surgical treatment is also used for refractory disease.

Several drugs can cause dizziness or a sensation similar to vertigo. Examples include antihypertensive agents, vasodilators and antiparkinsonian agents. A more serious degree of vestibular damage can be produced by aminoglycosides such as gentamicin (Ch. 51) and high doses of loop diuretics such as furosemide (Ch. 14). This type of vestibular toxicity can be reversible, but is often permanent.

FURTHER READING

Baloh RW (2003) Vestibular neuritis. *N Engl J Med* 348, 1027–1032

Bartlett N, Koczwara B (2002) Control of nausea and vomiting after chemotherapy: what is the evidence? *Int Med J* 32, 401–407

Gan TJ, Meyer T, Apfel CC et al (2003) Consensus guidelines for managing postoperative nausea and vomiting. *Anesth Analg* 97, 62–71

Gralla RJ (2002) New agents, new treatment, and antiemetic therapy. *Semin Oncol* 29(suppl 4), 119–124

Hain TC, Uddin M (2003) Pharmacological treatment of vertigo. *CNS Drugs* 17, 85–100

Saeed SR (1998) Diagnosis and treatment of Meniere's disease. *BMJ* 316, 368–372

Self-assessment

In questions 1 and 2, the first statement, in italics, is true. Are the accompanying statements also true?

1. *Nausea and vomiting can be caused by a number of different stimuli that may require different drugs to treat them.*

   a. Toxins need to cross the blood–brain barrier to cause vomiting by stimulating the CTZ (area postrema).
   b. Some antihistamines can be used for motion sickness.

2. *Dopamine antagonists such as metoclopramide used as antiemetics can cause extrapyramidal movement abnormalities, particularly in the elderly.* Metoclopramide decreases intestinal motility.

3. Choose the one <u>most appropriate</u> statement from the following concerning nausea and vomiting.

   A. Afferents from the stomach to the vomiting centre inhibit vomiting when stimulated.
   B. Selective $5HT_3$ receptor antagonists are particularly effective antiemetics against motion sickness.
   C. Metoclopramide inhibits the nausea and vomiting caused by opioids.
   D. Stimulation of NK_1 receptors on the CTZ inhibits nausea.
   E. Digoxin inhibits nausea.

4. Case history questions

   > A 35-year-old man was diagnosed with non-Hodgkin's lymphoma requiring many sessions of treatment with combined cytotoxic therapy, including cyclophosphamide, vincristine and prednisolone.

   a. Why was this man likely to experience nausea and vomiting?

   > Nausea and vomiting started several hours after each course of treatment and continued for 4 to 5 days.

   b. What planned antiemetic treatment prior to the first course of chemotherapy could be beneficial?
   c. How do the treatments you have chosen work?

   > This man became very distressed by the severity of the nausea and vomiting and developed intense nausea and vomiting prior to the administration of the chemotherapeutic agents.

   d. What treatment could be given?

   The answers are provided on pages 729–730.

Drug compendium

Antiemetic agents (all given orally)

Drug	Half-life (h)	Elimination	Comments
Antimuscarinics			
Hyoscine (scopolamine)	8	Metabolism	Used for motion sickness (given orally) and as premedication (given by subcutaneous or intramuscular injection); radiolabelled studies indicate very poor oral absorption (< 10%); hydrolysed to inactive product
Antihistamines			These drugs have sedating properties
Cinnarizine	3	Metabolism	Used for vestibular disorders and motion sickness; also used for peripheral vascular disease; given orally but very variable absorption; numerous metabolites which are eliminated in the urine and faeces
Cyclizine	20	Metabolism	Used for a wide range of indications; given orally or by intramuscular or intravenous injection; few data are available; demethylated metabolite has no activity
Meclozine (meclizine)	6	Metabolism	Used for motion sickness; undergoes extensive metabolism; few kinetic data available
Promethazine	7–14	Metabolism	Used for a wide range of indications; given orally; low bioavailability (25%); bile is a major route of elimination of the (inactive) metabolites
Dopamine receptor antagonists			
Chlorpromazine	8–35	Metabolism	Used for nausea and vomiting associated with terminal illness; given orally, rectally or by deep intramuscular injection; see Ch. 21
Domperidone	12–16	Metabolism	Used for a wide range of indications; given orally or rectally; low bioavailability (about 15%); oxidised in liver to metabolites, which are excreted in urine and faeces
Metoclopramide	3–5	Metabolism + renal	Used for a wide range of indications; given orally or by intramuscular injection or intravenous injection over 1–2 min; oral bioavailability is variable (40–100%); eliminated by N-sulphation (a rare reaction) and renal excretion
Perphenazine	9	Metabolism	Used for severe nausea and vomiting; low oral bioavailability (30–40%); undergoes extensive hepatic metabolism; see Ch. 21
Prochlorperazine	6–7	Metabolism	Given orally, rectally or by deep intramuscular injection; variable absorption of oral doses; see Ch. 21
Trifluoperazine	14 (7–18)	Metabolism	Oral bioavailability has not been defined; numerous metabolites formed; see Ch. 21
5HT$_3$ antagonists			
Dolasetron	0.1–0.3	Metabolism	Used to prevent nausea and vomiting induced by cytotoxic chemotherapy or surgery; given orally or by intravenous injection or infusion; undergoes extensive first-pass metabolism after oral dosage; the alcohol analogue, formed by reduction of the carbonyl group, is the major circulating metabolite; the alcohol metabolite has greater affinity for 5HT$_3$ receptors, is active in vivo and has a longer half-life (7 h), and is probably responsible for most of the activity

continued

Antiemetic agents (all given orally) *(continued)*

Drug	Half-life (h)	Elimination	Comments
5HT$_3$ antagonists (continued)			
Granisetron	4 (3–9)	Metabolism (+ some renal)	Used to prevent nausea and vomiting induced by cytotoxic chemotherapy or radiotherapy; given orally or by intravenous injection or infusion; oral bioavailability is 40–70%; metabolised by CYP3A4 with wide interindividual variability in kinetics
Ondansetron	3	Metabolism	Used to prevent nausea and vomiting induced by cytotoxic chemotherapy or radiotherapy; given orally, rectally, by intramuscular injection or by slow intravenous infusion; oral bioavailability is good (60%); oxidised in liver by CYP3A4 plus CYP2D6 (but no in vivo difference in kinetics between extensive and poor metabolisers of debrisoquine)
Tropisetron	6–7	Metabolism	Used to prevent nausea and vomiting induced by cytotoxic chemotherapy; given by slow intravenous injection or infusion followed by oral dosage; metabolised by CYP2D6, and poor metabolisers show an increased incidence of side-effects
Cannabinoids			
Nabilone	23	Metabolism	Used to prevent nausea and vomiting induced by cytotoxic chemotherapy which is unresponsive to conventional antiemetics; metabolised in the liver to active metabolites that contribute to the long duration of action
Other drugs used for treatment and prevention of nausea and vomiting			
Corticosteroids	–	–	See Ch. 44
Benzodiazepines	–	–	See Ch. 20
Betahistine	5 (metabolite)	–	Has been promoted as a specific treatment of Ménière's disease; undergoes almost complete first-pass metabolism to 2-pyridylacetic acid which has a half-life of 5 h

33

Dyspepsia and peptic ulcer disease

The spectrum of disease

Dyspepsia is the term used for a group of symptoms that arise from the upper gastrointestinal tract. They include heartburn, abdominal pain or discomfort, belching and nausea. Dyspepsia can occur alone or it can be associated with a number of upper gastrointestinal disorders.

Peptic ulcer disease

Peptic ulceration can occur in the stomach or duodenum. Characteristic features include epigastric pain (relieved by antacids or by food), nocturnal pain and vomiting. Peptic ulcer disease is more common in males and in smokers, and there is often a family history of the disorder. It is also more common in people who use non-steroidal anti-inflammatory drugs (NSAIDs; Ch. 29) or who have a heavy alcohol intake. Women more often have gastric rather than duodenal ulceration. Symptoms are a poor guide to the location of an ulcer, although gastric ulcer pain may be made worse by food and is more likely than duodenal ulcer to be associated with weight loss, anorexia and nausea.

A proportion of those who present with peptic ulcer symptoms, especially over the age of 45 years, will have a gastric cancer. Investigation by endoscopy above this age is important, since drug treatment can produce symptomatic improvement in early gastric cancer.

Aetiology of peptic ulceration

The precise aetiology of peptic ulceration is not known but there are many contributory factors (Fig. 33.1). A major risk factor associated with peptic ulceration is gastric and duodenal infection with *Helicobacter pylori*.

The presence of *H. pylori* on the gastric mucosa varies widely in the adult population worldwide, and about 10–15% of the UK population are infected; it is usually acquired in childhood and persists long-term unless treated. Only a small percentage of infected individuals develop *H. pylori*-associated disease. It is, however, an acknowledged risk factor for gastritis, peptic ulcer, gastric cancer and mucosa-associated lymphoid tissue (MALT) lymphoma. Infection with *H. pylori* is found in about 80% of people with duodenal ulcer and somewhat less with gastric ulcer. *H. pylori* prefers a microaerophil environment, and secretes the enzyme urease that contributes to its survival during brief exposure to acid by producing ammonia from urea.

The region of the stomach in which *H. pylori* infection and the associated gastritis is found appears to be associated with the site of peptic ulceration (duodenal or gastric ulcer, see below) and other host-related and environmental factors.

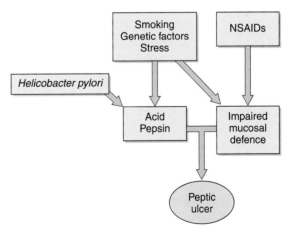

Fig. 33.1
Factors predisposing to peptic ulceration. NSAIDs, non-steroidal anti-inflammatory agents.

Both environmental and host factors appear to determine the distribution of colonisation of *H. pylori* in the stomach.

Duodenal ulceration

The duodenal mucosa is protected by a layer of viscoelastic mucus, but the mucosal cells are highly permeable, permitting absorption of luminal nutrients. The mucosal cells secrete HCO_3^-, which accumulates in the mucus layer (the mucosal barrier) and buffers the pulses of gastric acid entering from the stomach.

In duodenal ulceration, the *H.pylori* infection is predominantly in the *antral mucosa* and there is more often excess acid secretion. However, whether antral gastritis eventually leads to duodenal ulceration may also depend upon the virulence of the strain of *H. pylori*. Unless the *H. pylori* is eradicated, about 80% of duodenal ulcers will reoccur within a year after healing with proton pump inhibitors alone. The recurrence rate is low if *H. pylori* is eradicated.

Gastric metaplasia of duodenal mucosa occurs in response to excess acid secretion and allows colonisation of the gastric type cells in the duodenum by *H. pylori*. Duodenal bicarbonate secretion is deficient in duodenal ulceration. This appears to be related to duodenal *H. pylori* infection, and may be due to interference with nitric oxide synthase activity.

Gastric ulceration

The stomach is inherently resistant to acid digestion. There is an adherent layer of viscoelastic mucus that acts as a physical barrier, and HCO_3^- is is secreted into the mucus to neutralise acid locally. In addition, there is a high electrical resistance of, and tight junctions between, gastric mucosal cells, which result in relative impermeability to luminal contents. Gastric mucosal blood-flow provides an extra layer of defence, by delivering HCO_3^- to buffer H^+ ions that penetrate the mucosa. Many of these protective functions are dependent on the synthesis of prostaglandins (PG), especially PGE_2 and PGI_2 (Ch. 29), by gastric mucosal cells.

If a gastric ulcer is present, this is often associated with *H. pylori* infection of the corpus of the stomach or both the *corpus and antrum* (pangastritis). Moreover, unlike the situation in duodenal ulceration, there is a decrease or at least no change in acid secretion. This corporal pattern of infection is associated with gastric atrophy, gastric ulcers and eventually gastric cancer. The gastric atrophy and metaplasia of the gastric mucosa lead to gastric ulceration.

NSAID-induced gastric ulceration often occurs in the absence of *H. pylori*. The mechanisms are distinct, and relate to inhibition of prostaglandin formation and intracellular trapping of NSAID in gastric mucosa (Ch. 29).

In Western societies, the prevalence of non-*H. pylori*, non-NSAID-associated gastric ulcers appears to be increasing. The pathogenesis of these ulcers is poorly understood.

Gastro-oesophageal reflux disease

Gastro-oesophageal reflux disease (GORD) can produce heartburn, pain or difficulty in swallowing, and regurgitation of gastric contents into the mouth. If associated with oesophagitis, there may be more prolonged chest pain and chronic bleeding. Reflux is produced by transient lower oesophageal sphincter relaxations (TLOSRs) in the absence of swallowing. This allows gastric acid, pepsin and bile to come into contact with the vulnerable epithelium of the oesophagus. TLSORs are programmed responses from the brainstem in response to stimulation of gastric vagal mechanoreceptors. Oesophageal hypomotility and abnormal patterns of oesophageal contractility often coexist with GORD, and may reflect a sensory abnormality in the oesophageal mucosa. This reduces clearance of refluxed material. Oesophageal spasm is a distinct disorder, in which pain is often not accompanied by any change in luminal pH. Indeed, oesophageal pain often occurs without obvious dysmotility and this syndrome is probably due to a combination of local sensory disturbances and psychological factors.

Up to 50% of people with symptoms of GORD have no apparent oesophagitis at endoscopy, whereas severe oesophagitis may produce few symptoms unless complications such as stricture or anaemia arise. GORD has an association with asthma, through microaspiration into the lungs and triggering of vagal oesophagobronchial reflexes. GORD is also associated with chronic cough.

The relationship of *H. pylori* infection to GORD is not straightforward: antral infection appears to predispose to GORD by promoting greater amounts of gastric acid secretion, while corporal gastritis is protective partly because the acid content may be reduced. Symptoms in GORD are usually chronic and relapsing, with at least two-thirds of those diagnosed still taking continuous or intermittent treatment after 10 years. Relapse rates on stopping treatment are directly related to the initial severity of the disease. It is now believed that there are three distinct clinical groups of GORD rather than a steady progression of severity, possibly determined by genetic factors and the immunological response to reflux. The groups are:

- non-erosive reflux disease
- erosive oesophagitis, an acute inflammatory T helper cell 1 response (Ch. 38)
- Barrett's oesophagus (intestinal metaplasia of oesophageal mucosal cells) with increased risk of cancer; this is a T helper cell 2 type response (Ch. 38).

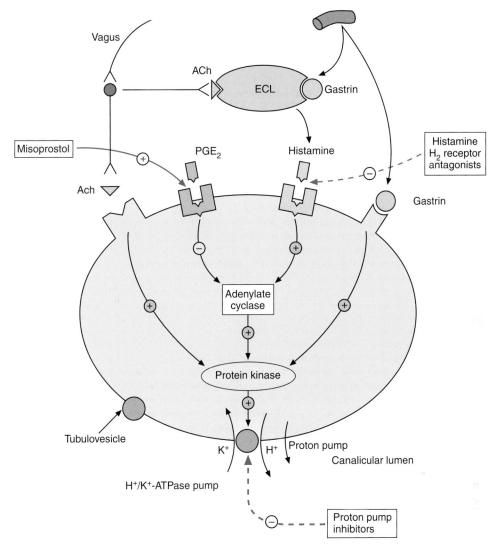

Fig. 33.2

Control of gastric acid secretion from the parietal cell. Acid secretion from the parietal cell is stimulated by acetylcholine (ACh), histamine and gastrin. Gastrin and ACh also reinforce acid secretion by causing the release of histamine from the enterochromaffin-like cells (ELC) which lie close to the parietal cells in the gastric pits. Prostaglandin E_2 (PGE$_2$) reduces acid secretion. The sites of action of the main drugs used to inhibit acid secretion from the parietal cell are shown. There are no useful inhibitors of gastrin action, and the muscarinic receptor inhibitor pirenzipine is no longer available in the UK.

Control of gastric acid secretion

Acid secretion into the canaliculi of gastric parietal cells is caused by the activity of a membrane-bound proton pump which exchanges K^+ and H^+ across the cell membrane (H^+/K^+-ATPase). Hydrogen ions are obtained from carbonic acid (H_2CO_3) using carbonic anhydrase, and HCO_3^- enters the plasma in exchange for Cl^-. Chloride ions are then secreted into the stomach lumen with H^+ via a symport carrier. The activity of the proton pump is controlled by several mediators, including histamine, gastrin and acetylcholine (Fig. 33.2).

Drugs for treating dyspepsia, peptic ulcer and gastro-oesophageal reflux disease

Antisecretory drugs

It is only necessary to raise intragastric pH above 3 for a few hours in the day to promote healing of most peptic ulcers; however, rapid healing requires acid suppression for a minimum of 18–20 h per day. The duration of acid suppression determines the rate of healing but not the eventual proportion of ulcers healed. Several classes of drug have antisecretory actions.

Proton pump inhibitors

Examples: omeprazole, lansoprazole, pantoprazole

Mechanism of action
Since the proton pump (H^+/K^+-ATPase) is the final common pathway for acid secretion in gastric parietal cells, inhibition of the pump almost completely blocks acid secretion (Fig. 33.2). Proton pump inhibitors are irreversible inhibitors of H^+/K^+-ATPase, and the return of acid secretion is dependent on the synthesis of new proton pumps. Acid production is inhibited by about 90% for approximately 24 h with a single dose.

Pharmacokinetics
Omeprazole is a prodrug that is unstable in acid, and is given orally as an enteric-coated formulation. Absorption is variable and incomplete, although it improves with repeated dosing. Omeprazole is also available in an intravenous formulation. Omeprazole is a weak base, and it is concentrated in the acid environment of the secretory canaliculi of the gastric parietal cell. Activation then occurs by protonation of the compound to the active sulfenamide, an irreversible inhibitor of the parietal cell proton pumps. Elimination is by hepatic metabolism. Omeprazole has a short plasma half-life, but, because of the irreversible mechanism of action, this bears no relationship to the long biological duration of action. Because the sulfenamide is only formed at acid pH, the drug is targeted to the parietal cell and not to other proton pumps in the body.

Lansoprazole is well absorbed from the gut. It is metabolised in the liver and has a short half-life, but also a long duration of action. Pantoprazole is available in both oral and intravenous formulations. It is well absorbed from the gut and undergoes extensive hepatic metabolism. Once again, the short half-life is not reflected in the long duration of action.

Unwanted effects
- gastrointestinal upset, such as abdominal pain, nausea and vomiting, diarrhoea
- headache
- hypersensitivity reactions, including skin rashes, urticaria, angioedema and anaphylaxis
- muscle and joint pains
- oedema
- blurred vision, dry mouth
- omeprazole induces the cytochrome P450 system in the liver but has few important drug interactions

apart from with warfarin or phenytoin (Ch. 2); lansoprazole, by contrast, is a weak enzyme inducer.

Concerns that substantial reductions of gastric acid, and the associated rise in gastrin secretion, might predispose to an increased incidence of gastric cancer (cf. the risk in pernicious anaemia) appear to be unfounded. These drugs do not completely abolish acid secretion and intragastric pH can still fall below 4 during part of the day, the critical pH below which bacterial populations are not thought to become established.

Histamine H₂ receptor antagonists

Examples: cimetidine, ranitidine

Mechanism of action
Histamine H_2 receptor antagonists act competitively at receptors on gastric parietal cells. They reduce basal acid secretion and pepsin production, and prevent the increase in secretin that occurs in response to several secretory stimuli. Overall, acid secretion is reduced by about 60% (Fig. 33.2).

Pharmacokinetics
Absorption of cimetidine and ranitidine from the gut is almost complete but both undergo limited first-pass metabolism. The drugs are mainly eliminated unchanged by the kidney, in part through active tubular transport. Their half-lives are short.

Unwanted effects

- diarrhoea and other gastrointestinal disturbances
- headache, dizziness
- confusion in the elderly
- gynaecomastia and impotence with cimetidine, through an antiandrogen effect
- cimetidine inhibits hepatic cytochrome P450; this creates the potential for important drug interactions with many drugs such as warfarin, phenytoin and theophylline (Ch. 2).

Antacids

Examples: aluminium hydroxide, magnesium trisilicate

Mechanism of action
Antacids neutralise gastric acid. Magnesium salts neutralise acid much more rapidly than aluminium salts. They have a more prolonged effect if taken after food; if used without food, the effect lasts no more than an hour because of gastric emptying. Antacids quickly produce

symptom relief in peptic ulcer disease, but large doses are required to heal ulcers. Liquids work more rapidly, but tablets are more convenient to use. Most antacids are relatively poorly absorbed from the gut.

Unwanted effects

- constipation can occur with aluminium salts, and diarrhoea with magnesium salts; mixtures may have less effect on stool consistency
- systemic alkalosis can occur with very large doses
- in advanced renal failure, requiring dialysis, retention of absorbed aluminium may contribute to metabolic bone disease and encephalopathy
- drug interactions: aluminium salts can bind other drugs and reduce their absorption, for example NSAIDs and tetracycline.

Alginic acid

Alginic acid is an inert substance. It is claimed that it forms a raft of high-pH foam which floats on the gastric contents and that alginic acid will protect the oesophageal mucosa during reflux. All proprietary preparations combine alginic acid with an antacid, which is probably responsible for much of the clinical effect. Some alginates contain a high sodium concentration and these should be used with caution in heart failure.

Cytoprotective drugs

Sucralfate

Mechanism of action

Sucralfate is a complex of aluminium hydroxide and sucrose octasulphate. It dissociates in an acid environment to its anionic form, which binds to the ulcer base and creates a protective barrier to pepsin and bile and inhibits the diffusion of gastric acid. Sucralfate also stimulates the gastric secretion of bicarbonate and prostaglandins.

Pharmacokinetics

Sucralfate is only slightly absorbed from the gut. The absorbed fraction is excreted unchanged by the kidney.

Unwanted effects

- constipation, diarrhoea, nausea
- rashes
- dry mouth
- dizziness, headache.

Bismuth salts

Example: tripotassium dicitratobismuthate

Mechanism of action

Bismuth salts precipitate in the acid environment of the stomach and then bind to glycoprotein on the base of an ulcer. The resulting complex adheres to the ulcer and has similar local effects to sucralfate. Bismuth salts, in combination with antibiotics, were the first effective anti-*Helicobacter* agents and this effect may have accounted for their ulcer-healing properties. They have now largely been superseded by proton pump inhibitor combinations for this purpose; a combination product with ranitidine (as ranitidine bismuth citrate) is still available.

Pharmacokinetics

Bismuth compounds are poorly soluble and only slightly absorbed from the gut. The absorbed fraction is excreted by the kidney, and has a very long half-life of 5 days.

Unwanted effects

- blackened stools and darkened tongue
- encephalopathy with overdose.

Prostaglandin analogues

Example: misoprostol

Mechanism of action

Misoprostol is an analogue of PGE_1 (Ch. 29) and has several potentially useful actions, including:

- increased gastric mucus production
- enhanced duodenal bicarbonate secretion
- increased mucosal blood flow, which aids buffering of H^+ that diffuses back across the mucosa
- inhibition of gastric acid secretion.

Misoprostol has both a direct effect on gastric acid secretion and it reduces endogenous histamine release. Misoprostol limits the damage caused by agents such as acid and alcohol to superficial mucosal cells, but is most widely used to reduce NSAID-induced gastric damage. It is available in tablet form, and as combination products with diclofenac or naproxen.

Pharmacokinetics

Misoprostol is well absorbed from the gut and undergoes extensive first-pass metabolism. The half-life is very short and elimination is mainly by hepatic metabolism.

Unwanted effects

- diarrhoea and abdominal cramps are common
- uterine contractions, therefore avoid in pregnancy
- menorrhagia and postmenopausal bleeding.

Prokinetic drugs

Example: metoclopramide

Mechanism of action

Metoclopramide is a dopamine receptor antagonist and is fully discussed in Chapter 32. It enhances gastric motility, increases the rate of gastric emptying and increases lower gastro-oesophageal sphincter tone.

Management of dyspepsia, peptic ulcer and gastro-oesophageal disease

Most people with dyspepsia do not have significant underlying disease (non-ulcer or functional dyspepsia). In all cases, efforts should be made to remove causative agents, for example smoking, excess alcohol or NSAIDs. For persistent symptoms, antacids provide symptomatic relief. Younger people (especially under 45 years of age) who do not have additional features such as anaemia, weight loss, dysphagia, early satiety or persistent vomiting, are often treated without initial investigation. Eradication of *H. pylori* may not confer any symptomatic benefit in this group; however, this continues to be a matter for debate among gastroenterologists. A histamine H_2 receptor antagonist or proton pump inhibitor is the usual first-line treatment, but should not be given for more than about 6 weeks in the absence of a confirmed diagnosis. Investigation should be carried out if symptoms fail to respond within 2 weeks or recur after stopping treatment. Accurate diagnosis can usually be obtained by gastroduodenoscopy, although more specialised tests may be required in some patients.

Confirmed peptic ulceration

Proton pump inhibitors produce the fastest rate of healing (over 90% of ulcers heal in 4 weeks). Histamine H_2 receptor antagonists usually give symptomatic relief for both gastric and duodenal ulcers within a week, but healing of the ulcer is much slower, requiring up to 8 weeks for duodenal ulcer or 12 weeks for gastric ulcer. Other agents such as colloidal bismuth and sucralfate will heal ulcers in a similar proportion of patients, but are less often used, since they do not improve symptoms as quickly.

If *H. pylori* infection is identified and eradicated, this enhances ulcer healing and reduces relapse, so that maintenance therapy with acid-suppressing drugs is often unnecessary for uncomplicated ulcers. If *H. pylori* is not eradicated, 80% of ulcers will re-occur within a year, whereas following successful eradication this is less than 20%.

Eradication of *H. pylori*

Several indications for eradication have been proposed (Box 33.1). Many eradication regimens are used: the highest eradication rates are achieved by treatment with high dosage of a proton pump inhibitor combined with two antibiotics (to maximise efficacy and minimise resistance) given for 1 week (Box 33.2). Treatment for 2 weeks has a higher eradication rate, but unwanted effects often reduce adherence, which reduces the success rate. The incidence of resistance to metronidazole (up to

---

Box 33.1

Indications for eradication of *Helicobacter pylori*

Recommended action
Proven peptic ulcer
Low-grade mucosa-associated lymphoid tissue (MALT) gastric lymphoma
Severe gastritis
After resection of early gastric cancer

Suggested action
Functional dyspepsia
Family history of gastric cancer
Non-steroidal anti-inflammatory drug (NSAID) therapy
Intended long-term proton pump inhibitor therapy

Box 33.2

Eradication regimens for *Helicobacter pylori*

- All regimens include a proton pump inhibitor, for example, esomeprazole, lansoprazole, omeprazole, pantoprazole or rabeprazole. If a proton pump inhibitor cannot be tolerated, then an H_2 receptor antagonist could be utilised.
- In addition to the proton pump inhibitor, two of amoxicillin, clarithromycin or metronidazole, in any combination, can be given for a period of 7 days. The choice of antibiotic combinations will depend upon acceptability and the sensitivity of the infective organism. This triple-therapy regimen should eradicate *H. pylori* in over 90% of cases.
- In resistant cases, tripotassium dicitratobismuthate plus a proton pump inhibitor plus two antibacterials are used.
- Tinidazole or tetracycline are also used occasionally for *H. pylori* eradication.

50% in some places) and clarithromycin is increasing. If in vitro clarithromycin resistance is detected, then this is always reflected in a reduced ability to clinically eliminate the bacterium; however, eradication may be successful even when laboratory resistance to metronidazole is demonstrated.

Resistance to amoxicillin is less common, and resistance to tinidazole is currently lower than to metronidazole.

For resistant bacteria, quadruple therapy can be used, comprising a proton pump inhibitor plus metronidazole or tinidazole plus amoxicillin with tetracycline or clarithromycin, for 7 days. This has an eradication rate of 93–98%. Maintenance therapy with acid-suppressant treatment is only required if symptoms continue despite eradication of *H. pylori* and after exclusion of more serious conditions.

Peptic ulceration associated with non-steroidal anti-inflammatory drugs

If the NSAID cannot be withdrawn, then ulcers will often heal if an ulcer-healing agent is co-prescribed. Continued use of NSAIDs can slow ulcer healing by histamine H_2 receptor antagonists, but probably not by proton pump inhibitors.

The prostaglandin analogue misoprostol provides effective prophylaxis against gastric or duodenal ulceration. However, a high dosage is necessary for prevention of ulcer recurrence and ulcer complications. At such doses, unwanted effects often reduce adherence to treatment. Proton pump inhibitors are effective for prophylaxis against recurrent gastric and duodenal ulcers. Standard doses of an histamine H_2 receptor antagonist protect against NSAID-induced duodenal ulcers, but not against gastric ulceration. Double doses of a histamine H_2 receptor antagonist or standard doses of a proton pump inhibitor protect against both gastric and duodenal ulceration, and are better tolerated than misoprostol.

Eradication of *H. pylori* infection is recommended if an NSAID must be continued in someone with previous peptic ulceration, although this may be more effective in preventing ulcers early in treatment with NSAIDs, and less effective during long-term use.

In the absence of previous ulceration, careful selection is recommended before prophylaxis against ulceration is given in the absence of symptoms. Those at higher risk are the elderly (>65 years), smokers, heavy alcohol users and people with a history of previous ulceration. The use of cyclo-oxygenase 2 (COX-2)-selective inhibitors has been advocated for those at higher risk of ulceration, but there has not been a comparison of this strategy against the use of a conventional NSAID with a proton pump inhibitor or misoprostol. There is no evidence to support the use of a COX-2-selective inhibitor with a proton pump inhibitor as a strategy to further reduce the risk of peptic ulceration, and this combination is not recommended. The combination of a COX-2 inhibitor with aspirin is particularly ulcerogenic and should be avoided.

Gastro-oesophageal reflux disease

Initial measures against GORD include avoidance of tight clothing, smoking, alcohol and caffeine, and encouraging weight loss. Raising the head of the bed by 15 cm on wooden blocks can aid symptom relief and mucosal healing. For mild persistent symptoms, reduction of gastric acid with antacids, with or without the addition of an alginate to provide a mechanical barrier, is often helpful. Alginates should be taken after meals to reduce clearance by rapid gastric emptying. Histamine H_2 receptor antagonists often relieve troublesome symptoms but may not produce mucosal healing; heartburn is relieved in up to 50% of cases after 4 weeks, but oesophagitis only heals in about 20%. Better response rates can often be achieved by using these drugs at high dosages, which will produce healing in 70–80% of patients by 8–12 weeks. Proton pump inhibitors are the most effective treatment for severe resistant or relapsing GORD. They will rapidly ease symptoms and heal oesophagitis in up to 85% of those treated by 8 weeks. Acid secretion may break through at night during treatment with a proton pump inhibitor. This may be important in severe erosive oesophagitis or Barrett's oesophagus. Failure to heal oesophagitis with a proton pump inhibitor often indicates biliary rather than acid reflux.

Eradication of *H. pylori* in GORD is controversial. If infection involves the body of the stomach, then eradication will increase gastric acid secretion and may make oesophagitis worse. However, if there is antral infection associated with duodenal ulceration, then eradication is beneficial. Current expert opinion advises *H. pylori* eradication, as proton pump inhibitors may accelerate gastric atrophy in colonised patients and increase the risk of gastric cancer.

An alternative approach to relief of symptoms is to enhance oesophageal motility with a prokinetic drug such as metoclopramide. This drug encourages normal peristalsis in the upper gastrointestinal tract and produces similar symptomatic relief to histamine H_2 receptor antagonists. However, metoclopramide does not heal oesophagitis, and should only be used alone for non-erosive disease.

Intermittent therapy with healing agents, or use of an alginate after healing, often controls recurrent symptoms. More severe disease requires continuous drug treatment. Long-term use of a proton pump inhibitor is the only effective treatment for severe or resistant reflux disease. About 60% of people will need only a low maintenance dose after healing has occurred.

Laparoscopic antireflux surgery is increasingly used, particularly if there is high-volume reflux.

Pain due to oesophageal spasm sometimes responds to smooth muscle relaxants such as calcium channel antagonists (Ch. 5), nitrates (Ch. 5) or sildenafil (Ch. 16). Local injection of botulinum toxin (Ch. 24) has also been successful in limited studies.

FURTHER READING

Belhoussine-Idrissi L, Boedeker EC (2002) *Helicobacter pylori* infection: treatment. *Curr Opin Gastroenterol* 18, 26–33

Chan FKL, Leung WK (2002) Peptic-ulcer disease. *Lancet* 360, 933–941

Hawkey CJ, Langman MJS (2003) Non-steroidal anti-inflammatory drugs : overall risks and management. Complementary roles for COX-2 inhibitors and proton pump inhibitors. *Gut* 52, 600–608

Nguyen NQ, Holloway RH (2003) Gastroesophageal reflux disease. *Curr Opin Gastroenterol* 19, 373–378

Seager JM, Hawkey CJ (2001) Indigestion and non-steroidal anti-inflammatory drugs. *BMJ* 323, 1236–1239

Stanghellini V, De Ponti F, De Giorgio R et al (2003) New developments in the treatment of functional dyspepsia. *Drugs* 63, 869–892

Storr M, Allescher H-D, Classen M (2001) Current concepts on pathophysiology, diagnosis and treatment of diffuse oesophageal spasm. *Drugs* 61, 579–591

Suerbaum S, Michetti P (2002) *Helicobacter pylori* infection. *N Engl J Med* 347, 1175–1186

Self-assessment

In questions 1–6, the first statement, in italics, is true. Are the accompanying statements also true?

1. *H. pylori infection induces a spectrum of consequences. Some infected individuals have persistently reduced acid secretion, whereas others may have enhanced acid secretion.*

   a. *H. pylori* infection is found in the duodenum in people with duodenal ulcers.
   b. Recurrence of duodenal ulcers following healing with proton pump inhibitors is approximately 20% over a year if *H. pylori* is not eliminated.
   c. *H. pylori* is a risk factor for the development of certain types of gastric cancer.
   d. Gastric acid inhibits bacterial growth.
   e. There is little risk of *H. pylori* developing resistance to antimicrobial treatment.
   f. Omeprazole is a prodrug.
   g. Histamine acts on H_1 receptors on the parietal cell to stimulate acid secretion.
   h. Vagal stimulation of the parietal cell increases acid secretion.

2. *An unwanted effect of antacids containing magnesium salts is diarrhoea.* Antacids are not effective in healing peptic ulcers.

3. *Therapeutic doses of cimetidine, but not ranitidine, can potentiate the effects of other drugs by inhibiting hepatic cytochrome P450 enzymes.*

   a. Ranitidine is associated with a lower incidence of gynaecomastia than cimetidine.

   b. Cimetidine reduces acid secretion by more than 90%.
   c. The active metabolite of omeprazole is a reversible inhibitor of the H^+/K^+-ATPase proton pump.

4. *Omeprazole is converted to its active form at acid pH. Omeprazole inhibits the cytochrome P450 system in the liver.*

5. *Misoprostil helps prevent mucosal damage by NSAIDs.*

   a. PGE_2 reduces gastric mucosal blood flow.
   b. Misoprostil causes constipation.
   c. Histamine H_2 receptor antagonists and proton pump inhibitors are not useful for treatment of ulcers induced by NSAIDs.

6. *Proton pump inhibitors are first-line drugs in the treatment of GORD.* Metoclopramide increases the rate of gastric emptying and raises lower oesophageal sphincter tone.

7. Choose the one <u>most appropriate</u> option from the following statements relating to peptic ulcer disease.

   A. *H. pylori* organisms are not found in the duodenum.
   B. Resistance to clarithromycin is not a problem in the treatment of *H. pylori* infection.
   C. Cimetidine increases the plasma levels of warfarin.
   D. One test for *H. pylori* is to incubate a gastric biopsy with a solution containing a pH indicator and urease.
   E. The biological half-life of omeprazole is about 2 h.

8. Case history questions

A 47-year-old man, Mr TK, was newly appointed as headmaster of a large comprehensive school and he was experiencing some difficulties with the increasing demands of the job. He increased his smoking from 5–20 cigarettes a day and he drank 10 units of alcohol a week. He had a good, varied diet. He had suffered intermittently from dyspepsia for some years, taking proprietary antacids when required. His symptoms then increased and the pain caused him to wake most nights. He bought a supply of ranitidine from the local chemist without consultation with the pharmacist. Following 2 weeks of treatment, his symptoms were successfully relieved and he was symptom-free for 3 months. His symptoms then returned and he took further treatment with ranitidine for 2 weeks. He was symptom-free for a further month, but when symptoms returned again he consulted his GP.

a. Why did his symptoms return?
b. Would his symptoms have been less likely to return following a short course of a proton pump inhibitor?

c. What should be the GP's course of action?

An endoscopic examination revealed a duodenal ulcer.

d. Why do some people infected with *H. pylori* develop gastric ulcer and some duodenal ulcer?
e. What eradication therapy for *H. pylori* should be given, and is a proton pump inhibitor beneficial when given with antimicrobial therapy?

The eradication therapy given was 7 days with omeprazole, metronidazole and clarithromycin. Mr TK was symptom-free for 6 weeks but then his symptoms returned.

f. What were the possible reasons for the return of the symptoms?
g. What treatment could be given?

The answers are provided on pages 730–731.

Drug compendium

Drugs used for dyspepsia and peptic ulcer disease (all given orally)

Drug	Half-life (h)	Elimination	Comments
Antisecretory agents			
Esomeprazole	1–2	Metabolism	PPI; the *S*-isomer of omeprazole; properties similar to omeprazole
Lansoprazole	1.3–1.7	Metabolism	PPI; weak correlation between blood levels and response, but local concentrations are of greater importance; induces cytochrome P450 enzymes
Omeprazole	1	Metabolism	PPI; given orally or by slow intravenous injection (over 5 min) or infusion; metabolised by CYP2C19; poor metabolisers have plasma AUC values 20-fold higher than fast metabolisers; no data available on plasma concentration–response relationship; induces cytochrome CYP1A2
Pantoprazole	0.7–1.4	Metabolism	PPI; given orally or by slow intravenous injection (over 2 min) or infusion; about 20% hepatic first-pass metabolism; unlike omeprazole, does not induce cytochrome P450 enzymes
Rabeprazole	1–2	Metabolism	PPI; shows limited activity against *H. pylori*; extensively metabolised in the liver to inactive products; induces cytochrome P450 less than omeprazole
Cimetidine	1–3	Renal	H2-antag; may be given orally, by intramuscular injection, or by slow intravenous injection or infusion; incomplete oral absorption; cleared by renal tubular secretion; weak relationship between blood levels and therapeutic response; inhibits cytochrome P450 enzymes
Famotidine	3–4	Renal + biliary	H2-antag; incomplete absorption; weak relationship between blood levels and response; does not affect cytochrome P450 enzymes
Nizatidine	1.5–1.6	Renal + metabolism	H2-antag; given orally or by intravenous infusion; blood levels correlate with response, but wide inter-individual variability in concentration–effect relationship; does not affect cytochrome P450 enzymes
Ranitidine	2–3	Renal + metabolism	H2-antag; may be given orally, by intramuscular injection, or by slow intravenous injection or infusion; oral bioavailability about 50%; cleared by renal tubular secretion and oxidation; no effect on cytochrome P450 enzymes
Cytoprotective agents			
Carbenoxolone	8–20	Metabolism	Used for oesophageal inflammation and ulceration; systemic levels correlate with hypokalaemia, but not with the therapeutic response; eliminated in bile as a glucuronide and undergoes enterohepatic circulation
Misoprostol	0.3 (acid)	Metabolism	A prostaglandin analogue; misoprostol is a methyl ester of misoprostol acid; misoprostol *per se* is not detectable in blood after oral dosage, because of essentially complete first-pass metabolism to misoprostol acid
Sucralfate	–	–	Minimal absorption (2% or less); no data on the fate of absorbed material (the high polarity would probably result in rapid renal excretion)

continued

Drug compendium

Drugs used for dyspepsia and peptic ulcer disease (all given orally) *(continued)*

Drug	Half-life (h)	Elimination	Comments
Cytoprotective agents (continued)			
Tripotassium dicitratobismuthate	–	–	Minimal absorption; absorbed bismuth is eliminated slowly in the urine
Prokinetic drugs			
Metoclopramide	3–5	Metabolism + renal	Major route of metabolism is by the formation of an *N*-sulphate conjugate (a rare metabolic reaction)
Other drugs			
Antacids	–	–	Antacids include aluminium hydroxide, magnesium trisilicate, hydrocalcite (mixed aluminium/magnesium preparation) and sodium carbonate; produce local effects within the stomach; their absorption and systemic fates are not of therapeutic importance
Alginic acid	–	–	Produces local effects within the stomach
Antimicrobials	–	–	See Ch. 51
Dimeticone	–	None	Antifoaming agent indicated for infantile colic; polysiloxane, which is chemically inert; excreted in faeces with minimal absorption

AUC, area under the curve for plasma concentration versus time; PPI, proton pump inhibitor; H2-antag, histamine H_2 receptor antagonist.

Crohn's disease and ulcerative colitis are chronic inflammatory disorders of the gastrointestinal tract which together are termed 'inflammatory bowel disease'. Their aetiology is unknown, although there is genetic predisposition and both conditions can occur in the same families. Hypotheses for increased risk in susceptible individuals include infective agents, local ischaemia and an altered immune state. Cigarette smoking increases the risk of Crohn's disease but slightly decreases the risk of ulcerative colitis. Inflammatory bowel disease can undergo periods of relapse and remission over many years.

Ulcerative colitis is a disorder that is confined to the mucosa and submucosa, and in which, inflammation is usually restricted to the large bowel. The extent of the colonic involvement varies, but the rectum is always involved and mucosal inflammation is continuous, not patchy. Symptoms include bloody diarrhoea, fever and weight loss. Ulcerative colitis can be associated with extracolonic manifestations such as uveitis, sacroileitis and various skin disorders.

Crohn's disease is a transmural granulomatous condition that can involve any part of the gut. The bowel involvement is discontinuous and segmental, often sparing the rectum. Fistula formation, small-bowel strictures, and perianal disease such as abscesses and fissures are common. Clinical features of colonic involvement include diarrhoea, abdominal pain and fatigue. Involvement of more proximal parts of the gut produces various symptoms depending on the site of the disease, and diarrhoea need not be present.

Treatment of both types of inflammatory bowel disease is intended to induce and maintain remission. The drugs used for these two conditions are broadly similar, but Crohn's disease is less responsive to some of the widely used drugs, especially when it involves the small intestine.

Drugs for inflammatory bowel disease

Aminosalicylates

Examples: sulfasalazine, mesalazine, olsalazine, balsalazide

Mechanism of action and effects
The active anti-inflammatory constituent of all the aminosalicylates is 5-aminosalicylic acid (5-ASA). The various products are formulated in a variety of ways to deliver the active agent to the lower bowel. Sulfasalazine was the first aminosalicylate shown to be effective in treating inflammatory bowel disease. Colonic flora cleave sulfasalazine into its constituent parts, 5-ASA and sulfapyridine. Sulfapyridine is probably responsible for many of the unwanted effects of this drug. 5-ASA can also be given without the sulfapyridine component (mesalazine). The mechanisms of action of aminosalicylates are not clear, but they may involve inhibition of leucocyte chemotaxis by reducing cytokine formation, reduced free radical generation and inhibition of the production of inflammatory mediators (such as prostaglandins, thromboxanes, leukotrienes and platelet-activating factor). Aminosalicylates are increasingly used as first-line treatment of mild to moderate ulcerative colitis, and are highly effective for reducing relapse rate in ulcerative colitis. Their efficacy in Crohn's disease is less well established, particularly for non-colonic disease.

Pharmacokinetics
Sulfasalazine is partially absorbed from the gut intact, but most reaches the colon, where it undergoes reduction by gut bacteria to sulfapyridine and 5-ASA. Sulfapyridine and about 20% of the 5-ASA are absorbed from the colon, and then metabolised in the liver. Both have intermediate half-lives in the circulation. Mesalazine must be given as an enteric-coated or modified-release formulation to limit absorption from

the small bowel. Olsalazine is a formulation of two 5-ASA molecules joined by an azo bond. It is not absorbed from the upper gut and 5-ASA is released after splitting of the azo bond by the colonic flora. Balsalazide is a prodrug in which 5-ASA is linked to a carrier molecule (4-amino-benzoyl-β-alanine) by an azo bond, which is cleaved by bacterial reduction in the large bowel.

Mesalazine and sulfasalazine can be given rectally (by suppository or enema) for distal disease in the colon.

Unwanted effects

Those caused by sulfapyridine are:

- headache, nausea, vomiting
- blood dyscrasias, especially agranulocytosis (these have also been reported with 5-ASA alone)
- oligospermia
- rashes.

Those caused by 5-ASA are:

- nausea, diarrhoea, abdominal pain, headache and flushing
- skin rashes, including urticaria
- nephrotoxicity (this is an unusual complication: 5-ASA can cause chronic interstitial nephritis and renal impairment).

Corticosteroids

Examples: prednisolone, hydrocortisone, budesonide

Corticosteroids (Ch. 44) are very effective for inducing remission in active inflammatory bowel disease. There is little evidence that they prevent relapse when used at doses that do not produce major unwanted effects. Newer corticosteroids formulated for topical use, such as budesonide (see also Ch. 44), have limited systemic unwanted effects and are useful alternatives to the older drugs. Topical treatment with liquid or foam enemas or suppositories is used for localised rectal disease, but oral or parenteral administration is needed for more severe or extensive disease.

Tumour necrosis factor alpha antibody

Example: infliximab

Mechanisms and uses

Infliximab is the first monoclonal antibody to be approved for the treatment of Crohn's disease. Other tumour necrosis factor alpha (TNFα) antibodies used for inflammatory arthritis (e.g. etanercept; Ch. 30) are not licensed for the treatment of inflammatory bowel

disease. Infliximab inhibits the binding of TNFα to its receptors. This probably reduces pro-inflammatory cytokine (e.g. interleukin-1 and interleukin-6) production, leucocyte migration and infiltration, and neutrophil and eosinophil activation. An infusion of infliximab can induce remission in Crohn's disease for up to 3 months. Long-term safety and efficacy have not yet been established. Intermittent administration with gaps of several weeks may reduce the severity of the disease. Antibody formation is a major problem and may cause allergic reactions and/or loss of efficacy. Corticosteroid pretreatment and maintenance immunosuppressive therapy both reduce this, but some authorities, particularly in the USA, advocate 2-monthly maintenance infusions of infliximab as the most effective way of avoiding antibody formation. UK practice is to use infliximab to induce remission, and to maintain remission with an immunosuppressant. Infliximab is also discussed in Chapter 30 under its role in arthritis. Unwanted effects of TNF$_\alpha$ antibodies are also discussed (Ch. 30).

Immunosuppressants

Azathioprine and, less often, mercaptopurine are useful in some cases of active inflammatory bowel disease and may enable corticosteroid doses to be reduced.

Azathioprine is a second-line drug and should be considered if control of inflammatory bowel disease requires more than two 6-week courses of oral corticosteroid therapy per year. Mercaptopurine is more frequently used in North America; it may be a little less effective but perhaps with a lower rate of nausea than found with azathioprine. Maximum efficacy is not achieved with either drug for 6–12 weeks. Nausea, vomiting, skin rashes and a hypersensitivity syndrome affect about 10% of individuals during the first 6 weeks of therapy. Pancreatitis and liver toxicity are rare but serious complications. Allopurinol dangerously potentiates the toxicity of these drugs. Both are considered safe in pregnancy.

Methotrexate is useful in Crohn's disease (an unlicensed indication in the UK). It needs to be given intramuscularly, requires special handling and disposal, and is teratogenic; it is therefore only used when azathioprine has failed. Ciclosporin and methotrexate are also being evaluated for Crohn's disease, but they appear to be less effective than azathioprine. Ciclosporin may induce remission in corticosteroid-resistant ulcerative colitis but has no long-term efficacy. More details of these drugs are found in Chapter 38.

Antimicrobials

Metronidazole (Ch. 51) is moderately effective in some cases of Crohn's disease, although the mechanism of action is uncertain. It is particularly useful in perianal disease. Data are emerging for similar benefit from other antimicrobials such as clarithromycin and ciprofloxacin.

Management of inflammatory bowel disease

Ulcerative colitis

Rectal drug delivery is often successful if the disease is limited to the rectum or left side of the colon (distal colitis). For mild symptoms, topical mesalazine or topical corticosteroid can be used. Foam enemas or suppositories will treat inflammation up to 12–20 cm, while liquid enemas are effective up to 30–60 cm (i.e. to the splenic flexure). An oral aminosalicylate is an alternative approach for more severe disease. Oral corticosteroids may be necessary to induce remission, with gradual dosage reduction when control is achieved, to minimise unwanted effects. Once symptoms are quiescent, maintenance treatment with topical mesalazine or an oral aminosalicylate is usually necessary. Indicators of disease severity are shown in Box 34.1.

More extensive colitis will respond to an oral aminosalicylate if symptoms are mild to moderate, but the response can take 6–8 weeks. Oral corticosteroids induce remission more quickly. Non-steroidal anti-inflammatory drugs (NSAIDs) and also selective cyclo-

oxygenase 2 (COX-2) inhibitors (Ch. 29), can exacerbate symptoms in severe colitis, while opioids (Ch. 35) should be avoided in the treatment of diarrhoea in extensive colitis since they can precipitate the life-threatening complication toxic megacolon.

Severe colitis requires intensive fluid and electrolyte replacement; anaemia should be corrected by transfusion, and large doses of parenteral corticosteroid should be given.

The indications for immunosuppressants in the treatment of ulcerative colitis are the same as for Crohn's disease. Azathioprine is the only agent with a good evidence base for long-term therapy of ulcerative colitis. Intravenous ciclosporin may induce remission in refractory cases.

Crohn's disease

Corticosteroid therapy is the mainstay of medical treatment for active Crohn's disease, usually with oral prednisolone. Maintenance corticosteroid therapy does not reduce the risk of relapse, and every effort should be made to withdraw the drug once the disease activity has been controlled. Immunosuppressive drugs such as azathioprine may be useful to aid this process, especially in chronically active Crohn's disease, where corticosteroid dependence occurs in 40–50% of people who take the drug to induce remission. Disease confined to the distal colon can respond to topical therapy with a corticosteroid, and an oral aminosalicylate such as sulfasalazine can also be useful.

Metronidazole is also effective in Crohn's disease, and is particularly useful for perianal disease, where it probably has both an antimicrobial and anti-inflammatory effect. Infliximab has been successfully used to induce remission in Crohn's disease that is resistant to conventional therapy.

Surgery may be necessary for disease refractory to medical therapy. Intestinal obstruction can require bowel resection, or abscesses may need drainage. A defunctioning ileostomy to 'rest' the bowel may allow active inflammation to settle with medical therapy in refractory disease, but colonic disease usually recurs after closure of the stoma. Surgery should be an integral part of the management plan and not seen as a failure or last resort.

Box 34.1

Indicators of severity of ulcerative colitis

More than 6–10 stools per day
Fever
Tachycardia
Anaemia
Nausea, vomiting
Abdominal tenderness
Abdominal distension with high-pitched bowel sounds
Rebound tenderness and reduction in bowel movements (toxic megacolon)

FURTHER READING

Elson CO (1996) The basis of current and future therapy for inflammatory bowel disease. *Am J Med* 100, 656–662

Ghosh S, Shand A, Ferguson A (2000) Ulcerative colitis. *BMJ* 320, 1119–1123

Hanauer SB (1996) Inflammatory bowel disease. *N Engl J Med* 334, 841–847

Longford CA, Klippel JH, Balow JE et al (1998) Use of cytotoxic agents and cyclosporine in the treatment of autoimmune

disease. Part 2: Inflammatory bowel disease, systemic vasculitis and therapeutic toxicity. *Ann Intern Med* 129, 49–58

National Institute for Clinical Excellence (2002) Full guidance on the use of infliximab for Crohn's disease. **http://www.nice.org.uk/page.aspx?o=31336** (accessed August 2004)

Rampton DS (1999) Management of Crohn's disease. *BMJ* 319, 1480–1485

Travis SPL, Jewell DP (1994) Salicylates for ulcerative colitis – their mode of action. *Pharmacotherapy* 63, 135–161

Self-assessment

In questions 1 and 2, the first statement, in italics, is true. Are the accompanying statements also true?

1. *Inflammatory bowel disease can be treated with prodrugs of 5-aminosalicylic acid (5-ASA).*

   a. The active constituent of sulfasalazine is 5-ASA.
   b. Mesalazine (5-ASA) can be given rectally.

2. *The aetiology of inflammatory bowel disease is unknown.*

   a. Cigarette smoking increases the risk of Crohn's disease.
   b. Mesalazine is equally useful in the treatment of Crohn's disease involving the colon or the small bowel.
   c. Corticosteroids are effective for maintaining remission in ulcerative colitis.
   d. Immunosuppressants such as azathioprine are ineffective for the treatment of Crohn's disease.

3. Choose the one <u>most appropriate</u> option from the following statements concerning treatment of inflammatory bowel disease.

   A. Crohn's lesions are transmural and confined only to the small bowel.
   B. Sulfapyridine is the active constituent in sulfasalazine that is used to treat inflammatory bowel disease.
   C. Azathioprine is the first-line drug of choice in treating mild Crohn's disease.

   D. Infliximab is antibody directed against interleukin-10.
   E. Antibiotics can be used in the treatment of inflammatory bowel disease.

4. Case history questions

   A 35-year-old man presented with a 3-week period of frequent diarrhoea with mucus but no blood in the stool. Stool analysis for infective agents was negative. Sigmoidoscopy indicated gross thickening of the mucosa, with inflammation and linear ulcers. Changes were present in restricted areas (skip lesions) with intervening normal mucosa. Histology was diagnostic of Crohn's disease and investigation suggested that the condition was confined to the sigmoid colon and rectum.

   a. What is the cause of Crohn's disease?
   b. How should this man be treated initially?
   c. How do corticosteroids act in Crohn's disease?
   d. How should the corticosteroid be given, and why?
   e. Why should the corticosteroid dosage be reduced slowly at the end of treatment?
   f. How can remission be maintained in this man?
   g. What alternative therapies can be given to try to reduce the risk of corticosteroid dependence?

   The answers are provided on pages 731–732.

Drugs used in inflammatory bowel disease (all drugs given orally, unless otherwise indicated)

Drug	Half-life (h)	Elimination	Comments
Aminosalicylates[a]			
Balsalazide	–	Metabolism	Used for mild to moderate ulcerative colitis; a prodrug which is converted to 5-aminosalicylate in the colon; half-life not reported due to wide inter-person variations
Mesalazine	0.5–1.0	Metabolism + renal + faecal	Used for mild to moderate ulcerative colitis; given orally, or rectally as a foam enema or a suppository; poorly absorbed from the gut; may be more effective than sulfasalazine in the presence of diarrhoea, because there is no requirement for reduction by the gut flora
Olsalazine	1	Metabolism + renal + faecal	Used for mild ulcerative colitis; only 3% absorbed in the upper intestine; bacterial azoreduction generates 5-aminosalicylate, which is partly absorbed and excreted in urine as parent drug and acetyl metabolite
Sulfasalazine	3–11 (parent drug)	Reductive metabolism	Used for mild to moderate and severe ulcerative colitis and for Crohn's disease; given orally or rectally as a retention enema or a suppository; about 20–30% absorbed in the small intestine; reduced by anaerobic intestinal bacteria to active metabolites (sulfapyridine and 5-aminosalicylate)
	6–17 (sulfapyridine)	Metabolism	Sulfapyridine has a local action; is absorbed and acetylated and oxidised in the liver; probably the cause of many of the unwanted effects
	4–10 (5-aminosalicylate)	Metabolism + renal + faecal	5-Aminosalicylic acid has a local action; is acetylated in the colonic wall and liver; poor absorption from the colon
TNFα antibodies			
Infliximab	9.5 days	Metabolism	Monoclonal antibody against tumour necrosis factor α; given by intravenous infusion (no oral preparation); no evidence of accumulation on repeated infusion; the place of etanercept (Ch. 40), another TNFα antibody used for arthritis, is unclear
Immunosuppressants			
Azathioprine	3–5	Metabolism	Used in resistant and frequently relapsing cases of ulcerative colitis or Crohn's disease; metabolism to 6-mercaptopurine represents a bioactivation process (see Ch. 38)
Ciclosporin	27	Metabolism	Used for short-term treatment of ulcerative colitis (an unlicensed indication in the UK); a lipid-soluble peptide oxidised by CYP3A4 (see Ch. 38)
Corticosteroids			See Ch. 44 (budesonide, hydrocortisone and prednisolone) – not suitable for maintenance treatment because of unwanted effects
Mercaptopurine	1–1.5	Metabolism	Used in resistant and frequently relapsing cases of ulcerative colitis or Crohn's disease; main use is as an anti-cancer drug (see Ch. 52); low oral bioavailability owing to first-pass metabolism (about 20%); bioactivated by intracellular phosphorylation; inactivated by xanthine oxidase (interaction with allopurinol – see Ch. 31)
Antibiotics			
Metronidazole	6–9	Metabolism + renal	May be beneficial for the treatment of active Crohn's disease; used in people who fail to respond to sulfasalazine; see Ch. 51

[a]The elimination half-life of the absorbed drug is not related to the amount at the site of action.

35

Constipation, diarrhoea and irritable bowel syndrome

> **Box 35.1**
>
> **Causes of constipation**
>
> Diet low in fibre or fluid
> Disease, e.g. colonic cancer, myxoedema, hypercalcaemia
> Drug-induced – frequent causes include:
>
> - opioid analgesics (this chapter and Ch. 19)
> - antimuscarinic agents, e.g. oxybutinin (Ch. 15), orphenadrine (Ch. 24), cyclizine (Ch. 32)
> - antacids containing calcium or aluminium salts (Ch. 33)
> - calcium channel blockers (Ch. 5)
> - iron salts (Ch. 47)
> - tricyclic antidepressants (Ch. 22)
> - phenothiazines (Ch. 21)
>
> Slow gut transit, especially in young women
> Immobility
> Hypotonic colon in the elderly or following chronic laxative abuse

---

Constipation

Humans normally defecate with a frequency ranging from once every 2 days (sometimes less often in women) to three times a day. Maintenance of 'regular' bowel habits is a preoccupation of Western societies, and is best achieved by increasing dietary fibre. Nevertheless, laxative drugs are widely prescribed, or taken without prescription, and are frequently abused.

Constipation affects 10% of the population, and is the passage of hard, small stools less frequently than the patient's own normal function. It is often associated with straining. There are many causes (Box 35.1). Constipation-predominant irritable bowel syndrome (IBS) is associated with frequent bowel movement but the sensation of incomplete evacuation. The symptoms vary from day to day, and urgency, intermittent diarrhoea, and abdominal pain and bloating are prominent (see below).

Underlying organic disease should be excluded when there is persistent constipation or if there has been a recent change in bowel habit.

Laxatives

The mechanisms of action of common laxatives are shown in Figure 35.1. There is overlap between the mechanisms by which the drugs are classified.

Bulking agents

Examples: bran, ispaghula, sterculia

Bulking agents include various natural polysaccharides, usually of plant origin, such as unprocessed wheat bran, ispaghula husk and sterculia, and methylcellulose, which are poorly broken down by digestive processes. They have several mechanisms of action:

- a hydrophilic action causing retention of water in the gut lumen, which expands and softens the faeces
- stimulation of colonic mucosal receptors by the increased bulk, promoting peristalsis
- proliferation of colonic bacteria, which further increases faecal bulk
- sterculia also contains polysaccharides that are broken down to fatty acids and have an osmotic effect.

Bulking agents take at least 24 h after ingestion to work. A liberal fluid intake is important to lubricate the colon and minimise the risk of obstruction. Bulking agents are useful for establishing a regular bowel habit in chronic constipation, diverticular disease and IBS, but they should be avoided if the colon is atonic or there is faecal impaction. Regular fibre intake may also be of benefit for diarrhoea.

Unwanted effects include a sensation of bloating, flatulence or griping abdominal pain.

415

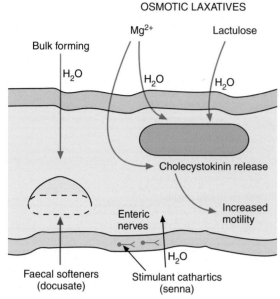

Fig. 35.1
Sites of action of the major types of laxative drug.

Osmotic laxatives

Examples: lactulose, macrogols, magnesium sulphate, sodium acid phosphate

Magnesium salts (sulphate [Epsom salts] and hydroxide) and lactulose are most frequently used. Magnesium salts are poorly absorbed, osmotically active solutes that retain water in the colonic lumen. They may also stimulate cholecystokinin release from the small-intestinal mucosa, which increases intestinal secretions and enhances colonic motility (Fig. 35.1). These actions result in more rapid transit of gut contents into the large bowel, where distension promotes evacuation within 3 h. About 20% of ingested magnesium is absorbed and has central nervous system (CNS) and neuromuscular-blocking activity if it is retained in the circulation in large enough amounts, as can occur in renal failure. Magnesium hydroxide is a mild laxative, while the action of magnesium sulphate can be quite fierce, associated with considerable abdominal discomfort.

Lactulose is a disaccharide of fructose and galactose. In the colon, bacterial action releases fructose and galactose, which are fermented to lactic and acetic acids with release of gas. The fermentation products are osmotically active. They also lower intestinal pH, which favours overgrowth of selected colonic flora and inhibits the proliferation of ammonia-producing bacteria. This is useful in the treatment of hepatic encephalopathy (Ch. 36). Unwanted effects include flatulence and abdominal cramps. Lactulose can take more than 24 h to act.

Macrogols (polyethylene glycols) are large, inert molecules that exert an osmotic effect; the available preparations also contain sodium salts. They are as effective as other osmotic agents, but the sodium content may be hazardous for those with impaired cardiac function.

Sodium acid phosphate and sodium citrate are osmotic preparations that are given as an enema or suppository, usually as bowel preparation before local procedures or surgery.

Irritant and stimulant laxatives

Examples: dantron, senna, bisacodyl, sodium picosulphate

Important examples are the anthraquinones senna and dantron, and the polyphenolic compounds bisacodyl and sodium picosulfate. They act by a variety of mechanisms, including stimulation of local reflexes through myenteric nerve plexuses in the gut, which enhances gut motility and increases water and electrolyte transfer into the gut. Stimulant laxatives are useful for more severe forms of constipation, but tolerance is common with regular use and they can produce abdominal cramps. Given orally, they stimulate defecation after about 6–12 h.

- Senna has the most gentle purgative action of this group. Given orally, it is hydrolysed by colonic bacteria to release the irritant anthracene glycoside derivatives sennosides A and B.
- Dantron is available as co-danthramer, a combination with the surface wetting agent poloxamer '188', and as co-danthrusate, a combination with the mildly stimulant agent docusate (see below). It is carcinogenic at high doses in animals, and it is recommended that its use in humans should be limited to the elderly or terminally ill.
- Bisacodyl can be given orally, or rectally for a more rapid action in 15–30 min; it undergoes enterohepatic circulation.
- Sodium picosulphate is a powerful irritant and is used to prepare the bowel for surgery or colonoscopy and generally acts in less than 6 h.

The chronic use of stimulant laxatives has been suspected to cause progressive deterioration of normal colonic function, with eventual atony ('cathartic colon'). It is now recognised that the condition probably arises from severe, refractory constipation, not from the treatment.

Faecal softeners

Example: docusate

Docusate sodium has detergent properties which may soften stools by increasing fluid and fat penetration into hard stool; it has some stimulant activity but overall it is a relatively ineffective compound. It is given rectally or is administered orally, alone or in combination with dantron (co-danthrusate). Arachis oil can be given rectally, or liquid paraffin orally. Liquid paraffin is not recommended since it impairs the absorption of fat-soluble vitamins, can cause anal seepage with anal pruritis, and accidental inhalation produces lipoid pneumonia.

Management of constipation

For simple constipation, adopting a high-fibre diet, supplemented by bulking agents when necessary, is recommended. Exercise and an adequate fluid intake are also important. For short-term use, a stimulant laxative such as senna or bisacodyl can be taken orally at night to give a morning bowel action. Suppositories will give a more rapid effect. For longer-term therapy, regular magnesium salts or macrogols are usually well tolerated and effective.

Senna, magnesium salts and docusate appear to be safe in pregnancy. Bisacodyl, co-danthramer and co-danthrusate are suitable for the elderly or for the terminally ill with opioid-induced constipation. Lactulose is useful as a second-line agent and specifically to treat constipation associated with hepatic encephalopathy (Chs 36 and 56). For those in whom neurological disease is the cause of constipation, a faecal softener should be used, with regular enemas or rectal washouts.

Refractory idiopathic constipation is a condition almost exclusively found in women, starting at a young age. Long-term use of stimulant laxatives, often at high dosage, may be necessary. Bulk laxatives are ineffective, and a high-fibre diet usually increases abdominal distension and discomfort. Biofeedback can help in up to 80% of cases. For those who fail with these approaches, surgical intervention with colectomy may be the only option.

Diarrhoea

Diarrhoea is frequent watery bowel movements, with or without gas and cramping. Severe acute diarrhoea is usually a result of gastrointestinal infection, and it can be the consequence of both reduced absorption of fluid and an increase in intestinal secretions. Viral gastroenteritis is much more common than bacterial causes of diarrhoea in children, but viral and bacterial causes are both important in adults. Traveller's diarrhoea is a particularly common problem because of exposure of the traveller to organisms which he or she has not encountered before. Common causes include enterotoxin-producing *Escherichia coli, Clostridium jejuni* and *Salmonella* and *Shigella* species. Parasites such as *Giardia lamblia, Cryptosporidium* species and *Cyclospora cayetanesis* are less commonly involved. Diarrhoea may result from local release of bacterial enterotoxins, which have a variety of actions on gut mucosal cells, including stimulation of intracellular cyclic adenosine monophosphate (cAMP), which causes excess Cl⁻ secretion into the bowel.

Drugs that can produce diarrhoea are magnesium salts (see above), cytotoxic agents (Ch. 52), α- and β-adrenoceptor antagonists (Chs 5 and 6), and broad-spectrum antibacterials, which produce diarrhoea by altering colonic flora (Ch. 51). Occasionally, antimicrobial treatment is associated with pseudomembranous colitis caused by overgrowth of toxin-producing *Clostridium difficile* in the bowel.

Chronic diarrhoea requires full investigation for non-infectious causes such as carcinoma of the colon, inflammatory bowel disease and coeliac disease. IBS is often accompanied by faecal frequency, loose stool and a sensation of incomplete evacuation.

Drugs for treating diarrhoea
Opioids

> Examples: codeine phosphate, diphenoxylate, loperamide

The antimotility action of opioids is a result of binding to μ-receptors (Ch. 19) on neurons in the submucosal neural plexus of the intestinal wall. This enhances segmental contractions in the colon, inhibits propulsive movements of the small intestine and colon, and prolongs the transit time of intestinal contents. These actions provide the opportunity for enhanced absorption of fluids. The opioids most often used to treat constipation are codeine, loperamide and diphenoxylate (used in combination with atropine as co-phenotrope). Most have short half-lives. Loperamide has a more rapid onset of action, and has an intermediate half-life, giving it a longer duration of action. It is more selective for the gut because high first-pass metabolism limits systemic absorption, and dependence is not a problem. Loperamide has additional antimuscarinic activity that also inhibits peristalsis (also achieved by atropine in co-phenotrope). Morphine is sometimes used to treat constipation in combination with kaolin (see below). Unwanted effects of opioid drugs are discussed in Chapter 19.

Adsorbent and bulking agents

Kaolin is an adsorbent that is relatively ineffective, and is not recommended for the treatment of acute diarrhoea. Ispaghula and methylcellulose are bulking agents that can help to control faecal consistency in diarrhoea-predominant IBS, or for ileostomy or colostomy. They are not recommended for treatment of acute diarrhoeas.

Management of diarrhoea

Hydration. In developed countries, most people with acute infective diarrhoea who are otherwise fit generally only require high oral fluid intake. Fluid and electrolyte balance are particularly important in young children and the elderly, as they can dehydrate more quickly. In severe dehydration, intravenous fluids may be required. Specially formulated powders containing electrolytes (particularly Na^+ and K^+) and glucose are available, which, when correctly reconstituted with clean water, provide a balanced rehydration solution. Replacement of electrolytes is as important as fluid replacement.

Antidiarrhoeal drugs. Opioids are useful for mild to moderate diarrhoea. They should be avoided in dysentery, when prolonging contact of the organism with the gut mucosa can be detrimental. In young children, ileus with severe abdominal distention can occur with opioids, and it is recommended that they are not used in this age group.

Traveller's diarrhoea. This can be prevented in people travelling to high-risk areas by antimicrobial prophylaxis. Co-trimoxazole or ciprofloxacin are most often recommended (Ch. 51), depending on the area to which the person is travelling. Alternatively, the antimicrobial can be taken at the first sign of illness, and it will usually shorten the duration of the attack to less than 24 h.

Antimicrobial-induced diarrhoea. Stopping the provoking drug usually leads to rapid resolution. In prolonged, severe cases, or when pseudomembranous colitis is suspected or *Clostridium difficile* toxin has been detected in the stool, treatment with oral metronidazole or vancomycin should be given (Ch. 51).

Inflammatory bowel disease. In this case, diarrhoea should be treated by management of the underlying condition. Antidiarrhoeals should not be used in active inflammatory bowel disease, because of the risk of precipitating toxic megacolon (see Ch. 34).

Irritable bowel syndrome

IBS is characterised by abdominal distension, bloating and alterations in bowel habit. There are two overlapping clinical presentations, constipation-predominant and diarrhoea-predominant. Abdominal discomfort may be relieved by defecation, but there is a sensation of incomplete evacuation and mucus is often passed per rectum. The cause is unknown, but a generalised motor and/or sensory disorder of the gastrointestinal tract is likely. A strong psychological component is also evident. IBS is said to occur in 15% of the population.

Drugs for treating irritable bowel syndrome

Antimuscarinic agents

Examples: dicycloverine, propantheline

Mechanism of action

Antimuscarinic drugs reduce colonic motility by inhibiting parasympathetic stimulation of the myenteric and submucosal neural plexuses. They also inhibit gastric emptying.

Pharmacokinetics

Oral absorption of dicycloverine is good and it is metabolised in the liver. The half-life is short. Propantheline is a poorly absorbed quaternary amine; most is hydrolysed in the bowel. Further details of these drugs are found in Chapter 4.

Other antispasmodic agents

Examples: alverine citrate, mebeverine, peppermint oil

Mechanism of action

These antispasmodic agents have direct smooth muscle relaxant properties (possibly by phosphodiesterase inhibition). They can relieve gut spasm and the associated pain.

Pharmacokinetics

Oral absorption of mebeverine is rapid and it undergoes extensive first-pass metabolism. The half-life of the main metabolite is short.

Unwanted effects

These are rare but include:

- gastrointestinal disturbances
- headache
- insomnia with mebeverine.

Management of irritable bowel syndrome

Drug therapy should form only part of the treatment, supplemented by counselling, relaxation and hypnotherapy where appropriate. Hypnosis is effective in up to 60% of individuals, but should be given by a properly trained therapist. Reduction in tea and coffee consumption and smoking, and modification of diet may be helpful. Constipation can be treated with bulking agents such as ispaghula husk, or if colonic transit time is very prolonged, an osmotic laxative may be effective. Diarrhoea can be ameliorated with an opioid. In true diarrhoea-predominant IBS, loperamide is useful as it has a rapid onset of action and enables individuals to control their bowels, particularly when out of their normal environment or in other circumstances where diarrhoea would be socially disruptive. Care has to be taken with other opioids because of the risks of dependency and opioid-induced abdominal pain.

These treatments for diarrhoea do not usually reduce the abdominal pain. There may be benefit from anti-spasmodic agents or low-dose tricyclic antidepressants or phenothiazines such as trifluoperazine (Ch. 22). Proton pump inhibitors (Ch. 33) may relieve diarrhoea by reducing the gastro-colic reflex.

Current treatment of IBS is unsatisfactory. Unfortunately, a promising approach, using agents that stimulate or block $5HT_3$ or $5HT_4$ receptors, is currently stalled, because of a high rate of ischaemic colitis in people who have taken the only compound so far licensed in other countries.

FURTHER READING

Clouse RE (2003) Antidepressants for irritable bowel syndrome. *Gut* 52, 598–599

De Ponti F, Tonini M (2001) Irritable bowel syndrome. New agents targeting serotonin receptor subtypes. *Drugs* 61, 317–332

Guerrant RL, Van Gilder T, Steiner TS et al (2001) Practice guidelines for the management of infectious diarrhea. *Clin Infect Dis* 32, 331–351

Lembo A, Camilleri M (2003) Chronic constipation. *N Engl J Med* 349, 1360–1368

Mertz HR (2003) Irritable bowel syndrome. *N Engl J Med* 349, 2136–2146

Talley NJ (2003) Pharmacologic therapy for the irritable bowel syndrome. *Am J Gastroenterol* 98, 750–758

Talley NJ, Spiller R (2002) Irritable bowel syndrome: a little understood organic bowel disease? *Lancet* 360, 555–564

Thielman NM (2004) Acute infectious diarrhea. *N Engl J Med* 350, 38–47

Self-assessment

In questions 1–4, the first statement, in italics, is true. Are the accompanying statements also true?

1. *Regulation of gastrocolonic motility involves the CNS, the enteric nervous system and gastrointestinal hormones.*

   a. Defecation once every 3 days in the absence of any organic disease requires investigation.
   b. The majority of cases of 'simple' constipation can be treated by lifestyle changes.
   c. Chronic intake of senna causes progressive hyperactivity of colonic motility.

2. *A drug history is important in investigation of people with chronic constipation or diarrhoea.*

   a. Antacids containing aluminium salts can cause constipation.
   b. All laxatives act to stimulate bowel movements within 3–6 h.

3. *The causes of diarrhoea are many but can be largely of psychological origin in some people.*

   a. In infants (<2 years), infectious diarrhoea is mainly caused by bacteria.
   b. Pseudomembranous colitis may result from the use of broad-spectrum antibacterial drugs.
   c. The use of antidiarrhoeal agents may increase the residence of entero-invasive bacteria in the gut.

4. *In industrialised countries, the use of antimicrobials to treat acute episodes of diarrhoea is rarely necessary.*

   a. There is little resistance among *Vibrio cholera* strains to tetracycline.
   b. Oral rehydration powders must be reconstituted with water to give a hypertonic solution.

5. Choose the one correct option from the following statements concerning laxatives.

   A. The use of bulk laxatives should be accompanied by drinking plenty of water.
   B. Magnesium sulphate acts as a laxative by inhibiting cholecystokinin release.
   C. Lactulose works by stimulating the enteric nerves.
   D. Aluminium hydroxide can cause diarrhoea.
   E. Sterculia acts as a laxative within 12 h.

6. Choose the one INCORRECT option from the following statements about diarrhoea.

   A. Rotavirus is an uncommon cause of diarrhoea in adults.
   B. *Campylobacter jejuni* is a Gram-negative microaerophilic bacterium.
   C. In developed countries, *Campylobacter jejuni* is the commonest cause of bacterial gastroenteritis.
   D. Loperamide decreases the gut residence time of the infective organism.
   E. In the UK, oral fluid replacement is all that is generally required for treating acute diarrhoea in otherwise healthy adults.

The answers are provided on pages 732–733.

Drugs used in constipation, diarrhoea and irritable bowel syndrome (all given orally unless indicated)

Drug	Half-life (h)	Elimination	Comments
Constipation			
Bulk and osmotic laxatives	–	–	Act because of their lack of absorption; uptake and systemic disposition is not relevant to their therapeutic effects (*brans, ispaghula husk, sterculia, lactitol, lactulose, macrogols [polyethylene glycol], magnesium salts and rectal phosphates or sodium citrate*); bulking agents may affect the absorption of nutrients and minerals
Gut stimulants	–	–	Some gut stimulants may undergo significant absorption and produce unwanted systemic effects, for example *dantron* and *oxyphenisatin* produce liver damage; *senna compounds* such as sennoside are degraded by the gut microflora and produce local effects; *bisocodyl* is a stimulant laxative that can be given orally or rectally; *sodium picosulfate* acts as a poorly absorbed softening agent
Faecal-softening agents	–	–	*Docusate sodium* probably acts as both a softening agent and a stimulant; *glycerol* or *arachis oil* may be given as a suppository or enema, respectively, to produce a local softening effect; oral liquid paraffin can be used to produce softening, but long-term treatment is not recommended and can result in anal leakage and irritation
Diarrhoea			Anti-motility drugs such as opioids should be used for treatment of acute uncomplicated diarrhoea in adults but not in young children
Adsorbants	–	–	Kaolin is given orally and acts because of its lack of absorption
Codeine	3–4	Metabolism	Opioid; codeine is oxidised to morphine (about 5%) by CYP2D6; see Ch. 19
Diphenoxylate	2–3	Metabolism + bile	Opioid; given as co-phenotrope (co-formulation with atropine); see Ch. 19
Loperamide	10–12	Metabolism	Opioid; main effect is from the parent drug prior to absorption; metabolites retain antidiarrhoeal activity; see Ch. 19
Morphine	1–5	Metabolism	Opioid; used in combination with kaolin for short-term treatment of diarrhoea; eliminated by conjugation with glucuronic acid; see Ch. 19
Irritable bowel syndrome			Treatment comprises antispasmodic drugs, including antimuscarinics (all are shown for completeness); all drugs are given orally unless otherwise stated
Alverine citrate	?	?	Smooth muscle relaxant used for irritable bowel disease, as an adjunct in disorders characterised by spasm, and also for dysmenorrhoea; lacks the serious side-effects of other antispasmodics; few data available

continued

Drugs used in constipation, diarrhoea and irritable bowel syndrome (all given orally unless indicated) *(continued)*

Drug	Half-life (h)	Elimination	Comments
Atropine	2–5	Metabolism + renal	Antimuscarinic used for symptom relief in disorders characterised by spasm of the gastrointestinal tract, also used for mydriasis and cycloplegia and as a premedication; good oral absorption; significant antimuscarinic unwanted effects limit use
Dicycloverine	9–10	Renal	Antimuscarinic used for symptom relief in disorders characterised by spasm of the gastrointestinal tract, including irritable bowel disease; less severe antimuscarinic unwanted effects than atropine; rapidly absorbed; oral bioavailability about 50%; eliminated in urine
Hyoscine	8	Metabolism	Antimuscarinic used for symptom relief in disorders characterised by spasm of the gastrointestinal tract and smooth muscle spasm in genitourinary disorders; can be given orally or by intramuscular or intravenous injection; poor oral absorption; antimuscarinic unwanted effects limit use
Mebeverine	?	Metabolism	Smoth muscle relaxant used for irritable bowel disease and in disorders characterised by spasm of the gastrointestinal tract; negligible absorption intact due to first-pass metabolism; metabolised rapidly by oxidation to mebeverine alcohol which is oxidised to the acid (half-life of 1 h)
Propantheline	1.5–2	Metabolism	Antimuscarinic used for symptom relief in disorders characterised by spasm of the gastrointestinal tract, including irritable bowel disease; incomplete oral absorption (10–25%); metabolites excreted as glucuronic acid conjugates

Drug compendium

Liver disease

Acute and subacute liver failure

Presenting symptoms of liver failure are often non-specific with malaise, nausea and abdominal pain. As the syndrome progresses, signs of impairment of brain function occur (hepatic encephalopathy) with initial confusion followed by drowsiness and coma. These clinical features reflect increased central nervous system (CNS) neuroinhibition, caused by endogenous toxins that the liver fails to remove, and alterations in neurotransmitter synthesis.

The syndrome of liver failure can be categorised by the speed of onset of encephalopathy after the onset of jaundice:

- hyperacute: onset within 7 days
- acute: onset between 7 and 28 days
- subacute: onset between 29 days and 12 weeks; in this form, ascites and renal failure may also be prominent.

Liver failure arises from a number of insults to liver cells, principally viral infection (such as hepatitis B) or the toxic effects of drugs and chemicals. In the UK, para-cetamol poisoning (Ch. 53) is the most common cause of acute liver failure.

Management

N-Acetylcysteine should be given if paracetamol was the precipitant (Ch. 53) and it may be useful in other forms of acute liver failure through beneficial effects on microcirculatory haemodynamics. Other management is supportive and includes:

- prevention of bacterial and fungal infection with broad-spectrum antibacterial and antifungal agents
- prevention of cerebral oedema by appropriate fluid management; if cerebral oedema arises, then mechanical ventilation and infusion of mannitol (Ch. 14) can reduce the resulting oedema
- prevention of hypoglycaemia with intravenous dextrose
- control of coagulopathy with intravenous vitamin K (Ch. 11), or fresh frozen plasma or cryoprecipitate if there is active bleeding
- treatment of shock, often with vasoconstrictors such as terlipressin (see below)
- artificial support for renal failure by maintaining circulating blood volume, and, if necessary, with haemofiltration or haemodialysis.

For many, liver transplantation is necessary.

Chronic liver disease and chronic hepatic encephalopathy

Many chronic liver diseases predispose to the neuro-psychiatric disturbance known as chronic hepatic encephalopathy. The clinical features are similar to those occurring in acute liver failure. Spontaneous bacterial peritonitis is a common cause of deterioration in pre-viously compensated liver failure. Nutritional support may be necessary, and malabsorption of fat-soluble vitamins can be a particular problem if there is cholestasis. Osteoporosis can result, made worse by the use of corticosteroids.

Management

- Lactulose (Ch. 35) can be given orally to reduce absorption of neurotoxins by decreasing intestinal transit time and increasing nitrogen fixation by colonic bacteria. The evidence that lactulose is effective has recently been challenged.
- Oral antimicrobials such as neomycin or metronidazole (Ch. 51) reduce bacterial ammonia

production in the colon. Neomycin is less favoured because of its potential to cause nephrotoxicity and ototoxicity, even though little is absorbed from the gut.

- Careful attention to nutrition is required, especially an appropriate carbohydrate and protein intake.
- Fat malabsorption can be treated with medium-chain triglyceride supplements, and sufficient calorie intake should be ensured. Fat-soluble vitamin supplements (A, D, E, K) may be needed. Metabolic bone disease may require treatment with bisphosphonates (Ch. 42).
- Potential sepsis should be treated with intravenous broad-spectrum antibacterial, such as cefuroxime with metronidazole (Ch. 51).

Variceal haemorrhage

Gastro-oesophageal varices are large collateral venous communications, often at the gastro-oesophageal junction in portal hypertension, but also at other places, for example the rectum. They arise from a combination of increased splanchnic blood flow and resistance to portal blood flow within the liver. Varices are found in 70% of people with cirrhosis and they carry a high risk of haemorrhage, from which mortality is 30–50%. Varices form after the hepatic venous pressure gradient rises above 10 mmHg, and the probability of rupture is high when the pressure gradient reaches 12 mmHg.

Management

Management of bleeding gastro-oesophageal varices

- Repletion of blood volume can be carried out with colloid solution, or preferably with whole blood. Impaired coagulation and thrombocytopenia are common findings in advanced liver disease, and transfusion of platelet concentrates and fresh frozen plasma may be necessary. The risk of bacterial infections is high in acute variceal bleeding, and short-term antibiotic prophylaxis with an agent such as ciprofloxacin (Ch. 51) should be given.
- Endoscopic variceal injection with a sclerosant is successful in up to 95% of cases. The main complications are oesophageal ulceration, increased risk of infections, and pleural effusions. Variceal band ligation is as effective as sclerosant therapy, and is now preferred in many centres.
- Balloon tamponade of the bleeding point achieves control in 80–90% of bleeding varices. It is often used

to treat re-bleeding after endoscopic sclerosant therapy or as a holding measure, and is rarely used as a first-line treatment.

- Transjugular intrahepatic portal-systemic shunting (TIPS) is used as rescue therapy when sclerosant therapy has failed.
- Terlipressin (N-triglycyl-8-lysine-vasopressin) is a synthetic vasopressin analogue (Ch. 43) that produces splanchnic vasoconstriction and reduces portal pressure. This reduces bleeding from varices. Terlipressin is a prodrug that is slowly converted to lypressin, and can be given by bolus injection. Unwanted effects are uncommon. It is mainly used when endoscopic sclerosant therapy is not immediately available. Vasopressin has also been used to treat varices, but has a shorter duration of action than terlipressin, and must be given by intravenous infusion. Systemic vasoconstriction causes ischaemic complications in up to 50% of those treated. It is therefore little used, although co-administration of the vasodilator glyceryl trinitrate (Ch. 5) reduces the systemic complication rate.
- Octreotide and somatostatin (Ch. 43) are probably as effective as vasopressin for stopping haemorrhage, but there is less convincing evidence compared with terlipressin. They work by reducing portal venous pressure and, therefore, flow in the splanchnic circulation and varices.

Prevention of variceal re-bleeding

- Splanchnic vasoconstrictors that lower portal flow and reduce portal pressure by at least 20% will reduce the risk of re-bleeding to about 10% at 2 years. This is most often achieved by the use of a non-selective β-adrenoceptor antagonist such as propranolol (Ch. 5). Sometimes, isosorbide mononitrate (Ch. 5) is added to vasodilate the portal circulation and further reduce portal flow; however, this can produce systemic hypotension and worsen salt and water retention.
- Local treatment of the varices, for example by banding, will reduce the risk of re-bleeding, but does not reduce portal pressure. In about 50% of cases, the varices will recur within 2 years. Banding is usually reserved for those who do not respond to drug therapy.
- TIPS is most commonly used for elective prevention of further bleeding. It can lead to chronic encephalopathy and other significant adverse effects, so is only undertaken in specialist centres. Surgical creation of a portal-systemic shunt is an alternative to TIPS. This is used when the previous treatments have failed.

Ascites

Ascites in chronic liver disease is largely a result of splanchnic vasodilation. The development of portal hypertension results in local production of vasodilators, eventually leading to a reduction in effective circulating blood volume, and salt and water retention in the kidney. The latter effect is due to activation of the renin–angiotensin system. The increased portal pressure combined with vasodilation leads to transudation of fluid into the peritoneal cavity. Spontaneous bacterial peritonitis can complicate ascites associated with liver disease and make the ascites resistant to treatment.

Management

The presence of ascites in chronic liver disease is associated with a poor prognosis, with a 5-year survival of 30–40%, unless there is liver transplantation. Management of ascites includes:

- reduction of salt intake
- diuretic therapy, starting with a potassium-sparing diuretic such as spironolactone or amiloride (Ch. 14); a low dose of furosemide can be added after a few days, with care taken to avoid hypovolaemia and consequent prerenal failure
- large-volume ascites usually requires drainage by paracentesis in addition to diuretics as maintenance therapy; paracentesis should be accompanied by plasma expansion with albumin to maintain circulating blood volume
- refractory ascites that fails to respond to high doses of diuretics, or recurs rapidly after paracentesis may need repeated large-volume paracentesis with intravenous albumin replacement.

Autoimmune liver disease

There are three principal forms of autoimmune liver disease: autoimmune hepatitis, primary biliary cirrhosis (PBC), and primary sclerosing cholangitis, which is less common. The pathogenesis of these diseases is poorly understood, but the occurrence of autoimmune phenomena (such as circulating autoantibodies) and histological evidence of immunogically competent cells in the inflammatory infiltrate in the liver has encouraged the use of immunosuppressive treatments. Without treatment, autoimmune hepatitis usually progresses to cirrhosis.

Management

There are several therapeutic options for autoimmune hepatitis.

- Corticosteroids, usually prednisolone (Ch. 44), induce remission in 85% of those with autoimmune hepatitis, but when used alone, up to 50% of those treated will still have cirrhosis within 10 years.
- Azathioprine (Ch. 38) has a corticosteroid-sparing action in autoimmune hepatitis and is widely used in combination with corticosteroids, both to induce remission and for maintenance therapy.
- Ciclosporin, tacrolimus or mycophenolate (Ch. 38) are used for autoimmune hepatitis that has not responded to corticosteroids. Evidence for their effectiveness is limited.
- Treatment of PBC is less satisfactory because immunosuppression is ineffective.Ursodeoxycholic acid is the only drug licensed for use in PBC. This is a bile acid that is produced by bacterial oxidation of chenodeoxycholic acid. It retards progression of the disease by a cytoprotective effect (by reducing nitric oxide synthesis), immune modulation and suppression of the cytotoxic effects of other bile acids. The main unwanted effect is diarrhoea. About one-third of those treated will have a response, with reduction in elevated liver enzymes, and a reduced risk of either death or the need for liver transplantation.
- Supportive therapy is necessary to reduce the complications that can arise from malabsorption of fat-soluble vitamins. Vitamin D (Ch. 42) and vitamin A supplements are most often needed.
- Primary sclerosing cholangitis is also responsive to ursodeoxycholic acid, but, unlike PBC, it may also respond to immunosuppression with prednisolone or azathioprine.
- Liver transplantation is necessary for end-stage disease in all autoimmune liver disease, and it has good long-term results.

Chronic viral hepatitis

There are two important hepatic viral infections that can cause chronic hepatitis: hepatitis B virus (HBV) and hepatitis C virus (HCV). The end result of the chronic inflammation produced by these viruses is cirrhosis.

Drugs for treatment of viral hepatitis

Interferon alfa

Mechanism of action and effects
Interferons are glycoprotein cytokines that are produced by virus-infected cells, and protect uninfected cells of the same type. Interferon alfa binds to cell surface receptors

and stimulates production of enzymes in the host cell that inhibit viral mRNA translation by host ribosomes. This inhibits viral replication, and augments clearance of infected hepatocytes (Ch. 51, Fig. 51.6). Interferon alfa-2a has lysine in position 23, while alfa-2b has methionine in this position. Interferons are obtained either by recombinant DNA technology or from virus-stimulated leucocytes.

Pharmacokinetics

Interferon alfa is given by subcutaneous injection three times a week for 4–6 months. It is metabolised in the kidney, and has a short half-life. Pegylated (polyethylene glycol-conjugated) derivatives of interferon alfa are available that prolong the presence of the interferon in the blood, and these are given once weekly.

Unwanted effects

- immediate effects are almost universal and include headache, myalgia, fever and rigors, usually occurring 4–6 h after injection. Tolerance occurs with repeated use
- delayed effects include fatigue and anorexia
- bone marrow suppression.

Lamivudine

Mechanism of action and use

Lamivudine is a nucleoside analogue that inhibits viral polymerase and suppresses viral replication. It has similar efficacy in chronic hepatitis B infection as interferon alfa. Resistance of the hepatitis B virus to lamivudine is found in 10–25% of those treated for 1 year.

Pharmacokinetics

Lamivudine is well absorbed from the gut. It is an inactive prodrug that is metabolised intracellularly to the active triphosphate derivative. It is eliminated by the kidney, and has an intermediate half-life.

Unwanted effects

- abdominal pain, nausea, vomiting, diarrhoea
- cough
- headache
- fatigue
- skin rashes
- muscle disorders.

Adefovir dipivoxil

Mechanism of action and use

Adefovir is used for treatment of hepatitis B virus. It is an adenosine nucleoside analogue that is a potent inhibitor of viral replication and is effective against viruses that have become resistant to lamivudine. Adefovir works in a similar way to lamivudine, with additional enhance-

ment of immune responsiveness through stimulation of the production of endogenous tumour necrosis factor alpha.

Pharmacokinetics

Adefovir dipivoxil is a prodrug for adefovir. It is well absorbed from the gut, and rapidly converted to adefovir, which is then phosphorylated intracellularly to the active derivative. Elimination is via the kidney by glomerular filtration and tubular secretion, and adefovir has an intermediate half-life.

Unwanted effects

- nausea, dyspepsia, abdominal pain, flatulence, diarrhoea
- headache
- fatigue
- renal failure.

Ribavirin

Mechanism of action and use

Ribavirin is a synthetic nucleoside analogue with activity against some RNA and DNA viruses. It inhibits viral RNA and protein synthesis, and it increases the production of antiviral cytokines. It has little effect on viral replication when used alone, but it enhances the efficacy of interferon alfa against hepatitis C virus. Ribavirin is also used by inhalation to treat respiratory syncytial virus infection.

Pharmacokinetics

Ribavirin is well absorbed from the gut but undergoes first-pass metabolism in the liver. It is phosphorylated intracellularly to active compounds. Ribavirin and its metabolite are excreted by the kidney; it has a long half-life of about 1–2 weeks.

Unwanted effects

- accumulation in red cells produces haemolysis
- anorexia, dyspepsia, nausea
- dizziness, insomnia, irritability
- dyspnoea.

Management of chronic viral hepatitis

Chronic hepatitis B. If there is evidence of active chronic infection with ongoing liver damage and high viral replication (usually, but not always, associated with hepatitis Be antigen [HBeAg] in plasma), then interferon alfa should be given. There is no role for this drug in the treatment of acute hepatitis B infection, which usually resolves spontaneously. Treatment is usually continued for 16 weeks, at which stage about 40% of those treated will show a conversion to low viral replication, and about 10% will have complete eradication. If cirrhosis is more advanced, or if interferon alfa therapy has been unsuccessful or poorly tolerated, then lamivudine is usually used. Complete eradication of the virus is unusual, but about two-thirds of those who take lamivudine will show viral suppression after 3 years of treatment. The relapse rate on withdrawal of lamivudine is high, with only about 10% of people showing long-term responses off treatment.

Emergence of viral strains with drug resistance to lamivudine is common and occurs progressively, with about 15–30% prevalence of resistant strains after 1 year of treatment. Adefovir is used to treat viruses that have developed resistance to lamivudine, or for those persons who cannot tolerate first-line treatment. Viral resistance to adefovir is unusual.

Chronic hepatitis C. The aim of treatment is eradication of the virus. If left untreated, then about 85% develop chronic infection, of whom up to 30% will develop cirrhosis. Treatment with interferon alfa alone can eradicate the virus, with a 15% sustained response rate. It can also prevent liver damage even if eradication is not successful. The addition of ribavirin increases the overall response rate to 40%, and is recommended for all those who can tolerate its combination with interferon alfa. Treatment duration and success depend on the viral genotype: for types 2 or 3, 24 weeks' treatment is sufficient for a maximal response, while treatment for type 1 should be continued for 48 weeks in those who have a response in the first 24 weeks. The overall response to combination treatment in genotypes 2 and 3 is about 70%, while that of genotype 1 is about 35%.

Pegylated interferons have up to a 10% higher response rate than the conventional interferons, and are recommended for moderate to severe hepatitis. For those who fail to respond to a combination of interferon alfa and ribavirin, there is no treatment currently available.

FURTHER READING

Bosch J, Garcia-Pagan JC (2003) Prevention of variceal rebleeding. *Lancet* 361, 952–954

Chapman R (2003) The management of primary sclerosing cholangitis. *Curr Gastroenterol Rep* 5, 9–17

Chin R, Locarnini S (2003) Treatment of chronic hepatitis B: current challenges and future directions. *Rev Med Virol* 13, 255–272

Ferguson JW, Tripathi D, Hayes PC (2003) Review article: the management of acute variceal bleeding. *Aliment Pharmacol Ther* 18, 253–262

Ginès P, Cárdenas A, Arroyo V et al (2004) Management of cirrhosis and ascites. *N Engl J Med* 350, 1646–1654

Gow PJ, Mutimer D (2001) Treatment of chronic hepatitis. *BMJ* 323, 1164–1167

Heathcote J (2003) Treatment of HBe antigen-positive chronic hepatitis B. *Semin Liver Dis* 23, 69–79

Lata J, Hulek P, Vanasek T (2003) Management of acute variceal bleeding. *Dig Dis* 21, 6–15

Medina J, Garcia-Buey L, Moreno-Otero R (2003) Review article: immunopathogenetic and therapeutic aspects of autoimmune hepatitis. *Aliment Pharmacol Ther* 17, 1–16

National Institute for Clinical Excellence (2004) Interferon alfa (pegylated and non-pegylated) and ribavirin for the treatment of chronic hepatitis C. h**ttp://www.nice.org.uk/pdf/ TA075guidance.pdf** (accessed August 2004)

Pearlman BL (2004) Hepatitis C treatment update. *Am J Med* 117, 344–352

Riordan SM, Williams R (1997) Treatment of hepatic encephalopathy. *N Engl J Med* 337, 473–479

Rossi SJ, Wright TL (2003) New developments in the treatment of hepatitis C. *Gut* 52, 756–757

Schiødt FV, Lee WM (2003) Fulminant liver disease. *Clin Liver Dis* 7, 331–349

Sharara AI, Rockey DC (2001) Medical progress: gastroesophageal variceal hemorrhage. *N Engl J Med* 345, 669–681

Talwalkar JA, Lindor KD (2003) Primary biliary cirrhosis. *Lancet* 362, 53–61

Self-assessment

1. A 45-year-old woman was admitted to the A&E department in a London hospital with acute liver failure. Choose the one **incorrect** statement concerning her condition.

   A. Paracetamol overdose should be excluded.
   B. Paracetamol-induced liver damage is not reversible once it has taken place.
   C. Mannitol could be used to reduce the cerebral oedema associated with acute liver failure.
   D. Warfarin could be used to manage the coagulopathy which can occur.
   E. Terlipressin could be given as a vasoconstrictor to treat shock.

2. Choose the one **incorrect** statement concerning the following antiviral treatments.

   A. Interferon alfa protects against viral hepatitis.
   B. Pegylated interferon alfa (polyethylene glycol conjugate with interferon alfa) is cleared from the plasma at the same rate as the non-pegylated interferon alfa.
   C. Pegylated interferon alfa is inactive if given orally.
   D. Lamivudine is a prodrug.
   E. Combination therapy with ribavirin and interferon alfa is recommended for the treatment of hepatitis C.

3. Case history questions

   > Mr S was a 61-year-old publican who presented 'feeling as though I am 9 months' pregnant'. His abdominal swelling was caused by ascites, which was drained. A liver biopsy was performed, which showed micronodular cirrhosis. He commenced treatment with oral spironolactone.

   a. Was this a good choice of diuretic?

   > He remained well on this regimen for 5 years but continued to imbibe large quantities of alcohol. He re-presented as an emergency, having had a haematemesis and melaena. At the time he was slightly jaundiced and demonstrated signs of hepatic encephalopathy. In addition, there was gynaecomastia and testicular atrophy. The liver edge was palpable 8 cm below the right costal margin. Investigations showed a bilirubin of 27 mmol l^{-1} (normal <17), an albumin of 30 g l^{-1} (normal 32–50). A gastroscopy was performed under sedation with intravenous diazepam, and revealed oesophageal varices.

   b. What evidence was there to indicate diminished hepatic reserve in this man?
   c. In what way(s) would the pharmacodynamics and pharmacokinetics of diazepam be altered in this man? Was diazepam a good choice?
   d. What alterations to the dosage of diazepam might be necessary when compared with its use in someone without liver disease?

   > It has been shown that the incidence of re-bleeding from oesophageal varices can be reduced by the oral administration of propranolol (by reducing portal venous pressure).

   e. What effect is this man's liver disease likely to have on the pharmacodynamics and pharmacokinetics of propranolol? Specifically, in what way will the free fraction of the drug in plasma be affected; how will its bioavailability be influenced and what, if any, would be the effects on the drug's half-life?
   f. People with hepatic cirrhosis are often treated with colestyramine and/or lactulose. How do these drugs work and what benefits are produced?
   g. What would you use for pain relief in someone with established liver cirrhosis?

   The answers are provided on pages 733–734.

Drug compendium

Drugs used in liver disease

Drug	Half-life (h)	Elimination	Comments
Adefovir dipivoxil	8 h (adefovir)	Hydrolysis	Used in chronic hepatitis B infection with *either* compensated liver disease with evidence of viral replication and histologically documented active liver inflammation and fibrosis, *or* decompensated liver disease; given orally; the drug is a diester prodrug which undergoes hydrolysis to adefovir; adefovir is an acyclic nucleotide analogue which is a prodrug that undergoes intracellular phosphorylation to the active diphosphate; adefovir is eliminated by the kidneys
Interferon alfa	3–4 h	Metabolism	Used in the treatment of chronic hepatitis B, but response rate is less than 50%; given by subcutaneous, intramuscular or intravenous injection; peak levels appear 4–8 h after subcutaneous or intramuscular injection; taken up by kidney and catabolised
Lamivudine	5–7 h	Renal (+ some metabolism)	Antiviral reverse transcriptase inhibitor used in the initial treatment of hepatitis B, and for decompensated liver disease; given orally; undergoes intracellular phosphorylation to an active triphosphate; eliminated by the kidneys and limited sulphoxidation
Peginterferon alfa	80 h	Metabolism	Used in combination with ribavirin for chronic hepatitis C; polyethylene glycol-conjugated form of interferon alfa, which gives more prolonged blood levels after dosage; given by subcutaneous injection; prolonged duration of action compared with interferon alfa
Ribavirin	7–21 days	Metabolisms + renal	Given orally; oral bioavailabaility is 50%; metabolised by hydrolysis of ribosyl group from triazole moiety, which is then excreted in urine; very slowly cleared from erythrocytes and tissue compartments (short half-lives are reported after single doses)

37

Obesity

Obesity is defined as a body mass index (BMI) above 30 kg m^2, compared with the ideal range of 18.5–24.9 kg m^2. A BMI of 25–29.9 kg m^2 is considered overweight. A simpler measure of obesity is the waist–hip ratio, which should not exceed 1.0 in men or 0.95 in women. Recent data suggest that waist circumference above 102 cm in males or 88 cm in females may be equally predictive of increased risk of obesity-related disease. Weight gain after the age of 20 years is more predictive of increased risk than obesity in childhood. The prevalence of obesity is increasing in the Western world; it varies from less than 10% in the Netherlands to about 50% in some parts of Eastern Europe. In the UK, it is currently about 15%, but over half the British population is now overweight.

The health consequences of obesity are considerable (Table 37.1). Weight loss reduces the associated morbidity, but it can be difficult to achieve and to maintain. Obesity is not caused by psychological disturbances, but these commonly arise in obese people. The social prejudice against obesity, concern about body image, and the depression and irritability that arise from dieting are all contributory factors.

Pathogenesis

Obesity results when energy input exceeds output, usually determined by the balance between energy intake and exercise, or muscular work. Obesity usually develops gradually, and small imbalances are all that is required for progressive weight gain. Excess calories are stored as fat in adipose tissue. Energy balance is regulated in the hypothalamus, which integrates neural, hormonal and circulating nutrient stimuli, and sends signals to higher centres to trigger feelings of satiety or hunger. The hypothalamus also regulates sympathetic nervous system function (lipolysis and thermogenesis) and pituitary hormones that help to regulate energy expenditure. The body has two types of adipose tissue: brown adipose tissue is responsible for thermogenesis, and white adipose tissue for lipolysis. White adipose tissue is also a target for insulin, and is resistant to the action of insulin in obese people.

The biochemical factors that underlie regulation of weight are increasingly well characterised. The long-term signals are provided by insulin and the hormone leptin that is produced by adipose tissue. Leptin signals via specific hypothalamic receptors to indicate the degree of filling of adipocytes and induces the sensation of satiety. Leptin inhibits several hypothalamic appetite-stimulating (orexigenic) neurotransmitters, including neuropeptide Y and agouti-related peptide. Leptin and insulin also stimulate pro-opiomelanocortin, generating

Table 37.1
Adverse health consequences of obesity

Metabolic consequences	Clinical consequences
Hypertension	Coronary artery disease (BMI >29 increases risk fourfold)
Hyperlipidaemia (raised very-low-density lipoproteins, reduced high-density lipoproteins)	Non-insulin-dependent diabetes mellitus (BMI >35 increase risk 40-fold)
	Stroke
Hyperuricaemia	Osteoarthritis
Insulin resistance	Sleep apnoea
	Large bowel and endometrial cancer (BMI >30 increases risk two to fivefold)
	Low self-esteem

BMI, body mass index

α-melanocyte stimulating hormone that decreases appetite. Circulating concentrations of leptin are usually high in obesity. This is interpreted by some as representing hypothalamic resistance to the hormone that may arise from saturation of the transport system for leptin across the blood–brain barrier. However, the high plasma leptin could simply reflect the excess fat accumulation; Hypothalamic resistance to satiety cues when faced with palatable food may be the principal cause of obesity.

Overall, the epidemic of obesity in stable populations suggests that a major factor is environmental (reduced activity and dietary change) rather than biological. However, for a few individuals, obesity arises from hormonal disturbances, or neurological conditions that lead to behavioural change.

Short-term appetite regulators include the peptides ghrelin and peptide YY_{3-36} (PYY). Ghrelin is released by the stomach pre-prandially, and stimulates orexigenic peptides. PYY is released from the small intestine and colon in response to carbohydrates and lipids, and inhibits orexigenic peptides. Several other neurotransmitters and hormones are known to influence appetite. These include the appetite inhibitors 5-hydroxytryptamine (5HT, serotonin), dopamine and cholecystokinin, while endogenous opioids and growth hormone-releasing hormone stimulate appetite.

Drugs for treatment of obesity

Pancreatic lipase inhibitors

Orlistat

Mechanism of action
By binding to pancreatic lipase in the gut and inhibiting its action, orlistat reduces triglyceride digestion and, therefore, energy intake from dietary fat. It achieves sustained weight loss when used as an adjunct to dietary restriction and exercise. Continuous use of orlistat for more than 2 years is not recommended.

Pharmacokinetics
Orlistat is minimally absorbed after oral administration and an effect on energy intake is seen after 24–48 h. The half-life of the absorbed fraction of orlistat is short.

Unwanted effects
Unwanted effects of orlistat include:

- gastrointestinal upset, including flatulence, faecal urgency and faecal soiling; these are most common with poor adherence to dieting while taking the drug
- reduced absorption of fat-soluble vitamins, especially vitamin D.

Centrally acting appetite suppressants

Sibutramine

Mechanism of action
Sibutramine inhibits the reuptake of noradrenaline and 5HT in the central nervous system. The increase in synaptic 5HT acts on the hypothalamus to produce appetite suppression. It is only licensed for use for up to 1 year, and rapid recurrence of weight gain often follows withdrawal. Several other centrally acting appetite suppressants, dexfenfluramine, fenfluramine and phentermine, have been withdrawn because of concerns over adverse affects of valvular heart disease and pulmonary hypertension.

Pharmacokinetics
Sibutramine is well absorbed from the gut and undergoes extensive first-pass metabolism in the liver, generating active derivatives. Elimination is by hepatic metabolism, and the active metabolites have long half-lives.

Unwanted effects

- constipation, anorexia, nausea, dry mouth
- insomnia, anxiety, headache
- tachycardia, palpitation, hypertension.

Fluoxetine

The selective serotonin reuptake inhibitor (SSRI) antidepressant fluoxetine (Ch. 22) causes weight loss, but it is not licensed in the UK for this use.

Miscellaneous agents

Methylcellulose is sometimes used to provide bulk in the gut, but there is little supportive evidence of its benefit in obesity.

Management of obesity

The cornerstone of management of obesity is to reduce energy intake by 500–600 kcal below daily requirements. Fat is 'energy dense' and should be particularly restricted. However, dietary restriction alone is usually inadequate to achieve weight loss, and increased exercise combined with diet is more effective than either alone. Exercise need not be vigorous, provided it is maintained long term; walking or cycling is usually enough if performed daily. Behaviour modification is essential for long-term adherence to treatment.

Drug treatment should be restricted to individuals with a BMI >27 kg m^2 who do not achieve target weight but who have lost at least 2.5 kg bodyweight by diet and exercise in the preceding month. There is no clear guidance on the choice of drug, but it may be more appropriate to choose sibutramine if control of eating is the main problem, or orlistat if fat intake is high (but only if fat intake can be modified to reduce unwanted effects with the drug). Surgery to restrict the size of the stomach (gastroplasty) or wiring the jaw to reduce solid food intake have been used in the morbidly obese (BMI >40 kg m^2), or those with a BMI >35 kg m^2 and an obesity-related medical condition.

Existing treatments for obesity can be expected to produce weight loss of about 10–15%, which is often enough to ameliorate the obesity-related metabolic disorders and their accompanying clinical manifestations. The management of obesity should be carried out by a multidisciplinary team, who can advise on lifestyle and other treatment options. There are several treatments under investigation that interfere with the many neurotransmitter systems that regulate weight. These promise to offer more effective pharmacotherapy than the current limited range of options. The National Institute for Clinical Excellence (NICE) has produced guidelines for the use of anti-obesity drugs.

FURTHER READING

Anon (1998) Executive summary of the clinical guidelines on the identification, evaluation and treatment of overweight and obesity in adults. *Arch Intern Med* 158, 1855–1867

Fernández-López J-A, Remesar X, Foz, M et al (2002) Pharmacological approaches for the treatment of obesity. *Drugs* 62, 915–944

Kushner RF, Manzano H (2002) Obesity pharmacology: past, present and future. *Curr Opin Gastroenterol* 18, 213–220

National Institute for Clinical Excellence (2004) NICE home page for access to guidance on treatment of obesity. **http://www.nice.org.uk/page.aspx?o=home** (accessed July 2004)

Yanovski SZ, Yanovski JA (2002) Drug therapy: obesity. *N Engl J Med* 346, 591–602

Self-assessment

Are the statements in questions 1–5 true or false?

1. Drug treatment for obesity should be restricted to those who fail to lose a realistic amount of weight by other means, for example diet and exercise.

2. Courses of appetite-suppressant drugs are virtually all followed by a rebound in weight gain.

3. The appetite suppressant sibutramine inhibits the actions of released noradrenaline.

4. One of the brain centres that controls appetite is in the posterior pituitary.

5. Leptin is a peptide that is produced in muscle cells and inhibits appetite.

6. Concerning drugs used in obesity, choose the one best answer from the following options.

   A. There is no association between obesity and symptoms of depression.
   B. An anti-obesity drug should only be considered for people with a BMI in excess of 27 kg m^2 who are losing weight but who are failing to reach target weight following a regimen managed by health professionals.
   C. Combination therapy with anti-obesity drugs should be tried if weight loss with one drug fails.
   D. Sibutramine causes virtually no unwanted effects.
   E. Orlistat acts centrally to inhibit naturally occurring appetite-stimulating neurotransmitters.

The answers are provided on page 734.

Self-assessment questions

Drug compendium

Principles of medical pharmacology and therapeutics

Drugs used in obesity

Drug	Half-life (h)	Elimination	Comments
Methylcellulose	–	Not absorbed	Taken before meals to produce a sense of satiety; preparations that swell should be taken carefully with water to avoid oesophageal obstruction; little evidence to support efficacy
Orlistat	1–2	Metabolism	Taken orally before, during or immediately after a meal; negligible absorption (about 1%) and low systemic exposure in clinical use; action is local within the intestine; no significant effects on the absorption of other drugs; systemic disposition is not important
Sibutramine	1	Metabolism	Neurotransmitter reuptake inhibitor; used in the adjunctive treatment of obesity for a maximum of 12 months; taken orally; undergoes extensive first-pass metabolism by CYP3A4 to a number of metabolites, two of which are active; the active metabolites have longer half-lives (about 15 h) than the parent drug

The immune system

38

The immune response and immunosuppressant drugs

Biological basis of the immune response[a]

The immune system is highly complex and the elucidation of many of its main aspects has been one of the triumphs of biomedical research.

Natural and adaptive immunity

The innate and adaptive responses of the immune system protect against pathogens, the innate system providing the initial general recognition and early response to the pathogen and producing signals to initiate the adaptive system, which then provides targeted defence specific to the particular pathogen.

Natural (innate) immune defences include:

- physicochemical barriers to infection (impermeable skin and mucous membranes, low pH in stomach, mucociliary escalator in airways, antibacterial agents in skin and tear secretions, e.g. lysozyme)
- non-specific mechanisms (alternative pathway of complement activation, stimulation of phagocytosis by bacterial cell wall lipopolysaccharides, activation of mast cells by tissue damage).

Adaptive immune responses are superimposed upon the innate mechanisms. They are evolutionarily more recent and depend on their exquisite specificity in recognising 'non-self' molecules, usually foreign proteins, either via the production of specific antibodies or via cell-mediated immunity (Figs 38.1 and 38.2). Examples include:

- classic (antibody-dependent) pathway of complement activation, leading to non-specific lysis of bacterial cells, and a powerful effect on recruitment and activation of phagocytic cells (neutrophils and monocytes)
- antibody-dependent activation of resident leucocytes (mast cells and macrophages), leading to recruitment of further phagocytes and phagocytosis of pathogens in an acute inflammatory response
- antibody-dependent cytolysis of virally infected cells.

Humoral immunity

Both innate immunity and adaptive immunity involve complex networks of soluble humoral components and cellular components. In adaptive immunity, the overall protective event occurring in response to exposure to a foreign protein is the production of specific antibodies to that foreign protein (antigen). The antigen is recognised by immunoglobulin (Ig) molecules specific to that antigen on the surface of a specific clone of B-lymphocytes. These are derived from a few of the millions of clones (cell lines) of B-cell precursors, each of which has surface Ig directed towards a specific foreign molecule (clonal selection; Fig. 38.1a).

The initiation of antibody production commences with antigens being presented to uncommited T-cells by antigen-presenting cells (APC), including macrophages, dendritic cells in the lung, and Langerhans cells in the skin (Fig. 38.1b). The antigen fragment is presented within the cleft of major histocompatibility complex (MHC) type II molecules on the APC surface and requires the presence of co-stimulatory cytokines such as interleukin (IL)-2. Proliferation of the B-cell clones can then occur and they becomes susceptible to cytokines from activated T-helper (Th) lymphocytes; supported by IL-1 from the APC, the Th-cell also undergoes clonal proliferation. This is perpetuated over numerous cell divisions by IL-2 from the Th-cells themselves. Activated Th-cells produce a number of cytokines, including interleukins that convert B-cells into active plasma cells that secrete antibodies of the IgG, IgM, IgA, IgD and IgE classes. The pattern of antibodies produced depends upon whether

---

[a]We are grateful to Dr Anthony Sampson, who wrote this section.

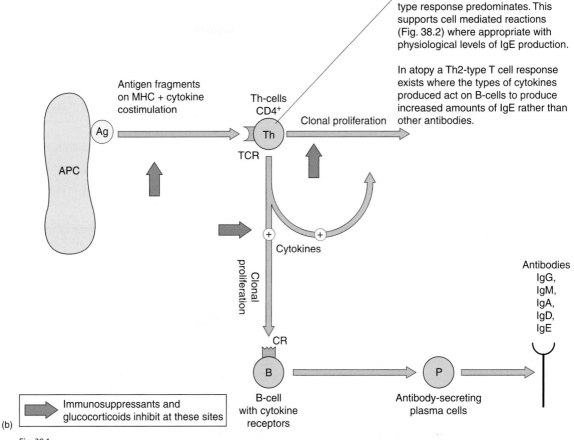

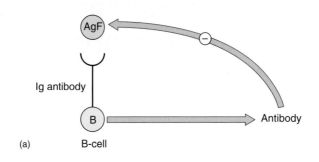

In non-atopic individuals a Th1-T cell type response predominates. This supports cell mediated reactions (Fig. 38.2) where appropriate with physiological levels of IgE production.

In atopy a Th2-type T cell response exists where the types of cytokines produced act on B-cells to produce increased amounts of IgE rather than other antibodies.

Antigen fragments on MHC + cytokine costimulation

Th-cells CD4⁺

Clonal proliferation

Ag

APC

TCR

Th

Clonal proliferation

+ +

Cytokines

CR

Antibodies IgG, IgM, IgA, IgD, IgE

B

P

B-cell with cytokine receptors

Antibody-secreting plasma cells

Immunosuppressants and glucocorticoids inhibit at these sites

(b)

Fig. 38.1

Aspects of humoral immunity. (a) There is production of specific antibodies to a foreign protein (AgF) after recognition of AgF by a selected group of B-cells carrying surface immunoglobulin (Ig) directed specifically towards AgF. (b) Adaptive immunity can result in production of antibodies (humoral response) or a cell-mediated response (Fig. 38.2). Antigen fragments can be presented on the major histocompatibility complex (MHC) to T-cells via a T-cell receptor (TCR) that recognises the antigen. T-cells undergo clonal proliferation, produce interleukins (IL) and stimulate B-cells to produce antibodies (IgG, IgM, IgA, IgD and IgE) – humoral immunity. In atopic individuals, the T-cells are tipped towards the Th2 type and produce IL-4, IL-5 and IL-13, which induce the B-cells to produce IgE. Th, T helper cell; P, plasma cell; Ag, antigen; CR, cytokine receptor; APC, antigen presenting cell.

the Th-cell is Th1 or Th2. In atopic individuals, the Th2-cell type is increased. This cell type secretes IL-4 and IL-13, which results in increased IgE synthesis (Fig. 38.1b).

High concentrations of monomeric IgG are found in the plasma and in tissue spaces. IgM circulates as pentamers linked by J chains, while IgA is secreted onto mucosal surfaces as dimers linked by a segment of its

receptor termed the secretory piece. IgD is involved in early-life processing of B-cells. IgE is important in immune responses to intestinal parasites and also in allergic hypersensitivity reactions such as hayfever and asthma. On encountering an antigen, the primary immune response consists of IgM, replaced later by IgG. On a further encounter with the antigen, the secondary

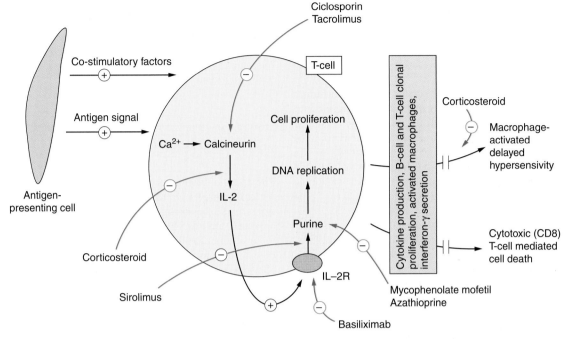

Fig. 38.2
Aspects of cell-mediated immunity. This shows in simplified form some steps in T-cell activation following antigen presentation to the T-cell receptor and subsequent events that may contribute to the aspects of cell-mediated immunity. Exogenous antigens are presented by antigen-presenting cells to the uncommitted CD4+ lymphocyte; under the influence of interleukin-2 (IL-2), Th1-cells are formed which activate macrophages, which are then responsible for some of the cell-mediated immune response. Antigens may also be presented to CD8+ lymphocytes, which mature into cytotoxic T-cells. Drugs used as immunosuppressants (red arrows) act at the sites shown. Corticosteroids act at many sites (see also Fig. 38.1 and Ch. 44). IL-2R, interleukin-2 receptor.

immune response occurs more rapidly and consists of large amounts of IgG produced by plasma cells derived from reactivation of memory B-cells.

Cell-mediated immunity

Not all adaptive immune responses involve antibodies. Cell-mediated immunity is largely T-cell driven, utilising Th1 and Tc (CD8) subtypes, and is involved in responses to viral infection, graft rejection, chronic inflammation, and tumour immunity (Fig. 38.2).

Virally infected host cells express fragments of viral proteins as antigens in association with MHC I molecules on the cell surface. These can be recognised by specific T-cell receptors (TCRs) on the surface of cytotoxic T-cells (Tc), which can kill the virus-infected host cell.

Delayed hypersensitivity also occurs. This aspect of cell-mediated immunity involves the regulation by antigen-specific T-lymphocyte clones of 'non-specific' inflammatory cells, including macrophages, neutrophils, eosinophils and basophils. Following recognition of antigens associated with MHC class II on the APC, Th-cells proliferate under the influence of IL-2, and secrete a number of cytokines that regulate leucocyte proliferation, recruitment and activation. The type of

response is determined by the profile of cytokines secreted. A subset of Th-cells, called Th1-cells, secrete interferon-gamma (IFN-γ) to activate macrophages, which in turn secrete IL-8 and other neutrophil chemo-attractants. This leads to macrophage/neutrophil-dependent inflammation, associated with immune responses to persistent infections such as tuberculosis. In contrast, cytokines derived from Th2-cells promote type 4 hypersensitivity reactions (e.g. asthma; see below).

Unwanted immune reactions

The processes of inflammation and immunity described above are essential to protect the host against pathogenic and other damage, but excessive, inappropriately prolonged or misdirected immune responses can cause disease, including hypersensitivity reactions, graft rejection and autoimmune diseases.

Hypersensitivity reactions

Hypersensitivity reactions were classified by Gell and Coombs in the late 1950s.

Type 1 (acute, immediate). This includes hayfever and acute asthma. IgE molecules on the surface of mast cells

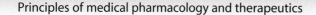

and basophils are cross-linked by harmless antigens (allergens such as pollens, house-dust mites), leading to synthesis and/or release of inflammatory mediators. These include cysteinyl leukotrienes, prostaglandins, histamine, platelet-activating factor, proteases and cytokines.

Type 2 (cytotoxic). Cell surface antigens, including microbial proteins and drug molecules haptenised onto cell surfaces, are recognised and bound by IgG and IgM antibodies (opsonisation), leading to activation of complement (classic pathway) and cytolysis of the target cell. Examples include destruction of red cells after incompatible blood transfusion, and haemolytic anaemia caused by binding of some drugs to host cells (see Ch. 53).

Type 3 (complex-mediated). Soluble antigens react with excess circulating antibodies to form complexes that precipitate in small blood vessels, causing vasculitis and organ damage. Pigeon fancier's lung and farmer's lung are systemic type 3 reactions, while the Arthus reaction is a local response to an injected antigen (e.g. non-human insulins).

Type 4 (cell-mediated, delayed-type hypersensitivity). Inappropriate regulation of cell-mediated immunity may cause damaging chronic inflammation, leading to fibrosis and granuloma formation. Cell-mediated immunity misdirected against harmless foreign proteins (allergens) can lead to chronic allergic inflammation (such as occurs in eczema), or cause contact sensitivity in the skin to haptenising metals and chemicals. In allergy, a subset of T-cells (Th2) secrete cytokines including IL-4, IL-5 and IL-13, which promote eosinophilic inflammation and overproduction of IgE by B-cells.

Transplant rejection

In blood transfusion, rejection usually occurs because non-self antigens on red blood cells (ABO system) trigger type 2 hypersensitivity reactions in the recipient. In immunodeficient patients, transfused T-cells react against recipient antigens (graft-versus-host reactions). For organ transplants, hyperacute rejection can occur if there is ABO incompatability, or host-versus-graft reactions can arise later with foreign MHC molecules (human leucocyte antigens, HLA). The latter can be reduced by HLA tissue-typing, which will reduce the rate of tissue destruction but not prevent chronic rejection. Rejection involves destruction of the graft by B-cells, T-cells and macrophages, and it can be immediate (days), acute (weeks) or chronic (years).

Autoimmunity

Normally the immune system is tolerant of 'self' antigens. If this tolerance breaks down, then autoimmune disorders result. Numerous mechanisms cause autoimmune diseases, including viral infection of host cells, binding of drug molecules to host cells (e.g. penicillin), antigens shared between host cells and microbes, and sequestered antigens liberated by cell damage. Examples include haemolytic anaemia, diabetes, Addison's disease, rheumatoid arthritis, myasthenia gravis, systemic lupus erythematosus and thyroiditis.

Immunosuppressant drugs

The immune system presents a large number of potential molecular targets for therapeutic intervention. Present drugs tend to be non-specific immunosuppressants with a range of adverse effects.

In addition to the drugs discussed in this chapter, others such as methotrexate and cyclophosphamide (Ch. 52) are also used for their immunosuppressant properties in various disease states. Methotrexate and cyclophosphamide have immunosuppressant properties at doses much lower than those required to treat malignancy (Ch. 52). These drugs are more fully discussed in other chapters. Corticosteroids (e.g. dexamethasone, prednisone) (Ch. 44) are highly effective anti-inflammatory drugs that can be used systemically to suppress type 4 hypersensitivity reactions, autoimmune diseases (e.g. rheumatoid arthritis) and graft rejection. Cushingoid unwanted effects are a drawback with systemic treatment; they are used topically for inflammatory skin disease and by inhalation for asthma (e.g. beclometasone, fluticasone; Ch. 12).

Inflammatory mediators released during immune reactions can be blocked by antagonists at their receptors on target cells, or by inhibiting their synthesis. Anti-mediator drugs include histamine H_1 receptor antagonists (antihistamines), cysteinyl-leukotriene receptor antagonists (LTRA) and cyclo-oxygenase inhibitors (non-steroidal anti-inflammatory drugs [NSAIDs]). Topical and systemic antihistamines (e.g. terfenadine, loratadine, cetirizine) are used in the control of hayfever and eczema (Ch. 39), while oral LTRAs (montelukast, zafirlukast) are used in asthma (Ch. 12). Oral NSAIDs block the synthesis of prostaglandins and are extensively used in rheumatoid arthritis (Chs 29 and 30).

Immunosuppressant drugs are widely used in many diseases; examples include rheumatoid arthritis, psoriasis and inflammatory bowel disease. Their benefit is both through modulation of the immune system and, in some cases, through their anti-inflammatory properties.

Calcineurin inhibitors

Examples: ciclosporin, tacrolimus

Ciclosporin

Mechanism of action

Ciclosporin is a fungal cyclic peptide which inhibits T-cell division. It binds in the cell cytoplasm to the protein cyclophilin, and the complex associates with and inhibits calcineurin, a calmodulin-Ca^{2+}-dependent phosphatase which is a key component in T-cell activation (Fig. 38.2). Activated calcineurin, which is produced in response to an antigenic signal at TCRs, dephosphorylates nuclear factor of activation in T-cells (NFAT), which then enters the cell nucleus and binds to a promoter region of the IL-2 gene. IL-2 stimulates T-cell division. By inhibiting calcineurin phosphatase, ciclosporin prevents dephosphorylation of NFAT, which remains in the cytoplasm. This inhibits IL-2 production and the T-cell cycle progression is inhibited between G_0 and G_1. Tacrolimus also ultimately inhibits the phosphatase activity of calcineurin, but acts in a somewhat different way.

Ciclosporin also inhibits other cellular mitogen-activated protein kinases triggered by the inflammatory cytokines tumour necrosis factor alpha (TNFα) and IL-1, and various other cellular factors. These include the jun-N terminal kinase and p38 kinases that phosphorylate transcription factors involved in upregulation of *c-fos*-mediated gene transcription.

Ciclosporin stimulates production of transforming growth factor beta (TGF-β), possibly by releasing an inhibitory effect of calcineurin on gene transcription. This may be responsible for some of the unwanted effects of ciclosporin.

Pharmacokinetics

Oral absorption of a standard formulation of ciclosporin is variable and incomplete, requiring initial dispersion by bile salts. For this reason, a microemulsion formulation has replaced it for oral use. This emulsifies when it comes into contact with water in the gut, increasing the surface area for absorption, which then becomes independent of bile production. After absorption, ciclosporin selectively concentrates in some tissues, including liver, kidney, several endocrine glands, lymph nodes, spleen and bone marrow. Ciclosporin is extensively metabolised in the liver by cytochrome P450 and has a long half-life. Ciclosporin can also be given by intravenous infusion. Trough plasma drug concentration monitoring has traditionally been used to guide dosage for optimal effectiveness and to minimise toxicity. However, recent evidence suggests that a blood concentration 2 h post-dose may be a better guide to graft survival and reduced toxicity.

Unwanted effects

- Nephrotoxicity almost always occurs, with a dose-dependent increase in serum creatinine in the first few weeks. The acute effect is due to intrarenal vasoconstriction that may persist and contribute to the less common long-term sequelae, which include interstitial fibrosis and tubular atrophy. Induction of TGF-β may be a contributory factor. The decline in renal glomerular function is usually reversible, but permanent renal impairment can result.
- Hypertension, often associated with fluid retention, occurs in up to 50% of people, and especially after heart transplantation. It usually responds to standard antihypertensive drug treatment.
- Hepatic dysfunction.
- Tremor, headache.
- Hypertrichosis (excessive hair growth) and gum hypertrophy are common.
- Gastrointestinal disturbance, including anorexia, nausea and vomiting.
- Hyperlipidaemia.
- Convulsions.
- Drug interactions can be dangerous and caution should be taken when ciclosporin is used with other nephrotoxic drugs, such as aminoglycoside antimicrobials and amphotericin (Ch. 51) and NSAIDs (Ch. 29). Drugs that induce hepatic cytochrome P450, such as phenytoin and carbamazepine, can reduce the plasma concentrations of ciclosporin to sub-therapeutic levels. Drugs that inhibit cytochrome P450, such as erythromycin or ketoconazole (Ch. 51), can increase ciclosporin concentrations and provoke toxicity.

Tacrolimus

Mechanism of action and effects

Tacrolimus inhibits calcineurin and, therefore, T-cell proliferation by arresting the cell cycle between G_0 and G_1 in a similar manner to ciclosporin. After binding to a receptor protein called FK-binding protein-12, the complex binds to calcineurin and inhibits Ca^{2+}-dependent calcineurin activation. Tacrolimus also inhibits jun-N terminal kinase and p38 kinases. Unlike ciclosporin, tacrolimus does not stimulate production of TGF-β.

Pharmacokinetics

Tacrolimus is more water soluble than ciclosporin and undergoes more predictable, though poor, absorption from the gut. It is metabolised by the liver and has an intermediate half-life.

Unwanted effects

These are similar to those of ciclosporin except that tacrolimus causes less hypertension, hirsutism or gum hyperplasia. Other effects that are more common with tacrolimus include:

- diabetes
- pleural and pericardial effusions
- cardiomyopathy in children, who should be monitored by echocardiography.

mTOR (target of rapamycin) inhibitors

Example: sirolimus

Mechanism of action and effects

Sirolimus (previously known as rapamycin) is a natural fungal fermentation product that inhibits T-cell proliferation by arresting the cell between the G_1 and S phases. It binds to intracellular FK-binding protein-12, and the complex inhibits the action of mTOR, a cytoplasmic kinase. mTOR is a key step in a series of intracellular Ca^{2+}-independent events that transduce signals from the cell surface IL-2 receptor and other growth factor receptors to cell cycle regulators that promote DNA and protein synthesis and mitogenesis. The action of sirolimus therefore differs from that of tacrolimus, despite binding to the same family of intracellular receptor.

Pharmacokinetics

Sirolimus is rapidly absorbed from the gut, and the absorption is modulated by P-glycoproteins. It is metabolised by intestinal and hepatic cytochrome P450 (CYP3A4), and has a very long half-life.

Unwanted effects

- lymphocoele
- abdominal pain, diarrhoea
- anaemia, thrombocytopenia
- hyperlipidaemia
- hypokalaemia
- arthralgia
- rash
- drug interactions: rifampicin reduces plasma sirolimus concentration by induction of CYP3A4; the antifungal agents itraconazole and ketoconazole increase plasma concentrations of sirolimus by enzyme inhibition.

Antiproliferative agents

Examples: mycophenolate mofetil, azathioprine

Mycophenolate mofetil

Mycophenolic acid reduces purine synthesis by inhibition of the enzymes inosine monophosphate (IMP) dehydrogenase and guanylate synthase. These enzymes are involved in the conversion of IMP to xanthylate, and then to guanylate. Guanylate is the precursor of guanosine triphosphate that is involved in RNA, DNA and protein synthesis. Inhibition of these enzymes depletes the cell of guanine nucleotides and inhibits cellular DNA synthesis. T- and B-lymphocytes and monocytes rely on de novo purine nucleotide synthesis, unlike neutrophils, which can re-use pre-formed guanine released from the breakdown of nucleic acids (the salvage pathway). Mycophenolate mofetil therefore shows specificity towards inhibition of lymphocyte function.

A further action of mycophenolate mofetil involves inhibition of smooth muscle proliferation in arterial walls. This may also be important in reducing graft rejection as a consequence of obliterative arteriopathy.

Pharmacokinetics

Mycophenolate mofetil is a prodrug ester of mycophenolic acid. It is almost completely absorbed from the gut, and hydrolysed rapidly to the acid derivative after absorption. Elimination of the active metabolite is via hepatic metabolism, and it has a long half-life. Mycophenolate mofetil can be given by intravenous infusion.

Unwanted effects

- gastrointestinal upset is very common, including nausea, vomiting, diarrhoea, abdominal cramps and, occasionally, pancreatitis; tolerance to the gastrointestinal symptoms often occurs
- hypertension, oedema, chest pain
- dyspnoea, cough
- dizziness, insomnia, headache
- bone marrow suppression resulting in leucopenia and anaemia
- opportunistic infections may be increased, especially with cytomegalovirus, herpes simplex, aspergillus and candida, as well as bacterial urinary tract infection and pneumonia
- lymphoproliferative disease and skin cancer.

Azathioprine

Mechanism of action

Azathioprine is widely used for immunosuppression. Most of the effects result from cleavage to the active derivative 6-mercaptopurine (Ch. 52). Both cell- and antibody-mediated immune reactions are suppressed (Figs 38.1 and 38.2). Effects on the immune response include impaired synthesis of immunoglobulins by B-lymphocytes, and inhibition of the infiltration of mononuclear cells into inflamed tissue. These arise from the antimetabolite action of 6-mercaptopurine, which interferes with purine biosynthesis, thus impairing DNA synthesis in the S-phase of the cell cycle (Fig. 52.1).

Pharmacokinetics

Oral absorption is almost complete. Azathioprine is a prodrug that is metabolised in the liver to produce the active compound 6-mercaptopurine, which is further metabolised to inactive compounds. The half-lives of azathioprine and 6-mercaptopurine are short. Azathioprine can be given by intravenous injection, but the solution is alkaline and very irritant.

Unwanted effects

- Dose-dependent bone marrow suppression, especially leucopenia and thrombocytopenia. Regular monitoring of the full blood count (at least every 3 months) is essential.
- Hypersensitivity reactions, with malaise, dizziness, vomiting, diarrhoea, fever, myalgia, arthralgia, rash and hypotension. The drug should be stopped immediately.
- Increased susceptibility to infection, often with 'opportunistic' organisms.
- Alopecia.
- There is a small risk of carcinogenicity, especially lymphomas.
- Drug interactions: the most important interaction is with allopurinol (Ch. 31); allopurinol inhibits the enzyme xanthine oxidase, which is involved in the metabolism of azathioprine. The dose of azathioprine should be reduced by 75% if the drugs are used together. Rifampicin may reduce the efficacy of azathioprine by inducing cytochrome P450.

Interleukin-2 receptor antibodies

Examples: basiliximab, daclizumab

Basiliximab is a chimeric monoclonal antibody with murine sequences in the hypervariable region that bind to the α-subunit of the IL-2 receptor and prevent T-cell proliferation. Daclizumab is a humanised antibody with fewer than 10% murine sequences, making it less immunogenic. Both drugs are used to prevent transplant rejection.

Pharmacokinetics
Basiliximab is given by intravenous infusion immediately before and again 4 days after surgery. Daclizumab is given immediately before surgery and then every 2 weeks for a total of five doses. Both drugs have very long half-lives (1–3 weeks).

Unwanted effects
Hypersensitivity reactions occur rarely.

Immunosuppression in organ transplantation

The immune response and its place in the rejection of a transplanted organ is complex. Graft destruction occurs as increased generation of B-cells, cytotoxic T-cells and monocyte/macrophages results in antibody production against the graft, lysis of cells and delayed hypersensitivity responses. This occurs as the antigens on the graft are recognised as foreign and the cascaded responses outlined in Figure 38.2 occur. Immunosuppressant drugs act at the steps of T-cell activation, proliferation and cytokine production (Fig. 38.2).

Effective immunosuppression has improved the early survival of kidney, liver, heart, heart–lung and haematopoietic stem-cell transplants. However, suppression of acute rejection is more effective than prevention of chronic rejection, which responds poorly to immunosuppressant therapy. Regimens for immunosuppression vary among transplant units and according to the immunogenicity of the transplanted tissue. Combination therapy with a corticosteroid, calcineurin inhibitor and an antiproliferative agent is commonly used.

For kidney transplantation, the corticosteroid prednisolone (Ch. 44) with ciclosporin (or sometimes tacrolimus) is widely employed. Some units add azathioprine to this regimen. Initial acute rejection is reduced by treatment with the IL-2 receptor antibodies basiliximab or daclizumab. With such regimens, more than 85% of cadaveric kidney grafts will survive beyond 1 year. Only half of those that fail are lost from rejection, and the rest from thrombosis. Progressive graft loss continues after the first year, with only 60% of grafts surviving at 10 years. Grafts from living donors have better survival rates of 95% at 1 year and 70% at 10 years. Most of the late graft losses are as a result of chronic vascular rejection. If this occurs, increasing the dosages of the primary immunosuppressant drugs may help. However, there is continuing uncertainty about whether chronic rejection reflects nephrotoxicity from long-term use of calcineurin inhibitors or inadequate immunosuppression. It is possible that drugs such as sirolimus or mycophenolate mofetil may reduce the incidence of chronic rejection, but there are few long-term data on outcome. Late acute rejection is a less common problem. It can sometimes be overcome by high-dose corticosteroid or the use of polyclonal antilymphocytic globulin or monoclonal antilymphocytic antibody (although the use of these is associated with an increased risk of opportunistic infection and long-term malignancy). Tacrolimus or mycophenolate mofetil can also be used successfully as a rescue treatment during late episodes of acute rejection.

In contrast to renal transplants, pancreatic transplants are more immunogenic and quadruple immunosuppressant regimens are widely used. Induction treatment with antilymphocytic globulin is then followed by ciclosporin, azathioprine and a corticosteroid. Mycophenolate mofetil is sometimes substituted for azathioprine, or tacrolimus for ciclosporin. Despite these treatments, 5-year graft survival is only about 60% and the risk of post-transplant infection is high.

Triple immunosuppressant therapy is used for heart (50% 10-year survival), heart–lung (30% 10-year survival), liver (70% 10-year survival) and intestinal (40–50% 3-year survival) transplants, often with initial use of an IL-2 antibody. In addition to prednisolone, tacrolimus is often included in these regimens in place of ciclosporin. The use of azathioprine is diminishing due to recent evidence that it may add little benefit but increase toxicity, and there is no consensus on the role of mycophenolate mofetil as an alternative.

With haematopoietic stem-cell transplantation, graft-versus-host disease (GVHD) is the major barrier. This usually begins at least 3 months after the transplant, and has three phases. The first phase involves damage to intestinal mucosa and the liver, with activation of host cells and release of inflammatory cytokines. These up-regulate major histocompatibility (MHC) antigens that are recognised by donor T-cells. The second phase involves activation and proliferation of donor T-cells, and the third phase includes tissue destruction by mono-cytes primed by inflammatory cytokines and lipopoly-saccharide from T-cells and damaged intestinal mucosa. GVHD can be prevented by inhibition of phase one, using a calcineurin inhibitor such as ciclosporin or tacrolimus, or possibly mycophenolate mofetil. Acute GVHD can be treated by corticosteroid with ciclosporin, and possibly daclizumab.

Immunosuppression in other disorders

Immunosuppression therapy is used in several diseases in which an autoimmune component may contribute to the pathogenesis. These include various connective tissue diseases such as vasculitis and systemic lupus erythematosus, certain types of glomerulonephritis, chronic active hepatitis, psoriasis, Crohn's disease and some haematological disorders. Drugs may be given alone or in combination. Those most widely used include corticosteroids, azathioprine, methotrexate and cyclophosphamide (Ch. 52). Ciclosporin and mycophenolate mofetil have also been studied in disorders such as asthma, inflammatory bowel disease and psoriasis, with some success.

FURTHER READING

Fernandez EJ, Lolis E (2002) Structure, function and inhibition of chemokines. *Annu Rev Pharmacol Toxicol* 42, 469–499

Formica RN, Friedmann AL, Lorber MI (2002) Evolving role of sirolimus immunosuppression after organ transplantation. *Curr Opin Organ Transplant* 7, 353–358

Jacobsohn DA, Vogelsang GB (2002) Novel pharmacotherapeutic approaches to prevention and treatment of GVHD. *Drugs* 62, 879–889

Jørgensen KA, Koefoed-Nielsen PB, Karamperis N (2002) Calcineurin phosphatase activity and immunosuppression. A review on the role of calcineurin phosphatase activity and the immunosuppressant effect of cyclosporin A and tacrolimus. *Scand J Immunol* 57, 93–98

Mascarell L, Truffa-Bachi P (2003) New aspects of cyclosporin A mode of action: from gene silencing to gene up-regulation. *Min Rev Med Chem* 3, 205–214

Meiser BM, Reichart B (2002) New agents and new strategies in immunosuppression after heart transplantation. *Curr Opin Organ Transplant* 7, 226–232

Moser MAJ (2002) Options for induction of immunosuppression in liver transplant recipients. *Drugs* 62, 995–1011

Neuhaus P, Klupp J, Langrehr JM (2001) mTOR inhibitors: an overview. *Liver Transpl* 7, 473–484

Pascual M, Theruvath T, Tatsuo K et al (2002) Medical progress: strategies to improve long-term outcomes after renal transplantation. *N Engl J Med* 346, 580–590

Vilatoba M, Contreras JL, Eckhoff DE (2003) New immunosuppressant strategies in liver transplantation: balancing efficacy and toxicity. *Curr Opin Organ Transplant* 8, 139–145

Self-assessment

In questions 1–3, the first statement, in italics, is true. Are the accompanying statements also true?

1. *Ciclosporin, tacrolimus and corticosteroids decrease maturation of cytotoxic T-cells by suppressing IL-2 transcription.*

   a. Ciclosporin does not cause bone marrow suppression.
   b. With ciclosporin administration, careful assessment of renal function is required.

2. *Immunosuppression induced by glucocorticoids involves their effects on T-cells and inflammation.* Tacrolimus enhances transformation of the glucocorticoid receptor.

3. *Using smaller doses than for cancer chemotherapy, drugs such as cyclophosphamide, methotrexate and azathioprine are immunosuppressant.* Azathioprine suppresses antibody-mediated immune responses.

4. Concerning the pharmacology of corticosteroids, choose the one <u>most appropriate</u> answer from the following.

Glucocorticoids:

A. Act within the nucleus to inhibit the expression of genes responsible for the generation of some inflammatory mediators.
B. Promote leukotriene synthesis in mast cells.
C. Reduce blood sugar by increasing glucose uptake into cells.
D. Promote growth in children.
E. Promote cytokine-mediated macrophage activation.

5. Case history questions

A 35-year-old woman was about to receive her second kidney transplant. The previous transplant lasted 5 years, but, despite immunosuppression with prednisolone and ciclosporin, it was eventually rejected.

   a. How might you reduce the chances of acute rejection of the second transplant?
   b. What were the long-term risks of combination chemotherapy with corticosteroids, tacrolimus and azathioprine?

The answers are provided on pages 734–735.

Drug compendium

Immunosuppressive drugs[a]

Drug	Half-life	Elimination	Comment
Azathioprine	3–5 h	Metabolism	Antiproliferative immunosuppressant used for transplant recipients, for autoimmune conditions and for rheumatoid arthritis; oral or intravenous dosage; converted to active metabolite, 6-mercaptopurine, which is converted to nucleoside and uric acid analogues (therefore interaction with allopurinol)
Basiliximab	7–11 days	Metabolism	Monoclonal antibody that prevents T-lymphocyte proliferation; used for prophylaxis to prevent kidney transplant rejection; given by intravenous infusion with ciclosporin and corticosteroid regimens; binding to interleukin-2 receptor α-chain maintained for 1 to 2 weeks after dosage
Ciclosporin	27 h (10–40)	Metabolism	A calcineurin inhibitor used in organ and tissue transplantation; oral or intravenous dosage; oral bioavailability is 40%; lipid-soluble cyclic peptide metabolised by CYP3A4 in liver and gut wall to at least 25 metabolites, some of which retain biological activity
Daclizumab	20 days	Metabolism	Monoclonal antibody that prevents T-lymphocyte proliferation; used for prophylaxis to prevent kidney transplant rejection; given by intravenous infusion with ciclosporin and corticosteroid regimens; normally given every 2 weeks for a total of five doses
Mycophenolate mofetil	18 h (as MPA)	Metabolism	Used for prophylaxis to prevent acute transplant rejection; oral or intravenous dosage; very rapidly hydrolysed (within minutes) to the active form mycophenolic acid (MPA); oral and intravenous doses undergo essentially quantitative conversion to MPA; MPA is eliminated as a glucuronide conjugate
Sirolimus	60 h	Metabolism	Potent non-calcineurin-inhibiting immunosuppressant; used for prophylaxis to prevent kidney transplant rejection; inhibits T-cell activation and proliferation; given orally as an oil solution; low bioavailability which is increased by giving with fatty food; substrate for and inhibitor of intestinal P-glycoprotein and metabolised by CYP3A4, which contributes to low oral bioavailablilty (see Ch. 2)
Tacrolimus	9 h (4–41)	Metabolism	Potent calcineurin-inhibiting immunosuppressant; used for prophylaxis to prevent kidney and liver transplant rejection; oral or intravenous dosage; substrate for P-glycoprotein in the intestine; metabolised by CYP3A4 in liver and gut wall; low bioavailability combined with low systemic clearance indicate that it undergoes extensive first-pass metabolism in the gut wall but not the liver; metabolites are mostly inactive

[a]Costicoseroids, such as prednisolone, have important immunosuppressive properties. Immunostimulants are covered in Chapter 52 (Chemotherapy of malignancy). See also the inflammatory arthritides (Ch. 30).

39

Antihistamines and allergic disease

Atopy, allergic disorders and anaphylaxis

Allergic responses occur in atopic individuals who are predisposed to produce antigen-specific immuno-globulin E (IgE) when exposed to common, normally harmless environmental allergens such as house-dust mite, grass pollen or animal dander. Re-exposure to the antigen then results in the antigen cross-linking IgE on mast cells and basophils and an allergic response as explained below. The control of antibody production in the immune response is shown in Figure 38.1(b). The key to the allergic reaction is that there is a prepon-derance of IgE production, rather than other antibodies. This is because when atopic individuals are exposed to allergens it provokes a type 2 helper (Th2) response, rather than the usually dominant Th1-cell response. The production of interleukin (IL)-4 and IL-13 by the Th2-cell type then causes the B-cells to produce IgE rather than IgG; this phenomenon is known as class switching. Dominance of Th1 or Th2 response is partially programmed in early life, with exposure to microbial antigens promoting the normal Th1 dominance.

Most allergic reactions are predominantly of the type 1 (immediate) hypersensitivity category (see Ch. 38 for definitions). Immediate hypersensitivity to an allergen in a person with atopy produces a weal and flare reaction in the skin, or sneezing and a runny nose, or wheezing within minutes. Pre-formed and newly synthesised mediators of the allergic response are released from mast cells and basophils after allergen cross-links IgE bound to cell surface receptors. The mediators include histamine, tryptase, platelet activating factor, prostag-landin D$_2$, and the cysteinyl leukotrienes LTC$_4$, LTD$_4$ and LTE$_4$ (Ch. 29). Tryptase activates receptors on endothelial and epithelial cells to upregulate adhesion molecules that attract inflammatory cells. Some allergic reactions, such as those that produce contact allergy and eczema, and a component of other allergic responses are driven by T-cell-mediated inflammatory processes. Many atopic individuals have coexisting allergic diseases such as asthma, hayfever and eczema, although these are not invariably associated.

A prolonged inflammatory reaction (delayed-type hypersensitivity) may follow the initial allergic response, reaching a peak 6–9 h later. This produces an oedematous, red, indurated swelling in the skin, sustained blockage in the nose, or further wheezing. This delayed reaction is associated with initial tissue accumulation of eosino-phils and neutrophils, followed by T-cells and basophils. Some delayed reactions can arise without an immediate phase, and may be triggered by activation of T-cells rather than mast cells. Chronic allergic inflammation is maintained by production of several Th2-type cytokines, such as IL-4, IL-5, IL-9 and IL-13, which promote the development of mast cells and eosinophils, stimulate adhesion molecules and enhance the production of IgE. Eosinophils release toxic basic proteins, cysteinyl leuko-trienes and platelet activating factor. T-cells, mast cells and eosinophils also produce neurotrophins that release neuropeptides such as substance P, calcitonin gene-related peptide and neurokinin A from sensory neurons. These contribute to the inflammatory response by producing vasodilation with increased vascular permeability, and smooth muscle contraction and mucus secretion in the lung.

Allergic reactions to antigens vary in severity. At the most severe end of the spectrum is anaphylaxis, a systemic allergic reaction which is life-threatening because of respiratory obstruction and/or hypotension. Severe anaphylactic reactions can occur within minutes of exposure to the allergen. There are several causes of anaphylaxis (Box 39.1). Drugs can also act directly on

---

Box 39.1

Causes of anaphylaxis

Foods: especially peanuts, tree nuts, fish, shellfish, eggs, milk
Drugs: especially penicillin, intravenous anaesthetic agents, aspirin and other non-steroidal anti-inflammatory drugs, intravenous contrast media, morphine
Bee and wasp stings
Latex rubber

447

mast cells to release mediators without the involvement of IgE. Such reactions are called anaphylactoid, and they present in the same way as true anaphylaxis. If the allergen exposure is via systemic injection, then hypotension and shock will predominate. Foods are more likely to cause facial and laryngeal oedema with prominent respiratory problems.

Histamine as an autacoid

Histamine is a heterocyclic amine that functions as a local hormone (autacoid). It is found in mast cells, particularly in tissues that come into contact with the outside world, for example skin, lungs and gut, where it forms part of the tissue defence mechanisms. It is also present in circulating basophils, where it may have a similar role. Histamine is found also in enterochromaffin-like cells in the stomach, where it participates in acid secretion (Ch. 33), and in the brain, where it acts as a neurotransmitter (Ch. 4).

Histamine is synthesised in mast cells and basophils from dietary histidine by decarboxylation. After release from the cells it is rapidly metabolised (see Ch. 4). Its effects are mediated by four distinct types of G-protein-coupled receptors known as H_1, H_2, H_3 and H_4. In general, H_1 receptors are involved in the 'defensive' actions of histamine and act through intracellular Ca^{2+} as a second messenger. Gastric acid secretion is mediated by H_2 receptors that generate cyclic adenosine monophosphate (cAMP) as a second messenger (Ch. 33). These receptors are also involved in cardiac function (stimulation of rate and force of contraction) and are inhibitory postsynaptic receptors in the brain. H_3 receptors are also involved in inhibitory neurotransmission, acting presynaptically on histamine-releasing neurons through inhibition of cAMP generation and by Ca^{2+} release. H_4 receptors may modulate the function of immune and inflammatory cells (such as T-cells, neutrophils and eosinophils) through Ca^{2+} release, and are also found in the intestines, lung and brain.

Allergic reactions involve the action of histamine at H_1 receptors. Histamine H_1 receptors are coupled to inositol phospholipid intracellular signalling pathways. They also activate the ubiquitous gene transcription factor nuclear factor kappa B (NF-κB) (Ch. 30). NF-κB stimulates production of pro-inflammatory cytokines (particularly tumour necrosis factor alpha [TNFα] and IL-6 and IL-8) and expression of epithelial and endothelial adhesion molecules (such as intercellular adhesion molecule [ICAM]-1) that attract inflammatory cells. The following are the major consequences of H_1 receptor stimulation.

- Capillary and venous dilation can produce marked hypotension. In the skin, histamine contributes to the weal and flare response; an axon reflex via H_1 receptors is responsible for the spread of vasodilation or flare from the oedematous weal.
- Increased capillary permeability can produce oedema. This can lead to urticaria, angioedema and laryngeal oedema. The consequent loss of circulating blood volume contributes to hypotension.
- Smooth muscle contraction can occur, especially in bronchioles and the intestine.
- Skin itching (in combination with kinins and prostaglandins).
- Pain from stimulation of nociceptors.

Histamine H_1 receptor antagonists (antihistamines)

Examples:
First-generation antihistamines: chlorphenamine, promethazine
Second-generation, non-sedating antihistamines: cetirizine, fexofenadine, mizolastine

Mechanisms of action and effects

The antihistamines are selective for histamine H_1 receptors (antagonists at other histamine receptors are traditionally not refered to as antihistamines). They are competitive inverse agonists (see Ch. 1) that reduce the basal level of spontaneous activity at histamine H_1 receptors as well as blocking the effects of histamine. Useful actions of antihistamines include:

- suppression of many of the vascular effects of histamine
- inhibition of inflammatory cell accumulation in tissues by second-generation antihistamines; this may result from downregulation of the activation of NF-κB in tissues at the site of an allergic response.

First-generation antihistamines have other actions that can be used therapeutically. They are lipophilic and cross the blood–brain barrier, producing sedation. They also have central antimuscarinic effects which may be clinically useful to suppress nausea in motion sickness (e.g. cyclizine, promethazine; Ch. 32).

Second-generation (non-sedating) antihistamines such as fexofenadine, loratadine, mizolastine and cetirizine are more hydrophilic or more ionised at physiological pH, do not penetrate the blood–brain barrier well, and have little sedative effect. They also have little antimuscarinic action.

Third-generation antihistamines are metabolites of second-generation drugs, such as desloratidine. They have similar efficacy to second-generation drugs but may have a different profile of unwanted effects.

Pharmacokinetics

Chlorphenamine is slowly absorbed from the gut, while promethazine is more rapidly absorbed. Both undergo considerable first-pass metabolism in the liver to inactive compounds and have short half-lives. An intravenous preparation of chlorphenamine is available for medical emergencies.

Most second-generation antihistamines are rapidly absorbed from the gut and metabolised in the liver to active compounds with long half-lives. Cetirizine undergoes little metabolism, and it is mainly eliminated unchanged by the kidney. It has an intermediate half-life.

Several topical formulations of antihistamines exist, including a nasal spray for allergic rhinitis, skin preparations for insect stings (but see unwanted effects) and eyedrops for allergic conjunctivitis.

Unwanted effects

- drowsiness or psychomotor impairment, especially with first-generation compounds, although paradoxical stimulation can occur in children and the elderly
- headache
- dry mouth, blurred vision, urinary retention and gastrointestinal upset from the antimuscarinic effects of first-generation compounds
- topical antihistamines for use on the skin should be avoided because hypersensitivity reactions are common.

Management of allergic disorders

Most allergic reactions involve a complex series of chemical processes. However, the mainstay of treatment for many conditions is based on the use of antihistamines. Their efficacy indicates the importance of histamine as a mediator of allergic responses. The contribution of the wider anti-inflammatory actions of these drugs that are most obvious at high blood concentrations is unclear.

Anaphylaxis

This is a medical emergency and requires rapidly acting treatments. The person should be laid flat with the feet raised if there is hypotension. Adrenaline (epinephrine) should be given intramuscularly and doses repeated every 10 min until the patient is stable. People known to have allergies that cause anaphylaxis can carry a preloaded adrenaline (epinephrine) syringe for emergencies, accompanied by detailed instructions on its appropriate use. Intravenous adrenaline (epinephrine) should only be given if there is profound shock, and then in a very dilute solution with close cardiac monitoring. Intra-venous use carries a risk of arrhythmias and intense vasoconstriction with myocardial ischaemic damage.

Once adrenaline (epinephrine) has been given, late relapse can be prevented by intramuscular injection or slow intravenous infusion of chlorphenamine and hydrocortisone (Ch. 44). Oxygen should be given in high concentration, and an inhaled β-adrenoceptor agonist such as salbutamol (Ch. 12) if there is marked bronchospasm. This can be particularly useful if a β-adrenoceptor antagonist has previously been taken, when adrenaline (epinephrine) may be less effective on the airways. If there is persistent hypotension, then intravenous fluid (a colloid such as gelatin or dextran if possible, or as saline if a colloid is unavailable) should be given rapidly.

Seasonal and perennial rhinitis

The symptoms of rhinitis include nasal obstruction, sneezing, itching and inflammation of the lining of the nose. These result from increased glandular secretion with nasal obstruction, mucous rhinorrhea and afferent nerve stimulation, which causes itching and sneezing. Allergies can cause both perennial (usually house-dust mite) and seasonal (pollens and moulds) rhinitis. The allergic response makes individuals more susceptible to the effects of non-specific irritants such as tobacco smoke or changes in temperature. Rhinitis also has several non-allergic causes, including acute infection and chronic sinus infection. Aspirin can produce rhinitis (as well as asthma [Ch. 12]) in sensitive subjects, probably by enhancing leukotriene generation. Prolonged use of nasal decongestants such as the α_1-adrenoceptor agonist oxymetazoline (see below) can also cause rhinitis. Less frequent causes include β-adrenoceptor antagonists (Ch. 5) and angiotensin-converting enzyme (ACE) inhibitors (Ch. 6).

Oral antihistamines are useful for reducing itching, sneezing and rhinorrhea, but they are less effective for nasal obstruction. They can also be useful if there is associated allergic conjunctivitis. Topical antihistamines (such as azelastine or levocabastine) are also available for use in the nose. For more severe allergic rhinitis, a topical intranasal corticosteroid (Ch. 44) is the treatment of choice, providing relief from most symptoms. Topical sodium cromoglicate or nedocromil (Ch. 12) can be useful in atopic subjects, but they are less effective than antihistamines or topical corticosteroids and are no longer preferred treatments. The antimuscarinic drug ipratropium bromide (Ch. 12) can also be used topically for relief of rhinorrhea. Nasal decongestants have a role early in treatment. These are solutions for topical application that contain α-adrenoceptor agonists such as ephedrine or xylometazoline. They work by producing local vasoconstriction, but prolonged use impairs ciliary activity in the nasal mucosa. They should not be given long-term because of the risk of rebound nasal congestion. Oral corticosteroids are reserved for the most severe symptoms. If drugs fail, then the possibility of structural abnormalities such as nasal polyps, hypertrophied inferior turbinates or a deviated nasal septum should be considered. In these situations, surgery may be helpful.

Urticaria

Acute urticarial reactions often occur to the same allergens that cause anaphylaxis. Antihistamines are the treatment of choice, with an oral corticosteroid (Ch. 44) for more severe episodes.

Chronic urticaria can be provoked by physical factors such as cold, sun, scratching the skin or exercise, or it can be caused by urticarial vasculitis in association with connective tissue diseases such as systemic lupus erythematosus. In some cases, the cause may be auto-immune, caused by IgG autoantibodies to the IgE receptors on mast cells and basophils. Antihistamines can be useful to suppress the itch from urticaria, but often they have little effect on the weal. About 15% of the histamine receptors in the skin are H_2, and a histamine H_2 receptor blocker (Ch. 33) may be useful in addition to an antihistamine. Leukotriene antagonists such as montelukast (Ch. 12) may be helpful in some individuals. Corticosteroids (Ch. 44) can be used in high dosage for severe symptoms, but long-term use should be avoided because of the unwanted effects. Immuno-suppression with ciclosporin (Ch. 38) has been used successfully for some severe autoimmune urticarias.

Allergic conjunctivitis

Topical treatment with antihistamines or mast-cell stabilisers is usually successful (see Ch. 50).

Contact and atopic eczema

Contact and atopic eczemas are considered in Chapter 49.

Asthma

Although asthma often has an allergic component, anti-histamines have little or no role. The management of asthma is considered in Chapter 12.

FURTHER READING

Charlesworth EN, Beltrani VS (2002) Pruritic dermatoses: overview of etiology and therapy. *Am J Med* 113(suppl 9A), 25S–33S

Ellis AK, Day JH (2003) Diagnosis and management of anaphylaxis. *CMAJ* 169, 307–311

Holgate ST, Canonica GW, Simons FE et al (2003) Consensus group on new-generation antihistamines (CONGA): present status and recommendations. *Clin Exp Allergy* 33, 1305–1324

Kaplan AP (2002) Chronic urticaria and angioedema. *N Engl J Med* 346, 175–179

Kay AB (2001) Advances in immunology: allergy and allergic diseases (second of two parts). *N Engl J Med* 344, 109–113

Leurs R, Church MK, Taglialatela M (2002) H_1-antihistamines: inverse agonism, anti-inflammatory actions and cardiac effects. *Clin Exp Allergy* 32, 489–498

Rosenwasser LJ (2002) Treatment of allergic rhinitis. *Am J Med* 113(suppl 9A), 17S–24S

Simons FER (2002) Comparative pharmacology of H_1 antihistamines: clinical relevance. *Am J Med* 113(suppl 9A), 38S–46S

Walsh GM, Annunziato L, Frossard N et al (2001) New insights into the second-generation antihistamines. *Drugs* 61, 207–236

Self-assessment

In questions 1 and 2, the first statement, in italics, is true. Are the accompanying statements also true?

1. *Antihistamines such as fexofenadine and loratadine are non-sedating.*

   a. Fexofenadine is associated with electrocardiographic (ECG) changes.
   b. Antihistamines reduce acid secretion from the gastric parietal cell.
   c. Fexofenadine reduces the release of histamine from mast cells.

2. *The allergic response in mast cells from atopic individuals can cause the release of leukotrienes, histamine and prostaglandins from sensitised mast cells.*

   a. Corticosteroids are ineffective for treating allergic rhinitis.
   b. Histamine is the only mediator that causes symptoms in rhinitis.

3. In an atopic individual, which one of the following would contribute to an allergic response to an allergen.

   A. Increased production of cytokines from Th1-cell response.
   B. Increased production of IgM.
   C. Stabilisation of mast cells.
   D. Histamine release acting on both H_1- and H_2-type receptors.
   E. Reduction in leukotriene production from mast cells.

4. Regarding the properties of antihistamines, choose the one correct answer from the following.

   A. First- and second-generation antihistamines are equally sedating.
   B. Second-generation antihistamines have less antimuscarinic activity than first-generation antihistamines.
   C. First-generation antihistamines are preferred treatment for cytotoxic drug-related vomiting.
   D. Second-generation antihistamines readily cross the blood–brain barrier.
   E. Antihistamines cause vasodilation.

5. Case history questions

A 10-year-old boy visited his doctor with his mother in the spring. He gave a history of repeated episodes of recurrent otitis media, rhinorrhoea, nasal congestion, sneezing and itching eyes occurring over a 3-year period, but predominantly in the spring and autumn. He had had three episodes of otitis media over the previous 2 years, the last being 6 months before, which were treated with antibiotics because of prolonged fluid in the middle ear. The boy had suffered from atopic dermatitis as an infant. He had no history of asthma; his mother had allergic rhinitis; they had two cats. Other than antibacterial drug treatment for his otitis media, he had taken no medication. Examination of the ears revealed healthy tympanic membranes with no current otitis media. He had no hearing loss. His current symptoms of rhinorrhoea, nasal congestion, sneezing and itching eyes were interfering with his schoolwork. He was otherwise fit.

   a. What was the likely diagnosis?
   b. Were the boy's symptoms related to the recurrence of otitis media?

Skin-test reaction showed him to be responsive to cat dander and house-dust mite.

   c. What treatment would you give?

The answers are provided on page 735.

Antihistamines[a]

Drug	Half-life (h)	Elimination	Comments
Non-sedating antihistamines			All drugs are given orally and used for symptomatic relief of allergic conditions such as hayfever and urticaria
Acrivastine	2	Renal + metabolism	Renal excretion of unchanged drug accounts for 60% of an oral dose, indicating high bioavailability; about 15% is converted to an active metabolite which has a half-life of 4 h
Cetirizine	9	Renal	Complete bioavailability; clearance is by both glomerular filtration and active renal tubular secretion; very slight metabolism
Desloratadine	20–30	Metabolism	The active metabolite of loratadine; undergoes oxidation in the liver and the product is conjugated with glucuronic acid and excreted in urine; slow metabolisers have been identified who show longer half-life and elimination via the urine rather than metabolism
Fexofenadine	14	Renal	The active metabolite of terfenadine; oral bioavailability has not been defined; about 1% only is metabolised (by CYP3A4)
Levocetirizine	–	–	The levo-isomer of cetirizine; properties similar to cetirizine (see above)
Loratadine	10	Metabolism	Oral bioavailability (about 10%) increased by food; it is a prodrug which undergoes extensive first-pass metabolism by CYP3A4 and CYP2D6 to an active metabolite which has a half-life of 28 h
Mizolastine	15	Metabolism	Oral bioavailability is about 70%; active metabolites have not been detected
Terfenadine	See fexofenadine	Metabolism	Essentially complete first-pass metabolism to the active metabolite, fexofenadine; negligible blood concentrations of parent drug after oral dosage; inhibition of first-pass metabolism by CYP3A4 linked to adverse cardiac effects (torsade de pointes)
Sedating antihistamines			All drugs given orally unless indicated
Alimemazine	4–7	Renal + metabolism	Used for urticaria and pruritis and as a premedication; minor metabolic pathways include S-oxidation and N-dealkylation (which produces an active metabolite)
Brompheniramine	25	Metabolism + renal	Used for symptomatic relief of hayfever and urticaria; main route of elimination is as inactive metabolites; bioavailability is probably about 50%, but it is reduced by food

continued

Antihistamines[a] *(continued)*

Drug	Half-life (h)	Elimination	Comments
Chlorphenamine	22	Renal + metabolism	Used orally for symptomatic relief of hayfever and urticaria and by slow intravenous injection as an adjunct to epinephrine (adrenaline) for the emergency treatment of anaphylaxis and angioedema; renal excretion is more important than metabolism; bioavailability is high (>80%)
Clemastine	21	Metabolism	Used for symptomatic relief of hayfever and urticaria; metabolised by oxidation; oral bioavailability is 40% (earlier data indicated a half-life of 4–6 h)
Cyproheptadine	1–4	Metabolism	Used for symptomatic relief of hayfever and urticaria and in the treatment of migraine; eliminated by oxidative metabolism; few kinetic data are available; duration of action is about 12 h
Diphenhydramine	3–9	Metabolism	Used in a variety of cough and decongestant preparations and for relief of temporary sleep disturbances; oral bioavailability is 40–60%; oxidised to a polar carboxylic acid (possibly by CYP2D6)
Diphenylpyraline	32	Metabolism	Used in a variety of cough and decongestant preparations; few kinetic data available
Doxylamine	10	Metabolism	Used in a variety of cough and decongestant preparations and in compound analgesics; metabolic fate has not been defined in humans
Hydroxyzine	20–30	Metabolism	Used for pruritis and for the short-term treatment of anxiety; metabolised to an active metabolite, cetirizine, which has a half-life determined by the half-life of hydroxyzine
Promethazine	7–14	Metabolism	Used orally for symptomatic relief of hayfever and urticaria and by slow intravenous injection as an adjunct to epinephrine (adrenaline) for the emergency treatment of anaphylaxis and angioedema; also used for motion sickness and as a premedication; can also be given by deep intramuscular injection; low oral bioavailability (25%); bile is the major route of elimination of the (inactive) metabolites
Triprolidine	3	Metabolism	Used in a variety of cough and decongestant preparations; well absorbed but oral bioavailability has not been defined; undergoes extensive oxidative metabolism in animals; fate in humans has not been defined (but only 1% is excreted unchanged in urine)

[a]Antihistamines may also be given topically in the eye, nose and on the skin. Drugs with antihistamine actions which are not used to treat allergic conditions, such as cinnarizine, cyclizine and meclozine (see Ch. 32), are used for the treatment of vestibular disorders and nausea and vomiting, especially motion sickness.

The endocrine system and metabolism

Diabetes mellitus

Control of blood glucose

Glucose occupies a central position in metabolism as the predominant substrate for energy production. Cells receive their supply of glucose from blood, and control mechanisms ensure that blood glucose concentrations remain within narrow limits. Glucose enters the blood by absorption from the gut and from breakdown of stored glycogen in the liver. At physiological concentrations, it leaves the blood almost entirely by active transport into the cells; in most tissues, this transfer is dependent on the action of the polypeptide hormone insulin.

Insulin is a protein which is rapidly secreted from the beta cells of the islets of Langerhans in the pancreas in response to a small rise in blood glucose; its secretion is inhibited by a fall in blood glucose. Insulin consists of two peptide chains, A and B, connected by two disulphide bridges.

Insulin is secreted under fasting conditions, with pulses every 10–14 min, and a slower cycle of release every 105–120 min. In response to a rise in plasma glucose (both the actual concentration and the rate of change), there is a superimposed biphasic pattern of insulin release.

- **Phase one** of release occurs within seconds, peaks at 3–5 min, and lasts for about 10 min. This is achieved by the release of a small pool of insulin in secretory vesicles.

- **Phase two** is more gradual, rising to a lower peak, and is partly due to release of a stored insulin pool, and partly to synthesis of new insulin.

Glucose stimulates insulin production by elevation of intracellular adenosine triphosphate (ATP) concentrations in the pancreatic beta cell. This leads to closure of inward rectifier K^+_{ATP} channels in the cell membrane, and reduced membrane K^+ permeability. The islet cell therefore depolarises and voltage-dependent Ca^{2+} channels in the cell membrane open. Calcium ion influx into the cell triggers exocytosis of insulin granules. In addition to glucose, many other factors influence insulin secretion (Fig. 40.1).

All peripheral tissues express specific cell surface receptors for insulin which are linked to the enzyme tyrosine kinase (Ch. 1). On activation of these receptors, the glucose transporter (Glut 4) is translocated to the cell surface, allowing glucose uptake. Metabolic effects of insulin include:

- inhibition of the conversion of amino acids to glucose (gluconeogenesis) in the liver, enhanced glucose storage as glycogen, and inhibition of the breakdown of glycogen (glycogenolysis); the overall effect is to increase glycogen stores

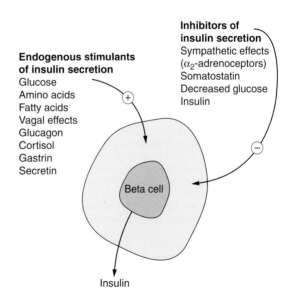

Fig. 40.1
Some physiological factors controlling insulin secretion.

- promotion of active transport of glucose into the cell, particularly in skeletal muscle, accompanied by potassium
- reduced plasma free fatty acids and increased adipocyte triglyceride storage; insulin does this by inhibiting lipases and preventing triglyceride breakdown in fat; it also increases hydrolysis of circulating triglycerides from lipoproteins by enhancing the activity of lipoprotein lipase; glucose entry into lipocytes provides glycerol phosphate for esterification of fatty acids.
- effects on protein metabolism, with inhibition of the catabolism of amino acids in the liver and, to a lesser extent, increased amino acid transport into muscle and enhanced protein synthesis.

The effects of insulin on different tissues are summarised in Table 40.1.

Several hormones naturally inhibit the anabolic action of insulin, particularly on carbohydrate metabolism, although effects on protein metabolism vary. These include glucagon, growth hormone, cortisol and catecholamines. Most of these hormones are released in stressful situations that require the breakdown of glycogen reserves for energy.

Diabetes mellitus

Failure to secrete sufficient insulin to maintain a normal level of blood glucose results in diabetes mellitus. The condition is diagnosed when the fasting plasma glucose concentration exceeds $7\,\text{mmol l}^{-1}$. The long-term consequences include increased risk of the development of vascular and neuropathic disease (Table 40.2). Two patterns of diabetes mellitus are recognised: type 1 and type 2.

Type 1 (or insulin-dependent) diabetes mellitus; IDDM

Type 1 diabetes represents a severe deficiency of insulin production and usually presents in youth. There is destruction of pancreatic beta cells, sometimes as part of an autoimmune process, although the cause in many cases is unknown. People with type 1 diabetes present with a history of feeling tired and unwell, together with weight loss; they develop polyuria and polydipsia, and are prone to ketoacidosis because of breakdown of fatty acids and amino acids in the liver.

Table 40.1
Metabolic effects of insulin

Liver	Increased glucose storage as glycogen
	Decreased protein catabolism
	Increased protein synthesis
	Decreased gluconeogenesis
Muscle	Increased protein synthesis
	Increased glycogen synthesis
	Increased glucose uptake
	Increased amino acid uptake
Adipose tissue	Increased triglyceride storage
	Increased triglyceride synthesis
	Decreased lipolysis

Table 40.2
Complications of diabetes

Complication	Consequences
Microvascular	
Nephropathy	Microalbuminuria, macroalbuminuria, renal failure
Retinopathy	Background retinopathy, proliferative retinopathy with blindness
Peripheral neuropathy	Loss of peripheral sensation
	Pain, ulceration
Autonomic neuropathy	Impotence
	Gastrointestinal disturbance
	Orthostatic hypotension
Macrovascular	
Cardiovascular disease	Hypertension
	Ischaemic heart disease
Cerebrovascular disease	Stroke

Type 2 (or non-insulin-dependent) diabetes mellitus; NIDDM

Type 2 diabetes, which usually presents later in life, is the consequence of a relative deficiency of insulin. It accounts for 90% of cases of diabetes in the Western world. In established type 2 diabetes, phase one of insulin secretion is absent or attenuated, and phase two is slowed. This beta-cell dysfunction precedes overt diabetes by up to 10 years. Overall, maximum insulin release is reduced by up to 50%, particularly in non-obese people with type 2 diabetes, in whom reduced insulin secretion is more important than tissue insulin resistance. Type 2 diabetics are often overweight (the average body mass index at diagnosis is 30 kg m^{-2}), and this increases cellular resistance to insulin in the liver and peripheral tissues. Insulin resistance characteristically precedes overt diabetes by several years, but for some time insulin secretion is sufficient to overcome it. Beta-cell dysfunction with loss of the early-phase insulin response to a glucose load results in loss of compensation for insulin resistance. There is both reduced tissue uptake of glucose and an inability to adequately suppress hepatic glucose output. In type 2 diabetes, postprandial hyperglycaemia is the major defect in blood glucose control.

Type 2 diabetics do not usually become ketotic. Sufficient glucose enters cells to permit adequate energy production for most situations. The main problem is excess glucose outside the cells rather than a shortage inside. The ideal approach to treatment would be an intervention that restores the early phase of insulin secretion in response to a glucose load.

Insulins and insulin analogues

Normal insulin secretion from the pancreas is into the portal circulation and is strictly related to metabolic needs. Sixty per cent of insulin released from the pancreas is extracted by the liver before reaching the systemic circulation. In contrast, therapeutic delivery of insulin is to the systemic circulation, and the relationship to metabolic needs can only be approximated by the dosages used and their timing in relation to meals.

Natural insulin formulations

Insulins for therapeutic administration were formerly extracted from either cattle or pig pancreas. Bovine insulin differs chemically from human insulin in three amino acid residues, and porcine in one, but their action is very similar to human insulin. Human-sequence insulin is pro-duced either by enzymatic modification of porcine insulin, or by recombinant DNA technology using bacteria or yeast. Human-sequence insulin preparations have largely superseded those of animal origin. All current insulin preparations have a low content of impurities that caused problems in the past, and have low immunogenic potential.

Pharmacokinetics

Currently available insulins must be given parenterally, as insulin is a protein and would otherwise be digested in the gut. Inhaled, nasal and orally acting insulins are in development, but, at present, subcutaneous injection is used for routine treatment, and intravenous infusion for emergency situations. The half-life of insulin in plasma is very short (about 8–16 min), and to avoid the need for frequent injections during maintenance treatment, the absorption of insulin from injection sites must be prolonged. Insulin is formulated either in a soluble preparation or is complexed with a substance to delay absorption from the injection site (Table 40.3). After subcutaneous injection, the maximum plasma concentration of soluble insulin (also called neutral insulin) is achieved about 2 h later, compared with minutes after intravenous injection. To limit the increase in plasma glucose concentration generated by a meal, subcutaneous insulin must be given at least 30 min before eating. The action of intravenous soluble insulin lasts less than an hour and is mainly terminated by degradation in the kidney. Continued absorption from a subcutaneous injection site prolongs the duration of action after injection to about 5 h.

Recommended subcutaneous injection sites include upper arms, thigh, buttocks or abdomen. Absorption is faster from the abdomen than from the limbs, although strenuous exercise can increase absorption from the limbs.

To generate intermediate- or long-acting insulin, it is complexed with:

- **Protamine**: to create the intermediate-acting isophane insulin. This can be given as a ready-mixed preparation with soluble insulin (biphasic isophane insulin). The ratio of soluble to isophane insulin in biphasic insulin varies from 10:90, through 20:80; 30:70, 40:60 to 50:50.
- **Zinc**: to create the intermediate-acting insulin zinc suspension or the long-acting crystalline insulin zinc suspension. Insulin molecules form dimers in solution. In the presence of zinc, these complex into hexamers. The size of these molecular aggregates determines the rate of diffusion from the site of injection. Such complexes act as modified-release formulations for subcutaneous administration (Table 40.3).
- **Protamine and zinc**: to create the long-acting protamine zinc insulin. This is now rarely used since

Table 40.3
Comparisons among insulins following subcutaneous administration

Type	Onset of action	Peak activity (h)	Duration (h)	
Insulin formulations				
Neutral (regular or soluble)	0.5 h	1–3	7	Short-acting
Isophane[a]	1 h	2–6	20	Intermediate/long-acting
Zinc	2 h	6–14	22	Long-acting
Protamine–zinc	4 h	12–24	30	Long-acting
Insulin analogues				
Insulin lispro	10–20 min	0.5–0.75	2–5	Short-acting
Insulin aspart	10–20 min	0.6–0.7	2–4	Short-acting
Insulin glargine	Plateau (4–24 h)		15–30	Long-acting
Insulin detemir	Plateau (7–24 h)		>20	Long-acting

[a]Sometimes called NPH insulin (neutral protamine Hagedorn).

it binds with soluble insulin if given in the same syringe.

Unwanted effects

- The main problem is an excessive action producing hypoglycaemia. Neuroglycopenia with confusion and coma can occur. Treatment is by intravenous injection of 20% or 50% glucose if the person is unconscious, or sugary foods or drinks, oral glucose or glucose gel (Hypostop®; 10–20 g) if conscious. Glucagon (see below) can be given intramuscularly if the person is unconscious and venous access is not available, followed by a sugary drink on waking. All people with diabetes who take insulin should carry a card with details of their treatment. Although most diabetics get warning symptoms of hypoglycaemia, some do not and are prone to sudden and severe hypoglycaemic coma. More frequent hypoglycaemic attacks reduce the awareness of their onset.
- Rebound hyperglycaemia can occur after an episode of hypoglycaemia, especially at night (Somogyi effect). This results from the compensatory release of hormones such as adrenaline, cortisol, glucagon and growth hormone. It can produce ketonuria, leading to a mistaken belief that too little insulin has been given.
- Animal insulins produce circulating antibodies, although this is less common with current highly purified preparations. These could diminish the activity of the insulin (insulin resistance) or produce local reactions (lipoatrophy) at injection sites.
- Insulins can cause local fat hypertrophy at the injection site; rotating the site of injection reduces this.

Insulin analogues

Examples: insulin aspart, insulin glargine, insulin lispro, insulin detemir

Mechanism of action and effects

The insulin analogues are recombinant chemical modifications of naturally occurring insulin.

- Insulin lispro has two changes in the amino acids at the C-terminal end of the polypeptide B chain (lysine and proline substituted at positions 28 and 29), which sterically hinders its ability to form dimers. Thus, insulin lispro is rapidly absorbed from an injection site.
- Insulin aspart has one amino acid substitution of aspartic acid for proline at position 28 of the B chain. The effect is similar to that of insulin lispro.
- Insulin glargine also has two amino acid changes (involving glycine and arginine, hence the name). This makes the molecule more soluble at acid pH, and less soluble at physiological pH. Insulin glargine precipitates after subcutaneous injection, slowly redissolves and is then absorbed.

These changes have no effect on the binding of the molecule to cellular insulin receptors.

Pharmacokinetics

Compared with standard soluble insulin, absorption of insulin aspart and lispro from a subcutaneous injection site occurs faster and leads to an earlier and high peak plasma concentration (Table 40.3). The duration of action is also shorter, at almost 3 h. Insulin aspart and lispro are usually given just before a meal, but can be used immediately after eating. They can be mixed with long-acting standard insulins, and are also available as biphasic formulations (insulin aspart with insulin aspart protamine in a 30:70 ratio; insulin lispro with insulin lispro protamine in a 25:75 ratio). Insulin aspart can be given by subcutaneous injection or infusion, and insulin lispro by subcutaneous injection or infusion, intravenous injection or intravenous infusion.

Insulin glargine is slowly and uniformly absorbed after subcutaneous injection, and avoids plasma insulin peaks. The plateau of action is 4–24 h. Insulin detemir, a long-acting synthetic insulin, binds to albumen. It is slowly released from albumen giving a plateau from 7–24 h, and less likelihood of hypoglycaemia.

Unwanted effects

- These are similar to those of other insulins. There is no reported excess of immunogenic reactions compared with standard insulin.
- There is a slightly reduced frequency of hypoglycaemia with insulin aspart or lispro compared with soluble insulin, because of the shorter duration of action.

Therapeutic regimens for insulin

The choice of regimen for insulin administration depends on the age, lifestyle, circumstances and preference of the patient. The general principle is to maintain a background (basal) level of insulin with boluses prior to meals to deal with the glucose load (basal-bolus regimens). Options include the following:

- **Single daily injections before breakfast or at bedtime**: used mainly for elderly people with type 2 diabetes who require insulin and in whom long-term complications of diabetes are less relevant. An intermediate- or long-acting insulin is used which can be combined with a short-acting one to optimise control.
- **Twice-daily injections before breakfast and evening meal**: suitable for people who have a reasonably stable pattern of activity and eating habits. Short- and intermediate-acting insulins are combined, either in fixed ratios provided by the manufacturers, or in varying ratios according to individual requirements. Fixed ratios vary from 10% short-acting with 90% intermediate-acting to a 50% mixture of each component.
- **Multiple injections before breakfast and evening meal and at bedtime** is increasingly used in younger,

active people who require more flexibility in their lifestyle. A number of tailored regimens can be employed using short- and intermediate-acting insulins. One regimen is that a short-acting insulin is given before breakfast, midday and evening meal, with an intermediate-acting insulin at bedtime to ensure a 'background' level during the night. A second regimen is that short-acting insulin is given before meals and the amount adjusted for the size of the meal. To ensure a 'background' effect of insulin throughout the 24 h, intermediate-acting insulin may be added at breakfast and at bedtime, depending upon individual insulin demands.
- **Continuous subcutaneous infusion** of a short-acting insulin via a portable infusion pump is sometimes used if there is a problem with recurrent or unpredictable hypoglycaemia despite optimisation of a multiple-injection insulin regimen
- **Intravenous infusion**: used for treatment of ketoacidotic crises, in labour, during and after surgery, or at other times when the person's usual routine cannot be adhered to. Short-acting insulin is infused in 5% dextrose solution with added potassium chloride (unless there is hyperkalaemia).
- **Intraperitoneal**: diabetics being treated for chronic renal failure by continuous ambulatory peritoneal dialysis can add their insulin to the dialysis fluid. Some implantable insulin pumps also use this route. This is the only therapeutic regimen in which insulin has direct access to the portal circulation.

Oral hypoglycaemic drugs

The main sites of action of oral hypoglycaemic drugs are shown in Figure 40.2.

Sulphonylureas

Examples: chlorpropamide, glibenclamide, gliclazide, glimepride, glipizide, tolbutamide

Mechanism of action

Sulphonylureas act mainly by increasing the release of insulin from the pancreatic beta cells in response to stimulation by glucose (Fig. 40.2). This is achieved by binding to and inhibiting the K^+_{ATP} channel in the cell membrane (see 'Control of blood glucose' above). The receptor for sulphonylureas is a regulator of the potassium-channel proteins. Glimepride and gliclazide bind less avidly than other sulphonylureas to cardiac K^+_{ATP} channels (that are very similar to those in the pancreas – see unwanted effects below).

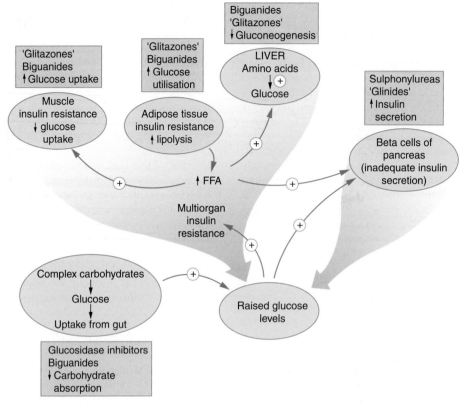

Fig. 40.2

Metabolic dysfunctions in type 2 diabetes and sites of drug action. The metabolic dysfunctions seen in type 2 diabetes are illustrated in green areas; these result from inadequate insulin secretion and tissue resistance to the effects of insulin. Drugs that are used to overcome the insulin resistance, 'insulin sensitisers', and increase insulin secretion, 'secretagogues', are shown in the light brown boxes.

Pharmacokinetics

Sulphonylureas are structurally related to sulphonamides. They are absorbed rapidly (although the rate of absorption is reduced when taken with food), are highly protein bound, and are metabolised by the liver. Compounds with a short duration of action are usually preferred when starting treatment with a sulphonylurea, to minimise the risk of hypoglycaemia. Tolbutamide, glipizide, glimepride and gliclazide have intermediate half-lives and a suitably short duration of action.

Chlorpropamide depends partly on the kidney for its elimination, and its very long half-life (about two days) may lead to accumulation. Glibenclamide has a longer duration of action than would be predicted from its short plasma half-life, through selective concentration in pancreatic islet cells. These long-acting drugs are not recommended for the elderly.

Unwanted effects

- Gastrointestinal disturbance, with nausea, vomiting, diarrhoea, constipation.
- Excessive (and particularly nocturnal) hypoglycaemia is most frequent with the longer-acting drugs or

with excessive dosage, especially in the elderly or if there is concurrent hepatic or renal impairment.

- Weight gain is almost inevitable unless dietary restrictions are observed.
- Hypersensitivity reactions (usually in the first 6–8 weeks of therapy) include skin rashes and, rarely, blood disorders.
- Chlorpropamide (and, less commonly, glipizide) increases renal sensitivity to antidiuretic hormone and can produce water retention with dilutional hyponatraemia.
- Chlorpropamide often produces flushing when alcohol is taken, through inhibition of aldehyde dehydrogenase (Ch. 54).
- Sulphonylureas (apart from glipizide) should be avoided in people with acute porphyria.
- Concerns were raised that sulphonylureas might increase cardiovascular mortality in type 2 diabetes, possibly as a result of inhibition of K^+_{ATP} channels in the heart. These have a cardioprotective role in ischaemic tissue, preventing cell depolarisation to conserve intracellular energy stores. Inhibition of the channels could lead to arrhythmias in diabetics with ischaemic heart disease (see Ch. 5). However, recent

clinical studies have failed to confirm the original concerns about cardiovascular mortality.

- There is some evidence that sulphonylureas may accelerate the rate of pancreatic beta-cell loss.

Meglitinides (also called 'glinides')

Examples: nateglinide, repaglinide

Mechanism of action

Nateglinide and repaglinide chemically resemble the sulphonylurea moiety of glibenclamide; this moiety is called meglitinide and the currently available glinides are derived from this; they bind to a different site on the beta cell from sulphonylureas. They stimulate insulin release by closing the K^+_{ATP} channel and restoring the early-phase postprandial insulin response to glucose. Nateglinide has an enhanced effect as the plasma glucose rises, unlike repaglinide, and therefore produces little stimulation of insulin secretion in the fasting state. However, the glycaemic control achieved with nateglinide is generally less than that with other oral hypoglycaemic drugs. The place of meglitinides in therapy, compared with sulphonylureas, is not yet established, although, in contrast to sulphonylureas, they hold out hope for preservation of beta-cell function.

Pharmacokinetics

Both nateglinide and repaglinide are rapidly and well absorbed from the gut, and are given immediately before a meal. They are metabolised in the liver to inactive metabolites and have short half-lives.

Unwanted effects

- gastrointestinal upset, including nausea, vomiting, abdominal pain, diarrhoea or constipation, with repaglinide
- hypoglycaemia, but much less than with sulphonylureas owing to the short duration of action; this also reduces the need to snack between meals, so that weight gain is not usual
- hypersensitivity reactions with rashes and urticaria.

Biguanides

Example: metformin

Mechanism of action and effects

Metformin does not affect insulin secretion. The major actions are as follows:

- Facilitation of glucose uptake in skeletal muscle and adipocytes. The full effect requires the presence of insulin. Metformin inhibits mitochondrial respiratory chain oxidation, which increases cell surface expression and activity of the membrane glucose transporters GLU1 and 4.
- Partial suppression of hepatic gluconeogenesis. Since some gluconeogenic activity remains, the risk of hypoglycaemia is minimal. Inhibition of mitochondrial respiratory chain oxidation underlies this effect as well.
- A reduction of glucose absorption from the small intestine, where high concentrations of metformin are found.
- An additional benefit is improvement in the adverse plasma lipid profile found in diabetes. Metformin reduces free fatty acid oxidation, which raises plasma high-density lipoprotein (HDL) cholesterol and reduces plasma triglycerides (Ch. 48). Enhanced free fatty oxidation in diabetes contributes to increased hepatic glucose production and the development of insulin resistance by inhibition of enzymes in the glycolytic pathway and attenuation of transmembrane glucose transport.

Metformin can suppress appetite and causes less weight gain than with sulphonylureas, which is useful in overweight diabetics. Metformin may have a cardioprotective effect in diabetes, with a 40% reduction in the risk of myocardial infarction and lower mortality when compared with treatment with a sulphonylurea. This is only partially explained by better glycaemic control, and various effects of metformin on atherogenic and thrombogenic factors have been proposed as explanations for this.

Pharmacokinetics

Metformin is slowly and incompletely absorbed from the gut and excreted unchanged by the kidney. It has a short half-life.

Unwanted effects

- Gastrointestinal upset, including anorexia, nausea, abdominal discomfort and diarrhoea (usually transient).
- Metallic taste.
- Decreased vitamin B_{12} absorption.
- Inhibition of pyruvate metabolism encourages lactate accumulation. In situations that lead to an increase in anaerobic metabolism (e.g. shock with hypoxaemia), lactic acidosis can result; metformin should be avoided in these situations. Lactic acidosis is more common in the presence of renal impairment, although the degree of renal impairment at which this becomes a significant risk is debated.

Thiazolidinediones (also called 'glitazones')

Examples: pioglitazone, rosiglitazone

Mechanisms of action and effects

Thiazolidinediones have no effect on insulin secretion and are referred to as 'insulin sensitisers'. They enhance glucose utilisation in peripheral tissues – especially adipocytes, but also skeletal muscle –and may also suppress gluconeogenesis in the liver by inhibition of the enzyme fructose-1,6-bisphosphatase. The effect is mediated through binding to peroxisome proliferator-activated receptor gamma (PPAR-γ) in the cell nucleus. PPAR-γ associates as a heterodimer with the retinoid X receptor (RXR) (Ch. 1) in the cell nucleus and binds to PPAR-γ response elements in the promoter domains of target genes. In the absence of a ligand, this heterodimer is further associated with a multiprotein co-repressor complex that contains histone deacetylase activity and inhibits gene transcription. When a PPAR ligand binds to the PPAR/RXR heterodimer, the co-repressor complex dissociates and a co-activator complex with histone acetylase activity is recruited. In the case of PPAR-γ, this results in the expression of genes that control adipocyte differentiation, and may increase the number of small adipocytes that are more insulin-sensitive. As a result, adipose tissue more readily takes up fatty acids from the blood.

As a secondary effect, reduced availability of fatty acids to muscle improves insulin sensitivity in muscle cells (see metformin above). Other effects on adipocyte cell signalling may also influence tissue insulin sensitivity. These include reduced synthesis of factors that interfere with the insulin signalling cascade, such as tumour necrosis factor alpha. Thiazolidinediones also increase the expression of cell glucose transporters GLU1 and 4, and may have direct effects on muscle insulin sensitivity.

In addition to reducing the plasma glucose concentration, thiazolidinediones also improve diabetic dyslipidaemia. Pioglitazone, in particular, decreases plasma triglyceride and increases plasma HDL cholesterol concentrations, due to increased lipolysis of triglycerides in very-low-density lipoprotein (VLDL). The plasma low-density lipoprotein (LDL) fraction may also become larger and less dense, which may further reduce atherogenesis (Ch. 48). Thiazolidinediones produce a small reduction in blood pressure, and reduce diabetic micro-albuminuria.

Pharmacokinetics

Pioglitazone and rosiglitazone are well absorbed from the gut and are metabolised in the liver. They have short half-lives. Since the mechanism of action involves gene transcription, the onset of the hypoglycaemic effect is gradual over 6–8 weeks.

Unwanted effects

- gastrointestinal disturbances
- headache
- anaemia
- fluid retention leading to oedema; this can cause decompensation in controlled heart failure
- weight gain because of fat-cell differentiation
- liver dysfunction has been reported rarely, and liver function tests should be monitored every 2 months during the first year of treatment, and periodically thereafter.

Glucosidase inhibitors

Example: acarbose

Mechanism of action and effects

Carbohydrate digestion in the intestine involves several enzymes that sequentially degrade complex poly-saccharides such as starch into monosaccharides like glucose. Initial digestion of carbohydrates in the gut lumen is carried out by amylases from the saliva and pancreas. The final digestion of oligosaccharides is carried out by β-galactosidases (including lactase) and various α-glucosidase enzymes (such as maltase, isomaltase, glucoamylase, and sucrase, which hydrolyses the disaccharide sucrose) in the small intestinal brush border. Acarbose competes with dietary oligosaccharides for α-glucosidase enzymes, and has a higher affinity for these enzymes. Binding to the enzymes is reversible, so that digestion and absorption of glucose after a meal is slower than usual but not prevented. As a result, the postprandial peak of blood glucose is reduced and blood glucose concentrations are more stable through the day. Acarbose has no effect on insulin secretion or its tissue action and is less effective for achieving glycaemic control than are other oral hypoglycaemic agents. Its use is limited by the high incidence of unwanted effects.

Pharmacokinetics

Oral absorption of acarbose is very poor. Only about 2% of the active parent drug reaches the circulation. Inactive metabolites are formed in the gut lumen by enzymic degradation. About one-third of the oral dose is absorbed as inactive metabolite and most of this is excreted in the faeces.

Unwanted effects

- gastrointestinal effects include flatulence, abdominal distension and diarrhoea, owing to fermentation of unabsorbed carbohydrate in the bowel. These effects are dose-related and often transient.
- abnormal liver function tests and hepatitis are rare complications.

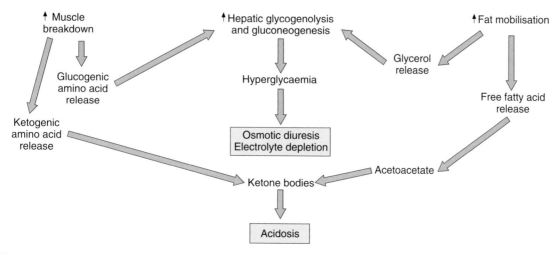

Fig. 40.3
Pathophysiology of diabetic ketoacidosis.

Drugs to increase plasma glucose levels

Glucagon

Mechanism of action and use
Glucagon is a polypeptide that is synthesised by the alpha cells of the pancreatic islets of Langerhans. It binds to specific hepatocyte receptors and activates membrane-bound adenylate cyclase. The consequent increase in intracellular cyclic adenosine monophosphate (cAMP) leads to inhibition of glycogen synthase. This blocks the effect of insulin on hepatocytes and mobilises stored liver glycogen. Glucagon is used to raise blood glucose in severe acute insulin-induced hypoglycaemia.

Pharmacokinetics
Glucagon must be given by intramuscular, subcutaneous or intravenous injection, and acts in 10–20 min. It is degraded rapidly by enzymes in the plasma, liver and kidney.

Unwanted effects
- nausea, vomiting and diarrhoea
- very occasionally, allergic reactions.

Management of type 1 diabetes

The aim of treatment is to maintain a plasma glucose concentration as close to normal as possible.

Maintenance treatment of type 1 diabetes should include an appropriate diet with a regulated carbohydrate intake distributed throughout the day. Excess dietary saturated fat should be avoided. The complications of type 1 diabetes can be reduced by close control of the blood sugar concentration using insulin in an appropriate regimen (see above).

The success of the chosen approach can be monitored by measurement of the blood sugar concentrations, often carried out on a finger-prick blood specimen using a blood glucose reagent strip. If peak or trough blood glucose estimations are outside an acceptable range, the insulin regimen should be adjusted, although this should not be done more than once or twice a week. Long-term control of diabetes is usually assessed by the plasma concentration of glycosylated haemoglobin (HbA_{1c}). A high concentration is a good marker for the risk of developing microvascular and neuropathic complications. An HbA_{1c} level greater than 7% carries a higher risk of complications (upper limit of normal, 6.0%). Hyperglycaemia leads to formation of glycosylation end products, which may be promotors of vascular and neurological damage. Several other mechanisms of vascular and neurological damage may also contribute to these complications.

The most dramatic complication of untreated or poorly controlled type 1 diabetes is diabetic ketoacidosis (Fig. 40.3), which can lead to coma if it is severe. In a treated type 1 diabetic, systemic infection, dietary indiscretion, or inappropriate dose reduction or omission can precipitate ketoacidosis. Apart from treatment of any precipitating cause, the management of ketoacidosis includes the following.

- Restoration of extracellular volume: hyperglycaemia leads to an osmotic diuresis with excessive urinary salt and water loss. Replacement by physiological (0.9%) saline is essential.
- Potassium replacement: the osmotic diuresis results in excessive urinary potassium loss. Potassium is also shifted from cells into extracellular fluid in exchange for hydrogen ions in the ketoacidotic state.

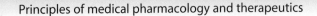

Correction of the extracellular acidosis reverses this shift and can produce profound hypokalaemia. Once a good urine flow has been established, intravenous potassium supplements are usually required.

- Intravenous insulin until the ketosis is abolished and the plasma glucose is below 15 mmol l^{-1}. The metabolic acidosis will usually correct with treatment of the hyperglycaemia and fluid replacement. Intravenous sodium bicarbonate is occasionally required if the arterial pH is less than 7.0, but should be used cautiously.

Management of type 1 diabetes in special situations

- Close attention to diabetic control is important before conception and during pregnancy since poor control will affect the fetus, leading to increased intrauterine and perinatal mortality.
- At times of intercurrent illness, the dose of insulin will need to be increased, guided by blood sugar monitoring, to counteract the hyperglycaemic action of hormones released during stress reactions.
- During and after surgery, soluble insulin should be given in 5% dextrose solution by intravenous infusion, dosage being guided by the blood glucose concentrations. Subcutaneous insulin can be restarted when the person is able to eat and drink.

Management of type 2 diabetes

The mainstays of treatment are lifestyle and dietary modifications. As for type 1 diabetes, close control of the blood sugar concentration in type 2 diabetes reduces the risk of microvascular complications, although the effect on macrovascular complications such as myocardial infarction is less convincing.

More than 75% of newly diagnosed type 2 diabetics are obese. Weight reduction not only improves blood glucose levels but also reduces other cardiovascular disease risk factors. Dietary advice should include:

- reducing energy intake if obese (an average weight loss of 18 kg is required to control blood sugar)
- eating small regular meals
- ensuring that more than half the total energy intake is from carbohydrates, total fat contributing less than 35% of total energy intake
- encouraging high-fibre foods and limiting sucrose and alcohol intake.

This should be combined with advice to exercise regularly and to stop smoking (because of the contribution to vascular disease) as appropriate. Underweight

people often require early treatment with an oral hypoglycaemic agent, usually a sulphonylurea. For obese people, lifestyle and dietary advice should initially be encouraged, with use of metformin if this fails. Combination therapy with a sulphonylurea and metformin can be useful if a single drug is insufficient to reduce the blood glucose concentration. According to expert advice from the National Institute for Clinical Excellence (NICE), the thiazolidinediones, such as pioglitazone, should only be considered if there is intolerance to combination therapy with metformin given together with a sulphonylurea (replacing the drug to which there is intolerance with a 'glitazone'). Use of the glitazones in triple therapy has not been evaluated. The metiglinides are used alone for non-obese diabetics or those in whom metformin is contraindicated, or it can be given in combination with metformin.

Within 3 years of onset, 50% of type 2 diabetics will need combination therapy to achieve glycaemic control. Failure of oral treatment usually implies 'beta-cell exhaustion', and up to 30% of people with type 2 diabetes require insulin with or without an oral hypoglycaemic drug. The most effective combination is a basal intermediate-acting insulin at bedtime combined with metformin during the day. A sulphonylurea can be used if metformin is contraindicated, but with a greater risk of hypoglycaemia and eventual loss of efficacy as beta-cell exhaustion develops. Combination therapy with insulin and a thiazolidinedione or a metiglinide is not well studied. There is some evidence that insulin therapy is more likely to be successful if used early in type 2 diabetes to preserve beta-cell function.

Acarbose is of limited value when used alone or in combination with metformin. It may be most effective in early diabetes, when there is still sufficient insulin secretion for it to influence glycaemic control.

Intensive management of risk factors for cardiovascular disease is of crucial importance because the major complications of type 2 diabetes are vascular. In particular, intensive control of raised blood pressure reduces both microvascular and macrovascular complications. There is little to choose between antihypertensive drugs except that thiazides and β-adrenoceptor antagonists may aggravate diabetes, whereas an angiotensin-converting enzyme (ACE) inhibitor or an angiotensin II receptor antagonist reduces the risk of overt renal failure when there is evidence of diabetic nephropathy (either overt or with microalbuminuria) (Ch. 6). Treatment of the abnormal atherogenic plasma lipid profile that is common in type 2 diabetes has been less fully studied than in people without diabetes, but if the calculated 10-year risk of cardiovascular disease is greater than 20%, treatment for a raised cholesterol should be started (Ch. 48). Once a diabetic person has developed coronary artery disease, intensive lipid lowering with a statin (Ch. 48) will reduce the risk of subsequent myocardial infarction or death.

FURTHER READING

Beckman JA, Creager MA, Libby P (2002) Diabetes and atherosclerosis. Epidemiology, pathophysiology, and management. *JAMA* 287, 2570–2581

De Witt DE, Dugdale DC (2003) Using new insulin strategies in the outpatient treatment of diabetes: clinical applications. *JAMA* 289, 2265–2269

De Witt DE, Hirsch IB (2003) Outpatient insulin therapy in type 1 and type 2 diabetes mellitus. *JAMA* 289, 2254–2264

Dornhurst A (2001) Insulinotropic meglitinide analogues. *Lancet* 358, 1709–1716

Gerich JE (2002) Novel insulins: expanding options in diabetes management. *Am J Med* 113, 308–316

Holmboe ES (2002) Oral antihyperglycaemic therapy for type 2 diabetes. Clinical applications. *JAMA* 287, 373–376

Inzucchi SE (2002) Oral antihyperglycaemic therapy for type 2 diabetes. Scientific review. *JAMA* 287, 360–372

Kirpichinikov D, McFarlane SI, Sowers JR (2002) Metformin: an update. *Ann Intern Med* 137, 25–33

Klein L, Gheorghiade M (2004) Management of the patient with diabetes mellitus and myocardial infarction: clinical trials update. *Am J Med* 116(suppl 5A), 47S–63S

Leahy JL (2003) What is the role for insulin therapy in type 2 diabetes? *Curr Opin Endocrinol Diabetes* 10, 99–103

Lenhard MJ, Reeves GD (2001) Continuous subcutaneous insulin infusion. *Arch Intern Med* 161, 2293–2300

Metchick LN, Petit WA Jr, Inzucchi SE (2002) Inpatient management of diabetes mellitus. *Am J Med* 113, 317–323

Mooradian AD (2003) Cardiovascular disease in type 2 diabetes. Current management guidelines. *Arch Intern Med* 163, 33–40

Mudaliar S, Henry RR (2002) PPAR agonists in health and disease: a pathophysiological and clinical overview. *Curr Opin Endocrinol Diabetes* 9, 285–302

Nathan DM (2002) Initial management of glycaemia in type 2 diabetes mellitus. *N Engl J Med* 347, 1342–1349

National Institute for Clinical Excellence (2003) Full guidance on the use of glitazones for the treatment of type 2 diabetes. **http://www.nice.org.uk/page.aspx?o=83265** (accessed August 2004)

Owens DR, Zinman B, Bolli GB (2001) Insulins today and beyond. *Lancet* 358, 739–746

Rosenstock J (2004) Basal insulin supplementation in type 2 diabetes: refining the tactics. *Am J Med* 116(suppl 3A), 10S–16S

Snow V, Weiss KB, Mottur-Pilson C et al (2003) Evidence for tight blood pressure control in type 2 diabetes mellitus. *Ann Intern Med* 138, 587–592

Vijan S, Hayward RA (2003) Treatment of hypertension in type 2 diabetes mellitus: blood pressure goals, choice of agents, and setting priorities in diabetes care. *Ann Intern Med* 138, 593–602

Wang C-HW, Weisel RD, Fedak PWM et al (2003) Glitazones and heart failure. *Circulation* 107, 1350–1353

Self-assessment

In questions 1–4, the first statement, in italics, is true. Are the accompanying statements also true?

1. *Oral hypoglycaemic drugs (sulphonylureas, biguanides, thiazolidinediones, acarbose) are only used in type 2 diabetes and act by different mechanisms to control glucose levels.*

   a. Glibenclamide is the drug of choice when there is no residual insulin secretion.
   b. Sulphonylureas should be administered in conjunction with a dietary regimen, particularly in obese people.
   c. Glibenclamide can cause hypoglycaemia, particularly in the elderly, and should be used very cautiously in this age group.

2. *Hyperglycaemia results from uncontrolled glucose output from the liver and reduced uptake of glucose into muscle and other tissues.* The oral hypoglycaemic drugs metformin and gliclazide can be taken together.

3. *Untreated diabetes during pregnancy results in increased intrauterine and perinatal mortality.*

   a. Oral hypoglyaemics given to a pregnant mother can cause hypoglycaemia in the fetus and are normally substituted with insulin in pregnancy.
   b. Sulphonylureas should not be given together with the antimicrobial trimethoprim.

4. *Different formulations of insulin are available that have varied peak effects and durations of action.* Insulin lispro has a longer duration of action than isophane insulin.

5. Ms JJ was a 55-year-old housewife with a body mass index of 35 kg m^{-2}. She was diagnosed with diabetes. Which one of the following statements is correct?

   A. The mainstay of treatment is diet and exercise.
   B. Diabetes presenting in this way is a medical emergency.
   C. A sulphonylurea would be the drug of first choice for Ms JJ.
   D. Rosigitazone would be the drug of first choice.
   E. Treatment with metformin can increase the risk of heart disease.

6. Case history questions

> A 35-year-old teacher, Mr JAH, was admitted to hospital as an emergency. He had developed a sore throat a week previously. His GP prescribed penicillin, but the soreness persisted and Mr JAH noticed profuse white spots on the back of his throat. He drank fluids copiously and passed more urine than usual. Two days before admission, he began to vomit. The day before admission, he became drowsy and confused. He had lost approximately 2 stones in weight, despite eating more than usual. His great uncle had diabetes mellitus. Mr JAH was clinically dehydrated and ketones could be smelt on his breath. Results of blood tests indicated that he had diabetic ketoacidosis.

a. Which type of diabetes did Mr JAH have?
b. What was the significance of his sore throat?
c. Was it significant that his great uncle suffered from diabetes mellitus?
d. Explain his polydipsia and polyuria.

e. What treatments should have been rapidly instituted?
f. After he had recovered from the acute illness, what general advice should have been given about diet?
g. Mr JAH was a 'three meals a day' man whose only exercise was walking a mile to work and back each day. Although insulin regimens vary widely, suggest a possible regimen and the types of insulin that could be given.
h. How long before meals should subcutaneous injection of soluble insulin have been given?
i. In addition to glucose levels, what other indicator could have been measured to signify good control in diabetes?
j. Mr JAH became more active, joined a health club and met a partner who liked to party. His eating became more irregular with hurried meals. His glycaemic control deteriorated. What alterations to his insulin regimen could have been helpful?

The answers are provided on pages 735–736.

Drugs used for diabetes mellitus

Drug	Half-life (h)	Elimination	Comments
Insulins			Normally given by subcutaneous injection; onset and duration of action depend on formulation used, many of which are combinations containing bovine, porcine or human insulin, e.g. insulin zinc suspension, isophane insulin, protamine zinc insulin, or recombinant human insulin analogues such as biphasic insulin aspart, biphasic insulin lispro and biphasic isophane insulin
Soluble insulin	See text	Metabolism	A sterile solution of bovine, porcine or human insulin; may also be given by intramuscular or intravenous injection or by i.v. infusion, depending on requirements
Insulin aspart	See text	Metabolism	A recombinant human insulin analogue; may also be given by i.v. injection or infusion, depending on requirements
Insulin lispro	See text	Metabolism	A recombinant human insulin analogue; may also be given by i.v. injection or infusion, depending on requirements
Insulin detemir	See text	Metabolism	Similar in action to insulin glargine
Insulin glargine	See text	Metabolism	A long-lasting recombinant human insulin analogue that has a longer duration of action than soluble insulin
Sulfonylureas			All are given orally for the treatment of type 2 diabetes mellitus
Chlorpropamide	25–60	Metabolism + renal	Complete oral bioavailability; eliminated by oxidative metabolism to inactive metabolites and by renal excretion (about 20%)
Glibenclamide	2–4	Metabolism	Complete oral bioavailability; metabolised in liver to active hydroxyl metabolites that have a longer duration of action than the parent drug (one study has reported a terminal half-life for the parent drug of 10 h)
Gliclazide	6–14	Metabolism (+ renal)	Variable absorption between patients, probably linked to differences in first-pass metabolism; eliminated largely by oxidative metabolism in the liver, with 10% excreted unchanged
Glimepiride	5–9	Metabolism	Complete bioavailability; oxidised by P450 to hydroxy and carboxy metabolites, the former of which retains activity; drug clearance increases at low creatinine clearance (probably because of decreased plasma protein binding)
Glipizide	2–4	Metabolism	Complete oral bioavailability; oxidised in the liver to inactive hydroxy metabolite
Gliquidone	17	Metabolism	Complete oral bioavailability; eliminated in bile as metabolites formed by oxidation and conjugation; parent compound responsible for most of activity
Tolbutamide	4–37	Metabolism	Complete oral bioavailability; about 1 in 500 people has severely impaired metabolism of tolbutamide; metabolised by the polymorphic CYP2C9

continued

Drug compendium

Drugs used for diabetes mellitus *(continued)*

Drug	Half-life (h)	Elimination	Comments
Meglitinides (also called 'glinides')			All drugs given orally
Nateglinide	1.5	Metabolism + some renal	Used for type 2 diabetes mellitus in combination with metformin, when metformin alone is inadequate; good oral bioavailability (70%); metabolised by CYP2C9 and CYP3A4, and metabolites eliminated as glucuronic acid conjugates
Repaglinide	1	Metabolism	Used for type 2 diabetes mellitus alone or in combination with metformin, when metformin alone is inadequate; good oral bioavailability (60%); eliminated by CYP3A4 oxidation to metabolites that are eliminated in the faeces
Biguanides			Given orally for the treatment of type 2 diabetes mellitus
Metformin	2–4	Renal	Oral bioavailability is 50–60% owing to incomplete absorption; eliminated largely unchanged by renal tubular secretion
Thiazolidinediones (also called 'glitazones')			All drugs given orally
Pioglitazone	3–7	Metabolism	Used for type 2 diabetes mellitus alone or in combination with metformin or a sulphonylurea only as a second-line drug when there is intolerance to one of these; metabolised by CYP2C8 and CYP3A4; metabolites contribute to in vivo activity due to their long half-lives (16–24 h)
Rosiglitazone	3–4	Metabolism	Used for type 2 diabetes mellitus alone or in combination with metformin or a sulphonylurea only as a second-line drug when there is intolerance to one of these; complete oral bioavailability; oxidised by CYP2C8 to hydroxy and demethylated metabolites
Other hypoglycaemics			All drugs given orally
Acarbose	3	Renal	Used for diabetes mellitus inadequately controlled by diet with or without other oral hypoglycaemic drugs; α-glycoside hydrolase inhibitor; negligible oral absorption (1–2%); main action is in the intestinal tract; the systemic disposition data given are largely irrelevant to therapeutic use
Guar gum	Not relevant	Not relevant	Inhibits glucose absorption
Treatment of hypoglycaemia			
Glucagon	5–10 min	Metabolism	Used for acute insulin-induced hypoglycaemia and *is not used* for chronic hypoglycaemia; given by subcutaneous, intramuscular or intravenous injection; rapidly and extensively degraded by liver and kidneys
Diazoxide	28	Renal (+ metabolism)	Used for chronic hypoglycaemia due to islet cell hyperplasia or tumour and *is not used* for acute hypoglycaemia; non-diuretic analogue of thiazides; given orally; good oral bioavailability; eliminated largely by glomerular filtration; long half-life is due to high protein binding (90%)

The thyroid and control of metabolic rate

Thyroid function

The term 'basal metabolism' refers to the energy-utilising chemical processes of the body at rest. Its rate is controlled by thyroid hormone, which stimulates tissue oxygen consumption and regulates energy and heat production, mainly by stimulating futile metabolic cycles. This creates a drain on energy reserves such as glycogen and fat. If thyroid function is normal, depletion of fat stores and breakdown of body protein is avoided by thyroid hormone-induced stimulation of thermogenic lipogenesis in brown fat in infants (although not in adults). Thyroid hormones also promote gluconeogenesis, obtaining the substrate for glycogen formation from tissues such as muscle and bone. Thyroid hormones, e.g. thyroxine, facilitate development of the nervous system, somatic growth and puberty. It also regulates the synthesis of proteins involved in hepatic, cardiac, neurological and muscular function. Thyroid hormones interact with the sympathetic nervous system, in particular enhancing the effects of β-adrenoceptor stimulation (Ch. 4).

There are two thyroid hormones, L-thyroxine (T_4) and tri-iodothyronine (T_3), of which T_3 is mainly responsible for effects at a cellular level, while T_4 is now considered to be a prohormone. T_3 and T_4 are synthesised in the thyroid gland (Fig. 41.1), where inorganic iodide is trapped with great avidity by an enzyme-dependent process. The iodide is then oxidised and incorporated into the tyrosyl residues of the glycoprotein thyroglobulin to form mono-iodotyrosine and di-iodotyrosine. Two di-iodinated tyrosine molecules or one di-iodinated molecule with one mono-iodinated tyrosine molecule are joined by a coupling reaction to form T_4 and T_3, respectively. The enzyme thyroxine peroxidase is important both in the initial oxidation and in the final combination steps of the synthetic process (Fig. 41.1). Proteolytic enzymes from thyroid lysosymes then degrade thyroglobulin and release thyroid hormone into the circulation.

Synthesis and release of thyroid hormones are controlled by the anterior pituitary hormone thyrotrophin (thyroid-stimulating hormone, TSH). This in turn is controlled by the hypothalamus, which secretes thyrotrophin-releasing hormone (TRH). Circulating T_3 and T_4 exert a negative feedback on both the hypothalamic and pituitary hormones (Fig. 41.2).

Circulating thyroid hormones are highly protein bound, mostly to thyroxine-binding globulin (TBG) (particularly T_4, of which less than 0.1% is free). Only the

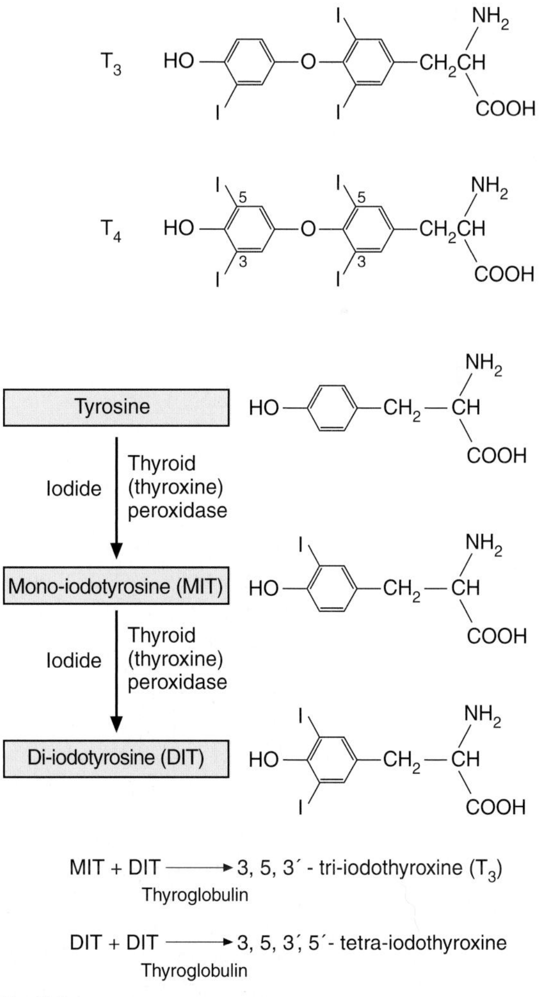

Fig. 41.1
The sequence of the synthesis of thyroid hormones. Peroxidation of iodide occurs after its incorporation into thyroglobulin, the colloidal substance that fills the lumen of the thyroid follicles.

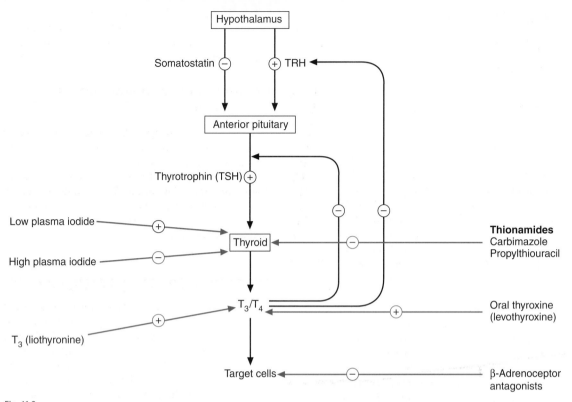

Fig. 41.2
Control of thyroid hormone synthesis and release, and sites of action of drugs acting on the thyroid. TRH = thyrotrophin-releasing hormone. Thyrotrophin (TSH, thyroid-stimulating hormone) is inhibited by circulating levels of T_3 and T_4. The actions of drugs used are shown by red arrows.

free fraction of hormone can bind to specific cell receptors. The thyroid secretes mainly T_4 (thyroxine) and a small amount of T_3. Most T_3 is derived from peripheral deiodination of T_4 by the enzyme thyroxine 5'-deiodinase, which is found in the liver, kidney, brain and brown adipose tissue. About 35% of T_4 is converted to T_3, while about 40% is converted to reverse T_3 (a metabolically inactive isomer of T_3). T_3 has a half-life in the circulation of about 1.5 days compared with about 7 days for T_4. Elimination of T_3 and T_4 is by conjugation, mainly in the liver.

The cellular actions of thyroid hormone are due to interaction with thyroid hormone receptors (Ch. 1) that belong to the superfamily of nuclear receptors. The receptor–T_3 complexes are nuclear transcription factors, which prompt the binding of accessory protein cofactors that activate or suppress genes and influence their transcription rate. Thyroid hormone receptors are expressed in most tissues, but there are three isoforms of the receptor, which differ in their tissue distribution. Recent evidence suggests that these isoforms mediate different effects of T_3. T_3 also has non-genomic actions that include stimulation of cellular uptake of amino acids and glucose, and interactions with G-protein-coupled membrane receptors with activation of the mitogen-activated protein kinase (MAPK) pathway.

Hyperthyroidism

The commonest form of hyperthyroidism (often, and interchangeably, called thyrotoxicosis) is Graves' disease, an autoimmune condition in which thyroid-stimulating IgG binds to thyrotrophin (TSH) receptors on thyroid cells and initiates signal transduction. There is often an immunologically mediated inflammatory reaction in the extrinsic muscles and fat of the orbit, causing swelling and the characteristic exophthalmos. Toxic multinodular goitre, thyroid adenomas (toxic nodule) and various forms of thyroiditis are much less common causes of hyperthyroidism. Rarely, the condition arises from ectopic production of thyrotrophin or thyroxine or it can be induced by treatment with amiodarone (Ch. 8). Symptoms of hyperthyroidism include weight loss, palpitation, sweating, fatigue, nervousness, heat sensitivity and tremor. These are in part mediated by the action of excess thyroid hormone, and partly by excess sensitivity of tissues to β-adrenoceptor stimulation. Signs are often less marked in the elderly, who are more likely to present with atrial fibrillation that is resistant to treatment.

Drugs for treatment of hyperthyroidism

Thionamides

Examples: carbimazole, propylthiouracil

Mechanism of action

Thionamides inhibit thyroxine peroxidase, and, therefore, synthesis of thyroid hormone (Fig. 41.2). The long half-life of T_4 means that changes in the rate of synthesis take 4–6 weeks to lower circulating T_4 and T_3 concentrations to normal. These drugs also appear to have an immunosuppressant effect in individuals with autoimmune thyroid disease. They reduce the levels of thyrotrophin receptor-stimulating antibody, although the clinical importance of this is uncertain.

Pharmacokinetics

Carbimazole is almost completely absorbed from the gut and rapidly converted by first-pass metabolism to the active derivative methimazole. Methimazole has a short half-life and is inactivated by hepatic metabolism. Propylthiouracil has only about one-tenth of the activity of methimazole and has a short half-life due to rapid liver metabolism. It is usually reserved for intolerance of carbimazole. Although the antithyroid drugs have short half-lives, they accumulate in the thyroid, which extends their duration of action.

Unwanted effects

- Gastrointestinal upset (especially nausea and epigastric discomfort), headache, arthralgia and pruritic skin rashes are common in the first 8 weeks of treatment.
- Allergic reactions, including vasculitis, a lupus-like syndrome, myopathy, cholestatic jaundice and nephritis. Some cross-sensitivity occurs between carbimazole and propylthiouracil.
- Bone marrow suppression, especially agranulocytosis, is an important unwanted effect and is probably immunologically mediated. A severe sore throat with fever is often the presenting complaint, and this, or any other infection, should be immediately reported to a doctor. The onset is sudden, and routine blood counts are unhelpful. The risk is higher with propylthiouracil than with carbimazole. The blood count usually recovers about 3 weeks after drug withdrawal.
- Placental transfer of the active metabolite of carbimazole can produce neonatal hypothyroidism, but propylthiouracil does not transfer in large enough quantities to cause problems. However, in Graves' disease, the thyroid-stimulating antibody crosses the placenta and causes fetal thyrotoxicosis;

therefore, carbimazole is the treatment of choice for maternal Graves' disease. Carbimazole is secreted in breast milk but rarely produces hypothyroidism in the infant.

Beta-adrenoceptor antagonists (β-blockers)

Beta-adrenoceptor antagonists are fully described in Chapter 5 (see also drug compendium of Ch. 8). Beta-adrenoceptor antagonists act on the target tissues to modulate the additive effects of thyroid hormones and β-adrenoceptor stimulation. They have immediate effects on symptoms such as anxiety, palpitation and tremor, but do not alter the rate of thyroid hormone synthesis or secretion.

Management of hyperthyroidism

Carbimazole is the drug of choice for Graves' hyperthyroidism, and will usually decrease the thyroid hormone concentration to normal levels over 4–12 weeks. It is usual to start treatment with a high dosage for 4–6 weeks, unless the thyrotoxicosis is mild, when smaller initial doses may be more appropriate. The dosage is then gradually reduced every 4–6 weeks, provided that the serum T_4 concentration remains within the normal range, to reach the lowest possible dose that controls the serum T_4. Initially, treatment should be continued for 12–24 months, then treatment can be tapered or withdrawn. Occasionally, a block–replace regimen is used, giving a high dosage of carbimazole in conjunction with thyroxine replacement for 6–12 months. This maintains normal thyroid function regardless of the dose of carbimazole. Beta-adrenoceptor antagonists are particularly useful for symptomatic relief from tremor, anxiety or palpitation during the early period of treatment with carbimazole.

Exophthalmos associated with Graves' disease usually responds poorly to treatment with antithyroid drugs, since it is caused by TSH receptor antibody. Severe thyroid eye disease can be helped by treatment with oral prednisolone if antithyroid treatment is not improving the condition.

Approximately 50% of people with Graves' disease have a single episode that is cured by drug treatment. Those who relapse will usually do so within 6 months, and then repeat relapses are common. Most are then offered definitive treatment by either a subtotal thyroidectomy (for a large goitre) or a therapeutic dose of radioactive iodine (^{131}I). Hypothyroidism, often delayed by several months or years, is common after both treatments.

Surgery in Graves' disease is used for poor response to antithyroid drugs, a very large goitre, for coexisting thyroid malignancy or if the person expresses a preference for this treatment. Before surgery, carbimazole is

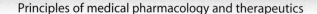

usually given to achieve a euthyroid state. Oral potassium iodide is reserved to achieve pre-operative control in resistant thyrotoxicosis. It is given for up to 2 weeks to inhibit thyroxine synthesis and release and to reduce the vascularity of the hyperplastic thyroid gland.

Radioiodine treatment can be used as first-line treatment for Graves' disease or for relapse after antithyroid drug treatment. Radioiodine may make thyroid ophthalmopathy worse, but this can be prevented by 2–3 months' treatment with a corticosteroid. Radioiodine is also used for toxic multinodular goitre. Before radioiodine treatment, it is often recommended that the thyrotoxicosis should be stabilised with carbimazole to reduce the risk of exacerbation of hyperthyroidism from radiation thyroiditis immediately after isotope treatment. However, antithyroid drug treatment must be stopped 3–4 days before radioactive iodine is given or it will prevent uptake of the radioiodine by the thyroid cells. Beta-adrenoceptor antagonists can be useful in this period to prevent symptomatic relapse. Carbimazole can be restarted 2–4 days after radioiodine to cover the few weeks before radioiodine is fully effective. Following radioiodine treatment, permanent hypothyroidism can occur: up to 1 year after treatment, the incidence is determined by the initial dose of radioactivity; thereafter, the risk is 2–3% annually. The theoretical increase in risk of cancer or leukaemia following radioiodine treatment has not been substantiated in clinical studies.

A solitary toxic thyroid nodule can be removed surgically, but radioactive iodine is extremely effective, because the isotope is taken up only by the abnormal tissue (the remainder is suppressed by the absence of thyrotrophin in the circulation). Multinodular toxic goitres are usually treated by radioiodine. Carbimazole is unsuitable as sole treatment for these conditions, since spontaneous remission does not occur. However, some elderly people may choose to continue treatment with carbimazole for life.

Treatment of amiodarone-induced thyroiditis (Ch. 8) depends on the clinical subtype. Type 1 is provoked by the iodide contained in the drug in people with an underlying multinodular goitre, and responds to antithyroid drug treatment. Type 2 is an inflammatory thyroiditis that arises from a direct toxic effect of the drug on the gland, and responds well to treatment with a corticosteroid.

Hypothyroidism

Hypothyroidism is usually caused by primary thyroid failure, and the low circulating T_4 concentration is accompanied by a raised plasma thyrotrophin (TSH) concentration. Autoimmune thyroiditis is the commonest cause, but hypothyroidism is occasionally congenital or can follow treatment for hyperthyroidism by surgery or radioiodine. Rarely, hypothyroidism can be secondary to pituitary or hypothalamic failure, when the circulating thyrotrophin concentrations will be low. Drug therapy with lithium (Ch. 22) or amiodarone (Ch. 8) can produce hypothyroidism. Typical symptoms of hypothyroidism are non-specific and include lethargy, slowing of mental processes, cold intolerance, dry skin, hoarseness, weight gain, constipation and menorrhagia. Severe hypothyroidism (myxoedema) produces marked coarsening of the facial appearance and may ultimately lead to a hypothermic, comatose state.

Management of hypothyroidism

Standard treatment is with oral thyroxine (levothyroxine, T_4) although its absorption is incomplete and variable. Sufficient T_3 will be formed by peripheral deiodination of T_4, but the proportion of circulating T_3 is usually lower than normal. Therefore, circulating levels of T_4 will often need to be higher than those in healthy subjects to obtain a satisfactory response. In some individuals, particularly those with ischaemic heart disease, a rapid increase in metabolic activity with thyroxine replacement can cause excessive cardiac stimulation, and thyroxine should be introduced gradually in those at risk of cardiac complications. In others, the anticipated weight-related maintenance dose can be given from the start. Because of its long half-life, steady-state plasma concentrations of thyroxine will not be achieved with constant dosage until about 4–5 weeks. The adequacy of thyroxine replacement therapy is best monitored by measurement of the serum thyrotrophin concentration 4–6 weeks after a change in dose of thyroxine. When the thyrotrophin concentration is within the normal range, the plasma T_4 will usually be slightly high or in the upper part of the normal range. Once the dose is correct, an annual check of serum thyrotrophin is sufficient, unless there are symptoms suggesting hypo- or hyperthyroidism. Problems with thyroid replacement preparations are uncommon, but allergic reactions have been reported, and transient scalp hair loss can occur in the first few weeks of treatment.

Some drugs interfere with the absorption of thyroxine from the gut. These include iron, calcium carbonate, mineral supplements, colestyramine (Ch. 48) and sucralfate (Ch. 33). The metabolism of thyroxine is accelerated by the concurrent use of the hepatic enzyme-inducing drugs phenobarbital, phenytoin, carbamazepine (Ch. 23) and rifampicin (Ch. 51). In all these situations, the therapeutic response to thyroxine may be impaired.

Liothyronine (T_3, triiodothyronine) is usually reserved for intravenous use in severe hypothyroidism (myxoedema coma), when its potency, more rapid effect and shorter half-life allow more rapid attainment of a therapeutic blood concentration. However, even in this situation, a large dose of thyroxine has been successfully used, and may be associated with a lower mortality.

FURTHER READING

Cooper DS (2003) Hyperthyroidism. *Lancet* 362, 459–468

Roberts CGP, Ladenson PW (2004) Hypothyroidism. *Lancet* 363, 793–803

Toft AD (2001) Subclinical hyperthyroidism. *N Engl J Med* 345, 512–516

Self-assessment

In questions 1 and 2, the first statement, in italics, is true. Are the accompanying statements also true?

1. *Synthesis and secretion of T_3 and T_4 are controlled by thyrotrophin and plasma iodide.*

    a. Most circulating T_3 and T_4 are highly bound to albumin.
    b. Thyroxine (T_4) has a long residence time in the body.
    c. At target cells, T_4 is converted to T_3, which then binds to specific nuclear receptors.
    d. Hyperthyroidism will be made worse by iodine administration.

2. *Severe hypothyroidism causes 'myxoedema' in adults and cretinism in children; its origins are immunological.*

    a. Therapy with ^{131}I can cause hypothyroidism.
    b. Hypothyroidism is treated with oral thyroxine.
    c. When thyroxine is taken, it reaches steady-state plasma concentrations after about 5 weeks.

3. Mr RH was diagnosed with thyrotoxicosis and was about to be started on carbimazole. Choose the one INCORRECT answer from the following.

    A. It will take 5 weeks to reduce the circulating T_4 and T_3 concentrations to normal.
    B. Carbimazole is a prodrug.
    C. An unwanted effect of carbimazole is bone marrow suppression.
    D. Carbimazole inhibits the stimulant action of thyrotropin on the thyroid.
    E. Carbimazole has a long duration of action.

4. Mrs JH was diagnosed with hypothyroidism and ischaemic heart disease and treatment for her hypothyroidism was started. Choose the one correct answer from the following statements about her condition and her treatment.

    A. Low circulating T_4 levels in hypothyroidism are accompanied by low levels of thyrotrophin.
    B. Treatment should be with oral levothyroxine.
    C. On regular dosing, steady-state plasma levels of levothyroxine are reached within 7 days.
    D. No special precautions are required when administering levothyroxine to Mrs JH.
    E. Oxygen consumption in metabolically active tissues is unaffected by levothyroxine.

5. Case history questions

    > A 45-year-old man suffered from weight loss, palpitations, tremor, anxiety and sweating, plus eyelid retraction, and orbital and ocular inflammation. Blood tests showed increased levels of free and bound T_3 and T_4. A diagnosis of Graves' thyrotoxicosis was made. An electrocardiogram showed atrial fibrillation.

    a. What is Graves' disease?
    b. What other blood tests could be done to confirm this diagnosis?
    c. Why were the free T_3 and T_4 measured?
    d. How could the symptoms be controlled?
    e. What drug could be given to control the hyperthyroidism?

    > With treatment, he became euthyroid, but relapsed in the following year. A decision was made to treat him with [131]I.

    f. What treatment should be given before administering the ^{131}I and what are the reasons for this?
    g. How long after treatment would you expect to see benefit?

    The answers are provided on pages 736–737.

Drug compendium

Thyroid and antithyroid drugs

Drug	Half-life	Elimination	Comments
Thyroid hormones			
Levothyroxine/thyroxine	6–7 days	Metabolism	Treatment of choice for maintenance therapy; given orally; oral bioavailability is 50–80% (with some variability between brands); metabolised by deiodination in peripheral tissues to T_3 (which has a half-life of 1–2 days)
Liothyronine (L-tri-iodothyronine)	1–2 days	Metabolism	More rapid onset of action than levothyroxine and can be used for severe hypothyroid states; given orally or by slow intravenous injection (for hypothyroid coma); almost complete oral bioavailability; metabolised by deiodination and conjugation with glucuronic acid and sulphate
Antithyroid drugs[a]			All drugs given orally once-daily, because of their long-term effects on the thyroid
Carbimazole	3–5 h (methimazole)	Metabolism	Complete absorption with complete presystemic metabolism to the active form methimazole; methimazole is eliminated by metabolism plus some renal excretion
Iodine and iodide	–	Renal	Used as an adjunct to antithyroid drugs for 10–14 days before partial thyroidectomy, but should not be given for long-term treatment; complete oral absorption; incorporated into thyroid hormones; excreted largely in urine
Propylthiouracil	1–3 h	Metabolism	Bioavailability is 50–75% due to poor absorption; the main metabolic route is formation of an *S*-glucuronide

[a]Beta-adrenoceptor antagonists, such as propranolol, can be used to treat the symptoms of thyrotoxicosis.

42

Calcium metabolism and metabolic bone disease

Regulation of calcium metabolism

Calcium ions play a part in a large number of cellular activities, including stimulus–response coupling in striated and smooth muscle, endocrine and exocrine glands. Calcium modulates the action of intracellular cyclic adenosine monophosphate (cAMP) and is a cofactor for numerous intracellular enzymes and for blood clotting. However, more than 98% of Ca^{2+} in the body is in the form of hydroxyapatite crystals deposited on the protein matrix of bone, which provides its mechanical strength.

Calcium circulates in plasma partly bound to protein (approximately 50%) and partly in the free ionised (and therefore 'active') form. The free fraction in plasma is precisely maintained within narrow limits principally by the actions of parathyroid hormone (PTH) and 1,25-dihydroxyvitamin D_3 (calcitriol). Calcitonin secretion also reacts to changing plasma Ca^{2+} concentrations but it is less important in overall control of Ca^{2+} homeostasis. Calcium in plasma is in constant flux with Ca^{2+} in the gut, renal tubules and bone. This is illustrated, with the main controlling factors, in Figure 42.1.

PTH is a polypeptide hormone which is the main physiological regulator of Ca^{2+} in blood. Its secretion from parathyroid chief cells is stimulated by a reduction of ionised Ca^{2+} in plasma, acting on the Ca^{2+}-sensing receptor. PTH secretion is inhibited when the plasma Ca^{2+} concentration rises.

The main actions of PTH relating to calcium homeostasis are that it:

- stimulates the synthesis of the biologically active form of vitamin D (calcitriol) in the kidney, which increases gut Ca^{2+} absorption and bone Ca^{2+} mobilisation
- facilitates reabsorption of Ca^{2+} from the kidney tubules and enhances urinary phosphate excretion
- mobilises calcium and phosphate from bone; this is by stimulation of bone resorption by osteoclasts, which increases bone turnover, although PTH also enhances osteoblastic activity, resulting in some bone repair.

The effect of PTH on the kidney occurs within minutes of PTH release, while that on bone begins after 1–2 h.

'Vitamin D' compounds (Box 42.1) have steroid nuclei. Ergocalciferol (vitamin D_2), a precursor of active vitamin D, is absorbed from the gut, but, given adequate sunlight, the major source of vitamin D is conversion of 7-dehydro-cholecalciferol in the skin to cholecalciferol (vitamin D_3). Therefore, cholecalciferol is really a skin-derived hormone rather than a vitamin, but this source was discovered after the dietary origins. Cholecalciferol is further metabolised in the liver to 25-hydroxy D_3, and then in the kidney to 1,25-dihydroxy D_3 (calcitriol). 1α-Hydroxylation is an essential step for activation of vitamin D; PTH stimulates 1α-hydroxylase activity in the kidney, increasing the formation of calcitriol. Vitamin D acts after binding to specific steroid receptors in the cell cytoplasm (Ch. 1), which then migrate to the nucleus and increase synthesis of an intracellular Ca^{2+}-binding protein. The main effect of active forms of vitamin D is to increase the plasma concentration of Ca^{2+} by stimulating its absorption from the gut. In the kidney, vitamin D promotes phosphate retention, in contrast to the action of PTH; and in bone, it increases osteoclastic activity. 1,25-Dihydroxy vitamin D_3 (calcitriol) also inhibits the transcription of the gene coding for PTH. These actions of vitamin D affect Ca^{2+} turnover in bone over periods of days to weeks.

The main actions of active forms of vitamin D relating to calcium homeostasis are that they:

- facilitate absorption of calcium from the small intestine
- enhance calcium mobilisation out of bone.

Calcitonin is a peptide secreted by the parafollicular cells of the thyroid when the Ca^{2+}-sensing receptor detects a rise in plasma Ca^{2+}. The main target cell for calcitonin

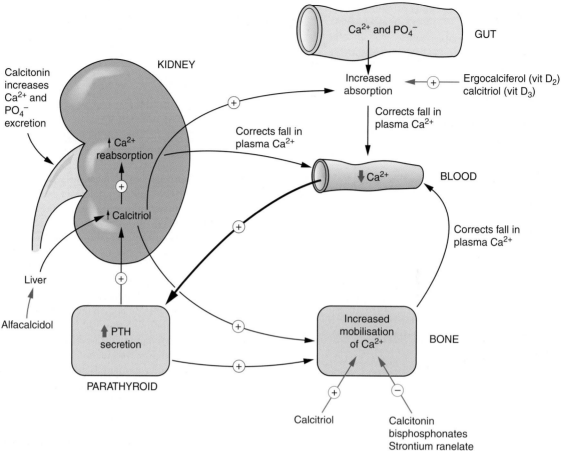

Fig. 42.1

Regulation of calcium metabolism. The primary response to a fall in plasma calcium is to stimulate parathyroid hormone (PTH) production from the parathyroid gland. This increases calcitriol (vitamin D_3) formation in the kidney. This in turn increases gut absorption of Ca^{2+}. PTH further increases bone mobilisation of Ca^{2+} to return plasma Ca^{2+} to normal. An increase in plasma Ca^{2+}, conversely, decreases PTH secretion. Calcitonin, secreted by the thyroid, decreases Ca^{2+} reabsorption from the kidney and decreases bone turnover. Drugs for hypercalcaemia are indicated by arrows in green. Drugs for hypocalcaemia are indicated by arrows in red.

Box 42.1

Vitamin D

The term vitamin D is used for a range of compounds. They include ergocalciferol (calciferol, vitamin D_2), cholecalciferol (vitamin D_3 – the approved drug name is colecalciferol), dihydrotachysterol, alfacalcidol (1α-hydroxycholecalciferol) and calcitriol (1,25-dihydroxycholecalciferol).

is the osteoclast, which it inhibits by stimulation of adenylate cyclase, thus reducing bone turnover. Calcitonin also decreases Ca^{2+} and phosphate reabsorption by the kidney thereby increasing their excretion.

Hypercalcaemia

The main causes of hypercalcaemia are:

- increased resorption of Ca^{2+} from bone – for example, primary hyperparathyroidism, secretion of parathyroid-related hormone by cancer cells, bony metastases
- increased absorption of Ca^{2+} from gut through excessive use of vitamin D or sarcoidosis
- reduced renal excretion of Ca^{2+} – for example, thiazide diuretics (Ch. 14).

Hypercalcaemia occurs when the mobilisation of Ca^{2+} into the extracellular space exceeds the capacity to remove it. Chronic moderate hypercalcaemia produces a progressive decline in renal function, formation of renal stones and ectopic calcification (e.g. cornea, blood vessels). Severe hypercalcaemia causes anorexia, nausea, vomiting, constipation, drowsiness and confusion, eventually leading to coma. Hypercalcaemia impairs the ability of the kidney to reabsorb salt and water; in conjunction with vomiting, this can lead to depletion of plasma volume and renal failure. Urgent treatment is indicated when the plasma Ca^{2+} concentration rises above 3.5 mmol l^{-1} (normal usually <2.6 mmol l^{-1}), since sudden death from cardiac arrest can occur

Antiresorptive drugs for hypercalcaemia

Bisphosphonates

> *eg*
> Examples: alendronic acid, sodium clodronate, disodium etidronate, disodium pamidronate, risedronate sodium

Mechanisms of action and effects

Bisphosphonates are pyrophosphate analogues that bind to hydroxyapatite crystals in bone matrix. They are preferentially deposited under osteoclasts, and are taken up by these cells and inhibit their resorptive action on bone. The cellular actions of the drugs on osteoclasts are:

- metabolism within the cell to form a toxic analogue of adenosine triphosphate (ATP) that induces osteoclast apoptosis (non-nitrogen-containing drugs: clodronate, etidronate)
- inhibition of the cholesterol synthetic pathway enzyme farnesyl diphosphate; this reduces the production of cholesterol and related lipids that are essential for osteoclast function, and eventually leads to apoptosis (nitrogen-containing drugs: alendronate, pamidronate, risedronate).

Etidronate is less potent than the other agents, and is given in larger doses. It is also deposited on bone formation surfaces and may affect the action of osteoblasts.

Pharmacokinetics

Bisphosphonates are poorly absorbed from the gut (less than 10% of the ingested dose). Oral formulations are best taken with the stomach empty, to avoid binding by Ca^{2+} in food. Alendronic acid, disodium etidronate and risedronate sodium are only available in an oral formulation; disodium pamidronate is only formulated for intravenous use. Removal of bisphosphonates from blood is rapid via the kidney, but their effect is prolonged since they remain bound to calcium salts in bone.

Unwanted effects

- gastrointestinal disturbance, particularly nausea, abdominal pain, diarrhoea or constipation with the oral treatments

- headache
- alendronic acid and risedronate sodium can cause severe oesophagitis and oesophageal strictures; to reduce the risk, the tablets should be taken whole with a full glass of water at least 30 min before food, and the person should then stand or sit, but not lie down, for at least 30 min after ingestion
- disodium pamidronate causes transient pyrexia and influenza-like symptoms after infusion
- continuous use of high doses of disodium etidronate impairs mineralisation of newly formed bone, with consequent risk of osteomalacia.

Calcitonin

Mechanism of action and effects

The actions of calcitonin on bone and the kidney to reduce the plasma calcium concentration have been discussed above. Calcitonin begins to act within a few hours of administration, with a maximum effect between 12 and 24 h; however, the hypocalcaemic effect produced by repeated administrations only lasts between 2 and 3 days. This loss of clinical response results from down-regulation of calcitonin receptors on osteoclasts leading to a rebound increase in bone resorption. Calcitonin is also used to treat Paget's disease of bone, and for the prevention and treatment of postmenopausal osteoporosis.

Pharmacokinetics

Salmon calcitonin (salcatonin) is now used exclusively, since it is less immunogenic than the earlier preparation of pork calcitonin. It is usually given by intramuscular or subcutaneous injection, although intravenous infusion can be used. A nasal spray formulation is also available. The half-life is short, and it is broken down to inactive fragments by enzymic degradation in plasma and in the kidney.

Unwanted effects

- facial flushing occurs in most people
- dizziness
- nausea, vomiting and diarrhoea
- tingling of the hands
- taste disturbance
- allergic reactions, including anaphylaxis.

Treatment of hypercalcaemia

When possible, the primary cause should be corrected, for example removal of a parathyroid adenoma or treatment of myeloma. Additional measures may include correction of dehydration, enhancing renal excretion of Ca^{2+} and inhibiting bone resorption.

Most people with severe hypercalcaemia are fluid depleted at presentation. Rehydration with intravenous saline is essential; this also promotes a sodium-linked Ca^{2+} diuresis in the proximal and distal renal tubules. Loop diuretics such as furosemide (Ch. 14) increase renal Ca^{2+} elimination but should be given with high volumes of intravenous saline and intensive monitoring of fluid balance to avoid dehydration.

A bisphosphonate, especially by intravenous infusion, is the drug treatment of first choice for severe hypercalcaemia. Initial intravenous rehydration is essential to avoid precipitation of calcium bisphosphonate in the kidney. Oral bisphosphonate treatment may be sufficient for less severe hypercalcaemia. Following a single intravenous infusion of bisphosphonate, the plasma Ca^{2+} concentration falls gradually, with a maximum effect after about a week, persisting for up to 4 weeks after treatment. Because of the delay in onset of action of the bisphosphonates, calcitonin can be given concurrently for an early effect. Glucocorticoids, such as prednisolone (Ch. 44), are effective for lowering Ca^{2+} when vitamin D excess is an important factor, for example in sarcoidosis, for acute treatment of vitamin D overdose or for hypercalcaemia associated with haematological malignancy such as myeloma. Glucocorticoids probably act by reducing the effect of vitamin D on intestinal Ca^{2+} transport, but can take several days to work.

Hypocalcaemia

There are two major underlying causes of hypocalcaemia:

- deficiency of PTH – for example, idiopathic hypoparathyroidism, after surgical parathyroid removal
- deficiency of vitamin D – for example, dietary deficiency, limited exposure to sunlight, renal failure (failure of 1α-hydroxylation).

Hypocalcaemia produces neuromuscular irritability with paraesthesiae of the extremities or around the mouth, muscle cramps and tetany. When severe, it can produce seizures. Chronic hypocalcaemia, especially in congenital hypoparathyroidism, is associated with mental deficiency, seizures, intracranial calcification (e.g. choroid plexus) and ocular cataracts.

Drugs for hypocalcaemia

Vitamin D compounds

> Examples: ergocalciferol (vitamin D_2), alfacalcidol (1α-hydroxycholecalciferol), calcitriol (1,25-dihydroxycholecalciferol)

Mechanism of action

This is discussed above. A dose-related increase in Ca^{2+} and phosphate absorption from the gut occurs at lower concentrations than those stimulating bone resorption. Ergocalciferol is inactive and can only be used if 1α-hydroxylation by the kidney is intact. In renal impairment, the hydroxylated active forms alfacalcidol or calcitriol should be used.

Pharmacokinetics

The fat-soluble D vitamins are well absorbed orally in the presence of bile. They can also be given intravenously. Both alfacalcidol and calcitriol are active forms of vitamin D; they have short half-lives and are excreted mainly in the bile.

Unwanted effects

- excessive dosing will produce hypercalcaemia
- excretion of vitamin D supplements in breast milk can cause hypercalcaemia in a suckling infant.

Treatment of hypocalcaemia

Mild hypocalcaemia can be treated with oral calcium supplements, taken between meals to avoid binding to dietary phosphate and oxalate, which are poorly absorbed. In the absence of reversible pathology such as malabsorption due to coeliac disease, the mainstay of treatment for more severe hypocalcaemia is vitamin D supplements. The few individuals who have vitamin D deficiency from inadequate diet or lack of exposure to sunlight (such as may be seen in Asian women in the UK) will respond to small doses of vitamin D. Most causes of hypocalcaemia, however, require much larger doses (usually given as ergocalciferol) to maintain normocalcaemia. Oral calcium supplements (as carbonate or citrate salts) are often used with vitamin D for treatment of chronic hypocalcaemia.

PTH is not readily available for replacement therapy, and alfacalcidol is given for treatment of hypoparathyroidism. Large doses of ergocalciferol could be used, but carry a risk of hypercalcaemia. The action of vitamin D begins after 2–4 weeks of treatment, because there is deficient renal hydroxylation of vitamin D in hypoparathyroidism, but the action of calcitriol is much more rapid, beginning after 1–2 days. Calcitriol is rarely required unless a very rapid onset of action is necessary.

Acute severe hypocalcaemia (sometimes occurring after parathyroidectomy) must be treated with intravenous calcium (as gluconate, gluceptate or chloride salt).

Metabolic bone disease

Osteomalacia

Osteomalacia is the bone disease resulting from failure of adequate bone mineralisation due to lack of vitamin D. Bone pain is prominent, and low plasma Ca^{2+} and phosphate concentrations produce muscle weakness. In developing children, the bones become distorted (rickets). Treatment is with vitamin D (ergocalciferol) supplements.

Osteoporosis

Osteoporosis is the loss of bone mass due to reduced organic bone matrix and, consequently, mineral content, which reduces the mechanical strength of bone. To some extent, it is a natural and inevitable part of the ageing process. In females, however, a marked increase in bone loss occurs after the menopause. Other predisposing factors include smoking, heavy alcohol intake and lack of exercise. Osteoporosis in younger people is associated with trabecular bone loss and predisposes to spontaneous vertebral fractures. In older people, cortical bone is also lost, increasing the risk of traumatic fracture, particularly of the neck of the femur. Sometimes osteoporosis is secondary to other conditions such as corticosteroid therapy (Ch. 44), myeloma or thyrotoxicosis. Once established, osteoporosis is extremely difficult to reverse, and emphasis should be placed on prevention where possible.

Prevention of osteoporosis

- The major opportunity for preventing osteoporosis is the use of hormone replacement therapy (HRT) with oestrogens (Ch. 45) in peri- and postmenopausal women. Unless a hysterectomy has been performed, progestogens must be given as well, to prevent endometrial hyperplasia and an increased risk of carcinoma. Five to 10 years of oestrogen therapy may be required, but the long-term use of HRT is no longer recommended, because of the increased risk of breast cancer and thromboembolic events.
- Oral calcium supplements probably also reduce the risk of vertebral fractures in postmenopausal women; the addition of vitamin D (ergocalciferol) may confer greater benefit.
- Raloxifene (Ch. 45) is a tissue-selective oestrogen receptor modulator which has oestrogenic effects on bone but oestrogen antagonist actions on breast and uterine receptors. It increases bone mineral density in postmenopausal osteoporosis, and reduces the risk of vertebral fractures. Unwanted effects include hot flushes, leg cramps and venous thromboembolism.

- Oral bisphosphonates are the treatment of choice for prevention of corticosteroid-induced osteoporosis.

Treatments for established osteoporosis

The choice of treatment depends on the clinical circumstances. Pain relief is important if there are fractures, but drug treatment to prevent bone loss can reduce the risk of further fractures by up to 50%. Options include the following.

- **Oral bisphosphonates** produce an increase in bone density. Most studies have been carried out in postmenopausal women. Oral etidronate, given for 2 weeks at 3-monthly intervals, usually with continuous calcium supplements, increases vertebral bone mineral content, and may reduce fractures. Alendronic acid has also been shown to reduce hip and wrist fractures. Bisphosphonates are also first-line treatment for the management of corticosteroid-induced osteoporosis.
- **Raloxifene** is useful for the management of vertebral fractures in postmenopausal women.
- **Oral fluoride supplements** increase bone formation in osteoporotic bone but also produce a defect in mineralisation of cortical bone. This can be minimised by giving calcium supplements, but the ability of fluoride to prevent fractures is unproven.
- **Salmon calcitonin** given subcutaneously or intranasally produces a modest increase in bone mass. Calcitonin can also produce pain relief when used for up to 3 months after a vertebral fracture.
- **Teriparatide** is a synthetic recombinant fraction of PTH (amino acids 1–34) that is effective for the treatment of postmenopausal osteoporosis. It is given daily by subcutaneous injection. The most common unwanted effects are nausea, oesophageal reflux, postural hypotension, dyspnoea, depression and dizziness. There is also evidence that it is effective for osteoporosis treatment in men.
- **Strontium ranelate** stimulates osteoblast activity and inhibits osteoclast differentiation and resorptive activity. It reduces the risk of both hip and vertebral fractures. It is taken orally and is eliminated by the kidneys with a long effective half-life of 60 hours. Unwanted effects include nausea, diarrhoea, headache and rashes.
- **Calcitriol** is effective when bisphosphonates are unsuitable, including for corticosteroid-induced osteoporosis.
- **Testosterone** (Ch. 46) is used for prophylaxis and treatment of corticosteroid-induced osteoporosis in men.

Paget's disease of bone

Paget's disease of bone is a disturbance of bone remodelling characterised by both excessive bone reabsorption by osteoclasts and an increase in formation of poor-quality bone. The new bone matrix is non-lamellar woven bone with areas of osteosclerosis, leaving bone that is structurally weakened. Paget's disease mainly affects the skull and long bones. The aetiology is unknown but a slow virus infection may initiate the disease.

About a third of the bone lesions are asymptomatic, but they can include bone pain and deformity, nerve entrapment and pathological fractures. Active treatment should be given if symptoms are present or a risk of complications is identified. Apart from symptomatic measures such as analgesics, two main treatments are used, as follows.

- **Bisphosphonates** are effective for treatment and primarily inhibit bone resorption, but long-term use can also impair bone mineralisation and produce

osteomalacia by creating secondary hyperparathyroidism. With intermittent treatment (e.g. 6 months out of every 12 months) prolonged remission of symptoms and reduction in complications can be achieved. Oral treatment is usually sufficient, with intravenous treatment reserved for severe disease. Calcium supplements may reduce the risk of osteomalacia.

- **Calcitonin**, by reducing osteoclastic bone resorption, can reduce pain and then improve the structural abnormalities in Pagetic bone. Pain relief usually begins within 2 weeks, but treatment may be necessary for several months to improve bone modelling. Approximately 50% of people will relapse on stopping treatment. Calcitonin is often reserved for initial treatment while awaiting a response to a bisphosphonate.

FURTHER READING

Bender IB (2003) Paget's disease. *J Endod* 29, 720–723

Burgess E, Nanes MS (2002) Osteoporosis in men: pathophysiology, evaluation and therapy. *Curr Opin Rheumatol* 14, 421–428

Hurtado J, Esbrit P (2002) Treatment of malignant hypercalcaemia. *Expert Opin Pharmacother* 3, 521–527

Marx SJ (2000) Medical progress: hyperparathyroid and hypoparathyroid disorders. *N Engl J Med* 343, 1863–1875

NIH Consensus Development Panel on Osteoporosis Prevention, Diagnosis, and Therapy (2001) Osteoporosis prevention, diagnosis, and therapy. *JAMA* 285, 785–795

Noor M, Shoback D (2000) Paget's disease of bone: diagnosis and treatment update. *Curr Rheumatol Rep* 2, 67–73

Reszka AA, Rodan GA (2003) Bisphosphonate mechanism of action. *Curr Rheumatol Rep* 5, 65–74

Rubin MR, Bilezikian JP (2002) New anabolic therapies in osteoporosis. *Curr Opin Rheumatol* 14, 433–440

Self-assessment

In questions 1 and 2, the first statement, in italics, is true. Are the accompanying statements also true?

1. *Hypocalcaemia develops when there is a deficiency in PTH or vitamin D, or when target organs do not respond to these hormones.*

   a. Vitamin D deficiency can lead to hypoparathyroidism.
   b. Calcitonin decreases Ca^{2+} resorption in the kidney.
   c. Bisphosphonates lower blood Ca^{2+} levels rapidly.

2. *Long-term oestrogen therapy (HRT) in postmenopausal women is no longer recommended, because of the risks of breast cancer and thromboembolic events.*

   a. Oestrogens maintain bone density by directly enhancing Ca^{2+} absorption from the intestine.
   b. Raloxifene stimulates oestrogen receptors on bone, breast and uterine tissue.

3. The following concern osteoporosis. Choose the one **incorrect** statement.

   A. High doses of oral prednisolone increase the risk of osteoporosis.
   B. Raloxifene has oestrogenic activity at all oestrogen receptors.
   C. Oral bisphosphonates reduce calcium mobilisation in bone.
   D. Raloxifene causes hot flushes in some women.
   E. Lack of exercise increases the risk of osteoporosis.

4. The following concern osteomalacia and rickets. Choose the one **incorrect** statement.

   A. Lack of sunlight can contribute to osteomalacia.
   B. Renal failure may reduce the effectiveness of ergocalciferol treatment in osteomalacia.
   C. Intestinal absorption of calcium will be decreased in osteomalacia.
   D. Low levels of PTH are associated with osteomalacia.
   E. Vitamin D promotes bone mineralisation.

The answers are provided on pages 737–738.

Drugs used to regulate calcium metabolism and in metabolic bone disease

Drug	Half-life	Elimination	Comments
Calcitonin (salmon)/salcatonin	12–21 min	Metabolism	Involved with parathyroid hormone in the regulation of bone turnover. Used to lower plasma calcium in hypercalcaemia and for the treatment of Paget's disease; given intranasally, by subcutaneous or intramuscular injection or by slow intravenous infusion; peak plasma concentrations are seen 15–45 min after subcutaneous injection; rapidly metabolised by the kidney (note, biological effects are prolonged for hours or days)
Teriparatide	5 min	Metabolism	A recombinant fragment of parathyroid hormone used for the treatment of postmenopausal osteoporosis; given by subcutaneous injection; clearance exceeds hepatic plasma flow, indicating a role for extrahepatic metabolism; the half-life from a subcutaneous injection is about 1 h owing to absorption rate-limited kinetics (see Ch. 2)
Bisphosphonates			All these drugs are adsorbed onto hydroxyapatite crystals and reduce bone turnover; there is an extremely long half-life of release from binding to bone and essentially all of the drugs share similar fates in the body; they are all used for osteoporosis; the drugs are highly polar and most of the dose is eliminated in the faeces after oral administration; elimination of absorbed drug is by renal excretion, and care should be taken in subjects with renal impairment
Alendronic acid (alendronate)	11 years (bone)	Renal	First-line option for the prevention and treatment of osteoporosis; given orally; very low oral bioavailability (<1%) reduced even further by food; the absorbed fraction is eliminated by glomerular filtration; about 40% of an intravenous dose is eliminated and the remainder retained and eliminated very slowly, due to binding to bone
Clodronate sodium	6 h	Renal	Used for hypercalcaemia of malignancy; given by intravenous infusion; the published half-life probably reflects the rate of bone uptake and renal excretion and does not reflect the release due to bone turnover (which is probably years)
Etidronate (disodium)	2–6 h (plasma), very long (bone)	Renal	Given orally; low absorption (1–9%); about 50% of intravenous dose is eliminated in the urine within 24 h, but the remainder is retained in bone and elimination is dependent on bone turnover (presumably about 11 years as for alendronate, see above)
Ibandronic acid	10–60 h	Renal	Potent bisphosphonate used for hypercalcaemia of malignancy; given by intravenous infusion; the published half-life probably reflects the rate of bone uptake and renal excretion and does not reflect the release due to bone turnover (which is probably years)
Pamidronate (disodium)	0.5 h (plasma), very long (bone)	Renal	Used for hypercalcaemia of malignancy and Paget's disease; given by slow intravenous infusion; the fate is similar to alendronate (see above) and the half-life given is the distribution from plasma to tissues; the half-life in bone depends on bone turnover (and has been reported to be about 2 years)

continued

Drug compendium

Drugs used to regulate calcium metabolism and in metabolic bone disease *(continued)*

Drug	Half-life	Elimination	Comments
Risedronate sodium	10 days	Renal	Potent bisphosphonate which is the drug of choice for the prevention and treatment of osteoporosis; given orally; high oral bioavailability (about 60%) due to the presence of a lipohilic pyridinyl side-chain; bioavailability is reduced if taken with food; the published half-life probably reflects the rate of bone uptake and renal excretion and does not reflect the release due to bone turnover (which is probably years)
Tiludronic acid	Very long (bone)	Renal	Used for Paget's disease; given orally; oral bioavailability is highly variable (between and within patients) and low (about 6%); see alendronate for probable fate in the body
Zoledronic acid	7 days	Renal	Used for hypercalcaemia of malignancy; given by intravenous infusion; see alendronate for probable fate in the body
Vitamin D			Used in the prevention or treatment of rickets; because vitamin D requires metabolic activation in the kidneys, alfacalcidol or calcitriol should be used in cases of severe renal impairment
Alfacalcidol	3 h	Metabolism	Given orally or by intravenous injection; 1α-hydroxycholecalciferol; high oral bioavailability; undergoes side-chain oxidation by a 25-hydroxylase to calcitriol, which is the active form
Calcitriol	24 h	Metabolism	Given orally or by intravenous injection; $1\alpha,25$-dihydroxycholecalciferol; rapidly and completely absorbed; oxidised to inactive metabolites
Colecalciferol (vitamin D_3)	Not defined	Metabolism	Given orally or by intravenous injection; high oral bioavailability; oxidised at 25-position to 25-hydroxycholecalciferol, which is oxidised to the active 1,25-dihydroxy compound in the kidney
Dihydrotachysterol	10 h (?)	Metabolism	Given orally; synthetic analogue of vitamin D_2; peak concentrations are at 4 h after dosage; few kinetic data available
Ergocalciferol (calciferol; vitamin D_2)	Not defined	Metabolism	Given orally or by intravenous injection; high oral bioavailability; metabolic precursor of cholecalciferol; metabolised to 1,25-dihydroxycholecalciferol (calcitriol) in liver and kidney
Strontium ranelate	60 h	Renal	Two atoms of stable strontium complexed with one molecule of ranelic acid. Bioavailability 25%; steady state achieved after two weeks of treatment

Anterior pituitary and hypothalamic hormones

Thyrotrophin and thyrotrophin-releasing hormone (TRH) are considered in Chapter 41.

Growth hormone

Growth hormone (GH), or somatotrophin, is a 191-amino acid peptide that is synthesised in specific cells in the anterior pituitary. Its secretion is controlled by the hypothalamus via a releasing hormone (GHRH) and dopamine (Fig. 43.1) and also modulated by a release-inhibiting hormone (GHRIH or somatostatin). GH is released in pulses repeatedly during both day and night. Like other peptide hormones, GH binds to cell surface receptors and activates adenylate cyclase. It has direct metabolic effects on several tissues, which are anabolic in relation to protein metabolism (especially in skeletal muscle and epiphyseal cartilage) and catabolic in relation to fat. The proliferating effects on epiphyseal cartilage stimulate bone growth. The anabolic effects on muscle and bone are mediated by insulin-like growth factor 1 (IGF-1, a somatomedin). Somatomedins are synthesised by the liver in response to GH stimulation. IGF-1 is highly protein bound in plasma.

Therapeutic uses of growth hormone

GH from human cadaveric pituitary origin (which could transmit the prion-mediated Creutzfeldt–Jakob disease) has been replaced since 1985 by biosynthetic human-sequence GH (somatropin) developed using recombinant DNA techniques. Therapeutic uses of somatropin include:

- children with proven GH deficiency (who usually lack GHRH: pituitary dwarfism) to improve linear growth
- chronic renal insufficiency before puberty
- Turner syndrome
- Prader–Willi syndrome.

To be effective, the hormone must be given before the closure of the epiphyses in long bones. If growth velocity does not increase by at least 50% from baseline, then treatment should be stopped.

Pharmacokinetics
Somatropin has a very short half-life, so plasma concentrations fluctuate widely following intramuscular or subcutaneous injection (although the latter gives more stable levels because of slower uptake into the circulation). By contrast, concentrations of IGF-1 are much more constant, due to its high protein binding. As a consequence, three doses of GH per week give good clinical results, although daily dosing is often used. GH is usually given by subcutaneous injection, although the intramuscular route can be used.

Unwanted effects
- headache, occasionally associated with visual problems, nausea and vomiting, and papilloedema, owing to benign intracranial hypertension
- fluid retention with peripheral oedema
- arthralgia, myalgia, carpal tunnel syndrome

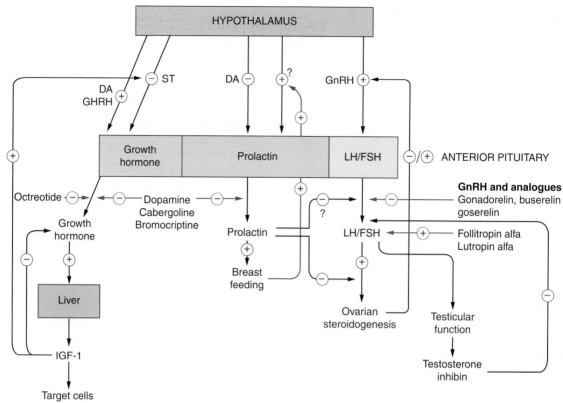

Fig. 43.1
Control mechanisms for the release of growth hormone, gonadotrophins and prolactin from the anterior pituitary. For control of other hormones, see Chapter 41 (thyroid) and Chapter 44 (adrenocorticotrophic hormones). Oestrogen effects on GnRH are shown as both positive and negative. Oestrogen suppresses LH secretion in the early follicular phase but enhances secretion around ovulation (Ch. 45). Gonadorelin is a GnRH analogue. Pulsatile administration enhances LH/FSH. On continued administration, it rapidly downregulates the GnRH receptors, inhibiting LH/FSH release. The actions of drugs are shown in red. DA, dopamine; FSH, follicle-stimulating hormone; GHRH, growth hormone-releasing hormone; GnRH = gonadotrophin-releasing hormone; IGF-1 = insulin-like growth factor-1; LH, luteinising hormone; ST, somatostatin; octreotide is synthetic somatostatin; ? = regulating hormone not yet established.
Note: Dopamine stimulates GH release in healthy individuals but paradoxically in acromegaly it inhibits release.

- there is a transient insulin-like action which occasionally produces hypoglycaemia
- if excessive doses are used (as may happen during illicit use by athletes), there is a risk of diabetes mellitus in predisposed individuals
- pain at the injection site.

Acromegaly

Acromegaly results from excessive production of GH, almost always by an adenoma in the anterior pituitary, which also secretes prolactin in one-third of cases (Fig. 43.1). The clinical features arise from excessive growth of bone and soft tissue. Complex metabolic consequences include insulin resistance with diabetes and hypertension. Occasionally, the tumour extends above the sella turcica, causing compression of the optic chiasm. This usually results in a bitemporal hemianopia, progressing eventually to complete loss of vision.

The morbidity and mortality of acromegaly vary according to its severity. Untreated acromegalic individuals have a life expectancy approximately half that of people without acromegaly, due to an excess incidence of cardiovascular and respiratory disease and of carcinoma of the colon. Acromegaly is therefore usually treated actively. Surgery by the trans-sphenoidal route is the usual treatment of choice, sometimes followed by external radiotherapy if the tumour was large. Three groups may be suitable for drug treatment:

- those in whom an excess of GH persists despite surgery and radiotherapy; after radiotherapy, the plasma GH concentration can take 1–2 years to fall
- those with mild acromegaly
- the elderly.

Drugs for acromegaly

Somatostatin analogues

Examples: lanreotide, octreotide

Mechanisms of action and uses

The synthetic derivatives of somatostatin (GHRIH) are both more potent and longer-acting than the native compound. Like somatostatin, they also inhibit the release of gastro-entero-pancreatic peptide hormones, such as insulin, glucagon and gastrin, via specific intestinal receptors which generate intracellular cyclic adenosine monophosphate (cAMP) and promote calcium influx into the cell.

Uses of somatostatin analogues include:

- management of acromegaly before pituitary surgery and for persistent acromegaly after surgery and radiotherapy; given by subcutaneous injection, they reduce GH release and pituitary tumour size
- management of other endocrine tumours, for example carcinoid tumours (to reduce flushing and diarrhoea), VIPoma (to reduce diarrhoea) and glucagonoma (to improve the characteristic necrolytic rash)
- octreotide is also used to stop bleeding from oesophageal varices (Ch. 36)
- octreotide has a limited role in the treatment of vomiting in palliative care.

Pharmacokinetics

Octreotide is given by subcutaneous injection. It has a short half-life but suppresses GH secretion for up to 8 h. A depot preparation has now been introduced in which octreotide is adsorbed onto microspheres and given by deep intramuscular injection. The duration of action of this preparation is about 4 weeks. The depot preparation is used once control has been achieved by the use of the conventional formulation three times daily. Lanreotide is formulated as a sustained-release preparation that is given by subcutaneous or intramuscular injection every 2–4 weeks, depending on the formulation.

Unwanted effects

- Gastrointestinal upset is common, especially anorexia, nausea, vomiting, abdominal pain, bloating and diarrhoea. It usually resolves with continued treatment
- Impaired postprandial glucose tolerance.
- Gallstones, from suppression of cholecystokinin secretion with decreased gallbladder motility. In addition, an increase in bowel transit time alters colonic flora and makes bile more lithogenic.
- Pain at the injection site.
- Pancreatitis, especially with abrupt withdrawal.

Dopamine receptor agonists

In healthy subjects, dopaminergic receptor stimulation increases secretion of GH, but in acromegaly there is a paradoxical decrease. Bromocriptine was originally used, but the clinical response was unpredictable and achieved control of IGF-1 in only about 20% of cases. It has been superseded by better-tolerated drugs such as cabergoline, which adequately suppress IGF-1 concentrations in about 40% of people with acromegaly. Further details of these drugs can be found in Chapter 24.

Adrenocorticotrophic hormone (ACTH)

ACTH is a straight-chain polypeptide with 39 amino acids, of which the 24 that form the N-terminal are essential for full biological activity. It promotes steroidogenesis in adrenocortical cells by occupying cell surface receptors and stimulating adenylate cyclase. Release of ACTH occurs in response to the hypothalamic peptide corticotrophin-releasing factor (CRF). CRF secretion is pulsatile and has a diurnal rhythm, with maximal release in the morning around the time of waking (Ch. 44). Other factors, including chemical (e.g. antidiuretic hormone, opioid peptides), physical (e.g. heat, cold, injury) and psychological influences, also affect release of CRF. The main inhibitory influence on ACTH release is negative feedback control by circulating glucocorticoids. This occurs at both hypothalamic and pituitary levels. Adrenal androgens, although stimulated by ACTH, play no part in feedback control.

Therapeutic uses of ACTH

ACTH preparations of animal origin have been replaced by a less allergenic, synthetic peptide analogue, tetracosactide (cosyntropin), which consists of the active N1–24 amino-acid section of the ACTH molecule. There are two formulations of tetracosactide.

- A rapid-acting form that increases steroidogenesis for about an hour and is suitable for tests of adrenocortical function. In adrenal insufficiency, there is a subnormal or no rise of plasma cortisol 30 min after intramuscular or intravenous injection of tetracosactide.
- A depot form that is absorbed slowly into the circulation over several hours and can be used as an alternative to exogenous corticosteroid therapy. However, the unpredictable response means that the therapeutic value of this drug is limited. Once absorbed into the circulation, tetracosactide is metabolised rapidly with a very short half-life.

Unwanted effects

Prolonged use will produce all the features of corticosteroid excess (Ch. 44).

Prolactin

Prolactin is a glycoprotein similar in structure to GH but secreted by distinct cells in the anterior pituitary (Fig. 43.1). The major hypothalamic control mechanism is inhibition by dopamine via D_2 receptors on the prolactin-secretory cells of the anterior pituitary (Ch. 45). The main target tissue for prolactin – a key hormone in lactation – is the breast, which secretes milk in response to prolactin if the mammary glands have been primed by ovarian and other hormones. At delivery, the maternal plasma prolactin concentration is high. Release of further prolactin continues as long as suckling continues. An intermediate may be production of a specific prolactin-releasing factor from the hypothalamus, and TRH may be involved. A high plasma concentration of prolactin leads to a failure of Graafian follicle growth and a low oestrogen state in the female. It may also interfere with gonadotrophin release. Plasma prolactin is raised during lactation, and this may explain the relative subfertility of women who are breastfeeding.

Hyperprolactinaemia

Persistent hyperprolactinaemia is usually caused by a microadenoma of the anterior pituitary or by the action of dopamine receptor antagonist drugs such as phenothiazines (Ch. 21). In younger women, hyperprolactinaemia can produce amenorrhoea, infertility, and signs and symptoms of oestrogen deficiency (e.g. vaginal dryness and dyspareunia, galactorrhoea and osteoporosis). In men it may cause hypogonadism. The dopamine receptor agonists bromocriptine and cabergoline (Ch. 24) can be used to suppress prolactin secretion.

Gonadotrophin-releasing hormone (GnRH, gonadorelin)

GnRH is a decapeptide that is synthesised in the hypothalamus and is transported by neuronal axons to the pituitary. It is then released in a pulsatile fashion into the capillaries of the pituitary-portal circulation and positively controls synthesis and release of both luteinising hormone (LH) and follicle-stimulating hormone (FSH) from the anterior pituitary (Fig. 43.1).

The surface receptors for GnRH are G-protein linked and are found widely in the body as well as on the gonadotrophic cells in the anterior pituitary. The receptors are induced by repeated stimulation with GnRH, but pulsatile exposure is essential to maintain responsiveness. There is rapid tolerance to constant-rate infusions of GnRH because of downregulation of cell surface receptors; both pulsatile stimulation and receptor downregulation are achieved with different patterns of therapeutic administration, and these have different clinical uses, as described below. There is negative feedback control of GnRH release via neural pathways and sex steroids (Fig. 43.1).

Synthetic GnRH (gonadorelin)

Synthetic GnRH is available for treatment of female infertility. In women with amenorrhoea due to impaired release of GnRH, repeated pulses of exogenous gonadorelin will often lead to normal pituitary–gonadal function, including a regular menstrual cycle and ovulation. The hormone is usually infused subcutaneously in pulses every 90 min (to avoid receptor downregulation) from a portable syringe-driving pump. Unwanted effects are unusual, but include nausea, headaches and abdominal pain.

Gonadorelin (GnRH) analogues

Examples: buserelin, goserelin

Mechanism of action

Structurally similar to the natural hormone, gonadorelin analogues (see Ch. 52) initially stimulate GnRH receptors, but rapidly promote receptor downregulation, which then inhibits further gonadotrophin production. This latter action underlies their clinical uses.

Pharmacokinetics

Buserelin can be given either by subcutaneous injection or by nasal spray. It has a short half-life. Goserelin must be given by subcutaneous injection and is available as an oily depot preparation. Depot formulations inhibit gonadotrophin production for up to 4 weeks after a single injection.

Unwanted effects

- menopausal effects in women, with hot flushes, sweating, vaginal dryness and loss of libido
- orchidectomy-like effects in men, with loss of libido, gynaecomastia and vasomotor instability
- headache
- hypersensitivity reactions, including skin rashes, asthma and anaphylaxis
- osteoporosis with repeated courses

- local reactions at injection sites, or intranasally with spray.

Clinical uses of gonadorelin analogues

- The main use is to reduce testosterone secretion to castration levels in men with prostatic cancer. An initial rise in testosterone from receptor stimulation can produce tumour 'flare' in the first 1–2 weeks of treatment (Ch. 52). An antiandrogen (Ch. 46) is usually given to counteract this effect.
- Treatment of endometriosis by reducing oestrogen secretion.
- Treatment of advanced breast cancer in women by reducing oestrogen secretion.
- To achieve reduction in endometrial thickness for 3–4 months prior to intrauterine surgery.
- For women undergoing preparation for assisted conception by methods such as in vitro fertilisation (IVF) (see below).

Gonadorelin (GnRH) antagonists

Examples: cetrorelix, ganirelix

Mechanism of action and uses
These drugs are competitive receptor antagonists that produce immediate, reversible suppression of gonadotrophin secretion. They are used in assisted reproduction techniques in the management of female infertility (IVF; see below). They have advantages compared with gonadorelin analogues in this role, since there is no initial surge of LH release (which can lead to cancellation of the IVF in about 20% of cycles).

Pharmacokinetics
Both cetrorelix and ganirelix are given by subcutaneous injection, and inactivated by hepatic metabolism. They have long half-lives.

Unwanted effects

- nausea
- headache
- injection-site reactions.

Gonadotrophins

LH and FSH are glycoproteins. Release of both hormones from the anterior pituitary is stimulated by pulsatile exposure to GnRH. Negative feedback by inhibin, a hormone of gonadal origin, selectively inhibits FSH secretion. In addition, both gonadotrophins are subject to negative feedback from gonadal steroids, including progesterone (Ch. 45).

In the male, LH acts on specific receptors on the surface of the Leydig cells in the testes and stimulates adenylate cyclase, leading to the production of testosterone. FSH acts in a similar way on the Sertoli cells of the seminiferous tubules, stimulating the formation of a specific androgen-binding protein.

In the female, receptors for FSH and LH are found in granulosa cells of ovarian follicles. FSH is responsible for follicular development. The rising oestradiol concentration in the late follicular phase has a positive-feedback effect on secretion of LH, and produces a short-lived surge of LH release. This triggers rupture of the follicle, release of the ovum, and formation of the corpus luteum (Ch. 45). Both FSH and LH, like human chorionic gonadotrophic hormone (HCG), are also produced in large quantities by the placenta during pregnancy.

Gonadotrophins for therapeutic use

- FSH and LH are extracted from urine obtained from postmenopausal women (known as human menopausal gonadotrophins: HMG).
- HCG is secreted by the placenta and extracted from the urine of pregnant women. It contains large quantities of LH. An alternative preparation is choriogonadotropin alfa.
- FSH alone is available as recombinant genetically engineered products known as follitropin alfa and beta (Fig. 43.1).
- LH alone is available as a recombinant genetically engineered product known as lutropin alfa (Fig. 43.1).

Gonadotrophins are given by intramuscular or subcutaneous injection.

Unwanted effects

- nausea and vomiting
- abdominal and pelvic pain
- headache
- in women, the most serious problem is ovarian hyperstimulation syndrome, in which the ovaries can become grossly enlarged as a result of multiple follicle stimulation, leading to considerable abdominal pain, ascites and even pleural effusions
- in men, the commonest problem is gynaecomastia or oedema with prolonged use.

Clinical uses of gonadotrophins
Clomifene

Mechanism of action and use
Clomifene is an agent with both oestrogenic and anti-oestrogenic properties. The latter are related to its ability

to block pituitary oestrogen receptors and increase gonadotrophin secretion. It is used to stimulate ovulation in anovulatory infertility.

Pharmacokinetics

Clomifene is well absorbed from the gut. It is metabolised in the liver, and has a very long half-life.

Unwanted effects

- reversible ovarian enlargement and cyst formation
- hot flushes
- adominal or pelvic pain
- nausea, vomiting
- breast tenderness, weight gain.

Drug treatment of female infertility

Infertility has several causes. If there is hyperprolactinaemia, then bromocriptine or one of the newer longer-acting dopamine agonists should suppress prolactin levels and permit ovulation in 70-80% of women. The management of polycystic ovary syndrome is considered below.

When deficiency of gonadal stimulation by gonadotrophin is the limiting factor, treatment with GnRH (gonadorelin) is given in a pulsatile fashion subcutaneously via a syringe pump. Conception rates are similar to those in the normal population.

If the hypothalamic–pituitary axis is normal, the antioestrogen clomifene blocks oestrogen receptors in the pituitary, which decreases the negative feedback on FSH, giving increased FSH concentrations that stimulate follicle growth. There is a small risk of ovarian hyperstimulation. If the hypothalamic–pituitary axis is not functioning, then FSH can be given. FSH, given alone (follitropin) or with LH (HMG), and HCG encourage the development of a single mature Graafian follicle. Again, ovarian hyperstimulation can be a problem.

Polycystic ovary syndrome

This is a common cause of infertility, affecting 5–10% of women of reproductive age. It is characterised by abnormal ovarian function with hyperandrogenism. Other complaints include menstrual disturbance, hirsutism and acne. It is often associated with obesity and insulin resistance in adipose and muscle tissue, conferring an increased risk of diabetes and cardiovascular disease in later life. Metformin (Ch. 40) is a first-line treatment, and the resulting improvement in insulin sensitivity reduces androgen concentrations. This leads to weight loss, reduction of the consequences of hyperandrogenisation, and improved fertility. If fertility is not restored, then clomifene can be added. In the absence of good safety data, metformin is usually stopped during pregnancy. There is potential for the use of newer insulin sensitisers such as the thiazolidinediones (Ch. 40) in polycystic ovary syndrome, and promising results have been obtained with these agents.

Preparation for assisted conception (IVF)

Ovulation is targeted on a particular date, and initial inhalation of a gonadorelin analogue or use of a gonadorelin antagonist will 'switch off' natural cyclical menstrual activity. Ovarian stimulation treatment is then begun to achieve maturation of oocytes at the time chosen for egg recovery prior to IVF. This involves giving large doses of HCG or HMG to stimulate the maturation of several follicles (superovulation treatment). These ova are then 'harvested' by aspiration of the follicles.

Male gonadotrophin deficiency

This requires long courses of gonadotrophin injections, initially to achieve external sexual maturation and then to maintain satisfactory sperm production. Spermatozoa take 70–80 days to mature, and a year or more of treatment may be needed to achieve optimal response. A combination of HMG and HCG is usually given.

Posterior pituitary hormones

Vasopressin

Vasopressin is a nonapeptide, sometimes referred to as arginine vasopressin (AVP) because human vasopressin has an arginine residue in position 8. It is also known as antidiuretic hormone (ADH). Vasopressin is released from neurosecretory cells of the hypothalamus and transported down the axons of the nerve cells that form the pituitary stalk. It is stored in the nerve endings in the posterior pituitary and released in response to stimulation of the hypothalamus via osmoreceptors, sodium receptors and volume receptors. Vasopressin has two main target tissues: vascular smooth muscle (via V1 receptors), leading to calcium influx into the cell, and the distal tubules of the kidney nephron (via V2 receptors), leading to intracellular cAMP production. A subtype of the V1 receptor (known as V1b or V3) is present on the pituitary. In the kidney, vasopressin facilitates water reabsorption specifically from the collecting ducts to produce a more concentrated urine. Vasoconstriction sufficient to raise blood pressure only occurs at high plasma vasopressin concentrations. Vasopressin is metabolised in many tissues, including the liver and kidney, and has a very short half-life of about 10 min. It is given therapeutically by subcutaneous or intramuscular injection or by intravenous infusion.

Vasopressin analogues

Examples: desmopressin, terlipressin

Vasopressin has a short duration of action. By deamination of residue 1 and substitution of D-arginine for L-arginine in position 8, the diuretic effect is increased, the pressor effect is reduced, and the action is prolonged. The resulting compound, known as des-amino-D-arginine vasopressin (DDAVP or desmopressin), is absorbed through the nasal mucosa and is most conveniently administered by a metered-dose nasal spray. It can also be given by subcutaneous, intramuscular or intravenous injection. An additional action of parenteral desmopressin is to increase clotting factor VIII concentration in blood (Ch. 11).

Terlipressin is also a vasopressin analogue that is used to treat bleeding oesophageal varices. It is fully discussed in Chapter 36.

Pharmacokinetics

Like the native hormone, desmopressin is metabolised in the liver and kidney, but it has a longer half-life than vasopressin.

Unwanted effects

- excessive water retention, producing dilutional hyponatraemia
- headache
- nausea, vomiting and abdominal pain.

Clinical uses of vasopressin and its analogues

- Treatment of cranial diabetes insipidus (see below), although the long-acting derivative desmopressin is usually used for maintenance treatment.
- Vasopressin can be given intranasally for primary nocturnal enuresis.

- To control bleeding from oesophageal varices in portal hypertension (Ch. 36). Aqueous vasopressin is infused intravenously to produce vasoconstriction. The analogue terlipressin is now preferred for this indication.
- Desmopressin by injection is used to boost factor VIII concentration and reduce bleeding in mild to moderate haemophilia.
- Desmopressin can be given to test for urine concentrating ability in suspected diabetes insipidus (see below).

Diabetes insipidus

Diabetes insipidus is usually caused by a failure of secretion of vasopressin in the hypothalamus ('cranial' diabetes insipidus). Tumours, inflammatory conditions, granulomatous conditions such as sarcoidosis, and trauma to the hypothalamus are the main causes. A distinct condition known as nephrogenic diabetes insipidus occurs when the kidney is unresponsive to vasopressin. It results from a hereditary deficiency of renal vasopressin receptors or sometimes arises as a consequence of drug therapy, particularly with lithium (Ch. 22) or the tetracycline demeclocycline. Diabetes insipidus presents clinically with thirst, polyuria, and a tendency to high plasma osmolality together with an inappropriately low urine osmolality. Vasopressin produces concentrated urine in patients with cranial diabetes insipidus, but the response in nephrogenic diabetes insipidus is impaired. Desmopressin is used for the long-term treatment of cranial diabetes insipidus.

Treatment of nephrogenic diabetes insipidus is more difficult. Paradoxically, thiazide diuretics (Ch. 14) can reduce the polyuria. Carbamazepine (Ch. 23) is also effective, by sensitising the renal tubule to the effect of vasopressin.

Oxytocin

Oxytocin is discussed in Chapter 45.

FURTHER READING

Baylis PH (1998) Diabetes insipidus. *J R Coll Physicians Lond* 32, 108–111

Bichet DG (1998) Nephrogenic diabetes insipidus. *Am J Med* 105, 431–442

Cahill DJ, Wardle PG (2002) Management of infertility. *BMJ* 325, 28–32

Colao A, Lombardi G (1998) Growth hormone and prolactin excess. *Lancet* 352, 1455–1461

Evers JLH (2002) Female subfertility. *Lancet* 360, 151–159

Harborne L, Fleming R, Lyall H et al (2003) Descriptive review of the evidence for the use of metformin in polycystic ovary syndrome. *Lancet* 361, 1894–1901 (**http://image.thelancet. com/extras/02art6157web.pdf**)

Huirne JAF Lambalk, CB (2001) Gonadotropin-releasing-hormone-receptor antagonists. *Lancet* 358, 1793–1803

Lamberts SWJ, de Herder WW, Van der Lely A-J (1998) Pituitary insufficiency. *Lancet* 352, 127–134

Melmed S, Casanueva FF, Cavagnini F et al (2002) Guidelines for acromegaly management. *J Clin Endocrinol Metab* 87, 4054–4058

Merza Z (2003) Modern treatment of acromegaly. *Postgrad Med J* 79, 189–193

Vance LE, Mauras N (1999) Growth hormone therapy in adults and children. *N Engl J Med* 341, 1206–1216

Self-assessment

In questions 1–3, the first statement, in italics, is true. Are the accompanying statements also true?

1. *The release of GH (somatotrophin) is reduced by somatostatin (GHRIH).*

   a. Somatostatin stimulates GH release.
   b. Somatostatin is produced only from the hypothalamus.
   c. The inhibition of GH release by bromocriptine in people with acromegaly is paradoxical.
   d. Octreotride is a useful drug for the treatment of acromegaly.

2. *Prolactin is an anterior pituitary hormone that is an essential hormone for milk secretion by the mammary gland; it also contributes to reduced fertility by suppressing steroidogenesis.*

   a. Bromocriptine reduces prolactin secretion.
   b. Continuous administration of analogues of gonadotrophin stimulates sex steroid synthesis.
   c. The gonadotrophin analogue gonadorelin has no clinical use in males.
   d. Gonadorelin is used for the treatment of endometriosis.
   e. Follitropin alfa is a genetically engineered FSH used in preparation for in vitro fertilisation.

3. *Vasopressin is an antidiuretic hormone and acts on the collecting ducts to facilitate water reabsorption. The response to vasopressin is impaired in nephrogenic diabetes insipidus.*

   a. Vasopressin is a peptide.
   b. Nephrogenic diabetes insipidus is a condition in which there is a failure of secretion of vasopressin (ADH).
   c. In nephrogenic diabetes insipidus, thiazide diuretics increase the polyuria.

4. Choose the one **incorrect** statement from the following options about GH.

   A. The release of GH is constant through a 24-h period.
   B. GH acts by stimulation of IGF-1 release.
   C. In acromegaly, the dopamine receptor agonist cabergoline inhibits IGF-1 levels.
   D. IGF-1 has a negative feedback effect on GH release.
   E. GH that is used in deficiency in children is obtained by recombinant DNA techniques.

5. Choose the one **incorrect** statement from these options about GnRH.

   A. GnRH used in treating IVF needs to be given by continuous high-dose infusion to stimulate sufficient gonadotrophin release.
   B. GnRH reduces testosterone secretion in men with prostate cancer.
   C. GnRH given in high dose cause a menopausal-like effect.
   D. Clomifene stimulates FSH secretion by having an anti-oestrogenic effect.
   E. GnRH produces a surge in gonadotrophins before blocking FSH and LH release.

6. Case history questions
   An assessment of a 10-year-old girl with short stature showed that she had abnormally low levels of GHRH and GH.

   a. Was this girl too old to benefit from treatment?
   b. If not, what treatment would you recommend and how would you administer it?
   c. What unwanted effects might occur?

   The answers are provided on page 738.

Pituitary and hypothalamic hormones

Drug	Half-life (h)	Elimination	Comments
Anterior pituitary hormones			
Chorionic gonadotrophin	30–35	Metabolism + renal	Glycoprotein extracted from the urine of pregnant women; given by subcutaneous or intramuscular injection; the half-life is longer after subcutaneous or intramuscular injection (30–35 h) because of slow release from the site of injection
Choriogonadotropin alfa	29	Metabolism + renal	Recombinant human chorionic gonadotrophin; given by subcutaneous injection; routes of metabolism have not been defined; about 10% is excreted in urine
Follitropin alfa and beta	24 (alfa), 30–40 (beta)	Metabolism + renal	Recombinant human follicle-stimulating hormone (FSH); given by subcutaneous or intramuscular injection
Human menopausal gonadotrophins (menotrophin)	7–10 (FSH) 3 (LH)	Metabolism	Contains a 1:1 mixture of pituitary-derived FSH and luteinising hormone (LH); given by deep intramuscular or subcutaneous injection; peak concentrations seen at 4–6 h after administration; metabolites eliminated in urine
Lutropin alfa	–	–	Recombinant human LH; given by subcutaneous injection; limited data available
Tetracosactide (cosyntropin)	0.2	Metabolism	Corticotrophin (ACTH) analogue; used largely as a test of adrenocortical function (formerly given by intramuscular injection for conditions such as Crohn's diseases and rheumatoid arthritis); given by intramuscular or intravenous injection; slower release from intramuscular injection; metabolised by endopeptidases in serum
Gonadotrophin-releasing hormone (GnRH) antagonists			Inhibit the release of gonadotrophins (LH and FSH); used to inhibit premature LH surges in the treatment of female infertility (under specialist supervision)
Cetrorelix	20–60	Metabolism	A synthetic decapeptide given by subcutaneous injection; metabolised by peptidases; some is eliminated unchanged in urine and bile
Ganirelix	16	Metabolism	Given by subcutaneous injection; metabolised by peptidases to oligopeptide products; some is eliminated unchanged in urine and bile
Anti-oestrogens			Used in the treatment of female infertility due to oligomenorrhoea or secondary amenorrhoea; they occupy oestrogen receptors and interfere with feedback mechanisms inducing gonadotrophin release

Drug compendium

continued

Pituitary and hypothalamic hormones *(continued)*

Drug	Half-life (h)	Elimination	Comments
Clomifene	5 days	Metabolism + bile	Anti-oestrogen given orally; a racemate with the more active isomer (zuclomifene) accumulating over the first few days of treatment; undergoes enterohepatic circulation
Tamoxifen	7 days	Metabolism	Main use is in breast cancer – see Ch. 52
Growth hormone			
Somatropin	0.5 (iv)	Metabolism	Synthetic form of growth hormone (somatotrophin); given by subcutaneous or intramuscular injection; serum half-life after subcutaneous administration (usual route) is 4 h due to absorption rate-limited elimination
Somatostatin (growth hormone release- inhibiting hormone – GHRIH) analogues			
Lanreotide	1.3	Renal + metabolism	Used for acromegaly and neuroendocrine tumours and for the treatment of thyroid tumours; given by intramuscular or deep subcutaneous injection; eliminated by renal excretion and probably by tissue uptake and metabolism
Octreotide	1.7	Renal + metabolism	Used for acromegaly and neuroendocrine tumours, and for reducing vomiting in palliative care and stopping oesophageal variceal bleeds; given by subcutaneous injection or by intravenous injection if a more rapid response is required; eliminated by renal excretion (about 40%) and probably by tissue uptake and metabolism
Hypothalamic hormones			
Gonadorelin	4 min	Metabolism (+ renal)	Gonadotrophin-releasing hormone (GnRH); given by subcutaneous or intravenous injection; very short half-life probably reflects tissue uptake and intracellular metabolism; synthetic analogues are used for endometriosis (Ch. 45) and breast and prostate cancer (Ch. 52)
Protirelin (TRH)	4 min	Metabolism	Thyrotrophin-releasing hormone; used for assessment of thyroid function; given by intravenous injection; rapidly metabolised by tissues and serum; half-life is for TRH
Sermorelin (GHRH)	1 (GHRH)	Metabolism	Analogue of growth hormone-releasing hormone (GHRH); used as a diagnostic test of secretion of growth hormone (GH); given by intravenous injection; half-life is for GHRH; the time for the release and removal of GH after GHRH are about 10 min and 20–30 min respectively

continued

Pituitary and hypothalamic hormones *(continued)*

Drug	Half-life (h)	Elimination	Comments
Posterior pituitary hormones and antagonists			
Desmopressin	0.5–2	Metabolism	Vasopressin analogue; used for treatment of pituitary diabetes insipidus; given orally, intranasally or by subcutaneous, intramuscular or intravenous injection; analogue of antidiuretic hormone (ADH); poor oral bioavailability due to presystemic metabolism; metabolised by liver, kidney and plasma to inactive products
Terlipressin	0.5	Metabolism	Used for treatment of oesophageal varices; given by intravenous injection; triglycyl prodrug of lysine-vasopressin which is metabolised by hydrolysis to the active form (which then has a formation rate-limited half-life of 0.5 h)
Vasopressin (ADH)	5–15 min	Metabolism	Used for treatment of pituitary diabetes insipidus and bleeding oesophageal varices; given by subcutaneous or intramuscular injection or by intravenous infusion; rapidly metabolised by kidney, liver, brain and placenta
Demeclocycline	10–15	Renal + bile	Has anti-ADH action possibly due to blockade of renal tubular effects of ADH; used for treatment of hyponatraemia resulting from inappropriate secretion of ADH; given orally; oral bioavailability is 66% (due to poor absorption)

Drug compendium

Corticosteroids (glucocorticoids and mineralocorticoids)

Structure and synthesis of steroid hormones

Steroid hormones comprise a range of compounds synthesised mainly in the adrenal cortex and the gonads. They are derived from cholesterol and share a common nucleus (Fig. 44.1). The steroid hormones responsible for phenotypic gender differences are known as the sex hormones; these compounds are considered in Chapters 45 and 46. The pathways of steroid hormone synthesis are shown in Figure 44.2.

This chapter considers steroid hormones derived predominantly from the adrenal cortex that are known as adrenal corticosteroids. They have two distinct classes of action, referred to as glucocorticoid and mineralocorticoid activity: glucocorticoid activity affects carbohydrate and protein metabolism, while mineralocorticoid activity affects water and electrolyte balance (see below and Table 44.1). The natural glucocorticoid cortisol (also known as hydrocortisone) and the natural mineralocorticoid aldosterone differ only in their constituents at position 17 and 18 of the steroid nucleus. Hydrocortisone has a hydroxyl grouping at position 17, and aldosterone an aldehyde grouping at position 18. There is overlap in activity of individual molecules, particularly when their structures are similar; for example, hydrocortisone has approximately equal glucocorticoid and mineralocorticoid activity. Synthetic corticosteroids have been modified structurally to enhance either the glucocorticoid or mineralocorticoid activity.

Glucocorticoid (and, to a lesser extent, mineralocorticoid) secretion is controlled by the hypothalamic–pituitary–adrenal axis (Fig. 44.3). An increase in glucocorticoid blood concentration feeds back to reduce corticotrophin-releasing factor (CRF) release.

Mode of action of steroid hormones

All steroid hormones share a common receptor mechanism, but have distinct receptors for the different structural variants. The distribution of these various receptors among tissues gives tissue specificity to each type of steroid hormone and defines its activity. In the circulation, steroid hormones are bound to specific globulins. Steroids are highly lipophilic and cross cell membranes by diffusion and bind to a specific cytoplasmic receptor (Ch. 1). In the absence of a steroid molecule, the receptor is retained in the cytoplasm and prevented from migrating to the cell nucleus because it is associated with a heat shock protein (HSP). Binding of the steroid to the receptor dissociates the complex from the HSP, and the steroid–receptor complex then enters the nucleus and binds to a steroid response element on the target genes (see Fig. 1.9). The binding usually involves the presence of other proteins, called chaperone proteins, and can lead to either increased or decreased transcription of proteins, depending on the target cell. Some genes are activated by simple interaction of the steroid receptor with the steroid response element, whereas others are modulated by interaction of the complex with various intranuclear co-activator complexes.

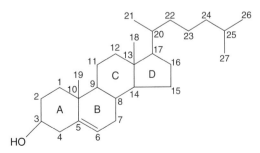

Fig. 44.1
The 'core' structure of steroid hormones is derived from the cholesterol molecule shown. Note: the four rings are each identified by a letter and each carbon atom by a number.

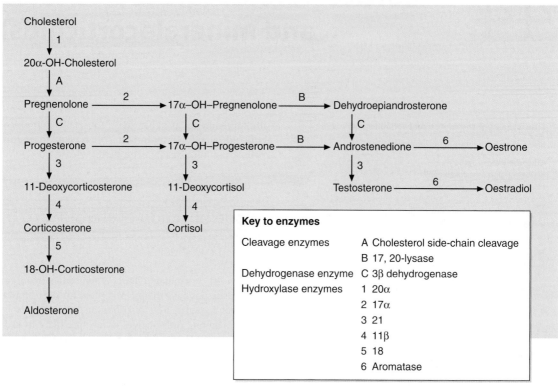

Fig. 44.2
Pathways of steroid hormone biosynthesis.

The corticosteroid receptor only interacts with the response element for a matter of seconds before dissociating, and appears to have a 'hit and run' effect on gene transcription. When corticosteroids are given for a therapeutic effect, the response is delayed by many hours due to the time taken for modulation of protein synthesis.

Glucocorticoids

Examples: betamethasone, dexamethasone, hydrocortisone, prednisolone

Hydrocortisone (cortisol) is the main natural glucocorticoid in humans. It is synthesised in the adrenal cortex in response to adrenocorticotrophic hormone (ACTH) secreted from the anterior pituitary. Glucocorticoid receptors are found in most tissues, giving hydrocortisone a wide range of actions. Glucocorticoids have important immunomodulatory actions that arise predominantly from inhibition of the activity of pro-inflammatory transcription factors such as activator protein-1 (AP-1)

Table 44.1
Relative glucocorticoid and mineralocorticoid activities of some natural and synthetic steroid hormones

	Glucocorticoid	Mineralocorticoid
Cortisol (hydrocortisone)	1	1
Prednisolone	4	0.8
Dexamethasone	30	Negligible
Betamethasone	30	Negligible
Aldosterone	0	80
Fludrocortisone	10	125

and nuclear factor kappa B (NF-κB) (transrepression). The activated glucocorticoid receptors recruit histone deacetylases to the transcription complex of genes that have been activated by inflammatory stimuli. The deacetylation of core histones at the transcription complex silences these genes. Glucocorticoids also activate anti-inflammatory genes (transactivation), which contributes to their immunomodulatory action. The effects on mediators which contribute to the anti-inflammatory consequences of glucocorticoid action include:

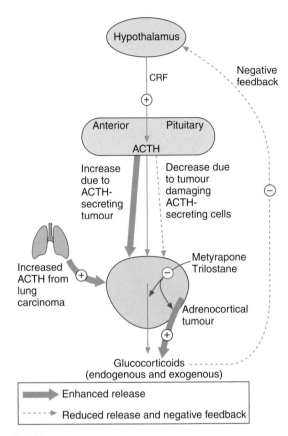

Fig. 44.3
Control of secretion of glucocorticoids and mineralocorticoids.
Stimulation by corticotrophin-releasing factor (CRF) and adrenocorticotrophic hormone (ACTH) increases the release of glucocorticoids and mineralocorticoids. The level of glucocorticoids in the blood feeds back and negatively controls the release of CRF and ACTH. Synthetic glucocorticoids have the same action, suppressing the hypothalamic–pituitary axis. In conditions in which excess corticosteroids are released, e.g. in ACTH-secreting tumours or adrenocortical tumours, corticosteroid synthesis and release can be reduced by drug therapy, shown in red. In patients with tumours that result in hormone-induced reduction in glucocorticoids, synthetic glucocorticoids can be administered.

- inhibition of synthesis of inducible cyclo-oxygenase (COX-2)
- inhibition of the inducible form of nitric oxide synthase
- inhibition of the synthesis of inflammatory cytokines such as interleukins (IL)-1, -2, -3, -4, -5, -6, -9, -12, -13, -16, -17 and -18, tumour necrosis factor alpha (TNFα) and many others
- inhibition of the synthesis of chemokines such as IL-8, RANTES (regulated on activation normal T-cell expressed and secreted), monocyte chemo-attractant proteins and eotaxin
- stimulation of the production of the intracellular protein annexin-1; this inhibits phospholipase A$_2$ and

therefore reduces the synthesis of prostaglandins and leukotrienes (Ch. 29); it is also involved in the negative feedback of glucocorticoids on the hypothalamus.

Glucocorticoids also transactivate other genes for enzymes involved in metabolic control. These actions are probably responsible for many of the non-immunomodulatory effects of glucocorticoids.

Actions of glucocorticoids

Anti-inflammatory effects (see also Ch. 12)

- Inhibition of mononuclear cell and neutrophil leucocyte migration and their adhesion to inflamed capillary endothelium. The ability of these inflammatory cells to phagocytose and destroy micro-organisms and to release oxygen free radicals is also reduced.
- Reduced synthesis of inflammatory prostaglandins and leukotrienes (Ch. 29).
- Impaired fibroblast activity, which reduces tissue repair.
- Capillary permeability is decreased, which has a protective effect on blood volume and raises blood pressure. The sensitivity of vascular walls to the vasoconstrictor actions of catecholamines is also enhanced.

Immunological actions

- The main immunological effect is reduced proliferation of T lymphocytes. This is largely due to reduced production of the cytokine IL-2 (Ch. 38).
- Decreased IgG production.

Metabolic effects

The metabolic effects of glucocorticoids are on carbohydrate and protein metabolism.

- Gluconeogenesis is increased and leads to increased storage of glycogen in the liver and, to a lesser extent, in muscle. Tissue uptake and utilisation of glucose is impaired. These actions promote hyperglycaemia.
- Protein is degraded, particularly in muscle, to enable synthesis of glucose and to increase the available pool of amino acids, while protein synthesis is inhibited. As a result, there is an overall negative nitrogen balance.
- Fat is redistributed from the corticosteroid-sensitive fat stores in the limbs to the corticosteroid-resistant stores in the face, neck and trunk. This action results from enhancement of the lipolytic response to catecholamines.

- Osteoblast formation is decreased. The function of mature osteoblasts is inhibited. These actions decrease bone mineralisation.

Central nervous system effects

Plasma cortisol concentrations rise to a peak at the time of awakening and are lowest during sleep. In general, high circulating concentrations of hydrocortisone are associated with alertness, but severe disturbances of mood may occur with abnormally high levels of glucocorticoid. Low concentrations produce a feeling of lethargy.

Mineralocorticoid effects

Natural glucocorticoids also have mineralocorticoid activity (see below). Synthetic glucocorticoid compounds are altered structurally to change the relationship between the amount of mineralocorticoid and glucocorticoid activity (Table 44.1).

Pharmacokinetics of glucocorticoids

Both hydrocortisone and synthetic glucocorticoids are used in clinical practice. They are readily absorbed from the gut. Hydrocortisone binds to corticosteroid-binding globulin and to albumin in the blood; it is extensively metabolised in the gut wall and liver. Synthetic glucocorticoids are more potent than hydrocortisone and more slowly metabolised in the liver, giving them a longer duration of action. Substantial amounts are excreted via the kidney as metabolites. They bind to albumin but not to corticosteroid-binding globulin.

Prednisone is a synthetic glucocorticoid which is effectively a prodrug because most of its activity results from conversion in the liver to prednisolone; the latter compound is preferred in clinical practice. Of the many synthetic glucocorticoids, dexamethasone is the most potent and has the least mineralocorticoid activity.

Most glucocorticoids are available in formulations for parenteral use. This does not appreciably shorten the time to onset of action, which is delayed by up to 8 h while protein synthesis is modulated intracellularly. Glucocorticoids can also be delivered topically to reduce their systemic actions (see below). Some glucocorticoids (e.g. beclometasone, budesonide and fluticasone by inhaler for asthma) have preparations for local use, but systemic adverse effects can occur, particularly with high doses (see Chs 12 and 34 for example).

The plasma half-lives vary, but their biological (i.e. effective) half-lives are long (varying from 12 h for hydrocortisone to two days for dexamethasone) because of their mechanism of action via protein synthesis.

> **Box 44.1**
>
> **Examples of diseases for which systemic glucocorticoid therapy is useful**
>
> *Replacement therapy in corticosteroid deficiency*
> *Acute inflammatory disease*
>   Bronchial asthma
>   Anaphylaxis and angioedema
>   Acute fibrosing alveolitis
>
> *Chronic inflammatory disease*
>   Connective tissue disorders, e.g. systemic lupus erythematosus, polymyositis, vasculitides
>   Renal disorder, e.g. glomerulonephritis
>   Hepatic disorders, e.. chronic active hepatitis
>   Bowel disorders, e.g. inflammatory bowel disease
>   Eye disorders, e.g. posterior uveitis
>
> *Neoplastic disease*
>   Myeloma
>   Lymphomas
>   Lymphocytic leukaemias
>
> *Miscellaneous disorders*
>   Bell's palsy
>   Sarcoidosis
>   Organ transplantation

Clinical uses of systemically administered glucocorticoids

Box 44.1 shows some of the uses of systemic glucocorticoids.

Physiological replacement therapy for corticosteroid deficiency. Hydrocortisone or an equivalent synthetic glucocorticoid is given orally twice or three times daily in doses as close as possible to the amount normally secreted by the adrenal cortex. In stressful situations, for example intercurrent infection, the dose must be doubled or tripled. Acute adrenal insufficiency requires immediate treatment with high-dose intravenous hydrocortisone. Conditions that can give rise to corticosteroid deficiency are shown in Box 44.3.

Therapeutic uses. The anti-inflammatory and immunosuppressive effects of glucocorticoids are used for various inflammatory diseases (especially those which are immunologically mediated) and neoplastic conditions, particularly when they involve lymphoid tissue (Box 44.1). Powerful glucocorticoids such as prednisolone with little mineralocorticoid activity are usually chosen.

For uses of ACTH and analogues, see Chapter 43.

Table 44.2
Examples of topical corticosteroid administration

Disease	Mode of administration	Chapter
Asthma	Aerosol	12
Vasomotor rhinitis	Aerosol	39
Eczema	Ointment or cream	49
Superficial ocular inflammation	Aqueous solution	50
Ulcerative colitis	Aqueous solution or foam enema	34
Proctitis	Suppository	34
Arthritis	Aqueous solution by intra-articular injection	30

Topical administration of glucocorticoids

Topical use of glucocorticoids can deliver high concentrations to a target site and reduce systemic unwanted effects. However, significant absorption into the blood can occur at higher doses. Examples of the clinical uses of topical corticosteroids are given in Table 44.2.

Unwanted effects of glucocorticoids

Pharmacological doses of glucocorticoids given over long periods will produce the typical features of adrenocortical overactivity (Cushing's syndrome). Unwanted glucocorticoid actions are shown in Box 44.2.

Cushing's syndrome

Cushing's syndrome is characterised by excessive glucocorticoid effects (Box 44.2). There are four causes (Box 44.3).

Management of Cushing's syndrome

The definitive treatment for excessive pituitary secretion of ACTH (usually from an adenoma) and for unilateral adrenal tumours is surgery, with subsequent radiotherapy for some pituitary tumours.

Drug treatment to reduce corticosteroid secretion is desirable for several weeks before surgery, to reverse the excessive tissue catabolism and correct the metabolic disturbances. This is usually achieved with metyrapone. This drug reduces corticosteroid biosynthesis by competitive inhibition of 11β-hydroxylase (Figs 44.1, 44.2 – enzyme 4). It also inhibits cytochrome P450 in the liver, which can produce important drug interactions (Ch. 2). Oral absorption of metyrapone is variable, and extensive metabolism occurs in the liver. Gastrointestinal upset is the main unwanted effect. Trilostane is an alter-

native to metyrapone, and is a reversible inhibitor of the earlier enzymatic step of 3β-dehydrogenation (Fig. 44.2 – enzyme C). The antifungal agent ketoconazole (Ch. 51) reduces cortisol synthesis by inhibition of 11β-hydroxylase, but its onset of action is slower than that of metyrapone. It also inhibits sex steroid production, and therefore often causes gynaecomastia and decreased libido in males, and

Box 44.2

Unwanted effects of glucocorticoids

- Central obesity with 'buffalo hump', moon face and abdominal striae.
- Loss of supporting tissue in skin with skin atrophy, bruising, and poor wound healing. Local atrophy can be marked at the site of topical corticosteroid application.
- Osteoporosis due to catabolism of protein matrix in the bone and defective mineralisation.
- Proximal (i.e. shoulder and hip girdle) muscle wasting and weakness.
- Hyperglycaemia, which may lead to overt diabetes mellitus (Ch. 40).
- Peptic ulceration due to gastrointestinal prostaglandin inhibition (Ch. 33).
- Mood changes, including euphoria and occasionally psychosis.
- Posterior capsular cataracts in the eye, and exacerbation of glaucoma.
- Increased susceptibility to infection with bacteria, viruses or fungi. Activation of latent infection such as tuberculosis can also occur.
- Growth retardation in children, with reduced linear bone growth and premature epiphyseal closure.
- After long-term treatment, sudden withdrawal can produce an acute adrenal crisis due to suppression of the hypothalamic–pituitary–adrenal axis and adrenal atrophy. Recovery of adrenal responsiveness can take several months. Basal cortisol secretion is restored before maximal responses, leaving patients at risk during stress and intercurrent infection.
- Mineralocorticoid effects (which vary among the different drugs).

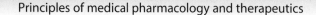

hirsutism in females. It can be used alone, or in combination with metyrapone.

Ectopic ACTH secretion is not usually amenable to surgical cure but palliative drug treatment with metyrapone can be helpful (Fig. 44.3).

Mineralocorticoids

Example: fluorocortisone

Aldosterone is the principal mineralocorticoid and is secreted from the zona glomerulosa of the adrenal cortex. Aldosterone secretion is regulated by several factors, of which angiotensin II (Ch. 6), a low plasma Na$^+$ and a high plasma K$^+$ are the most important. Angiotensin II acts via specific angiotensin receptors (AT$_1$ and AT$_2$) (see Ch. 4 and Ch. 6), of which the AT$_1$ receptor induces aldosterone release. ACTH has some stimulatory effect on aldosterone secretion. Mineralocorticoid receptors are found in fewer tissues than are glucocorticoid receptors. The main target cells are in the distal renal tubule and

collecting duct, where aldosterone increases the permeability of the luminal tubular membrane to Na$^+$ by increasing the number of Na$^+$ channels. It also stimulates the Na$^+$/K$^+$-ATPase pump in the basolateral membrane, which leads to active Na$^+$ reabsorption and loss of K$^+$ into tubular urine (Ch. 14). Water is passively reabsorbed with Na$^+$, so extracellular fluid volume and blood pressure are increased. Target cells for aldosterone contain the enzyme 11β-hydroxysteroid dehydrogenase which degrades hydrocortisone to compounds that have very low affinity for the mineralocorticoid receptor. This ensures that aldosterone-responsive tissues are not stimulated by glucocorticoids.

Fludrocortisone

Pharmacokinetics
Aldosterone is almost completely inactivated at its first passage through the liver and is therefore unsuitable for oral administration. 9α-Fluorohydrocortisone (fludrocortisone) is a synthetic alternative which is well absorbed from the gut; about 10% escapes first-pass metabolism. The half-life is short due to hepatic metabolism.

Unwanted effects
Excessive Na$^+$ retention and K$^+$ loss can occur with pharmacological doses of fludrocortisone. Hypertension can result; however, the expansion of blood volume stimulates cardiac stretch receptors, leading to secretion of natriuretic peptides. The resulting natriuresis initiates an 'escape' mechanism which establishes a new equilibrium between Na$^+$ intake and excretion at a higher blood volume. Consequently, oedema does not usually occur.

Clinical uses of fludrocortisone

- Fludrocortisone is given as replacement therapy for defective aldosterone production. This is usually the result of primary adrenal pathology with destruction of all three zones of the cortex (Addison's disease).
- Expansion of blood volume by fludrocortisone can be used to raise blood pressure in postural hypotension resulting from autonomic neuropathy; however, it often produces supine hypertension without fully eliminating the postural fall in blood pressure.

Primary hyperaldosteronism (Conn's syndrome)

Autonomous oversecretion of aldosterone causes hypertension and a hypokalaemic alkalosis. Most cases are caused by an adenoma in the zona glomerulosa of the adrenal cortex and are treated surgically. The remainder are usually the result of hyperplasia of both zonae glomerulosa; these cases are usually less severe clinically and a potassium-sparing diuretic (usually spironolactone) is the treatment of choice (Ch. 14).

FURTHER READING

Adcock IA (2003) Glucocorticoids: mechanisms and future agents. *Curr Allerg Asthma Rep* 3, 249–257

Canalis E (2003) Mechanisms of glucocorticoid-induced osteoporosis. *Curr Opin Rheumatol* 15, 454–457

Lipworth BS (1999) Systemic adverse effects of inhaled corticosteroid therapy. *Arch Intern Med* 159, 941–955

Lovas K, Husebye ES (2003) Replacement therapy in Addison's disease. *Expert Opin Pharmacother* 4, 2145–2149

Morris D, Grossman A (2002) The medical management of Cushing's syndrome. *Ann N Y Acad Sci* 970, 119–133

Young WF Jr (2003) Minireview: primary aldosteronism – changing concepts in diagnosis and treatment. *Endocrinology* 144, 2208–2213

Self-assessment

In questions 1–4, the first statement, in italics, is true. Are the accompanying statements also true?

1. *In maximum recommended doses, inhaled corticosteroids can cause systemic unwanted effects.*

   a. Oral fludrocortisone is a useful anti-inflammatory steroid in severe asthma.
   b. Beclometasone is not used orally.

2. *Corticosteroids take many hours to produce their clinical effect because they act by modulating cellular production of proteins.*

   a. Hypoglycaemia is common during glucocorticoid administration.
   b. If prolonged administration of prednisolone results in unwanted effects, it is appropriate to withdraw the drug slowly.

3. *Mineralocorticoid secretion is decreased in Addison's disease. Examples are primary adrenal insufficiency (predominantly autoimmune) or secondary insufficiency, e.g. due to a pituitary tumour or following prolonged glucocorticoid treatment.*

   a. Aldosterone secretion is inhibited by angiotensin II.
   b. Aldosterone and cortisol secretion are regulated by ACTH.

4. *Glucocorticoids affect all inflammatory responses caused by infection, chemical or altered immune stimuli.*

   a. Dexamethasone causes vomiting.
   b. Glucocorticoids delay wound healing.
   c. Before giving an intra-articular injection of glucocorticoid in gout, infection of the joint should be excluded.

5. Case history 1 questions

   > A 35-year-old female showed signs of cortisol excess, including centripetal obesity, muscle weakness, easy bruising and amenorrhoea.

   a. What were the possible causes?

   > She was not taking corticosteroids, eliminating an iatrogenic cause. The cortisol level in a 24-h urine collection was elevated. Plasma ACTH levels were also high.

   b. What did these results indicate?

   > A single high dose of dexamethasone was administered and resulted in only marginal suppression of plasma cortisol.

   c. What did this result indicate?

   > A computed tomography scan and other tests showed an inoperable carcinoma of the bronchus.

   d. What treatment could be given?

6. Case history 2 questions

   > Mr BFG, a 69-year-old man, suffered from late-onset asthma, which was poorly controlled by β_2-adrenoceptor agonists. His GP prescribed a corticosteroid aerosol (low dose) which helped him initially.

   a. Which corticosteroids could have been given by aerosol?
   b. What were the possible unwanted effects of inhaled corticosteroid?

   > Mr BFG then had a particularly severe attack (acute severe asthma or status asthmaticus) which led to his admission to hospital as an emergency.

c. Amongst the drugs he was given was a corticosteroid. Which drug was likely to have been given, by what route, and what was the objective of its use?

> Mr BFG's status asthmaticus resolved and he was then prescribed a course of oral corticosteroid while in hospital and subsequently sent home with high-dose inhaled corticosteroid.

d. Which corticosteroid could have been used for oral therapy?
e. Comment on the principles that should be followed for the initiation and duration of the course of treatment with the oral corticosteroid.
f. Compare the unwanted effects resulting from high-dose oral corticosteroid with those of the low-dose aerosol.

> Mr BFG's asthma was poorly controlled by high-dose inhaled corticosteroid and it was decided to recommence oral therapy.

g. Why would oral therapy likely to have been better than inhaled therapy in more severe asthma?
h. How would you have determined the dose to be used and monitor its appropriateness?

> After many months of this therapy, Mr BFG started to complain of apparently unrelated problems, including: recurrent minor infections; minor epigastric discomfort, especially on an empty stomach; weight gain and increased appetite; a tendency to bruise easily; and severe back pain after a minor fall.
>
> Examination revealed a cushingoid appearance, and investigation showed a raised plasma glucose level and decreased plasma levels of cortisol and ACTH.

i. Discuss the reasons for Mr BFG's symptoms.

The answers are provided on pages 738–739.

Corticosteroids. The durations of action ('biological half-lives') of corticosteroids greatly exceed their chemical half-lives because of their mechanism of action

Drug	Half-life (h)	Elimination	Comments
Glucocorticoids			
Betamethasone	35–55	Metabolism	Used for suppression of inflammatory and allergic disorders, congenital adrenal hyperplasia and cerebral oedema; given orally, topically, by intramuscular or slow intravenous injection, or by intravenous infusion; phosphate ester prodrug used for injections; ester prodrugs hydrolysed to betamethasone, which is inactivated by metabolism
Cortisone acetate	1–2 (HC)	Metabolism	Formerly used for replacement therapy; given orally; oral bioavailability is 20–90%; rapidly hydrolysed and converted to cortisol (hydrocortisone; HC) which is inactivated by oxidation to cortisone and reduction to tetrahydrocortisol
Deflazacort	1	Metabolism	Used for suppression of inflammatory and allergic disorders; given orally; bioavailability not affected by food (absolute bioavailability not defined); hydrolysed to the active 21-desacetyl metabolite (21-hydroxy-compound)
Dexamethasone	2–4	Metabolism	Used for suppression of inflammatory and allergic disorders, congenital adrenal hyperplasia and cerebral oedema and diagnosis of Cushing's disease; given orally, by intramuscular or slow intravenous injection, or by intravenous infusion; phosphate ester prodrug used for injections; high but variable oral bioavailability possibly due to intestinal CYP3A metabolism; metabolised in the liver by CYP3A4-mediated oxidation to the 6-hydroxy compound
Hydrocortisone (cortisol)	1–2	Metabolism	Numerous anti-inflammatory and anti-allergic uses; given orally, by intramuscular or slow intravenous injection, or by intravenous infusion; phosphate ester prodrug used for injections, variable absorption (30–90%) due to first-pass metabolism; metabolised by oxidation to cortisone and reduction to dihydro- and tetrahydro-cortisol
Methylprednisolone	1–3	Metabolism	Used for suppression of inflammatory and allergic disorders, cerebral oedema and rheumatic disease; given orally, by intramuscular or slow intravenous injection, or by intravenous infusion; injectable forms are lipid-soluble esters in solvents; high oral bioavailability (80–90%); esters are very rapidly hydrolysed; metabolised in liver and kidney by reduction to 20-hydroxy compound
Prednisolone	2–4	Metabolism	Used for suppression of numerous inflammatory and allergic disorders; given orally, topically and by intramuscular injection; injectable form is the acetate ester as an aqueous suspension; high oral bioavailability (70–80%); extensively metabolised but all pathways have not been defined
Triamcinolone	2–5	Metabolism	Used for suppression of inflammatory and allergic disorders; given by deep intramuscular injection as an aqueous suspension; metabolised by oxidation
Mineralocorticoids			
Fludrocortisone acetate	0.5	Metabolism	Mineralocorticoid used in combination with hydrocortisone for adrenocortical insufficiency; given orally; low bioavailability (10%) due to first-pass metabolism; hydrolysed to fludrocortisol, which is reduced and eliminated as conjugated metabolites

continued

Drug compendium

Corticosteroids. The durations of action ('biological half-lives') of corticosteroids greatly exceed their chemical half-lives because of their mechanism of action *(continued)*

Drug	Half-life (h)	Elimination	Comments
Inhibitors of steroid metabolism			
Metyrapone	?	Metabolism	Competitive inhibitor of 11β-hydroxylation in the adrenal cortex; used to control the symptoms of Cushing's syndrome, especially prior to surgery; given orally; an old drug with few kinetic data available; eliminated by hepatic metabolism; inhibitor of CYP isoenzymes
Trilostane	?	Metabolism	Reversible inhibitor of 3β-hydroxysteroid dehydrogenase, causing inhibition of the synthesis of both glucocorticoids and mineralocorticoids; used in Cushing's syndrome (but is less effective than metyrapone) and primary hyperaldosteronism; given orally; eliminated by oxidation to a keto-analogue which has slightly more activity than the parent drug

Corticosteroids are also covered extensively in Chapters 12, 34, 38 and 39.

Female reproduction

ovulation at the expense of the remaining antral follicles, which regress. The regression possibly results from the lack of gonadotrophin receptors on the unsuccessful follicles.

The developing Graafian follicle is driven by FSH and LH to convert the androgens produced by thecal cells of the follicle into oestradiol within granulosa cells. Oestrogen secretion from the follicle slowly rises as the follicle matures. In the window of time between the early to mid follicular phase of the menstrual cycle, the modest concentration of oestrogen secreted exerts a negative feedback on both hypothalamic and pituitary gonadotrophin secretions. The low concentrations of progesterone also weakly suppress gonadotrophin secretion in the early follicular phase. Although circulating FSH levels are low, oestradiol enhances the effectiveness of the action of gonadotrophin on the ovary to stimulate further oestradiol synthesis.

In the late follicular phase, a cohort of granulosa cells in the maturing Graafian follicle differentiates under the influence of FSH and starts to express LH receptors. These granulosa cells can then be stimulated by LH to secrete progesterone and are destined to become the

Physiology of the menstrual cycle

The endocrine function of the hypothalamic–pituitary–ovarian axis acts through a series of feedback loops to control the reproductive processes of the menstrual cycle (Fig. 45.1). Following the shedding of the endometrium (days 1 to 3–5 of the menstrual cycle), a group of follicles in the ovary start to develop and mature under the influence of the gonadotrophic hormones follicle-stimulating hormone (FSH) and luteinising hormone (LH) secreted from the anterior pituitary. Release of the gonadotrophic hormones (FSH and LH) is controlled by pulsatile release of gonadotrophin-releasing hormone (GnRH), which is secreted from the hypothalamus. The prolonged release of low levels of FSH and LH results in the selection and ongoing maturation of a single Graafian follicle; this is prepared for

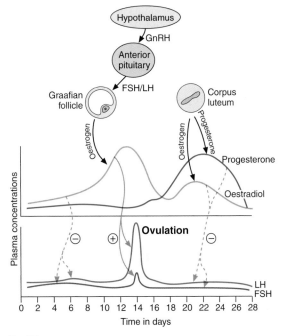

Fig. 45.1
Endocrine control of the menstrual cycle. - - -, Negative feedback; ——, positive feedback.

corpus luteum. The elevated circulating oestradiol levels in the mid-to late-follicular phase eventually reach a critical concentration of about 200 pg ml^{-1} for 48 h. This sustained concentration of oestradiol and the relatively rapid rate of increase in oestradiol triggers a switch from a negative feedback to a positive feedback of oestradiol upon the pituitary and hypothalamus. As a result, the midcycle surge of LH and, to a lesser extent, FSH that is essential for ovulation begins.

Following ovulation, the plasma LH levels fall rapidly and remain low throughout the secretory phase. The reason for this is that granulosa cells containing LH receptors proliferate in the corpus luteum and produce increasing concentrations of progesterone; this in turn suppresses LH and FSH production by negative feedback on the hypothalamus and pituitary. Plasma levels of oestrogen rise due to production by the corpus luteum. If implantation of a fertilised ovum does not occur, the corpus luteum regresses after about 10 days, possibly under the influence of local synthesis of vasoconstrictor prostaglandin (PG) $F_{2\alpha}$, although there is little direct confirmation of this in humans.

From day 1 to late in the menstrual cycle, gradually increasing plasma concentrations of oestrogen and progesterone produced as the menstrual cycle progresses result in proliferation and vascularisation of endometrial cells, which are able to secrete a variety of fluids and nutrients aimed at making the endometrium receptive for implantation. The temporal precision of the change in receptivity is critical if successful implantation is to occur. Oestrogens and progesterone cause the endometrium to become oedematous, and glands secrete increasing quantities of amino acids, sugars and glycoproteins in a viscous liquid. At the end of the menstrual cycle, the decreasing circulating levels of progesterone and oestrogen eventually no longer support the endometrium. Deprived of hormonal support, the endometrial spiral arteries go into spasm and the endometrial cells die, producing digestive enzymes. As a consequence of this and other changes, the endometrium is shed during menstruation.

The cervical mucus is also influenced by oestrogen and progesterone concentrations. Under the dominant influence of progesterone, cervical mucus is viscid and less penetrable by sperm, whereas at ovulation, the high plasma oestradiol concentration results in a thinner, elastic mucus that is easily penetrable by sperm. Progesterone also inhibits the motility of the fallopian tube, altering the transport of sperm, and the fertilised or unfertilised oocyte. Excess progesterone may alter the chance of fertilisation occurring or the embryo may reach the uterine cavity when the endometrium is not receptive to implantation. Oestrogens have the opposite action, increasing tubal motility, and may accelerate the transport of the ovum into the uterine cavity.

Pregnancy is accompanied by considerable hormonal changes. The combined feto-placental unit produces progressively greater quantities of oestrogen and progesterone which reach the maternal circulation. The placenta also produces human chorionic gonadotrophin (HCG) (Ch. 43) from early in pregnancy, which reaches a peak circulating concentration at about 50–60 days of gestation, then falls. HCG stimulates progesterone and oestrogen production from the corpus luteum. The corpus luteum is essential for the maintenance of pregnancy during the first 6–8 weeks, after which, placental production of hormones takes over. The increasing placental production of oestrogens, progesterone and human placental lactogen as pregnancy advances results in the development of duct and milk-secreting cells in the breast. The precise balance of sex steroids also contributes to quiescence of the uterus during pregnancy and the onset of labour at term.

Mechanism of action of oestrogens and progestogens

In common with other steroid hormones, both oestrogens and progestogens act by influencing gene transcription. They passively diffuse into the cell and associate with specific receptors either in the cytoplasm or cell nucleus (see Fig 1.9). The receptors are probably associated with 'chaperone' molecules when in their unbound state, which are displaced by the hormone. Oestrogen binds to two specific cytoplasmic receptors (ERα and ERβ), and the steroid–receptor complex enters the cell nucleus to act. The complex then associates with the oestrogen response elements of oestrogen-related genes on DNA. This leads to recruitment of co-activator or co-repressor molecules to the complex, and, therefore, gene activation or repression. In the absence of oestrogen, the receptor can also cyclically bind to the gene, but is then chemically modified without affecting gene transcription and degraded. Progesterone has two specific receptors (PR-A and PR-B) that regulate progestogen-responsive genes.

Steroidal contraceptives

Oral contraceptives ('the pill') are the most widely used form of contraception and contain either a combination of a synthetic oestrogen and a progestogen (a C-19 synthetic progesterone derivative) or a progestogen alone. The failure rate during perfect usage is 0.2–3 pregnancies per 100 women-years of use. The oestrogen component of the combined pill is usually ethinylestradiol (an oestrogen that is alkylated at C17 to slow its metabolism) but is occasionally mestranol, a compound that is metabolised in the liver to ethinylestradiol. Over the years since the oral contraceptive was introduced, the dose of the oestrogen component has been reduced. 'Second-generation' pills (to differentiate them from first-generation pills with a high oestrogen content) have 20–35 µg ethinylestradiol, although higher oestrogen concentrations are available for special uses. The progestogen component of the second-generation contraceptives is either levonorgestrel or norethisterone, which possess progestational but also androgenic activity.

'Third-generation' pills contain modified progestogens, such as desogestrel, gestodene, norgestimate and drospirenone, with less androgenic acitivity, and are used if there are unacceptable unwanted effects with other progestogens. Other differences and similarities between second- and third-generation contraceptives are discussed later.

Mechanisms of contraception

Elevated circulating levels of synthetic oestrogen and progestogen prevent the precise cyclic pattern of hormone-related events seen in the normal menstrual cycle.

- The combination of oestrogen and progestogen exerts its contraceptive effect mainly through suppression of mid-cycle FSH release, and inhibition of the LH surge that causes ovulation.

- The sustained levels of oestrogen, and, to a lesser extent, progestogen, suppress LH and FSH secretion and follicular development.
- Progestogen produces asynchronous development of the endometrium with stromal thinning, which makes it less receptive to implantation. Fallopian tube motility is increased by oestrogens and decreased by progestogens; this may affect fertility by altering the rate of transport of the gamete.
- Progestogen alters cervical mucus, making it thicker and less copious, thereby creating an environment more hostile to sperm penetration. Ovulation is inhibited with the oral progestogen-only pill in only about 25% of women. Contraception must therefore rely upon the other actions of the hormone (Fig. 45.2).

'Combined' oral contraceptive

Monophasic preparations

Monophasic preparations contain fixed amounts of oestrogen and progestogen. They are taken daily for the first 21 days of the menstrual cycle, followed by 7 days without contraceptive. To improve adherence, 28-day packs ('every day' preparations) are available that include an inactive substance, such as lactose, during the 7 contraceptive-free days. The oestrogen and progestogen concentration should be the lowest that main-

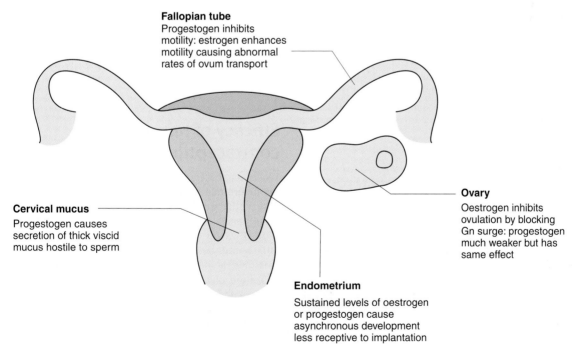

Fallopian tube
Progestogen inhibits motility: estrogen enhances motility causing abnormal rates of ovum transport

Cervical mucus
Progestogen causes secretion of thick viscid mucus hostile to sperm

Endometrium
Sustained levels of oestrogen or progestogen cause asynchronous development less receptive to implantation

Ovary
Oestrogen inhibits ovulation by blocking Gn surge: progestogen much weaker but has same effect

Fig. 45.2
The contraceptive actions of the synthetic oestrogen and progestogen in the contraceptive pill. Gn, gonadotrophin (LH and FSH).

tains good cycle control and produces minimal unwanted effects. There are several preparations to choose from:

- low-strength preparations contain 20 µg ethinylestradiol
- standard-strength preparations contain 30 or 35 µg ethinylestradiol, or mestranol.

The combined oral contraceptive pill contains one of several progestogens: levonorgestrel, norethisterone, norgestimate, desogestrel or gestodene (see above). Preparations are also available that contain different amounts of the same progestogen; for example, Microgynon 30® contains 150 µg levonorgestrel, and Eugynon 30® 250 µg levonorgestrel. In some women it may be necessary to change the formulation to reduce minor unwanted effects such as breakthrough bleeding or weight gain during the menstrual cycle. The androgenic or antiandrogenic properties possessed by different progestogens may influence the suitability of an individual preparation for a particular woman.

A transdermal formulation of low-strength ethinylestradiol with norelgestromin is also available, applied weekly for 3 weeks followed by a 7-day patch-free interval.

Biphasic and triphasic preparations

Biphasic and triphasic preparations are designed to mimic more closely the changes in sex hormone concentrations that occur during the natural menstrual cycle. The total sex hormone intake through the cycle is no less than with monophasic preparations. Several preparations are available, all of which contain ethinylestradiol in combination with either levonorgestrel, norethisterone or gestodene. In most preparations, the ethinylestradiol dose is kept constant as in the monophasic pills, although in some it is increased during days 7–12. Progestogen doses are increased once (biphasic) or twice (triphasic) as the menstrual cycle proceeds. Biphasic and triphasic preparations containing second- or third-generation progestogens are available.

Progestogen-only contraceptive

Oral progestogen

The progestogen-only pill is particularly useful for women in whom the administration of oestrogen is considered to be undesirable, for example if there is a history of thromboembolic disorders (see below). It is as effective as combined pills containing 30 µg of ethinylestradiol, although some reports say that pregnancy rates are slightly higher. Tablets containing desogestrel, ethynodiol, levonorgestrel or norethisterone are given continuously, without a break, and must be taken within 3 h of the usual time every day. Because the dose of progestogen is low, bleeding does occur at approximately monthly intervals but may be irregular. Breakthrough bleeding occurs in up to 40% of women; this is much higher than with the combined oral contraceptive. Some women become amenorrhoeic. Ectopic pregnancy may be increased in women taking the progestogen-only pill, due to impaired tubal transport, but its occurrence is extremely rare.

Parenteral progestogen-only contraceptive

Intramuscular injection of a progestogen, either medroxyprogesterone acetate or norethisterone, can provide contraception for up to 8–12 weeks. Ovulation is reliably inhibited, unlike with the oral progestogen-only contraceptives, and therefore there is a low incidence of ectopic pregnancy. The contraceptive effect is fully reversible, but there is a high incidence of amenorrhoea when its effect wears off.

A subcutaneous implant of etonorgestrel provides contraception for up to 3 years, after which time it should be replaced; the progestogen is released from a flexible rod inserted subdermally on the lower surface of the upper arm. Unwanted effects are the same as those experienced with the progestogen-only oral contraceptive, but lower doses of progestogen are needed, because first-pass metabolism is avoided.

Intrauterine progestogen-only device

A copper intrauterine contraceptive device (IUCD) with a levonorgestrel-releasing system from a silicone reservoir provides effective contraception with reduced menstrual blood loss compared with IUCDs that do not contain a progestogen. The progestogen is released from the device for a period of 5 years.

Efficacy of hormonal contraception

When taken according to the recommended schedule, the failure rate for the combined oral contraceptive is 0.2%. With the combined oral preparations, contraceptive protection is lost if there is a delay of more than 12 h in taking the daily dose. In such circumstances, the missed pill should be taken and additional contraceptive measures should be used for 7 days.

Failure of the progestogen-only pill is age-related and is up to 5% in young women, falling with decreasing fertility to about 0.3% at the age of 40 years. With the progestogen-only contraceptive, other contraceptive precautions should be taken for 7 days if there is a delay of only 3 h or more after the normal time of taking the pill.

Emergency contraception

This can be carried out with 1.5 mg levonorgestrel taken as soon as possible after unprotected intercourse. The mechanism of action may be to accelerate transport of the fertilised ovum so that it reaches the uterine cavity before the endometrium is receptive. The treatment is successful in up to 99% of cases. If used between 72 and 120 h after unprotected intercourse, the efficacy is greatly reduced. Nausea is a frequent unwanted effect, occurring in up to 22% of people; vomiting can occur and an anti-emetic (Ch. 32) may be needed. Absorption takes 3 h, and vomiting after this time will not affect the efficacy of treatment. In the UK, levonorgestrel can be purchased without prescription by women over the age of 16 years. This is the only preparation listed in the British National Formulary; in other countries, preparations containing levonorgestrel and ethinylestradiol are also available with prescription. Insertion of a copper IUCD is an alternative strategy that is equally effective, and retains its efficacy when inserted up to 120 h after unprotected intercourse.

Pharmacokinetics of contraceptive steroids

The synthetic oestrogens, like the naturally occurring oestradiol-17β, are well absorbed orally but are less rapidly degraded and undergo a variable amount of enterohepatic cycling. There is considerable inter-individual variation in plasma levels of oestrogen and progestogen after ingestion of the combined oral contraceptive pill. Progesterone itself is inactive orally because of extensive hepatic metabolism.

The pharmacokinetics of individual synthetic oestrogens and progestogens vary widely and data on ethinylestradiol and norethisterone only are summarised.

Ethinylestradiol is absorbed rapidly from the gut. It undergoes considerable first-pass metabolism (although this is reduced compared with estradiol) and has an intermediate half-life (Ch. 2). Enterohepatic cycling of ethinylestradiol is responsible for maintaining effective plasma concentrations with low-dose formulations. Norethisterone is rapidly and completely absorbed from the gut and also undergoes extensive first-pass metabolism in the intestinal wall and liver. It has an intermediate half-life.

Beneficial and unwanted effects of contraceptive steroids

Beneficial effects

- Cancer: there is a 50% reduction in the risk of ovarian cancer, seen after 5 years of use and persisting for up to 20 years after stopping. This may be a result of suppression of ovulation. Endometrial cancer may also be reduced after a similar duration of use.
- Acne can be treated with oral contraceptives, since they reduce the concentration of free testosterone (Ch. 49).
- Dysfunctional uterine bleeding is reduced by the combined oral contraceptive.

Unwanted effects

Both oestrogen and progestogen have a number of minor and major unwanted effects, but the incidence of the major effects, although important, is relatively low.

- Thromboembolism: the incidence of venous thromboembolic disease is increased by taking the combined oral contraceptive. The mechanism is complex but includes procoagulant activity from increased production of clotting factors X and II and decreased production of the protective antithrombin (Ch. 11). Fibrinolysis is impaired, while reduced prostacyclin generation enhances platelet aggregation (Ch. 11). The risk increases with age, is increased in women who smoke (because smoking increases the risk of thrombogenesis) and is increased in those with a thrombophilic tendency such as deficiency of protein C or protein S or the presence of factor V Leiden. The baseline risk of venous thromboembolism in women of reproductive age is 5 or less per 100 000. The excess risk in women taking second-generation pills is 6–12 per 100 000 (depending on age) and in those taking pills containing desogestrel or gestodene (third-generation) is 16–30 per 100 000. Publication of the increased risk for the third-generation pills resulted in many women ceasing to take the oral contraceptive pill, and an increase in pregnancy rate. It is important that these risks are put into context: the risk of venous thrombosis in pregnancy is 60 per 100 000.
- Ischaemic heart disease and ischaemic stroke: analysis of data in women largely taking the second- and third-generation pills has indicated that there is no significantly increased risk of myocardial infarction or ischaemic stroke for women who are non-smokers and have normal blood pressure, irrespective of age. There is an increased risk of myocardial infarction and cerebrovascular disease in

women taking the combined oral contraceptive who smoke or who are hypertensive, particularly in those over the age of 35 years. The excess risk in those over 40 years is 20 per 100 000 for smokers and 29 per 100 000 for hypertensives. It has been suggested that enhanced thrombogenesis rather than premature atherogenesis is responsible for the excess cardiovascular risk with the oral contraceptive. It is uncertain whether the risk is different for the newer progestogens. If older women use the combined contraceptive pill, then the lowest possible dose of oestrogen should be given.

- Increase in blood pressure: a small increase in blood pressure is frequently found during use of the combined oral contraceptive, but a significant rise can occur in about 5% of previously normotensive women; regular monitoring of blood pressure is important. A rise in blood pressure occurs in up to 15% of women with pre-existing hypertension. The mechanism is probably an increase in plasma renin activity (Ch. 6) produced by oestrogen and, to a lesser extent, progestogen. Blood pressure may remain elevated for some months after the combined contraceptive has been stopped.

- Cancer: despite numerous studies, the question of an association between combined oral contraceptives and breast cancer remains unresolved, and a small excess risk cannot be ruled out. The effect on the incidence of cervical cancer is uncertain, but it may be increased by oral contraceptives in the presence of human papilloma virus infection.

- Nausea, mastalgia, depression, headache and provocation of migraine can occur. They are probably related to the oestrogen content of the pill and can often be minimised by prescribing contraceptives with a low oestrogen content.

- Breakthrough bleeding occurs frequently in some women, whereas in others withdrawal bleeding fails to occur. Gestodene-containing pills or triphasic preparations probably give the best cycle control. Amenorrhoea after stopping the combined contraceptive can last beyond a few months in about 5% of women, and a small number can experience amenorrhoea for more than a year. A history of irregular periods before taking the pill increases the chance of prolonged amenorrhoea.

- Metabolic effects: oestrogens alone increase protective plasma high-density lipoprotein (HDL) cholesterol, decrease low-density lipoprotein (LDL) cholesterol and increase plasma triglycerides. When used in combination with progestogens in the second-generation pills, HDL cholesterol is reduced possibly due to the effect of the progestogen component (see also Ch. 48). Oestrogens increase vascular prostacyclin and nitric oxide synthesis, inhibit platelet adhesion, and suppress smooth muscle cell proliferation. They also reduce cholesterol accumulation in the arterial walls of cholesterol-fed animals. Some progestogens such as norethisterone and medroxyprogesterone acetate may oppose the beneficial effects of oestrogens on the arterial wall. The third-generation pills containing gestodene and desogestrel increase plasma triglycerides but, unlike the progestogens in the second-generation pills, they increase HDL cholesterol. Although the latter could be advantageous, the benefit may be illusory, as there is little evidence that the second-generation pills promote atherosclerosis.

- Increased skin pigmentation can occur in some women given oestrogens. The androgenic progestogens can sometimes cause or aggravate hirsutism and acne or produce weight gain. In women with hyperandrogenaemia, the third-generation pills would be preferred, as gestogene and desogestrel have little androgenic activity.

- Effects on the liver are occasionally seen. Cholestatic jaundice can be produced by progestogens, and oestrogens increase the risk of gallstones.

- Drug interactions: drugs that alter the metabolism of oestrogen may cause a reduction in the efficacy of the combined pill, which may result in breakthrough bleeding and contraceptive failure. Contraceptive failure may occur if there is concomitant treatment with anticonvulsants (e.g. barbiturates, carbamazepine or phenytoin), antiretroviral drugs such as nelfinavir, nevirapine or ritonavir, or the antibacterials rifampicin and rifabutin (Ch. 51) which induce liver cytochrome P450 enzymes. A pill containing 50 μg of ethinylestradiol should be used if these drugs are given long term. Some antibacterials, for example ampicillin and doxycycline (Ch. 51), alter the gut flora and thereby decrease the enterohepatic circulation of ethinylestradiol. Alternative methods of contraception should be used for the duration of a course of these broad-spectrum antibacterials and for 7 days after (4 weeks in the case of rifampicin).

Non-contraceptive uses of steroidal contraceptives

The combined oral contraceptive can be used:

- to reduce excessive blood loss from menorrhagia
- to reduce the pain of dysmenorrhoea
- to treat premenstrual tension
- to treat endometriosis.

Dysmenorrhoea

Primary dysmenorrhoea (pain associated with menstruation) is of unknown aetiology; many explanations have been proposed, including uterine hyperactivity, prostaglandin or leukotriene generation, and excessive production of vasopressin. Excess prostaglandin concentrations have been measured in endometrial curettings. A variety of non-steroidal anti-inflammatory drugs (NSAIDs) (Ch. 29) have been used for the relief of dysmenorrhoea, including ibuprofen, indometacin and mefenamic acid. All NSAIDs are useful for the relief of primary dysmenorrhoea, with approximately 70% of subjects being relieved of their symptoms. However, there are differences among the NSAIDs which are poorly understood, and their efficacy in dysmenorrhoea does not seem to be simply related to their analgesic activity.

The combined oral contraceptive and the progestogen-only contraceptive are effective in reducing symptoms of dysmenorrhoea. Small studies also suggest that calcium channel antagonists and β_2-adrenoceptor agonists have some beneficial effect.

Menorrhagia

Excessive menstrual blood loss is a common gynaecological problem. Menstrual loss can be reduced variably by NSAIDs (Ch. 29), and numerous different NSAIDs have been used. They are administered only during the time of menstruation. The combined oral contraceptive and the progestogen-only contraceptives can also reduce excessive menstrual loss. For the progestogen-only contraceptive to be useful, it has to be administered for 3 weeks at a fairly high dose. A more effective way of administering the progestogen is from an IUCD, where reduction in blood loss of up to 90% can be expected within a 12-month period.

The antifibrinolytic agent tranexamic acid (Ch. 11) can also reduce blood loss by up to 50%. Its effect is rapid in onset and therapy is only required during the time of menstruation.

Endometriosis

This is the presence and proliferation of endometrial tissue outside the uterine cavity. It may arise from retrograde menstrual flow through the fallopian tubes. The main consequences are pelvic pain, dysmenorrhoea, dyspareunia and infertility. Treatment is either medical or surgical. Medical treatment creates a hypo-oestrogenic anovulatory state, and does not restore fertility. If fertility is the major problem, then treatment involves surgery or in vitro fertilisation techniques (Ch. 43).

Symptoms often improve in pregnancy, and medical treatment is often successful with the combined oral contraceptive pill, or continuous progestogen. Alternative strategies include induction of a pseudo-postmenopausal state with the use of danazol (Ch. 46) or GnRH agonists (Ch. 43). Treatment is usually necessary for at least 6 months.

Hormone replacement therapy (HRT)

The consequences of oestrogen deficiency include the following.

- Symptoms such as vasomotor instability (hot flushes and night sweats), and altered sexual and urinary function. Vasomotor instability results from resetting of the hypothalamic temperature set-point so that it perceives that the body is warmer than it is. Vasodilation and sweating represent an attempt to disperse heat. The mechanism is uncertain but may be due to either reduced oestrogen or increased gonadotrophins leading to a reduction in 5-hydroxytryptamine (5HT) concentrations in the brain, and an imbalance of $5HT_{1A}$ and $5HT_2$ receptors. Loss of connective tissue in the vagina and trigone of the bladder underlies many of the other problems. Other postmenopausal symptoms such as irritability and depression are less clearly related to oestrogen deficiency.
- Bone loss leading to osteoporosis (Ch. 42) and an increased susceptibility to fracture occur after the menopause. The ERβ receptor is present in higher concentrations in developing cancellous bone (such as vertebrae), and the ERα receptor in developing cortical bone (such as the hip). Oestrogen deficiency increases bone turnover, with bone resorption increasing more than formation.
- Cardiovascular and cerebrovascular disease are increased. The cause is uncertain. Unfavourable changes in lipids may be part of the explanation, due to a reduced HDL_2 cholesterol subfraction and increased LDL cholesterol (Ch. 48). However, an independent effect of oestrogen in reducing plasma fibrinogen (a factor in thrombogenesis) may be more important. Oestrogen receptors are found on the cells of the arterial wall, and stimulation decreases arterial resistance and increases vessel compliance, which may also be relevant.

Treatment with oestrogens during the peri- and postmenopausal period is often advocated to try to reverse the effects of oestrogen deficiency, but recent evidence of lack of efficacy or potential harm has limited their use (see benefits and risks below).

Oral hormone replacement therapy

Examples: estradiol-17β, tibolone, raloxifene

For HRT, oestrogens are given at a much lower concentration than is used for contraception. If treatment is given for more than a few weeks to a woman who has a uterus, then cystic hyperplasia of the endometrium can occur. Progestogen, given concurrently, avoids this, and is used for 12 days each calendar month or continuously if withdrawal bleeding is to be avoided. The majority of oral HRT preparations contain the natural estradiol-17β as the oestrogen, although preparations with conjugated equine oestrogens are also available. The progestogens used are dydrogesterone, medroxyprogesterone, norethisterone or levonorgestrel. Oral oestrogen replacement will reduce the symptoms of postmenopausal oestrogen deficiency, although relief may take up to 3 months. Treatment for symptom relief probably should be given for at least 6 months to perimenopausal women, after which, withdrawal can be attempted to see if symptoms have spontaneously resolved.

Tibolone

Tibolone is a synthetic molecule with combined weak oestrogenic, progestogenic and andogenic properties. The global effects are predominantly oestrogenic, although in breast tissue it inhibits the enzyme responsible for activation of its metabolites, giving a low incidence of breast tenderness. In the endometrium it activates progesterone and androgen receptors, and the effects are mainly progestogenic, without stimulation of the endometrium or producing bleeding. Given orally, it reduces postmenopausal symptoms and it prevents postmenopausal bone loss. Vaginal bleeding can occur in women who still produce some endogenous oestrogen and therefore tibolone is not usually given to women who are within 12 months of their last period.

Pharmacokinetics

Tibolone is a prodrug that is well absorbed from the gut, and metabolised in the liver to active metabolites.

Unwanted effects

- headache
- dizziness
- nausea
- rash
- weight gain
- increased risk of breast cancer, but less than with combined HRT.

Raloxifene

Raloxifene is a selective oestrogen receptor modulator. It shows tissue specificity, since although it binds to both oestrogen receptors, it is an antagonist of ERβ by recruiting co-repressor molecules, but a partial agonist of ERα. Raloxifene has oestrogen receptor agonist effects on bone and lipids but acts as an anti-oestrogen on the breast and endometrium. It is, therefore, used for reduction of the risk of osteoporosis (Ch. 42) and does not reduce menopausal vasomotor symptoms. Raloxifene reduces the risk of breast cancer, but its effects on pre-existing breast cancer are unknown.

Pharmacokinetics

Raloxifene is well absorbed orally, and is metabolised in the liver. Enterohepatic cycling gives it a long half-life.

Unwanted effects

- hot flushes
- leg cramps
- raloxifene increases the risk of venous thromboembolism, particularly during the first 4 months of treatment.

Vaginal oestrogen

Oestrogen cream (usually estradiol-17β) or pessaries can be used to treat vaginal atrophy and dyspareunia and can relieve perimenopausal urinary symptoms such as frequency and dysuria. Considerable systemic absorption occurs with some formulations, and oral progestogen may be needed to prevent endometrial hyperplasia. Creams or pessaries are used daily for 2–3 weeks initially and then applied twice weekly for as long as required.

Subcutaneous oestrogen implants

Estradiol can be surgically implanted as pellets which release drug for up to 6 months. The major use for this option is when tolerance of oral oestrogen is poor, perhaps because of nausea. Oral progestogen must also be given for 10–12 days each month if the woman has a uterus, and continued for up to 2 years after stopping oestrogen, to prevent vaginal bleeding from persistent high oestrogen levels.

Transdermal oestrogen/progestogen

A variety of patch-delivered sex steroids are available. In some preparations, oestrogen alone is delivered by patches twice weekly for 2 weeks, followed by patches delivering oestrogen plus progestogen for 2 weeks. In other regimens, progestogen is taken orally for at least 12 days of the cycle while continuing with the patch-delivered oestrogen. Patches delivering continuous oestrogen plus progestogen (levonorgestrel or norethisterone) are also available. Avoidance of first-pass metabolism means that a lower dose of progestogen can be used transdermally, which might reduce unwanted effects. Estradiol gels applied twice daily are also available and require 12 days progestogen per month in women with a uterus. It is recommended that patches are applied below the waistline, and not close to the breasts.

Benefits and risks of hormone replacement therapy

The benefits and risks of HRT are highly individual for the patient. For most women, it is recommended that HRT is reserved for short-term alleviation of menopausal symptoms. If used, treatment should be reviewed at least annually. Alternative approaches to the treatment of menopausal symptoms should be considered. These include tibolone, clonidine (Ch. 6) and selective serotonin reuptake inhibitors for vasomotor symptoms, although unwanted effects often limit acceptability. Atrophic vaginitis may respond to a short course of topical oestrogen.

HRT reduces the risk of osteoporotic fractures of both the hip and vertebrae. However, because of the potential risks of treatment, HRT is not considered to be first-line treatment except for women with early natural or surgical menopause before the age of 45 years. It is not recommended that treatment should continue beyond age 50 years if osteoporosis is the main concern. Raloxifene decreases vertebral, but not hip, fractures, which is consistent with its receptor selectivity. Tibolone is a second-line treatment for postmenopausal osteoporosis.

Unwanted effects of hormone replacement therapy

- Breakthrough bleeding can be troublesome, and regular withdrawal bleeds during the cycle are common. These may be preceded by symptoms of premenstrual tension.
- Breast pain and abdominal or leg cramps due to the oestrogen or progestogen component.
- Nausea and vomiting.
- Headache, dizziness.
- Depression, irritability, loss of energy and poor concentration due to progestogen.
- Transdermal delivery can cause contact sensitisation.
- Increased risk of venous thromboembolism, especially in the first year. The excess risk after 5 years of use is about twofold (excess risk 4 cases per 1000 if aged 50–60 years). Limited evidence suggests that transdermal oestrogen replacement may not increase the risk of venous thromboembolism.
- Increased risk of stroke of about 30% in women aged 50–60 years after 5 years treatment (the excess risk is 1 case per 1000).

- HRT does not prevent coronary heart disease, and may increase the risk in the first year of treatment.
- Increased risk of breast cancer within 1–2 years of starting use, increasing further with duration of use. The excess risk is lost 5 years after stopping HRT. Taking combined HRT for 10 years leads to a 60% increase in the risk of developing breast cancer in women aged 50–65 years (the excess risk is 19 cases per 1000). Oestrogen-only HRT carries about one-quarter of this excess risk.
- Increased risk of endometrial cancer by threefold over 10 years (excess risk 10 cases per 1000).

The onset and induction of labour

The aetiology of the induction of labour is still uncertain (Fig. 45.3). The actual onset may be multifactorial in nature and it is probable that prostaglandins, oxytocin, progesterone, oestrogen and corticosteroids are among

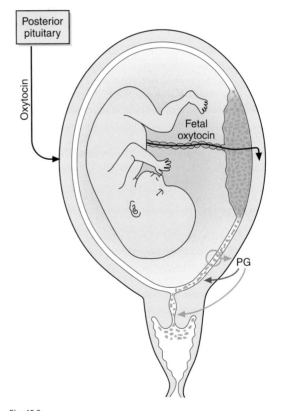

Fig. 45.3
Induction of labour. The mechanisms involved in the onset of labour in man are uncertain but it is likely to be multifactorial. Prostaglandin (PG) is synthesised by the amnion and the decidua and can act to stimulate the uterus and soften the cervix. Fetal and maternal oxytocin and prostaglandins may be involved in the processes of labour; their role in the **initiation** of labour is uncertain.

the agents involved. Our lack of knowledge is directly reflected in our poor ability to prevent preterm labour, where at best we can delay labour for short periods of time (see below).

Prostaglandins

$PGF_{2\alpha}$ and PGE_2 have many actions that could contribute to labour. They are synthesised by the cells of the amnion and decidua. The levels of these prostaglandins increase progressively in the amniotic fluid during labour and have been shown to be elevated before the discernible onset of labour. Uterine sensitivity to prostaglandins increases at term, when it is approximately 10-fold higher than in earlier pregnancy. The contractility of the uterus during labour commences at the uterotubular junction and progresses through the body of the uterus to the cervix, thus promoting efficient labour. This type of contractile pattern, which is not seen in early pregnancy, is caused by prostaglandins and oestrogens promoting the synthesis of gap junctions. These are specialised connections between the smooth muscle cells allowing excitatory impulses to pass between cells. Only in uterine muscle cells that are rich in gap junctions can the 'right type' of uterine contraction occur and result in efficient progress of labour. The progesterone-dominated uterus has few gap junctions. Prostaglandins also increase the synthesis of oxytocin from the posterior pituitary. PGE_2 softens the cervix, an essential prerequisite for the smooth passage of labour. Indometacin has been used experimentally to inhibit preterm labour in limited trials. The concern in using indometacin is its ability to close the ductus arteriosus prematurely in the fetus by inhibiting prostaglandin synthesis.

Oxytocin

Oxytocin is a peptide produced by the posterior pituitary. It has a marked uterotonic action at term but is much less effective earlier in pregnancy. The reason for this is that there is a marked increase in the expression of uterine oxytocin receptors from about 35 weeks of pregnancy onwards. Oxytocin levels in the maternal circulation do not increase during labour until the second stage. Interestingly, there are higher levels of oxytocin in the fetal circulation than in the mother during labour. Inhibitors of the oxytocin receptor have been produced and limited data suggest partial usefulness in the inhibition of preterm labour.

Steroid hormones

Oestrogens and progesterone both increase during pregnancy, and overall the actions of oestradiol promote uterine contractility while those of progesterone diminish it. Although in some animals there is a clear pre-labour decrease in progesterone which may contribute to the onset of labour, there is little evidence for this effect in humans. It has been suggested that a decrease in progesterone concentrations may occur only at a local uterine level which might not be reflected in the maternal circulation. A role for progesterone in the control of uterine contractility is suggested as the anti-progesterone drug mifepristone does increase the rate of spontaneous labour. Oestradiol increases the number of uterine oxytocin receptors and increases oxytocin release from the posterior pituitary. It increases gap junctions, and fundal dominance of uterine contractility is increased by an effect on the functional pacemaker at the uterotubular junction. Oestradiol increases the synthesis of prostaglandins and increases the sensitivity of the uterus to their effects. Oestradiol also has a softening effect on the cervix. In contrast, progesterone decreases gap junctions and diminishes pacemaker activity. It also decreases the sensitivity of the uterus to oxytocin and prostaglandins.

Drugs used for inducing labour

Oxytocin and prostaglandins are the only drugs used to induce labour.

Oxytocin

Oxytocin is used for the induction of labour and to augment contractions in inadequate labour. It is given by slow intravenous infusion to induce labour. The concentration given depends upon the response of the patient: the aim is to produce regular coordinated contractions at intervals of approximately 1.5–2 min with complete relaxation between contractions. Oxytocin is an effective uterine stimulant in women at term, and labour will usually proceed well if the cervix is partially dilated and softened prior to its use. Inappropriately high concentrations of oxytocin can cause hypertonus, in which the uterus does not relax between contractions, and fetal distress can occur. As labour progresses and the woman's 'endogenous' induction mechanisms come into play, the concentration of oxytocin may need to be reduced. Following delivery, postpartum haemorrhage can be reduced by increasing the concentration of oxytocin or giving oxytocin combined with ergometrine intramuscularly (see below). Oxytocin, unlike prostaglandins, does not soften the cervix and is now often used after intravaginal prostaglandin (usually dinoprostone) has been given for this purpose (see below). Oxytocin in high doses has a weak antidiuretic activity as it is related to vasopressin (Ch. 43).

Dinoprostone

Dinoprostone (the name for exogenous PGE_2) causes contractions of both the non-pregnant and the pregnant uterus. Like oxytocin, in correct doses it can produce contractions that are indistinguishable from spontaneous labour, but prostaglandins have the advantage of softening the cervix. Thus, they can be used for induction of labour before term. Dinoprostone is given as vaginal tablets, pessaries or gels for induction of labour or for priming of the uterus prior to rupture of membranes and induction by oxytocin. Dinoprostone frequently causes uterine contractions; in some women it will only result in cervix softening, whereas others will go into labour. Intravenous dinoprostone is now far less commonly used for induction of labour.

Unwanted effects

- gastrointestinal disturbances, particularly nausea, vomiting and diarrhoea
- uterine hypertonus
- flushing
- bronchospasm.

Induction of abortion

Prostaglandins are widely used for the induction of abortion. In the *second trimester*, their use results in fewer complications than with dilatation and curettage or other surgical techniques. Gemeprost (PGE_1 analogue), given by the intravaginal route, is used for the medical induction of late therapeutic abortion. Misoprostol (Ch. 33) is also used for induction of abortion, but this is an unlicensed use in the UK. Extra-amniotic dinoprostone is now rarely used for induction of abortion. The mechanism of action of these drugs is to produce prolonged uterine contraction. Gemeprost is also given as a pessary to ripen and soften the cervix prior to surgical abortion and together with mifepristone for early abortion (see below).

Mifepristone

Mechanism of action and uses

Mifepristone is a potent progesterone antagonist that binds to the progesterone receptor. It sensitises the uterus to prostaglandin-induced contractions and softens the cervix. It is used for the termination of early and mid-trimester pregnancy, when it is given in combination with the PGE_1 analogue gemeprost or misoprostol. In early pregnancy, up to 20 weeks' gestation, mifepristone is given as a single oral dose followed 36 hours later by vaginal gemeprost. Oral or vaginal misoprostol (Ch. 33) can be used as an alternative to gemeprost.

The softening effect on the uterine cervix can also be used for cervical ripening prior to the induction of labour at term, although there is little information on fetal outcome or maternal unwanted effects and it is not licensed in the UK for this purpose.

Pharmacokinetics

Mifepristone is well absorbed from the gut and metabolised slowly by the liver, generating an active metabolite. The half-life, therefore, is long.

Unwanted effects

- nausea, vomiting
- vaginal bleeding
- uterine pain (that can be severe)
- malaise, faintness, headache.

Postpartum haemorrhage

Ergometrine should be given by intramuscular injection, together with oxytocin by intramuscular injection, on delivery of the anterior shoulder, for the reduction of postpartum haemorrhage. Following delivery of the baby, postpartum haemorrhage can also be reduced by increasing the concentrations of intravenous oxytocin being administered. This causes hypertonic contraction of the uterus and compresses intrauterine blood vessels. If bleeding continues, the prostaglandin carboprost (15-methyl $PGF_{2\alpha}$) is given by intramuscular injection.

Ergometrine maleate

Ergometrine is not used for induction of labour as it causes hypertonic contractions of the uterus and fetal distress. The action of ergometrine on the uterus is partially through stimulation of α-adrenoceptors (see ergotamine Ch. 26), and it produces vasoconstriction, which further limits haemorrhage.

Pharmacokinetics

Ergometrine is given intramuscularly, and works within 2–7 mins. Elimination is by hepatic metabolism.

Unwanted effects

- nausea, vomiting
- headache, dizziness, tinnitus
- abdominal or chest pain
- peripheral vasoconstriction.

Myometrial relaxants and preterm labour

Prematurity is the largest cause of neonatal morbidity and mortality, but we have few pharmacological tools for preventing it.

β₂-Adrenoceptor agonists

Examples: terbutaline, ritodrine, salbutamol

β₂-Adrenoceptor agonists inhibit uterine contractility, and thus premature labour, for about 48 h. They are used for uncomplicated premature labour between 24 and 33 weeks of gestation. The use of β₂-adrenoceptor agonists alone does not improve fetal morbidity or mortality, but they provide a limited time for treatment with corticosteroids to enhance lung maturation (Ch. 13). β₂-Adrenoceptor agonists can be administered intravenously or orally. Unwanted effects include nausea, vomiting, flushing and maternal tachycardia with hypotension (see also Ch. 12).

Atosiban

Atosiban is a peptide analogue of oxytocin and is an oxytocin receptor antagonist. It has similar indications as β₂-adrenoceptor agonists, with fewer unwanted effects.

Pharmacokinetics

Atosiban is given by intravenous injection or infusion. It is metabolised to an active derivative, and has a short half-life.

Unwanted effects

- nausea, vomiting
- headache, dizziness
- tachycardia, hypotension
- hyperglycaemia.

Other agents for preterm labour

Magnesium sulfate is widely used in the USA for treating women in preterm labour. It may work by inhibiting Ca^{2+} availability. It is as effective as β₂-adrenoceptor agonists, and unwanted effects are minor.

The NSAID indometacin (Ch. 29) can be successful for delaying delivery, but there are concerns about transient neonatal renal impairment and premature closure of the ductus arteriosus.

Uterine and vaginal infection is also thought to be an important risk factor for preterm labour in a subgroup of women, and some data have demonstrated the effectiveness of antimicrobials in delaying delivery.

FURTHER READING

Bygdeman M, Danielsson KG (2002) Options for early therapeutic abortion. *Drugs* 62, 2459–2470

Chamberlain G, Zander L (1999) Induction. *BMJ* 318, 995–998

Child TJ, Tan SL (2001) Endometriosis. Aetiology, pathogenesis and treatment. *Drugs* 61, 1735–1750

Davison S, Davis SR (2003) Hormone replacement therapy: current controversies. *Clin Endocrinol* 58, 249–261

Franco V, Oparil F (2002) Hormone replacement therapy and hypertension. *Curr Opin Nephrol Hypertens* 11, 229–235

Greendale GA, Lee NP, Arriola ER (1999) The menopause. *Lancet* 353, 571–580

Gruber CJ, Tschuggel W, Schneeberger C et al (2002) Production and actions of estrogens. *N Engl J Med* 346, 340–352

Nelson HD, Humphrey LL, Nygren P et al (2002) Postmenopausal hormone replacement therapy. Scientific review. *JAMA* 288, 872–881

Norwitz ER, Robinson JN, Shallis JRG (1999) The control of labor. *N Engl J Med* 341, 660–666

Petitti DB (2003) Combination estrogen–progestin oral contraceptives. *N Engl J Med* 349, 1443–1450

Prentice A (1999) Medical management of menorrhagia. *BMJ* 319, 1343–1345

Riggs BL, Hartmann LC (2003) Selective estrogen-receptor modulators. Mechanisms of action and application to clinical practice. *N Engl J Med* 348, 618–629

Stearns V, Ullmer L, Lopez JF et al (2002) Hot flushes. *Lancet* 360, 1851–1861

Westhoff C (2003) Emergency contraception. *N Engl J Med* 349, 1830–1835

Self-assessment

In the questions 1–10, the first statement, in italics, is true. Are the accompanying statements also true?

1. *The mid-cycle surge in LH and FSH is essential for ovulation to occur.*

   a. Oestrogen has a negative feedback effect on LH and FSH secretion from the anterior pituitary throughout the follicular phase.
   b. The elevated level of progesterone in the secretory phase is under the control of gonadotrophins.

2. *Progesterone causes cervical mucus to be viscous and hostile to the passage of sperm. This is an important contraceptive action of the oral progestogen-only pill.*

   a. The oral progestogen-only pill inhibits ovulation in 90% of women.
   b. Both oestrogen and progesterone inhibit the motility of the fallopian tube, altering the rate of transport of sperm and the oocyte.
   c. The functioning corpus luteum is essential for the maintenance of pregnancy for about the first 6–8 weeks following implantation.

3. *The second generation of combined contraceptives refers to those that have low concentrations of ethinylestradiol and generally either levonorgestrel or norethisterone as the progestogenic component. The third generation of combined contraceptives contains the progestogens such as gestodene or desogestrel.*

   a. There is little to choose between the different progestogens in contraceptive pills in terms of their androgenic activity.
   b. The combined oral contraceptives administered in a biphasic or triphasic pattern result in the overall administration of less oestrogen and progestogen.
   c. Plasma concentrations of administered ethinylestradiol are lower than anticipated because ethinylestradiol undergoes enterohepatic recycling.
   d. With the combined oral contraceptive pill and the progestogen-only pill, effective protection may be lost if there is a delay of more than 12 h in taking the daily dose.

4. *The antibacterials rifampicin and ampicillin can lower the effective concentrations of ethinylestradiol in the plasma. Antiepilepsy drugs such as carbamazepine can reduce the plasma concentrations of oestrogens and progestogens.*

5. *There is no significant increased risk of myocardial infarction irrespective of age in women who are non-smokers taking the combined contraceptive pill.*

   a. Mortality from venous thromboembolism is increased in women who smoke, particularly those over the age of 35 years.
   b. The second- and third-generation oral contraceptives can decrease glucose tolerance.

6. *In women who have not had a hysterectomy, unopposed oestrogen treatment can result in endometrial hyperplasia and an increased risk of endometrial cancer.*

   a. Postmenopausal women taking continuous therapy containing both oestrogen and progestogens do not experience breakthrough bleeding.
   b. Oestrogens and progestogens can be given by skin patches to reduce the level of first-pass metabolism.
   c. Raloxifene is a selective oestrogen receptor modulating agent.
   d. Tibolone reduces bone loss in postmenopausal women.

7. *Unlike oxytocin, the prostaglandins have a softening effect on the cervix.*

   a. Oxytocin is preferred to prostaglandins for the induction of labour in a woman at 34 weeks' gestation.
   b. Progesterone increases the number of gap junctions in the uterus.
   c. Natural prostaglandins are produced from the posterior pituitary during labour.

8. *For the induction of abortion, mifepristone should be given 24–48 h before the administration of prostaglandins.*

   a. Prostaglandins given for the induction of labour do not produce hypertonic uterine activity.
   b. Ergometrine can be used for the induction of labour.

9. *NSAIDs are used in treating dysmenorrhoea. The combined oral contraceptive is ineffective for relieving the symptoms of dysmenorrhoea.*

10. *β_2-Adrenoceptor agonists do not reduce fetal mortality or morbidity in preterm labour.* Magnesium sulfate inhibits uterine motility.

11. You are discussing the benefits and drawbacks of oral contraception with a 35-year-old woman who smokes 40 cigarettes a day and, despite treatment, has not been able to stop smoking. Choose the one <u>most appropriate</u> option from the following.

Self-assessment questions

A. The combined oral contraceptive pill will be suitable for her contraception.
B. The combined contraceptive pill increases the risk of endometrial cancer.
C. The intrauterine contraceptive device has a higher failure rate than the oral contraceptive pill.
D. The progestogen-only pill does not increase the risk of thromboembolic disease.
E. An injection of medroxyprogesterone acetate will give contraceptive protection for more than 6 months.

12. You are discussing with a medical student the drugs that are used during labour and abortion. Choose the one **incorrect** option from the following.

A. Mifepristone acts to induce abortion and is an antagonist at progesterone receptors.
B. PGE_2 is preferred to oxytocin for induction of labour at 35 weeks of gestation in a woman with intact membranes.
C. Oxytocin has a lower potential than prostaglandins to cause uterine hypertonus.
D. β_2-Adrenoceptor agonists are ineffective in reducing morbidity or mortality in children born pre-term.
E. Ergometrine reduces postpartum haemorrhage by acting on uterine blood vessel α_1-adrenoceptors to cause vasoconstriction.

The answers are provided on pages 739–741.

Drugs acting on the female reproductive system

Drug	Half-life (h)	Elimination	Comments
Oestrogens			Components of oral contraceptives and for HRT; other uses are specified
Conjugated oestrogen equine	–	Metabolism	Given as sulphate conjugates of >10 equine oestrogens; components are absorbed both intact and after hydrolysis; excreted as sulphate conjugates
Estradiol	1	Metabolism	Metabolised to estrone, which undergoes P450 oxidation
Estradiol valerate	–	Metabolism	Assumed to be a prodrug for estradiol
Ethinylestradiol	8–24	Metabolism	Component of oral contraceptive pill; has been replaced by other oestrogens for the treatment of menopausal symptoms; limited use for the management of hereditary haemorrhagic telangiectasia; undergoes both oxidation and direct conjugation with glucuronic acid and sulphate
Mestranol	8–24	Metabolism	More than 50% is converted to ethinylestradiol
Progestogens			Components of oral contraceptives and for HRT; other uses are specified
Desogestrel	30	Metabolism	Component of oral contraceptive pill; termed a *third-generation progestogen*; undergoes P450-mediated oxidation in gut wall and liver
Dydrogesterone	–	–	Progesterone analogue used for the treatment of endometriosis, infertility, recurrent miscarriage, premenstrual syndrome, amenorrhoea and dysmenorrhoea; kinetic data not identified
Etonogestrel	29	Metabolism	Etonogestrel-releasing implant can be inserted subdermally to give prolonged contraception; activity of metabolites is unknown
Gestodene	18	Metabolism	Component of oral contraceptive pill; termed a *third-generation progestin*; undergoes oxidation plus reduction reactions; oxidation of ethinyl side-chain causes 'suicide inactivation' of CYP3A4
Levonorgestrel	8–30	Metabolism	Component of oral contraceptive pill; effective emergency contraception if used within 72 h of unprotected intercourse; also present in an intrauterine device that is used for contraception and for primary menorrhagia; undergoes reduction plus oxidation followed by conjugation
Medroxyprogesterone acetate	30	Metabolism	A long-acting progestogen given as an aqueous suspension by deep intramuscular injection; undergoes oxidation and reduction reactions to give 26 essentially inactive metabolites
Norethisterone	5–12	Metabolism	Testosterone analogue used for the treatment of endometriosis, premenstrual syndrome, dysmenorrhoea and postponement of menstruation; reduction of unsaturated A ring and ketone group are major routes of metabolism
Norethisterone acetate	10 (NEth)	Hydrolysis	Component of oral contraceptive preparations; hydrolysed to norethisterone (NEth)
Norethisterone enantate	10 (NEth)	Hydrolysis	A long-acting progestogen given as an oil solution by very slow deep intramuscular injection; prodrug of norethisterone (NEth)

continued

Drug compendium

Drugs acting on the female reproductive system (continued)

Drug	Half-life (h)	Elimination	Comments
Norgestimate	12–30 (17DAN)	Metabolism	Component of oral contraceptive preparations; a prodrug; active metabolites include the 17-dimethylnorgestimate (17DAN), the 3-keto analogue and levonorgestrel
Norgestrel	20	Metabolism	Component of oral contraceptive preparations; undergoes hepatic metabolism
Progesterone	5 min	Metabolism	Given as rectal or vaginal pessaries for the treatment of infertility, premenstrual syndrome and postnatal depression, or by injection for the treatment of dysmenorrhoea; metabolised in the liver to pregnanediol and conjugated with glucuronic acid
Drugs used primarily for endometriosis			Other uses are specified
Danazol	4–5	Metabolism	Antigonadotrophic drug with androgenic, anti-oestrogenic and anti-progestogenic effects; anti-gonadotrophic effects are due to parent drug; also used for severe pain in benign fibrocystic breast disease and hereditary angioedema; synthetic steroid given orally; metabolised by oxidation in the liver
Gestrinone	27	Metabolism	Actions are similar to danazol; given orally; oxidised to less active products, which are excreted as conjugates
Gonadorelin	4 min	Metabolism + renal	Complex peptide given by intravenous injection for assessment of pituitary function, but of questionable value; the half-life probably reflects tissue distribution and binding at therapeutic doses rather than excretion and metabolism; see Ch. 43
Gonadorelin analogues			Produce downregulation of gonadotrophin-releasing hormone receptors and thereby reduce the release of gonadotrophins; used for endometriosis, infertility, and before intrauterine surgery; other uses are specified.
Buserelin	3–6 min	Metabolism + excretion	Given nasally for endometriosis and by subcutaneous injection for prostate cancer (see Ch. 52); complex peptide (see gonadorelin above concerning half-life)
Goserelin	4	Metabolism	Given by subcutaneous implant for prostate cancer and early and advanced breast cancer (see Ch. 52); complex peptide; metabolised by cell peptidases
Leuprorelin acetate	3	Metabolism	Given by subcutaneous or intramuscular injection for prostate cancer (see Ch. 52); complex peptide; metabolised by proteases
Nafarelin	4	Metabolism	Given as a nasal spray for endometriosis; slow hydrolysis; inactive metabolites have long half-lives (85 h)
Triptorelin	3	Metabolism	Given by intramuscular injection for prostate cancer (see Ch. 52); metabolism and routes of elimination are not known
Drugs used for menopausal symptoms and/or osteoporosis			Given orally
Raloxifene	28	Metabolism	Used for the treatment and prevention of postmenopausal osteoporosis; does not affect menopausal vasomotor symptoms; undergoes extensive first-pass conjugation with glucuronic acid and enterohepatic cycling

continued

Drugs acting on the female reproductive system *(continued)*

Drug	Half-life (h)	Elimination	Comments
Tibolone	Unknown	Metabolism	Used for the short-term treatment and prevention of menopausal vasomotor symptoms and postmenopausal osteoporosis; shows oestrogenic, progestogenic and weak androgenic activities; metabolised by reduction of 3-keto group, and isomerisation to three active metabolites
Anti-oestrogens			Induce gonadotrophin release
Clomifene	5 days	Metabolism	Given orally for the treatment of female infertility associated with oligomenorrhoroea or secondary amenorrhoea; exists as two isomers of which the Z (cis) is active and the E (trans) is inactive; Z-isomer is eliminated more slowly and is detectable in plasma one month after treatment; see Ch. 43
Tamoxifen	7 days	Metabolism	Main use is in breast cancer – see Ch. 52
Drugs used to treat mastalgia			
Bromocriptine	–	–	See Chs 24 and 43
Danazol	–	–	See above
Tamoxifen	–	–	See Ch. 52
Prostaglandins and oxytocics			
Carboprost	–	–	Given by deep intramuscular injection for postpartum haemorrhage due to uterine atony; no relevant published kinetic data
Dinoprostone (PGE$_2$)	30 s	Metabolism	Given intravaginally (or rarely by intravenous injection) for the induction of labour; metabolised by dehydrogenation
Ergometrine (ergonovine)	2	Metabolism	Given by intramuscular injection to prevent and treat postpartum haemorrhage; eliminated by hepatic metabolism
Gemeprost	–	Metabolism	Given intravaginally to soften the cervix in labour induction and to induce abortion; systemic half-life not known; very rapidly hydrolysed (within minutes) and subsequently oxidised
Oxytocin	2–10 min	Metabolism	Given by slow intravenous injection or infusion for the induction of labour; rapid metabolism via reduction of the intramolecular disulphide bond followed by peptidase hydrolysis
Drugs used for effects on ductus arteriosus			
Alprostadil (PGE$_1$)	30 s	Metabolism	Given as an intravenous infusion to maintain patency in neonates with congenital heart defects; metabolised by dehydrogenation
Indometacin	3–5	Metabolism	Given by intravenous injection to close the ductus arteriosus in premature babies; metabolised by conjugation and oxidation

continued

Drug compendium

Drugs acting on the female reproductive system *(continued)*

Drug	Half-life (h)	Elimination	Comments
Drugs used primarily for therapeutic abortions			
Mifepristone	12–72	Bile + metabolism	Given orally or vaginally prior to therapeutic abortion to sensitise the uterus to the actions of prostaglandins; undergoes extensive enterohepatic cycling
Myometrial relaxant drugs			
Atosiban	0.25	Metabolism	An oxytocin receptor antagonist given by intravenous injection or infusion for the inhibition of uncomplicated premature labour between 24 and 33 weeks of gestation; metabolised to an active derivative
Ritodrine	15–20	Metabolism	β_2-Adrenoceptor agonist given orally or by intravenous infusion for the inhibition of uncomplicated premature labour between 24 and 33 weeks of gestation; conjugated with sulphate and glucuronic acid
Salbutamol	3–5	Metabolism + renal	β_2-Adrenoceptor agonist given by intravenous infusion and then orally for the inhibition of uncomplicated premature labour between 24 and 33 weeks of gestation; eliminated in urine as the sulphate conjugate
Terbutaline	14–18	Renal + metabolism	β_2-Adrenoceptor agonist given orally or by subcutaneous or intravenous infusion for the inhibition of uncomplicated premature labour between 24 and 33 weeks of gestation; see Ch. 12

Some oestrogens (diethylstilbestrol and ethinylestradiol), progestogens (gestonorone, medroxyprogesterone, megestrol and norethisterone) and oestrogen receptor antagonists (tamoxifen and toremifene) are used for the treatment of malignant disease – see Ch. 52.

Androgens and anabolic steroids

- Sexual differentiation in the fetus.
- Sexual development of the male testis, penis, epididymis, seminal vesicles and prostate at puberty, and maintenance of these tissues in the adult.
- Spermatogenesis in the adult.
- Stimulation and maintenance of sexual function and behaviour.
- Metabolic actions. Testosterone is a powerful anabolic agent producing a positive nitrogen balance with an increase in the bulk of tissues such as muscle and bone. In the skin, sebum production is increased, which can provoke acne. Growth of axillary, pubic, facial and chest hair is stimulated. In the liver, testosterone increases the synthesis of several proteins, including clotting factors, but decreases high-density lipoprotein (HDL) synthesis (Ch. 48). Testosterone also induces several liver enzymes, including steroid hydroxylases.
- Haematological actions. Testosterone stimulates production of erythropoietin by the kidneys, leading to a higher haemoglobin concentration in men than in women.

Androgens

Naturally occurring androgens are 19-carbon steroid hormones that are synthesised in the adrenal cortex and gonads (see Fig. 44.2). They have characteristic actions on the reproductive tract and other tissues as well as an anabolic effect on metabolism. A number of synthetic androgenic steroids have been developed. The substance is described as an 'anabolic steroid' when the predominant action is anabolic rather than reproductive. Although there are a few medical uses for such compounds, they have achieved notoriety because of their abuse by athletes to enhance muscle development.

Testosterone is the most powerful and the major androgen. It is secreted by the Leydig cells of the testis, and its synthesis and release are stimulated by the gonadotrophin luteinising hormone (Ch. 43). The androgens released from the adrenal cortex, in response to stimulation by adrenocorticotrophic hormone (ACTH), are mainly dehydroepiandrosterone and androstenedione (see Fig. 44.2). The cellular mechanism of action of steroid hormones is discussed in Chapters 1 and 44.

Male sex hormones

Examples: mesterolone, testosterone

Actions of testosterone

The actions of testosterone are in part due to its metabolite dihydrotestosterone. The latter is produced in the prostate, skin and reproductive tissues by the action of the enzyme 5α-reductase. Dihydrotestosterone has a higher affinity for the androgen receptor than testosterone. Actions of androgens include the following:

Pharmacokinetics

Oral preparations. Testosterone is well absorbed from the gut but is almost completely degraded by first-pass metabolism in the gut wall and liver. Esterification of testosterone creates hydrophobic compounds, such as testosterone undecanoate, which can be given orally because they are absorbed via lacteals into the lymphatic system, thus avoiding hepatic metabolism. Mesterolone is a testosterone derivative that has a greater oral bioavailability than testosterone.

Testosterone esters for depot injection. The most popular form of replacement therapy for hypogonadal men is an intramuscular injection of a testosterone ester, usually in oily solution, every 2–3 weeks. Testosterone is absorbed gradually after ester hydrolysis at the site of injection. Examples include testosterone enantate, isocaproate, propionate and undecanoate.

Transdermal delivery. A transdermal delivery patch containing testosterone can be used to treat hypogonadism. It is usually applied to the back, abdomen, upper arm or thigh, rotating the site daily to avoid skin irritation. Testosterone gel is an alternative way to deliver the drug transdermally.

Buccal delivery. A buccal-delivered tablet which softens to a gel and adheres to the mucosa has recently been introduced for transmucosal delivery and gives sustained slow release of testosterone.

Subcutaneous implant. A pellet of pure crystalline testosterone provides a reservoir for gradual absorption of testosterone into the systemic circulation for up to 4 months. A minor surgical procedure is necessary, and therefore this method of delivery is rarely used.

Circulating androgens are bound largely to a specific transport protein, sex hormone-binding globulin (SHBG), which has a greater affinity for androgens than for oestrogen. Testosterone is metabolised in the liver to androstendione, and then to inactive compounds. Some testosterone undergoes conversion in specific organs by 5α-reductase to dihydrotestosterone, and a small amount is aromatised to oestrogenic derivatives. Mesterolone is not metabolised to oestrogenic compounds. The half-life of testosterone is short.

Unwanted effects

- In hypogonadal adolescents, initial nitrogen retention and a spurt in linear growth is followed by premature epiphyseal closure and short stature. A short course can be used for treatment of delayed puberty without inducing epiphyseal closure.
- Headache.
- Anxiety, depression.
- Nausea, gastrointestinal bleeding.
- Sodium retention with oedema and hypertension.
- Hirsutism, male-pattern baldness, acne. Virilisation occurs in women given testosterone.
- Conversion to oestrogens by aromatase can produce gynaecomastia (see Fig. 44.2). This is less likely to occur with mesterolone.
- Suppression of gonadotrophin release with diminished testicular size and reduced spermatogenesis. Hypogonadal men will not regain fertility while taking androgens.
- Cholestatic jaundice. Liver tumours are a rare complication.

Clinical uses of testosterone

- The main clinical use for testosterone is as replacement therapy for primary hypogonadism in adult males.
- It can be used briefly in constitutionally delayed puberty, even in the absence of hypogonadism.
- Androgens are occasionally beneficial for promoting erythropoiesis in some forms of aplastic anaemia.

Danazol

Mechanism of action

Danazol is an androgen derivative described as an 'impeded' androgen. It is weakly androgenic on peripheral tissues and is not converted into an oestrogen. Its main property is feedback inhibition of gonadotrophin

and gonadotrophin-releasing hormone secretion. It therefore has anti-oestrogenic and anti-progestogenic actions.

Pharmacokinetics

Danazol is well absorbed orally, metabolised in the liver and has a short half-life.

Unwanted effects

- nausea, epigastric pain
- acne, hirsutism, oedema, hair loss or deepening of voice, due to androgenic effects
- depression, anxiety
- dizziness, headache
- vaginal dryness, reduction in breast size, changes in libido, amenorrhoea, hot flushes.

Clinical uses of danazol

- treatment of endometriosis (Ch. 45)
- treatment of menorrhagia (Ch. 45)
- management of gynaecomastia
- long-term management of hereditary angioedema.

Anabolic steroids

Example: nandrolone

Anabolic steroids are most frequently encountered as drugs of abuse to improve athletic performance. In medical practice, there are few indications for these compounds, and there is little evidence for efficacy in many conditions where their use has been advocated.

Pharmacokinetics

Nandrolone is given as a decanoate ester depot formulation by intramuscular injection every 3 weeks.

Unwanted effects

Androgenic effects may be troublesome in women.

Clinical uses

- promotion of erythropoiesis in aplastic anaemias
- itching associated with chronic biliary obstruction in palliative care.

Abuse of anabolic steroids

The ability of androgens to promote an increase in muscle mass has led to their abuse to improve physical performance by athletes, weightlifters and bodybuilders. Often, several different androgens are used for prolonged periods, perhaps with a brief 'drug-free' period. Abused compounds include testosterone, nandrolone, oxymetholone, stanozolol and many that are licensed only for veterinary use. The consequences of abuse include:

- weight gain from muscle hypertrophy and fluid retention
- acne in adolescent and young men
- decreased testicular size and reduced sperm count
- hepatotoxicity with cholestasis, hepatitis or, occasionally, hepatocellular tumours
- atherogenic changes in the plasma lipids with a rise in plasma LDL cholesterol and a fall in HDL cholesterol (Ch. 48); this may predispose to premature vascular disease
- psychological disturbance, including changes in libido, increased aggression and psychotic symptoms.

Antiandrogens

Bicalutamide and flutamide

Mechanism of action
Flutamide is a relatively pure antiandrogen without significant glucocorticoid or progestogenic actions.

Pharmacokinetics
Bicalutamide and flutamide are well absorbed orally, and are metabolised in the liver. Bicalutamide has a very long half-life of 7–10 days, while that of flutamide is short. The major metabolite of flutamide, 2-hydroxy-flutamide, is more active than the parent compound and also has a short half-life.

Unwanted effects

- anti-androgenic effects, for example gynaecomastia
- gastrointestinal upset
- insomnia.

Cyproterone acetate

Mechanism of action
Cyproterone acetate, a 21-carbon steroid, is a progestogen, a weak glucocorticoid (Ch. 44), and at high doses has an inhibitory action on peripheral androgen receptors. Its progestational activity includes feedback inhibition of gonadotrophin secretion.

Pharmacokinetics
Cyproterone acetate is well absorbed orally, metabolised in the liver, and has a long half-life of 2 days.

Unwanted effects

- antiandrogenic effects, for example gynaecomastia
- inhibition of spermatogenesis
- reduction in libido and potency in males
- hepatotoxicity with long-term use, causing hepatitis and, occasionally, hepatic failure.

Clinical uses of antiandrogens

- The main use of antiandrogens is in the treatment of carcinoma of the prostate (Ch. 52), usually in conjunction with a gonadorelin analogue (Chs 43, 45).
- Cyproterone acetate is used in male sexual offenders as 'chemical castration'.
- Cyproterone acetate can be given for manifestations of hyper-androgenisation in females, such as acne and hirsutism, in conjunction with ethinylestradiol (Ch. 45).

5α-Reductase inhibitors

Examples: dutasteride, finasteride

Mechanism of action and effects
5α-Reductase is an enzyme associated with androgen-dependent target cells. It is responsible for the conversion of testosterone to dihydrotestosterone (DHT), which is the hormone responsible for prostatic growth. In the adult male, finasteride can produce regression of benign prostatic hypertrophy and improve the symptoms of prostatism (Ch. 15).

FURTHER READING

Conway AJ, Handelsman DJ, Lording DW et al (2000) Use, misuse and abuse of androgens. *Med J Aust* 172, 220–224

Rhoden EL, Morgentaler A (2004) Risks of testosterone-replacement therapy and recommendations for monitoring. *N Engl J Med* 350, 482–492

Schneider HPG (2003) Androgens and antiandrogens. *Ann N Y Acad Sci* 997, 292–306

Self-assessment

In questions 1 and 2, the first statement, in italics, is true. Are the accompanying statements also true?

1. *Mature men with androgen deficiency may have decreased libido, impotence, reduced muscle mass and reduced body hair.*

   a. Testosterone cannot be given orally.
   b. Testosterone alone cannot stimulate spermatogenesis.
   c. Nandrolone causes less virilisation in women than androgens.

2. *The antiandrogen cyproterone acetate is used as an adjunct to the treatment of prostate cancer and hirsutism.* Antiandrogens can cause gynaecomastia.

3. Regarding drugs that affect androgenic and anabolic activities, choose the one <u>most appropriate</u> option from the following.

   A. 5α-Reductase inactivates dehydrotestosterone.
   B. Cyproterone acetate promotes spermatogenesis.
   C. Nandrolone reduces muscle mass.
   D. Danazol is used in the treatment of endometriosis.
   E. Testosterone has marked anti-anabolic activity.

   The answers are provided on page 741.

Drugs acting on the male reproductive system

Drug	Half-life	Elimination	Comment
Androgens			
Danazol	3 h	Metabolism	Clinical uses are *not* related to its weak androgenic activity (see compendium for Ch. 45); given orally; metabolites are inactive
Mesterolone (methyltestosterone)	3 h	Metabolism	Used for androgen deficiency and male infertility associated with hypogonadism; given orally; eliminated as glucuronide and sulphate conjugates; oral bioavailability is 50%
Testosterone and esters	See comments	Metabolism	Used for androgen deficiency and breast cancer in women; given orally (as undecanoate), by intramuscular injection (as enantate or propionate), as an implant (as testosterone) or as patches (as testosterone); testosterone per se is inactive orally; testosterone is very rapidly cleared from blood and the different dosage methods act as 'sustained-release' preparations that maintain blood testosterone concentrations despite its rapid elimination
Anabolic steroids			
Nandrolone decanoate	5–17 days (from injection)	Metabolism	Used for aplastic anaemia, and has been used for osteoporosis in postmenopausal women; given as deep intramuscular injection (sustained release – see testosterone); the in vivo half-life is dependent on release from the depot injection, since the half-life for hydrolysis and the elimination of nandrolone from the circulation is only 4 h
Antiandrogens[a]			
Bicalutamide	7–10 days	Metabolism	Used for advanced prostate cancer; given orally; undergoes oxidation and conjugation, with the metabolites excreted in urine and bile
Cyproterone acetate	2 days	Metabolism	Used as an adjunct for prostate cancer, for hirsutism and acne in women, and for severe hypersexuality and sexual deviation in men; given orally; hydrolysed and conjugated with glucuronic acid and sulphate; metabolites eliminated in urine and bile
Dutasteride[b]	5 weeks	Metabolism	Used for benign prostatic hyperplasia; selective inhibitor of type I and II 5α-reductase; given orally; oral bioavailability about 60%; metabolised by CYP3A4 to largely inactive products; long half-life results in slow accumulation to steady-state (by about 6 months)
Finasteride[b]	5–6 h	Metabolism	Used for benign prostatic hyperplasia and male-pattern baldness in men; given orally; selective inhibitor of type II 5α-reductase; metabolised by hepatic oxidation
Flutamide	8 h	Metabolism	Used for advanced prostate cancer; acts by inhibition of the uptake and/or nuclear binding of testosterone and dihydrotestosterone by prostatic tissue; given orally; essentially complete oral bioavailability; rapid oxidation in the liver to an active hydroxy metabolite

[a]Note: the gonadorelin analogues (buserelin, goserelin, leuprorelin and triptorelin) given in the drug compendium for Chapter 45 are used for their antiandrogenic properties.
[b]Inhibitor of 5α-reductase, which converts testosterone to 5α-dihydrotestosterone (DHT), the primary androgen that stimulates the development of prostate tissue.

47

Anaemia and haematopoietic colony-stimulating factors

Anaemia

The definition of anaemia is rather arbitrary, and the absolute normal ranges vary between laboratories. In adults, anaemia equates to a blood concentration of haemoglobin in males below about 135 g l^{-1} (normal is about 154 g l^{-1}) or in females below about 115 g l^{-1} (normal is about 135 g l^{-1}). Lower concentrations can be normal in children. Anaemia causes symptoms such as shortness of breath and fatigue. Many individuals, however, have concentrations below these arbitrary values without apparent detriment. There are many causes of anaemia (Box 47.1).

Anaemias are classified by red cell size and haemoglobin content (Box 47.2).

Iron

Dietary iron is absorbed from the duodenum and upper jejunum. Most iron is absorbed from meat in an omnivorous diet, and is present as haem, i.e. as the ferrous form complexed with a porphyrin ring. Haem is readily absorbed from the gut, but non-haem iron, which is mainly in the ferric state, is inefficiently absorbed. Gastric acid increases the solubility of ferric iron, which then binds to mucoprotein. Conversion of ferric to ferrous iron is then aided by reducing agents such as ascorbic acid, fructose and some amino acids. Intestinal absorption of non-haem iron is mediated by the divalent metal transporter (DMT-1); expression of the transporter is increased in iron deficiency and in hereditary haemochromatosis.

In the circulation, ferric iron is bound to the globulin transferrin and transported to the bone marrow and

---

Box 47.1

Causes of anaemia

Reduced red cell production
    Defective precursor proliferation, e.g. iron deficiency, anaemia of chronic disorder, marrow aplasia or infiltration
    Defective precursor maturation, e.g. vitamin B$_{12}$ or folate deficiency, myelodysplastic syndrome, toxins

Increased rate of red cell destruction
    Haemolysis

Loss of circulating red cells
    Bleeding

Box 47.2

Classification of anaemias by red cell characteristics

Hypochromic, microcytic (small size cells)
    Genetic, e.g. thalassaemia, sideroblastic anaemia
    Acquired, e.g. iron deficiency, sideroblastic anaemia

Normochronic, macrocytic (large size cells)
    With megalobastic marrow: vitamin B$_{12}$ or folate deficiency
    With normoblastic marrow: alcohol, myelodysplasia

Polychromatophilic, macrocytic
    Haemolysis

Normochromic, normocytic (normal size cells)
    Chronic disorders, e.g. infection, malignancy, autoimmune disease
    Renal failure
    Bone marrow failure

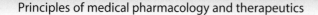

iron stores. Cellular iron uptake occurs via transferrin receptors, and within most cells, iron is stored complexed to the protein ferritin. In some tissues, iron is also found as the insoluble degraded form of ferritin, known as haemosiderin. Two-thirds of the iron in the body is present in circulating red cells, and about half of the remainder is stored. The rest is in myoglobin or associated with various enzymes. When ageing red cells are broken down by the reticuloendothelial system, most of the released iron is recycled. Iron loss from the body is small, and occurs through shedding of mucosal cells containing ferritin.

Iron deficiency

The main cause of iron deficiency in the UK is abnormal loss of blood, particularly from the gut or exaggerated menstrual loss. Iron malabsorption can result from disease of the upper small intestine, for example coeliac disease, or following partial gastrectomy. Dietary deficiency is rarely a major cause in Western societies, although, worldwide, a vegetarian diet low in absorbable iron is the commonest contributory cause of iron deficiency.

Therapeutic iron preparations

Oral iron

Oral supplements are preferred and are given as ferrous salts, for example sulphate, fumarate or gluconate. Tablets are normally used, but some people find a syrup more acceptable. In anaemia, a daily dose of 100–200 mg of elemental iron produces the maximum rate of rise of haemoglobin (200 mg ferrous sulphate = 65 mg elemental iron); about one-third of this dose will be absorbed. Gastrointestinal intolerance to oral iron is common, but unwanted effects can be minimised by taking iron supplements with food or by reducing the dose. Modified-release iron formulations have been developed to improve tolerance, but much of the iron is released beyond the site where it is best absorbed. These formulations should only be used when other methods for improving iron tolerance are ineffective.

Unwanted effects

- Gastrointestinal intolerance, especially nausea and dyspepsia. The prevalence of these effects depends both on the dose of elemental iron and on psychological factors, rather than the iron salt used. Diarrhoea or constipation also occur, but are not dose related.
- Oral iron turns stools black.

Parenteral iron

Parenteral iron preparations are used if there are intractable unwanted effects from oral preparations, if there is severe uncorrectable malabsorption or continuing heavy blood loss, and when adherence to oral treatment is poor. Parenteral iron does not raise the haemoglobin concentration any faster than oral iron, except in severe renal failure during dialysis.

Intravenous: iron dextran or iron sucrose

Iron dextran is a complex of ferric hydroxide with dextrans that is not bound to transferrin but accumulates in reticuloendothelial cells. It is usually given as a 'total dose' intravenous infusion, when the approximate total body deficit (haemoglobin and body stores) is estimated from the person's size and haemoglobin concentration, then replaced with a single slow iron infusion. Iron sucrose (ferric hydroxide with sucrose) is an alternative formulation.

Unwanted effects

- nausea, vomiting, diarrhoea
- flushing, fever
- headache
- bronchospasm
- chest pains, arthralgia, myalgia
- urticaria
- anaphylactoid reactions, including cardiovascular collapse; facilities for resuscitation should always be available.

Therapeutic use of iron

The cause of iron deficiency should always be sought before resorting to symptomatic treatment with iron. If this is not done, serious disorders, such as gastrointestinal malignancy, can be overlooked. Oral iron supplements are adequate for most mild or moderate iron deficiency anaemias, and, after an initial delay of a few days, should raise the haemoglobin concentration by about 20 g l^{-1} over 3–4 weeks. After the haemoglobin concentration has been restored, oral iron supplements should be continued for three months to replenish tissue iron stores.

Failure to respond to oral iron can be caused by several factors:

- incorrect diagnosis, e.g. anaemia of chronic disorder, thalassaemia
- poor adherence to prescribed iron therapy
- inadequate iron dosage, e.g. in some modified-release formulations
- continuing excessive blood loss
- malabsorption
- concurrent deficiency of other haematinics (substances that increase haemoglobin).

Iron supplements are occasionally given for prophylaxis against iron deficiency at times of high demand for iron, e.g. pregnancy, menorrhagia, or if there is a poor diet. The reduced iron absorption after subtotal or total gastrectomy may also be overcome by long-term iron supplements.

Folic acid

Folic acid (pteroylglutamic acid) is ingested as conjugated folate polyglutamates, found mainly in fresh leaf vegetables (in which it is heat labile) and in liver (where it is more heat stable). Before absorption, the polyglutamates are deconjugated to the monoglutamate, then methylated and reduced to 5-methyltetrahydrofolate by dihydrofolate reductase. 5-Methyltetrahydrofolate is absorbed principally in the duodenum and jejunum. Tetrahydrofolate is essential for the synthesis of pyrimidines and purines and hence of DNA (see also Ch. 52)

Folate deficiency

The most obvious consequence of folate deficiency is a macrocytic anaemia with the presence of megaloblasts in the marrow, a feature it shares with vitamin B_{12} deficiency. Folate deficiency can arise for a number of reasons (Box 47.3).

Therapeutic use of folic acid

Folate deficiency almost always responds to oral folic acid supplements. Folic acid is a poor substrate for dihydrofolate reductase, and is largely absorbed unchanged and then converted to tetrahydrofolic acid in the plasma and liver. Treatment is usually given for 4 months to correct the anaemia and replace folate stores.

Box 47.3

Causes of folate deficiency

- Poor diet: folate stores are adequate for a few weeks only. Lack of folate is uncommon in Western diets, but may be more common in the diet of elderly people or in alcoholism.
- Increased requirements: e.g. pregnancy, malignancies, haemolytic anaemias, exfoliative dermatitis.
- Malabsorption: e.g. coeliac disease, tropical sprue.
- Drugs that interfere with folate metabolism; anticonvulsants (especially phenytoin, Ch. 23), methotrexate (Ch. 52), pyrimethamine (Ch. 51)

Folic acid is given prophylactically in pregnancy. It is given in higher doses if there is a history of neural tube defect in a previous pregnancy, when it may protect against recurrence. Folic acid is also given prophylactically during renal dialysis, to premature infants, and in chronic haemolytic anaemia.

Treatment of deficiencies in both vitamin B_{12} and folate using only folic acid may correct the anaemia, but neurological damage can be precipitated (see below). Therefore, vitamin B_{12} deficiency must be excluded before folic acid is used, or both vitamin B_{12} and folic acid should be administered if the extent of the deficiency is uncertain.

For folate deficiency produced by drugs that inhibit the enzyme dihydrofolate reductase (e.g. methotrexate, Ch. 52), it is necessary to 'bypass' this enzyme blockade by giving the synthetic tetrahydrofolic acid, folinic acid (5-formyl tetrahydrofolic acid), given as calcium folinate, disodium folinate or calcium levofolinate; this is the basis of 'leucovorin rescue' discussed in Chapter 52.

Vitamin B_{12}

The term vitamin B_{12} refers to a group of cobalt-containing compounds, also known as cobalamins. Bacteria are the only organisms that can synthesise cobalamins de novo. Humans obtain vitamin B_{12} from meat (particularly liver), from animal products (milk, cheese, eggs, etc.) or from vegetables contaminated by bacteria. Absorption is by an unusual mechanism: dietary vitamin B_{12} binds in the stomach to a glycoprotein called intrinsic factor that is produced by gastric parietal cells. This complex is absorbed principally from the terminal ileum after binding to receptors on the luminal membranes of ileal cells.

In plasma, most vitamin B_{12} is bound to a glycoprotein, transcobalamin I, from which it is rapidly taken up by the tissues, especially the liver, where about 50% of the body content of vitamin B_{12} is stored. A second protein, transcobalamin II, is mainly responsible for rapid transport to tissues, and for enhancing vitamin B_{12} uptake by the bone marrow via specific receptors. Vitamin B_{12} is essential as a coenzyme in nucleic acid synthesis, and in other metabolic pathways in conjunction with folate. Effects of vitamin B_{12} include isomerisation of methylmalonyl coenzyme A to succinyl coenzyme A, isomerisation of α-leucine to β-leucine, and methylation of homocysteine to methionine.

Vitamin B_{12} deficiency

Impairment of vitamin B_{12}-dependent reactions affects DNA synthesis. The major organs affected by vitamin

B_{12} deficiency are those with a rapid cell turnover, i.e. bone marrow and the gastrointestinal tract.

Vitamin B_{12} deficiency presents with a macrocytic anaemia and a megaloblastic bone marrow. The tongue becomes smooth, and changes to the lining of the small bowel can lead to malabsorption. Damage to the posterior and lateral neuronal tracts in the spinal cord can also occur, leading to a condition known as subacute combined degeneration of the cord. The biochemical basis for the neurological damage is poorly understood: it may not be fully reversible after correction of vitamin B_{12} deficiency.

Causes of vitamin B_{12} deficiency include:

- diet: strict vegetarians (vegans) only
- intestinal malabsorption due to damage to the terminal ileum, for example Crohn's disease, lymphoma
- deficiency of intrinsic factor: pernicious anaemia (destruction of gastric parietal cells with achlorhydria and failure of intrinsic factor production), total and subtotal gastrectomy.

Therapeutic use of vitamin B_{12}

Most people with vitamin B_{12} deficiency have problems absorbing it from the gut, and treatment is usually by intramuscular injection of vitamin B_{12} in aqueous solution. Hydroxocobalamin is the form of vitamin B_{12} used for treating anaemia, and has completely replaced cyanocobalamin, because it is more highly bound to transcobalamins and less is excreted in the urine. Following initial injections on alternate days for 2 weeks to replenish stores, maintenance injections every 3 months for life are adequate. In the rare dietary causes of vitamin B_{12} deficiency, oral cyanocobalamin supplements can be given, but otherwise oral treatment is never indicated.

Erythropoietin

Examples: epoetin, darbepoetin

Erythropoietin is a glycosylated protein hormone, produced mainly by the kidney, which regulates red cell production by stimulating differentiation and proliferation of erythroid precursors. Deficiency of erythropoietin in end-stage renal disease contributes to the anaemia that characterises this disorder. Human erythropoietin has been synthesised using recombinant DNA technology (epoetin): it is produced in two forms, alpha and beta, which have identical clinical effects. Erythropoetin is also available as a hyperglycosylated derivative, darbepoetin, which has a longer half-life.

Pharmacokinetics

Epoetin can be given intravenously or, more conveniently, subcutaneously, when a 25–50% lower dose can be used. The red cell response is most rapid after intravenous use, but ultimately greater after subcutaneous injection. Doses of epoetin are normally given two or three times weekly. Darbepoetin is given once a week. Adequate iron stores are essential, since erythropoiesis demands large amounts of iron, and iron supplements may improve the response. The route of elimination is uncertain, but may be largely by receptor-mediated uptake in the bone marrow and subsequent intracellular degradation.

Unwanted effects

- influenza-like symptoms early in treatment.
- hypertension, which is dose-dependent and can be severe, leading to encephalopathy with seizures.
- thrombosis of arteriovenous shunts.
- pure red cell aplasia occurs rarely during subcutaneous administration in renal failure; this is usually associated with formation of antibodies to epoetin and treatment must be discontinued if this occurs.

Therapeutic uses of epoetin

- Anaemia of end-stage renal disease. Other causes of anaemia should be excluded, and iron supplements may be needed to maximise the response. Anaemia can be corrected in more than 90% of those treated, and treatment improves quality of life. Epoetin also modulates lipid metabolism, creating a less atherogenic plasma lipid profile, which may reduce the high cardiovascular mortality in renal failure.
- To increase red cell production prior to surgery. Autologous blood transfusion is becoming more popular to reduce the use of banked blood. Epoetin given twice weekly for 3 weeks before surgery can increase the number of units of blood that can be obtained.
- Anaemia associated with human immunodeficiency virus (HIV) infection or acquired immunodeficiency syndrome (AIDS).
- Anaemia associated with cytotoxic chemotherapy of non-myeloid malignant disease (Ch. 52).
- Epoetin is sometimes abused by athletes to increase haematocrit and improve performance. This abuse is associated with an increased risk of arterial and venous thromboses.

Drug treatment in other anaemias

Certain other anaemias require specific drug therapy.

> **Box 47.4**
>
> **Causes of aplastic anaemia**
>
> Drugs:
> - cytotoxic agents
> - chloramphenicol
> - sulphonamides
> - NSAIDs (especially phenylbutazone)
> - gold salts
> - carbimazole
> - phenytoin
> - carbamazepine
> - phenothiazines
> - chlorpropamide
>
> Radiation
> Infections, e.g. hepatitis, Epstein–Barr virus
> Inherited, e.g. Fanconi anaemia
> Malignant, e.g. myelodysplastic syndrome

> **Box 47.5**
>
> **More common causes of sideroblastic anaemia**
>
> Congenital
> Acquired
> Myelodysplastic syndrome
> Drugs:
> - isoniazid
> - chloramphenicol
> - alcoholism
> - lead poisoning

> **Box 47.6**
>
> **Drugs causing haemolysis in glucose-6-phosphate dehydrogenase deficiency**
>
> Antimalarials
>   Primaquine
>   Pamaquine
>
> Analgesics
>   Aspirin (high dose)
>
> Others
>   Sulphonamides
>   Nalidixic acid
>   Dapsone

Aplastic anaemia. Failure of haemopoietic stem cell production has many causes, including certain drugs (Box 47.4). Drugs do not have a major role in treatment. The anabolic steroid oxymetholone (available in the UK only on a named-patient basis) is sometimes used, but its effectiveness is unpredictable. Antilymphocyte globulin is helpful in some acquired aplastic anaemias, perhaps in combination with ciclosporin (Ch. 39).

Sideroblastic anaemia. This can also be caused by drugs (Box 47.5). It is characterised by accumulation of iron in erythroblasts, particularly in the mitochondria which lie in a ring around the nucleus. Staining for iron reveals the characteristic ring sideroblasts. Pyridoxine supplements can increase the haemoglobin concentration in idiopathic acquired and hereditary forms of the disorder. They can also be useful for reversible sideroblastic anaemia associated with pregnancy, haemolysis, alcohol dependence or during treatment with the antituberculous drug isoniazid (Ch. 51).

Autoimmune haemolytic anaemia. This can respond to immunosuppression with corticosteroids (Ch. 44).

β-Thalassaemia major. This is a genetic disorder of haemoglobin synthesis with a hyperplastic bone marrow and refractory anaemia. Blood transfusions or excessive iron supplements lead to iron overload, with damage to the liver, heart and pancreas. Iron overload can be prevented with infusions of desferrioxamine (Ch. 53) together with vitamin C, which enhances iron excretion. An oral iron chelator, deferiprone, is used when desferrioxamine is poorly tolerated or contraindicated, but it can cause neutropenia.

Sickle cell anaemia. This inherited disorder occurs when more than 80% of the haemoglobin is HbS; fetal haemoglobin (HbF) forms the remainder. Hydroxycarbamide (see Ch. 52) raises the HbF concentration and also reduces the number of young red cells, which are those most likely to adhere to endothelium and occlude blood vessels. Hydroxycarbamide reduces the frequency and severity of sickle cell crises.

Drugs as a cause of anaemia

- Iron deficiency: especially drugs causing bleeding from the upper gut, e.g. non-steroidal anti-inflammatory drugs (NSAIDs).
- Aplastic anaemia (Box 47.4).
- Sideroblastic anaemia (Box 47.5).
- Haemolysis in glucose-6-phosphate dehydrogenase (G6PD) deficiency (Box 47.6). G6PD is involved in generating reduced glutathione, which protects red cells against oxidative stresses. Oxidant drugs produce haemolysis in deficient individuals, who are usually male (Ch. 53).

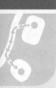

Neutropenia

Leucocytes are part of the first-line defence against pathogens. They include phagocytic cells (neutrophils, monocytes and eosinophils) and non-phagocytic cells (lymphocytes and basophils). In addition to their role in acute inflammation, all these cells participate in regulation of cellular and humoral immunity through production of cytokines (Ch. 38). A reduction in the number of circulating neutrophils (neutropenia) in particular increases the risk of serious infection. There are several causes of neutropenia (Box 47.7).

Drugs for neutropenia

Colony-stimulating factors

Colony-stimulating factors are molecules produced by many cells, such as endothelial cells, monocytes and fibroblasts, which stimulate maturation of pluripotent stem cells in the bone marrow. Several of these factors have now been produced by recombinant DNA technology, including granulocyte–macrophage colony-stimulating factor (GM-CSF) and granulocyte colony-stimulating factor (G-CSF), which acts only on neutrophil cell lines. Therapeutic agents include:

- filgrastim (unglycosylated recombinant human granulocyte colony-stimulating factor, rhG-CSF)
- lenograstim (glycosylated rhG-CSF)
- pegfilgrastim (polyethylene glycol-conjugated [pegylated] derivative of filgrastim)
- molgramostim (recombinant human granulocyte–macrophage colony-stimulating factor, rhGM-CSF).

The molecules are glycosylated in their natural state, but this does not seem to be a prerequisite for effectiveness.

A transient fall in circulating white cell numbers occurs within minutes of the injection, followed a few hours later by a substantial rise. After treatment with G-CSF, circulating neutrophils increase, while after GM-CSF, there is also a smaller rise in monocyte and eosinophil counts.

Pharmacokinetics

Colony-stimulating factors are given by prolonged intravenous infusion or subcutaneous injection to achieve sufficient stimulation of the bone marrow. After chemotherapy, daily injections are given until there is an adequate neutrophil response. Pegfilgrastim has a longer duration of action than filgrastim, and is only given once after chemotherapy. Filgrastim, lenograstim and molgramostim are eliminated both by the kidney and by neutrophil uptake. Pegfilgrastim is not eliminated by the kidney, and has a prolonged effect in neutropenia, since few neutrophils are available to contribute to its elimination.

Unwanted effects

rhGM-CSF (molgramostim) has more unwanted effects than rhG-CSF (filgrastim, lenograstim, pegfilgrastim).

- musculoskeletal or bone pain
- headache
- fever
- fatigue
- anorexia, nausea, vomiting , diarrhoea
- myeloproliferative disorders with long-term treatment
- osteoporosis with long-term treatment.

Therapeutic use of colony-stimulating factors

The use of these drugs remains controversial in many indications.

Congenital neutropenia. There is concern over the risk of promoting myeloid malignancy with prolonged use in this condition. Molgramostim is ineffective.

Chemotherapy-induced neutropenia. The duration of neutropenia may be reduced, with a reduction in associated sepsis. However, there is no evidence that long-term survival is improved.

Mobilisation of progenitor cells into peripheral blood for harvesting prior to bone marrow transplantation. The white blood cell count rises 7–12 days after treatment, and the cells are obtained via a cell separation machine.

Box 47.7

Causes of neutropenia

Inherited
  Congenital agranulocytosis
  Cyclical neutropenia

Acquired
  Viral infection, e.g. hepatitis, influenza, rubella, infectious mononucleosis
  Bacterial infection
  Radiotherapy
  Drugs, especially cytotoxic drugs, carbimazole
  Autoimmune
  Hypersplenism
  Marrow infiltration

FURTHER READING

Crawford J, Dale DC, Lyman GH (2004) Chemotherapy-induced neutropenia: risks, consequences and new directions for its management. *Cancer* 100, 228–237

Frewin R, Henson A, Provan D (1997) Iron deficiency anaemia. *BMJ* 314, 360–363

Glaspy JA (2003) Haematopoietic management in oncology practice. Part 1. Myeloid growth factors. *Oncology (Huntingt)* 17, 1593–1603

Henry DH, Bowers P, Romano MT et al (2004) Epoietin alpha. Clinical evolution of a pleiotropic cytokine. *Arch Intern Med* 164, 262–276

Hoffbrand V, Provan D (1997) Macrocytic anaemias. *BMJ* 314, 430–433

Hubell K, Engert A (2003) Clinical applications of granulocyte colony-stimulating factor: an update and summary. *Ann Haematol* 82, 207–213

Macdougall IC (2003) Erythropoetin and renal failure. *Curr Haematol Rep* 2, 459–464

Muirhead N (1997) The clinical impact of recombinant human erythropoietin. *J R Coll Physicians Lond* 31, 125–129

Ng T, Marx G, Littlewood T et al (2003) Recombinant erythropoetin in clinical practice. *Postgrad Med J* 79, 367–376

Provan D, Weatherall D (2000) Red cells II: acquired anaemias and polycythaemias. *Lancet* 355, 1260–1268

Weatherall D, Provan D (2000) Red cells I: inherited anaemias. *Lancet* 355, 1169–1175

Weiss MJ (2003) New insights into erythropoietin and epoetin alpha: mechanisms of action, target tissues, and clinical applications. *Oncologist* 8(suppl 3), 18–29

Self-assessment

In questions 1–4, the first statement, in italics, is true. Are the accompanying statements also true?

1. *Pernicious anaemia is caused by reduced vitamin B_{12} absorption due to autoimmunity that inhibits intrinsic factor release from the parietal cell.*

   a. Vitamin B_{12} is absorbed from the stomach.
   b. In vitamin B_{12} deficiency, treatment is required for life.
   c. The blood film in pernicious anaemia shows macrocytosis.

2. *The most common causes of megaloblastic anaemias are vitamin B_{12} or folate deficiency.*

   a. Both vitamin B_{12} and folate are essential for DNA synthesis. A product of folate is necessary for purine and pyrimidine synthesis, and vitamin B_{12} is also necessary for the formation of a cofactor in the synthesis of purines and pyrimidines.
   b. Folate deficiency can be associated with drug therapy, examples of which are methotrexate, trimethoprim and phenytoin.
   c. Folic acid cannot be given orally.

3. *Erythropoietin is a product of the kidney that stimulates progenitor cells to generate erythrocytes.* Chronic renal failure can result in a deficiency in erythropoietin.

4. *Colony-stimulating factors (CSFs) are formed from many cells and control the formation and survival of neutrophils, monocytes and eosinophils.* CSFs reduce the release of progenitor cells of neutrophils from bone marrow into the circulation.

5. Concerning the properties of erythropoetin, choose the one correct answer from the following.

   A. Erythropoetin is synthesised mainly by the adrenal glands.
   B. Erythropoetin can correct anaemia in end-stage renal disease.
   C. Erythropoetin is an effective sole treatment of anaemia even if iron levels are low.
   D. Erythropoetin can reduce athletic performance in long-distance runners.
   E. Erythropoetin can be given orally.

6. Concerning the usage and properties of folic acid and its metabolites, choose the one **incorrect** answer from the following.

   A. Tetrahydrofolate is a product of folic acid metabolism involved in the synthesis of the bases in DNA.
   B. Administration of folate to correct folate deficiencies requires months of treatment.
   C. Folate is absorbed in the duodenum.
   D. To correct the folate deficiency caused by methotrexate, tetrahydrofolic acid is given rather than folic acid.
   E. Deficiency in vitamin B_{12} and folic acid both cause macrocytic megaloblastic anaemia.

7. Case history questions

   A 40-year-old woman complained to her GP of fatigue and heavy menstrual periods lasting 7 days and occurring every 28 days. Her GP noted that she was pallid; her haemoglobin level was 67 g l^{-1} and mean cell volume (MCV) was 61 fl. Other blood measurements of platelets and white cell counts were unremarkable.

Self-assessment questions

a. How would you interpret these data and what were the possible reasons?
b. What biochemical tests could have helped the diagnosis?

The tests confirmed iron deficiency anaemia.

c. What pharmaceutical preparation should have been given?

Several iron formulations were tried, as the woman felt unwell taking ferrous sulphate.

d. What unwanted effects might she have experienced?
e. Where was the iron absorbed?
f. In what dietary form would iron have been optimally absorbed?

After 2 months of oral iron therapy, the haemoglobin value was 80 g l^{-1}.

g. Was this a sufficient response?

The woman was intolerant of oral iron.

h. What could have been the reasons for the poor response?
i. What alternative treatment could have been administered?

Her haemoglobin rose to 115 g l^{-1} over 2–3 weeks.

The answers are provided on page 741.

Anaemia and haematopoietic colony-stimulating factors

Drug	Half-life	Elimination	Comments
Iron			
Oral formulations			
Ferrous sulphate Ferrous fumarate Ferrous gluconate Ferrous glycine sulphate Polysaccharide-iron complex Sodium feredetate	–	–	Often given as co-formulations with folic acid; extent of absorption depends on form, the presence of food, and iron status; water-soluble forms are the sulphate and gluconate, whereas the fumarate and glycine sulphate are only sparingly soluble
Parenteral formulations			
Iron dextran	–	–	A complex of ferric hydroxide with sucrose containing 5% iron; given by slow i.v. injection or infusion; extensive uptake by macrophage-rich spleen with effective release for erythrocyte formation
Iron sucrose	–	–	A complex of ferric hydroxide with sucrose containing 2% iron; given by slow i.v. injection or infusion; extensive uptake by macrophage-rich spleen with effective release for erythrocyte formation
Drugs for megaloblastic anaemias			Hydroxocobalamin has completely replaced cyanocobalamin as the drug of choice
Cyanocobalamin	Dose-dependent	Renal + metabolism	Given orally or by intramuscular injection; dose-dependent absorption and elimination; free cyanocobalamin is eliminated by glomerular filtration (and, like creatinine, can be used to determine GFR); the excretion increases with dose, from 5% after 25 mg to 85% after 1000 mg; metabolism gives cobalamin
Folic acid	Dose-dependent	Renal	Has few indications for long-term therapy, since folate deficiency responds to a short course of treatment; usually given with hydroxocobalamin; given orally; 70–80% absorption; low doses are retained in cells and higher doses are eliminated in urine; folic acid *per se* does not occur naturally in food
Hydroxocobalamin	Dose-dependent	Renal + metabolism	Given by intramuscular injection; elimination by glomerular filtration, with 25% excreted at 500 mg and 29% at 1000 mg; excretion is complete by 24 h after dosage
Drugs used in hypoplastic, haemolytic and renal anaemias			
Darbepoetin alfa	20	Metabolism + renal	Recombinant form of renal erythropoietin that is used for anaemia associated with chronic renal disease and anaemia in adults receiving chemotherapy for non-myeloid malignancies; a hyperglycosylated derivative of epoetin with a longer half-life; given by i.v. or s.c. injection; eliminated largely by undefined metabolism; half-life is longer after s.c. dosage (30–90 h)

continued

Drug compendium

Anaemia and haematopoietic colony-stimulating factors *(continued)*

Drug	Half-life	Elimination	Comments
Drugs used in hypoplastic, haemolytic and renal anaemias *(continued)*			
Epoetin alfa and beta	4–6	Metabolism	Used for anaemia associated with chronic renal disease, to increase autologous blood in normal subjects and for anaemia in adults receiving chemotherapy for malignancies; given by s.c. or i.v. injection; catabolised by target cells after internalisation
Treatment of iron overload			
Deferiprone	1.5	Renal + metabolism	Used for iron overload in thalassaemia major for subjects intolerant to desferrioxamine; given orally; eliminated by renal excretion plus some conjugation with glucucronic acid
Desferrioxamine mesilate (deferoxamine mesilate)	6	Metabolism + renal	Used for iron overload in thalassaemia major, and for haemochromatosis in subjects in whom repeated venesection is contraindicated; given by s.c. infusion; chelating agent used for iron overload (or aluminium in dialysis patients); eliminated unchanged in urine (15–65%) and by metabolism to inactive products
Drugs used in neutropenia			All drugs are recombinant stimulating factors which have to be given parenterally; all drugs are for specialist use only
Filgrastim	3.5	Renal excretion + some neutrophil uptake	Unglycosylated rhG-CSF; used for reduction in the duration of neutropenia, for example following cytotoxic chemotherapy of malignancy, and for severe congenital neutropenia; given by s.c. injection or by s.c. or i.v. infusion; mostly eliminated by the kidneys (90% in animal studies)
Lenograstim	2.5–3.5 (s.c.); 1 (i.v.)	Renal excretion + neutrophil uptake	Glycosylated rhG-CSF; used for reduction in the duration of neutropenia, for example following cytotoxic chemotherapy of malignancy; given by s.c. injection or i.v. infusion
Molgramostin	1–1.5	Renal excretion + neutrophil uptake	rhGM-CSF; used for reduction in the severity of neutropenia, for example following cytotoxic chemotherapy of malignancy (ineffective in congenital neutropenia); given by s.c. injection or i.v. infusion
Pegfilgrastim	15–80	Slow elimination mostly by neutrophil uptake	Polyethylene glycol-conjugated (pegylated) derivative of filgrastim; used for reduction in the duration of neutropenia, for example following cytotoxic chemotherapy of malignancy; given by s.c. injection; clearance by neutrophil uptake depends on both the dose and the neutrophil count

i.v., intravenous; rhG-CSF, recombinant human granulocyte-colony stimulating factor; rhGM-CSF, recombinant human granulocyte–macrophage colony-stimulating factor; s.c., subcutaneous.

48

Lipid disorders

Lipids and lipoproteins

Lipid and lipoprotein metabolism is complex and the following account is a very brief summary, sufficient to establish the mechanism of action of drugs used to correct lipid abnormalities.

Cholesterol and triglycerides

Cholesterol is a vital structural component of cell membranes and a precursor of many other steroids, including bile salts and steroid hormones. Fatty acids are an important energy source: in plasma they are esterified with glycerol to form triglycerides, and fatty acids are released from triglycerides in periods of reduced calorie intake.

Cholesterol is a sterol that is mainly synthesised in the liver but is also obtained in the diet. Its synthesis in the liver involves several enzymes, but the rate-limiting step is catalysed by HMG-CoA (β-hydroxy-β-methylglutaryl-coenzyme A) reductase. Intracellular cholesterol causes negative feedback on HMG-CoA reductase to reduce further hepatic cholesterol synthesis. Cholesterol leaves hepatocytes either by transport into the circulation or by secretion into the bile after incorporation into bile salt micelles (Figs 48.1 and 48.2). Some cholesterol is absorbed from the gut, following either dietary ingestion or enterohepatic circulation of bile salts and cholesterol (Fig. 48.2).

Triglycerides are the major dietary fat, and can also be synthesised from intermediary metabolites formed in the liver from excess carbohydrate in the diet. Triglycerides are stored in adipose tissue, from which they can be mobilised as non-esterified free fatty acids to act as an energy substrate during periods of fasting.

A simplified account of lipoprotein metabolism

Lipids (triglycerides and esters of cholesterol) circulate in plasma encased in a coat of polar phospholipids, cholesterol and apolipoproteins. The apolipoprotein–lipid complexes are termed lipoproteins. They are usually classified according to the density of the particles into very-low-density (VLDL), low-density (LDL) intermediate-density (IDL) and high-density (HDL) lipoproteins. In healthy individuals, about 70% of plasma cholesterol is carried by LDL and 20% by HDL. The lipoproteins can be fractionated according to the triglyceride/cholesterol ratio they carry, their apolipoprotein constitution and their density (Table 48.1). The least dense and largest diameter particles, known as chylomicrons, are exclusively concerned with the transport of dietary lipid from the intestine to the liver. Their low density and large size reflect their high content of triglycerides (Table 48.1), and they almost completely disappear from blood after a 12-h fast. VLDL carries about 60% of plasma triglyceride in the fasting state. The source of the lipoproteins and their associated apolipoproteins are shown in Table 48.1.

Processing of lipids absorbed from the gut (Fig. 48.1)

Chylomicrons contain triglycerides and cholesterol with associated apolipoproteins; chylomicrons are formed in gut mucosal cells after absorption of cholesterol and triglycerides in micelles with bile salts. They pass into the lymphatic system and then into the circulation. Hydrolysis of triglycerides in the chylomicrons is carried out by a *lipoprotein lipase* (LPL, attached to endothelium of capillaries perfusing muscle and adipose tissue) and requires the chylomicron-associated apolipoprotein C (the subtype C-II) as a cofactor (Table 48.1). Free fatty acids are released by hydrolysis from chylomicrons and also from VLDL (synthesised by the liver, see below), and can then be utilised by muscle and liver as an energy source or stored as triglycerides in adipose tissue. After removal of triglycerides from the chylomicrons, the remaining surface lipoprotein and lipid fractions leave the particles to enter the HDL pool as 'nascent HDL' (Fig. 48.1). The chylomicron remnants are

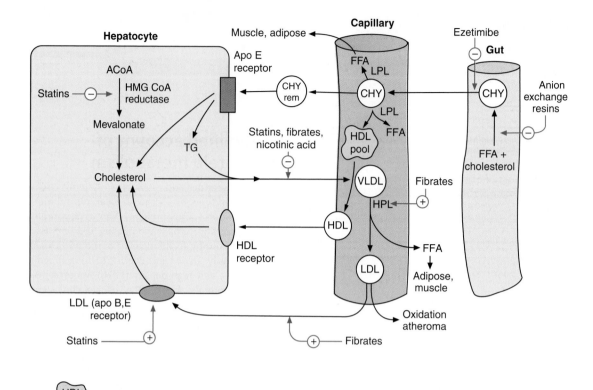

Fig. 48.1
Some steps in lipoprotein formation and metabolism. Apo, apolipoprotein; CHY, chylomicron; CHY rem, chylomicron remnant; FFA, free fatty acid; HPL, hepatic lipoprotein lipase; LPL, lipoprotein lipase; +, increases activity; −, decreases activity. The HDL pool is also referred to as nascent HDL and is an important source of mature HDL. It is derived from the chylomicron following the action of LPL. Drugs used and their targets are shown in red arrows.

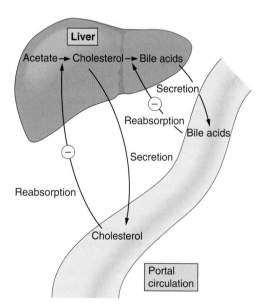

Fig. 48.2
Enterohepatic recycling of cholesterol and bile acids. They are secreted into the duodenum via the bile duct and are then returned to the liver by the portal circulation.

taken into hepatocytes by specific chylomicron remnant (apo E) receptors.

Plasma transport and liver processing of lipids

Liver cholesterol (as esters) and triglycerides in the liver that are surplus to synthetic and oxidative requirements are released into the circulation complexed to VLDL, which is synthesised by the liver. Peripheral LPL acts on VLDL to release free fatty acids, and the IDL is formed (not shown in Fig. 48.1); the enzyme *cholesterol ester transfer protein* (CETP) can transfer cholesterol from HDL to VLDL in exchange for triglycerides. The extent of these transfers depends on the concentration of circulating triglycerides. Triglycerides in IDL are hydrolysed by hepatic lipase to generate LDL. LDL therefore contains a higher concentration of cholesterol and a lower concentration of triglyceride compared with VLDL (Table 48.1). LDL is removed from the circulation by uptake into liver cells (75%) and peripheral tissues (25%). Some 70% of this uptake is by specific receptors for the apoproteins type B and E (Fig. 48.1), while the

Table 48.1
Apoliprotein and lipid composition of some lipoproteins and their sources

Lipoprotein	Major associated apolipoproteins[a]	Cholesterol (%)	Triglycerides (%)	Source
Chylomicrons	Apo A/Apo B/Apo B$_{48}$/Apo C/Apo E	3	90	Intestine
VLDL	Apo C/Apo B$_{100}$/Apo E	20	50	Liver
LDL	Apo B$_{100}$	50	7	VLDL
HDL	Apo A	40	6	Chylomicrons, VLDL, liver, intestine

[a]The associated apolipoproteins supply essential structural integrity without which the lipoprotein cannot be synthesised or secreted. Individual apolipoproteins also have roles in controlling enzymes involved in lipoprotein metabolism and as receptor ligands. For example, Apo B$_{100}$ and Apo E are the binding ligands for LDL and the chylomicron remnants, respectively (Fig. 48.1). Apo CI is associated with HDLs, and Apo CII activates lipoprotein lipase.
HDL, high-density lipoproteins, LDL, low-density lipoproteins, VLDL, very-low-density lipoproteins.

rest is by non-receptor-mediated pathways. The circulating levels of LDL rise if there is excess LDL or deficient receptor numbers, and non-receptor-mediated uptake of cholesterol in peripheral tissues such as arterial walls will then increase. This is followed by oxidation of LDL cholesterol, which leads to formation of lipid-rich deposits in arterial walls as atheromatous plaques (see below).

HDL carries cholesterol mobilised from peripheral tissues, and transports it to the liver. The efflux of cholesterol from peripheral cells is facilitated by *cholesterol efflux regulatory protein* (CERP). This cholesterol is bound to nascent HDL, then the cholesterol is esterified by the circulating enzyme *lecithin-cholesterol acyltransferase* (LCAT) to create mature HDL. HDL is believed to protect against atheroma by this reverse cholesterol transport from peripheral tissues to the liver.

Hyperlipidaemias and atheroma

Abnormalities of plasma lipoprotein metabolism produce an excess of circulating cholesterol and/or triglyceride concentrations. Their clinical importance lies in their relationship to the production of atheroma (mainly cholesterol with a contribution from triglycerides) and pancreatitis (triglycerides >12 mmol l^{-1}).

Injury to endothelium (possibly due to LDL as well as other atherogenic factors such as smoking or hypertension) encourages monocyte attachment and cholesterol accumulation from LDL. In the arterial wall, the cholesterol undergoes oxidation to produce a cytotoxic and chemotactic lipid that increases endothelial injury and attracts monocytes. Oxidised LDL is taken up into macrophages (derived from circulating monocytes), which migrate into the arterial wall. The lipid-rich

macrophages (foam cells) form the fatty streaks of atherosclerosis. Cytokine release from these cells enhances LDL binding to smooth muscle cells in the arterial wall, while the endothelial injury initiates platelet activation and smooth muscle cell proliferation over the lipid-based plaque.

Atherogenic patterns of lipoproteins can result from the following.

- Dietary factors.
- Primary (inherited) disorders of enzymes or receptors involved in lipid metabolism. Most inherited hyperlipidaemias are polygenic, but an important inherited defect is familial hypercholesterolaemia, a single recessive gene disorder that affects 1 in 500 of the population, who have reduced synthesis of LDL receptors.
- Secondary lipid disorders, when hyperlipidaemia results from diseases that affect lipid metabolism, for example liver disease, nephrotic syndrome, hypothyroidism.

A classification for the various phenotypic patterns of primary hyperlipidaemia adopted by the World Health Organization is shown in Table 48.2.

Drugs for hyperlipidaemias

HMG-CoA reductase inhibitors ('statins')

Examples: atorvastatin, pravastatin, simvastatin

Mechanism of action and effects
HMG-CoA reductase inhibitors competitively inhibit the enzyme that catalyses the rate-limiting step in the synthesis of cholesterol by the liver (Fig. 48.1). The fall in

Table 48.2
The Fredrickson classification of dyslipidaemias

Type	Triglyceride	Total cholesterol	LDL cholesterol	Raised lipoprotein	Atheroma risk
I	+++	+	N	Chylomicrons	N
IIa	N	++	++	LDL	+++
IIb	++	++	++	LDL/VLDL	+++
III	++	+	N	VLDL and chylomicron remnants	++
IV	++	N/+	N	VLDL	++
V	+++	+	N	VLDL/chylomicrons	N

N = Normal; + = slightly raised; ++ = moderately raised; +++ = extremely raised.

Box 48.1

Non-lipid effects of statins

- Restored function to vascular endothelium that has been functionally damaged by hypercholesterolaemia. It is not known whether this is a direct effect or a consequence of reduction in plasma LDL cholesterol
- Stabilisation of atherosclerotic plaques by altered smooth muscle proliferation and migration (inhibited by simvastatin, unchanged by pravastatin)
- Changes in haemostasis: pravastatin decreases plasma fibrinogen and enhances fibrinolysis
- Reduction of inflammatory cell infiltration into atherosclerotic plaques

cholesterol available for bile acid synthesis produces a compensatory upregulation in the number of LDL receptors on the hepatocyte surface, with increased clearance of circulating LDL cholesterol. Statins also reduce the hepatic production of VLDL and, therefore, reduce circulating triglycerides, although the mechanism of this effect is unclear. A modest increase in HDL cholesterol is often seen. Statins also have several other actions, some of which may be distinct from their ability to reduce plasma lipids (Box 48.1). The contribution of these to the beneficial actions of statins is unknown.

Pharmacokinetics
The statins are well absorbed from the gut. Simvastatin is a prodrug (Ch. 2) which is activated by first-pass metabolism in the liver by cytochrome P450 (CYP3A). Further metabolism inactivates the drug and little active compound reaches the circulation. Atorvastatin undergoes first-pass metabolism, in part to active derivatives, and has a very long half-life. Pravastatin is a hydrophilic drug that is eliminated mainly by the kidneys; its half-life is short.

Unwanted effects

- Gastrointestinal upset, including nausea, vomiting, abdominal pain, flatulence and diarrhoea.
- Central nervous system effects, such as dizziness, blurred vision, headache.
- Transient disturbance of liver function tests, and, rarely, hepatitis.
- Myalgia or myositis, and, occasionally, rhabdomyolysis. The mechanism is uncertain, but reduced activation of muscle regulatory proteins that depend on the production of intermediates in the cholesterol synthetic pathway may be responsible. There is an increased risk when a statin is used in combination with a fibrate, nicotinic acid or ciclosporin (Ch. 38).

Specific cholesterol absorption inhibitors

Example: ezetimibe

Mechanism of action
Ezetimibe acts at the brush border of the small intestinal mucosa to specifically inhibit cholesterol absorption. Cholesterol absorption is reduced by about 50%, but it has no effect on the absorption of triglycerides, bile acids or fat-soluble vitamins. Given alone, ezetimibe reduces plasma total cholesterol by about 15% and LDL cholesterol by about 18%. When taken with a low dose of statin, the combination is as effective as three doublings of the statin dose.

Pharmacokinetics
Ezetimibe is rapidly but incompletely absorbed from the gut, and metabolised in the gut wall and the liver. It undergoes enterohepatic circulation, which gives it a long effective half-life. About 80% is excreted in the faeces.

Unwanted effects

- diarrhoea, abdominal pain
- headache
- angioedema.

Bile acid-binding (anion-exchange) resins

Example: colestyramine

Mechanism of action

Bile acid-binding resins are insoluble, non-absorbable polymers that bind bile salts in the gut and prevent enterohepatic circulation of bile acids. The taste and texture limit acceptability; consequently, they are no longer widely used. Bile acids are synthesised from cholesterol in the liver, a process that is initiated by the enzyme cholesterol 7α-hydroxylase. They are secreted into the duodenum to aid absorption of dietary fat, reabsorbed in the terminal ileum and returned to the liver in the portal circulation (Fig. 48.2). When reabsorption is impaired, there is a compensatory increase in bile acid synthesis in the liver, leading to a reduction in cholesterol. Intracellular cholesterol depletion in the liver results in upregulation of LDL receptors, and, as a result, LDL cholesterol in blood is cleared more rapidly, with a fall in circulating levels by 15–20%. Stimulation of VLDL synthesis produces a small rise in plasma triglycerides. There is a small rise in HDL cholesterol, but the mechanism is unclear.

Unwanted effects

- unpalatability: sachets containing several grams of powder have to be taken, usually mixed with food
- constipation, or, occasionally, diarrhoea
- interference with the absorption of certain acidic drugs, for example digoxin (Ch. 7), warfarin (Ch. 11) and thyroxine (Ch. 41); these drugs should be given at least 1 h before or 4 h after taking a resin.

Fibrates

Examples: bezafibrate, gemfibrozil, ciprofibrate

Mechanism of action

The main effect of these drugs is to activate a gene transcription factor known as peroxisome proliferator-activated receptor alpha (PPAR-α), which encodes for proteins that control lipoprotein metabolism. The mechanism of PPAR-mediated drug action is described in more detail in Chapter 40 (under thiazolidinediones). PPAR-α is expressed in several tissues, including the liver, heart and kidney. There are several consequences of PPAR-α activation:

- Increased free fatty acid uptake by the liver due to induction of the fatty acid transport protein in the cell membrane. In the liver, conversion to acyl-coenzyme A derivatives is enhanced as a result of increased acyl-CoA synthetase activity. The esterified fatty acids are less available for hepatic triglyceride synthesis.
- Increased mitochondrial free fatty acid uptake in the heart and skeletal muscle, with enhanced oxidation.
- Increased lipoprotein lipase activity, which enhances the clearance of triglycerides from lipoproteins in the plasma (Fig. 48.1).
- Increased plasma HDL because of enhanced apolipoprotein A-I and A-II production in the liver.

Pharmacokinetics

Fibrates are well absorbed from the gut and highly protein bound in the plasma. Excretion is primarily by the kidney, although some metabolism occurs in the liver. The half-lives of bezafibrate and gemfibrozil are short, whereas other fibrates have long half-lives.

Unwanted effects

- gastrointestinal upset
- rash or pruritis
- dizziness, headache
- increased lithogenicity of bile theoretically increases the risk of gallstones, but this has not been a problem with the drugs mentioned here
- myalgia or myositis are uncommon, unless there is impaired renal function or the fibrate is used in combination with a statin
- drug interactions include inhibition of the effect of warfarin (Ch. 11).

Nicotinic acid and derivatives

Examples: nicotinic acid, acipimox

Mechanism of action

Nicotinic acid is a B vitamin which, when used in pharmacological doses, has effects on lipids. It reduces lipolysis and, therefore, free fatty acid mobilisation from adipocytes, by acting at a high-affinity inhibitory G-protein-coupled membrane receptor, and reducing intracellular cyclic adenosine monophosphate (cAMP) generation. This leads to decreased free fatty acid availability to the liver and reduced hepatic triglyceride synthesis and VLDL secretion from the liver. Circulating triglycerides are substantially reduced by up to 35% and LDL cholesterol modestly reduced by up to 15%. HDL cholesterol is increased by up to 25%, as a result of reduced hepatic uptake of the HDL molecule. A decrease in the activity of hepatic lipase also shifts the distribution of HDL subfractions, with a predominant elevation of HDL_2, which has greater protective effect than HDL_3.

Pharmacokinetics

Nicotinic acid is well absorbed from the gut. Hepatic metabolism occurs via two pathways. Oxidation is a high-affinity, low-capacity pathway that is readily saturable and the products of which are thought to be responsible for high-dose niacin-induced hepatotoxicity. The other pathway is a low-affinity, high-capacity conjugation pathway. Very large doses of nicotinic acid are excreted unchanged in the urine. Nicotinic acid has a very short half-life.

Acipimox is a synthetic derivative of nicotinic acid that is longer-acting but rather less effective for lowering LDL cholesterol.

Unwanted effects

Nicotinic acid is often poorly tolerated, but unwanted effects can be reduced by gradual dosage increases. A modified-release formulation that minimises the risk of saturating hepatic metabolism, and acipimox, are better tolerated.

- cutaneous vasodilation (mediated by prostaglandins) is particularly troublesome and causes flushing and itching; a small dose of aspirin taken 30 min before nicotinic acid, or taking the drug with food, will reduce this
- gastrointestinal upset and peptic ulceration
- headache, dizziness
- glucose intolerance with high doses of nicotinic acid (not with acipimox)
- exacerbation of gout
- hepatotoxicity, which is less common with a modified-release formulation of niacin.

Omega-3 fatty acids

There are three long-chain polyunsaturated omega-3 fatty acids: alpha-linoleic acid, which is found in plants, and eicosapentaenoic acid (EPA) and docosahexaenoic acid (DHA), which are found in high quantities in oily fish such as mackerel and sardines. They have several potential cardioprotective effects.

- Since they are poor substrates for enzymes that synthesise triglycerides, they lead to production of triglyceride-poor LDL and reduce triglycerides in plasma, although cholesterol is increased. They also increase conversion of VLDL to LDL, and increase circulating HDL cholesterol.
- Reduction of plasma fibrinogen, decreasing thrombogenesis.
- Impairment of platelet aggregation (Ch. 11).
- Retardation of growth of atherosclerotic plaques by reduced expression of endothelial adhesion molecules and an anti-inflammatory action.
- Promotion of nitric oxide-mediated vasodilation.

- Membrane stabilisation in heart muscle, with reduced susceptibility to ventricular arrhythmias and sudden cardiac death.

Unwanted effects

- gastrointestinal upset with nausea, belching, diarrhoea or constipation
- prolonged bleeding time.

Management of hyperlipidaemias

Cardiovascular disease is the major risk associated with a raised LDL cholesterol. The relationship with raised LDL cholesterol is strongest for coronary atherosclerosis and peripheral vascular atherosclerosis, and to a lesser extent for cerebrovascular disease and atherothrombotic stroke. HDL cholesterol is protective against atherosclerosis; an HDL cholesterol of less than 1.0 mmol l^{-1} is associated with the highest risk of disease. The ratio of total cholesterol:HDL cholesterol provides a much more sensitive – and reliable – indicator of relative risk of cardiovascular disease than does total cholesterol alone.

While a high total cholesterol:HDL cholesterol ratio predicts the relative risk of cardiovascular disease, the absolute risk (i.e. the numbers of individuals in the population under study who will develop disease in unit time) will be determined by the coexistence of other risk factors (see below).

Raised plasma triglycerides are an independent predictor of the risk of atherosclerosis, but less so than raised plasma cholesterol. Nevertheless, when raised triglycerides coexist with an atherogenic cholesterol profile, the overall risk is enhanced. A markedly raised plasma triglyceride concentration (>12 mmol l^{-1}) confers a progressively increasing risk of acute pancreatitis. Isolated hypertriglyceridaemia should be treated intensively for this reason alone.

Before embarking on management of hyperlipidaemia, secondary causes such as diabetes, hypothyroidism and nephrotic syndrome should be excluded or treated.

Primary prevention of cardiovascular disease

Coronary atheroma has a multifactorial aetiology, and any strategy for primary prevention must consider all relevant treatable factors. Treatment of hyperlipidaemia with drugs for primary prevention should only be considered if there is a high absolute risk of disease, and should not be based on the lipid level alone. Important factors to consider in risk management include the following.

Smoking. Smoking doubles the risk of coronary artery disease. Stopping smoking reduces risk to that of a non-smoker in 3–5 years (see Ch. 5).

Physical activity. A physically active lifestyle reduces risk of myocardial infarction by up to 50%, compared with a sedentary lifestyle.

Maintaining ideal bodyweight. Obesity (see Ch. 37) increases the risk of myocardial infarction by up to 50%.

Mild-to-moderate alcohol consumption. A modest alcohol intake (see Ch. 54) can reduce the risk of myocardial infarction by about one-third. A high alcohol intake increases blood pressure, and thus increases cardiovascular risk.

Hypertension (see Ch. 6). Although treating hypertension is more effective for prevention of stroke, it also reduces the risk of myocardial infarction, especially in older people.

Control of diabetes. There is increasing evidence that close control of plasma glucose reduces vascular events. Since the risk of ischaemic heart disease in diabetes is at least twice that of non-diabetics, intensive management of coexistent risk factors in diabetics should also be undertaken.

Low-dose aspirin. This is less effective for primary prevention than for secondary prevention (Ch. 11) but is useful in selected high-risk individuals, especially those with hypertension.

Cholesterol. This is a powerful predictor of future cardiovascular disease, especially in young people. The greatest risk is present when there is familial hypercholesterolaemia (FH), a dominantly inherited genetic defect that predisposes to premature coronary heart disease even in the absence of other risk factors. Heterozygous FH is associated with reduced LDL receptors on liver cells, and the total serum cholesterol is usually greater than 7.5 mmol l^{-1} in adult life. Lipid-lowering therapy in FH, usually with a statin, should normally begin in late teens in males and early twenties in females (because of the later onset of disease).

For other forms of hypercholesterolaemia, the risk of cardiovascular disease should first be estimated using risk tables that assess the contribution of the cholesterol profile, systolic blood pressure, smoking, presence of diabetes, and preferably the presence of left ventricular hypertrophy on the electrocardiogram. The question exercising the minds of health economists is not whether treatment is effective, but when it becomes cost-effective. As part of a multiple risk factor intervention strategy, drug therapy has a role for those at higher absolute risk, usually because several other risk factors coexist or there is a history of premature coronary artery disease in a first-degree relative. Specialist societies in the UK concerned with coronary heart disease prevention believe that a raised cholesterol should be treated if the ten-year coronary heart disease risk is greater than 15% (equivalent to a cardiovascular disease risk that includes stroke of 20%). Once treatment is started, the target plasma cholesterol should be no greater than 5 mmol l^{-1} (LDL cholesterol less than 3 mmol l^{-1}) and, on the basis of the latest evidence, it should be 4 mmol l^{-1} (LDL cholesterol less than 2 mmol l^{-1}) to minimise risk.

Dietary management should be advised initially for all people with hypercholesterolaemia who do not have evidence of vascular disease. This involves a reduction in saturated-fat intake and an increase in mono-unsaturated fats. Increasing antioxidants in the diet by eating more fresh fruit and vegetables reduces oxidation of LDL cholesterol and therefore makes it less atherogenic. However, in most cases (and always in FH), drug therapy will be necessary in addition to dietary management. The ability of cholesterol-lowering drugs (and particularly statins) to prevent ischaemic heart disease has been demonstrated in many trials. Reducing plasma total cholesterol by 25–30% (with a reduction in LDL cholesterol of 30–35%) using a statin reduces the subsequent risk of myocardial infarction or vascular death by about 30%.

Secondary prevention of cardiovascular disease

Once cardiovascular disease is clinically apparent, the subsequent risk of death from vascular events is high. People with clinical evidence of vascular disease are at much greater absolute risk of a further event than those without clinical coronary artery disease who have similar, or even higher, plasma cholesterol concentrations. Recent myocardial infarction or an episode of unstable angina confers the highest risk. At slightly lower absolute risk are those with stable angina pectoris, peripheral vascular disease or ischaemic stroke. Reduction of even 'normal' plasma cholesterol concentrations (as low as 4.0 mmol l^{-1}) in people with vascular disease reduces the subsequent risk of both fatal and non-fatal cardiovascular events. Current evidence supports the use of statins as first-line therapy; trials with fibrates have shown less marked benefit unless the major lipid abnormality is a low HDL cholesterol (see also Ch. 5). The target cholesterol concentration is the same as for primary prevention. There is also strong evidence that the use of omega-3 fatty acids after myocardial infarction has a cardioprotective effect that may not entirely relate to their effects on plasma lipids. Lowering plasma cholesterol for secondary prevention of coronary artery disease should be only one aspect of a comprehensive strategy for improving prognosis. This is discussed more fully in Chapter 5.

Mechanisms of prevention of coronary events

There is a close relationship between the degree of LDL cholesterol reduction and the reduced risk of coronary events. Overall, there is a 2–3% reduction in risk for every 1% reduction in plasma total cholesterol concentration. Reducing plasma cholesterol probably stabilises existing atheromatous plaques by preventing lipid accumulation in their core and therefore reducing the risk of plaque rupture. Statins prevent the growth of existing coronary artery plaques and reduce the formation of new plaques. Other actions of statins, such as reduction in thrombogenicity of blood and inhibition of smooth muscle proliferation in atheromatous plaques, may also contribute to the clinical benefit, but their role remains speculative.

Management of hypertriglyceridaemia

When triglycerides are markedly raised, non-pharmacological methods of treatment are often useful. These include control of diabetes, weight loss and reduction of alcohol intake. If these are insufficient, then drug therapy may be necessary. Modest hypertriglyceridaemia in association with hypercholesterolaemia will usually respond to a statin.

Extremely high plasma triglyceride concentrations usually respond well to a fibrate or to nicotinic acid. Combination therapy with a statin and a fibrate may be necessary in some high-risk individuals, to achieve an acceptable lipid profile.

FURTHER READING

Balk EM, Lau J, Goudas LC et al (2003) Effects of statins on nonlipid serum markers associated with cardiovascular disease. *Ann Intern Med* 139, 670–682

Cannon CP, Braunwald E, McCabe CH et al (2004) Comparison of intensive and moderate lipid lowering with statins after acute coronary syndromes. *N Engl J Med* 350, 1495–1504

Durrington P (2003) Dyslipidaemia. *Lancet* 362, 717–731

Gami AS, Montori VM, Erwin PJ et al (2003) Systematic review of lipid lowering for primary prevention of coronary heart disease in diabetes. *BMJ* 326, 528–529

Harper CR, Jacobson TA (2001) The fats of life. The role of omega-3 fatty acids in the prevention of coronary heart disease. *Arch Intern Med* 161, 2185–2192

Heart Protection Study Collaborative Group (2002) MRC/BHF Heart Protection Study of cholesterol lowering with simvastatin in 20 536 high-risk individuals: a randomised placebo-controlled trial. *Lancet* 360, 7–22

Lee C-H, Olson P, Evans RM (2003) Minireview: lipid metabolism, metabolic diseases, and peroxisome proliferator-activated receptors. *Endocrinology* 144, 2201–2207

McKenney J (2004) New perspectives on the use of niacin in the treatment of lipid disorders. *Arch Intern Med* 164, 697–705

Mudaliar S, Henry RR (2002) PPAR agonists in health and disease: a pathophysiological and clinical overview. *Curr Opin Endocrinol Diabetes* 9, 285–302

Rizos ED, Mikhailidis DP (2002) Are high-density lipoprotein and triglyceride levels important in secondary prevention: impressions from the BIP and VA-HIT trials. *Int J Cardiol* 82, 199–207

Rosenson RS (2004) Current overview of statin-induced myopathy. *Am J Med* 116, 408–416

Schillinger M, Exner M, Mlekusch W et al (2004) Statin therapy improves cardiovascular outcome of patients with peripheral vascular disease. *Eur Heart J* 25, 742–748

Snow V, Aronson MD, Hornbake R et al (2004) Lipid control in the management of type 2 diabetes mellitus: a clinical practice guideline from the American College of Physicians. *Ann Intern Med* 140, 644–649

Thompson PD, Clarkson P, Karas RH (2003) Statin-associated myopathy. *JAMA* 289, 1681–1690

Vijan S, Hayward RA (2004) Pharmacologic lipid-lowering therapy in type 2 diabetes mellitus: background paper for the American College of Physicians. *Ann Intern Med* 140, 650–658

Walsh JME, Pignone M (2004) Drug treatment of hyperlipidaemia in women. *JAMA* 291, 2243–2253

Wood D (1998) European and American recommendations for coronary heart disease prevention. *Eur Heart J* 19(suppl 1A), A12–A19

Self-assessment

In questions 1 and 2, the first statement, in italics, is true. Are the accompanying statements also true?

1. *Different drug classes available for treating hyperlipidaemia act at differing steps in the lipoprotein metabolic pathway.*

   a. In individuals with high HDL cholesterol, there is a lowering in the risk of coronary disease if the HDL cholesterol levels are reduced.
   b. An important contributor to the development of hypercholesterolaemia is a genetic defect.
   c. Anion-exchange resins act by enhancing the absorption of bile acids from the gut.

2. *Statins reduce cholesterol levels by inhibiting the rate-limiting enzymatic step (HMG-CoA reductase) in its synthesis.*

   a. Decreased hepatic cholesterol synthesis results in increased numbers of HDL receptors.
   b. Simvastatin lowers serum LDL cholesterol by 5%.
   c. Co-administration of bile acid-binding resins and statins has no greater effect than giving each drug separately.

3. The following statements concern the physiological and pharmacological control of plasma lipids. Choose the one correct answer.

   A. In a lipoprotein, the outer coat is phospholipid in structure.
   B. VLDL has a greater percentage of cholesterol than does HDL.
   C. Lowering of plasma cholesterol by statins is not related to the dose of statin administered.
   D. Raising plasma cholesterol has a positive effect on liver cholesterol synthesis.
   E. Fibrates decrease the uptake of LDL cholesterol from the plasma.

4. Case history questions

   > A 58-year-old man recovered from an anterior myocardial infarction. His fasting plasma cholesterol was 7.8 mmol l^{-1}. You want to reduce his risk of a further myocardial infarction by lowering his cholesterol.

   a. What advice would you have given him?
   b. What drug would you have recommended and why?
   c. What reduction in plasma cholesterol would you have expected, and when would you have expected an adequate response?
   d. How do statins work?
   e. What target total cholesterol would you have aimed for?
   f. What unwanted effects would you have warned him about?
   g. If the target cholesterol was not attained, how could you have reduced his cholesterol further?
   h. How did the additional drugs you have recommended work?

   The answers are provided on page 742.

Drug compendium

Drugs used to treat hyperlipidaemias (all drugs given orally unless otherwise stated)

Drug	Half-life (h)	Elimination	Comments
HMG-CoA reductase inhibitors			
Atorvastatin	32–36	Metabolism	Used for primary hypercholesterolaemia, heterozygous familial hypercholesterolaemia, or mixed hyperlipidaemia in individuals who have not responded to dietary measures; bioavailability is 14% (as drug) and 30% (as HMG-CoA reductase inhibition) because the first-pass metabolites are active; bioavailability is lower if taken with food or in the evening; oxidised by CYP3A4 to metabolites that are responsible for much of the activity
Fluvastatin	1	Metabolism	Used as an adjunct to diet in primary hypercholesterolaemia and mixed hyperlipidaemias in those who have not responded to dietary measures, and for prophylaxis of coronary atherosclerosis; bioavailability is 30%; extensive hepatic uptake and oxidation; metabolites are conjugated and excreted in bile; parent drug is the active form
Pravastatin	1–2	Renal + metabolism	Used as an adjunct to diet in primary hypercholesterolaemia in those who have not responded to dietary measures, and for prophylaxis of coronary atherosclerosis; low oral bioavailability (17%), which is decreased by food and is due to poor absorption plus first-pass metabolism; eliminated by renal tubular secretion plus oxidative metabolism; parent drug is the active form
Rosuvastatin	20	Bile + renal	Used in primary hypercholesterolaemia, mixed dyslipidaemia and homozygous familial hypercholesterolaemia in those who have not responded to diet or alternative treatments; bioavailability is 20% and nearly all activity is due to the parent compound; limited metabolism by CYP2C isoenzymes and little potential for drug interactions; about two-thirds of absorbed dose is eliminated in bile and the rest in faeces
Simvastatin	2 (activity)	Metabolism	Used as an adjunct to diet in primary hypercholesterolaemia and mixed hyperlipidaemias in those who have not responded to dietary measures, and for prophylaxis of coronary atherosclerosis; a lactone prodrug which is converted to the active ring-opened acid analogue; oral bioavailability as the acid is low (about 5%); metabolised by hepatic CYP3A4 to active products
Bile acid-binding resins			
Colestyramine	Not relevant	Not absorbed	Used for hyperlipidaemias in individuals not responding to diet and other measures, for primary prevention in men aged 35–59 with primary hypercholesterolaemia not responding to other measures, and to treat pruritis associated with biliary obstruction; not absorbed
Colestipol	Not relevant	Not absorbed	Used for hyperlipidaemias in people not responding to diet and other measures; not absorbed
Fibrates			Used for hyperlipidaemias types IIa, IIb, III, IV and V in people who have not responded adequately to diet; most fibrates are carboxylic acid derivatives that are eliminated unchanged and as acyl glucuronides formed largely in the kidneys

550

continued

Drugs used to treat hyperlipidaemias (all drugs given orally unless otherwise stated) *(continued)*

Drug	Half-life (h)	Elimination	Comments
Bezafibrate	1–5	Renal + metabolism	Complete oral bioavailability; eliminated equally by renal excretion (unchanged) and by metabolism (conjugation and oxidation)
Ciprofibrate	27–28	Metabolism	Not used in type V hyperlipidaemia; complete oral bioavailability; eliminated by glucuronidation, but very low clearance (about 40 ml h^{-1}); contraindicated in severe renal dysfunction
Fenofibrate	20–27 (FA)	Metabolism	Ester prodrug of fenofibric acid (FA); good oral bioavailability (60–90%) as FA (negligible ester absorbed intact); FA is eliminated mainly as the acyl glucuronide
Gemfibrozil	1–2	Renal + metabolism	Complete oral bioavailability; about one-half of the dose is excreted unchanged, with the remainder as hydroxylated metabolites and their conjugates
Nicotinic acid and derivatives			
Acipimox	1–2	Renal	Used for hyperlipidaemia types IIa, IIb, and IV in people who have not responded adequately to diet; complete oral bioavailability; polar pyridine-N-oxide derivative which has a low volume of distribution; undergoes limited reduction to the pyridine analogue (<5%) and is eliminated by renal excretion
Nicotinic acid (niacin)	0.3–0.8	Metabolism + renal	Used to reduce both cholesterol and triglycerides, but limited by vasodilation and hepatic effects; rapidly and completely absorbed; at therapeutic doses, about one-third is excreted unchanged and the remainder is oxidised or conjugated with glycine
Other treatments			
Ezetimibe	22	Metabolism	Used as an adjunct to dietary measures and a statin in primary and homozygous familial hypercholesterolaemia; inhibits intestinal absorption of cholesterol; given orally; metabolised by formation of a pharmacologically active glucuronide, which undergoes biliary excretion and enterohepatic circulation
Ispaghula	Not relevant	Not relevant	Soluble fibre which probably acts by reducing the reabsorption of bile acids in the bowel; acts as a bulk laxative (see Ch. 35)
Omega-3-acid ethyl esters	Not relevant	Not relevant	Used as an adjunct for treating hypertriglyceridaemias in those at a special risk of ischaemic heart disease
Omega-3 marine triglycerides	Not relevant	Not relevant	Used as an adjunct for treating hypertriglyceridaemias, but can aggravate hypercholesterolaemia

The skin and eyes

49

Skin disorders

Topical applications

Topical preparations for the treatment of skin disorders usually have two components: a base and the active ingredient, such as a corticosteroid or an antifungal agent. Four types of base are used:

- ointments, which are greases such as white or yellow soft paraffin
- pastes, which are suspensions of powder in an ointment and will stay where they are put on the skin; their main use is to apply noxious chemicals that should be confined to one area of the skin
- creams, which are emulsions of water with a grease; they are less greasy than ointments, are absorbed more quickly into the skin and are often used as a vehicle for active ingredients
- lotions, which are any kind of liquid; they are used on wet surfaces and hairy areas and their main advantage is that they do not make a mess.

The choice between an ointment or cream depends on individual preference, unless the skin is very dry, when an ointment is better.

Atopic and contact dermatitis

Dermatitis describes eczematous inflammation triggered by external factors.

Atopic dermatitis (eczema). This is often associated with asthma and hayfever and has a familial tendency. The pathogenesis is determined by genetic, environmental, pharmacological and immunological factors. There are two forms of atopic dermatitis: the extrinsic type (70–80% of cases) is associated with IgE-mediated sensitisation, while the intrinsic type, which is less common, is not. Most people with atopic dermatitis have an eosinophilia in the peripheral blood, with a raised IgE concentration. Circulating mononuclear cells have a reduced ability to produce interferon gamma, which normally inhibits IgE production and T-helper type 2 (Th2)-cell proliferation. Production of cytokines that stimulate eosinophil activation and adhesion to vascular walls is increased. As a result of the changes in the immune regulation, Th2-cells proliferate. Dominance of Th1 or Th2 response is partially programmed in early life, with exposure to microbial antigens promoting the normal Th1 dominance. Th1-cell responses, induced by infections, antagonise the development of Th2-cells, and therefore it is possible that the increasing use of antibacterials in childhood may partially explain the rise in atopic dermatitis (Chs 38 and 39).

Affected skin is red, scaly and extremely dry. The dryness is a consequence of the inflammation, but the permeability barrier function of the skin is also impaired, resulting in increased transepidermal water loss. There may be vesicles and weeping and crusting over the skin surface. Scratching produces excoriation and thickening of the skin. The affected skin is infiltrated with activated T-cells, with selective recruitment of Th2-cells, and eosinophils. Increased skin carriage of *Staphylococcus aureus* on the affected skin may also maintain skin inflammation by activating T-cells and macrophages.

Contact dermatitis. Two main types are recognised.

- Due to an external agent inducing direct irritation.
- Resulting from immunological sensitisation involving a delayed hypersensitivity response (Ch. 39). Once the skin has been sensitised, the potential for further reaction persists indefinitely. Sterilisation can arise in response to topical application of drugs.

Treatment of atopic dermatitis

- Emollients (substances that soften the skin) are helpful as hydrophobic agents that seal the surface of the skin and reduce water loss. Paraffin derivatives are most effective but are greasy and not well accepted by most people. Alternatives, such as aqueous creams, are more cosmetically acceptable.
- Avoidance of irritants, such as soaps, detergents, alcohols and astringents. Wet dressings may help to prevent skin fissuring and reduce scratching.
- Identification of allergens by patch tests and their subsequent elimination.

- Topical corticosteroid ointment (Ch. 44) is effective, but, whenever possible, the least potent corticosteroids should be used, in order to minimise unwanted effects. The anti-inflammatory effect of these drugs makes them the mainstay of treatment, but tachyphylaxis (diminished effectiveness with prolonged use) limits their long-term value. Tachyphylaxis may be delayed by twice-weekly application of the corticosteroid.
- Topical calcineurin inhibitors, such as tacrolimus (Ch. 38) and pimecrolimus, inhibit the intracellular phosphatase calcineurin. The end result is reduced activation of many of the inflammatory cells involved in the pathogenesis of the dermatitic lesions, including T-cells, dendritic cells, mast cells and keratinocytes. Local burning is the major unwanted effect.
- Sedative antihistamines (Ch. 39), taken orally at night, assist sleep, although they have little effect on itching. Recently, a topical formulation of the tricyclic antidepressant doxepin (see Ch. 22) has been introduced to treat itch. It is uncertain whether its antihistamine activity is the major mode of action.
- Immunosuppressant therapy with azathioprine, ciclosporin or mycophenolate mofetil (Ch. 38) can be tried for treatment-resistant dermatitis. Apart from unwanted effects, the main problem is rapid relapse when treatment is stopped.
- Phototherapy with natural sunlight is helpful, but sweating can increase pruritis. Broad- or narrowband ultraviolet B (UVB) or broadband ultraviolet A (UVA) (see psoriasis) are useful alternatives.
- Tar bandages on the limbs are messy, but have anti-inflammatory and antipruritic effects.
- Systemic antimicrobials are given for secondary infection. Anti-staphylococcal agents are often helpful if the skin lesions are poorly controlled.

Treatment of contact dermatitis

- Provision of a barrier to an irritant, for example wearing gloves, or removing an allergen may be sufficient.
- Dilute topical corticosteroid ointment (Ch. 44).
- Potassium permanganate soaks can help to dry up exudative lesions.

Psoriasis

Psoriatic skin lesions are produced by a very rapid proliferation of epidermal cells. Cell turnover time is decreased from about 28 days to 3–4 days, which prevents adequate maturation. Instead of producing a normal keratinous surface layer, the skin thickens, forming a silvery scale with dilated upper dermal blood vessels. Inflammatory cells such as T-lymphocytes infiltrate into the dermis and then the epidermis. The process is driven by an immune reaction in the dermis which is initiated by an unknown antigen. Epidermal antigen-presenting cells in the dermis mature after contact with the antigen, migrate to regional lymph nodes and activate T-cells. T-cells then proliferate and enter the circulation and extravasate into the skin at sites of inflammation, assisted by local chemokine production. In the dermis, interaction with the initiating antigen results in Th1 responses, with secretion of cytokines such as interferon gamma, interleukin 2 and tumour necrosis factor alpha (TNFα). The cytokines stimulate proliferation and impair maturation of keratinocytes, and produce vascular changes in the skin. There is a genetic component to psoriasis, which interacts with the unknown environmental factors to produce the lesions.

Psoriatic plaques usually affect the elbows, knees, lower back, buttocks, scalp and nails. Various subtypes of the condition present with different clinical manifestations. An inflammatory arthritis occurs in up to 40% of people with psoriasis (see Ch. 30). There are several treatments for the skin lesions, both topical and systemic, but none produces long-term remission.

Psoriasis can be provoked or exacerbated by several drugs, including lithium, chloroquine, hydroxychloroquine, β-adrenoceptor antagonists, non-steroidal anti-inflammatory drugs and angiotensin-converting enzyme inhibitors.

Topical therapy

Emollients (see atopic dermatitis above). These reduce scaling and itching and may be sufficient in mild psoriasis. They can also be used with a keratolytic.

Keratolytics. Keratolytics such as salicylic acid break down keratin and soften skin, which improves penetration of other treatments. Salicylic acid ointment is most frequently used.

Vitamin D analogues (e.g. calcipotriol). Vitamin D regulates epidermal proliferation and differentiation. It also has immunosuppressant properties. Vitamin D analogues are clean and simple to apply and are particularly useful for chronic plaque psoriasis, although complete clearing of the plaques is unusual. Ointment has greater emollient effect than cream, but is more messy. Calcipotriol should not usually be used for the face, where it often causes irritation; this is less troublesome elsewhere. Excessive use can lead to hypercalcaemia. The ease of use of these compounds makes them a popular choice if a keratolytic is insufficient.

Topical retinoids (e.g. tazarotene). Retinoids are discussed more fully under systemic treatments. Tazarotene gel can be applied to plaque psoriasis and has minimal systemic absorption. Unlike other retinoids, tazarotene is selective for retinoic acid receptor (RAR) proteins, with no affinity for retinoid X receptors (RXR) see below. This may reduce unwanted effects, which are mainly local irritation of healthy skin with pruritis. It should be avoided for 1 month before conception, because of potential teratogenic effects.

Dithranol. This anthraquinone decreases cell division and is very effective for healing psoriatic plaques. In hospital, it is applied in a stiff paste so that the dithranol does not come into contact with, and burn, normal skin. It is left in contact with the plaque for 24 h. At home, dithranol is used as a cream that is applied to the plaque for 30 min and then washed off. The oxidation products of dithranol stain the skin brown, leaving discoloration of healed areas for a few days. They also stain bedding and clothes a mauve colour that will not wash out. Since dithranol irritates normal skin, it should not be used in flexures.

Coal tar preparations. Crude coal tar is a mixture of a large number of hydrocarbons that have a cytostatic action. It enhances the healing effect of UVB radiation on psoriatic lesions. The main disadvantage is messiness, and its efficacy when used alone is modest. More refined tar preparations have greater acceptability, but are even less effective.

Phototherapy. Ultraviolet light produces improvement by inhibiting DNA synthesis and depleting intra-epidermal T-lymphocytes. It should not be used on individuals who are very fair and who burn in the sun. UVB ('sunburn' wavelength 290–320 nm), administered at least three times per week, is very useful for extensive small plaques of psoriasis. It is now recognised that the greatest benefit is derived from narrowband UVB (around 311 nm) rather than broadband UVB. Long-wavelength UVA (320–400 nm) requires more specialised equipment and prior administration of an oral photosensitising drug such as psoralen (a process called photochemo-therapy or PUVA). Psoralen probably locates between pyrimidine base pairs in the DNA helix and inhibits cell replication. PUVA is usually reserved for severe, resistant psoriasis and it is more effective than treatment with UVB. Psoralen can produce nausea, and headache acutely. The long-term risks of PUVA include accelerated skin ageing and an increased incidence of skin cancer.

Topical corticosteroid preparations. These should be used sparingly on limited areas. Unwanted effects can be troublesome (Ch. 44). Withdrawal of a high-potency corticosteroid can produce a rebound phenomenon and even generalised pustular psoriasis.

Systemic treatments

Apart from emollients and corticosteroids, which are most useful for chronic plaque psoriasis, topical treatments should be avoided in more inflammatory forms of the condition because they can cause troublesome skin irritation. Systemic treatment is reserved for the most severe forms of disease.

Methotrexate (Chs 38 and 52). This is a very effective treatment at low dosages for resistant and widespread disease. Its main actions are cytostatic and immunosuppressant. Oral or intramuscular dosing is commonly used once a week. Bone marrow depression and hepatotoxicity with liver fibrosis are the main complications; blood counts must be checked every 2–3 months and liver biopsies performed every 1–2 years to monitor treatment.

Retinoids. This term covers vitamin A (retinol) and therapeutically useful synthetic vitamin A derivatives, such as acitretin, the active metabolite of etretinate, which is no longer used. Given orally, they are anti-inflammatory and cytostatic. Vitamin A, and its metabolites all-*trans*-retinoic acid and 9-*cis*-retinoic acid, are involved in epithelial cell growth and differentiation. Retinoids enter cells by endocytosis and interact with two forms of retinoic acid nuclear receptor, RARs and RXRs, that are related to steroid/thyroid hormone receptors (Ch. 1). The retinoid receptor complex initiates gene transcription and may affect cell growth and differentiation by modulation of growth factors and their receptors. Response of psoriatic lesions is delayed by up to 2 months. The half-life of etretinate is very long (up to 6 months) because of sequestration in subcutaneous fat; the half-life of acitretin is about 2 days. Elimination of retinoids is by hepatic metabolism. Unwanted effects are almost universal and include dry lips and nasal mucosa, dryness of the skin with localised peeling over the digits, and transient thinning of hair. These effects are dose-dependent and reversible. Longer-term problems include ossification of ligaments, increased plasma triglycerides and, to a lesser extent, increased plasma cholesterol. There is a high risk of teratogenesis, and women must use adequate contraception during treatment and stop treatment for 2 years before conception, even with acitretin.

Ciclosporin or tacrolimus (Ch. 38). These immunosuppressants are effective in psoriasis at lower doses than those required for prevention of allograft rejection. However, remissions induced by these drugs are usually short.

TNFα antibodies. Etanercept and infliximab (Chs 30 and 34) are intravenous therapies that are highly effective in treatment-resistant psoriasis. Blocking TNFα inhibits the production of chemokines and endothelial adhesion molecules that attract activated lymphocytes into the skin. Infliximab produces a more rapid response than etanercept. These drugs are the first of several 'biological' agents undergoing trial for the management of severe psoriasis.

Fumaric acid esters. This is an oral treatment for severe psoriasis that probably works by promoting a Th2-like lymphocyte response in place of the Th1-dominated response found in psoriasis. Fumaric acid is poorly absorbed from the gut, and is therefore given as an ester. This is rapidly hydrolysed by esterases to monomethylfumarate, the active compound, and further metabolised in cells to water and carbon dioxide in the citrate cycle. Monomethylfumarate has a very long half-life of about 36 h. Unwanted effects include gastrointestinal upset in more than two-thirds of people, and flushing in one-third.

Acne

Acne most commonly arises in adolescence and often regresses in the late teens or early twenties. Acne affects areas of skin with large numbers of sebaceous glands: the face, back and chest. There is increased production of sebum, which distends the pilosebaceous duct, producing a small closed papule (comedo) called a whitehead. Hyperkeratosis at the mouth of the hair follicle blocks the duct. If the duct then opens, compacted follicular cells at the tip give comedones the appearance of a blackhead. A resident anaerobic bacterium, *Propionibacterium acnes*, degrades triglycerides in sebum to free fatty acids and glycerol. It also produces chemotactic factors and inflammatory mediators. These, and the irritant free fatty acids, produce inflamed lesions of pustules, nodules or multilocular cysts if the lesions coalesce. The inflammatory lesions can scar, with permanent disfigurement.

There is a genetic background to acne, which determines the rate of sebum production, particularly in response to androgens. Androgens, which are produced at puberty, induce hypertrophy of sebaceous glands, and the excess secretion rate in predisposed individuals triggers the acne.

Treatment of acne

There are several effective treatments for acne. The choice will depend on the nature of the lesions and their severity. Topical treatments do not influence the rate of production of sebum.

Topical treatment

- Benzoyl peroxide has antibacterial activity against *P. acnes* and a keratolytic action, both of which reduce the numbers of comedones. It produces scaling and skin irritation, which may limit its use to short treatment periods.
- Topical antibacterials, for example clindamycin, erythromycin and tetracycline (Ch. 51), are less effective than oral antibacterials but have fewer unwanted effects. Their efficacy is similar to that of benzoyl peroxide, with less skin irritation; tetracycline is least likely to cause bacterial resistance. Combination therapy with benzoyl peroxide reduces the problem of bacterial resistance. Topical antibacterials are used for mild to moderate acne,

and are particularly useful in pregnant women since there is no systemic absorption.
- Isotretinoin (13-*cis*-retinoic acid) is a vitamin A derivative that has a keratolytic action which unblocks the pilosebaceous follicles and allows flow of sebum to extrude the plug. The mechanism of action is similar to that of acitretin (see under psoriasis). It also reduces sebum production by up to 90% by decreasing sebocyte proliferation (this action is probably independent of effects on nuclear retinoid receptors). Topically, it produces erythema and scaling, which can be minimised by starting with a low concentration. Adapalene is an extensively modified retinoid that has a faster onset of action and produces less skin irritation.
- Azelaic acid is an aliphatic dicarboxylic acid that has an antibacterial action against propionibacteria and is effective against bacteria that have become resistant to erythromycin and tetracycline. It also inhibits the division of keratinocytes, which may reduce follicular plugging and prevent the development of comedones. It is applied topically; the most frequent unwanted effects are local burning, scaling or itching, although hypopigmentation can also be a problem. Azelaic acid is most effective for mild to moderate non-inflammatory comedonal acne, especially of the face.

Systemic treatment

- Oral antibacterials that are active against *P. acnes* are used for inflammatory acne (papules/pustules). Penetration into sebaceous follicles is poor, but they produce some improvement after 2–3 months, requiring 4–6 months of treatment for maximal benefit. Treatment should be given for extended periods, since relapse is common if it is stopped. Among the more useful antibacterial agents are tetracyclines, for example oxytetracycline and doxycycline. Alternatives include ciprofloxacin and cotrimoxazole (Ch. 51). Resistance to erythromycin makes it a less suitable choice than in the past.
- The antiandrogen cyproterone acetate (Ch. 46) is useful in women with moderate or severe acne and is usually given in combination with ethinylestradiol (Ch. 45). The combination reduces sebum flow by 40%. Alternatively, oestrogen can be given with a non-androgenic progestogen such as norgestimate or desogestrel. Improvement can take 2–4 months.
- Isotretinoin is used orally in severe acne and gives an almost 100% probability of complete remission. High doses can produce prolonged remission. Unwanted effects include dry lips, nose and eyes, increased plasma triglycerides, and, less commonly, myalgia. Teratogenesis is a major problem, and, although the half-life of the metabolites is less than 2 days, conception should be avoided during and for one menstrual cycle after stopping treatment.

Choice of treatment for acne

Initially, management of non-inflammatory comedones is by topical treatment such as azelaic acid or retinoids. For early inflammatory lesions, a topical antibacterial or benzoyl peroxide can be considered, alone or in combination. More severe inflammatory acne usually requires topical or systemic antibacterials with topical retinoid. Systemic treatment with isotretinoin is used for more severe and unresponsive acne. Oestrogen and antiandrogen therapy are alternatives for women, and oral contraceptives can be of benefit. Overall, the most common reason for treatment failure is probably non-adherence to the recommended regimen.

Wound healing

Becalpermin

Mechanism of action and use

Becalpermin is a human recombinant platelet-derived growth factor (PDGF). Endogenous PDGF is synthesised by megakaryocytes, macrophages, fibroblasts, smooth muscle cells and endothelial cells. Platelets release PDGF after tissue injury. PDGF contributes to tissue healing by encouraging cell chemotaxis and activation of inflammatory cells, and by increasing extracellular matrix deposition, cell mitogenesis and cell protein synthesis. This enhances granulation tissue in wounds. Becalpermin can be used to enhance healing of chronic neuropathic diabetic foot ulcers.

Pharmacokinetics

Belcalpermin is applied topically as a gel. There is negligible systemic absorption.

Unwanted effects

A local erythematous rash can occur. Concern over the possibility of local carcinogenesis appears unfounded in short-term studies.

FURTHER READING

Barnetson R, Rogers M (2002) Childhood atopic eczema. *BMJ* 324, 1376–1379

Haider A, Shaw JC (2004) Treatment of acne vulgaris. *JAMA* 292, 726–735

Kupper TS (2003) Immunologic targets in psoriasis. *N Engl J Med* 349, 1987–1990

Lebwohl M (2003) Psoriasis. *Lancet* 361, 1197–1204

Leung DYM, Bieber T (2003) Atopic dermatitis. *Lancet* 361, 151–160

Leyden JJ (2003) A review of the use of combination therapies for the treatment of acne vulgaris. *J Am Acad Dermatol* 49, S200–S210

Mrowietz U, Christophers E, Altmeyer P (1999) Treatment of severe psoriasis with fumaric acid esters: scientific background and guidelines for therapeutic use. *Br J Dermatol* 141, 424–429

Reynolds NJ, Al-Daraji WI (2002) Calcineurin inhibitors and sirolimus: mechanisms of action and application in dermatology. *Clin Exp Dermatol* 27, 555–561

Webster GF (2002) Acne vulgaris *BMJ* 325, 475–479

Zouboulis CC, Piquero-Martin J (2003) Update and future of systemic acne treatment. *Dermatology* 206, 37–53

Self-assessment

In questions 1–3, the first statement, in italics, is true. Are the following statements also true?

1. *Atopic dermatitis is the most common form of dermatitis and is an inflammatory condition with a familial tendency. It involves acute and chronic inflammation.*

   a. Topical corticosteroids should not be used in atopic dermatitis.
   b. Antihistamines given orally can reduce itching in atopic dermatitis.

2. *Dominance of Th1-type lymphocytes is important in psoriasis.*

   a. In severe resistant psoriasis, immunosuppressant drugs are contraindicated.
   b. Retinoids reduce cell growth and differentiation.

3. *Severe inflammatory acne should be treated with topical or systemic antibacterials and a topical retinoid.*

   a. Suitable topical antibacterials for inflammatory acne are erythromycin or clindamycin.
   b. Antibacterial resistance in *Propionibacterium acnes* does not occur.

4. You have discussed with 50-year-old Mr PP the treatment options for his widespread psoriasis. He was also taking medication for high blood pressure. Choose the one correct option from the following.

A. Mr PP thought that the atenolol he was taking as part of the regimen to lower his blood pressure did not affect his psoriasis.
B. Mr PP would not go on holiday to Spain because he had heard that sunshine would make his psoriasis worse.
C. Mr PP was pleased that he had been prescribed methotrexate; it helped his condition and he had read that it had few unwanted effects.
D. You recommended the vitamin D analogue calcipotriol applied topically, because it would help improve his condition.
E. Using a TNFα antibody would be of little benefit in psoriasis resistant to other treatments.

5. Case history questions

> A 7-year-old girl with a history of asthma developed a red, scaly and dry rash in her knee and elbow flexures and on her arms and cheeks. The rash was extremely itchy and she was scratching the affected areas, causing excoriation and weeping. Her mother had atopic dermatitis when she was young.

   a. What was the possible diagnosis?
   b. What treatments should have been tried initially?
   c. What other factors should have be considered in the treatment of this young girl?

The answers are provided on pages 742–743.

Drugs used in the treatment of skin disorders

Drug[a]	Half-life (h)[b]	Elimination	Comments
Corticosteroids			Given topically for inflammatory skin conditions
Alclometasone dipropionate	–	Metabolism	Synthetic corticosteroid; about 3% of the applied dose is absorbed across the skin over a period of 8 h; fate of absorbed compound has not been defined
Beclometasone dipropionate	–	Metabolised and eliminated in faeces	Use is restricted to severe conditions, such as eczemas unresponsive to less potent drugs; only about 2% is absorbed from the forearm but much higher absorption occurs from the forehead (7%), scrotum (36%), eyelids (40%) and from inflamed skin; hydration of the skin increases drug uptake and absorption
Betamethasone esters	–	Metabolism	Use is restricted to severe conditions, such as eczemas unresponsive to less potent drugs; poor absorption with variations between different sites (see beclometasone)
Clobetasol propionate	–	Metabolism	Use is restricted to short-term treatment of severe resistant conditions, such as eczemas unresponsive to less potent drugs; very poor absorption (see beclometasone); suppression of adrenocortical function is possible in people with psoriasis
Clobetasone butyrate	–	Metabolism	Poorly absorbed (see beclometasone)
Desoximetasone	–	Metabolism (?)	Used for severe acute inflammatory, allergic and also chronic skin disorders, and for psoriasis; few data available; possible reduction in plasma cortisol in people with psoriasis given long-term treatment suggests the possibility of significant absorption under such circumstances (a similar result was not obtained when intact skin was treated)
Diflucortolone valerate	–	Metabolism	Use is restricted to severe conditions, such as eczemas unresponsive to less potent drugs, and for psoriasis; few data available; transdermal absorption is probably similar to beclometasone; only weak adrenocortical effects compared with clobetasol propionate
Fludroxycortide	–	Metabolism	No published data have been identified; the route of elimination is predicted as no data are available
Fluocinolone acetonide	–	Metabolism	Poorly absorbed (see beclometasone); the route of elimination is predicted as no data are available
Fluocinonide	–	Metabolism	Use is restricted to severe conditions, such as eczemas unresponsive to less potent drugs, and for psoriasis; poorly absorbed (see beclometasone); the route of elimination is predicted as no data are available
Fluocortolone	–	Metabolism	Use is restricted to severe conditions, such as eczemas unresponsive to less potent drugs, and for psoriasis; few data available after topical dosing (not surprisingly, it causes cortisol suppression after oral dosage, but comparable topical data are not available)
Fluticasone propionate	2–5	Metabolism	Use is restricted to severe conditions, such as eczemas unresponsive to less potent drugs, and for psoriasis; poorly absorbed transdermally (see beclometasone); half-life is following inhalation exposure

continued

Drugs used in the treatment of skin disorders (continued)

Drug[a]	Half-life (h)[b]	Elimination	Comments
Halcinonide	–	Metabolism	Use is restricted to short-term treatment of severe conditions, such as eczemas unresponsive to less potent drugs, and for psoriasis; poorly absorbed (see beclometasone); higher risk of cortisol suppression than with betamethasone valerate (but better response) especially with occlusion; the route of elimination is predicted as no data are available
Hydrocortisone	1.5	Metabolism	Poorly absorbed transdermally (see beclometasone); probably undergoes metabolism within the skin; see Ch. 44
Hydrocortisone butyrate	1.5	Metabolism	Use of the butyrate ester is restricted to severe conditions, such as eczemas unresponsive to less potent drugs; prodrug; poorly absorbed transdermally (see beclometasone); the ester group is completely hydrolysed during transdermal absorption; half-life is for hydrocortisone
Mometasone furoate	–	Metabolism	Use is restricted to severe conditions, such as eczemas unresponsive to less potent drugs, and for psoriasis; very poor absorption (see beclometasone); extensively metabolised, with metabolites eliminated in urine and bile
Triamcinolone acetonide	2–5	Metabolism	Use is restricted to severe conditions, such as eczemas unresponsive to less potent drugs, and for psoriasis; poorly absorbed from the skin (see beclometasone); rapidly eliminated from the blood by oxidation and then conjugation
Drugs for eczema and/or seborrhoeic dermatitis			Topical corticosteroids and antibacterial agents may also be given orally
Gamolenic acid	–	Metabolism	Taken orally; metabolised to dihomogammalinolenic acid (DGLA), which is incorporated into cell membranes; scant evidence to support its value in atopic eczema
Ichthammol	–	–	A sulphonated shale oil that is used as an ointment or cream
Lithium succinate	–	–	Used as an ointment with zinc sulphate; high concentration used (8%) but absorption has not been defined
Pimecrolimus	30–40 (oral)	Metabolism	Calcineurin inhibitor; used for mild to moderate atopic eczema; very limited absorption across the skin and no skin-mediated metabolism; absorbed drug is metabolised by CYP3A
Tacrolimus	9 (oral)	Metabolism	Calcineurin inhibitor; used topically for moderate to severe atopic eczema unresponsive to other treatments; limited absorption across the skin; see Ch. 38
Drugs for psoriasis			
Acitretin	50	Metabolism	Retinoid given orally for severe extensive and resistant psoriasis; teratogenic risk; long half-life owing to low hepatic extraction and metabolism
Calcipotriol (calcipotriene)	–	Metabolism	Vitamin D analogue used for plaque psoriasis; about 5% absorbed after topical application; few data available (very short plasma half-life in animal studies)

continued

Drugs used in the treatment of skin disorders (continued)

Drug[a]	Half-life (h)[b]	Elimination	Comments
Drugs for psoriasis (continued)			
Calcitriol	–	–	Vitamin D analogue used for mild to moderate plaque psoriasis; see Ch. 42
Ciclosporin	27	Metabolism	Given orally for short-term treatment of severe atopic dermatitis and severe psoriasis; bioavailability is about 30%; oxidised by intestinal and hepatic CYP3A4; see also Ch. 38
Coal tar	–	Metabolism	Also used occasionally for chronic atopic eczema; coal tar contains polycyclic aromatic hydrocarbons which are oxidised (and activated) by CYP1A2; high transdermal absorption
Dithranol (anthralin)	–	Metabolism	Used for subacute and chronic psoriasis; poorly absorbed across the skin; metabolised within the skin
Methotrexate	8–10	Metabolism	Folate antagonist used in the treatment of severe uncontrolled psoriasis, rheumatoid arthritis (see Ch. 30) and malignant disease (see Ch. 52); given orally; good oral absorption (20–95%); metabolised by the formation of polyglutamates (which are active and retained intracellularly) and by oxidation
Psoralen (8-methoxypsoralen)	–	Metabolism	Unlicensed product given before ultraviolet A irradiation to increase effectiveness (PUVA treatment)
Salicylic acid	–	–	Used with coal tar and dithranol preparations as a keratolytic in scaly psoriasis; see Ch. 29
Tacalcitol	–	Metabolism	Vitamin D_3 analogue (1,24-dihydroxyvitamin D_3) used for plaque psoriasis; negligible absorption after topical dosage
Tazarotene	18 (TA)	Metabolism	Retinoid used for mild to moderate plaque psoriasis; poorly absorbed across the skin; hydrolysed in skin to tazarotenic acid (TA), which is further metabolised; TA is responsible for binding to retinoid receptors
Drugs for acne and rosacea			In addition to the topical preparations given below, antibiotics such as clindamycin, doxycycline, erythromycin, minocycline, oxytetracycline, tetracycline and trimethoprim may be given in the treatment of acne
Adapalene	–	–	Retinoid-like drug; binds to nuclear but not cytosolic retinoid receptors; very low topical absorption; very few data available
Azelaic acid	0.75	Renal	Low absorption (about 4%); eliminated unchanged in the urine (plus some limited β-oxidation); as for most topical drugs, absorption rate-limited kinetics result in a half-life after topical dosage (2 h) that is considerably longer than the elimination half-life
Benzoyl peroxide	–	Metabolism	Powerful oxidising agent that is reduced to benzoic acid; about 5% of the benzoic acid is absorbed
Co-cyprindiol	NA	NA	A mixture of cyproterone acetate and ethinylestradiol used for the treatment of severe acne unresponsive to antibiotics, and hirsutism in women at low risk of thromboembolism (which is increased by this treatment)

continued

Drug compendium

Drugs used in the treatment of skin disorders (continued)

Drug[a]	Half-life (h)[b]	Elimination	Comments
Isotretinoin	10–20	Metabolism	Given topically; retinoid (13-*cis*-retinoic acid); isomerises to all-*trans*-retinoic acid; may be given orally but known to be a human teratogen; activity is largely owing to all-*trans*-retinoic acid
Tretinoin	1–2	Metabolism	Given topically; retinoid (all-*trans*-retinoic acid); metabolised by oxidation and formation of an acyl glucuronide; half-life is derived from studies following its formation from vitamin A

Key NA – not applicable as the 'drug' is a combination preparation.
[a] The majority of treatments are given topically and show very slow and limited absorption. All drugs are given topically unless otherwise stated.
[b] The systemic half-lives (when given) are not an indication of duration of action of topical formulations.

50

The eye

Vision depends upon the eye converting light falling on the retina into an electrical signal to be carried to the brain through the optic nerve. The eye must focus objects sharply on the retina, a process called accommodation. To adjust the innate focus to achieve this, the ciliary muscle alters the shape of the lens, allowing the eye to accommodate to objects at different distances. The iris determines the size of the pupil and the amount of light entering the eye. The autonomic nervous system innervates the ciliary muscles and the iris.

Accommodation. The ciliary muscle is a circular (constrictor) smooth muscle that is attached to the lens by suspensory ligaments. The ciliary muscle receives parasympathetic innervation only. When the muscle is relaxed, tension on the suspensory ligaments stretches and flattens the lens inside its capsule, which adjusts visual acuity for distant vision. Paralysis of the ciliary muscle by drugs to maintain the relaxed state is known as cycloplegia. Parasympathetic stimulation contracts the ciliary muscle, which relaxes the suspensory ligaments, and the lens assumes a more globular shape, which accommodates the eye for near vision (Fig. 50.1).

Pupil size. This is determined by the relative tone in the two smooth muscles of the iris. The circular (constrictor) muscle is the more powerful and receives parasympathetic nervous innervation, releasing acetylcholine, which acts on muscarinic receptors. The radial (dilator) muscle is sympathetically innervated, releasing noradrenaline and adrenaline, which act on α_1-adrenoceptors. Constriction of the pupil is known as miosis; dilation is called mydriasis. Accommodation for near vision is accompanied by a response in the parasympathetic nervous system producing pupillary constriction. The light reflex also reduces pupil size. Dilation of the pupil is caused by shortening of the radial muscle, which also has the effect of moving the iris towards the cornea and narrows the angle between the iris and the cornea.

Drainage of aqueous humour. The space between the cornea, at the front of the eye (Fig. 50.1), and the lens is filled with a clear liquid known as aqueous humour. Contraction of the ciliary muscle aids drainage of aqueous humour through the trabecular meshwork into the episcleral veins. Pressure in the eye is maintained by a balance between the production of aqueous humour and its drainage. The intraocular pressure rises if drainage of the aqueous humour is impaired. High pressure is one of the factors that can damage retinal ganglion cells, leading to progressive loss of vision (glaucoma). If the anterior chamber of the eye is abnormally shallow, dilation of the pupil may restrict drainage of aqueous humour through the trabecular meshwork. This can result in an acute rise in pressure (acute angle-closure glaucoma) (Fig. 50.1). Conversely, constriction of the iris makes the pupil smaller and moves the iris away from the trabecular meshwork of Schlemm's canal, facilitating drainage.

Topical application of drugs to the eye

Drugs applied in solution to the anterior surface of the eye can penetrate to the anterior chamber and the ciliary muscle, principally via the cornea. The high water content of the cornea makes lipid solubility less important for adequate penetration of a drug than it is for transdermal drug delivery, but formulation of the carrier is important to avoid irritation of the conjunctiva. There is little diffusion to the more posterior structures of the eye.

Systemic absorption of drug following topical application to the surface of the eye can occur either via conjuctival vessels or from the nasal mucosa after drainage of excess drug via the tear ducts. Topical administration of drugs to the eye may, therefore, produce systemic effects. Drainage can be reduced by shutting the eyes for at least 1 min after putting the drops in and by compressing the nasolacrimal duct at the medial corner of the eye with a finger. Both eye-drops and ointments are usually administered into the pocket (the lower fornix) that can be formed by gently pulling the lower eyelid downwards.

Microbial contamination is a potential problem once eye preparations are opened. Multiple-application containers have preservative added to reduce the risk, but it is not advisable to use any eye preparation more than a month after it has been opened.

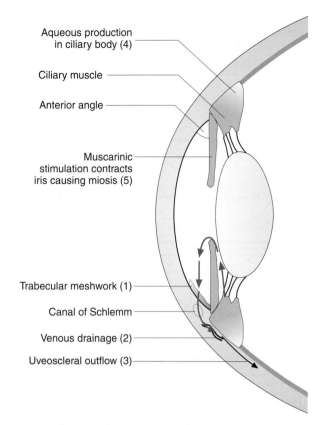

Cholinergic agonists, e.g. pilocarpine
(i) constrict iris (5)
    open anterior angle
(ii) constrict ciliary muscle
    enhance aqueous drainage (1,2)

Carbonic anhydrase inhibitors,
e.g. acetazolamide, decrease
aqueous production (4)

Beta adrenoceptor antagonists,
e.g. timolol, reduce aqueous
production (4), increase outflow (1)

Selective stimulants of α_2-adrenergic
receptors decrease aqueous
production (4) e.g. apraclonidine,
brimonidine

Prostaglandin $F_{2\alpha}$ analogues,
e.g. latanoprost, enhance uveoscleral
outflow (3)

⟶ Route of drainage of aqueous humour

Fig. 50.1
The route of drainage of aqueous humour from the eye and the sites and mechanisms of action of drugs used in the treatment of glaucoma.

Glaucoma

Glaucoma is a group of disorders, characterised by loss of retinal ganglion cells. In some cases, the intraocular pressure is raised, and ischaemia of the optic nerve head may be the cause. In many cases, however, the pressure in the anterior chamber of the eye is normal and a genetic susceptibility to ganglion cell apoptosis is responsible. Progressive visual defects occur, initially as scotomas (blind spots) in the peripheral visual field. These scotomas enlarge, resulting in tunnel vision and finally total blindness. Glaucoma is the second most common cause of blindness in the UK.

Aqueous humour is constantly secreted by the ciliary body. Most flows through the pupil to the anterior chamber, and leaves the eye via the trabecular meshwork that drains to the episcleral veins through the canal of Schlemm (Fig. 50.1). Some aqueous humour drains through the sclera (uveoscleral outflow). Production is influenced by innervation from the autonomic nervous system. α_2-Adrenoceptor stimulation of the ciliary body reduces the production of aqueous humour, while β_1-adrenoceptor stimulation increases its production.

Outflow of aqueous humour is also influenced by innervation from the autonomic nervous system, and by prostaglandins. **Open-angle glaucoma** is caused by obstruction in the trabecular meshwork in the absence of a reduced drainage. **Angle-closure glaucoma** is less common, usually acute in onset, and results from the iris blocking the drainage angle and preventing drainage through the trabecular meshwork. This usually arises in people with a shallow anterior chamber, such as occurs in long-sighted individuals. Chronic angle-closure glaucoma is rare.

Drugs for glaucoma

Beta-adrenoceptor antagonists

Examples: timolol, betaxolol

Beta-adrenoceptor antagonists reduce the formation of aqueous humour. They have no effect on accommodation or pupil size, which makes them a treatment of first choice for glaucoma. However, systemic absorption can produce the typical unwanted effects associated with these compounds, particularly bronchospasm, bradycardia and worsening of uncontrolled heart failure (Ch. 5). The contraindications for topical use in the eye are the same as those for oral use. Timolol is a nonselective β-adrenoceptor antagonist; betaxolol is 'cardioselective', but this does not influence its benefits in the eye.

Sympathomimetics

Examples: brimonidine, apraclonidine, dipivefrine

Dipivefrine is converted to adrenaline (epinephrine) in the eye, and has greater penetration than adrenaline (epinephrine) through the cornea. It is mydriatic (dilates the pupil) by stimulating α_1-adrenoceptors in the radial muscle of the iris, and should not be used in angle-closure glaucoma. It improves drainage through the trabecular meshwork and decreases aqueous humour production by α_2-adrenoceptor stimulation. Dipivefrine should be used with care in people with hypertension and heart disease, because of the potential to cause systemic vasoconstriction.

Apraclonidine and brimonidine are selective α_2-adrenoceptor agonist drugs that decrease ciliary body aqueous humour production and are not mydriatic.

Carbonic anhydrase inhibitors

Examples: acetazolamide, dorzolamide

The mechanism of action of the carbonic anhydrase inhibitors is discussed in Chapter 14. Carbonic anhydrase in the eye plays a key role in controlling aqueous humour production. It is responsible for about 70% of the Na^+ that enters the anterior chamber, which is followed by water to maintain isotonicity. Therefore, inhibition of the enzyme reduces aqueous humour production.

Acetazolamide is taken orally. Dorzolamide and brinzolamide are topical preparations for the eye with fewer systemic unwanted effects; they have a duration of action in the eye of 6–12 h, but a very long plasma half-life due to retention within erythrocytes.

Prostaglandin analogues

Examples: latanoprost, travoprost

These drugs are analogues of prostaglandin $F_{2\alpha}$ that increase uveoscleral outflow of aqueous humour. This may result in part from an increase in extracellular matrix metalloproteinases in ciliary smooth muscle cells, and from remodelling of the uveal meshwork. The prostaglandin analogues also increase blood flow to the optic nerve, and this may contribute to neuroprotection in the retina. The reduction in intraocular pressure is greater than that achieved by β-adrenoceptor antagonists. The major disadvantage of prostaglandin analogues is an increase in brown pigmentation of the iris and growth of eyelashes. A rare complication in people who have no lens in the eye (aphakia) is the development of cystoid macular oedema, which responds to treatment with nonsteroidal anti-inflammatory drugs. The prostaglandin analogues have a long duration of action of 1–2 days.

Miotic drugs (muscarinic agonists)

Example: pilocarpine

Pilocarpine (see also Ch. 4) is usually given for angle-closure glaucoma to contract the sphincter muscle of the iris to produce miosis and open up the drainage channels in the anterior chamber of the eye. The miotic effect lasts for about 4 h, and more prolonged miosis can be achieved by the use of a gel delivery system. Ciliary muscle spasm is an undesirable consequence and produces blurred vision and an ache over the eye (especially in younger people). Pilocarpine can be used together with other drugs in simple open-angle glaucoma.

Treatment of glaucoma

In open-angle glaucoma, reducing intraocular pressure can slow the rate of disease progression sufficiently to prevent significant visual impairment. A target pressure reduction of at least 30% below the presenting pressure is usually set.

In primary open-angle glaucoma, a topical β-adrenoceptor antagonist or a prostaglandin analogue is the treatment of choice when there are no contraindications, because of their lack of ocular unwanted effects. If either treatment alone is insufficient, then a combination can give an additive effect. If these agents cannot be used, then choice of a second-line drug lies between pilocarpine, a topical carbonic anhydrase inhibitor or a sympathomimetic agent. Surgery may also be considered at this point. Laser burns applied to the trabecular meshwork can produce a temporary increase in aqueous humour outflow, but drug treatment may still be required. Drainage surgery is the alternative and can often bring about long-term pressure control. In the future, it is likely that neuroprotective drugs will be used to retard neuronal degeneration in the retina.

Angle-closure glaucoma is treated by laser peripheral iridotomy or surgical peripheral iridectomy to provide a channel for aqueous humour to flow through the iris. If drug therapy is required after surgery, then a topical treatment with a prostaglandin analogue or a β-adrenoceptor antagonist can be used.

Mydriatic and cycloplegic drugs

Antimuscarinics

Examples: atropine, homatropine, cyclopentolate, tropicamide

Antimuscarinic drugs (see also Ch. 4) are both mydriatic (dilating the pupil) and cycloplegic (paralysing the ciliary muscle). Tropicamide is weak and short-acting (about 3 h), which makes it useful for dilating the pupil for fundal examination. Cyclopentolate and homatropine both last for up to 24 h and are more powerful; the former has a more rapid onset of action. Atropine is long-acting, the effect persisting for up to 7 days. The longer-acting compounds are used to prevent adhesions (posterior synechiae) in anterior uveitis (often in combination with phenylephrine). Dark irises are more resistant to pupillary dilation wth these drugs, as the pigments adsorb the applied drug.

The degree of cycloplegia will depend on the dose of drug; small doses produce pupil dilation with insufficient diffusion to reach the ciliary muscle and much affect accommodation. The law does not specifically ban driving after pupil dilation, but many people find that their vision is impaired for several hours. Care must be taken using these drugs in individuals predisposed to acute angle-closure glaucoma. Local irritation in the eye is the most common unwanted effect, but systemic effects occasionally occur in children or the elderly (see Ch. 4).

Sympathomimetics

Example: phenylephrine

Phenylephrine is a relatively selective α_1-adrenoceptor agonist that stimulates the radial muscle of the iris and produces mydriasis. It does not affect the ciliary muscle, and therefore does not affect accommodation. It is a vasoconstrictor, and can decrease vascular congestion of the conjunctiva and eyelid oedema in allergic conjunctivitis. In this role, it is often combined with an antihistamine in over-the-counter preparations. Local

irritation is the most common unwanted effect, although systemic vasoconstriction with hypertension or coronary artery spasm can occur occasionally.

Other topical applications for the eye

Several other drugs are used topically in the eye.

Antibacterial agents (Ch. 51). These are given for local infections such as blepharitis, conjunctivitis or trachoma (caused by chlamydial infection). Aqueous solutions are rapidly diluted or flushed away by lacrimation and should initially be used every 1–2 h; ointments are often given for longer action, for example at night. Examples of broad-spectrum agents are gentamicin, chloramphenicol, ciprofloxacin, fusidic acid, neomycin and chlortetracycline (the last for trachoma).

Antiviral agents (Ch. 51). These are mainly used for herpes simplex infection, which causes dendritic corneal ulcers. Aciclovir is most frequently used.

Corticosteroids. Local inflammatory conditions of the anterior part of the eye, such as uveitis and scleritis, are treated with corticosteroids, for example dexamethasone or prednisolone (Ch. 44). Care must be taken to exclude a viral dendritic ulcer and glaucoma before using them, since these conditions can be exacerbated by corticosteroids. Prolonged use of corticosteroids can lead to thinning of the sclera or cornea, or formation of a 'steroid cataract'.

Antiallergic agents. Topical antihistamines such as antazoline (usually given in combination with the sympathomimetic xylometazoline) or levocabastine (Ch. 39) can be given for allergic conjuctivitis. Topical sodium cromoglicate or nedocromil (Ch. 12) are generally less effective than antihistamines.

Local anaesthetics. Oxybuprocaine or lidocaine eyedrops provide surface anaesthesia (Ch. 18) for tonometry (measurements of pressure in the anterior chamber). For minor surgical procedures, such as removal of cataracts, tetracaine gives more profound anaesthesia and may be combined with injection of a small amount of lidocaine into the anterior chamber.

Artificial tears. Hypromellose is most commonly used to treat dry eyes, such as occurs in Sjögren's syndrome. It may need to be reapplied every hour. The surface mucin in the eye is often abnormal when there is tear deficiency, and the mucolytic agent acetylcysteine is often added to hypromellose. Carbomers, synthetic high-molecular-weight polymers of acrylic acid, cling better to the surface of the eye than does hypromellose and need less frequent application.

FURTHER READING

Alward WLM (1998) Medical management of glaucoma. *N Engl J Med* 339, 1298–1307

Bielory L (2002) Ocular allergy guidelines. *Drugs* 62, 1611–1634

Coleman AL (1999) Glaucoma. *Lancet* 354, 1803–1810

Hylton C, Robin AL (2003) Update on prostaglandin analogs. *Curr Opin Ophthalmol* 14, 65–69

Saw S-M, Gazzard G, Friedman DS (2003) Interventions for angle-closure glaucoma. An evidence-based update. *Ophthalmology* 110, 1869–1879

Self-assessment

In questions 1 and 2, the first statement, in italics, is true. Are the accompanying statements also true?

1. *The production of aqueous humour is not altered in glaucoma but drainage is reduced.*

   a. Adrenaline (epinephrine) is the drug of choice in patients with angle-closure glaucoma.
   b. Stimulation of α_2-adrenoceptors in the ciliary body reduces aqueous humour production.
   c. Tropicamide should be avoided if there is glaucoma in the eye.

2. *Accommodation of the lens is controlled by the parasympathetic autonomic nervous supply to the ciliary muscle.*

   a. Cocaine is a local anaesthetic that does not alter pupil size when administered topically.
   b. Cyclopentolate is a longer-acting mydriatic drug than tropicamide.
   c. Pilocarpine causes accommodation for near vision.

3. Extended-matching questions

   A. Cocaine
   B. Pilocarpine
   C. Aproclonidine
   D. Phenylephrine
   E. Tetracaine
   F. Tropicamide
   G. Timolol
   H. Atropine.

From the list A–H above, choose the <u>most appropriate</u> option in response to the statements 1–5 given below. Each option may be used more than once in answer to each question or not at all.

1. An antagonist of receptors in the ciliary body that will reduce aqueous production in glaucoma and has no effect on pupil size.
2. An agonist of receptors in the ciliary body that will reduce aqueous production in glaucoma and has no effect on pupil size.
3. A drug that will dilate the pupil without affecting accommodation.
4. A relatively short-acting drug that will dilate the pupil and is weakly cyclopegic.
5. A long-acting drug that can be used to prevent adhesions (posterior synechiae) in anterior uveitis and is stongly cycloplegic.

4. Case history questions

   During a routine eye examination, the optician noted a chronically raised intraocular pressure in a 56-year-old woman. Further tests revealed she had open-angle (simple) glaucoma.

   a. What could be the common cause of open-angle glaucoma?
   b. What drugs could have been used for this condition?
   c. What precautions should have been taken when using these drugs?

   The answers are provided on page 743.

Drug compendium

Drugs used in the eye[a]

Drug	Half-life (h)[b]	Elimination	Comments
Antibacterials			See Ch. 51 – systemic treatment may be necessary in some cases
Chloramphenicol	5 (2–12)	Metabolism	Broad spectrum; used for a wide range of infections; drug of choice for superficial eye infections; eliminated mainly by glucuronidation
Ciprofloxacin	3–4	Renal + metabolism	Broad spectrum; used for a wide range of infections, including *Pseudomonas aeruginosa*; used for corneal ulcers; eliminated by glomerular filtration, renal tubular secretion plus metabolism (15%)
Framycetin	–	–	Broad spectrum; used for a wide range of infections; no relevant kinetic data are available
Fusidic acid	9	Metabolism	Used for staphylococcal infections; metabolised in liver and metabolites excreted in bile
Gentamicin	1–4	Renal	Broad spectrum; used for a wide range of infections, including *Pseudomonas aeruginosa*; eliminated by glomerular filtration
Neomycin	2	Renal	Broad spectrum; used for a wide range of infections; eliminated by glomerular filtration
Ofloxacin	6–7	Renal (+ metabolism)	Broad spectrum; used for a wide range of infections, including *Pseudomonas aeruginosa*; eliminated by kidneys plus limited metabolism (<5%)
Polymyxin B	4–6	Renal	Used for Gram-negative organisms; elimination is prolonged in subjects with renal impairment
Propamidine isetionate	–	–	Principal use is for treatment of the rare but devastating condition *Acanthamoeba* keratitis; no relevant kinetic data available
Antivirals			
Aciclovir	3	Renal (+ metabolism)	Used for local treatment of herpes simplex infections; eliminated largely by renal tubular secretion + filtration; only about 10% is metabolised to inactive excretory products; see Ch. 51
Ganciclovir	4	Renal	Used for acute herpetic keratitis; given orally or by intravenous infusion; eliminated largely by glomerular filtration; see Ch. 51
Corticosteroids			The drugs shown below are used locally for short-term treatment of inflammation (oral corticosteroids are given for treating anterior segment inflammation – see. Ch. 44)
Betamethasone	35–55	Metabolism	Phosphate ester hydrolysed to betamethasone, which is inactivated by metabolism
Dexamethasone	2–4	Metabolism	Metabolised in the liver by CYP3A4-mediated oxidation to the 6-hydroxy compound
Fluorometholone	–	Metabolism	Only used topically; metabolism probably occurs locally in the eye; systemic disposition has not been defined

continued

Drugs used in the eye[a] *(continued)*

Drug	Half-life (h)[b]	Elimination	Comments
Hydrocortisone acetate	1–2	Metabolism	Metabolised by oxidation to cortisone and reduction to dihydro- and tetrahydrocortisol
Prednisolone	2–4	Metabolism	Extensively metabolised but all pathways have not been defined
Rimexolone	1–2	Metabolism (+ bile)	The elimination half-life has been estimated by the fact that steady-state levels are achieved after 5–7 h; few other data available
Other anti-inflammatory preparations			Many are histamine H_1 receptor antagonists – see also Ch. 39
Antazoline	–	–	Used for allergic conjunctivitis; histamine H_1 receptor antagonist; no relevant kinetic data are available
Azelastine	17	Metabolism	Used for allergic conjunctivitis; histamine H_1 receptor antagonist; metabolised by hepatic P450 to active desmethyl metabolite
Emedastine	3–4	Metabolism	Used for seasonal allergic conjunctivitis; histamine H_1 receptor antagonist; eliminated in urine largely as oxidised metabolites plus about 5% as the unchanged drug
Ketotifen	22	Metabolism	Used for seasonal allergic conjunctivitis; antihistamine and mast cell stabiliser; rapid onset of action after application to the eye and negligible systemic exposure; metabolised by formation of an *N*-glucuronide
Levocabastine	35–40	Renal (+ metabolism)	Used for seasonal allergic conjunctivitis; histamine H_1 receptor antagonist; extensive absorption (30–60%) has been found following ocular administration; elimination is largely as the unchanged compound (plus the acyl glucuronide) in urine
Lodoxamide	8	Renal	Used for allergic conjunctivitis; mast cell stabiliser; eliminated largely in the urine as the parent drug; few data available
Nedocromil	2	Renal	Used for allergic conjunctivitis; mast cell stabiliser; highly polar compound showing slow absorption across membranes; once in the blood it is eliminated rapidly by renal excretion (a slower late phase with a half-life of 14 h has been reported but this is probably of little clinical relevance)
Olopatadine	3	Renal + metabolism	Used for seasonal allergic conjunctivitis; antihistamine and mast cell stabiliser; detectable plasma levels after administration into the eye which persist for up to 2 weeks
Sodium cromoglicate	1–1.5	Renal	Used for allergic conjunctivitis; mast cell stabiliser; highly polar drug that shows limited absorption across cell membranes; absorbed drug is eliminated largely in the urine
Mydriatics and cycloplegics			
Atropine	2–5	Metabolism + renal	Used for refraction procedures in children and for anterior uveitis; longer-acting antimuscarinic; probably well absorbed; undergoes limited hydrolysis, plus oxidation and conjugation; about 30% of the dose is excreted unchanged in the urine

continued

Drug compendium

Drugs used in the eye[a] *(continued)*

Drug	Half-life (h)[b]	Elimination	Comments
Mydriatics and cycloplegics (continued)			
Cyclopentolate	2	?	Used for refraction procedures in children; longer-acting antimuscarinic; peak plasma concentrations occur about 30 min after giving eye-drops; method of elimination has not been described
Homatropine	–	–	Used for treatment of anterior segment inflammation; antimuscarinic; probably well absorbed; no relevant kinetic data are available
Phenylephrine	2–3	Metabolism + renal	Sympathomimetic α_1-selective adrenoceptor agonist; eliminated in urine as glucuronic acid and sulphate conjugates and as parent compound (15–20% after intravenous dosage)
Tropicamide	0.3 (or less)	?	Used to facilitate examination of the fundus; short-acting antimuscarinic; rapidly absorbed after ophthalmological dosage; peak plasma concentration occurs at 5 min, decreasing rapidly to undetectable levels by 2 h
Local anaesthetics			See Ch. 18
Lidocaine	2	Metabolism	Metabolised by dealkylation, catalysed by CYP3A4, followed by hydrolysis
Oxybuprocaine	–	Metabolism	Widely used; few kinetic data available; about 90% recovered in urine as parent drug and metabolites within 9 h (therefore half-life is 3 h or less)
Proxymetacaine	–	–	Causes less initial stinging and is useful for children; few relevant kinetic data available
Tetracaine	Very short (?)	Metabolism	Widely used; produces a more profound anaesthesia and is suitable for minor procedures; any absorbed drug would be very rapidly hydrolysed by plasma pseudocholinesterase.
Treatment of glaucoma			
Miotics			
Carbachol	–	–	Muscarinic agonist; no relevant kinetic data are available
Pilocarpine	1	Metabolism	Muscarinic agonist; ocular effects persist for 4–14 h; few details available; oxidised to an acid analogue
Sympathomimetics			
Apraclonidine	8	–	Used short-term before or after surgery; agonist at α_2-adrenoceptors; measurable systemic absorption

continued

Drugs used in the eye[a] *(continued)*

Drug	Half-life (h)[b]	Elimination	Comments
Sympathomimetics *(continued)*			
Brimonidine	3	Metabolism	Used alone or in combination with a β- adrenoceptor antagonists for ocular hypertension and alone for open-angle glaucoma if β-adrenoceptor antagonists are ineffective or inappropriate; agonist at α_2-adrenoceptors; metabolised by human liver preparations to oxidised products; relative importance of metabolism and other routes of elimination have not been defined
Dipivefrine	–	–	A produg of adrenaline (epinephrine) that passes more rapidly through the cornea; few data available
Beta-adrenoceptor antagonists			Effective in chronic simple glaucoma
Betaxolol	13–24	Metabolism (+ some renal)	Selective for β_1-adrenoceptors; oxidised in liver, and metabolites eliminated in urine
Carteolol	3–7	Renal + metabolism	Mostly eliminated in urine unchanged; the main metabolite (8-hydroxycarteolol) is a more potent β-adrenoceptor antagonist
Levobunolol	5–8	Metabolism + renal	Eliminated in urine as parent drug (about 15%), as a reduced metabolite and as conjugates of the parent drug and metabolite
Metipranolol	5	Metabolism	Various pathways of metabolism, including deacetylation giving a highly active metabolite (which is responsible for in vivo activity on cardiac β-adrenoceptors); the role of local metabolism in relation to ocular effect is not known
Timolol	2–5	Metabolism (+ some renal)	Non-selective β-adrenoceptor antagonist, eliminated by metabolism and renal excretion (20%)
Carbonic anhydrase inhibitors			
Acetazolamide	6–9	Renal	Used for open-angle, secondary and pre-operative angle-closure glaucoma; given orally or by intravenous injection as an adjunct to other treatments; not recommended for long-term use; eliminated in urine without detectable metabolism
Brinzolamide	11 days	Renal + some metabolism	Used topically in combination with a β-adrenoceptor antagonist for ocular hypertension and open-angle glaucoma if β-adrenoceptor antagonists alone are ineffective, or alone if β-adrenoceptor antagonists are inappropriate; distributes into erythrocytes where it has a very long half-life (111 days)
Dorzolamide	Weeks	Renal (+ metabolism)	Used topically in combination with a β-adrenoceptor antagonist for ocular hypertension, and open-angle and pseudo-exfoliative glaucoma if β-adrenoceptor antagonists alone are ineffective, or alone if β-adrenoceptor antagonists are inappropriate; blood concentrations are not detectable after ophthalmological use; an active de-ethylated metabolite has been reported; retained in red blood cells, which gives rise to an elimination half-life on cessation of the treatment of weeks

continued

Drugs used in the eye[a] *(continued)*

Drug	Half-life (h)[b]	Elimination	Comments
Prostaglandin analogues			Used to reduce pressure in ocular hypertension and open-angle glaucoma
Bimatoprost	45 min (intravenous)	Metabolism	Used alone or as adjunctive therapy; rapid absorption with peak blood levels within 10 min, which decrease rapidly over the next hour; metabolised by oxidation and conjugation
Latanoprost	0.3 (acid)	Metabolism	Analogue of $PGF_{2\alpha}$; the parent compound can be measured in the plasma during the first hour after ophthalmological administration; metabolised to an active acid metabolite, which has a half-life of 0.3 h; the reduction of intraocular pressure occurs at about 8–12 h (so systemic disposition gives no indication of therapeutic effect)
Travoprost	–	Hydrolysis	A synthetic analogue of $PGF_{2\alpha}$; a prodrug that is hydrolysed by esterases in the eye to the active form, travoprost acid

[a] Drugs are usually given topically to reduce systemic unwanted effects.
[b] The half-life data in this table refer to the systemic fate following absorption into the general circulation – the duration of action will depend on the rate of uptake by, and removal from, the eye.

Chemotherapy

51

Chemotherapy of infections

Antimicrobial agents are natural or synthetic chemical substances that suppress the growth of, or destroy, micro-organisms, including bacteria, fungi and viruses. The term antibiotic is widely used, but strictly should be reserved for those antimicrobial agents that are derived from micro-organisms. The term antimicrobial or the more restrictive terms antibacterial, antifungal and antiviral are used in this book.

Effective antimicrobial agents have certain key attributes. In order to avoid unwanted effects in humans, most are designed to have actions on processes that are unique to the pathogen. They must also be able to reach the site of infection. Micro-organisms can acquire resistance to an antimicrobial and will then no longer be affected by the drug. To keep 'ahead' of the micro-organism, there is a continuing effort to discover and develop antimicrobial agents that avoid or overcome these mechanisms of resistance.

Bacterial infections

Classification of antibacterial agents

Antibacterial agents can be classified in several overlapping ways.

Firstly, they can be bacteriostatic or bactericidal. This categorisation depends largely on the concentration of drug that can be safely achieved in plasma without causing significant toxicity in the person who takes the drug. Bacteriostatic antibacterials inhibit bacterial growth, but do not destroy the micro-organism at concentrations in plasma that are safe for humans, and the natural immune mechanisms of the body are used to eliminate the organism. Such drugs will be less effective in immunocompromised individuals or when the micro-organisms are dormant and not dividing. Bactericidal antibacterials kill micro-organisms at safe plasma concentrations, but even then, immune mechanisms will play a role in elimination of the micro-organism. Some bactericidal agents are more effective when cells are actively dividing; therefore, by preventing cell division, a bacteriostatic agent that is taken with a bactericidal drug may make the bactericidal drug less effective. For antibacterials to be bactericidal, they must be present at adequate concentration; too low a concentration may render them bacteriostatic.

Secondly, antibacterials can be grouped according to their mechanisms of action (Fig. 51.1):

- agents that inhibit the synthesis of peptidoglycans of the cell wall of the micro-organism, or activate enzymes that disrupt the cell wall (e.g. β-lactams)
- agents that act directly on the cell phospholipid membrane and affect its permeability, leading to leakage of intracellular contents (e.g. polymyxins)

577

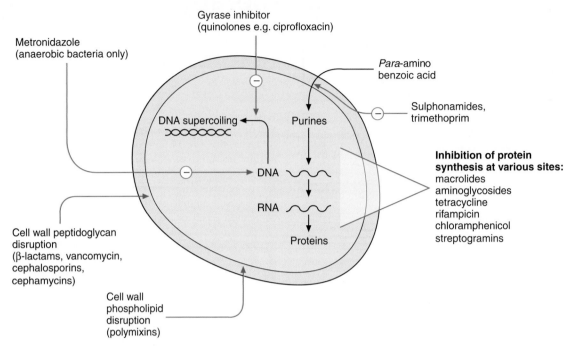

Fig. 51.1
A simplified scheme of the sites of action of the main classes of antibacterial drugs.

- agents that alter ribosomal function, producing a reversible inhibition of protein synthesis (e.g. aminoglycosides, macrolides); it is possible to achieve a high degree of selectivity of such drugs for bacteria because bacterial 70S ribosomes differ structurally from the 80S ribosomes in humans
- agents that block metabolic pathways that are essential for the life of the micro-organism (e.g. trimethoprim)
- agents that interfere with replication of DNA or RNA in the micro-organism (e.g. quinolones).

Thirdly, antibacterials may be classified according to whether their spectrum of activity against micro-organisms is limited (narrow spectrum) or extensive (broad spectrum).

Finally, they can be classified by chemical structure. In the following text, the antimicrobial agents are grouped according to their mechanism of action and then by their chemical structure. However, cross-referencing to other methods of classification is necessary. The drug compendium is organised to accord with the *British National Formulary* (BNF).

Antimicrobial resistance

When an antimicrobial is ineffective against a micro-organism in doses that can be used safely in humans,

the organism is said to be resistant to the antimicrobial agent. Resistance to antimicrobial agents can be intrinsic to the micro-organism or can be acquired by modification of its genetic structure. There are four general processes by which a micro-organism can acquire resistance to antimicrobial drugs (Fig. 51.2):

- modification of the micro-organism such that it produces enzymes that inactivate the drug; for example, β-lactamase enzymes inactivate penicillin and acetylating enzymes can inactivate aminoglycosides
- modification of the micro-organism such that penetration of the drug is reduced or it is pumped out faster than it can enter; for example, absence of the membrane protein D2 porin in resistant *Pseudomonas aeruginosa* prevents penetration of the β-lactam antibacterial imipenem
- structural change in the target molecule for the antimicrobial drug; for example, low affinity of mutated penicillin-binding proteins in resistant enterococci reduces binding of cephalosporins; mutation may also prevent the binding of aminoglycosides to the previously sensitive 30S unit of ribosomes
- production of a bypass pathway to overcome the effect of the antimicrobial drug; for example, resistant organisms can develop a mutant dihydrofolate reductase that is not inhibited by trimethoprim (see Fig. 51.4).

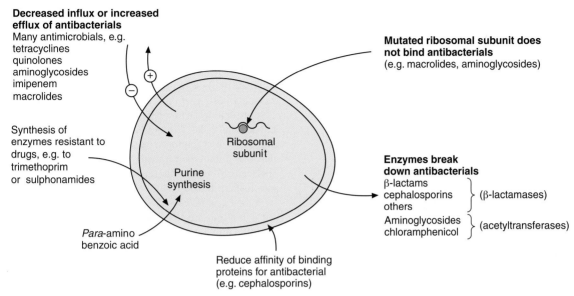

Decreased influx or increased efflux of antibacterials
Many antimicrobials, e.g.
tetracyclines
quinolones
aminoglycosides
imipenem
macrolides

Mutated ribosomal subunit does not bind antibacterials
(e.g. macrolides, aminoglycosides)

Synthesis of enzymes resistant to drugs, e.g. to trimethoprim or sulphonamides

Ribosomal subunit

Purine synthesis

Para-amino benzoic acid

Enzymes break down antibacterials
β-lactams
cephalosporins   } (β-lactamases)
others
Aminoglycosides
chloramphenicol   } (acetyltransferases)

Reduce affinity of binding proteins for antibacterial (e.g. cephalosporins)

Fig. 51.2
Mechanisms by which bacteria can resist antibacterial drugs.

Resistance is a major problem for infections with bacteria, protozoa (e.g. malaria) and viruses (e.g. human immunodeficiency virus [HIV]), but is less significant in fungal infections (apart from in people with immuno-deficiency). Resistance in protozoa and viruses is discussed below in the individual sections.

The major mechanisms by which bacteria acquire resistance to antibacterial drugs are spontaneous mutation, conjugation, transduction and transformation.

Spontaneous mutation. In this process, a single-step genetic mutation in a bacterial population leads to selective growth of the resistant strain in the presence of an antibacterial drug.

Conjugation. Direct cell-to-cell contact is a way of exchanging genetic material that confers antibacterial resistance. It usually involves transfer of self-replicating circular fragments of DNA called plasmids, which can contain multiple resistance genes. The resistance genes are found on sections of DNA that can jump from one plasmid to another (a transposon). Transposons can remain outside the genome of the micro-organism or can be incorporated into it, when they are more stable but less transmissible. Conjugation is by far the most important source of extrinsic DNA transfer between bacteria.

Transduction. Bacteria are susceptible to infection by viruses known as bacteriophages. During replication of the bacteriophages, the host cell's DNA (containing resistance genes) may be replicated along with viral DNA and taken into the virus. The phage carrying the resistance genes can then infect other bacterial cells and spread resistance.

Transformation. Uptake of DNA from dead bacteria by live bacteria can spread resistance genes.

Antibacterial agents

The antibacterial agents described are grouped by their mechanism of action and then by their chemical structure.

Agents affecting the cell wall: β-lactam antibacterials

This group of drugs all have a β-lactam ring in common, which is responsible for their activity (Fig. 51.3). The β-lactams include penicillins, cephalosporins and cephamycins, monobactams and carbapenems. Some are susceptible to attack by bacterial enzymes that split the β-lactam ring – β-lactamases (penicillinases) – but some are structurally modified to confer resistance to the β-lactamases.

Penicillins

Examples:
Penicillins: benzylpenicillin, phenoxymethylpenicillin
Aminopenicillins: amoxicillin, ampicillin, flucloxacillin
Ureidopenicillins: piperacillin
Amidinopenicillin: pivmecillinam
Carboxypenicillin: ticarcillin

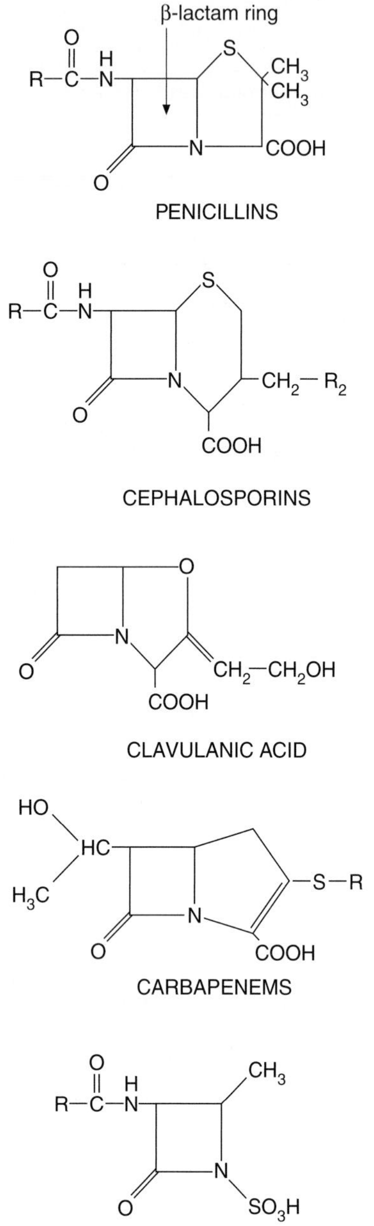

β-lactam ring

PENICILLINS

CEPHALOSPORINS

CLAVULANIC ACID

CARBAPENEMS

MONOBACTAMS

Fig. 51.3
The structural backbone of β-lactam antibacterial agents and the β-lactamase inhibitor clavulanic acid.

Mechanism of action

Penicillins consist of a thiazolidine ring connected to a β-lactam ring to which is attached a side-chain (Fig. 51.3). The side-chain determines many of the antibacterial and pharmacological characteristics of a particular penicillin. The β-lactam antibacterials inhibit synthesis of the peptidoglycan layer of the cell wall which surrounds certain bacteria and which is essential for their survival. The β-lactam ring contains structural similarities to one of the constituents of the peptidoglycan layer of the bacterial cell wall. Peptidoglycan synthesis occurs in three stages. The last stage of cross-linking in the cell wall is inhibited by β-lactam antibacterials, which bind to the transpeptidase enzymes in the cross-linking process; these are amongst a number of penicillin-binding proteins in bacterial cells. The antibacterial effect of β-lactam antibacterials is confined to dividing cells, which are unable to maintain their transmembrane osmotic gradient. This leads to cell swelling, which is followed by rupture and death of the bacterium.

Some bacterial cells also contain enzymes that cause cell lysis if they are activated. The β-lactam antibacterials bind to a number of specific penicillin-binding proteins within bacteria. Such binding reduces the action of the natural inhibitor of these lytic enzymes, leading to lysis of the bacterial cell wall.

Spectrum of activity

Penicillins differ considerably in their spectrum of activity (Table 51.1).

Benzylpenicillin (penicillin G) is active against many aerobic Gram-positive bacteria, Gram-negative cocci and many anaerobic micro-organisms. Gram-negative bacilli are not sensitive to benzylpenicillin. Benzylpenicillin is inactivated by the action of β-lactamase (see below).

The addition of an acyl side-chain to the β-lactam ring produces derivatives such as flucloxacillin, which prevent access of β-lactamase to the β-lactam ring. However flucloxacillin is generally less effective than benzylpenicillin against those bacteria that do not produce β-lactamase. Therefore, flucloxacillin is usually reserved for treating β-lactamase-producing staphylococci, which are particularly common in hospitals.

Ampicillin and amoxicillin are aminopenicillins that have an extended spectrum of activity to include many Gram-negative bacilli. However, they are less effective than benzylpenicillin against Gram-positive cocci. Both drugs are inactivated by β-lactamase.

Other extended-spectrum penicillins include ureidopenicillins (e.g. piperacillin), which are active against *Pseudomonas aeruginosa*, and amidinopenicillins (e.g. pivmecillinam), which are active mainly against Gram-negative bacteria. Carboxypenicillins (e.g. ticarcillin) are not widely used now, but have activity against *Pseudomonas* species, *Proteus* species and *Bacteroides fragilis*.

Clavulanic acid is a potent inhibitor of β-lactamase that is structurally related to the β-lactam antibiotics, although it has little intrinsic antibacterial activity (Fig. 51.3). When given in combination with penicillins that are destroyed by β-lactamase, such as amoxicillin and ticarcillin, they can be used to treat infections caused by β-lactamase-producing organisms that are otherwise insensitive to penicillins. Tazobactam has similar properties to clavulanic acid.

Table 51.1
Example of penicillins and their properties

	β-Haemolytic streptococci	Staphylococcus aureus		Enterobacteriaceae (coliforms)	Pseudomonas aeruginosa	Bacteroides fragilis
		β-Lactamase negative	β-Lactamase positive			
Benzylpenicillin/ phenoxymethylpenicillin	++	+	0	0	0	++
Broader spectrum Amoxicillin/ampicillin	++	+	0[a]	++	0	0
β-Lactamase resistant Flucloxacillin	+	+	+[b]	0	0	0
Antipseudomonal Ticarcillin	++	+	0[a,c]	+	+	+/0
Azlocillin	++	+	0[a]	+	+	+/0
Piperacillin	++	+	0[a]	+	+	+/0

++, active; +, variable activity; 0, inactive.
[a]Can be used combined with a β-lactamase inhibitor, e.g. tazobactum.
[b]Resistance is developing.
[c]Ticarcillin only available with clavulanic acid.

Resistance

Resistance to penicillins is most often due to the production of β-lactamases which hydrolyse the β-lactam ring (Fig. 51.3). Some Gram-positive bacteria release extracellular β-lactamases, particularly *Staphylococcus aureus*. In Gram-negative bacteria, the β-lactamases are located between the inner and outer cell membranes in the periplasmic space. The β-lactamases produced by various organisms have different spectra of activity against antimicrobials. The information for β-lactamase production is often encoded in a plasmid and this may be transferred by conjugation to other bacteria.

An alternative type of penicillin resistance occurs in gonococci and in meticillin-resistant *Staphylococcus aureus* (MRSA), which develop mutated penicillin-binding proteins that do not bind to β-lactams. Meticillin is now discontinued.

Pharmacokinetics

Benzylpenicillin and phenoxymethylpenicillin. Only about one-third of an orally administered dose of benzylpenicillin is absorbed, the rest is destroyed by acid in the stomach. Benzylpenicillin is, therefore, restricted to intramuscular or intravenous routes of administration. The phenoxymethyl derivative (penicillin V) is more stable in an acid environment and is better absorbed from the gut. Maximum concentrations in blood occur rapidly in 30–60 min. Penicillins are widely distributed throughout the body, although transport across the meninges is poor unless they are acutely inflamed (e.g. in meningitis), when penetration by the antibacterial is improved. The half-lives of most penicillins are short because they are very rapidly eliminated by the kidney, mainly by active tubular secretion chiefly in the proximal tubule. Effective plasma concentrations of penicillins are usually maintained by frequent dosing or by intravenous infusion, but sometimes by complexing with other agents (see below).

Flucloxacillin, amoxicillin and ampicillin. Flucloxacillin and amoxicillin are rapidly and almost completely absorbed from the gut, but ampicillin is incompletely absorbed. These drugs are eliminated by the kidney in a similar way to benzylpenicillin and have short half-lives. They can also be given intramuscularly or intravenously.

Other penicillins. The amidinopenicillin pivmecillinam is a prodrug for oral use. The carboxypenicillin ticarcillin is only available in combination with clavulanic acid for intravenous use. These drugs are excreted renally. The ureidopenicillin piperacillin is given intravenously in combination with the β-lactamase inhibitor tazobactam. Biliary excretion is responsible for the elimination of about a quarter of piperacillin.

Unwanted effects

Penicillins are normally very safe antibacterials with a high therapeutic index.

- Nausea, vomiting.
- Hypersensitivity reactions in 1–10% of exposed individuals. Manifestations of allergy to penicillins include rashes, fever, vasculitis, serum sickness,

exfoliative dermatitis, Stevens–Johnson syndrome and anaphylactic shock. Cross-allergy is widespread among various penicillins and to a lesser extent with cephalosporins. Penicillins and their breakdown products bind to proteins and act as haptens, stimulating the production of antibodies that mediate the allergic response (Chs 38 and 53).

- Aminopenicillins (e.g. amoxicillin) frequently produce a non-allergic maculopapular rash in people with glandular fever.
- Reversible neutropenia and eosinophilia can occur with prolonged high doses.
- Encephalopathy with excessively high cerebrospinal fluid (CSF) concentrations of penicillin. This occurs in severe renal failure, or after intrathecal injection (which should never be given).
- Diarrhoea or antibiotic-associated colitis can occur as a result of disturbance of normal colonic flora, especially with broad-spectrum penicillins.
- Cholestatic jaundice can occur with flucloxacillin or clavulanic acid.

Cephalosporins

> Examples:
> 'First generation': cefadroxil, cefalexin
> 'Second generation': cefaclor, cefuroxime
> 'Third generation': cefotaxime, cefixime, ceftazidime, ceftriaxone

Mechanism of action

Cephalosporins, like penicillins, have a β-lactam ring. To this ring is fused a dihydrothiazine ring, which makes them more resistant to hydrolysis by β-lactamases (Fig. 51.3). They inhibit bacterial cell wall synthesis in a manner similar to that of the penicillins.

Spectrum of activity

Cephalosporins are often classified by 'generations'. The members within each generation share similar anti-bacterial activity. However, the pharmacokinetics of individual drugs within each generation vary, and each generation of cephalosporins includes examples that can only be given parenterally. Succeeding generations tend to have increased activity against Gram-negative bacilli, usually at the expense of Gram-positive activity, and increased ability to cross the blood–brain barrier (Table 51.2).

- First-generation oral cephalosporins (e.g. cefadroxil or cefalexin) have activity against staphylococci and most streptococci, but not enterococci. They cross the blood–brain barrier poorly.
- Second-generation oral cephalosporins (e.g. cefuroxime) have additional activity against some Gram-negative bacteria such as *Haemophilus influenzae* and *Neisseria gonorrhoea*.
- Third-generation oral cephalosporins have improved β-lactamase stability and are able to penetrate the CSF in useful quantities. They also have greater Gram-negative activity than the other two generations. Cefixime adds *Proteus* and *Klebsiella* species to its spectrum, but it has no activity against staphylococci (Table 51.2). Ceftazidime has good activity against *Pseudomonas* species.

Resistance

The earlier generations are relatively more sensitive to β-lactamase-mediated enzymatic hydrolysis of the β-lactam ring, but susceptibility is considerably less with the later generations (Table 51.2).

Pharmacokinetics

The pharmacokinetics of the cephalosporins vary greatly. First-generation oral cephalosporins are usually well absorbed. Several second- and third-generation drugs, for example cefuroxime and cefotaxime, are acid-labile and must be given by a parenteral route. Cefuroxime has been formulated as a prodrug (cefuroxime axetil) for oral use, which has good absorption and is hydrolysed at first pass through the liver to cefuroxime. Most cephalosporins are primarily excreted by the kidney and have short half-lives. Cefixime is mainly eliminated by biliary excretion and has an intermediate half-life.

Unwanted effects

- Nausea, vomiting, abdominal discomfort.
- Headache.
- Skin rashes, including erythema multiforme and toxic epidermal necrolysis.
- Cephalosporins can produce hypersensitivity reactions similar to those observed with the penicillins. About 10% of people who are allergic to penicillins show cross-allergy to cephalosporins. A history of a serious reaction to penicillins precludes the administration of cephalosporins.
- Diarrhoea or antibiotic-associated colitis can be caused by disturbance of normal bowel flora. This is more common with oral cephalosporins.

Cephamycins

> Example: cefoxitin

Cefoxitin is a β-lactam cephalosporin-type antibacterial having a 7-methoxy group and possessing marked resistance to the action of β-lactamases from Gram-positive and Gram-negative bacteria.

Spectrum of activity

Cefoxitin has greater activity than cefaclor against Gram-negative bacteria, especially *Bacteroides fragilis*.

Table 51.2
Examples of cephalosporins and their spectra of activity

	Staphylococcus aureus	Haemophilus influenzae	Enterobacteriaceae (coliforms)	Pseudomonas aeruginosa	Bacteroides fragilis	Ability to cross blood–brain barrier	Resistance to β-lactamase
First generation							
Cefadroxil/cefradine (oral)	+	0	+/0	0	0	+/0	+
Cefalexin (oral)	+	0	+/0	0	0	+/0	+
Second generation							
Cefuroxime axetil (oral)	++	++	++	0	+[a]	++	++
Cefuroxime (parenteral)	++	++	++	0	+	++	++
Third generation							
Cefixime (oral)	0	+++	++	0	0	++	++
Cefotaxime (parenteral)	+	+++	+++	0	+	++	++
Ceftazidime (parenteral)	0	0	+	++	0	+/0[b]	++

Staphylococcus aureus is a Gram-positive staining organism. Other illustrative bacteria are Gram-negative staining.
+++, very active; ++, active; +, variable activity; 0 inactive or poor activity.
[a]Cefoxitine (a cephamycin) is active.
[b]Some cephalosporins penetrate better into the CNS in the presence of inflamed meninges.

This makes it useful for the treatment of intra-abdominal sepsis.

Resistance

Cefoxitin is resistant to the action of β-lactamase, in common with some cephalosporins, although reports of resistant strains are increasing.

Pharmacokinetics

Cefoxitin is given by deep intramuscular or by intravenous injection. It is excreted unchanged by the kidney and has a short half-life.

Unwanted effects

These are similar to those of cephalosporins.

Monobactams

Example: aztreonam

Aztreonam is a β-lactam antibacterial related to the penicillins but with a single ring structure ('monocyclic β-lactam') (Fig. 51.3). It has little cross-allergenicity with the penicillins and has been successfully given to people with proven penicillin allergy. Its spectrum of activity is limited to Gram-negative bacteria, including *Pseudomonas aeruginosa*, *Neisseria meningitidis*, *Neisseria gonorrhoeae* and *Haemophilus influenzae*, with no activity against Gram-positive bacteria or anaerobes. Aztreonam is given intramuscularly or intravenously and is β-lactamase resistant. It is excreted by the kidney and has a short half-life. Unwanted effects are similar to those of other β-lactam antibacterials.

Carbapenems

Examples: ertapenem, imipenem, meropenem

Imipenem is a β-lactam agent that has an extremely broad spectrum of bactericidal activity. It has potent activity against Gram-positive cocci, including some β-lactamase-producing pneumococci; Gram-negative bacilli, including *Pseudomonas aeruginosa*, *Neisseria suppurans* and *Bacteroides* species; and also many anaerobic bacteria. Imipenem can penetrate the blood–brain barrier and is resistant to β-lactamases. Narrow-spectrum resistance to imipenem in *Pseudomonas aeruginosa* occurs from a mutation that results in loss of a specific cell membrane uptake pathway. Imipenem is rapidly metabolised by dihydropeptidases in the kidney and so is given in combination with cilastatin, a compound that inhibits dihydropeptidase-induced destruction. Meropenem is not inactivated by the renal

enzyme and can be given alone. Both imipenem and meropenem are given intravenously; imipenem can also be given by deep intramuscular injection. Ertapenem has a broad spectrum of activity against Gram-positive and Gram-negative bacteria, but is inactive against *Pseudomonas* species. It is given intravenously. These drugs are mainly excreted by the kidney and have short half-lives. Unwanted effects are similar to those of other β-lactam antibacterials.

Other agents affecting the cell wall

Glycopeptides

Examples: vancomycin, teicoplanin

Mechanism of action

Vancomycin and teicoplanin are high-molecular-weight glycopeptide compounds that act by inhibiting bacterial cell wall synthesis. They achieve this by inhibiting the linkages of peptidoglycan constituents (Fig. 51.1). Glycopeptides are bactericidal.

Spectrum of activity

Vancomycin and teicoplanin are active only against Gram-positive bacteria, particularly multi-resistant staphylococci. They do not penetrate the cell wall of Gram-negative bacteria. Both are usually reserved for treatment of serious staphylococcal infection or for bacterial endocarditis that is not responding to other treatments. Vancomycin given orally is also effective against *Clostridium difficile*, which colonises the colon when normal flora are disturbed, causing antibiotic-associated colitis. Metronidazole is preferred for this indication, but some strains are resistant to metronidazole.

Resistance

Acquired resistance is uncommon. Vancomycin-resistant *Staphylococcus aureus* develops as a result of a multi-step genetic acquisition of a thickened peptidoglycan cell wall. This traps the drug and prevents it reaching its target on the cytoplasmic membrane. For other organisms, plasmid-mediated resistance involves incorporation of D-lactate into the cell wall in place of D-alanine. This modification prevents binding of the antibacterial.

Pharmacokinetics

Both vancomycin and teicoplanin are very poorly absorbed orally and are given by intravenous infusion. Teicoplanin can also be given by intramuscular injection. Oral vancomycin is only used for treating antibiotic-associated colitis. Both drugs are excreted by the kidney; vancomycin has an intermediate half-life, teicoplanin a long half-life.

Unwanted effects

- ototoxicity, often starting with tinnitus
- nephrotoxicity, which may be enhanced if vancomycin or teicoplanin are used in combination with an aminoglycoside
- thrombophlebitis at the site of infusion
- rashes, including Stevens–Johnson syndrome and toxic epidermal necrolysis; rapid intravenous injection of vancomycin produces upper body flushing, the 'red man' syndrome
- blood disorders, including neutropenia, thrombocytopenia
- nausea.

Polymyxins

Example: Colistin (colistimethate sodium)

Mechanism of action

Polymyxins bind to bacterial membrane phospholipids and alter permeability of the membrane to K^+ and Na^+. The cell's osmotic barrier is lost, and susceptible bacteria are killed by lysis (Fig. 51.1).

Spectrum of activity

Polymyxins have bactericidal action against Gram-negative bacteria, including *Pseudomonas* species, but are inactive against Gram-positive bacteria.

Resistance

Acquired resistance is rare.

Pharmacokinetics

Colistin is very poorly absorbed from the gut and is usually given by inhalation or topically to the skin. Penetration into joint spaces or CSF is poor. It is excreted unchanged by the kidney and has an intermediate half-life. It is sometimes given by mouth for bowel sterilisation.

Unwanted effects

Substantial toxicity limits the use of polymyxins by systemic administration.

- Nephrotoxicity produces a dose-related reversible renal impairment.
- Neurotoxicity produces dizziness, circumoral and peripheral paraesthaesiae, and confusion. Rarely, neuromuscular blockade can produce respiratory paralysis with apnoea.
- Bronchospasm or sore throat after inhalation.

Agents affecting bacterial DNA
Quinolones (fluoroquinolones)

Examples: ciprofloxacin, levofloxacin, moxifloxacin, norfloxacin

Mechanism of action

Quinolones inhibit replication of bacterial DNA. They block the activity of bacterial DNA gyrase and DNA topoisomerase, the enzymes that form DNA supercoils and are essential for DNA replication and repair (Fig. 51.1). The effect is bactericidal.

Spectrum of activity

Ciprofloxacin has a broad spectrum of activity and is active against many micro-organisms resistant to penicillins, cephalosporins and aminoglycosides. Its spectrum includes Gram-positive bacteria, but with only moderate activity against *Streptococcus pneumoniae* and *Enterococcus faecalis*. It is active against most Gram-negative bacteria, including *Haemophilus influenzae*, *Pseudomonas aeruginosa*, *Neisseria gonorrhoea*, and *Enterobacter* and *Campylobacter* species. Its spectrum extends to chlamydia and some mycobacteria, but not anaerobes.

Levofloxacin has greater activity against pneumococci than has ciprofloxacin. Moxifloxacin has a broad spectrum of activity against Gram-positive and Gram-negative bacteria, but is inactive against *Pseudomonas aeruginosa*. It has greater activity than ciprofloxacin against pneumococci. Norfloxacin is mainly useful for urinary tract pathogens.

Resistance

Resistance to ciprofloxacin is relatively uncommon but can be produced by a mutation that results in a DNA gyrase that is less susceptible to the drug's action, or by increased active drug efflux from the cell (Fig. 51.2). Plasmid-mediated resistance has not been found.

Pharmacokinetics

Oral absorption of ciprofloxacin is variable but adequate. It is widely distributed in body tissues and fluids, but CSF penetration is poor unless there is meningeal inflammation. The majority of the drug is eliminated unchanged by the kidney, partly by tubular secretion, but about 20% is excreted in the bile and a similar amount is metabolised in the liver. Ciprofloxacin has a short half-life. Levofloxacin has a longer half-life than ciprofloxacin, and continues to inhibit bacterial growth even if concentrations of drug have fallen to undetectable levels (post-antibiotic effect). Intravenous formulations of ciprofloxacin and levofloxacin are available. Moxifloxacin is well absorbed from the gut, is metabolised in the liver and partially excreted unchanged in the urine, and has a long half-life. Norfloxacin is moderately well absorbed from the gut, is eliminated by a combination of metabolism and renal excretion, and has a short half-life.

Unwanted effects

- Nausea, vomiting, abdominal pain, diarrhoea.
- Central nervous system (CNS) effects: dizziness, headache, tremor, seizures (especially in those with a prior history of epilepsy).
- Rashes.
- Pain and inflammation in tendons, occasionally with tendon rupture (especially in the elderly or with concomitant use of corticosteroids).
- Moxifloxacin prolongs the Q–T interval on the electrocardiogram (ECG) and predisposes to ventricular arrhythmias. The risk is greater if it is used in combination with other pro-arrhythmic drugs (Ch. 8).
- Drug interactions: the plasma concentrations of theophylline (Ch. 12), warfarin (Ch. 11) and ciclosporin (Ch. 38) are increased by ciprofloxacin and norfloxacin, through inhibition of hepatic cytochrome P450; this can produce toxicity. The absorption of quinolones from the gut is decreased by oral iron salts.

Metronidazole and tinidazole

Mechanism of action

Metronidazole is bactericidal only after it has been degraded to an intermediate transient toxic metabolite, which inhibits bacterial DNA synthesis and breaks down existing DNA. Only some anaerobes and some protozoa contain the oxidoreductase enzyme that converts metronidazole to its antibacterial derivative. The intermediate metabolite is not produced in human cells, or in aerobic bacteria. The effect of metronidazole is bactericidal. It is equally active against dividing and non-dividing cells.

Spectrum of activity

Metronidazole and tinidazole are mainly active against anaerobic bacteria and protozoa, including *Bacteroides fragilis, Clostridium* species, *Gardnerella vaginalis* and *Giardia lamblia*. They are also amoebicidal with activity against *Entamoeba histolytica*. Metronidazole is an important drug for treating antibiotic-induced colitis (pseudomembranous colitis) caused by *Clostridium difficile*. Metronidazole or tinidazole are important constituents of the triple or quadruple therapy utilised for the elimination of *Helicobacter pylori* (Ch. 33).

Resistance

Acquired resistance is not high but is developing. For example, in some countries, a significant percentage of strains of *Helicobacter pylori* are resistant to metronidazole and some types of *Clostridium difficile*-induced colitis,

too, are resistant. Resistance can result from by-pass mechanisms, when bacteria develop alternative oxido-reductases that do not act on metronidazole, or from induction of oxidative stress mechanisms that inhibit the action of the drug.

Pharmacokinetics

Metronidazole is well absorbed orally and can also be given intravenously, or by rectal suppositories. Rectal absorption is high, and this route is often preferable to intravenous administration if the drug cannot be taken by mouth. Metronidazole penetrates well into body fluids, including vaginal, pleural and cerebrospinal fluids, and can cross the placenta. It is mainly metabolised by the liver and has an intermediate half-life. Tinidazole is similar, but has a long half-life.

Unwanted effects

- nausea, vomiting, metallic taste
- intolerance to alcohol can occur by a mechanism that is similar to the disulfiram reaction (Ch. 54)
- rashes.

Nitrofurantoin

Mechanism of action

Nitrofurantoin is probably activated by reduction to unstable metabolites inside bacteria, which produces DNA disruption. It is bactericidal, especially to bacteria in acid urine.

Spectrum of activity

Nitrofurantoin is active against most Gram-positive cocci and *Escherichia coli. Pseudomonas* species are naturally resistant, as are many *Proteus* species. Its use is confined to infections of the lower urinary tract.

Resistance

Chromosomal resistance occurs but is not common.

Pharmacokinetics

Nitrofurantoin is well absorbed from the gut. The half-life is short in the plasma, and therapeutic concentrations are not achieved. It is excreted unchanged in the urine by both glomerular filtration and tubular secretion, but also appears in the bile. Urinary concentrations are high enough to treat lower urinary tract infections, but the low tissue concentrations are often inadequate for the treatment of acute pyelonephritis.

Unwanted effects

- gastrointestinal upset is common, including anorexia, nausea and vomiting
- pulmonary toxicity with long-term use produces acute allergic pneumonitis or chronic interstitial fibrosis
- peripheral neuropathy.

Agents affecting bacterial protein synthesis

Macrolides

Examples: azithromycin, clarithromycin, erythromycin, telithromycin

Mechanism of action

Macrolides interfere with bacterial protein synthesis by binding reversibly to the 50S subunit of the bacterial ribosome. This causes dissociation of the peptidyl transfer RNA (tRNA) from its translocation site. The action is primarily bacteriostatic (Fig. 51.1).

Spectrum of activity

Erythromycin has a similar spectrum of activity to broad-spectrum penicillins, and is often used for treatment in people who are penicillin-allergic. It is effective against Gram-positive bacteria and gut anaerobes, but has poor activity against *Haemophilus influenzae*. It is also used for infections by *Legionella*, *Mycoplasma*, *Chlamydia*, *Mycobacteria* and *Campylobacter* species and for *Bordetella pertussis*. Although erythromycin is primarily bacteriostatic, it is bactericidal at high concentrations for some Gram-positive species, such as group A streptococci and pneumococci. Azithromycin has less activity than erythromycin against Gram-positive bacteria, but enhanced activity against *Haemophilus influenzae*. Clarithromycin has slightly greater activity than erythromycin and is also used as part of the multidrug treatment of *Helicobacter pylori* (Ch. 33). Telithromycin is a ketolide derivative of erythromycin that is active against penicillin- and erythromycin-resistant *Streptococcus pneumoniae*.

Resistance

Bacteria become resistant to macrolides by activation of an efflux mechanism. To a lesser extent, there is also a gene mutation that encodes for a methyltransferase that modifies the target site on the ribosome.

Pharmacokinetics

Erythromycin is adequately absorbed from the gut. It is destroyed at acid pH and is, therefore, given as an enteric-coated tablet or as an ester prodrug (erythromycin ethyl succinate), which is acid-stable. Erythromycin can also be administered intravenously. Clarithromycin is acid-stable and well absorbed from the gut, but undergoes first-pass metabolism in the liver. Erythromycin and clarithromycin are metabolised in the liver and have short half-lives.

Azithromycin is poorly absorbed from the gut. It is widely distributed and released slowly from the tissues. Azithromycin is excreted unchanged in the bile and has

a very long half-life of about 2 days. Telithromycin is fairly well absorbed from the gut, is metabolised in the liver, partly by CYP450, and has an intermediate half-life.

Unwanted effects

- Epigastric discomfort, nausea, vomiting and diarrhoea are common with the oral preparation of erythromycin. Azithromycin and clarithromycin are better tolerated.
- Rashes.
- Cholestatic jaundice with erythromycin, usually if treatment is continued for more than 2 weeks.
- Prolongation of the Q–T interval on the ECG, with a predisposition to ventricular arrhythmias (Ch. 8).
- Erythromycin and clarithromycin inhibit P450 drug-metabolising enzymes and can elevate levels of drugs requiring these enzymes for metabolism. Examples include carbamazepine (Ch. 23) and ciclosporin (Ch. 38).

Aminoglycosides

Examples: amikacin, gentamicin, netilmicin, streptomycin, tobramycin

Mechanism of action

The aminoglycosides are similar in their properties but there are some important differences that can be exploited in particular clinical circumstances, as illustrated below. Aminoglycosides inhibit protein synthesis in bacteria by binding irreversibly to the 30S ribosomal subunit (Fig. 51.1). This inhibits translation from messenger RNA (mRNA) to protein and also increases the frequency of misreading of the genetic code. Aminoglycosides are bactericidal.

Spectrum of activity

Aminoglycosides are active against many Gram-negative bacteria (including *Pseudomonas* species) and some Gram-positive bacteria. They are inactive against anaerobes, which are unable to take up the aminoglycosides. Aminoglycosides are particularly useful for serious Gram-negative infections, when they have a complementary and synergistic action with agents that disrupt cell wall synthesis (e.g. penicillins). Gentamicin is the most widely used aminoglycoside. Streptomycin is mainly used as part of the drug regimen to treat *Mycobacterium tuberculosis* (see below).

Resistance

Resistance is increasingly a problem with the aminoglycosides and can occur by several mechanisms. It is transferred by plasmids and is principally caused by production of enzymes that acetylate, phosphorylate or adenylate aminoglycosides in the bacterial periplasmic space. Bacterial uptake of the modified drug is poor (Fig. 51.2). Amikacin is less susceptible to these enzymes, and is effective against many gentamicin-resistant Gram-negative bacilli. Changes in the ribosomal proteins in resistant bacteria can also reduce drug binding and antibacterial effectiveness, particularly for streptomycin. Netilmicin remains effective against many of these gentamicin-resistant bacteria. Resistance resulting from reduced penetration of the drug can be overcome by co-administration of antibacterials that disrupt cell wall synthesis, such as penicillins.

Pharmacokinetics

Aminoglycosides are poorly absorbed from the gut, and, therefore, are given parenterally. They have short half-lives and are rapidly excreted by the kidney. They do not cross the blood–brain barrier; however, they cross the placenta and can damage the VIIIth cranial nerve in the fetus (see below). Blood concentrations should always be measured to guide dosing. Peak concentrations, measured 1 h after dosing, and trough concentrations immediately before the next dose are important, both to ensure bactericidal efficacy and to minimise the risk of toxic effects. Once-daily dosage regimens for aminoglycosides are becoming more popular and are no more toxic than multiple daily dosages.

Tobramycin is also available as a preservative-free solution for administration by nebuliser for the management of people with cystic fibrosis whose respiratory tracts are colonised by *Pseudomonas aeruginosa*.

Unwanted effects

Most unwanted effects of aminoglycosides are dose related and many are reversible; they are probably related to high trough concentrations of the drug.

- Ototoxicity can lead to both vestibular and auditory dysfunction. Prolonged treatment or high plasma drug concentrations lead to accumulation of aminoglycoside in the inner ear, resulting in often irreversible disturbances of balance or deafness. Ototoxicity can be enhanced by loop diuretics (Ch. 14). Netilmicin causes less ototoxicity than the other aminoglycosides.
- Renal damage occurs through retention of aminoglycosides in the proximal tubular cells of the kidney. It is usually reversible and is manifest initially by a defect in the concentrating ability of the kidney, with mild proteinuria followed by a reduction in the glomerular filtration rate.
- Acute neuromuscular blockade can occur, usually if the aminoglycoside is used with anaesthetic agents (Ch. 17), and they can enhance the effects of other neuromuscular-blocking agents (Ch. 27). This action is the result of inhibition of prejunctional acetylcholine release, and also reduced postsynaptic sensitivity. It is reversed by intravenous Ca^{2+} salts.

Tetracyclines

Examples: oxytetracycline, doxycycline, minocycline

Mechanism of action

Tetracyclines enter bacteria mainly by an active uptake mechanism that is not found in human cells. They are bacteriostatic and inhibit bacterial protein synthesis by binding reversibly to the 30S subunit of ribosomes.

Spectrum of activity

Tetracyclines have a broad spectrum of activity against many Gram-positive and Gram-negative bacteria and in infections caused by rickettsiae, amoebae, *Chlamydia psittici, Trachomatis coxiella, Vibrio cholerae,* and *Mycoplasma, Legionella* and *Brucella* species. They are useful in acne (Ch. 49). Minocycline is active against *Neisseria meningitidis,* unlike other tetracyclines.

Resistance

Resistance is carried by plasmids and is usually due to increased pumping of the drug out from the bacterium (Fig. 51.2). An alternative mechanism is decreased binding of tetracyclines to bacterial ribosomes. Resistance to the tetracyclines develops slowly, but in the UK is now widespread among most Gram-positive and several Gram-negative bacteria. Micro-organisms that have developed resistance to one tetracycline frequently display resistance to the others.

Pharmacokinetics

Tetracyclines are incompletely absorbed from the gut, particularly if taken with food. Absorption of oxytetracycline is further impaired by milk, aluminium, calcium or magnesium salts (antacids; Ch. 33), iron and increased intestinal pH; tetracyclines bind to divalent and trivalent cations, forming inactive chelates (Ch. 56).

The tetracyclines diffuse reasonably well into sputum, urine, and peritoneal and pleural fluid, and cross the placenta. They have poor penetration into CSF. All of the tetracyclines have intermediate or long half-lives, with doxycycline and minocycline having the longest. Tetracyclines are concentrated in the liver and some drug is excreted via the bile into the small intestine, from where it is partially reabsorbed. Drug concentrations in the bile may be three to five times higher than in the plasma.

Tetracyclines are mainly eliminated unchanged in the urine, with the exception of doxycycline, which is largely eliminated in the bile.

Unwanted effects

- Nausea, vomiting, epigastric discomfort and diarrhoea.

- Tetracyclines in children produce permanent yellow–brown discoloration of the growing teeth by chelating with Ca^{2+}. They can also cause dental hypoplasia. Tetracyclines should be avoided during the latter half of pregnancy and in children in the first 12 years of life.
- Anti-anabolic effects can occur in human cells from inhibition of protein synthesis (not seen with doxycycline or minocycline). If there is pre-existing impairment of renal function, this can lead to uraemia.
- Benign intracranial hypertension, with headache and visual disturbances.

Chloramphenicol

Mechanism of action
Chloramphenicol inhibits protein synthesis in bacteria by binding reversibly to the 50S subunit of bacterial ribosomes (Fig. 51.1). It inhibits peptide bond formation by impairing the reading of mRNA. The effect is mainly bacteriostatic, but can be bactericidal in some micro-organisms.

Spectrum of activity
Chloramphenicol is a broad-spectrum antibacterial, active against many Gram-positive cocci (both aerobic and anaerobic) and Gram-negative bacteria. The sensitivities of all bacteria are variable, but it has a bactericidal effect on *Escherichia coli*, *Streptococcus pneumoniae*, *Haemophilus influenzae*, *Neisseria meningitidis*, *Bordetella pertussis*, *Vibrio cholerae* and *Salmonella*, *Shigella* and *Bacteroides* species. Some streptococci and staphylococci are inhibited.

Because of its toxicity, chloramphenicol is reserved for life-threatening infections, particularly with *Haemophilus influenzae* or *Salmonella typhi*. It is used topically for conjunctivitis (Ch. 50).

Resistance
Resistance is caused by the production of a plasmid-mediated enzyme that inactivates the drug by acetylation. The enzyme is produced by many Gram-negative bacteria but can also be induced in Gram-positive bacteria. Resistant bacteria may also show reduced uptake of the drug.

Pharmacokinetics
Chloramphenicol is well absorbed orally, and can also be given intravenously. It is widely distributed into many tissues, including CSF and the biliary tree; it crosses the placenta and is present in breast milk. Chloramphenicol is almost completely metabolised by glucuronidaton in the liver and has a short half-life.

Unwanted effects
- The most important unwanted effect is bone marrow toxicity. Reversible anaemia, thrombocytopenia or neutropenia can occur, particularly in people receiving high or prolonged dosing. Aplastic anaemia is rare, but usually fatal.
- Peripheral neuritis, optic neuritis, headache.
- Rashes.
- Premature infants and babies of less than 2 weeks of age have immature hepatic enzymes, particularly glucuronyl transferase, and reduced renal drug elimination. Chloramphenicol can accumulate in neonates, causing the 'grey baby syndrome'. Initial symptoms include vomiting and cyanosis, followed by hypothermia, vasomotor collapse and an ashen grey discoloration of the skin. There is a high mortality.

Lincosamides

Example: clindamycin

Mechanism of action
Clindamycin inhibits bacterial protein synthesis in a similar manner to the macrolide antibacterials.

Spectrum of activity
Clindamycin is used for staphylococcal bone infection such as osteomyelitis, and as prophylaxis for endocarditis in individuals who cannot take penicillins. It is also effective against Gram-positive cocci.

Resistance
Resistance develops by modification of the ribosomal binding site.

Pharmacokinetics
Clindamycin is well absorbed orally. It undergoes metabolism in the liver and has a short half-life.

Unwanted effects
- nausea, vomiting, abdominal discomfort, diarrhoea and sometimes pseudomembranous colitis
- rashes
- jaundice and abnormal liver function tests
- neutropenia, thrombocytopenia.

Fusidic acid

Mechanism of action
Fusidic acid is a steroid compound that inhibits bacterial protein synthesis. It forms a complex, binds to the ribosome and inhibits translocation of peptidyl-tRNA.

Spectrum of activity
Fusidic acid is a narrow-spectrum antibacterial, mainly active against Gram-positive bacteria. It is most commonly used for treatment of penicillin-resistant

Staphylococcus aureus, especially in the treatment of osteomyelitis. It is bactericidal.

Resistance

Resistance occurs either by mutation or by plasmid conjugation. Resistance occurs rapidly when fusidic acid is used alone; consequently, it is usually given in combination with another drug.

Pharmacokinetics

Oral absorption is complete, but an intravenous formulation is available. Penetration into synovial fluid and soft tissues is good, and the drug concentrates in bone. Fusidic acid is extensively metabolised in the liver and has an intermediate half-life.

Unwanted effects

- thrombophlebitis with intravenous infusions
- cholestatic jaundice
- nausea, vomiting.

Streptogramins

Examples: quinupristin with dalfopristin

Mechanisms of action and use

Streptogramins are isolated from *Streptomyces pristinae spiralis*. Quinupristin and dalfopristin bind to the 50S subunit of the bacterial ribosome and inhibit the late phase of protein synthesis.

Spectrum of activity

The combination of quinupristin with dalfopristin acts synergistically and is effective against aerobic Gram-positive bacteria, including MRSA and vancomycin-resistant *Enterococcus faecium*, but not *Enterococcus faecalis*. It should be reserved for serious infections. There is little activity against Gram-negative bacteria

Resistance

This occurs by modification of the ribosomal binding site.

Pharmacokinetics

The streptogramins are given intravenously; their metabolism is complex and several active metabolites are formed by cytochrome P450 enzymes. The main route of elimination is faecal. The half-lives of both quinupristin and dalfopristin are very short.

Unwanted effects

- nausea, vomiting, diarrhoea
- headache
- arthralgia, myalgia
- injection site reactions
- hepatitis

- prolongation of the Q–T interval on the ECG, with a risk of ventricular arrhythmias (Ch. 8).

Oxazolidinones

Example: linezolid

Mechanisms of action

The oxazolidinones are active against non-replicating bacteria. They have a unique mechanism of action, inhibiting protein synthesis through binding to the ribosomal 50S subunit and preventing initiation of tRNA transcription.

Spectrum of activity

Linezolid is active against a range of Gram-positive organisms, including MRSA and also vancomycin-resistant *Enterococcus faecium*.

Resistance

Resistance is due to mutation leading to modification of the ribosomal target for the drug. This can develop with prolonged treatment, or with inadequate doses.

Pharmacokinetics

Linezolid is well absorbed orally. It is mainly metabolised in the liver, but one-third is excreted by the kidney. Linezolid has a short half-life.

Unwanted effects

- headache
- nausea, vomiting, taste disturbances, diarrhoea.

Agents affecting bacterial metabolism

Sulphonamides

Examples: sulfadiazine, sulfamethoxazole

The global therapeutic importance of the sulphonamides has diminished because of the spread of resistance, and there are now only a few situations (nonetheless important) in which they are first-choice drugs. Sulfamethoxazole is only used in combination with trimethoprim, as co-trimoxazole (see below).

Mechanism of action

Unlike humans, bacteria cannot utilise pre-formed folate, a nutrient that is essential for cell growth and is used to manufacture purines for incorporation into DNA. Bacteria must synthesise folate from para-aminobenzoic acid (PABA). Sulphonamides are structurally similar to

The Folic Acid Pathway:

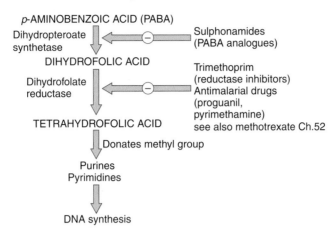

Fig. 51.4
Mechanism of action of the sulphonamides, trimethoprim and antimalarial drugs in the folic acid pathway.

PABA and inhibit the enzyme dihydropteroate synthetase in the synthetic pathway for folic acid (Fig. 51.4).

Spectrum of activity
Sulphonamides have a bacteriostatic action against a wide range of Gram-positive and Gram-negative bacteria and are also active against *Toxoplasma*, *Chlamydia* and *Nocardia* species. Because of the frequency of resistance, sulphonamides are given as sole therapy only for the treatment of nocardiosis or toxoplasmosis.

Resistance
Resistance is common and occurs through production of a mutated dihydropteroate synthetase that has reduced affinity for binding of sulphonamides (Figs 51.2 and 51.4). Resistance is transmitted among Gram-negative bacteria by plasmids. Resistance in *Staphylococcus aureus* occurs as a result of excessive synthesis of PABA. Some resistant bacteria have reduced uptake of sulphonamides.

Pharmacokinetics
Sulphonamides are well absorbed orally; a parenteral preparation of sulfadiazine is available. They are widely distributed in the body and cross the blood–brain barrier and placenta.

Sulphonamides are metabolised in the liver, initially by acetylation, which shows genetic polymorphism (Ch. 2). The acetylated product has no antibacterial action but retains toxic potential. Substantial amounts of parent drug and *N*-acetyl metabolite are excreted by the kidney. Most sulphonamides have intermediate half-lives.

Unwanted effects

- nausea and vomiting
- rashes, including toxic epidermal necrolysis and Stevens–Johnson syndrome
- haemolysis in people with glucose 6-phosphate dehydrogenase deficiency (Chs 47, 53)
- neutropenia, thrombocytopenia
- sulphonamides should not be used in the last trimester of pregnancy or in neonates, because the drug competes for bilirubin-binding sites on albumin; this can raise the concentration of unconjugated bilirubin and increases the risk of kernicterus.

Trimethoprim

Trimethoprim can be combined with the sulphonamide sulfamethoxazole, as co-trimoxazole.

Mechanism of action
Trimethoprim inhibits dihydrofolate reductase, which converts dihydrofolate to tetrahydrofolate (Fig. 51.4). The bacterial enzyme is inhibited at much lower concentrations than its mammalian counterpart. The combination of trimethoprim with sulfamethoxazole (co-trimoxazole) acts synergistically to prevent folate synthesis by bacteria. However, resistance to the sulfamethoxazole component, and the incidence of unwanted effects, limit the value of this combination.

Spectrum of activity
Trimethoprim has wide-spectrum bacteriostatic activity against Gram-positive and Gram-negative bacteria. The combination with sulfamethoxazole is also effective against the protozoan *Pneumocystis carinii*, which causes pneumonia in patients with acquired immunodeficiency syndrome (AIDS), and this is now its major indication (see below). In many urinary and respiratory tract infections, trimethoprim alone gives results similar to the combination with sulfamethoxazole.

Resistance

Resistance to trimethoprim occurs in a variety of ways, including the production of mutated dihydrofolate reductases insensitive to trimethoprim.

Pharmacokinetics

Trimethoprim is well absorbed from the gut. Most is excreted unchanged by the kidney and it has an intermediate half-life. Both trimethoprim and co-trimoxazole are available for intravenous use.

Unwanted effects

- nausea, vomiting and diarrhoea, which are usually mild
- rashes
- bone marrow depression
- folate deficiency, leading to megaloblastic changes in the bone marrow, is rare, except in people with depleted folate stores.

Agents used for tuberculosis

Tuberculosis is usually treated with a multidrug regimen because of the rapid development of resistance.

Rifamycins

Examples: rifampicin rifabutin

Mechanism of action and spectrum of activity

Rifamycins act by inhibition of DNA-dependent RNA polymerase and inhibit transcription in the bacterium. They have a bactericidal action. Rifampicin (rifampin) has a broad spectrum of activity and is used in the treatment of mycobacterial infections (*M. tuberculosis* and *M. leprae*), brucellosis, *Legionella* infections and serious staphylococcal infections. In tuberculosis, it is considered an essential drug in the UK. Rifabutin is also used for prophylaxis against *Mycobacterium avium* complex infection, most commonly occurring in people who are infected with HIV.

Resistance

Resistance develops rapidly, which limits the wider use of rifampicin as an antibacterial agent apart from the treatment of tuberculosis. It is acquired by a one-step genetic mutation of the DNA-dependent RNA polymerase.

Pharmacokinetics

Oral absorption is good, and an intravenous formulation of rifampicin is also available. Rifampicin is metabolised in the liver and has a short half-life, although it undergoes some enterohepatic cycling. Rifabutin is also metabolised in the liver and has a very long half-life.

Unwanted effects

- nausea and anorexia
- pseudomembranous colitis with rifampicin
- hepatotoxicity, usually only producing a transient rise in plasma transaminases; regular monitoring is recommended
- orange coloration of tears, sweat, urine;
- various 'toxicity syndromes' occur, commonly with intermittent use, owing to sensitisation; they include renal failure, a shock-like syndrome and acute haemolytic anaemia
- drug interactions: induction of drug-metabolising enzymes in the liver (Ch. 2) can reduce the levels of plasma oestrogen in those taking oral contraceptives (Ch. 45), and reduce plasma levels of phenytoin (Ch. 23), warfarin (Ch. 11) and sulphonylureas (Ch. 40).

Isoniazid

Mechanism of action

Isoniazid is an important and specific drug for the treatment of *Mycobacterium tuberculosis*. Isoniazid is a prodrug that is activated by catalase-peroxidase activity within susceptible cells. Isoniazid acts on enzymes in the cell to inhibit synthesis of long-chain mycolic acids, which are unique to the cell wall of *Mycobacteria* species. It is bactericidal against dividing organisms, but bacteriostatic on resting organisms. In the UK, it is considered an essential drug for treatment of tuberculosis along with rifampicin.

Resistance

Resistance may be due to mutations in enzymes responsible for the synthesis of mycolic acid, making them less susceptible to the drug. Resistance occurs rapidly through mutation if isoniazid is used alone. It is uncommon in developed countries, but can be troublesome in developing countries.

Pharmacokinetics

Oral absorption is good but reduced by food. Isoniazid is metabolised by acetylation in the liver, which is subject to genetic polymorphism (Ch. 2). Rapid acetylators show extensive first-pass metabolism, and blood isonizaid concentrations in slow acetylators are twice those in rapid acetylators. The half-life is short, but varies according to acetylator status.

Unwanted effects

- Nausea, vomiting, constipation.
- Peripheral neuropathy with high doses. This can be prevented by prophylactic use of oral pyridoxine supplements in people at high risk, for example those with diabetes, alcoholism, chronic renal failure, malnutrition or HIV infection. Neuropathy is more common in slow acetylators.

- Hepatitis is rare, but regular monitoring with liver function tests is recommended.
- Systemic lupus erythematosus-like syndrome. Positive antinuclear antibodies are found in 20% of people during long-term treatment, but fewer develop symptoms.

Pyrazinamide

Mechanism of action
Pyrazinamide is a prodrug that acts through metabolites formed by the enzyme pyrazinamidase, which is found in *Mycobacterium tuberculosis*. The product pyrazinoic acid lowers intracellular pH, inactivates a vital enzyme in fatty acid synthesis and destroys the bacterium. It is bactericidal to semi-dormant cells.

Resistance
Resistance results from a point mutation in the gene that codes for pyrazinamidase. It develops rapidly if pyrazinamide is used as a sole treatment for tuberculosis.

Pharmacokinetics
Oral absorption is good and metabolism occurs in the liver. Pyrazinamide has a long half-life.

Unwanted effects

- hepatotoxicity: a rise in plasma bilirubin usually requires cessation of treatment; regular monitoring is recommended
- nausea and vomiting
- arthralgia
- sideroblastic anaemia.

Ethambutol

Mechanism of action
It is uncertain how ethambutol acts, but it probably functions as an arabinose analogue, and inhibits arabinosyl transferase, resulting in impaired synthesis of the cell wall of mycobacteria. Ethambutol is primarily bacteriostatic. It is effective against *Mycobacterium tuberculosis* and several other mycobacteria, including *Mycobacterium avium*, which can cause lung infections.

Resistance
Resistance may be due to gene mutations that inhibit the binding of ethambutol to its target enzyme. It develops slowly, but is common during prolonged treatment of tuberculosis if ethambutol is used alone.

Pharmacokinetics
Oral absorption is good. It is mainly eliminated unchanged by the kidney. The half-life is long.

Unwanted effects

- optic neuritis produces initial red/green colour blindness, then reduced visual acuity; it is dose-related but usually reversible
- peripheral neuritis.

Streptomycin

Streptomycin was discussed above (see aminoglycosides). It is not used in the UK as first-line treatment for tuberculosis because of its toxicity and the need for parenteral administration.

Other drugs used in the treatment of tuberculosis

Other drugs can be used as second-line treatments in multidrug-resistant tuberculosis. These include cycloserine, capreomycin, amikacin, ciprofloxacin, azithromycin, clarithromycin and para-aminosalicylic acid. Drugs used in countries other than the UK include thiacetazone and protionamide.

Agents used for leprosy

The drugs recommended for treatment of leprosy, which is caused by *Mycobacterium leprae*, are rifampicin (see above), dapsone and clofazimine.

Dapsone

Mechanism of action
Dapsone is similar to the sulphonamides and acts by inhibition of folate synthesis. It is the most active drug against *Mycobacterium leprae*.

Resistance
Resistance can develop as for sulphonamides (see above).

Pharmacokinetics
Dapsone is well absorbed from the gut, is metabolised in the liver and undergoes enterohepatic cycling. It has a long half-life.

Unwanted effects

- blood disorders: haemolysis and methaemoglobinaemia, although these are rare at the doses used for treatment of leprosy (Ch. 53)
- neuropathy
- anorexia, nausea, vomiting
- allergic dermatitis.

Clofazimine

Clofazimine is a dye that interferes with DNA and is used as a second-line drug in the event of dapsone intolerance in those with leprosy. It is a long-acting drug that tends to accumulate. Unwanted effects include gastrointestinal upset, brownish-black discoloration of the skin, and acne.

Principles of antibacterial therapy

The following guidelines outline the principles that should be considered in the choice of a safe and effective therapy.

Presumptive treatment. Most antibacterial therapy is started 'blind' without prior identification of the organism and its antibacterial drug sensitivities. Such treatment should be guided by the clinical diagnosis and a knowledge of the most common pathogenic bacteria in the current situation. Local information about patterns of antibacterial resistance should be considered.

Drug spectrum. A drug with a narrow spectrum of activity should be used in preference to a broad-spectrum drug whenever possible. Unnecessary use of broad-spectrum drugs encourages the broader development of resistant bacteria. This can present problems for the individual by the selection of resistant pathogens or overgrowth of resistant commensal micro-organisms. For the community, the selection of resistant pathogens can create problems by rendering standard antibacterial therapy less reliable. Broad-spectrum antibacterial cover is sometimes appropriate, for example in a seriously ill person when the infecting bacterium is unknown and a variety of bacteria could be causing the condition being treated.

Combination therapy. Treatment with more than one antibacterial agent should not be used routinely. It may, however, be valuable to provide broad-spectrum cover in serious illness when the organism is unknown, for example the combination of cefotaxime and metronidazole to cover aerobic and anaerobic organisms in suspected Gram-negative septicaemia. When resistance is likely to develop readily to the first-choice drug during protracted treatment, the use of combination therapy can minimise that risk, for example in the treatment of infective endocarditis or tuberculosis.

Bactericidal versus bacteriostatic drugs. In some situations, bactericidal drugs are preferred to bacteriostatic agents, for example for the treatment of infective endocarditis or when the person being treated is immunocompromised. In most other situations, the choice is probably not important.

Site of infection. This may determine the choice of drug; for example, some antibacterials only achieve low concentrations in the biliary tree, urine, bone or CSF.

Mode of administration. Oral therapy is usually preferred to parenteral treatment. Exceptions include the treatment of serious infections when reliable blood concentrations are essential, if the drug is only available in parenteral formulation, or if gastrointestinal absorption may be unreliable, for example after abdominal surgery.

Duration of therapy. This should be as short as is compatible with adequate treatment of the infection. The decision is often arbitrary, for example 7–10 days in many infections. Some infections can be effectively treated over much shorter periods; for example, courses of 1–3 days are usually adequate for lower urinary tract infections. For a few infections, long periods of treatment may be necessary to eliminate semi-dormant organisms or those in 'privileged sites' to which antibacterial drug penetration is poor. Examples include infective endocarditis, osteomyelitis and tuberculosis.

Chemoprophylaxis. The use of chemoprophylaxis to prevent infection is important in many situations. Common examples include prevention of meningococcal meningitis in close contacts of an infected person, prevention of infective endocarditis in people with diseased or artificial heart valves undergoing surgery or dental treatment, and pre-operative prophylaxis before gut, biliary, thoracic or orthopaedic surgery.

Treatment of specific bacterial infections

This section is not intended to be comprehensive. It will outline the approach to antibacterial therapy in several common bacterial infections. The choice of antibacterial agent for these infections will depend on factors such as local patterns of bacterial resistance, which make universal recommendations impossible.

Upper respiratory tract infections

Most upper respiratory tract infections are caused by viruses, producing symptoms of the common cold. Symptomatic treatment is all that should be offered, with an antihistamine (e.g. chlorpheniramine; Ch. 39) or an anticholinergic spray (e.g. ipratropium; Ch. 12) to reduce rhinorrhoea and sneezing. An α-adrenoceptor agonist given orally or nasally (e.g. xylometazoline; Ch. 4) can reduce nasal congestion, but prolonged use can provoke a rebound effect (rhinitis medicamentosa). A non-steroidal anti-inflammatory drug (NSAID; Ch. 29) can be used to reduce associated headache and malaise. Antibacterial drugs are widely prescribed for upper respiratory tract symptoms but have no benefit.

Sinusitis and otitis media

Sinusitis and otitis media accompany catarrhal conditions in childhood and frequently follow an upper respiratory tract infection. Sinusitis produces headache, facial pain, fever and purulent rhinorrhoea. A nasal decongestant such as an α-adrenoceptor agonist can be helpful, in conjunction with an analgesic. An antimicrobial is often not beneficial in acute sinusitis unless there is marked facial swelling and pain, or failure to resolve after 10–14 days. The most common infecting organisms are *Haemophilus influenzae* (which often produces β-lactamase), *Streptococcus pneumoniae* and *Moraxella catarrhalis*. Suitable antibacterial drugs include co-amoxiclav (amoxicillin plus clavulanic acid), cefuroxime axetil and erythromycin. Chronic sinusitis usually requires correction of an anatomical obstruction in the nose.

Otitis media is very common in childhood. When associated with an effusion, increased pressure in the middle ear causes pain and perforation of the eardrum. The organisms responsible are similar to those causing acute sinusitis. In more than 80% of children, the condition is self-limiting over 2–3 days without treatment. An antibacterial should be used for protracted episodes of otitis media. Surgery is occasionally necessary for recurrent infections.

Lower respiratory tract infection

Acute bronchitis

This is recent, often productive, cough without evidence of pneumonia. It is usually caused by a viral infection, which often takes 2–4 weeks to resolve without treatment. Antibacterial treatment is inappropriate and does not alter the course of the illness: even if there is an underlying risk factor for bacterial infection, such as chronic obstructive airways disease, the evidence for benefit of antibacterial drugs is negligible. In such cases, *Streptococcus pneumoniae* (pneumococcus), *Haemophilus influenzae* or *Moraxella catarrhalis* are commonly found in the sputum, but are often isolated in remissions as well. If an antibacterial drug is used, then amoxicillin, co-amoxiclav or erythromycin will be effective against the most likely pathogens. Quinolones other than ciprofloxacin (which is poorly active against pneumococci) are an alternative.

Pneumonia

Primary community-acquired pneumonia is most commonly caused by *Streptococcus pneumoniae*, followed by *Haemophilus influenzae* and staphylococci. 'Atypical' micro-organisms can also cause pneumonia, such as *Mycoplasma pneumoniae* or *Chlamydia pneumoniae*. *Legionella* species are sometimes also considered in this category. Appropriate antibacterial treatment will be dictated by the most likely infecting agent.

If pneumococcus is suspected, amoxicillin is the treatment of choice. For people who are penicillin-sensitive, erythromycin will cover most likely micro-organisms, including 'atypical' micro-organisms. For community-acquired pneumonia requiring admission of the person to hospital, oral amoxicillin combined with erythromycin is often used, or intravenous ampicillin or benzylpenicillin combined with intravenous clarithromycin. Severe community-acquired pneumonia is treated with intravenous therapy comprising a β–lactamase-resistant antimicrobial such as co-amoxiclav or cefuroxime, with intravenous clarithromycin. A fluoroquinolone with activity against pneumococci, such as levofloxacin, would be an alternative choice. Adjunctive treatment of pneumonia may include supplemental oxygen via a facemask, pain relief for pleurisy, and ensuring adequate hydration.

Secondary pneumonias occur in patients with other concurrent diseases, often during a stay in hospital (nosocomial or hospital-acquired pneumonia). A wide range of pathogens may be involved and parenteral drug treatment is usually necessary. A cephalosporin, such as cefotaxime, or an anti-pseudomonal penicillin (e.g. azlocillin) is usually used. An aminoglycoside is added if the infection is severe.

Pneumocystis carinii pneumonia

Pneumonia caused by *P. carinii* in people with AIDS is treated with high doses of co-trimoxazole as the first-line treatment. Some individuals have adverse reactions to co-trimoxazole, or it is ineffective. Second-line drugs that can be given include pentamidine, atovaquone and trimetrexate (see drugs for protozoal infections, p. 611).

Chronic lung sepsis

This encompasses lung abscess, bronchiectasis and empyema. The pathogens in lung abscesses vary according to the immune status of the individual. Ideally, the antibacterial treatment should be directed by isolation and sensitivity testing of the bacteria. Bronchiectasis is most frequently associated with colonisation by *Haemophilus influenzae*, followed by *Pseudomonas* species, then *Streptococcus pneumoniae*. A fluoroquinolone such as levofloxacin is a reasonable empirical treatment choice. Empyema requires drainage, and then specific antibacterial therapy directed at the cultured pathogen.

Urinary tract infections

Urinary tract infections are more common in women than men, because of their shorter urethra. Infections can occur in structurally normal urinary tracts or in association with a structural genitourinary abnormality that impairs drainage of urine or acts as a focus for infection, such as a stone in the urinary tract. An indwelling urinary catheter is often associated with bacterial colonisation of the urine that is almost impossible to eradicate.

The most frequent bacterial cause of urinary tract infection is *Escherichia coli*. Hospital-acquired infections are often caused by *Klebsiella*, *Enterobacter* and *Serratia* species or by *Pseudomonas aeruginosa*, because these organisms can be selected as resistant bacteria following antibacterial usage. *Proteus mirabilis* is often found if there are stones in the urinary tract. Less commonly, staphylococci, especially *Staphylococcus saprophyticus*, are responsible.

Uncomplicated urinary tract infection is confined to the bladder (cystitis) and can be treated by short courses

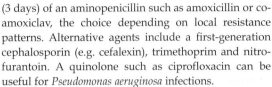

(3 days) of an aminopenicillin such as amoxicillin or co-amoxiclav, the choice depending on local resistance patterns. Alternative agents include a first-generation cephalosporin (e.g. cefalexin), trimethoprim and nitrofurantoin. A quinolone such as ciprofloxacin can be useful for *Pseudomonas aeruginosa* infections.

Complicated urinary tract infections also involve the kidney (pyelonephritis), or the prostate in males, and require longer courses of treatment. For pyelonephritis, initial intravenous therapy is usually started with broad-spectrum agents such as aztreonam, ciprofloxacin or cefuroxime; treatment is usually continued for 14 days. If there is associated prostatitis, oral treatment with trimethoprim or ciprofloxacin for at least 4 weeks is recommended.

If infection occurs with an indwelling urinary catheter, then treatment is only recommended if there are systemic symptoms of infection, for example fever or rigors.

Long-term antibacterial prophylaxis against urinary tract infections may be necessary to prevent recurrent infection if there are underlying urinary tract abnormalities. Suitable agents, usually given at low dosage, include trimethoprim, nitrofurantoin and cefalexin.

Gastrointestinal infection

Gastroenteritis (a syndrome that includes nausea, vomiting, diarrhoea and abdominal discomfort) can result from ingestion of bacterial pathogens. Severe disease of the large intestine can cause dysentery, an inflammatory disorder often associated with fever, abdominal pain, and blood and pus in the faeces.

'Food poisoning' of bacterial origin can occur from ingestion of a pre-formed bacterial toxin (e.g. from *Clostridium botulinum* or *Staphylococcus aureus*), with onset of symptoms usually within hours, or it can be caused by ingested bacteria in the bowel (e.g. *Campylobacter* or *Salmonella* species).

The most common cause of bacterial diarrhoea (especially in children in developing countries) is *Escherichia coli*, which produces powerful enterotoxins. In other circumstances, *Salmonella* species, *Campylobacter* species, *Vibrio cholerae*, *Shigella* species or various other organisms are responsible. However, in the UK, diarrhoea in adults is usually caused by viruses and is self-limiting.

If diarrhoea is severe, fluid replacement is often necessary. Antimicrobial treatment is not usually recommended even if bacterial infection is suspected, unless there are systemic symptoms such as fever, rigors and hypotension. Ciprofloxacin or erythromycin can be useful for *Campylobacter* enteritis. Salmonella infections or shigellosis can be treated with ciprofloxacin or trimethoprim, unless *Salmonella typhi* is suspected, when ciprofloxacin, cefotaxime or chloramphenicol is used.

Antibacterial agents can themselves cause diarrhoea (antibiotic-associated diarrhoea), which usually resolves

rapidly when the drug is withdrawn. However, if it is complicated by *Clostridium difficile* infection or pseudomembranous colitis, then oral metronidazole or oral vancomycin can be used.

Biliary tract infection

Acute cholecystitis and cholangitis are often caused by *Escherischia coli* and most often occur if there is biliary obstruction. Supportive treatment with fluid and electrolytic replacement is usually required. Antibacterial therapy with a cephalosporin or gentamicin is usually effective. Combination therapy with both agents is recommended if the infection is severe; alternatively, a ureidopenicillin such as piperacillin can be given alone. Treatment is usually given for 7–10 days.

Osteomyelitis

Infection of bone produces necrotic tissue and generates an avascular privileged site for bacteria that antibacterial drugs penetrate to only a limited extent. Organisms involved include *Staphylococcus aureus*, which adheres readily to bone matrix, various streptococci, *Serratia* species, *Pseudomonas aeruginosa* and enteric Gram-negative rods.

Early antibacterial treatment is essential, with intravenous therapy for 6 weeks to achieve a cure. Surgical intervention may be necessary to remove necrotic tissue. The choice of drug depends on the suspected organisms. First-line treatment is often with clindamycin or flucloxacillin, combined with fusidic acid if a prosthesis is present or the infection is severe. If *Haemophilus influenzae* is identified, then amoxicillin or cefuroxime is usually used. Acute infections are treated for 4–6 weeks, but chronic infections for at least 12 weeks. If long-term therapy is necessary for chronic refractory osteomyelitis, then an oral quinolone such as ciprofloxacin can be substituted.

Septic arthritis

The standard treatment is with flucloxacillin together with fusidic acid or rifampicin. For people who are penicillin-allergic, then clindamycin is used alone. Vancomycin is used for MRSA, combined with fusidic acid or rifampicin if a prosthesis is present or the infection is severe. Treatment should be continued for 6–12 weeks.

Cellulitis

This usually complicates a wound, ulcer or dermatosis. In most cases, the infecting organism is *Staphylococcus aureus* or streptococci. Treatment should be given with β-lactam antimicrobials that are active against β-lactamase-producing *Staphylococcus aureus*. Benzylpenicillin (or phenoxymethylpenicillin for oral use) with flucloxacillin is normally used. Erythromycin is used alone for people who are penicillin-allergic.

Septicaemia

Septicaemia is a bacterial infection involving the bloodstream and can present with fever, or, if more severe, can result in circulatory collapse, hypotension and shock. This is a medical emergency requiring intensive fluid replacement, plasma volume expansion and electrolyte correction. There have been many advances in our understanding of the pathogenesis of sepsis and the associated immune activation. A recent adjunctive therapy for severe sepsis is with recombinant activated protein C, an anticoagulant. This agent blocks the interaction between the coagulation system and the inflammatory cascade. Its use is usually restricted to those with sepsis and severe organ compromise.

If the source of infection is not clinically apparent, then empirical antibacterial therapy is given to cover as wide a range of potential infecting organisms as possible. Suitable treatment would be with an aminoglycoside such as gentamicin combined with a broad-spectrum penicillin (e.g. amoxicillin) or a broad-spectrum cephalosporin (e.g. cefotaxime, or ceftazidime if *Pseudomonas* infection is suspected). Alternatively, a carbapenem such as meropenem or imipenem with cilastin can be used alone. If anaerobic infection is suspected, then metronidazole is added.

Immunocompromised individuals are at particularly high risk from septicaemia. A combination of gentamicin with a broad-spectrum penicillin or cephalosporin could be given in this situation. Other authorities recommend gentamicin combined with either piperacillin (plus tazobactam) or with meropenem. If anaerobic infection is suspected, then metronidazole is usually added; flucloxacillin or vancomycin is added if Gram-positive infection is suspected. Failure to respond to such triple therapy may indicate a fungal infection, for which amphotericin can be added (see below).

Infective endocarditis

The majority of cases of infective endocarditis are caused by bacterial pathogens, most commonly oral streptococci, followed by enterococci, *Staphylococcus aureus* and coagulase-negative staphylococci. Endocarditis usually arises on the endothelial surface of a pre-existing heart defect (e.g. valvular heart defect, ventricular septal defect) or on a prosthetic heart valve. It arises when micro-organisms enter the bloodstream and become established on the endocardium, where they may adhere to pre-existing fibrin–platelet vegetations. Bacteria enter the blood during dental procedures, vigorous teeth cleaning or during some surgical procedures.

Untreated infection can destroy the infected heart valve and produce severe haemodynamic disturbance. Systemic complications can also arise from embolisation of vegetation from the valve, from bacteraemia or through immune complexes that form in response to the infection.

When infection is suspected, treatment should be started and blood cultures taken. Prior to identification of the organism, treatment is usually started with intravenous benzylpenicillin combined with low-dose gentamicin. If the organism is sensitive to penicillin, then the benzylpenicillin is continued for 4 weeks and the gentamicin stopped after 2 weeks. Vancomycin is substituted for benzylpenicillin in individuals with penicillin-allergy. If renal function is impaired, then ceftriaxone is often used as single therapy. For staphylococcal endocarditis, flucloxacillin is given in combination with either gentamicin or fusidic acid; for people who are penicillin-allergic, vancomycin is used alone.

Antibacterial prophylaxis prior to dental treatment or certain surgical or other procedures is extremely important for individuals with a cardiac lesion that places them at risk of endocarditis. A single large dose of amoxicillin should be given immediately before the procedure, or clindamycin if the individual is allergic to penicillin or has taken penicillin in the previous month. For high-risk individuals (e.g. with a prosthetic valve or previous endocarditis), amoxicillin is combined with gentamicin, and a second dose of amoxicillin is given after the procedure.

Meningitis

Bacterial meningitis is a medical emergency. The most likely organism depends on the age of the person (Table 51.3). Empirical selection of therapy is usually necessary, and treatment should be started at the first suspicion of bacterial meningitis. A single dose of benzylpenicillin can be given if the person is outside hospital, but cefotaxime is the preferred treatment in hospital. Chloramphenicol is an option for individuals who have an allergy to both penicillin and cephalosporins. Treatment is given for 5 days for meningococcus, and 10 days for *Haemophilus influenzae* or pneumococcus.

Table 51.3
Organisms causing bacterial meningitis

Age	Organism
<1 month	Group B streptococci
1 month to 4 years	*Haemophilus influenzae*
>4 years to young adult	*Neisseria meningitidis* (meningococcus)
Older adults	*Streptococcus pneumoniae* (pneumococcus)

If the meningitis was caused by meningococcus or *Haemophilus influenzae*, rifampicin is given for 2–4 days before hospital discharge. Close contacts of subjects with meningococcal or *Haemophilus influenzae* meningitis are usually given rifampicin as prophylaxis against infection.

Tuberculosis

Mycobacterium tuberculosis readily develops resistance to single-drug therapy. Three or four drugs are used in the 'initial phase' for the first 2 months to rapidly reduce the bacterial population until bacterial sensitivities are known, when treatment is continued with two drugs for a further 6 months ('continuation phase') to achieve a cure. In some cases, more prolonged treatment may be necessary, especially for tuberculous meningitis or for resistant mycobacteria. A standard regimen in the UK includes rifampicin, isoniazid and pyrazinamide for 2 months (or until bacterial sensitivities are known), followed by rifampicin and isoniazid for a further 4 months. Ethambutol is added as a fourth drug if there is an increased risk of resistance to isoniazid (e.g. after previous treatment for tuberculosis, immunosuppression, contact with drug-resistant myobacteria). Ethambutol is not used for treatment of young children because of difficulty in monitoring for eye toxicity.

Streptomycin is used in some countries in the initial phase of treatment. In countries that cannot afford rifampicin, thiacetazone is often used with isoniazid and initially streptomycin. Compliance can be a major problem in the treatment of tuberculosis, and combination tablets are often used to maximise this. In developed countries, directly observed treatment (DOT) has been instituted to improve compliance. This can result in major improvements in eradication rates.

Fungal infections

Fungi usually infect skin or superficial mucous membranes, but can, more rarely, involve internal organs. Most fungal infections occur because of an underlying defect in host resistance. Fungi grow readily in immunosuppressed individuals or following the suppression of normal flora with antibacterials. Treatment with general measures such as good hygiene and avoidance of sources of infection is an important complement to the use of antifungal agents.

Compared with antibacterial drugs, fewer agents have been developed that have activity against fungi, and many of these are toxic to humans. A simplified outline of the ways in which antifungal drugs work is shown in Figure 51.5.

Antifungal agents

Polyene antifungal agents

Examples: nystatin, amphotericin

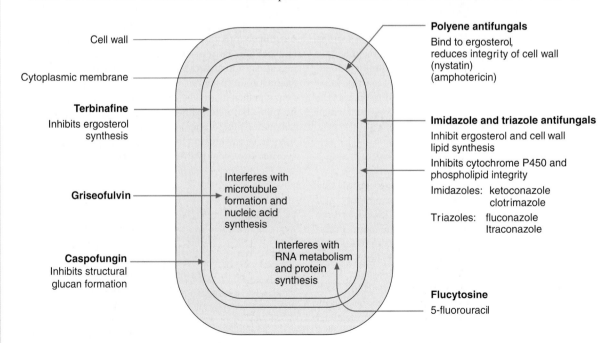

Fig. 51.5
Sites at which antifungal drugs exert their actions on fungi.

Mechanism of action

Polyenes bind to ergosterol in the cell wall of fungi and form aqueous pores that promote leakage of intracellular ions and disruption of membrane active transport mechanisms. They can be fungistatic or fungicidal.

Spectrum of activity

Nystatin is particularly effective against infections with *Candida* species. Amphotericin is active against all common fungi that cause systemic infection (*Candida*, *Aspergillus*, *Mucor* and *Cryptococcus* species).

Resistance

Acquired resistance is rare but can occur in immuno-suppressed people. Moulds and yeasts develop a mutation that permits synthesis of the cell membrane without using ergosterol.

Pharmacokinetics

Nystatin is too toxic for systemic use and is not absorbed from the gastrointestinal tract. It is therefore used topically, for example as cream for skin infection or as vaginal pessaries, or orally for buccal and bowel infections.

Amphotericin is poorly absorbed from the gut and is usually given intravenously for treatment of serious systemic fungal infections. An oral formulation is used for buccal and intestinal candidiasis. Amphotericin can also be given intrathecally for fungal meningitis. Amphotericin binds to steroid molecules in human tissue, and is released slowly and eliminated via the biliary tract and kidney. It has a very long half-life. Lipid delivery vehicles for amphotericin have been developed to reduce its nephrotoxicity. These formulations alter drug distribution and help to concentrate it at the site of infection. Formulations include liposomal spheres in which the drug is dissolved (phospholipid membrane vesicles), lipid complexes in which the lipid exists in ribbons interspersed with amphotericin, and a colloidal dispersion of lipid discs that incorporate the drug. The lipid component is probably cleared from the blood by mononuclear phagocytes.

Unwanted effects

Nystatin is virtually free of both toxic and allergic unwanted effects when used topically. Used orally for intestinal infection, it can cause gastrointestinal upset. Host toxicity with amphotericin is due to binding to cholesterol rather than ergosterol. Intravenous infusion of amphotericin is commonly associated with:

- fever and rigors during the first week of therapy
- anorexia, nausea, vomiting, diarrhoea
- muscle and joint pain
- dose-related nephrotoxicity, which is the major limiting factor in treatment; it presents with reduced glomerular filtration rate and produces hypokalaemia

and hypomagnesaemia through tubular leakage of K^+ and Mg^{2+}; lipid formulations substantially reduce the risk of nephrotoxicity and are particularly useful to treat people with pre-existing renal impairment.

Imidazoles

Examples: clotrimazole, ketoconazole, miconazole

Mechanism of action

The imidazoles alter the cell membrane fluidity of fungi by inhibiting lanosterol 14α-demethylase, which participates in the conversion of lanosterol to ergosterol. This alters cell membrane synthesis, reduces the activity of membrane-associated enzymes and increases cell wall permeability. Accumulation of ergosterol precursors in the cell causes growth arrest. The enzyme inhibited is a form of cytochrome P450. Although the human equivalent enzyme is much less sensitive to the effects of the drug, inhibition of cytochrome P450 enzymes can occur in human tissues, especially with ketoconazole.

Spectrum of activity

The imidazoles are active against a wide variety of filamentous fungi and yeasts, including *Candida* species. They are less active against *Candida krusei*. Clotrimazole and miconazole are used for vaginal candidiasis and for dermatophyte infections (e.g. ringworm [tinea]; causative species vary geographically, but generally are *Trichophyton*, *Microsporon* or *Epidermophyton* species). Miconazole is also used to treat oral and intestinal fungal infections. Ketoconazole can be used for systemic mycoses, resistant mucocutaneous candidiasis, resistant vaginal candidiasis and resistant dermatophyte infections.

Resistance

The development of resistance is rare, except during long-term use in people with AIDS. The mechanism involves a point mutation in the target enzyme, or development of an active pump that removes drug from the cell, especially in *Candida* species.

Pharmacokinetics

Absorption of imidazoles from the gastrointestinal tract is poor, and only ketoconazole achieves blood concentrations that are high enough to treat systemic infection. Clotrimazole is only used in topical formulations for superficial infections, for example skin and vagina. The imidazoles are metabolised in the liver; ketoconazole has an intermediate half-life.

Unwanted effects

These are unusual with topical formulations, although oral miconazole can cause gastrointestinal upset. Oral ketoconazole causes:

- nausea, vomiting, abdominal pain
- rash, urticaria, pruritis
- hepatitis: asymptomatic elevation of liver enzymes is common; more severe hepatic reactions are unusual but can be fatal; liver function tests must be monitored during systemic use of ketoconazole
- high doses of ketoconazole suppress androgen production in males and can cause oligospermia or gynaecomastia
- drug interactions: ketoconazole can inhibit metabolism of drugs that are eliminated by cytochrome P450; examples include ciclosporin, tacrolimus (Ch. 38) and warfarin (Ch. 11); if co-prescribed with terfenadine (Ch. 39), the increase in plasma terfenadine concentration can lead to ventricular arrhythmias through prolongation of the Q–T interval on the ECG (Ch. 8).

Triazoles

> Examples: fluconazole, itraconazole, voriconazole
>
>

The triazoles have a similar mechanism of action and spectrum of activity to the imidazoles (see above). Fluconazole is used for candidiasis or for cryptococcal infection. Itraconazole is used for mucocutaneous candidiasis and for dermatophyte infections such as pityriasis versicolor (caused by an organism known as *Malassezia furfur* or *Pityriasis orbiculare*) and tinea corporis or pedis (ringworms). Voriconazole is used for invasive aspergillosis, serious infections caused by *Scedosporium* species, *Fusarium* species, or invasive fluconazole-resistant *Candida krusei*.

Pharmacokinetics

Oral absorption is good. Intravenous (fluconazole, voriconazole) and topical (itraconazole) formulations are also available. The triazoles are metabolised in the liver and have very long half-lives. Fluconazole penetrates well into CSF, which is useful for treatment of fungal meningitis.

Unwanted effects

- nausea, abdominal pain and diarrhoea
- headache, dizziness
- abnormalities of liver function and, occasionally, hepatitis or cholestasis. These are more common during prolonged treatment with itraconazole; monitoring of liver function tests during systemic treatment is essential
- rashes, including Stevens–Johnson syndrome.

Terbinafine

Mechanism of action

Terbinafine is an allylamine that inhibits squalene epoxidase, an enzyme that converts squalene to ergosterol in the cell wall, and consequently, cell wall synthesis is impaired; the intracellular accumulation of squalene is probably cytotoxic (Fig. 51.5).

Resistance

Resistance is rare, but similar to that for imidazole antifungals.

Pharmacokinetics

Terbinafine penetrates well into the stratum corneum and hair follicles after topical use. After oral administration, it is metabolised in the liver and has a long half-life.

Unwanted effects

Unwanted effects are unlikely with topical use of the drug.

- nausea, taste disturbance, abdominal discomfort and diarrhoea
- headache
- rashes, which are occasionally severe.

Caspofungin

Mechanism of action

This drug inhibits fungal cell wall synthesis, targeting the glucans that are found in fungal but not human cell walls (Fig. 51.5). Caspofungin inhibits the enzyme β1,3-glucan synthase, and prevents production of the main structural polymer in the fungal cell wall. It is used to treat invasive aspergillosis as a second-line agent, and invasive candidiasis.

Resistance

This is uncommon at present, but can occur from a point gene mutation coding for a structural change in the enzyme, which no longer binds the drug.

Pharmacokinetics

Caspofungin is only given by intravenous infusion. It is metabolised in the liver and has a long half-life.

Unwanted effects

- nausea, vomiting, abdominal pain, diarrhoea
- flushing, fever
- headache
- rashes.

Flucytosine

Mechanism of action

Flucytosine is converted to 5-fluorouracil (5-FU) selectively in fungal cells by the enzyme cytosine deaminase. This acts as an antimetabolite that competes with uracil for incorporation into fungal RNA. 5-FU is metabolised to compounds that inhibit enzymes involved in DNA synthesis (Fig. 51.5).

Flucytosine is only active against yeasts such as *Candida, Aspergillus* and *Cryptococcus* species. It is used for systemic infections.

Resistance

Resistance occurs readily and arises through a mutation that produces a deficiency of the enzyme which metabolises flucytosine or through excessive synthesis of uracil, which competes with the antimetabolite. For this reason, flucytosine is only used in combination with amphotericin or fluconazole.

Pharmacokinetics

Flucytosine is only available for intravenous use. It is mainly eliminated unchanged in the urine and has a short half-life.

Unwanted effects

- nausea, abdominal pain and diarrhoea
- rashes
- high concentrations produce reversible bone marrow depression.

Griseofulvin

Mechanism of action

Griseofulvin inhibits dermatophyte mitosis by impairing the polymerisation of microtubule protein. It is active against dermatophytes such as *Microsporum, Epidermophyton* and *Trichophyton* species (Fig. 51.5).

Resistance

Resistance has not been shown.

Pharmacokinetics

Griseofulvin is well absorbed from the gut and is selectively concentrated in skin and nail beds; only low concentrations are found in plasma. Elimination is by metabolism in the liver and the half-life is long.

Unwanted effects

- nausea, vomiting
- headache, dizziness, fatigue
- rashes, including photosensitivity.

Treatment of some specific fungal infections

Aspergillosis

This is an invasive fungal infection that most commonly affects the lung. However, in immunocompromised individuals, it can invade more widely and infect the heart, brain, sinuses and skin. The treatment of choice is amphotericin. If this fails, then itraconazole or voriconazole can be used. Caspofungin is reserved for infections that have failed to respond to standard treatments, or for those persons who cannot tolerate the other drugs.

Candidiasis

For oral candidiasis, amphotericin or nystatin is often used. If there is oropharyngeal disease that is refractory to topical treatment, then an absorbed drug such as fluconazole or itraconazole is used. Vulvovaginal infection is treated with cream and pessaries, and imidazole drugs, such as clotrimazole, are usually the first choice. Nystatin is an alternative for vulvovaginal candidiasis, but stains clothing yellow. For recurrent vulvovaginal infections, intermittent oral fluconazole or itraconazole should be taken for 6 months. Superficial candidal infections of the skin are treated topically with cream, usually containing an imidazole. Terbinafine or nystatin can also be used topically.

Cryptococcus

Infection usually occurs in people who are immunocompromised. It can cause life-threatening meningitis, and is treated with intravenous amphotericin. Fluconazole is an alternative, and can be given orally for prophylaxis against relapse.

Skin and nail infections

Topical therapy is usually suitable for infections with most dermatophytes. Ringworm infection of the scalp (tinea capitis), body (tinea corporis), groin (tinea cruris), hand (tinea manuum), foot (tinea pedis) or nail (tinea unguium) will respond to most azoles. Griseofulvin is usually reserved for treatment of scalp infections. Nail infection usually requires systemic treatment, with terbinafine or itraconazole.

Pityriasis versicolor can be treated topically or orally wth itraconazole, or with oral fluconazole.

Prophylaxis in immunocompromised individuals

People who are immunocompromised are at greater risk of fungal infection. Prophylaxis is often given with oral fluconazole, since this has better oral absorption than most azoles, and is less toxic than ketoconazole.

Viral infections

Viruses are small infective particles consisting of either DNA or RNA, inside a protein coating (capsule), which

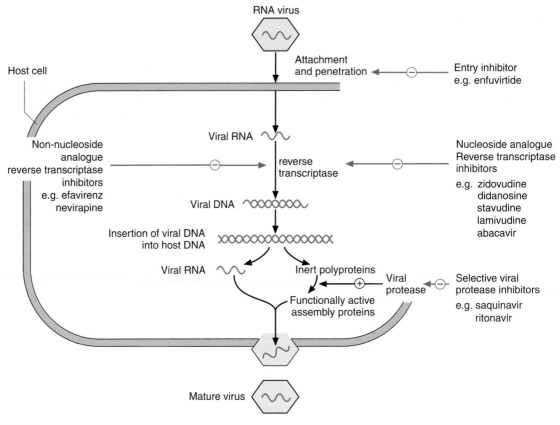

Fig. 51.6
Principles of RNA virus replication and sites of action of antiviral drugs. For details, see text.

in some viruses may be further surrounded by a lipo-protein coating. The proteins can have antigenic pro-perties. Viruses lack any inherent metabolic machinery and must attach parasitically to and enter host cells in order to survive and replicate. To do this, some viruses produce enzymes to facilitate their own replication, and in the process they can acquire phospholipids of host cell origin. Viruses access host cells after binding to recognition sites that are endogenous receptors for normal cellular constituents, for example adrenoceptors, cytokine receptors, etc.

The host will normally eliminate the virus by killing the infected cell. Cytotoxic T-lymphocytes recognise the viral surface proteins that are expressed by infected cells. The host can also produce antibodies that bind to and inactivate virus particles extracellularly. Vaccination is designed to mimic this approach.

Since viruses share many of the host's metabolic processes, this makes it difficult to damage the virus without damaging the host. Importantly, antiviral drugs are only effective while the virus is replicating, so the

earlier they are given in the course of the infection the more likely they are to work. An outline of the repli-cation of RNA and DNA viruses is shown in Figures 51.6 and 51.7. Since the replicative mechanisms involved may be distinctive to one type of virus, some antiviral drugs are specific for one or another class of virus.

New antiviral drugs are being introduced into clinical practice at an increasing rate. Currently, drugs are available to treat infection by RNA viruses (e.g. HIV and influenza viruses) and DNA viruses (e.g. herpes viruses, cytomegalovirus [CMV] and hepatitis viruses).

Resistance to antiviral drugs occurs readily. This relates to the high rate of natural occurrence of mutations in the viral genome and production of quasi-species of the virus. Viral polymerases have a high inherent error rate (especially RNA viruses) and viruses tolerate a large number of nucleoside mutations without losing their infectivity. Normally, the large variety of viral quasi-species will be dominated by the variant most selected for survival. However, use of an antiviral drug will select for growth of resistant variants.

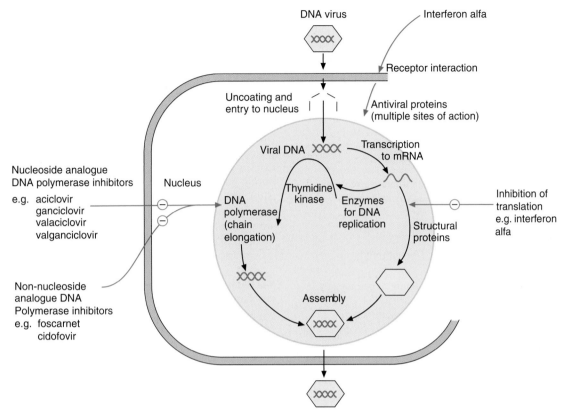

Fig. 51.7
Principles of DNA virus replication and sites of actions of antiviral drugs. For details, see text.

Antiviral agents

HIV reverse transcriptase inhibitors

The reverse transcriptase inhibitors are active against the RNA virus HIV. They prevent viral RNA being transcribed as viral DNA in the host cell (Fig. 51.6).

Nucleoside analogue HIV reverse transcriptase inhibitors

Examples: abacavir, didanosine, lamivudine, stavudine, zidovudine

Mechanism of action
The HIV reverse transcriptase inhibitor drugs (Fig. 51.6) are activated by intraviral phosphorylation to the 5'-triphosphate form. The nucleoside reverse transcriptase inhibitors are analogues of precursors of the natural purines and pyrimidines involved in DNA transcription

initiated by the virus. Zidovudine and stavudine are analogues of thymidine, one of the constituents of the base pairs in DNA (Fig. 51.6). Didanosine is an analogue of deoxyadenosine, lamivudine is an analogue of cytidine, and abacavir an analogue of deoxyguanosine.

These drugs inhibit RNA viral replication by reversible inhibition of the viral enzyme HIV reverse transcriptase, which generates viral DNA for insertion into the host DNA sequence. The inhibition is achieved by competitive binding of the activated drug to the enzyme–template–primer complex in place of the natural 5'-deoxynucleoside triphosphates, thus terminating further DNA chain elongation.

Mechanisms of resistance
Resistant quasi-species emerge rapidly, within weeks or months, through mutation of the drug-binding site on the transcriptase enzyme that increases the affinity for natural substrate compared with the drug. Because of rapid development of resistance, multiple drug therapy is used for treatment.

Pharmacokinetics
These drugs are almost completely absorbed from the gut. Elimination of abacavir, didanosine and zidovudine

is by hepatic metabolism and the half-lives are short. Stavudine is mainly eliminated unchanged by the kidney; lamivudine is largely excreted unchanged by the kidney but its full metabolic fate is not well characterised. Both have short half-lives.

Unwanted effects

These are often severe enough to prompt withdrawal of therapy. The mechanism is believed to be related to inhibition of mitochondrial enzymes, with impaired generation of adenosine triphosphate (ATP).

- neutropenia and anaemia are the most frequent unwanted effects (usually occurring in those with advanced AIDS)
- nausea, vomiting, diarrhoea
- headache, insomnia
- myalgia or myositis, especially with high doses
- severe potentially life-threatening hepatomegaly with steatosis and lactic acidosis
- peripheral neuropathy and pancreatitis are particular problems with zalcitabine, stavudine and didanosine.

Non-nucleoside reverse transcriptase inhibitors

Examples: efavirenz, nevirapine

Mechanisms of action and resistance

This group of drugs inhibit HIV reverse transcriptase by binding at a site remote from the active site. They produce a conformational change in the enzyme that prevents substrate binding. They have greater antiviral activity than nucleoside inhibitors, and are better tolerated. Resistance still emerges rapidly by single point gene mutations, unless they are used in combination with at least two other antiretroviral drugs.

Pharmacokinetics

Oral absorption of nevirapine is very good, while that of efavirenz is less so. They are metabolised by hepatic cytochrome P450, and also induce the enzyme. They have very long half-lives of about 2 days.

Unwanted effects

- rash (severe in 10%)
- nausea, vomiting, abdominal pain, diarrhoea
- headache, drowsiness, fatigue
- hepatotoxicity with nevirapine, which can cause potentially fatal fulminant hepatitis
- drug interactions with drugs that are metabolised by hepatic cytochrome P450.

HIV protease inhibitors

Examples: ritonavir, saquinavir

Mechanism of action

In HIV infection, there are some steps in viral replication that differ from the processes in host cells. RNA is translated into inert polyproteins rather than the functional proteins that are the products in host cells. Proteases that are found only in viruses cleave the polyproteins during budding from the infected cell to the functionally active proteins required by the viruses for their continued existence (Fig. 51.6). Protease enzyme inhibitors are specific for the enzymes found in HIV. They block the infectivity of the viruses but do not affect virus activity in host cells that are already infected.

Mechanism of resistance

Resistance occurs by mutation in the amino acid sequence of the HIV protein that forms the target for the enzyme. Multiple mutations are required for high-level resistance, but over one-third of the amino acid residues in HIV protein can be changed without altering viral function. High plasma drug concentrations delay the onset of resistance, as does the combination of a protease inhibitor with two reverse transcriptase inhibitors. Sequential use of more than one protease inhibitor encourages high-level resistance.

Pharmacokinetics

Oral absorption is high, but bioavailability varies among the drugs, being very low with saquinavir owing to high first-pass metabolism and transport back into the gut lumen by intestinal P-glycoprotein (see Ch. 2); bioavailability is higher with ritonavir. They are all metabolised by the P450 enzyme CYP3A4 in the liver and have short half-lives. They are inhibitors of human cytochrome P450 enzymes.

Unwanted effects

- Nausea, vomiting, abdominal pain, diarrhoea.
- Metabolic disturbance, e.g. hyperlipidaemia, insulin resistance with glucose intolerance, lipodystrophy, fat redistribution (buffalo hump), breast enlargement. This may be due to inhibition of regulatory proteins in adipocytes.
- Hepatic dysfunction.
- Pancreatitis.
- Circumoral and peripheral paraesthesiae with ritonavir.
- Drug interactions (Ch. 56): inhibition of the P450 enzyme CYP3A4 (Ch. 2) can enhance the unwanted effects of protease inhibitors; the concurrent use of inducers of CYP3A4 can lower plasma concentrations of the protease inhibitor and encourage viral

resistance. Inhibition of the enzyme by ritonavir can increase the clinical effect of other antiretroviral drugs, a useful action that allows less frequent dosing. It also inhibits the metabolism of drugs such as warfarin (Ch. 11) and carbamazepine (Ch. 23). The use of protease inhibitors with simvastatin (Ch. 48) should be avoided because of an increased risk of myopathy.

HIV binding-fusion-entry inhibitors

Example: enfuvirtide

Mechanism of action

In order to enter a host cell, HIV fuses with the host cell membrane. This fusion is facilitated by a conformational change in a glycoprotein in the viral cell membrane. Enfuvirtide is a 36-amino-acid peptidomimetic that binds to the glycoprotein and prevents the conformational change. Enfuvirtide is used when there is resistance or intolerance to other antiretroviral drugs.

Mechanism of resistance

This occurs by gene mutation that modifies the glycoprotein target.

Pharmacokinetics

Enfuvirtide is given by subcutaneous injection. It is expected to undergo catabolism to its constituent amino acids, but the metabolic fate has not been elucidated.

Unwanted effects

- injection site reactions
- headache, insomnia
- eosinophilia.

Viral DNA polymerase inhibitors

Nucleoside analogue DNA polymerase inhibitors

Examples: aciclovir, ganciclovir, valaciclovir, valganciclovir

Mechanism of action

Aciclovir and the other drugs in this class are guanosine analogues that inhibit the synthesis of viral DNA (Fig. 51.7). They all require phosphorylation by viral enzymes that are not present in uninfected host cells, before they can exert their antiviral activity; the dependency on viral enzymes prevents cytotoxic effects in human tissue. The phosphorylating enzymes, however, are not present in all DNA viruses.

Aciclovir is activated by conversion to a monophosphate following phosphorylation of the drug by herpes virus thymidine kinase. The monophosphate is then converted to a triphosphate derivative by other intracellular enzymes. The triphosphate derivatives are potent inhibitors of viral DNA polymerase. This terminates viral DNA synthesis and thus inhibits viral replication (Fig. 51.7).

Ganciclovir has some differences from aciclovir in its mechanisms of action; it does suppress viral DNA replication, but, unlike aciclovir, it does not act as a DNA chain terminator.

Spectrum of activity

Aciclovir is most active against herpes viruses (both simplex and zoster). It is only active against CMV at high doses. Ganciclovir has much greater activity than aciclovir against CMV, possibly because it is a better substrate for the CMV protein kinase, which activates it by phosphorylation.

Mechanisms of resistance

Viral mutants are selected that are unable to phosphorylate the drugs. Thymidine kinase-deficient mutants of herpes virus usually develop in immunocompromised individuals, for example those with AIDS or after bone marrow transplantation, when resistance rates average 5–10%.

Pharmacokinetics

Aciclovir can be given orally, intravenously, or topically to the skin or eye. Absorption from the gut is poor. The drug is widely distributed, but concentrations in the CSF are low compared with those in plasma. Most is eliminated by the kidney, and the half-life is short. Valaciclovir is an ester of aciclovir with higher oral bioavailability. Ganciclovir is given intravenously for acute infections since it is poorly absorbed from the gut; oral dosage forms for maintenance therapy are available; it penetrates into the CSF moderately well. It is eliminated by the kidney and has a short half-life. Valganciclovir is an oral prodrug of ganciclovir with better absorption.

Unwanted effects

Most unwanted effects occur with intravenous use, and are much more frequent with ganciclovir than with aciclovir.

- severe local phlebitis at an infusion site
- nausea, vomiting, abdominal pain, diarrhoea
- rashes
- encephalopathy
- nephrotoxicity is caused by crystallisation of the drug in the kidney; it can be limited by a high fluid intake

- bone marrow suppression is the most frequent serious unwanted effect with ganciclovir, with neutropenia occurring in up to 40% of people, and thrombocytopenia less frequently; the neutropenia can be prevented by the use of granulocyte or granulocyte–macrophage colony-stimulating factor (Ch. 47)
- azoospermia with ganciclovir.

Non-nucleoside analogue DNA polymerase inhibitors

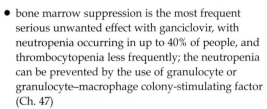

Examples: foscarnet sodium, cidofovir

Mechanisms of action

Foscarnet is an inorganic pyrophosphate compound that binds to the pyrophosphate-binding sites of viral DNA polymerase, preventing DNA chain elongation. Affinity for the viral DNA polymerase is a hundred times greater than for the host cell DNA polymerase. Cidofovir is similar in structure to aciclovir but contains a phosphate moiety. Its action is similar to that of foscarnet. Neither foscarnet nor cidofovir relies on intracellular activation for its antiviral activity (Fig. 51.7). These drugs are reversible inhibitors of CMV and herpes simplex replication.

Pharmacokinetics

Because both foscarnet and cidofovir are highly polar molecules, they are only given intravenously; they are eliminated by the kidney and have intermediate half-lives. Cidofovir is given with probenecid (Ch. 2) (and adequate hydration) to inhibit its renal tubular secretion and minimise nephrotoxicity.

Unwanted effects

- nausea, vomiting
- neutropenia
- headache, tremor, dizziness, mood disturbances with foscarnet
- both agents are highly nephrotoxic, causing a rise in plasma creatinine; good hydration reduces kidney damage
- iritis or uveitis with cidofovir.

Other antiviral drugs

Drugs for treating viral hepatitis

Ribavirin, adefovir and lamivudine are used in the treatment of infections with hepatitis B and C viruses and respiratory syncytial virus (RSV). They are discussed in Chapter 36.

Idoxuridine

The phosphorylated metabolite of idoxuridine is incorporated into viral DNA and impairs transcription. It is now little used. Idoxuridine has been used topically to treat superficial eye and skin infections caused by herpes simplex. For use on the skin, penetration is enhanced by dissolving it in dimethyl sulfoxide (DMSO).

Influenza virus neuraminidase inhibitor

Example: zanamivir

Mechanism of action

Influenza virus neuraminidase is a surface glycoprotein that cleaves sialic acid from a sugar residue. This promotes the spread of the virus by increasing penetration into respiratory epithelial cells, releasing virions from infected cells, promotes viral activation and induces cellular apoptosis. Zanamivir binds and inhibits only the neuraminidases of influenza A and B and is effective against isolates resistant to amantidine.

Pharmacokinetics

Zanamivir is administered by inhalation, when systemic absorption is low. Absorbed drug is excreted unchanged and the half-life is short.

Unwanted effects

- gastrointestinal disturbance
- bronchospasm.

Immunomodulators

Interferon alfa

Interferon alfa is used in the treatment of hepatitis B infection, and is discussed in Chapter 36. Clinical uses of interferon alfa include the treatment of:

- chronic hepatitis
- condylomata acuminata
- AIDS-related Kaposi's sarcoma
- hairy cell leukaemia
- recurrent or metastatic renal cell carcinoma (Ch. 52).

Palivizumab

Mechanism of action and use

Palivizumab is a humanised monoclonal antibody with human and murine antibody sequences produced by recombinant DNA technology. It has potent neutralising and fusion-inhibiting activity against RSV. It reduces the ability of RSV to replicate and infect cells by binding to an antigenic site on the surface of RSV. RSV is a common cause of mild respiratory illness in infants but can produce more severe illness in premature infants or those with congenital heart disease or bronchopulmonary dysplasia. Palivizumab is given to at-risk children under the age of 2 years prior to commencement of the RSV season (October to April in the Northern Hemisphere) and monthly thereafter.

Pharmacokinetics

Palivizumab is given intramuscularly into the anterolateral aspect of the thigh. It has a long half-life of 20 days. The routes of metabolism and elimination are unknown.

Unwanted effects

- fever
- injection site reactions.

Treatment of specific viral infections

HIV infection

There are several principles of antiviral therapy for HIV (retroviral) infection which are now widely adopted. The most frequently used treatment regimens include a protease inhibitor (e.g. saquinavir) or a non-nucleoside reverse transcriptase inhibitor (e.g. nevirapine or efavirenz) combined with two nucleoside analogue reverse transcriptase inhibitors (e.g. zidovudine or stavudine with lamivudine or didanosine). A low dose of ritonavir is often added to this regimen, not for its antiviral effect but to prolong the action of the other drugs and simplify the treatment regimen. Such combinations are referred to as highly active antiretroviral therapy (HAART). This treatment involves complex regimens that require adherence by the individual and careful assessment of the progress of viral suppression. Key principles include the following.

- Combination drug treatment should be started before substantial immunodeficiency is present. The goal is to suppress the virus before resistant mutants emerge or irreversible immune damage occurs. The current recommendation is to start treatment at the onset of an acute HIV syndrome, or within 6 months of seroconversion. Failing these, treatment is given if symptoms occur as a result of HIV infection.
- When resistance occurs, changes in drug therapy should involve the addition or change of at least two drugs. However, if toxicity limits the tolerability of one drug, a single substitution of a similar agent is a reasonable option.
- Optimal treatment should reduce the viral load to below detectable limits, and achieve a rise in CD4 lymphocyte count. This may take 6 months of adequate therapy to achieve.
- Failure to achieve full suppression of viral load should prompt a change in therapy if adherence is believed to be good. Poor adherence with therapy is likely to encourage the development of drug resistance (see above) and thus treatment failure. Drug therapy is ideally guided by patterns of resistance in the virus.

Prophylaxis after accidental exposure to the virus is now recommended. The regimen depends on the level of risk: two drugs are often used for moderate risk, or three drugs if the risk is high.

Varicella–zoster virus infections

Varicella–zoster virus (VZV) is a herpes virus responsible for both chickenpox and shingles (zoster). Shingles arises from reactivation of the virus, which lies dormant in a dorsal root ganglion after the primary chickenpox infection. Chickenpox is rarely treated with antiviral therapy, although the use of oral aciclovir reduces lesion formation and results in quicker healing.

Zoster is most commonly found in the elderly and immunosuppressed people. The rash is often preceded by pain for 1–4 days. Oral antiviral drug therapy reduces pain and accelerates healing but must be given while the virus is still replicating. Oral aciclovir is often used and is particularly indicated for those older than 55 years (who are at greater risk of complications), for ophthalmic infections or in immunosuppressed people. Complications occur in 15–20% of those with zoster and include meningoencephalitis, motor nerve paralysis, ocular complications and postherpetic neuralgia. The use of aciclovir has little effect on the risk of developing postherpetic neuralgia but does reduce the risk of motor nerve damage. Corticosteroids have no value as an adjunctive treatment to aciclovir. Valaciclovir may be more effective for resolving symptoms than aciclovir, through its higher blood concentrations. Analgesics are often required in the early phases of zoster, and postherpetic neuralgia may require specific therapy (Ch. 19).

Herpes simplex virus infections

Herpes simplex virus exists in two forms: type 1 produces either oral or genital ulceration, and type 2 produces genital ulceration. Oral herpes infection will respond to early topical application of aciclovir. Primary genital herpes produces multiple painful lesions and responds to oral aciclovir given for five days. Recurrent lesions occur from reactivation of latent virus in the dorsal root ganglia, producing symptoms that are usually less severe than with primary episodes. After initial therapy with aciclovir, continuous prophylactic therapy can be given to prevent further relapses.

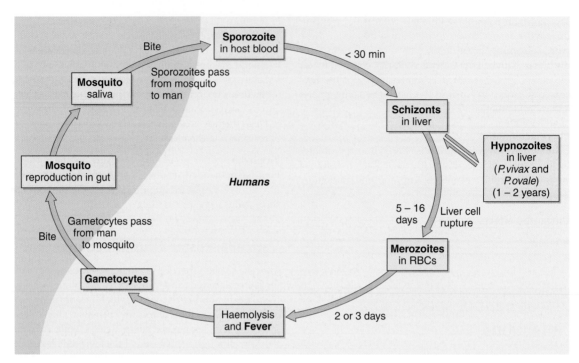

Fig. 51.8
Life-cycle of malarial parasite.

Cytomegalovirus infection

CMV infection is common and usually produces mild symptoms. However, it can be devastating in immuno-suppressed people. Troublesome complications in this group include retinitis (which can threaten sight), gastrointestinal manifestations (including oesophagitis, gastritis, cholecystitis or colitis), pneumonia and CNS involvement.

Intravenous ganciclovir is the treatment of choice for severe manifestation of CMV infection. Foscarnet can be used as an alternative to ganciclovir, or cidofovir if both are contraindicated. For CMV retinitis, oral valganciclovir is used both for treatment and to prevent relapse. Oral valganciclovir or valaciclovir may be of particular value for the prevention of CMV infection, especially in renal transplant recipients or bone marrow transplant recipients in whom CMV pneumonia is a major potential compli-cation. Combined therapy with ganciclovir and CMV immunoglobulin may be more effective than ganciclovir alone for treatment of pneumonia in this group.

Influenza

The use of a neuraminidase inhibitor, such as zanamavir, reduces the duration of uncomplicated disease by about one day. This is not recommended by the National Institute for Clinical Excellence (NICE) in the UK, unless the individual is at risk of complications. These are people with chronic respiratory disease, significant cardiovascular disease, chronic renal disease, diabetes mellitus or who are immunocompromised. Treatment must be started within 48 h of the onset of an influenza-like illness. There is little evidence on the ability of these drugs to prevent the complications of influenza. Neura-minidase inhibitors are also effective for prevention of influenza during an epidemic, reducing the likelihood of developing the illness by 70–90%. They are only adjuncts to an effective vaccination campaign.

Protozoal infections

Malaria

Four species of the protozoan *Plasmodium* produce malaria in humans: *P. vivax*, *P. ovale*, *P. malariae* and *P. falciparum*. Sporozoites are formed by repeated division of oocysts in the body of the mosquito and are transferred into host blood in the anopheles mosquito saliva during a blood meal. The parasite is sequestered in the liver and divides to form tissue schizonts (Fig. 51.8). When the pre-erythrocytic (liver) sexual cycle is complete, the liver cells rupture and 20 000–40 000 merozoites escape into the blood and invade erythrocytes. They then undergo the erythrocytic cycle, multiplying asexually in the erythrocytes. The red cells then rupture and release merozoites to invade other red cells. Merozoites in the plasma at this stage are termed gametocytes. A mosquito biting an infected individual ingests gametocytes, which then go through a development cycle in the mosquito to form sporozoites.

At the pre-erythrocytic stage in the liver, some schizonts from *P. vivax* and *P. ovale*, rather than being released as merozoites, remain in the liver, forming hypnozoites. These form a reservoir of parasites that are difficult to eradicate and can emerge to give relapses months or years after the initial infection. Release of merozoites in the human every 2–3 days causes repeated bouts of tertian or quartan fever. The duration of the infection varies with the parasite. Because *P. vivax* and *P. ovale* continue to multiply in the liver as hypnozoites, drugs that treat only the erythrocytic phase will not produce a radical cure (elimination of all parasites), and relapsing infection can occur.

P. falciparum and *P. malariae* only multiply in erythrocytes, but disease can recrudesce if parasites are not completely eliminated from the blood.

Clinical symptoms include chills as merozoites enter blood from ruptured erythrocytes. Nausea, vomiting and headache are common. A fever follows, and the attack concludes with sweating. *P. falciparum* produces the most severe symptoms because it causes agglutination of red cells, which produces capillary thrombosis, especially in the brain, leading to cerebral malaria.

Antimalarial drugs

Chloroquine

Mechanism of action

Erythrocytes infected by malaria parasites concentrate chloroquine more than 100-fold, since it binds to a breakdown product of haemoglobin induced by the parasite, and interferes with the haem degradative pathway.

- Chloroquine is digested by the erythrocyte-resident parasite, and this raises lysosomal pH, which will reduce the ability of the parasite to digest haemoglobin and inhibit its growth.
- Chloroquine interacts with ferriprotoporphyrin IX, which is formed during digestion of haemoglobin, an action that prevents further degradation of haemoglobin by the parasite.

Chloroquine (and its close relative hydroxychloroquine) also possesses slow-onset anti-inflammatory activity, which is useful in the treatment of rheumatoid arthritis (Ch. 30).

Pharmacokinetics

Chloroquine is a 4-aminoquinoline that is completely absorbed from the gut, or it can be given intravenously. It has a very high volume of distribution because of selective concentration in melanin-containing tissues, for example the retina of the eye, and in the liver, spleen and kidney. Approximately half is converted in the liver to active metabolites, the rest is excreted unchanged by the kidney. The half-life is very long during chronic dosing; an initial half-life of up to 6 days is followed by a second slow phase of tissue elimination with a half-life of greater than 1 month.

Unwanted effects

- Nausea, vomiting, diarrhoea, abdominal pain, which may be caused by anticholinesterase activity (Chs 27 and 28).
- Cardiovascular depression after intravenous use, with hypotension and heart block; these are quinidine-like effects (Ch. 8).
- Retinopathy with cumulative doses, producing retinal pigmentation and visual field defects. Visual function should be monitored.
- Rashes and pruritis.

Mefloquine

Mechanism of action

Mefloquine has a similar mode of action to chloroquine.

Pharmacokinetics

Mefloquine is an amino alcohol that is well absorbed from the gut and has a high affinity for lung, liver and lymphoid tissue. Extensive metabolism occurs in the liver, but the elimination half-life is very long, in excess of 3 weeks.

Unwanted effects

- CNS effects: dizziness, vertigo, headache. Less commonly, severe psychiatric disturbance can occur, and mefloquine should not be given to individuals with a previous history of psychiatric disorder.
- Gastrointestinal effects occur that are similar to those seen with chloroquine.

Primaquine

Mechanism of action

Unlike structurally related drugs, primaquine only affects the exoerythrocytic parasite. It enters the parasite in the liver and may inhibit mitochondrial respiration. It is used after treatment with chloroquine, to eradicate *P. vivax* or *P. ovale* from the liver.

Pharmacokinetics

Primaquine is an 8-aminoquinolone that is completely absorbed from the gut and rapidly metabolised in the

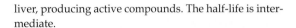

liver, producing active compounds. The half-life is intermediate.

Unwanted effects

- intravascular haemolysis in people with glucose 6-phosphate dehydrogenase (G6PD) deficiency (Chs 47 and 53); G6PD activity in erythrocytes should be checked before initiating treatment
- gastrointestinal effects are similar to those seen with chloroquine.

Quinine

Mechanism of action
Quinine is similar to chloroquine in its action.

Pharmacokinetics
Quinine is well absorbed from the gut but can also be given by intravenous infusion. Metabolism in the liver is extensive and the half-life is intermediate in healthy people, becoming long in severe malaria.

Unwanted effects

- 'cinchonism': tinnitus, headache, nausea, visual disturbances with vertigo and hearing loss if severe
- stimulation of insulin secretion, producing hypoglycaemia
- quinidine-like effects on the heart (Ch. 8), with bradycardias, heart block or ventricular tachycardia; this most often occurs with intravenous loading doses.

Pyrimethamine

Mechanism of action
Selective inhibition of dihydrofolate reductase in the parasite reduces folic acid synthesis (Fig. 51.4). Pyrimethamine should only be given in combination with a sulphonamide-like drug, either sulfadoxine or dapsone.

Pharmacokinetics
Pyrimethamine is well absorbed from the gut and undergoes extensive hepatic metabolism. The half-life is very long, approximately 2–6 days.

Unwanted effects
Pyrimethamine is usually well tolerated; occasional effects are:

- photosensitive rashes
- megaloblastic anaemia due to inhibition of human folate metabolism (with chronic therapy).

Proguanil

Mechanism of action
Proguanil inhibits plasmodial dihydrofolate reductase (Fig. 51.4), mainly through its active metabolite, which inhibits folate production in both pre-erythrocytic and erythrocytic parasites. It is usually used for malaria prophylaxis, in combination with chloroquine.

Pharmacokinetics
Absorption of proguanil from the gut is good, and extensive metabolism occurs in the liver to cycloguanil, a potent active derivative. The half-life of proguanil is long; that of cycloguanil is short.

Unwanted effects

- mouth ulcers
- epigastric discomfort, diarrhoea.

Treatment of malaria

Chemotherapy of malaria falls into three categories:

- rapid-acting blood schizonticides (to kill schizonts in acute malaria): chloroquine, quinine, mefloquine
- slow-acting blood schizonticides (to prevent blood infections): pyrimethamine, proguanil
- tissue schizonticides (to eliminate liver parasites): primaquine.

The recommended drug to use within each category depends on the type of parasite and the pattern of resistance where the infection was acquired. If the infecting organism is unknown, it is assumed to be *P. falciparum*, which carries the greatest risk. Latest recommendations should be obtained from tropical-disease advisory centres.

Examples are given for current recommended treatments for acute attacks of high- and low-risk malaria.

For *P. falciparum*, chloroquine resistance is common. Oral quinine or mefloquine is given initially (intravenous quinine is used for serious infections). Alternative options are proguanil with atovaquone (see below) or artemether with lumefantrine (see compendium). Initial treatment is followed by pyrimethamine with sulfadoxine for 7 days or by doxycycline (see Antibacterials above) if the plasmodia are resistant to sulfadoxine.

For benign malaria, chloroquine is given initially. For *P. vivax* and *P. ovale*, primaquine is then given to destroy hepatic parasites.

Prophylaxis against malaria

The recommendations for prophylaxis depend on patterns of resistance in the area to be visited. Where resistance is low, chloroquine or proguanil is often recommended. For many areas, a combination of both

Table 51.4
Selected protozoan infections and antiprotozoal drugs

Protozoa	Disease	Drug examples
Plasmodium	Malaria	Chloroquine, halofantine, mefloquine, primaquine, quinine, proguanil, pyrimethamine
Entamoeba histolytica	Amoebic dysentery	Metronidazole, tinidazole, diloxanide
Trichomonas vaginalis	Vaginitis	Metronidazole, tinidazole
Giardia lamblia	Gastrointestinal dysfunction	Metronidazole, tinidazole, mepacrine
Leishmania	Cutaneous or visceral (kala-azar) leishmaniasis	Stibogluconate, pentamidine
Trypanosomes	Trypanosomiasis, Chagas' disease, sleeping sickness	Suramin, nifurtimax, benznidazole, eflornithine, pentamidine, melarsoprol
Toxoplasma gondii	Encephalomyelitis, toxoplasmosis	Pyrimethamine plus sulfadiazine, trimetrexate
Pneumocystis carinii	Pneumocystis pneumonia	Co-trimoxazole, pentamidine, atovaquone, trimetrexate

drugs is desirable. Mefloquine, doxycycline or proguanil with atovaquone are recommended in some areas when there is a high risk of chloroquine-resistant malaria. Prophylaxis must also take into account the unwanted effects of the drugs and other factors such as pregnancy and renal or hepatic impairment. Prophylaxis must be started 1 week before travel (3 weeks for mefloquine) and continued for 1 month after leaving a malarious area, to protect against infection acquired immediately prior to departure.

Other protozoal infections

Details of the natural history of other protozoal infections are not given in this book. Important drugs available in the UK for these conditions are discussed below. An outline of therapeutic uses is given in Table 51.4.

Atovaquone

Indications
Atovaquone is used for treatment of *Pneumocystis carinii* and *Toxoplasma gondii* infections as well as for malaria.

Mechanisms of action
Atovaquone is used as a second-line agent for treatment of *P. carinii* infections and for treating *T. gondii* infection (see above). In *P. carinii*, atovaquone does not inhibit folate but interferes with DNA synthesis by inhibiting pyrimidine synthesis. It is selective for protozoa, which cannot utilise pre-formed pyrimidines. It is able to kill *Pneumocystis* rather than just delaying growth. It is also active against *Plasmodium* species, *Entamoeba histolytica* and *Trichomonas vaginalis*.

Pharmacokinetics
Oral absorption of atovaquone is poor but is improved with food. It is excreted unchanged in the bile, but undergoes enterohepatic cycling, which gives it a very long half-life of 60 h.

Unwanted effects

- diarrhoea, nausea, vomiting
- rash
- headache, insomnia
- neutropenia.

Pentamidine

Indications
Pentamidine is used in *Pneumocystis carinii* pneumonia, leishmaniasis and trypanosomiasis.

Mechanism of action and uses
Pentamidine undergoes active uptake into the cell, where it probably inhibits DNA synthesis and ribosomal synthesis of protein and phospholipid. It is cytotoxic to *P. carinii* in the non-replicating state. Because of its toxicity, pentamidine is usually reserved for people who are intolerant of co-trimoxazole, which is the drug of first choice for pneumocystis pneumonia (see Antibacterials, p. 595).

Pharmacokinetics
Pentamidine is given intravenously or inhaled as an aerosol for pneumocystis pneumonia. It can be given by deep intramuscular injection for leishmaniasis or trypanosomiasis. Inhalation is particularly useful for pneumocystis pneumonia (which affects immunocompromised patients, especially those with AIDS), since lung concentrations are low after intravenous administration. Pentamidine is metabolised in the liver and has a long half-life.

Unwanted effects

- Inhaled pentamidine produces bronchial irritation with cough and bronchospasm.

- Intravenous pentamidine is nephrotoxic, and can produce irreversible hypoglycaemia and life-threatening arrhythmias such as ventricular tachycardia.

Sodium stibogluconate

Indications
Sodium stibogluconate is used to treat visceral leishmaniasis.

Mechanism of action
Sodium stibogluconate is an organic pentavalent antimony derivative that may act by binding to thiol groups in the parasite.

Pharmacokinetics
Sodium stibogluconate must be given parenterally, either by intramuscular injection or slow intravenous infusion. It has a short half-life and is eliminated by the kidney.

Unwanted effects

- anorexia, nausea, vomiting
- headache
- lethargy
- myalgia
- cough and substernal pain during intravenous infusion.

Diloxanide furoate

Indications
Diloxanide is used to treat chronic amoebiasis in asymptomatic individuals who are excreting cysts of *Entamoeba histolytica* in the stool. Acute infection is treated with metronidazole or tinidazole (see above).

Mechanism of action
The mechanism of action is unknown.

Pharmacokinetics
Hydrolysis in the gut liberates diloxanide and furoic acid; 90% of the diloxanide is then absorbed and rapidly conjugated in the liver. Diloxanide has a short half-life. The unabsorbed fraction of diloxanide may contribute to the drug's effectiveness in amoebic dysentery.

Unwanted effects

- flatulence, anorexia, nausea and diarrhoea
- urticaria, pruritis.

Helminth infections

Details of the natural history of helminth infections are not given here, but an outline of the more commonly encountered conditions is given in Table 51.5. Drugs specifically for helminth infections are discussed below.

Antihelminthic agents

Ivermectin

Indications
Ivermectin is used to treat filariasis (especially onchocerciasis), hookworm and *Strongyloides stercoralis* infection.

Mechanism of action
Ivermectin is a macrocyclic lactone. It produces an influx of Cl⁻ via an action on cell membrane ion channels, generating hyperpolarisation of the filariae and muscle paralysis. In the UK, it is an unlicensed drug, available on a 'named-patient' basis only. It is the drug of choice for onchocerciasis.

Table 51.5
Helminth infections

Helminth	Common name	Drug examples
Enterobius vermicularis	Threadworm	Mebendazole, piperazine
Ascaris lumbricoides	Roundworm	Mebendazole, piperazone, levamisole
Toxocara canis	Dog roundworm	Tiabendazole, diethylcarbamazine
Taenia species	Tapeworm	Niclosamide, praziquantel
Ancylostoma species, *Necator* species	Hookworm	Mebendazole, ivermectin, albendazole
Microfilariae (e.g. *Loa loa, Wuchereria bancrofti, Brugia malayi*)		Diethylcarbamazine, ivermectin
Strongyloides stercoralis		Tiabendazole, albendazole, ivermectin
Echinococcus granulosa	Hydatid disease	Albendazole

Pharmacokinetics

Ivermectin is well absorbed from the gut and is excreted mainly in the faeces. It undergoes some hepatic metabolism and has a long half-life. Treatment with a single dose reduces microfilarial levels for several months, and it can be repeated every 6–12 months if necessary.

Unwanted effects

- itching
- skin rash.

Diethylcarbamazine

Indications

Diethylcarbamazine is used to treat filariasis.

Mechanism of action

The mechanism of action of diethylcarbamazine is not well understood. It may inhibit arachidonic acid metabolism in the filariae. It also triggers exposure of antigens on the surface coat, leading to antibody-mediated destruction. Diethylcarbamazine is not on the UK market.

Pharmacokinetics

Oral absorption is good, and approximately half the drug is metabolised in the liver; the rest is excreted unchanged by the kidney. The half-life is intermediate. Treatment is usually required for 2–3 weeks to eliminate the microfilariae.

Unwanted effects

Most problems are caused by release of antigens from dying filariae. The onset is about 2 h after dosing and is almost diagnostic of the disease. The reaction is occasionally severe and life-threatening. The reaction includes:

- fever
- headache
- nausea
- muscle and joint pains
- itching
- postural hypotension.

Benzimidazoles

Examples: tiabendazole, mebendazole, albendazole

Indications

Tiabendazole: *Strongyloides stercoralis*, hookworm (cutaneous larva migrans)
Mebendazole: threadworm, roundworm, hookworm
Albendazole: hydatid cysts, *Strongyloides stercoralis*.

Mechanism of action

The benzimidazoles bind to tubulin, preventing its polymerisation into the cytoskeletal microtubules. The effect is selective for parasitic tubulin and the drugs are active against the adults, larvae and eggs. Tiabendazole is available in the UK on a 'named-patient' basis.

Pharmacokinetics

Oral absorption of tiabendazole is almost complete and metabolism in the liver is extensive. The half-life is short. Oral absorption of mebendazole and albendazole is very poor; the little drug that is absorbed is metabolised in the liver. These drugs act principally from within the gut.

Unwanted effects

- gastrointestinal effects are common with tiabendazole and include anorexia, nausea, vomiting and diarrhoea; they are less severe with the other agents
- dizziness and drowsiness can occur with tiabendazole.

Piperazine

Indications

Piperazine is used to treat threadworm and roundworm infections.

Mechanism of action

Piperazine competitively inhibits the effect of acetylcholine on the smooth muscle of the worm, producing a reversible flaccid paralysis.

Pharmacokinetics

Absorption of piperazine is rapid from the gut, but little is known about its handling after absorption.

Unwanted effects

Gastrointestinal upset can occur.

Niclosamide

Indications

Niclosamide is used to treat tapeworm infection.

Mechanism of action

Niclosamide inhibits generation of ATP by preventing phosphorylation of adenosine diphosphate (ADP) in mitochondria. It is ineffective against larval worms. Purgatives are usually given after niclosamide to remove viable ova from the gut. Niclosamide is available in the UK on a 'named-patient' basis.

Pharmacokinetics

Some oral absorption (up to 20%) occurs, with subsequent liver metabolism.

Unwanted effects

- gastrointestinal upset, nausea, abdominal pain
- lightheadedness
- pruritis.

Praziquantel

Indications

Praziquantel is used to treat tapeworm infection and schistosomiasis.

Mechanism of action

It is not well understood how praziquantel acts; it is known to interfere with Ca^{2+} homeostasis in the parasite, causing muscular paralysis and increasing cell membrane permeability. Praziquantel is unlicensed in the UK and is available only on a 'named-patient' basis.

Pharmacokinetics

Praziquantel is well absorbed from the gut and penetrates well into most tissues; it is extensively metabolised by the liver and has a short plasma half-life.

Unwanted effects

- dizziness, headache, lassitude
- gastrointestinal upset.

FURTHER READING

Antibacterial agents

Barker AF (2002) Bronchiectasis. *N Engl J Med* 346, 1383–1391

Bartlet JG (2002) Antibiotic-associated diarrhoea. *N Engl J Med* 346, 334–339

British Thoracic Society Standards of Care Committee (2001) BTS guidelines for the management of community-acquired pneumonia in adults. *Thorax* 56(suppl IV), iv1–iv64

Chan ED, Iseman MD (2002) Current medical treatment of tuberculosis. *BMJ* 325, 1282–1286

Ewig S, Bauer T, Torres A (2001) The pulmonary physician in critical care 4: nososcomial pneumonia. *Thorax* 57, 366–371

Fihn SD (2003) Acute uncomplicated urinary tract infection in women. *N Engl J Med* 349, 259–266

Frieden TR, Sterling TR, Munsiff SS et al (2003) Tuberculosis. *Lancet* 362, 887–899

Garcia D, Torre I (2003) Advances in the management of septic arthritis. *Rheum Clin North Am* 29, 61–75

Hirschmann JV (2002) Antibiotics for common respiratory tract infections in adults. *Arch Intern Med* 162, 256–264

Mansharamani NG, Koziel H (2003) Chronic lung sepsis: lung abscess, bronchiectasis and empyema. *Curr Opin Pulm Med* 9, 181–185

Moreillon P, Que Y-A (2004) Infective endocarditis. *Lancet* 363, 139–149

Mukherjee JS, Rich ML, Socci AR et al (2004) Programmes and principles for treating multidrug-resistant tuberculosis. *Lancet* 363, 474–481

Quagliarello VJ, Scheld WM (1997) Treatment of bacterial meningitis. *N Engl J Med* 336, 708–716

Ray PS, Simonis RB (2002) Management of acute and chronic osteomyelitis. *Hosp Med* 63, 401–407

Rovers MM, Schilder AGM, Zielhuis GA et al (2004) Otitis media. *Lancet* 363, 465–473

Sefton AM (2002) Mechanisms of antimicrobial resistance. *Drugs* 62, 557–566

Swartz MN (2004) Cellulitis. *N Engl J Med* 350, 904–912

The Task Force on Infective Endocarditis of the European Society of Cardiology (2004) Guidelines on prevention, diagnosis and treatment of infective endocarditis. Executive summary. *Eur Heart J* 25, 267–276

Turnidge J (2001) Responsible prescribing for upper respiratory tract infections. *Drugs* 61, 2065–2077

Viscoli C, Castagnola E (2002) Treatment of febrile neutropenia: what is new? *Curr Opin Infect Dis* 15 377–382

Westphal J-F, Brogard J-M (1999) Biliary tract infections. *Drugs* 57, 81–91

Antifungal agents

Balkis MM, Leidich SD, Mukherjee PK et al (2002) Mechanisms of fungal resistance. *Drugs* 62, 1025–1040

Hart R, Bell-Syer SE, Crawford F et al (1999) Systematic review of topical treatments for fungal infections of the skin and nails of the feet. *BMJ* 319, 79–82

Kontoyiannis DP, Lewis RE (2002) Antifungal drug resistance of pathogenic fungi. *Lancet* 359, 1135–1144

Leather HL, Wingard JR (2002) Prophylaxis, empirical therapy, or pre-emptive therapy of fungal infections in immunocompromised patients; which is better for whom? *Curr Opin Infect Dis* 15, 369–375

Rubin EA, Somani J (2004) New options for the treatment of invasive fungal infections. *Semin Oncol* 31(suppl 2), 91–98

Sobel JD (2003) Management of patients with recurrent vulvovaginal candidiasis. *Drugs* 63, 1059–1066

Antiviral agents

Burger DM, Aarnoutse RE, Hugen PWH (2002) Pros and cons of the therapeutic drug monitoring of antiretroviral agents. *Curr Opin Infect Dis* 15, 17–22

Carr A, Cooper DA (2000) Adverse effects of antiretroviral therapy. *Lancet* 356, 1423–1430

Clavel F, Hance AJ (2004) HIV drug resistance. *N Engl J Med* 350, 1023–1035

Couch RB (2000) Drug therapy: prevention and treatment of influenza. *N Engl J Med* 343, 1778–1787

Gnann JW, Whitley RJ (2002) Herpes zoster. *N Engl J Med* 347, 340–346

Nicholson KG, Wood JM, Zambon M (2003) Influenza. *Lancet* 362, 1733–1745

Snoek R, De Clercq E (2002) New treatments for genital herpes. *Curr Opin Infect Dis* 15, 49–55

Thorner AR, Rosenberg ES (2003) Early versus delayed antiretroviral therapy in patients with HIV infection. *Drugs* 63, 1325–1337

Yeni PG, Hammer SM, Hirsch MS et al (2004) Treatment for adult HIV infection: 2004 recommendations of the International AIDS Society-USA Panel. *JAMA* 292, 251–265

Antiprotozoal agents

Kremsner PG, Krishna S (2004) Antimalarial combinations. *Lancet* 364, 285–294

Montoya JG, Liessenfeld O (2004) Toxoplasmosis. *Lancet* 363, 1965–1977

Nosten F, Brasseur P (2002) Combination therapy for malaria. *Drugs* 62, 1315–1329

Stanley SL Jr (2003) Amoebiasis. *Lancet* 361, 1025–1034

Antihelminthic agents

de Silva N, Guyatt H, Bundy D (1997) Antihelminthics. *Drugs* 53, 769–788

Self-assessment

In questions 1–7, the first statement, in italics, is true. Are the accompanying statements also true?

1. *Resistance to antibacterials can be generated by bacteria increasing efflux or decreasing uptake of drugs, producing enzymes that metabolise drugs, replacing essential microbial enzymes that could be inhibited by antibacterials with mutant enzymes that are no longer inhibited, or developing mutated ribosomal subunits that do not bind antibacterials.*

   a. Benzylpenicillin has a short half-life as it is rapidly excreted by the kidneys.
   b. Broad-spectrum penicillins do not disturb normal colonic flora.
   c. The antipseudomonal penicillin azlocillin is resistant to β-lactamase.
   d. Penicillins are bactericidal by binding to bacterial ribosomal-binding sites.

2. *A number of cephalosporins exist that show a range of activities against Gram-positive and Gram-negative bacteria and have high CNS penetration.*

   a. Cefotaxime is a third-generation cephalosporin. It crosses the blood–brain barrier and is not broken down by β-lactamases.
   b. People who are allergic to penicillins cannot be given cephalosporins.

3. *The carbapenem imipenem is a broad-spectrum β-lactamase-resistant drug that is effective against many Gram-positive and Gram-negative bacteria.*

   a. Imipenem is rapidly metabolised.
   b. Imipenem shows only bacteriostatic activity.

4. *The quinolone ciprofloxacin is active against many Gram-negative and Gram-positive bacteria but has weak activity against streptococci and staphylococci. It has a relatively low incidence of unwanted effects.*

   a. Ciprofloxacin can be used for *Pseudomonas aeruginosa* infections in people with cystic fibrosis.
   b. Ciprofloxacin can safely be given together with theophylline in people with asthma.

5. *Macrolide antibiotics (e.g. erythromycin, clarithromycin) can be used as part of the regimen to eliminate* Helicobacter pylori *and* Legionella *infection.*

   a. Erythromycin commonly causes gastrointestinal disturbances.
   b. Gentamicin has a low incidence of unwanted effects.
   c. Gentamicin is not active when given orally.

6. *Metronidazole can be used as part of the regimen for eradicating* Helicobacter pylori *and for treatment of pseudomembranous colitis resulting from overgrowths with* Clostridium difficile.

   a. Antibacterials do not reduce the development of serious illness for the majority of people with sore throat.
   b. Tetracyclines should be avoided during pregnancy and in young children.
   c. Vancomycin is active against β-lactamase-producing Gram-positive bacteria.

7. *Because of problems with resistance,* Mycobacterium tuberculosis *is always treated with at least two drugs acting at different sites.*

   a. Rifampicin is an important drug for the treatment of tuberculosis and also serious Legionnaire's disease and leprosy.
   b. Isoniazid is active against a wide range of bacteria.
   c. Co-trimoxazole is the drug of choice for hospital-acquired acute urinary tract infection.
   d. Trimethoprim administration can result in folate deficiency.

8. Case history 1 questions

> Mr JW, age 40 years, living at home was previously healthy, but saw his GP in August, 5 days after returning from a conference abroad where he had stayed in a large hotel and indulged his passion for frequent whirlpool baths. He had characteristic symptoms of pneumonia, including pleuritic chest pain and sudden development of fever and cough, producing yellow sputum. Physical examinations and chest radiograph corroborated the diagnosis.

  a. Before the results of the microbiological test were available, what treatment would you have commenced and what route of administration would you have used?
  b. How do the drugs you are proposing to give work?

9. Case history 2 questions

> Mr RH, age 80 years, had influenza and was admitted to hospital when he developed symptoms similar to Mr JW and became seriously ill. A chest radiograph showed multiple abscesses.

  a. What treatment would you have commenced before microbiological results were available?
  b. What antibacterial could be used if the organism was not treatable by β-lactamase-resistant penicillins?

10. Case history 3 questions

> A 31-year-old homosexual man was admitted with shortness of breath, cough and generalised chest discomfort. Chest radiograph revealed diffuse bilateral opacities and a blood gas analysis demonstrated an arterial partial oxygen pressure (PaO_2) of 8.0 kPa (normal range 11.0–14.0). Sputum culture was non-contributory. A bronchoalveolar lavage was performed and transbronchial biopsies taken.

  a. What was the likely clinical diagnosis?
  b. What microscopic investigation could have been useful and what might it have shown?
  c. How could this man have been managed and what factors needed to be considered?
  d. What drug treatment could have exposed him to the increased risk of opportunistic infection similar to that which had already occurred?
  e. What needed to be considered after initial treatment?

11. Case history 4 questions

> Twenty-four hours after attending a convention, a 36-year-old man became ill with a temperature, abdominal pain, vomiting and diarrhoea. Faeces were collected and inoculated onto culture plates with several different types of culture medium. Pale-coloured colonies that were non-lactose fermenting were identified.

  a. What organisms could have been causing this infection?
  b. How should this man have been managed?
  c. What food was most likely to have caused this infection?

The answers are provided on pages 743–745.

Drug compendium

Drugs used for infections

Drug	Half-life (h)	Elimination	Comments
Antibacterial drugs			
Penicillins			
Amoxicillin	1	Renal + metabolism	Used for urinary tract infections, otitis media, sinusitis, bronchitis, uncomplicated community-acquired pneumonia, *Haemophilus influenzae* infections, invasive salmonellosis and listerial meningitis; broad-spectrum penicillin; given orally, by intramuscular injection or by intravenous injection or infusion; good oral bioavailability (90%) not influenced by food; rapid renal excretion
Ampicillin	1–2	Renal + metabolism	See amoxicillin for uses; broad-spectrum penicillin; given orally, by intramuscular injection or by intravenous injection or infusion; low oral bioavailability which is reduced if taken with food; eliminated largely by renal clearance
Benzylpenicillin (penicillin G)	0.5–1	Renal + metabolism	Used for throat infection, otitis media, streptococcal endocarditis, meningococcal disease, pneumonia and anthrax; given by intramuscular injection, slow intravenous injection or infusion; unreliable oral absorption owing to hydrolysis by gastric acid; rapidly eliminated by renal excretion; depot formulation (procaine benzylpenicillin) is available as intramuscular injection
Flucloxacillin (floxacillin)	0.8–1.2	Renal + metabolism	Used for infections caused by β-lactamase-resistant staphylococci; given orally, by intramuscular injection, or by intravenous injection or infusion; high oral bioavailability (80%); absorption delayed by food; cleared largely by the kidneys
Phenoxymethyl penicillin (penicillin V)	0.5	Renal + metabolism	Used for tonsillitis, otitis media, erysipelas, rheumatic fever and pneumococcal infection prophylaxis; given orally; rapidly but incompletely (60%) absorbed from the gut; eliminated equally by renal excretion unchanged and as the penicilloic acid metabolite
Piperacillin	0.7–1.3	Renal (+ bile)	Antipseudomonal used for infections of lower respiratory tract, urinary tract, abdomen and skin; given by intramuscular injection, or by intravenous injection (over 3–5min) or infusion; poorly absorbed from the gut, therefore not given orally; not metabolised
Pivmecillinam	–	Hydrolysis	Antipseudomonal and active against many Gram-negative bacteria; used for urinary tract infections; given orally; rapidly and extensively hydrolysed prodrug for mecillinam; mecillinam has a half-life of 1–2 h
Ticarcillin	1	Renal	Antipseudomonal active also against *Proteus* species; given by intravenous infusion in combination with clavulanic acid; excreted mostly in the urine unchanged

continued

Drug compendium

Drugs used for infections *(continued)*

Drug	Half-life (h)	Elimination	Comments
Cephalosporins and other β-lactams			
Aztreonam	1.7	Renal	Active only against Gram-negative bacteria and used for infections by *Pseudomonas aeruginosa*, *Haemophilus influenzae* and *Neisseria meningitides*; given by deep intramuscular injection, or by intravenous injection (over 3–5 min) or infusion; not given orally as very poor absorption (<1%); rapidly eliminated by renal clearance without metabolism
Cefaclor	0.5–1	Renal + metabolism	Used for sensitive Gram-negative or Gram-positive infections of urinary tract (unresponsive to other drugs), respiratory tract and soft tissues, and for otitis media and sinusitis; given orally; rapidly and extensively absorbed; eliminated largely by the kidneys plus limited metabolism (15%)
Cefadroxil	1–2	Renal	For uses, see under cefaclor; given orally; rapidly and completely absorbed (not affected by food); eliminated unchanged (>90%)
Cefalexin	1	Renal	For uses, see under cefaclor; given orally; rapidly and completely absorbed; eliminated unchanged
Cefixime	2.5–3.8	Renal + bile	For uses, see under cefaclor (but acute infections only), also used for gonorrhoea; given orally; absorbed slowly and incompletely (50%); excreted more slowly than other cephalosporins (not eliminated by renal tubular secretion)
Cefotaxime	0.9–1.3	Renal + metabolism	For uses, see under cefaclor, also used for gonorrhoea, surgical prophylaxis, *Haemophilus epiglottitis* and meningitis; given by deep intramuscular injection, or by intravenous injection (over 3–5 min) or infusion; renal excretion (with some tubular secretion) is major route of elimination but metabolism accounts for 20% of dose
Cefoxitin (a cephamycin)	1	Renal	For uses, see under cefaclor, also used for surgical prophylaxis; given by deep intramuscular injection, or by intravenous injection (over 3–5 min) or infusion; eliminated by glomerular filtration plus extensive tubular secretion
Cefpirome	1.4–2.3	Renal	For uses, see under cefaclor; given by intravenous injection or infusion; eliminated by glomerular filtration with negligible secretion
Cefpodoxime	1.9–3.2	Renal	Used for upper and lower respiratory tract infections, skin and soft tissue infections, uncomplicated urinary tract infections and uncomplicated gonorrhoea; given orally as the proxetil derivative prodrug, which is absorbed rapidly and quantitatively hydrolysed to cefpodoxine; only about 50% of the dose is absorbed and the fraction absorbed is increased by low gastric pH; cefpodoxine is eliminated by glomerular filtration and secretion
Cefprozil	1.0–1.4	Renal + metabolism	Used for upper respiratory tract infections, skin and soft tissue infections, and otitis media; given orally; rapidly and completely absorbed; eliminated by glomerular filtration (main route) and renal tubular secretion plus metabolism

618

continued

Drugs used for infections *(continued)*

Drug	Half-life (h)	Elimination	Comments
Cephalosporins and other β-lactams (continued)			
Cefradine	?	Renal	For uses, see under cefaclor, also used for surgical prophylaxis; given orally, by deep intramuscular injection, or by intravenous injection (over 3–5 min) or infusion; completely absorbed but rate affected by food; eliminated unchanged in urine
Ceftazidime	1.8–2.2	Renal	For uses, see under cefaclor, also used for surgical prophylaxis; given by deep intramuscular injection, or by intravenous injection (over 3–5 min) or infusion; eliminated unchanged by glomerular filtration
Ceftriaxone	6–9	Renal + bile	For uses, see under cefaclor, also used for surgical prophylaxis and prophylaxis of meningococcal meningitis; given by deep intramuscular injection, or by intravenous injection (over 3–5 min) or infusion; eliminated unchanged; long half-life is probably a result of extensive plasma protein binding (95%)
Cefuroxime	1.2	Renal	For uses, see under cefaclor, also used for surgical prophylaxis; given orally (as cefuroxime axetil), by deep intramuscular injection, or by intravenous injection (over 3–5 min) or infusion; the oral formulation is the axetil derivative prodrug, which is quantitatively hydrolysed to cefuroxime and absorbed better if taken after food; cefuroxime is eliminated equally by renal filtration and secretion
Ertapenem	4.5	Renal + metabolism	Broad-spectrum active against both Gram-negative and Gram-positive organisms; used for abdominal and acute gynaecological infections and for community-acquired pneumonia; given by intravenous infusion; eliminated in urine as equal amounts of parent drug and an inactive metabolite
Imipenem (with cilastatin)	1	Renal + metabolism	Active against aerobic and anaerobic Gram-negative and Gram-positive organisms; used for hospital-acquired septicaemia and for surgical prophylaxis; given by deep intramuscular injection or intravenous infusion; eliminated unchanged in urine and also hydrolysed by a renal enzyme; always given with cilastatin, which inhibits the renal enzyme (although this does not have a major impact on half-life or clearance)
Meropenem	1	Renal + metabolism	Used for aerobic and anaerobic Gram-negative and Gram-positive infections; given by intravenous injection (over 5 min) or intravenous infusion; eliminated by kidneys (80%) and hepatic metabolism (20%)
β-Lactamase inhibitors			Given with some β-lactam antibacterial agents that are susceptible to hydrolysis
Clavulanic acid	1	Metabolism + renal	Given orally, or by slow intravenous injection or infusion in combination with amoxicillin, or intravenously with ticarcillin; undergoes extensive metabolism (pathways are not known) and glomerular filtration

continued

Drugs used for infections (continued)

Drug	Half-life (h)	Elimination	Comments
Tazobactam	0.7–1.5	Renal + metabolism	Given by slow intravenous injection or infusion in combination with piperacillin; eliminated via renal tubular secretion and filtration; the one identified metabolite is inactive
Quinolones			
Ciprofloxacin	3–4	Renal + metabolism	Active against Gram-positive and especially Gram-negative organisms, including *Salmonella*, *Shigella*, *Campylobacter*, *Neisseria* and *Pseudomonas* species, and used for infections of respiratory tract (but not pneumococcal pneumonia), of the urinary and gastrointestinal tracts, chronic prostatitis and gonorrhoea and septicaemia; given orally or by intravenous infusion; good bioavailability (50–80%); eliminated by glomerular filtration, renal tubular secretion, plus biliary excretion and metabolism (15%); the relatively long half-life results from a high apparent volume of distribution (3 l kg^{-1}), not low clearance
Levofloxacin	6–8	Renal + metabolism	Similar activity to ciprofloxacin, but more active against pneumococci; used for bronchitis, community-acquired pneumonia, and infections of urinary tract, skin and soft tissues; given orally or as an intravenous infusion; complete bioavailability (unaffected by food); eliminated largely unchanged by the kidneys
Moxifloxacin	12	Metabolism + renal	Similar activity to ciprofloxacin, but more active against pneumococci but not active against *Pseudomonas aeruginosa* or MRSA; used for bronchitis, community-acquired pneumonia, and sinusitis; given orally; high bioavailability (90%); metabolised by conjugation with glucuronic acid and sulphate
Nalidixic acid	1.5	Metabolism	Used in uncomplicated urinary tract infections; given orally; essentially complete bioavailability; eliminated by hepatic metabolism (oxidation + conjugation)
Norfloxacin	3	Renal + metabolism	Used in uncomplicated urinary tract infections; given orally; bioavailability has not been defined, but absorption is reduced by 30% if taken with food; eliminated by kidneys (filtration + secretion) plus metabolism (about 10%)
Ofloxacin	6–7	Renal + metabolism	Used for infections of the urinary tract and lower respiratory tract, and for gonorrhoea, and non-gonococcal urethritis and cervicitis; given orally or as intravenous infusion; rapid and complete oral absorption; eliminated by kidneys plus limited metabolism (<5%)
Macrolides			
Azithromycin	40–60	Bile	Used for respiratory tract infections, otitis media, skin and soft tissue infections, uncomplicated chlamydial infections, non-gonococcal urethritis and moderate typhoid due to multiple antibiotic-resistant organisms; given orally; bioavailability is 37% (owing to poor absorption) and is reduced by food; eliminated largely by biliary excretion of the parent drug (mol. wt. 785 Da); does not induce P450 isoenzymes

continued

Drugs used for infections (continued)

Drug	Half-life (h)	Elimination	Comments
Macrolides (continued)			
Clarithromycin	3	Metabolism + renal	Used for respiratory tract infections, otitis media, mild to moderate skin and soft tissue infections, and for *Helicobacter pylori* eradication; given orally or by intravenous infusion; bioavailability is 55% (owing to first-pass metabolism); eliminated by metabolism and renal excretion; half-life increased to 9 h at high doses; induces CYP3A4
Erythromycin	1–1.5	Metabolism (+ bile + urine)	Spectrum is similar to penicillins and used for patients hypersensitive to these drugs; used for *Campylobacter* enteritis, pneumonia, Legionnaires' disease, syphilis, non-gonococcal urethritis, chronic prostatitis, diphtheria and whooping cough prophylaxis and for acne vulgaris and rosacea; given orally or by intravenous infusion; oral formulations are as ester prodrugs; eliminated largely by CYP3A4 in the liver (plus gut wall after oral dosage?); inhibits CYP3A4
Spiramycin	6–8	Bile	Used on a named-patient basis for toxoplasmosis
Telithromycin	10	Metabolism + renal + bile	Used for community-acquired pneumonia, bronchitis, sinusitis, β-haemolytic streptococcal pharyngitis, or tonsillitis when β-lactams are inappropriate; given orally; good bioavailability (60%); metabolised by CYP3A4 and other enzymes
Aminoglycosides			All are bactericidal and active against Gram-negative and Gram-positive organisms; gentamicin is the aminoglycoside of choice in the UK and is used for serious infections
Amikacin	2	Renal	Used for serious Gram-negative infections resistant to gentamicin; given by intramuscular injection, slow intravenous injection or intravenous infusion; eliminated by glomerular filtration
Gentamicin	1–4	Renal	Used for septicaemia and neonatal sepsis, CNS infections (including meningitis), biliary tract infections, acute pyelonephritis and prostatitis, endocarditis, pneumonia in hospital, and as an adjunct in listerial meningitis; given by intramuscular injection, slow intravenous injection, intravenous infusion or by intrathecal injection; eliminated by glomerular filtration
Neomycin	2	Renal	Too toxic for parenteral use and restricted to skin infections and for bowel sterilization before surgery; given orally; very poor absorption (<5%); eliminated by glomerular filtration
Netilmicin	2.5	Renal	Used for serious Gram-negative infections resistant to gentamicin; given by intramuscular injection, slow intravenous injection or intravenous infusion; eliminated by glomerular filtration
Tobramycin	2–3	Renal	For uses, see under gentamicin; given by intramuscular injection, slow intravenous injection or intravenous infusion; eliminated by glomerular filtration

continued

Drug compendium

Principles of medical pharmacology and therapeutics

Drugs used for infections *(continued)*

Drug	Half-life (h)	Elimination	Comments
Tetracyclines			Broad-spectrum antibiotics but with increasing resistance; remain drugs of choice for infections caused by *Chlamydia*, *Rickettsia* or *Brucella*, and for Lyme disease; all given orally; no parenteral formulations are available
Demeclocycline	10–15	Renal + bile	Main uses are given above; oral bioavailability is 66% (owing to poor absorption); equal amounts excreted unchanged in urine and bile
Doxycycline	18–22	Bile + urine	Main uses are given above, also used for chronic prostatitis, sinusitis, syphilis, pelvic inflammatory disease, anthrax, malaria, rosacea and acne vulgaris; also used with quinine in the treatment of malaria (see below); high oral bioavailability (>90%); eliminated in bile (20–40%) and urine (20–26%)
Lymecycline	8–10	Hydrolysis	Main uses are given above; degraded in gastrointestinal tract into tetracycline, lysine and formaldehyde
Minocycline	12–16	Bile + urine + metabolism	Main uses are given above, also used for meningococcal carrier state and acne vulgaris; oral bioavailability is >90%; bile is major route of elimination; only 30% has been recovered in excreta (possibly chemical decomposition in vivo rather than metabolism?)
Oxytetracycline	9	Urine + bile	Main uses are given above, also used for acne vulgaris and rosacea; variable absorption (up to 60%); renal excretion is major route of elimination
Tetracycline	9	Bile + urine	Main uses are given above, also used for acne vulgaris and rosacea; irregular and incomplete absorption; eliminated in bile and urine, with some metabolism
Sulphonamides			Their importance has decreased due to increasing resistance and the availability of better alternatives
Sulfadiazine	7–12	Metabolism + renal	Used for prevention of rheumatic fever recurrence; given orally or by intravenous infusion (silver sulfadiazine cream is available for topical use); completely absorbed from the gut, but first-pass metabolism reduces the bioavailability to 60–90%; metabolised by acetylation, and parent drug and acetyl metabolite eliminated by kidney
Sulfamethoxazole	9 (6–20)	Metabolism + renal	Used only in combination with trimethoprim (see below) and restricted to *Pneumocystis carinii* (where it is the drug of choice), toxoplasmosis, nocardiasis and for acute exacerbations of infections shown to be susceptible; given orally or by intravenous infusion; eliminated mainly by acetylation
Trimethoprim	9–17	Renal + metabolism	Used with sulfamethoxazole (see above) and alone for urinary tract infections and bronchitis (when it is given orally); essentially complete absorption and bioavailability; eliminated largely by the kidneys (filtration + secretion) with some oxidative metabolism (20%)

continued

Drugs used for infections (continued)

Drug	Half-life (h)	Elimination	Comments
Other antibacterial drugs			
Chloramphenicol	5 (2–12)	Metabolism	Potent but toxic broad-spectrum compound with use limited to life-threatening infections, especially *Haemophilus influenzae* and typhoid fever; given orally or by intravenous injection or infusion; high oral bioavailability (80–90%); eliminated mainly by glucuronidation
Clindamycin	2.5	Metabolism (+ renal)	Use limited to staphylococcal bone and joint infections and for peritonitis, because of serious toxicity; given orally, by deep intramuscular injection or by intravenous infusion; rapidly and extensively absorbed after oral dosage; mostly eliminated by hepatic metabolism, with two of the metabolites being active; elimination in saliva may give a bitter taste
Colistin (Colistimethate sodium)	4–8	Renal	Used for infections by Gram-negative organisms, including *Psuedomonas aeruginosa*; given orally (for bowel sterilisation only), by intravenous injection or infusion, or by inhalation (nebuliser); not absorbed orally; eliminated by renal excretion
Fusidic acid (sodium fusidate)	9	Metabolism	Narrow spectrum with use restricted to penicillin-resistant staphylococcal infections; given orally or by intravenous infusion; essentially completely bioavailable after oral dosage; metabolised in liver and metabolites excreted in bile
Linezolid	5	Metabolism + renal	Used for pneumonia and complicated skin and soft tissue infections caused by Gram-positive organisms; given orally or by intravenous infusion; eliminated by oxidative metabolism (not P450) to inactive carboxylic acid metabolites; about 30% is excreted unchanged in urine
Methenamine	?	Metabolism	Used for prophylaxis and long-term treatment of lower urinary tract infections; given orally for urinary tract infections; broken down in acid stomach contents, so given as enteric-coated formulation; gives rise to urinary excretion of formaldehyde; half-life is 6 h (or less) because 90% is eliminated in 24 h
Metronidazole	6–9	Metabolism + renal	Active against anaerobic bacteria and used for surgical and gynaecological sepsis, antibiotic-associated colitis and eradication of *Helicobacter pylori*; given orally, rectally or by intravenous infusion; complete oral bioavailability; metabolites are eliminated slowly, primarily in the urine
Nitrofurantoin	0.3–1	Renal + metabolism	Used for urinary tract infections, when it is given orally; complete oral bioavailability; over 40% is excreted rapidly unchanged by filtration and renal tubular secretion; about 20% metabolised by nitroreduction

continued

Drugs used for infections (continued)

Drug	Half-life (h)	Elimination	Comments
Other antibacterial drugs (continued)			
Quinupristin plus dalfopristin	0.5–1.0	Metabolism	Used for serious Gram-positive infections where no alternative antibiotic is suitable; given by intravenous infusion; treatment reserved for MRSA or patients who cannot be treated with other regimens; both drugs are rapidly cleared from the blood and converted into active metabolites which are eliminated in the bile
Teicoplanin	32–176	Renal	Used for Gram-positive infections, including endocarditis, peritonitis and for prophylaxis in orthopaedic surgery; given by intramuscular injection, intravenous injection or infusion; slowly eliminated in urine without metabolism; slower elimination than vancomycin because its higher lipid solubility gives a higher volume of distribution, and because renal excretion is limited by extensive reabsorption and high plasma protein binding (90%)
Tinidazole	12–14	Metabolism + renal	Uses and actions similar to metronidazole; given orally; complete oral bioavailability; about 25% excreted unchanged and the remainder metabolised and eliminated via urine and bile
Vancomycin	5–11	Renal	Used for prophylaxis and treatment of endocarditis and other serious infections of Gram-positive cocci and for antibiotic-associated colitis; given orally (for colitis) or by intravenous infusion; negligible absorption from the gut; eliminated by glomerular filtration
Antituberculous drugs			
Capreomycin	?	Renal + ?	Used in combination with other drugs when resistance to first-line drugs occurs; given by deep intramuscular injection; about 50% is eliminated by renal excretion; old drug with few data available
Cycloserine	4–30	Renal + metabolism	Used in combination with other drugs when resistance to first-line drugs occurs; given orally; high oral bioavailability (> 90%); 60–70% excreted in urine and the remainder is metabolised
Ethambutol	10–15	Renal + metabolism	First-line drug (initial phase only) which is included in treatment regimen if resistance to isoniazid is suspected; given orally; good oral bioavailability (80%); cleared by glomerular filtration + renal tubular secretion, plus < 10% metabolism
Isoniazid	0.5–2 RA 2–6.5 SA	Metabolism	First-line drug; given orally or by intramuscular or intravenous injection; high oral bioavailability; eliminated largely by acetylation, with slow acetylators (SA) having higher blood concentrations than rapid acetylators (RA); other minor metabolites may be linked to hepatotoxicity
Pyrazinamide	10–24	Metabolism + renal	First-line drug (initial phase only) which is particularly useful in tuberculous meningitis; given orally; high oral bioavailability; metabolised in liver to the active compound pyrazinoic acid, which is eliminated in urine

continued

Drugs used for infections (continued)

Drug	Half-life (h)	Elimination	Comments
Antituberculous drugs (continued)			
Rifabutin	35–40	Metabolism (+ renal)	New drug that is an analogue of and alternative to rifampicin (see below); given orally; bioavailability is 20%, decreasing to 12% (owing to autoinduction); eliminated largely by CYP3A, which it induces during chronic treatment; only about 5% is excreted unchanged
Rifampicin (rifampin)	1–6	Metabolism + renal + bile	Key component of any regimen (also used for brucellosis, Legionnaires' disease and serious staphylococcal infections); given orally or by intravenous infusion; high oral bioavailability (percentage not defined); eliminated by a number of routes; potent inducer of CYP3A4
Streptomycin	2–9	Renal	Use is mainly restricted to resistant organisms (also used as an adjunct in the treatment of brucellosis); given by deep intramuscular injection because of poor and highly variable oral bioavailability (0–40%); eliminated by kidney (50–60%) but the fate of the remainder not known (metabolites?)
Drugs used in leprosy			
Clofazimine	10 days	Bile	Given orally; bioavailability is variable (20–85%), dependent on formulation and food (which enhances absorption); slowly eliminated unchanged in bile; urinary excretion is negligible (but enough to make urine red)
Dapsone	27	Metabolism + renal	Given orally; bioavailability is > 90%; undergoes polymorphic acetylation and *N*-glucuronidation (a rare reaction); metabolites undergo enterohepatic circulation; about 10% eliminated in urine unchanged
Rifampicin	–	–	See above
Antifungal agents			
Amorolfine	–	–	Used for fungal infections of skin and nails; applied as a cream or nail lacquer; limited transdermal absorption (<10% across 100 cm^2); very slow elimination may be because of a build-up of drug in the skin
Amphotericin	24–48	Renal	Active against most fungi and yeasts; given orally (for intestinal candidiasis) or by intravenous infusion for systemic infections; negligible oral absorption; slow renal excretion; the half-life given is following a single dose; the elimination half-life after chronic administration is up to 2 weeks, probably reflecting detectable plasma concentrations due to drug released from the tissues
Caspofungin	40–50	Metabolism	Used for invasive aspergillosis unresponsive to amphotericin or itraconazole and for invasive candidiasis; given by intravenous infusion; metabolised by hydrolysis and *N*-acetylation in the liver; metabolites are eliminated in bile

continued

Drug compendium

Drugs used for infections (continued)

Drug	Half-life (h)	Elimination	Comments
Antifungal agents (continued)			
Clotrimazole	–	Metabolism	Used for fungal skin infections and vaginal candidiasis; applied as a cream, powder or spray; negligible absorption across the skin; 5–10% is absorbed after vaginal use and fungicidal concentrations are maintained locally for up to 3 days
Econazole	–	–	Used for fungal skin infections and vaginal candidiasis; applied as a cream; negligible absorption across the skin; data on absorption after vaginal use are not available (see clotrimazole)
Fluconazole	30	Renal + some metabolism	Used for local and systemic fungal infections; good penetration of blood–brain barrier makes it useful for fungal meningitis; given orally or by intravenous infusion; high oral bioavailability (90%); renal excretion accounts for 80% of clearance, with oxidation and conjugation a further 11%; weak inhibitor of CYP3A4
Flucytosine	3	Renal	Used for systemic fungal and yeast infections, sometimes in combination with amphotericin; given by intravenous infusion; eliminated by glomerular filtration; about 1% is deaminated to 5-fluorouracil (which may explain the bone marrow toxicity)
Griseofulvin	10–21	Metabolism	Used for widespread or intractable dermatophyte infections of the skin, scalp and nails where topical treatment has been ineffective; given orally; variable absorption, which is increased by ingestion with fatty foods (bioavailability not defined); eliminated by glucuronidation
Itraconazole	20	Metabolism	Used for numerous local and systemic fungal infections; given orally; oral bioavailability is 55%; eliminated by hepatic metabolism followed by biliary excretion; metabolised by and is a competitive inhibitor of CYP3A4
Ketoconazole	6–10	Metabolism + bile	Used for systemic mycoses and for a range of serious and resistant infections; given orally; incomplete bioavailability owing to first-pass metabolism (absolute bioavailability has not been reported); metabolised by CYP3A4 and inhibits CYP3A4 metabolism of other drugs
Miconazole	24	Metabolism	Used for oral and intestinal infections; given orally; poorly absorbed from the gut; data indicate that up to 50% is absorbed from the gut but blood levels are too low to give a therapeutic effect
Nystatin	–	–	Principally used for *Candida albicans* infections of skin and mucous membranes; given orally or topically (for vaginal and skin infections); not absorbed from the gastrointestinal tract or from intact skin
Sulconazole	–	Renal	Used for fungal skin infections; applied as a cream; limited absorption across the skin (5–15%); absorbed drug is eliminated in the urine; half-life will be limited by the absorption rate

continued

Drugs used for infections *(continued)*

Drug	Half-life (h)	Elimination	Comments
Antifungal agents *(continued)*			
Terbinafine	11–17	Metabolism	Drug of choice for fungal nail infections (also used for ringworm infections); given orally; good oral bioavailability (80%); numerous pathways of metabolism; does not inhibit P450 isoenzymes
Tioconazole	–	–	Used for fungal nail infections; applied as a solution; negligible systemic absorption after topical treatment
Voriconazole	6	Metabolism	Used for invasive aspergillosis and other serious infections; given orally or by intravenous infusion; high oral bioavailability (96%); metabolised mainly by the polymorphic enzyme CYP2C19; poor metabolisers have fourfold higher blood levels
Antiviral agents			
Reverse transcriptase inhibitors			Each drug is used for the treatment of HIV infection in combination with other antiretroviral drugs (any other indications are given under the individual drug)
Abacavir	1.5	Metabolism	Given orally; good oral bioavailability (80%); metabolised by alcohol dehydrogenase and glucuronidation; does not inhibit P450 isoenzymes
Didanosine	0.6–1.4	Renal + metabolism	Given orally; absorption is approximately 20–40% but affected by gastric acidity and food; about one-half of the absorbed fraction is excreted unchanged in the urine and the remainder metabolised (pathways not known)
Efavirenz	40–70	Metabolism	Non-nucleoside drug; given orally; variable and incomplete absorption; metabolised by CYP3A4 and CYP2B6, which it induces; half-life is shorter after regular dosage (40–55 h) compared with the first dose (50–75 h) (because of autoinduction)
Emtricitabine	10	Renal + metabolism	Given orally; rapidly and essentially completely absorbed; forms an intracellular triphosphate which has a half-life of about 40 h; eliminated largely by renal secretion and by S-oxidation and conjugation with glucuronic acid
Lamivudine	5–7	Renal + metabolism	Also used for chronic hepatitis B with evidence of viral replication; given orally; rapid and nearly complete absorption as parent drug (90%); eliminated largely in the urine unchanged; the intracellular half-life of the active triphosphate metabolite (11–16 h) is longer than that of the parent drug in the plasma
Nevirapine	45	Metabolism	Used in advanced disease in combination with at least two other drugs; given orally; high bioavailability (90%); eliminated by hepatic metabolism via CYP3A4; half-life is reduced to 25–30 h after chronic treatment, owing to induction of its own metabolism

continued

Drugs used for infections (continued)

Drug	Half-life (h)	Elimination	Comments
Antiviral agents (continued)			
Stavudine	1–1.6	Renal + metabolism	Given orally; high oral bioavailability (> 80%); approximately equal amounts eliminated unchanged and by metabolism through normal pathways of pyrimidine biochemistry
Tenofovir disoproxil	17	Renal	Given orally; rapidly converted to tenofovir in the gut, giving a bioavailability of 25%; forms active intracellular diphosphate metabolite; eliminated by glomerular filtration and renal tubular secretion
Zalcitabine	1–2	Renal + metabolism	Given orally; high oral bioavailability (80–90%); about 75% is eliminated unchanged; metabolism is by normal pathways for pyrimidines (including phosphorylation)
Zidovudine	1	Metabolism + renal	Also used for prevention of maternal–fetal HIV transmission; given orally or by intravenous infusion; oral bioavailability is about 65% owing to first-pass metabolism; most of the dose is metabolised by glucuronidation, with limited excretion unchanged (about 20%); intracellular phosphorylation may be saturable, which may explain the apparent non-linear dose–response relationship
Protease inhibitors			Each drug is used for the treatment of HIV infection in combination with other antiretroviral drugs (any other indications are given under the individual drug); all are given by oral route only
Amprenavir	7–10	Metabolism	Used in patients treated previously with other antiretroviral drugs; metabolised by CYP3A4 to numerous metabolites that are eliminated in bile
Indinavir	2	Metabolism (+ renal)	Used in combination with nucleoside reverse transcriptase inhibitors; oral bioavailability is only 18–20% owing to metabolism by CYP3A4 in gut wall and liver, and by efflux from enterocytes back into the gut lumen by the P-glycoprotein transporter (saturation of which results in increased absorption at high doses); eliminated solely by CYP3A4 metabolism; metabolites eliminated via the faeces
Lopinavir (with ritonavir)	5–6	Metabolism	The extent of absorption is increased markedly by a high-fat meal; metabolised by CYP3A4 to numerous metabolites that are eliminated in bile
Nelfinavir	3.5–5	Metabolism + bile	Oral bioavailability in humans is not known; metabolised in liver by CYP3A4, with a major metabolite as active as the parent drug; metabolites plus parent drug (about 20%) are eliminated via the faeces
Ritonavir	3–5	Metabolism	Used for progressive and advanced HIV infection in combination with nucleoside reverse transcriptase inhibitors, and low doses are used to increase the effect of some protease inhibitors; oral bioavailability in humans is not known, but is very high (>70%) in test animals; metabolised by CYP3A4 and is an inhibitor of the enzyme (more potent than other protease inhibitors); one of the metabolites is as active as the parent drug; metabolites eliminated in the faeces

continued

Drugs used for infections *(continued)*

Drug	Half-life (h)	Elimination	Comments
Antiviral agents *(continued)*			
Saquinavir	5–7	Metabolism	Oral bioavailability is low and variable (1–30%) (see indinavir for reasons) and is considerably influenced by food; metabolised by CYP3A4, and metabolites are eliminated in the faeces (different papers have reported average half-lives of between 1 and 7 h after oral dosage, and 10–15 h after intravenous dosage, which suggests this inconsistency is an artifact of analytical sensitivity)
Viral DNA polymerase inhibitors			
Aciclovir	3	Renal (+ metabolism)	Used for herpes simplex and varicella–zoster infections; given orally, topically or by intravenous infusion; slowly and poorly absorbed from the gut (bioavailability = 10–20%); eliminated largely by renal tubular secretion + filtration; only about 10% is metabolised to inactive excretory products
Cidofovir	3	Renal	Used for CMV in people with AIDS; given by intravenous infusion; phosphorylated analogue of aciclovir; undergoes further intracellular phosphorylation to mono-, di- and triphosphates, which have longer half-lives; eliminated by renal tubular secretion + filtration
Famciclovir (prodrug for penciclovir)	2 (penciclovir)	Metabolism	Used for treatment of herpes zoster, acute genital herpes simplex and suppression of recurrent genital herpes infections; given orally; inactive prodrug for penciclovir; negligible oral absorption intact, but extensive conversion to penciclovir (77%); penciclovir is eliminated largely by renal excretion; triphosphate formed intracellularly has a longer half-life
Foscarnet	3–7	Renal	Used for CMV retinitis in people with AIDS and mucocutaneous herpes simplex infections unresponsive to aciclovir in immunocompromised subjects; given by intravenous infusion; highly polar compound; eliminated by glomerular filtration and renal tubular secretion + filtration
Ganciclovir	4	Renal	Used for life-threatening or sight-threatening CMV infections in immunocompromised patients only; given by intravenous infusion; very low oral bioavailability (3–7%), which is enhanced by food; eliminated largely by glomerular filtration
Valaciclovir	3 (aciclovir)	Metabolism	Uses similar to aciclovir; given orally; rapidly and well absorbed (bioavailability 55%); rapidly and extensively metabolised to aciclovir; aciclovir is eliminated by the kidneys
Valganciclovir	4 (as ganciclovir)	Metabolism to ganciclovir	Used for CMV retinitis in people with AIDS and for prevention of CMV infection following transplantation from an infected donor; L-valyl ester prodrug of ganciclovir; given orally; nearly completely converted to ganciclovir by intestinal and hepatic esterases giving a 'bioavailability' as ganciclovir of 60% (compared with 3–7% when the parent drug itself is given)

continued

Drugs used for infections *(continued)*

Drug	Half-life (h)	Elimination	Comments
Other antivirals			
Adefovir dipivoxil	8 (adefovir)	Hydrolysis	Used for chronic hepatitis B infection with either compensated liver disease and evidence of viral replication or decompensated liver disease; given orally; after oral dosage, diester prodrug extensively converted to adefovir, which is eliminated by filtration plus active renal tubular secretion
Amantidine	10–15	Renal	Used for herpes zoster and influenza A; given orally; slowly but completely absorbed from the gut; eliminated by active renal tubular secretion plus filtration
Enfuvirtide	4	Metabolism	Used for the treatment of HIV infection in combination with other antiretroviral drugs for resistant infection or in subjects intolerant to other drugs; given by subcutaneous injection; a peptide that undergoes hepatic hydrolysis
Idoxuridine	?	?	Used for topical infections with herpes simplex and herpes zoster, but is of little value; given as a 5% solution; few data available
Inosine pranobex	?	?	Used for mucocutanous herpes simplex, genital warts and subacute sclerosing panencephalitis; given orally; very few data available; complex that probably decomposes to *p*-acetamidobenzoic acid, *N,N*-dimethylamino-2-propanol and inosine
Oseltamivir	1–3	Hydrolysis	Used to treat influenza in at-risk subjects if started within 48 h of onset of symptoms; given orally; undergoes almost complete first-pass metabolism to the carboxylic acid analogue (the active form), which has a longer half-life (6–10 h) and is excreted by the kidneys
Palivizumab	20 days	?	Used for prevention of serious lower respiratory tract infection by RSV in neonates and children under 2 years; given by intramuscular injection; humanised monoclonal antibody; very few published kinetic data available
Ribavirin (tribavirin)	7–21 days	Metabolism + renal	Used for severe RSV bronchiolitis in infants and children, and with interferon alfa or peginterferon alfa for chronic hepatitis C infection; given orally or by inhalation; oral bioavailability is 50%; metabolised by hydrolysis of ribosyl group from triazole moiety, which is then excreted in urine; very slowly cleared from erythrocytes and tissue compartments (shorter half-lives are reported after single doses)
Zanamivir	2–5	Renal	Used to treat influenza in at-risk subjects if started within 48 h of onset of symptoms; given by inhalation for influenza; very low oral absorption (1–5%), therefore not given by this route; eliminated in urine
Antiprotozoal drugs			
Antimalarials			
Artemeter with lumefantrine	?	?	Used for the treatment of acute uncomplicated falciparum malaria; given orally; few data available

continued

Drugs used for infections *(continued)*

Drug	Half-life (h)	Elimination	Comments
Antimalarials (continued)			
Atovaquone	3 days	Faeces + urine	Given orally with proguanil for the treatment of acute uncomplicated falciparum malaria and for prophylaxis of falciparum malaria; also used for mild to moderate *Pneumocystis carinii* pneumonia; poor and variable absorption influenced by food; most eliminated in faeces
Chloroquine	30–60 days	Renal + metabolism	Used for chemoprophylaxis and treatment of malaria and also used for rheumatoid arthritis and lupus erythematosus; given orally or by intravenous infusion; complete oral bioavailability; limited metabolism (about 20%) but metabolite retains activity; mostly eliminated by filtration in the kidney; the very long half-life results from the very high volume of distribution (200 l kg^{-1}) and low renal clearance
Mefloquine	15–33 days	Metabolism + renal	Used for chemoprophylaxis and treatment of uncomplicated falciparum and chloroquine-resistant vivax malaria; given orally; good bioavailability (80%); metabolised by hydrolysis and metabolites eliminated in urine and bile; renal clearance accounts for about 10% of total
Primaquine	4–10	Metabolism (+ renal)	Used as an adjunct for eradication of the liver stages of vivax and ovale malaria; given orally; rapidly absorbed, with almost complete bioavailability; metabolised to carboxyprimaquine, which retains antimalarial activity and is implicated in haemolysis
Proguanil (prodrug for cycloguanil)	12–24	Metabolism	Used for chemoprophylaxis of malaria; given orally (alone or with atovaquone); high oral bioavailability; it is a prodrug for cycloguanil (which accounts for 19% of an oral dose), which has a short half-life (2 h), so plasma concentrations of the active metabolite are usually less than those of the parent drug
Pyrimethamine	2–6 days	Metabolism	Used for malaria but only in combination with sulfadoxine; given orally; well absorbed (human bioavailability is not known); numerous metabolites eliminated mainly in the faeces
Quinine	6–47	Metabolism (+ renal)	Used for treatment but not chemoprophylaxis of falciparum malaria, or when the infection is either mixed or not known; also used in combination with doxycycline (see above); given orally or by intravenous infusion; high oral bioavailability (80–90%); eliminated largely by metabolism by CYP3A4; also binds to and inhibits CYP2D6; may also be metabolised by CYP1A2, because smoking (which does not induce CYP3A4) increases its clearance
Sulfadoxine	240	?	Used for malaria but only in combination with pyrimethamine (see above); given orally
Other antiprotozoals			
Diloxanide furoate	–	Metabolism	Used for amoebiasis and is drug of choice for asymptomatic *Entamoeba histolytica* infections; given orally; completely hydrolysed in the gut lumen and mucosa to diloxanide, which is incompletely absorbed; absorbed diloxanide is conjugated with glucuronic acid

continued

Drug compendium

Drugs used for infections *(continued)*

Drug	Half-life (h)	Elimination	Comments
Other antiprotozoals (continued)			
Mepacrine	?	?	Used for giardiasis and discoid lupus erythematosus; given orally; few published data available
Metronidazole	6–9	Metabolism + renal	Used for intestinal and extra-intestinal amoebiasis and for urogenital trichomoniasis and giardiasis; also has antibacterial actions (see above); given orally; complete oral bioavailability; metabolites are eliminated slowly in urine
Pentamidine	13 days	Metabolism + renal	Used for *Pneumocystis carinii* pneumonia, leishmaniasis and trypanosomiasis; given by inhalation (nebuliser), by deep intramuscular injection or by intravenous infusion; metabolised by oxidation, and conjugation with sulphate and glucuronic acid
Stibogluconate	6	As pentavalent antimony	Used for leishmaniasis; given by intravenous injection (over at least 5 min); pentavalent antimony compound; pentavalent antimony eliminated in urine; very slow minor late elimination phase reported (half-life of 76 h) but chemical form of pentavalent antimony not defined
Tinidazole	12–14	Metabolism + renal	Uses are similar to metronidazole; also has antibacterial actions (see above); given orally; complete oral bioavailability; about 25% excreted unchanged and the remainder metabolised and eliminated via urine and bile

Antihelminthic drugs

Drug	Half-life (h)	Elimination	Comments
Albendazole	8–12	Metabolism	Used on a named-patient basis either alone or as an adjunct to surgery for *Echinococcus* infections and for cutaneous hookworm larval infections; given orally; low oral bioavailability (parent drug not usually detectable); metabolised by *S*-oxidation; the parent compound and sulphoxide (SO) are active, while the sulphone $(SO)_2$ is inactive
Diethylcarbamazine	?	?	A filaricide (not available in the UK); no data available
Ivermectin	12	Metabolism	Used on a named-patient basis as the drug of choice for onchocerciasis, also used for cutaneous hookworm larval infections and for chronic *Strongyloides* infections; given orally; bioavailability is not defined; eliminated as metabolites in faeces
Levamisole	4–6	Metabolism	Used on a named-patient basis as the drug of choice for *Ascaris lumbricoides* infection; given orally; bioavailability 60–70%; oxidised in liver and conjugated with glucuronic acid
Mebendazole	3–9	Metabolism	Used for threadworm, roundworm, whipworm and hookworm infections; given orally; low bioavailability (20% for solutions, 2% for tablets); metabolites excreted in urine
Niclosamide	?	?	Used on a named-patient basis for tapeworm infections; given orally; few data available

continued

Drugs used for infections *(continued)*

Drug	Half-life (h)	Elimination	Comments
Antihelminthic drugs *(continued)*			
Piperazine	?	Renal	Used for threadworm and roundworm infections; given orally; 5–30% of an oral dose is excreted in urine unchanged within 24 h; few data available
Praziquantel	2	Metabolism	Used on a named-patient basis for tapeworm infections and bilharziasis; given orally; probably extensive first-pass metabolism; rapidly metabolised and excreted
Tiabendazole	1.2	Metabolism	Used on a named-patient basis as the drug of choice for *Strongyloides* infection and used for cutaneous hookworm larval infections; given orally; rapidly and extensively absorbed; metabolised by oxidation and conjugation

Key AIDS, acquired immunodeficiency disease; CMV, cytomegalovirus; HIV, human immunodeficiency virus; MRSA, methicillin-resistant *Staphylococcus aureus*; RSV, respiratory syncytial virus.

Drug compendium

Chemotherapy of malignancy

Approximately 20–25% of people in the Western world die from cancer. Surgery and radiotherapy are valuable for treating localised cancers but are less effective in prolonging life once the tumour has spread to produce metastases. The successful treatment of cancer frequently involves a multidisciplinary approach, which also includes necessary psychological and social support. The introduction of cytotoxic chemotherapy to kill rapidly proliferating neoplastic cells has had a major impact on the successful treatment of malignant disease, especially diffuse tumours.

A wide range of different chemicals, with a variety of mechanisms and sites of action within the cell, has been introduced into clinical practice since the 1970s. Although the agents may differ in their specific cellular targets, they nearly all rely on the rapid rate of growth and division of cancer cells to provide a degree of selectivity between normal and malignant tissue. The drugs share a number of generic properties and characteristics, both beneficial and adverse, which will be discussed first. The major classes of drug will then be discussed, with information on mechanisms of action and general toxic effects.

The rate of introduction of new anticancer drugs decreased in the 1990s, largely because effective agents were already available. A placebo-controlled clinical trial (Ch. 3) of a new antineoplastic drug given as sole treatment is now unethical, and the efficacy of any new agent usually has to be assessed by its addition to the best available current therapy. Therefore, a successful new agent would have to show a clinically significant effect above that of current treatment. There are a number of in vivo animal tests for detecting antineoplastic activity, but these frequently overpredict the likely effectiveness of a compound in clinical use, because the animal tumours used as models have a much higher growth fraction (see below). For all these reasons, many recent advances in cancer chemotherapy have arisen from the more effective use of existing agents, by optimising drug combinations and regimens, and by minimising toxicity, rather than the introduction of novel compounds. Recent developments in molecular biology are resulting in the discovery of new potential targets for drug action, and a resurgence of drug development. The ability of molecular biological approaches to define the mechanisms of cell–cell communication, apoptosis, angiogenesis etc., will undoubtedly prove a major stimulus for the production of new drugs with greater selectivity for cancer cells.

Molecular origins of cancer

Most cancers probably arise from a combination of genetic mutations in a cell, with sequential gene defects resulting in progressive changes in the cell through initial metaplastic and dysplastic phases, and then to invasive and ultimately metastatic cancer.

The genetic changes that result in cancer lead to activation of oncogenes (cell factors that cause cells to divide), and suppression or deletion of tumour suppressor genes. As a result, there is unregulated cell proliferation, and also a delay in programmed cell death (apoptosis). Normal cells are regulated by numerous external factors that control cell growth and death. These include growth factors, cytokines and hormones that activate or suppress the genes controlling cell division. Gene mutations that activate oncogenes lead to the excessive production of proteins that inhibit cell death, and that allow cell growth in the absence of stimulation by an external regulator. Genetic changes also result in low activity of tumour suppressor genes, which would normally inhibit cell division and cause programmed cell death. Genetic changes in cancer cells can give rise to metabolic changes or transporters such as P-glycoprotein that confer resistance to chemotherapy. Growth factors secreted by cancer cells promote angiogenesis and increase blood supply to the tumour. Other secreted factors can impede the host's immune response to the cancer cells.

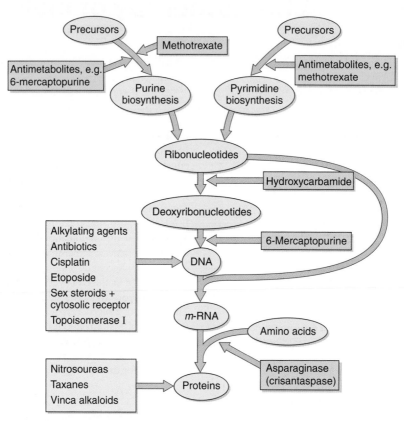

Fig. 52.1
Sites of action for the main groups of anticancer drugs.

Proto-oncogenes are normal gene sequences that control cell proliferation and differentiation. They are capable of being activated to oncogenes, the expression of which leads to tumour development. Considerable attention is currently being given to the products of proto-oncogene activation, since these are often linked to cell growth factors and may provide useful targets for drug development. Identification of the protein sequence and tertiary structure of the growth factors may allow new drug molecules to be designed to interact specifically with the growth factor (analogous to recent developments in the field of receptor pharmacology). However, whether this will increase the selectivity of drugs for neoplastic cells compared with normal cells is unknown, because selectivity may still be based on rates of growth and division. Other possible future approaches for therapy are to increase the effectiveness of tumour suppressor genes.

Antineoplastic agents

Mechanisms of action

The majority of antineoplastic agents act on the process of DNA synthesis within the cancer cell, as summarised in Figure 52.1. Therefore, selectivity of these drugs for cancer cells compared with normal tissues is determined by the rate of DNA synthesis and cell division. Resting cells, that is those in the G_0 phase (Fig. 52.2), are resistant to many antineoplastic drugs. Some antineoplastic drugs, such as the antimetabolites, work effectively only when the cells are in the appropriate phase of the cell cycle at the time of treatment with the drug; these are termed cell cycle-specific agents (Fig. 52.2). Other drugs, such as the alkylating agents, nitrosoureas and cisplatin, have a 'hit and run' action on the DNA, and it is not critical when the cell is exposed, because the drug effect becomes apparent later when the cells attempt to undergo division.

Therefore, the sensitivity of a cancer to treatment depends on its growth fraction – that is, the fraction of cells undergoing mitosis at any time. For example, in Burkitt's lymphoma, almost 100% of neoplastic cells are undergoing division, and the tumour is very sensitive to chemotherapy, showing a dramatic response to a single dose of cyclophosphamide. In contrast, the growth fraction in a carcinoma of the colon represents less than 5% of cells, resulting in its relative resistance to chemotherapy. However, metastases from colonic carcinoma deposited in the liver and elsewhere initially have a high growth fraction and are sensitive to anticancer

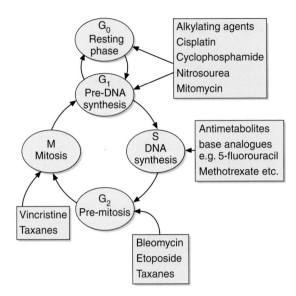

Fig. 52.2
Sites of action for the main groups of cell cycle-specific anticancer drugs.

drugs; therefore, chemotherapy is frequently given following surgical removal of the primary tumour.

Using in vitro cancer cell lines, it has been shown that:

- antineoplastic drugs produce a proportional cell kill; in other words, a proportion, such as 95% of the cells present, may be eliminated during a single course of treatment; consequently, multiple treatments may be necessary to eradicate the cancer, with each treatment producing an exponential decrease in the number of residual viable cancer cells
- essentially complete eradication of tumour cells is necessary to prevent regrowth
- efficacy of chemotherapy is increased if treatment with cell cycle-specific drugs is timed to coincide with the appropriate phase of cell division within the cell population.

While these concepts apply to in vivo therapy of cancers, risk–benefit considerations can change with successive treatments and preclude complete eradication of the tumour. In addition, the immune system probably contributes to the final removal of residual malignant cells, and yet most antineoplastic drugs compromise immunoresponsiveness, which will reduce this removal process. Finally, the periodicity of doses is less critical in vivo because cancer cell cycles are not synchronised within the target cell population between treatments.

Resistance

Resistance to chemotherapeutic agents may develop in a number of ways (further explanations are given later in the text under the individual agents).

- Reduced drug uptake into cancer cells, e.g. methotrexate enters cells by the high-affinity transport system used for reduced folate (tetrahydrofolic acid), and downregulation of the transporter limits the uptake of methotrexate and confers resistance to the drug.
- Use of alternative metabolic pathways and salvage mechanisms to circumvent a blocked biochemical process; such mechanisms are usually drug-specific, e.g. induction of asparagine synthesis in cells exposed to crisantaspase (asparaginase).
- Alteration of intracellular drug targets, e.g. production of topoisomerase II with reduced sensitivity to the inhibitory effects of anthracyclines.
- Increased inactivation of the compound within the cancer cell, e.g. high intracellular levels of glutathione-S-transferase inactivate cisplatin and alkylating agents.
- Reduced activation of prodrugs, e.g. low intracellular levels of deoxycytidine kinase reduces activation of cytarabine (cytosine arabinoside).
- Increased removal of the drug from the cancer cell. This involves the possibility of increased transcription of the gene for proteins which act as carriers for the elimination from the cell of complex foreign chemicals (see Ch. 2), including a number of cytotoxic compounds. There are several such proteins, including P-glycoprotein and the multidrug resistance protein (MRP1). The increased production of the carrier confers multidrug resistance to a number of structurally unrelated natural compounds, or their derivatives, including vinca alkaloids, etoposide, taxanes, anthracyclines, dactinomycin (actinomycin D), mitomycin C and mitoxantrone. The carrier can be blocked by calcium channel antagonists, such as nifedipine or verapamil, or by ciclosporin and tamoxifen. These drugs may be added to cytotoxic drug regimens to minimise resistance.

Unwanted effects

Cytotoxic antineoplastic drugs are among the most toxic compounds given to humans. Many have a therapeutic index of approximately 1 – that is, the therapeutic dose usually is the toxic dose. Because drug selectivity is for tissues with a high growth fraction, it is not surprising that a number of normal non-malignant tissues are also affected. In addition to effects that occur in all rapidly dividing tissues, many chemotherapeutic drugs also have specific toxic effects on other tissues. Dosage regimens are usually designed so that normal tissues, especially bone marrow and gut, can recover between doses (Fig. 52.3).

Gastrointestinal tract. Mucosal cells have a rapid turnover. Toxicity can produce anorexia, mucosal

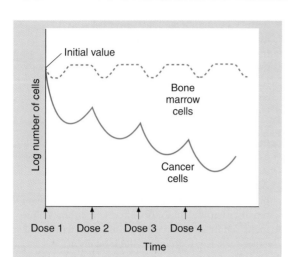

Fig. 52.3
Hypothetical dosing schedule to allow recovery of normal tissues.
The malignant cells show a greater proportional kill because a greater fraction are in division at any time. Theoretically, the response of the malignant cells to dose 2 would be greater than for dose 1 if cell cycles became synchronised and dose 2 was given during the correct phase of the growth cycle. A typical dose interval would be 3–4 weeks. A minimum of 10^9 tumour cells are usually present when tumours are first detectable.

ulceration or diarrhoea. Nausea and vomiting are common, especially with alkylating agents and cisplatin, and this may limit an individual's ability to tolerate an optimal dosage regimen.

Bone marrow. Myelosuppression is a serious consequence of treatment and can lead to severe leucopenia, thrombocytopenia and, sometimes, anaemia. These haematological consequences may limit the drug dosage that the person being treated is able to tolerate. There is a high risk of both infection and haemorrhage following cytotoxic chemotherapy (see the drug compendium table).

Hair follicle cells. Partial or complete alopecia may occur, but this is usually temporary.

Reproductive organs. Both sexes are affected and sterility can result, particularly after therapy with cyclophosphamide or cytarabine; women frequently have dysmenorrhoea or amenorrhoea. Because of the mechanisms of action of cytotoxic drugs, most would be expected to exhibit teratogenic activity. Pregnant women should not be exposed to cytotoxic drugs for treatment or as members of the healthcare team. Drugs that mimic or affect the activity of sex hormones are frequently used for the treatment of breast or prostate cancer, and these produce adverse effects on sexual function.

Growing tissues in children. Of particular concern in children is the possibility that intensive cytotoxic chemotherapy can impair growth. Children treated with cytotoxic drugs for malignancy also have an increased risk of the subsequent development of a second malignancy (about 10%), which is often leukaemia.

Drug combinations

It is common practice to treat many cancers with a mixture of different antineoplastic drugs simultaneously, and there are numerous permutations used clinically. Criteria for selecting ideal combinations are:

- each drug should be an active antineoplastic drug in its own right (e.g. a second drug would not be given simply to increase the formation of an active metabolite of the first)
- each drug should have a different mechanism of action and target site within the cancer cell: this will increase efficacy while reducing the likelihood of resistance
- each drug should have a different site for any organ-specific toxicity (some common toxicity is almost inevitable because nearly all agents affect tissues with a high growth factor).

Specific antineoplastic agents

The drug compendium table gives the uses of individual drugs and notes any unusual or limiting toxicity.

Agents affecting nucleic acid function

Alkylating agents

Examples: cyclophosphamide, melphalan, busulfan, chlorambucil

The nitrogen mustards were developed from the sulphur mustard gases used in the trenches in World War I. These chemical warfare gases caused bone marrow suppression in addition to the respiratory toxicity for which they were developed. Replacement of the divalent sulphur atom by trivalent nitrogen allowed the introduction of a complex side-chain, which resulted in a range of more stable non-volatile agents that could be given therapeutically under controlled conditions. Alkylating agents contain side-chains (for example -CH_2CH_2Cl) which undergo a metabolic activation step that involves loss of part of the molecule (for example the Cl is lost from -CH_2CH_2Cl) and yields a highly reactive product which binds to DNA or proteins. Many alkylating agents are bifunctional (i.e. have two reactive groups).

Mechanism of action
The reactive alkylating group(s) in the molecule may be:

- *nitrogen mustard* N-CH$_2$CH$_2$Cl (Cl is the leaving group), e.g. carmustine (BCNU), chlorambucil, chlormethine, cyclophosphamide, estramustine, ifosfamide, lomustine (CCNU), melphalan
- *sulphonate ester* -CH$_2$OSO$_2$CH$_3$ (SO$_2$CH$_3$ is the leaving group), e.g. bulsulfan, treosulfan
- *nitrosourea* -N-N=O, e.g. carmustine, lomustine
- *cyclic nitrogen derivative* (a three-membered ring with CH$_2$, CH$_2$ and N as the three components), e.g. thiotepa (which has three of these rings attached to a central P-S group).

The mechanism of action is by covalent binding to DNA (nitrogen mustards, sulphonate esters and cyclic nitrogen compounds), which prevents DNA and RNA synthesis, by binding to proteins (nitrosoureas), which blocks DNA repair processes such that the DNA damage cannot be repaired and the cell is killed. Because of the covalent nature of the product, these effects are not cell cycle-specific (Fig. 52.2).

The alkylating agents are highly reactive and produce a chemical species that binds covalently to sites within DNA, such as N-7 of guanine. The alkylated guanine in DNA may either be repaired, in which case the cell survives, or it may interfere with DNA replication by:

- being misread
- undergoing further metabolism via ring opening
- cross-linking to another guanine (bifunctional drugs, via the remaining reactive group).

Alkylating agents have numerous clinical uses in cancer chemotherapy.

Pharmacokinetics

The pharmacokinetic characteristics of the alkylating agents depend on the nature of the reactive group(s) and the third non-reactive substituent on the N-atom. The original and simplest drug is chlormethine, which is a nitrogen mustard with a simple methyl group and two -CH$_2$CH$_2$Cl groups attached to the N-atom; it is very unstable, and solutions have to be injected soon after preparation because decomposition occurs within minutes. Care is necessary when handling the toxic dosing solutions, and chlormethine is now used much less commonly. A major advance in the use of nitrogen mustards was achieved with the introduction of cyclophosphamide, which is a chemically stable solid chemical that can be given orally. It is a prodrug that undergoes metabolic activation to produce two toxic metabolites: acrolein (CH$_2$=CHCHO) and phosphoramide mustard, which contains the N-(CH$_2$CH$_2$Cl)$_2$ group. Ifosfamide undergoes similar metabolism to cyclophosphamide, and toxic metabolites of both cyclophosphamide and ifosfamide are excreted in the urine. Melphalan and chlorambucil, which have an aromatic substituent, undergo rapid metabolism and have short half-lives.

Unwanted effects

- Alkylating agents are highly cytotoxic and cause bone marrow suppression and neutropenia. Amifostine is a compound used to reduce the severity of cyclophosphamide- (and cisplatin-) induced neutropenia in advanced ovarian cancer. It is a prodrug that is metabolised in cells by alkaline phosphatase to a free thiol metabolite that binds to the reactive metabolites of the cytotoxic drugs. Selective protection of normal tissue may result from a higher alkaline phosphatase activity.
- Fertility is reduced through impaired gametogenesis.
- A particular problem with the long-term use of alkylating agents, especially if combined with radiotherapy, is the development of acute myeloid leukaemia.
- Busulfan, carmustine and treosulfan can cause pulmonary fibrosis.
- Busulfan and treosulfan commonly cause skin pigmentation.
- Cyclophosphamide and ifosfamide cause bladder toxicity with haemorrhagic cystitis; this is due to acrolein and can be prevented by prior treatment with mesna (mercaptoethane sulphonic acid; Ch. 53), which provides free thiol groups in the urinary bladder. Bladder cancer may develop years after cyclophosphamide therapy.

Platinum compounds

Examples: cisplatin, carboplatin, oxaliplatin

Mechanism of action

The platinum drugs enter cells and generate a reactive complex that cross-links between guanine units in DNA. The result is similar to that of alkylating agents that break the DNA chain. Cisplatin and carboplatin are particularly useful for ovarian and testicular tumours. Oxaliplatin is used for advanced colorectal cancer.

Pharmacokinetics

These drugs are poorly absorbed from the gut and are given by intravenous infusion. They are mainly excreted by the kidney as platinum compounds and have a long half-life, largely owing to extensive protein binding.

Unwanted effects

- severe nausea and vomiting
- nephrotoxicity with irreversible renal impairment; hydration is important to minimise the risk
- hypomagnesaemia
- ototoxicity with hearing loss and tinnitus
- peripheral neuropathy (especially oxaliplatin)
- myelosuppression (more marked for carboplatin).

Most effects are more marked for cisplatin than for carboplatin. Amifostine (see above) is used to reduce the severity of cisplatin-induced neutropenia in advanced ovarian cancer. It also reduces the nephrotoxicity of cisplatin.

Topoisomerase I inhibitors

Examples: irinotecan, topotecan

These are semi-synthetic derivatives of a cytotoxic alkaloid isolated from the Chinese tree *Camptotheca acuminata*.

Mechanism of action
The drugs inhibit topoisomerase I, which is important in DNA transcription and translation. The enzyme produces single-strand breaks that relieve the torsional strain in DNA; under normal cell conditions, the strands are then religated. The drugs bind to the DNA–topoisomerase I complex and prevent religation. Although this binding is readily reversible, the consequences are irreversible, because cell death occurs when a double-strand break is produced at the DNA replication fork during S phase. Inhibition of DNA repair increases the sensitivity of the cell to ionising radiation. Topoisomerase I inhibitors are given as second-line treatments for metastatic colorectal or ovarian cancer (see the drug compendium table).

Pharmacokinetics
They are large complex molecules that are given by intravenous infusion and are eliminated mainly by hepatic metabolism.

Unwanted effects
- general cytotoxicity, with dose-limiting myelosuppression
- diarrhoea; cholinergic stimulation produces early diarrhoea, but other toxicity can result in delayed onset.

Cytotoxic antibiotics

Examples: bleomycin, dactinomycin, doxorubicin, epirubicin, mitomycin, mitoxantrone

The cytotoxic antibiotics represent a diverse range of chemical structures.

- The 'rubicin' drugs are all quinone-containing four-ringed structures (planar anthraquinones) that contain an amino sugar group.
- Mitoxantrone has a three-ringed planar quinone structure with amino-containing side-chains, and mitomycin is a non-planar tricyclic quinone.

- Bleomycin and dactinomycin are complex peptide or glycopeptide derivatives.

Mechanisms of action
Although these antibiotics affect normal nucleic acid function, they also have a number of other mechanisms of action.

- Intercalation. This is shown particularly by the rubicins, with the planar ring system intercalating between DNA bases, and the amino sugar part binding to the deoxyribose phosphate groups. Intercalation blocks reading of the DNA template and also stimulates topoisomerase II-dependent DNA double-strand breaks.
- Free radical attack. The metabolism of the drugs gives rise to superoxide and hydroxyl radicals and hydrogen peroxide, which cause DNA damage and cytotoxicity.
- Membrane effects. Interference with membrane function can occur either directly or via oxidative damage.

In general, the mechanisms of action are not cell cycle-specific, although some members of the class are reported to show greatest activity at certain phases of the cycle, for example S phase (doxorubicin, mitoxantrone), G_1 and early S phase (mitomycin), and G_2 phase and mitosis (bleomycin).

Pharmacokinetics
The cytotoxic antibiotics are poorly absorbed from the gut and are given intravenously. They are eliminated by metabolism, and some have very long half-lives.

Unwanted effects
Many of these drugs have radiomimetic properties. They should not be used at the same time as radiotherapy, since toxicity can be greatly increased.

- general cytotoxicity
- doxorubicin, epirubicin and mitoxantrone produce dose-related irreversible myocardial damage leading to cardiomyopathy, through free radical release and oxidative stress; liposomal formulations of doxorubicin may reduce the cardiac toxicity
- painful skin eruptions with liposomal doxorubicin
- bleomycin often causes skin pigmentation
- bleomycin and mitomycin produce dose-related pulmonary fibrosis.

Antimetabolites

Antimetabolites interfere with normal metabolic pathways. They can be divided into folate antagonists and analogues of purine or pyrimidine bases (Fig. 52.1).

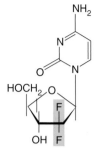

Fig. 52.4
The structure of some antimetabolites, illustrating their similarity to normal bases and nucleotides (structural changes are highlighted).

Fludarabine (F replaces
H of adenosine and ribose
is replaced by arabose)

5-Fluorouracil
(F replaces H
of uracil)

Gemcitabine
(F replaces H and
OH on ribose ring)

6-Mercaptopurine
(sulphur substitute
in purine)

Folic acid antagonists

Example: methotrexate

An astute clinical observation, that the administration of folic acid to children with leukaemia exacerbated their condition, led to the development of a folate antagonist, methotrexate. This represented an important landmark in cancer chemotherapy.

Mechanism of action and uses

Folic acid in its reduced form (tetrahydrofolic acid; THF) is an important biochemical intermediate. It is essential for synthetic reactions that involve the addition of a single carbon atom during a biochemical reaction, such as the introduction of the methyl group into thymidylate and the synthesis of the purine ring system. During such reactions, THF is oxidised to dihydrofolic acid (DHF), which has to be reduced by dihydrofolate reductase back to THF before it can accept a further 1-carbon group, and be reused.

Methotrexate has a very high affinity for, and inhibits the active site of, mammalian dihydrofolate reductase. This blocks purine and thymidylate synthesis and inhibits the synthesis of DNA, RNA and protein. Methotrexate blocks dihydrofolate reductase and the 1-carbon cycle. It may show selectivity for cancer cells because these rely more on de novo synthesis of purines and pyrimidines, whereas normal tissues use salvage pathways (for preformed purines and pyrimidines) to a greater extent. Methotrexate is specific for S phase and slows G_1 to S phase.

Methotrexate is given for acute lymphoblastic leukaemia, non-Hodgkin's lymphomas and various other malignancies. It is also used in non-malignant conditions such as inflammatory joint diseases and psoriasis (Chs 30 and 49).

Pharmacokinetics

Methotrexate is well absorbed from the gut but can also be given intravenously or intrathecally. It is eliminated by renal excretion, but a small amount may be retained for longer periods both strongly bound to the dihydrofolate reductase and intracellularly as polyglutamate conjugates.

Unwanted effects

- toxicity to normal rapidly dividing tissues (especially the bone marrow)
- hepatotoxicity can follow chronic therapy (as in psoriasis).

Toxicity is increased in the presence of reduced renal excretion, and methotrexate should be avoided if there is significant renal impairment. Folinic acid (leucovorin) is frequently administered shortly after high-dose methotrexate, to reduce mucositis and myelosuppression. Non-steroidal anti-inflammatory drugs such as aspirin can reduce renal excretion of methotrexate and increase its toxicity.

Base analogues

Examples: capecitabine, cladribine, cytarabine, fludarabine, fluorouracil, gemcitabine, mercaptopurine, ralitrexed, tegafur, tioguanine (6-thioguanine)

A number of useful chemotherapeutic agents have been produced by simple modifications to the structures of normal purine and pyrimidine bases (Fig. 52.4). These act in a number of ways to interfere with DNA synthesis (Table 52.1).

Table 52.1
Mechanisms of action of base analogues

Analogue	Metabolism	Action	Cell cycle effect
Cladribine	Phosphorylated intracellularly by deoxycytidine kinase	The main action is by incorporation of the triphosphate into DNA and blocking DNA polymerase and DNA ligase	Not specific
Cytarabine	Phosphorylated intracellularly by deoxycytidine kinase	The main action is by incorporation of the triphosphate into DNA and blocking DNA polymerase and DNA ligase	Specific: mostly active is S phase
Fludarabine	Phosphorylated intracellularly by deoxycytidine kinase	The main action is by incorporation of the triphosphate into DNA and blocking DNA polymerase and DNA ligase	Specific: mostly active in S phase
5-Fluorouracil	Phosphorylated intracellularly to fluorouridine monophosphate (FUMP) and the deoxy analogue (FdUMP)	FdUMP inhibits thymidylate synthase, is converted to the triphosphate and is incorporated into DNA. FUMP is converted to the triphosphate and is incorporated into RNA	Some selectivity for G_2 and S phases
Gemcitabine	Converted to a triphosphate	Trihosphate is incorporated into DNA and blocks elongation and promotes apoptosis	Specific for S phase
6-Mercatopurine	Phosphorylated to mono- and triphosphate	Monophosphate inhibits de novo purine synthesis. Triphosphates are incorporated into DNA and/or RNA giving cytotoxicity	Specific for S phase
Ralitrexed	–	Inhibits thymidylate synthase	
Tioguanine	Converted to intracellular nucleotides	Main action arises from incorporation of triphosphates into DNA and RNA. The nucleotides cause 'pseudo' feedback inhibition of the synthesis of other purines and inhibit purine nucleotide interconvensions	Active in G_1 and S phases

Pharmacokinetics

Base analogues tend to be absorbed and metabolised by the pathways involved with the corresponding normal (unmodified) base. Oral absorption is often erratic, and most are given intravenously. The urine is a minor route of elimination (up to 1% of the parent drug) and half-lives are short to intermediate. Tegafur is a prodrug of fluorouracil, and is given in combination with uracil, which inhibits the breakdown of fluorouracil.

Unwanted effects

- typical cytotoxic effects are common; myelosuppression, in particular, can be severe and prolonged after cladribine, cytarabine and fludarabine
- drug interaction: allopurinol (Ch. 31) interferes with the metabolism of 6-mercaptopurine, and the dose should be reduced if these drugs are used concurrently.

Agents affecting microtubule function

Vinca alkaloids and etoposide

Examples: vinblastine, vincristine, vinorelbine, etoposide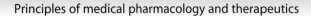

The vinca alkaloids are complex natural chemicals isolated from the periwinkle plant (*Vinca rosea*). Etoposide is a synthetic derivative of a compound that is extracted from the mandrake root (*Podophyllum peltatum*) and is sometimes called a 'podophyllotoxin'.

Mechanism of action and uses

Vinca alkaloids bind to tubulin and cause depolymerisation of microtubules, thus producing metaphase arrest. They are therefore cycle-specific. The vinca alkaloids are used for various lymphomas and for acute leukaemia. They are also effective in some solid tumours.

Etoposide is active during the G_2 phase and binds to the complex of DNA and topoisomerase II (an enzyme involved in the uncoiling and coiling of DNA during repair). The etoposide-bound complex prevents DNA replication and causes strand breaks.

Pharmacokinetics

The absorption of oral doses of vinca alkaloids is unpredictable and they are usually given intravenously. Etoposide can be given orally. Elimination is largely by metabolism, with little renal excretion. They have long half-lives.

Unwanted effects

The spectrum of unwanted effects differs between different drugs, despite their close structural similarities.

- General cytotoxicity. Myelosuppression is dose-limiting for vinblastine and vinorelbine, but unusual with vincristine.
- Neurotoxicity is dose-limiting with vincristine. It causes peripheral paraesthesiae, loss of tendon reflexes, abdominal pain and constipation; motor weakness occasionally accompanies the sensory neuropathy
- Severe tissue damage if the drugs extravasate from the infusion site.

Taxanes

Examples: docetaxel, paclitaxel

The clinically used drugs are produced from taxane, which is a diterpenoid extracted from the bark of the Pacific Yew tree (*Taxus bretifolia*).

Mechanism of action

Taxanes promote the assembly of microtubules and inhibit their depolymerisation, leading to the formation of stable and non-functional microtubular bundles in the cell. They bind to a different site to that used by vinca alkaloids. Microtubules are essential for numerous cellular functions, including maintenance of cell shape, motility, transport between organelles and cell division.

The cell is inhibited during G_2 and M phases of the cell cycle. Taxanes are also radiosensitisers, since cells in the G_2 and M phases are more sensitive to radiation. The drugs are used for ovarian and breast cancer.

Pharmacokinetics

These drugs are given intravenously because of poor oral absorption. They are extensively metabolised in the liver and have short half-lives.

Unwanted effects

- General cytotoxicity.
- Severe hypersensitivity reactions can occur, with hypotension, angioedema and bronchospasm. Routine premedication with histamine (H_1 and H_2) receptor antagonists (Chs 33 and 39) combined with a corticosteroid (Ch. 44) is recommended.
- Neutropenia is dose-limiting.
- Arthalgia/myalgia syndrome.
- Paclitaxel causes peripheral sensory neuropathy, with motor neuropathy at high dosages.
- Docetaxel causes persistent leg oedema due to fluid retention.

Miscellaneous anticancer drugs

Examples: amsacrine, bexarotene, crisantaspase (asparaginase), dacarbazine, hydroxycarbamide, imatinib, pentostatin, porifimer sodium, procarbazine, temoporfin, temozolomide, tretinoin

These drugs represent a mixture of compounds with a variety of mechanisms of action. Further details are given in the drug compendium table.

Mechanisms of action

Most potential biochemical sites within the process of cell division have been investigated as targets for anticancer drugs. Actions of different drugs include:

- removal of asparagine for protein synthesis (crisantaspase)
- inhibition of incorporation of thymidine and adenine into DNA (procarbazine)
- inhibition of adenosine deaminase, which causes a build up of deoxyadenosine triphosphate (dATP), which inhibits the formation of other deoxyribonucleotide triphosphates (pentostatin)
- inhibition of reduction of ribonucleotides to deoxyribonucleotides (hydroxycarbamide)
- intercalation between DNA base pairs (amsacrine)
- alkylating action, especially on thiol groups, to inhibit DNA repair (dacarbazine and temozolomide)
- increased cell differentiation by action on retinoid receptors (RAR and RXR) (bexarotene, tretinoin) (Ch. 49)
- photodynamic activation in superficial tumours by laser light to produce cytotoxic oxygen free radicals (porfimer sodium, temoporfin).

Pharmacokinetics

The drugs show a diverse array of pharmacokinetic characteristics (see the drug compendium table).

Unwanted effects

See the drug compendium table.

Other drugs used for the treatment of cancer

Other drugs used in cancer therapy act to suppress cell division; for example, drugs such as corticosteroids, antibiotics, cytokines or drugs acting to control the division of cells sensitive to sex hormones. Cancers that arise from cell lines possessing steroid receptors that promote their growth and cell division are frequently susceptible to inhibitory steroids.

Glucocorticoids. Glucocorticoids (Ch. 44) suppress lymphocyte mitosis and are used in leukaemia and lymphoma; they are also helpful in reducing oedema around a tumour.

Oestrogens. Oestrogens (Ch. 45) suppress prostate cancer cells, both locally and in metastases, and provide symptomatic improvement; gynaecomastia is a common unwanted effect.

Progestogens. Progestogens (Ch. 45) suppress endometrial cancer cells and kidney cancer metastases.

Oestrogen antagonists. Cells in breast cancer can be suppressed by oestrogen antagonists (e.g. tamoxifen). Tamoxifen is active orally and binds competitively to oestrogen receptors. It shows both oestrogenic effects (on bone) and anti-oestrogenic effects (on breast tissue). Tamoxifen inhibits oestrogen-regulated genes and reduces the secretion of growth factors by tumour cells. Tumour cells are affected mainly in the G_2 phase of the cell cycle. Tamoxifen is extensively metabolised in the liver and has active metabolites with long half-lives; therefore, several weeks of treatment are necessary to achieve steady-state concentrations. Unwanted effects include hot flushes and amenorrhoea in premenopausal women and vaginal bleeding in postmenopausal women. Tamoxifen inhibits CYP3A4 and, therefore, reduces the metabolism of other substrates, such as warfarin.

Androgen antagonists. These drugs (e.g. flutamide; Ch. 46) suppress prostate cancer cells.

Gonadorelin analogues. These drugs (e.g. buserelin; Ch. 43) suppress prostate cancer cells.

Aromatase inhibitors. Aromatase is the enzyme that converts androgens to oestrogens. Inhibitors of aromatase (e.g. formestane) reduce oestrogen production in postmenopausal women, who produce oestrogen mainly from androstenedione and testosterone in many tissues such as adipose tissue, skin, muscle and liver. Aromatase is also present in the cells of two-thirds of breast carcinomas, and many breast cancers are oestrogen-dependent.

Interferon. Interferon alfa has proved to be a disappointing agent despite the vast resources committed to its isolation in sufficient amounts for early clinical trials. It is used for certain lymphomas and solid tumours but is not the 'natural, side-effect-free' agent that was hoped for when it was first isolated.

Aldesleukin (interleukin-2). Interleukin-2 is a lymphokine produced by T-lymphocytes that activates cytotoxic killer cells (Ch. 38). Aldesleukin, made by recombinant DNA technology, has been given by intravenous infusion for the treatment of patients with metastatic renal carcinoma. Its efficacy has yet to be established, but toxic effects include hypotension and oedema owing to capillary leakage, influenza-like symptoms, nausea, vomiting, diarrhoea, anaemia and thrombocytopenia.

Monoclonal antibodies. Several monoclonal antibodies have been developed that have highly specific effects. Unwanted effects are common, especially during the first infusion, with fever, chills, nausea, vomiting and allergic reactions (tumour lysis syndrome) or severe dyspnoea with bronchospasm (cytokine release syndrome). Examples of monoclonal antibodies include:

- alemtuzumab: produces lysis of B-lymphocytes in treatment-resistant or rapidly relapsing chronic lymphocytic leukaemia
- rituximab: produces lysis of B-lymphocytes in chemotherapy-resistant advanced follicular lymphoma
- trastuzumab: used for metastatic breast cancer when the tumour overexpresses human epidermal factor receptor 2 (HER-2).

Clinical use of antineoplastic agents

Different forms of cancer vary in their sensitivity to chemotherapy. The most responsive include lymphomas, leukaemias, choriocarcinoma and testicular carcinoma, while solid tumours such as colorectal, adrenocortical and squamous cell bronchial carcinomas generally show a poor response. An intermediate response is shown by other cancers, for example those of the bladder, head and neck, oat cell bronchogenic tumours and sex-related cancers (breast, ovary, endometrium and prostate). In addition, the sensitivity of an individual tumour can change during treatment with antineoplastic agents, because of the development of resistance.

Anticancer drug therapy for specific malignancies

The following discussion selects certain important cancers and outlines the role of chemotherapeutic drugs in their management. Trials produce a continuing flow of improved therapeutic options, and this is a field of medicine that changes rapidly.

Oesophageal cancer

Oesophageal cancer usually presents with advanced disease, with 50% being unresectable, or having radiological metastases at presentation. If the disease is localised, then surgical resection is the treatment of choice. Therapy with cisplatin and fluorouracil before surgery improves short-term survival. However, chemotherapy after surgery has no benefit. Chemotherapy with the same regimen given at the same time as radiotherapy may improve long-term survival.

Gastric cancer

Surgery can be curative for early disease, but about 90% of patients present with advanced disease. For these people, neoadjuvant chemotherapy in order to reduce tumour bulk before surgical resection is undergoing trials; an example of the drugs chosen is the combination of epirubicin, cisplatin and long-term intravenous infusion of fluorouracil. Adjuvant chemotherapy after surgery has not yet been shown to improve survival, however, it can be palliative in advanced disease, using fluorouracil combined with cisplatin or methotrexate and doxorubicin. This has a 65% response rate. Radiotherapy is used for palliation of bone metastases.

Pancreatic cancer

Most pancreatic cancers present late and 5-year survival is rare because of liver metastases. Surgical resection is the treatment of choice. Chemotherapy with fluorouracil plus radiotherapy may shrink larger tumours and make subsequent surgery possible. Adjuvant chemotherapy combined with radiotherapy after resection in people with resection margins free of tumour only produces a marginal improvement in survival. For people with liver metastases, chemotherapy with gemcitabine may offer greater palliation than with fluorouracil. Several trials of more intensive adjuvant chemotherapy are under way.

Colorectal cancer

Surgery is the treatment of choice for people with colorectal cancer without metastatic disease, and palliative surgery is often used even if spread has occurred. About 50% of colorectal tumours are cured by surgery; the recurrence rate of rectal tumour is higher than that of colonic tumour. Adjuvant chemotherapy is often given, with fluorouracil modulated by the use of folinic acid. This regimen has improved survival by 10–15% for locally invasive tumours. Chemotherapy with fluorouracil plus radiotherapy is preferred for rectal cancer. The major benefit of these adjuvant treatments is reduction of metastatic spread rather than of local recurrence. Once a patient has survived for 5 years, life expectancy is similar to that in the general population.

In advanced colorectal cancer, prolonged intravenous infusion of fluorouracil combined with irinotecan or oxaliplatin more than doubles survival and improves quality of life. In rectal cancer, this treatment can be combined with radiotherapy.

Lung cancer

There are four principal types of lung cancer. Non-small-cell cancers (adenocarcinoma, squamous cell cancer and large-cell cancer) account for about three-quarters of cases, with small-cell cancer responsible for the remainder.

For non-small-cell lung cancer, superficial lesions are amenable to several treatments, including photodynamic therapy with porfimer sodium. Surgical resection can be curative in the early stages. Radiotherapy is used after surgery when the tumour is not fully resectable, or for palliation of metastases. Neoadjuvant therapy is under investigation. Chemotherapy has a limited place for advanced or recurrent disease but is mainly palliative. Regimens including agents such as cisplatin, doxorubicin and cyclophosphamide produce only a small survival advantage. Current interest is focusing on chemoradiotherapy, which is a combination of cyclical multidrug chemotherapy followed by radiotherapy. In these studies, cisplatin is often combined with one or more additional drugs.

Small-cell lung cancer is more sensitive to chemotherapy, and has an initial response rate of 60–70%, with complete remission in 20–30%. Cisplatin combined with etoposide is often used, and various other combinations are being studied. Radiotherapy is also given for limited-stage disease.

Melanoma

Survival in melanoma is related to tumour thickness, falling from >95% 5-year survival with superficial tumours to <50% survival if the depth is greater than 4 mm. Wide surgical excision is the treatment of choice. Postsurgical adjuvant chemotherapy does not improve survival or disease-free outcome. Immunotherapy with Bacillus Calvette Guérin (BCG) may produce a benefit for people who had a negative tuberculin skin test before therapy. The use of granulocyte–macrophage colony-stimulating factor (GM-CSF) has shown promising preliminary results. Currently, interferon alfa is the only agent shown to increase disease-free survival. For metastatic disease, current therapy rests mainly on single-agent chemotherapy with dacarbazine or the vinca alkaloids (vincristine or vinblastine), which produces responses in 10–20% of patients. Combination chemotherapy increases toxicity with no improvement in response. Immunotherapy with interferon alfa has produced similar response rates to chemotherapy, and a combination of interferon alfa and dacarbazine may have additive or synergistic effects.

Renal cancer

Nephrectomy is the treatment of choice for early-stage renal cancer. However, up to one-third of people have metastases at the time of diagnosis. Options for chemotherapy include the following.

- Chemotherapy with a combination of the antimetabolites 5-fluorouracil and gemcitabine; the response is generally low, with fewer than 15% partial or complete responses.
- Progestogens produce a response in about 10% of those treated.
- Immunotherapy with interferon alfa produces a response rate of about 10%; aldesleukin (interleukin-2) has a slightly higher success rate of about 15%. Combination therapy with low doses of both agents is now the treatment of choice for disseminated disease.
- Renal cancer is very vascular. Thalidomide is an immunomodulatory drug with anti-angiogenic properties that is being studied with other anti-angiogenic agents.

Bladder cancer

Superficial bladder tumours are removed surgically, but recurrence rates are high. Intravesical immunotherapy with BCG vaccine is used to limit recurrence in superficial disease. For more advanced disease, neoadjuvant chemotherapy with gemcitabine and cisplatin improves survival. Several other regimens have been used or are under investigation. Bladder-sparing chemoradiation, using transurethral resection followed by cisplatin, methotrexate and vinblastine with irradiation, has given promising results for those who do not want cystectomy.

Prostate cancer

Treatment is largely determined by the extent of spread of the cancer. There are several options.

- 'Watchful waiting' for localised disease confined to the prostate. This is usually used for individuals with a life expectancy under 10 years, since many tumours do not progress in this time.
- Radical prostatectomy for localised disease, usually in men under 70 years. Impotence is a common sequel, occurring in 35–60%.

- Radiotherapy for localised disease or locally advanced disease in older men. Impotence follows therapy in 40–70%.
- Interstitial implantation of radioisotope for localised disease or locally advanced disease.
- Hormonal therapy for lymph node or distant metastases. Prostate cancer is hormone-dependent for growth. Testosterone reduction can be achieved by bilateral orchidectomy or the use of gonadotrophin-releasing hormone (GnRH) analogues such as goserelin (Ch. 43). Tumour flare reactions are prevented by the use of antiandrogen therapy (e.g. with flutamide or cyproterone acetate; Ch. 46) to block adrenal androgen activity.
- Hormone-refractory disease can be treated by combination chemotherapy with drugs such as estramustine with either vinblastine, etoposide, docetaxel or paclitaxel. Response rates of about 50% can be achieved. Painful metastatic deposits can be treated with radiotherapy or with strontium-89, which is taken up by sclerotic metastases.

Testicular cancer

Testicular tumours are either seminomas or non-seminomatous germ cell tumours, depending on the tissue of origin. Cure rates are now greater than 95%.
For seminomas, treatment choice includes:

- radiotherapy for localised disease
- for more advanced disease, chemotherapy with cisplatin, bleomycin and etoposide.

For non-seminomatous germ cell tumours, treatment includes:

- chemotherapy for early disease, with a regimen containing cisplatin
- for more advanced or recurrent disease, combination chemotherapy with cisplatin, etoposide and bleomycin, which, combined with surgery, produces an 85% complete remission rate.

Ovarian cancer

Initial surgery for ovarian cancer is followed by chemotherapy for all disease that is not localised to the ovary (which occurs in 80% of cases). About 70% of these women respond to chemotherapy, with complete remission in 10–20%. Options include:

- carboplatin or cisplatin alone: this is the most widely used first-line treatment
- for tumours that are refractory to standard chemotherapy, the addition of paclitaxel achieves palliation in 25–35% of cases.

The role of intraperitoneal drug delivery and more intensive combination chemotherapy is the subject of several current studies.

Cervical cancer

Surgery is the mainstay for local disease, but if there are poor prognostic predictors or advanced disease, then chemoradiation is used. Cisplatin is most frequently used, and improves survival by 30%. For recurrent disease, the combination of cisplatin and paclitaxel has a small advantage over cisplatin alone.

Endometrial cancer

Surgery is the usual initial treatment for endometrial cancer. Subsequent irradiation is used for extrauterine metastases. Disseminated disease can be treated by hormone therapy with progestogens, but responses are low (less than one-third of those treated) and may depend on the presence of progesterone receptors on the tumour cells. Adjuvant chemotherapy has a palliative role in advanced disease, with agents such as doxorubicin, cyclophosphamide, fluorouracil, cisplatin or paclitaxel.

Breast cancer

Limited surgery is the treatment of choice for very early disease and oestrogen receptor-positive tumours; it is usually followed by local radiotherapy. The risk of invasive recurrence is low and this is treated by mastectomy followed by chemotherapy. Chemotherapy or hormonal therapy is used for larger locally invasive tumours or distant spread, with neoadjuvant treatment started before surgery. Determination of the hormone receptor status of the tumour is an important guide to chemotherapy. Options for hormonal therapy for oestrogen receptor-positive tumours include the following.

- For postmenopausal women, non-steroidal aromatase inhibitors such as anastrazole are more effective than tamoxifen, which was long considered the treatment of choice. They can also be used as neoadjuvant therapy to reduce the extent of surgical resection.
- Anti-oestrogen therapy, e.g. with tamoxifen, is often considered second-line treatment for hormone-responsive cancer.
- The selective oestrogen receptor downregulator (SERD) fulvestrant should be available in the future as an alternative second-line treatment.
- The steroidal aromatase inhibitor exemestane is used for third-line treatment.
- Progestogens such as megestrol acetate are also used as a third-line treatment.
- GnRH analogues such as goserelin (Ch. 43) are a fourth-line treatment.
- For premenopausal women, tamoxifen remains the cornerstone of treatment, with or without chemotherapy.

Treatment is usually given for 5 years. The 10–20% of women who become unresponsive to one hormonal treatment may still benefit from use of an alternative class of drug.

Chemotherapy is used for oestrogen receptor-negative tumours, or hormonally unresponsive disease,. An example of a current regimen is doxorubicin combined with docetaxel and cyclophosphamide, which produces response rates of up to 40%. Trastuzumab added to chemotherapy for cancers that express HER-2 improves survival by 25%, and can be used as first-line therapy without cytotoxic drugs.

Acute myeloid leukaemias

The acute myeloid leukaemias are a heterogenous group of disorders (Box 52.1) that are differentiated on morphological grounds. Acute myeloid leukaemia is responsible for up to 15% of childhood leukaemias and is the commonest leukaemia of adult life. Complications result from bone marrow failure, and management of serious infection or bleeding are important issues in supportive care. The risk of infection is amplified by chemotherapy. The initial aim of chemotherapy is to reduce 'blast' cells in the marrow to below 5% of the total cell population (remission) with induction therapy and then to eradicate the leukaemic cells with consolidation therapy.

In the induction phase, cyclical intravenous chemotherapy with three or more drugs is used to reduce the development of resistance, usually giving four courses with 3–5 weeks between courses. A typical regimen consists of daunorubicin, cytarabine and either tioguanine or etoposide in younger people (under 60 years of age). Consolidation is achieved with further courses of similar therapy. Bone marrow transplantation may be considered after remission is achieved. In children, treatment for the central nervous system is also given with intrathecal methotrexate.

For acute promyelocytic leukaemia, the best initial response is obtained with tretinoin, a vitamin A derivative

---

Box 52.1

Simplified classification of acute myeloid leukaemias

Acute myeloid leukaemia
Acute myeloblastic leukaemia
Acute promyelocytic leukaemia
Acute myelomonocytic leukaemia
Acute monocytic/monoblastic leukaemia
Acute erythroleukaemia
Acute megakaryoblastic leukaemia

(see Ch. 49), and consolidation achieved by the addition of daunorubicin.

Acute lymphoblastic leukaemia

Acute lymphoblastic leukaemia is most common in children under 10 years of age, with a few cases occurring after age 40 years. Supportive therapy is similar to that for acute myeloid leukaemia.

Remission is achieved with vincristine, crisantaspase (asparaginase), prednisolone and often doxorubicin or daunorubicin. Consolidation therapy is initially with at least two multidrug intensification modules, using a combination of cytarabine, tioguanine, daunorubicin, vincristine, prednisolone and etoposide. Continuation therapy is continued after the first 5 months with vincristine and prednisolone for at least 2 years. Eradication of cranial disease is important, using intrathecal methotrexate or cranial irradiation. Selective use of haematopoietic stem cell transplantation can further improve outcome.

The results of treatment in childhood are excellent, with about 80% 5-year survival; this falls to 40% if the disease occurs in adult life.

Chronic myeloid leukaemia

Chronic myeloid leukaemia occurs in all age groups but is rare in children. Most treatments involve an initial chronic course, lasting 3–4 years, followed by transformation to an accelerated phase, when survival is just 3–6 months. In younger people, allogeneic bone transplantation is the treatment of choice after high-dose chemotherapy.

For older people, the goal of treatment is to suppress the abnormal clone of Philadelphia chromosome-positive cells. Initially, hydroxycarbamide is given to reduce the white cell count. Once symptoms are relieved, treatment with interferon alfa is substituted and can achieve remission in up to 80% of people. Survival is prolonged by up to 20 months with this regimen. Busulfan is an alternative chemotherapeutic agent for individuals who cannot tolerate hydroxycarbamide. The most recent innovation is the use of imatinib for disease that is resistant to interferon alfa, producing a response in 40–50% of those treated.

For advanced disease, combination chemotherapy can be considered, such as the regimen used for acute myeloid leukaemia.

Chronic lymphocytic leukaemia

Chronic lymphocytic leukaemia is predominantly a disease of the elderly. Cure is unusual and median survival is 5–8 years. Treatment may not be necessary if the disease is causing few problems, but oral chlorambucil, often combined with prednisolone, can be given for up to 6 months to regress the disease. Transformation of the disease to a more aggressive form can occur after several years, when combination chemotherapy should be considered.

Fludarabine is the second-line treatment of choice. It is used intravenously for relapse after treatment with chlorambucil. Response rates of about 50% have been reported, with remissions lasting, on average, 8 months. The monoclonal antibody rituximab has efficacy similar to that of fludarabine, and may have additive effects in combination.

Malignant lymphomas

The malignant lymphomas are a diverse group of disorders comprising Hodgkin's disease and a variety of non-Hodgkin's lymphomas, which are classified by histopathological and cytochemical techniques. Low-grade non-Hodgkin's lymphomas are managed in a similar way to chronic lymphocytic leukaemia and have a similar prognosis. Non-Hodgkin's lymphomas of intermediate grade are curable in about 40% of people, using courses of combination chemotherapy with cyclophosphamide, doxorubicin, vincristine and prednisolone ('CHOP' therapy, named after a combination of the initials of the generic and proprietary names of the drugs). Rituximab may improve survival when added to standard chemotherapy, and radiotherapy is sometimes used as adjunctive treatment. More frequent, intensive therapy is required for high-grade, aggressive non-Hodgkin's lymphomas.

For Hodgkin's disease, radiotherapy is curative if the tumour is located. For more extensive disease, combination chemotherapy is the usual approach. The most frequently used regimens are chlormethine, vincristine, procarbazine and prednisolone (MOPP), and doxorubicin, bleomycin, vinblastine and dacarbazine (ABVD).

Multiple myeloma

Multiple myeloma is mainly a disorder of the elderly. Treatment is aimed at suppression of the monoclonal protein in the blood. Supportive therapy is often required to treat hypercalcaemia, renal impairment and infection. Rehydration and analgesia for bone pain are often required.

Chemotherapy is usually with oral melphalan and prednisolone in pulses for 4–6 weeks. This reduces the myeloma protein in blood by more than 50% in half of those treated. Median survival with this treatment is 3 years.

High doses of intravenous melphalan or combination therapy with vincristine, doxorubicin and dexamethasone, or cyclophosphamide, vincristine, doxorubicin and methylprednisolone, produce a response rate of up to 70% and may be justifiable in younger people who tolerate the associated toxicity better. Bortezomib is expected to be available shortly for the treatment of relapsed disease. This is the first drug in a new class of agents called proteasome inhibitors.

Autologous bone marrow transplantation is increasingly used as salvage therapy after intensive chemotherapy and can produce 30–50% complete remission.

FURTHER READING

Drugs and drug action

Ambudkar SV, Dey S, Hrycyna CA, Ramachandra M, Pastan I, Gottesman MM (1999) Biochemical, cellular, and pharmacological aspects of the multidrug transporter. *Annu Rev Pharmacol Toxicol* 39, 361–398

Dubowchik GM, Walker MA (1999) Receptor-mediated and enzyme-dependent targeting of cytotoxic anticancer drugs. *Pharmacol Ther* 83, 67–123

Franks ME, Macpherson GR, Figg WD (2004) Thalidomide. *Lancet* 363, 1802–1811

Gottesman MM (2002) Mechanisms of cancer drug resistance. *Annu Rev Med* 53, 615–627

Griffioen AW, Molema G (2000) Angiogenesis: potentials for pharmacologic intervention in the treatment of cancer, cardiovascular diseases, and chronic inflammation. *Pharmacol Rev* 52, 237–268

Hofseth LJ, Hussain SP, Harris CC (2004) p53: 25 years after its discovery. *Trends Pharmacol Sci* 25, 177–181

Links M, Lewis C (1999) Chemoprotectants: a review of their clinical pharmacology and therapeutic efficacy. *Drugs* 57, 293–308

Marsh S, McLeod HL (2004) Cancer pharmacogenetics. *Br J Cancer* 90, 8–11

Njar VC, Brodie AM (1999) Comprehensive pharmacology and clinical effcacy of aromatase inhibitors. *Drugs* 58, 233–255

Pizzolato JF (2003) The camptothecins. *Lancet* 361, 2235–2242

Bowel cancer

Allum WH, Griffin SM, Watson A et al (2002) Guidelines for the management of oesophageal and gastric cancer. *Gut* 50(suppl V), v1–v23

Enzinger PC, Mayer RJ (2003) Esophageal cancer. *N Engl J Med* 349, 2241–2252

Hohenberger P, Gretschel S (2003) Gastric cancer. *Lancet* 362, 305–315

Labianca RF, Beretta GD, Pessi MA (2001) Colorectal cancer. *Drugs* 61, 1751–1764

Roch Lima CMS, Centeno B (2002) Update on pancreatic cancer. *Curr Opin Oncol* 14, 424–430

Lung cancer

Booton R, Jones M, Thatcher N (2003) Lung cancer 7: management of lung cancer in elderly patients. *Thorax* 58, 711–720

Cullen M (2003) Lung cancer 4: chemotherapy for non-small cell lung cancer: the end of the beginning. *Thorax* 58, 352–356

Price A (2003) Lung cancer 5: state of the art radiotherapy for lung cancer. *Thorax* 58, 447–452

Spira A, Ettinger DS (2004) Multidisciplinary management of lung cancer. *N Engl J Med* 350, 379–392

Urogenital cancer

Borden LS, Clark PE, Hall MC (2003) Bladder cancer. *Curr Opin Oncol* 15, 227–233

Bott SR, Birtle AJ, Taylor CJ et al (2003) Prostate cancer management: 1. An update on localised disease. *Postgrad Med J* 79, 575–580

Bott SR, Birtle AJ, Taylor CJ et al (2003) Prostate cancer management: 2. An update on locally advanced and metastatic disease. *Postgrad Med J* 79, 643–645

Dearnaley DP, Huddart RA, Horwich A (2001) Managing testicular cancer. *BMJ* 322, 1583–1588

Harris KA, Reese DM (2001) Treatment options in hormone-refractory prostate cancer. *Drugs* 61, 2177–2192

Hellerstedt BA, Pienta KJ (2002) Testicular cancer. *Curr Opin Oncol* 14, 260–264

Hernandez J, Thompson IM (2004) Diagnosis and treatment of prostate cancer. *Med Clin North Am* 88, 267–279

Southcott BM (2001) Carcinoma of the endometrium. *Drugs* 61, 1395–1405

Waggoner SE (2003) Cervical cancer. *Lancet* 361, 2217–2225

Whang YE, Godley PA (2003) Renal cell carcinoma. *Curr Opin Oncol* 15, 213–216

Breast cancer

Morrow M, Gradishar W (2002) Breast cancer. *BMJ* 324, 410–414

Sayer HG, Kath R, Kliche K-O et al (2002) Premenopausal breast cancer. *Drugs* 62, 2025–2038

Smith IE, Dowsett M (2003) Aromatase inhibitors in breast cancer. *N Engl J Med* 348, 2431–2442

Melanoma

Eggermont AMM (2002) European approach to the treatment of malignant melanoma. *Curr Opin Oncol* 14, 205–211

Acute leukaemias

Pui C-H, Relling MV, Downing JR (2004) Acute lymphoblastic leukemia. *N Engl J Med* 350, 1535–1548

Ravandi F, Kantarajian H, Giles F et al (2004) New agents in acute leukemia and other myeloid disorders. *Cancer* 100, 441–454

Chronic leukaemias

Goldman JM, Melo JV (2003) Chronic myeloid leukemia – advances in biology and new approaches to treatment. *N Engl J Med* 349, 1451–1464

Schriever F, Huhn D (2003) New directions in the diagnosis and treatment of chronic lymphocytic leukaemia. *Drugs* 63, 953–969

Lymphomas

Evans LS, Hancock BW (2003) Non-Hodgkin lymphoma. *Lancet* 362, 139–146

Yung L, Linch D (2002) Hodgkin's lymphoma. *Lancet* 361, 943–951

Multiple myeloma

Sirohi B, Powles R (2004) Multiple myeloma. *Lancet* 363, 875–887

Self-assessment

1. What are the criteria for combination chemotherapy of cancer? How well do the following treatment regimens meet the criteria?

   a. Acute lymphoblastic leukaemia (ALL; initial phase for induction of remission): intravenous vincristine (1.5 mg m^{-2}), subcutaneous crisantaspase (asparaginase; 6000 units m^{-2}) and oral prednisolone (40 mg m^{-2}).

   b. Hodgkin's lymphoma (MOPP regimen): intravenous chlormethine (6 mg m^{-2}), intravenous vincristine (1.5 mg m^{-2}), oral procarbazine (100 mg m^{-2}) and oral prednisolone (40 mg m^{-2}).

   c. Testicular teratoma (in an adult): intravenous etoposide (120 mg m^{-2}), intravenous bleomycin (30 mg) and intravenous cisplatin (20 mg m^{-2}).

2. Why are the doses of anticancer drugs corrected to surface area rather than simply bodyweight (e.g. mg kg^{-1} bodyweight)? Does the use of surface area correction result in higher or lower doses for children compared with simple bodyweight correction (Table 52.2)?

Surface area is calculated using a nomogram or the equation:

$$A = 71.84 \ W^{0.425} \ H^{0.725}$$

where A is surface area (in cm^2), W is weight (in kg) and H is height (in cm).

The answers are provided on pages 745–746.

Table 52.2
Examples of surface area calculation

Age (years)	Body weight (kg)	Height (cm)	Body surface area (m^2)
0.5	7.4	65.8	0.350
1.0	9.9	74.7	0.434
3	14.5	96.0	0.613
6	21.5	116.8	0.835
Adult			
Male	72.1	175.3	1.874
Female	60.3	167.6	1.681

Drugs used in the treatment of cancer

Drug	Half-life (h)	Elimination	Comments	Unusual or limiting toxicity[a]
Alkylating agents				
Busulfan	2–3	Metabolism	Mainly used for effects on the bone marrow (e.g. chronic myeloid leukaemia); given orally or by intravenous infusion; 'metabolism' is largely by interaction with thiol groups, such as cysteine, the products of which are further metabolised and eliminated	Myelosuppression and irreversible bone marrow aplasia; rare pulmonary fibrosis
Carmustine (BCNU)	0.4–0.5	Metabolism	Used for myeloma, lymphoma and brain tumours; given intravenously; unstable reactive molecule that cross-links DNA and the nitroso function inactivates DNA repair; crosses blood–brain barrier; metabolites eliminated in urine	Renal damage; delayed pulmonary fibrosis
Chlorambucil	1–2	Metabolism	Used mainly in lymphocytic leukaemia, non-Hodgkin's lymphoma and Hodgkin's disease; given orally, usually after fasting; 'metabolised' at alkylating groups owing to reactivity and in the liver by β-oxidation of the carboxylic acid side-chain	Vomiting
Chlormethine (mustine)	–	Metabolism	Used in some regimens for management of Hodgkin's disease; (it is the M in the MOPP [MVPP] regimen); given intravenously as a freshly prepared solution by a fast-running infusion; extremely unstable and reactive; volatility poses occupational risk	–
Cyclophosphamide	4–10	Metabolism	Widely used for leukaemias, lymphomas and solid tumours; given orally or by intravenous injection; good penetration of blood–brain barrier; metabolic oxidation by CYP2B1 and CYP3A4 leads to bioactivation; wide intersubject variability	Haemorrhagic cystitis (see mesna antidote)
Estramustine	20–24	Metabolism	Used for prostate cancer; given orally (an oestrogen molecule linked to a nitrogen mustard group); acts as an alkylating agent especially on microtubule proteins, and increases circulating oestrogen levels; the phosphate ester, which is given orally, is dephosphorylated to the active drug, which is oxidised in the steroid ring	–
Ifosfamide	4–15	Metabolism	Uses similar to cyclophosphamide; given by intravenous injection; metabolic fate is similar to cyclophosphamide	Cystitis (see mesna antidote)
Lomustine (CCNU)	1–5 (4-OH)	Metabolism	Mainly used for Hodgkin's disease and some solid tumours; given orally; bifunctional drug similar to carmustine; oxidised to 4-hydroxy compound (4-OH) completely in the gut wall and liver during first-pass metabolism	Permanent bone marrow damage

continued

Drugs used in the treatment of cancer *(continued)*

Drug	Half-life (h)	Elimination	Comments	Unusual or limiting toxicity[a]
Alkylating agents (continued)				
Melphalan	1.5	Metabolism	Used mainly for multiple myeloma, ovarian adenocarcinoma, advanced breast cancer and neuroblastoma; given orally or by intravenous injection; oral absorption is incomplete and variable; does not cross blood–brain barrier in useful amounts; pathways of metabolism are not well defined	–
Thiotepa	1–3 thiotepa 10–21 TEPA	Metabolism	Used for bladder cancer; given by intravesicular injection; extensively absorbed from bladder lumen; bioactivated by CYP2B and CYP2C to TEPA (the active form), in which sulphur is replaced by oxygen	–
Treosulfan	1–2	Non-enzymatic	Used mainly for ovarian cancer; given orally or by intravenous injection; high oral bioavailability; 'metabolised' by loss of reactive groups through non-enzymatic reactions; leaving groups are eliminated as methylsulphonic acid	Allergic alveolitis; pulmonary fibrosis
Cytotoxic antibiotics				
Aclarubicin	1–9	Metabolism	Used for acute non-lymphocytic leukaemia in relapsed/resistant disease; given intravenously; rapidly taken up by cells; crosses blood–brain barrier in useful amounts; metabolised to active (M1 – which has a half-life of 10–20 h) and inactive metabolites; activity linked to parent drug and M1	Bone marrow suppression
Bleomycin	2–4	Metabolism + renal	Used for testicular cancer, lymphomas and squamous cell carcinoma; given intravenously or intramuscularly; slow uptake by tissues; hydrolysed by enzyme 'bleomycin hydrolase', which largely inactivates the drug; low levels of the hydrolase correlate with cytotoxicity	Dermatological effects; progressive pulmonary fibrosis
Dactinomycin (actinomycin D)	36	Renal + bile	Mainly used for paediatric solid tumours; given intravenously; negligible metabolism	Bone marrow toxicity; gastrointestinal toxicity
Daunorubicin	24–48	Metabolism + bile	Used for acute leukaemias and AIDS-related Kaposi's sarcoma (as a liposome preparation which has a half-life of 5 h); given intravenously; undergoes metabolic reduction and redox cycling, giving toxic superoxide radicals and H_2O_2; long half-life owing to slow release from tissues; metabolite retains activity	Bone marrow toxicity
Doxorubicin	2–10	Metabolism	Widely used for leukaemias, lymphomas and a variety of solid tumours; given intravenously; reduced in liver to doxorubicinol, which is further metabolised and excreted, largely in the bile; does not cross blood–brain barrier	Myelosuppression; cardiotoxicity

continued

Drugs used in the treatment of cancer *(continued)*

Drug	Half-life (h)	Elimination	Comments	Unusual or limiting toxicity[a]
Cytotoxic antibiotics (continued)				
Epirubicin	11–69	Metabolism (+ renal)	Uses are similar to doxorubicin; given intravenously; reduced to epirubicinol and also conjugated in amino sugar ring; very wide inter-subject variability in kinetics; does not cross blood–brain barrier	Myelosuppression; cardiotoxicity (less than doxorubicin)
Idarubicin	12–35	Metabolism	Used mainly for acute leukaemias and advanced breast cancer (non-responsive to first-line treatments); given orally or intravenously; oral bioavailability is low and variable (4–50%); metabolised by reduction to idarubicinol (which has a longer half-life of 50–70 h and retains activity) and by hydrolysis of the amino sugar moiety	Myelosuppression
Mitomycin	0.5–1.5	Metabolism	Mainly used for upper gastrointestinal and breast cancers and by bladder instillation for superficial bladder tumours; given intravenously; reduced to a hydroquinone, which gives rise to a highly unstable alkylating species that cross-links DNA; metabolism gives toxic superoxide and hydroxyl radicals	Myelosuppression; nephrotoxicity; lung fibrosis
Mitoxantrone	4–220	Renal + metabolism	Used to treat metastatic breast cancer and non-Hodgkin's lymphoma and non-lymphocytic leukaemia; given by intravenous infusion; metabolised in the liver by side-chain oxidation to inactive metabolites; extremely wide inter-individual variability in half-life; long half-life may result from high tissue uptake and affinity	Myelosuppression; cardiotoxicity
Antimetabolites				
Capecitabine	0.5–1	Hydrolysis	Used as monotherapy for metastatic colorectal cancer; given orally; metabolised to fluorouracil	–
Cladribine	7	Metabolism	Used for hairy cell leukaemia; given by intravenous infusion; chlorine-substituted purine; undergoes intracellular phosphorylation to the active triphosphate form	Myelosuppression; neurotoxicity
Cytarabine (cytosine arabinoside)	1–3	Metabolism	Main use is for induction of remission in acute myeloblastic leukaemia; given intravenously, subcutaneously or intrathecally; undergoes intracellular phosphorylation to the active triphosphate form; metabolism to uracil arabinoside gives inactivation	Myelosuppression

continued

Drugs used in the treatment of cancer (continued)

Drug	Half-life (h)	Elimination	Comments	Unusual or limiting toxicity[a]
Antimetabolites (continued)				
Fludarabine phosphate	7–20	Renal + metabolism	Used for B-cell chronic lymphocytic leukaemia; given orally or by intravenous injection or infusion; fluorine-substituted purine riboside; phosphate is rapidly hydrolysed to give fludarabine, which enters the cell and is phosphorylated to a triphosphate	Myelosuppression
Fluorouracil	0.25	Metabolism	Used for cancers of the gastrointestinal tract and malignant and pre-malignant skin lesions; given topically or by intravenous injection or infusion or intra-arterial infusion; fluorine-substituted uracil; converted to fluorouracil monophosphate intracellularly and then to di- and triphosphates; catabolised in the liver by dihydropyrimidine dehydrogenase	Relatively low toxicity (not usually the limiting drug given in a combination)
Gemcitabine	0.2–0.5	Metabolism	Used for palliative treatment of non-small-cell lung and pancreatic cancer; given intravenously; deoxycytidine analogue with two fluorine atoms in the deoxyribose moiety; bioactivated by intracellular conversion to the active triphosphate; inactivated by deamination to difluorodeoxyuridine	Limited toxicity
Mercaptopurine	1–1.5	Metabolism	Used almost exclusively for maintenance therapy for acute leukaemias; (also used in inflammatory bowel disease); given orally; sulphur-substituted purine; poor oral bioavailability owing to first-pass metabolism (about 20%); bioactivated by intracellular phosphorylation; inactivated by xanthine oxidase (interaction with allopurinol)	Limited toxicity
Methotrexate	8–10	Renal + metabolism	Used for maintenance therapy for childhood acute lymphoblastic leukaemia, choriocarcinoma, non-Hodgkin's lymphoma and some solid tumours; (also used for rheumatoid arthritis and psoriasis); given orally, intravenously, intramuscularly or intrathecally; folate analogue; taken up into cells by the reduced folate carrier and undergoes polyglutamate formation (like folate); the polyglutamates are retained for months (the half-life refers to the non-glutamate form); eliminated mainly by the kidneys with some as a hydroxy metabolite; contraindicated in renal impairment	Myelosuppression (folinic acid is an 'antidote'– see below)

continued

Drugs used in the treatment of cancer (continued)

Drug	Half-life (h)	Elimination	Comments	Unusual or limiting toxicity[a]
Antimetabolites (continued)				
Raltitrexed	10–12 days	Renal + some metabolism	Used for palliation of metastatic colon cancer when fluorouracil cannot be used; given intravenously; prolonged retention within cells gives prolonged inhibition of thymidylate synthase and 3-weekly dosage intervals; forms polyglutamates intracellularly	Myelosuppression
Tegafur with uracil	8	Metabolism	Used with folinate for management of metastatic colorectal cancer; given orally; a racemate that is metabolised to 5-fluorouracil; the *R*-isomer is more rapidly metabolised and determines the formation rate-limited half-life of 5-fluorouracil; the half-life of the parent compound is determined by the *S*-isomer	–
Tioguanine	3–6	Metabolism + renal	Used for acute leukaemia and chronic myeloid leukemia; given orally; bioavailability is 25–50%; rapidly taken up by cells; converted to corresponding nucleotide intracellularly, which is retained within cells; methylation of the 6-thio group is the major route of metabolism	Myelosuppression
Vinca alkaloids and etoposide				
Etoposide	4–8	Metabolism	Used for small-cell carcinoma of the bronchus, lymphomas and testicular cancer; given orally or by slow intravenous infusion; oral absorption is 25–75%; eliminated in urine and bile mainly as metabolites	Myelosuppression; alopecia
Vinblastine	20–80	Metabolism	Used for acute leukaemias, lymphomas and non-solid tumours (e.g. breast and lung); given by intravenous injection; metabolised by hepatic CYP3A4, and metabolites eliminated in bile and urine	Myelosuppression
Vincristine	85	Metabolism	Used for acute leukaemias, lymphomas and non-solid tumours (e.g. breast and lung); given by intravenous injection; metabolised in liver; metabolites eliminated mainly in the bile	Neurotoxicity – peripheral and autonomic neuropathy (recovery is slow but complete)
Vindesine	25	Metabolism + renal	Used for acute leukaemias, lymphomas and non-solid tumours (e.g. breast and lung); given by intravenous injection; metabolised by CYP3A4, and metabolites are eliminated in bile and urine; up to 10% excreted unchanged in urine	Myelosuppression

continued

Drug compendium

Drugs used in the treatment of cancer *(continued)*

Drug	Half-life (h)	Elimination	Comments	Unusual or limiting toxicity[a]
Vinca alkaloids and etoposide (continued)				
Vinorelbine	28–44	Metabolism	Used for advanced breast and non-small-cell lung cancer; given intravenously; semi-synthetic vinca alkaloid made from vinblastine; metabolised by CYP3A4, and metabolites are eliminated in bile and urine	Myelosuppression
Platinum compounds				
Carboplatin	1.5	Renal	Used for ovarian cancer and some other solid tumours; given by intravenous injection; active form produced by interaction with water; eliminated by glomerular filtration; good correlation between AUC in blood (see Ch. 2), creatinine clearance and myelosuppression; the excretion of total platinum (Pt) (equivalent to 'metabolites') is much slower than that of the parent compound	Myelosuppression (plus some nausea and vomiting – less than cisplatin)
Cisplatin	24–60	Renal	Used for solid tumours such as ovarian cancer and metastatic seminoma and testicular teratoma; given by intravenous injection; active form produced by interaction with water; eliminated by kidney; some sources give the half-life as up to 60 h, and these values relate to total Pt not cisplatin per se	Nausea and vomiting; nephrotoxicity; myelosuppression; ototoxicity
Oxaliplatin	27	Renal	Used for metastatic colorectal cancer; given intravenously; has a 1,2-diaminocyclohexane ligand (which increases the formation of DNA adducts) and an oxalate ligand on the Pt atom; half-life relates to free Pt because the parent drug undergoes rapid hydration and ligand-exchange reactions	Neurotoxicity
Taxanes				
Docetaxel	11	Metabolism (+ renal)	Used for advanced or metastatic anthracycline-resistant breast cancer; given by intravenous infusion; metabolised by CYP3A4-mediated oxidation; metabolites eliminated in the bile; a small amount (<10%) excreted unchanged in urine	Hypersensitivity reactions; myelosuppression; peripheral neuropathy; fluid retention
Paclitaxel	19	Metabolism	Used for advanced ovarian cancer and as secondary treatment for breast and non-small-cell lung cancer; given by intravenous infusion; metabolised by CYP2C8 and CYP3A4 to different metabolites, which are eliminated in bile	Hypersensitivity reactions; myelosuppression; peripheral neuropathy

continued

Drugs used in the treatment of cancer (continued)

Drug	Half-life (h)	Elimination	Comments	Unusual or limiting toxicity[a]
Topoisomerase I inhibitors				
Irinotecan	6	Metabolism + renal	Used for metastatic colorectal cancer; given by intravenous infusion; metabolised by esterase to a highly active metabolite and by CYP3A4 to largely inactive metabolites; activity resides in parent drug and esterase product; some renal excretion (10–20%)	Myelosuppression; gastrointestinal effects
Topotecan	2–3	Renal + hydrolysis	Used for metastatic ovarian cancer when first-line treatment has failed; given by intravenous infusion; undergoes pH-dependent hydrolysis of the lactone ring, which results in inactivation; enzymatic metabolism is only a minor route of elimination	Myelosuppression; gastrointestinal effects
Miscellaneous anticancer drugs				
Amsacrine	4–7	Metabolism	Used for acute myeloid leukaemia; action and toxicity similar to doxorubicin; given as intravenous infusion; metabolites formed in the liver and eliminated as bile	Myelosuppression (fatal arrhythmias when there is hypokalaemia)
Bexarotene	7	Metabolism	An agonist at retinoid X receptors; used for skin manifestations of cutaneous T-cell lymphoma; given orally; oxidised in the liver by CYP3A4, and products conjugated and excreted	Leucopenia
Crisantaspase (asparaginase)	7–13	Metabolism	Used for acute lymphoblastic leukaemia; given by intramuscular or subcutaneous injection; enzyme isolated from *Erwinia chrysanthemi*; taken up by reticuloendothelial system and degraded	Anaphylaxis; CNS depression; nausea; hyperglycaemia
Dacarbazine	5	Renal	Used for metastatic melanoma and soft tissue sarcomas; given intravenously; activated by P450-mediated metabolism to a cytotoxic and alkylating metabolite; about 50% is excreted in the urine unchanged	Myelosuppression; intense nausea and vomiting
Hydroxycarbamide	2–6	Urine	Used for chronic myeloid leukaemia; given orally; eliminated by glomerular filtration	Myelosuppression
Imatinib	18	Metabolism	Used for newly diagnosed chronic myeloid leukaemia (under special circumstances); a protein-tyrosine kinase inhibitor; given orally; rapidly and completely absorbed; metabolised by CYP3A4 to an active metabolite which has a longer half-life (40 h) and contributes to in vivo activity	Gastrointestinal effects

continued

Drugs used in the treatment of cancer (continued)

Drug	Half-life (h)	Elimination	Comments	Unusual or limiting toxicity[a]
Miscellaneous anticancer drugs (continued)				
Pentostatin	3–15	Renal	Used for hairy cell leukaemia; given intravenously; eliminated by kidneys with negligible metabolism; clearance correlates with creatinine clearance	Myelosuppression; immunosuppression
Porfimer	40–50	Bile	Used in photodynamic treatment of small-cell lung cancer and for oesophageal cancer; given by intravenous injection; breakdown products eliminated in bile; the photosensitising product has a very long half-life (250 h)	Photosensitivity
Procarbazine	0.1	Metabolism (+ renal)	Used in Hodgkin's disease (part of MOPP regimen); given orally; very rapidly eliminated by hepatic metabolism via CYP1A2, which gives rise to methyl radicals; limited renal excretion (5% of dose); crosses blood–brain barrier; ingestion with alcohol may give a disulfiram-like effect	Nausea; myelosuppression; rash
Razoxane (dexrazoxane)	2–4	Metabolism	It is of limited value for leukaemias; the dextroisomer is approved by the FDA to prevent cardiac complications associated with cases of chemotherapy (by chelating iron and preventing redox cycling with, for example, doxorubicin); given orally; metabolised in the liver	–
Trastuzumab	25 days	?	Used for metastatic breast cancer; given by intravenous infusion; few details available	Cardiotoxicity, especially if used with anthracyclines (cytotoxic antibiotics – see above)
Temoporfin	Days?	?	Used in photodynamic treatment of advanced refractory head and neck squamous cell carcinoma; given by intravenous injection; few data available; animal studies indicate kinetics may be similar to porfimer	Photosensitivity
Temozolomide	2	Metabolism	Used as a second-line treatment for malignant glioma; given orally; structural analogue of dacarbazine (see above) and converted to the same active compound non-enzymatically; eliminated as metabolites	Myelosuppression
Tretinoin (all-*trans*-retinoic acid)	1–2	Metabolism	Used for remission of acute promyelocytic leukaemia; given orally; eliminated by oxidation, conjugation with glucuronic acid, and isomerisation to the less active *cis*-isomer	Numerous symptoms (highly teratogenic)

continued

Drug compendium

Drugs used in the treatment of cancer *(continued)*

Drug	Half-life (h)	Elimination	Comments	Unusual or limiting toxicity[a]
Antidotes (chemoprotectants)				
Folinate (leucovorin) and levofolinate	0.75	Metabolism	Given 24 h after methotrexate to speed recovery from myelosuppression; given orally or by intramuscular or intravenous injection; formyl group is used for thymidate synthesis and folate enters body pool	–
Amifostine	<0.2	Metabolism	Used prior to cytotoxic treatment to reduce the risk of neutropenia-related infection in people treated with cisplatin or cyclophosphamide, and to reduce cisplatin nephrotoxicity; given by intravenous infusion; rapidly cleared by uptake into normal tissues, where it is hydrolysed	Hypotension
Mesna (mercaptoethane sulphonic acid)	1	Renal + metabolism	Given either before (oral) or with (intravenous) cyclophosphamide or ifosfamide treatment, to prevent urothelial toxicity; given orally or by intravenous injection; highly polar molecule that contains a sulfhydryl (SH) group; eliminated in the urine; some dimerisation of SH group to a disulphide, which is eliminated in the urine and reduced back to mesna	–
Other drugs used for the treatment of cancer			The drugs given below are those that affect the cancer per se; other drugs used in the management of people with cancer (e.g. antiemetics) are described in the appropriate chapter	
Aldesleukin (interleukin-2)	0.5–6	Metabolism	Use restricted to metastatic renal cell carcinoma; given by subcutaneous injection; recombinant interleukin-2; taken up and degraded by the kidneys; the half-life is that seen after intravenous dosage; subcutaneous dosage gives prolonged low plasma levels with a half-life of 3–12 h	Severe toxicity; pulmonary oedema; hypotension; bone marrow, hepatic, renal, thyroid and CNS toxicity
Alemtuzumab	12 days	?	Unconjugated, humanised monoclonal antibody against antigen CD52 used for chronic lymphocytic leukaemia unresponsive to an alkylating agent; monoclonal antibody that causes lysis of B-lymphocytes; given by intravenous infusion; few data available	Cytokine release syndrome (characterised by severe dyspnoea)
Diethylstilbestrol	2–3 days	Metabolism	Used (but very rarely) for prostate cancer, and occasionally for breast cancer; given orally; eliminated by conjugation with glucuronic acid; undergoes enterohepatic cycling	Nausea; fluid retention; thrombosis; impotence and gynaecomastia in men; hypercalcaemia and bone pain in women
Ethinylestradiol	8–24	Metabolism	May be used for breast cancer (unlicensed indication in the UK); given orally; see contraceptive hormones (Ch. 45)	See contraceptive hormones (Ch. 45)

continued

Drug compendium

Drugs used in the treatment of cancer *(continued)*

Drug	Half-life (h)	Elimination	Comments	Unusual or limiting toxicity[a]
Other drugs used for the treatment of cancer (continued)				
Gestonorone caproate	–	Metabolism	Progestogen used to treat endometrial cancer and for benign prostatic hypertrophy; given by intramuscular injection; few kinetic data available; probably undergoes hydrolysis of the caproate ester group to liberate the steroid	Usually mild effects only
Interferon alfa	3–4	Metabolism	Used for certain lymphomas and solid tumours; given by subcutaneous or intravenous injection; catabolised by kidney; slow absorption from subcutaneous dosage with peak concentrations at 4–8 h	Nausea; lethargy; ocular effects; depression; myelosuppression; cerebrovascular, liver and kidney problems
Medroxy-progesterone acetate	30	Metabolism	Progestogen used for breast and endometrial cancer, and rarely for prostate and renal cancer; given orally or by deep intramuscular injection; complete oral bioavailability; eliminated as conjugated metabolites	Glucocorticoid effect at high doses
Megestrol acetate	15–20	Metabolism	Progestogen used for breast and endometrial cancer; given orally; complete oral bioavailability; metabolised largely by oxidation followed by conjugation	Usually mild
Norethisterone	5–12	Metabolism	Progestogen used for breast cancer; given orally; complete oral bioavailability; metabolised by reduction of the ketone group to an alcohol, which is conjugated	–
Prednisolone	2–4	Metabolism	Has a marked antitumour effect in acute lymphoblastic leukaemia, Hodgkin's disease and non-Hodgkin's lymphoma (also used in palliative care); given orally, topically and by intramuscular injection; injectable form is the acetate ester as an aqueous suspension; high oral bioavailability (70–80%); extensively metabolised but all pathways have not been defined	See corticosteroids (Ch. 44)
Rituximab	60	Metabolism	Used for chemotherapy-resistant advanced follicular lymphoma; given by intravenous infusion; monoclonal chimeric mouse/human antibody that causes lysis of B-lymphocytes; the elimination of the peptide has a shorter half-life for the first infusion compared with subsequent dosage	Fever; chills; nausea; allergic reactions; cytokine release syndrome (characterised by severe dyspnoea)
Drugs for breast cancer			See also drugs listed above	

continued

Drugs used in the treatment of cancer (continued)

Drug	Half-life (h)	Elimination	Comments	Unusual or limiting toxicity[a]
Drugs for breast cancer (continued)			See also drugs listed above	
Aminoglutethimide	12	Renal + metabolism	Aromatase inhibitor which has been largely replaced by selective aromatase inhibitors but still sometimes used for treatment of prostate cancer; eliminated in urine unchanged (50%) and as *N*-acetyl and other metabolites	Drug fever; drowsiness; adrenal hypofunction
Anastrozole	40–50	Metabolism (+ renal)	Selective aromatase inhibitor used as adjunct for oestrogen receptor-positive early breast cancer, and for advanced metastatic breast cancer in postmenopausal women; given orally; metabolised by oxidation and formation of an *N*-glucuronide (rare reaction); a small amount is excreted unchanged	Hot flushes; vaginal dryness and bleeding; gastrointestinal effects
Exemestane	24	Metabolism	Used for advanced breast cancer in postmenopausal women in whom anti-oestrogen therapy has failed; given orally; bioavailability is about 40% and increased markedly by a fatty meal; metabolised by CYP3A4-mediated oxidation and by reduction to essentially inactive metabolites	–
Letrozole	2 days	Metabolism	Selective non-steroidal aromatase inhibitor used for advanced metastatic breast cancer in postmenopausal women that is not responsive to other anti-oestrogens; given orally; high oral bioavailability; oxidised in the liver by CYP3A4 to an inactive metabolite	Hot flushes; nausea; gastrointestinal effects
Tamoxifen	7 days	Metabolism	Non-steroidal anti-oestrogen used for oestrogen receptor-positive breast cancer; given orally; high bioavailability; oxidised by CYP2C and CYP3A isoenzymes	Exacerbation of pain from bone metastases
Toremifene	5 days	Metabolism	Non-steroidal oestrogen receptor antagonist used for hormone-dependent metastatic breast cancer in postmenopausal women; given orally; metabolised by CYP3A4-mediated demethylation; metabolite retains weak activity; undergoes enterohepatic circulation	Hot flushes; vaginal bleeding and discharge plus numerous other effects
Drugs for prostate cancer				
Bicalutamide	7–10 days	Metabolism	Antiandrogen used for advanced prostate cancer; used to cover the 'flare' associated with administration of gonadorelin analogues; given orally; undergoes oxidation and conjugation; metabolites excreted in urine and bile	Hot flushes; pruritus; gynaecomastia plus rare serious hepatic and cardiovascular effects

continued

Drugs used in the treatment of cancer *(continued)*

Drug	Half-life (h)	Elimination	Comments	Unusual or limiting toxicity[a]
Drugs for prostate cancer (continued)				
Buserelin	3–6 min	Metabolism + renal	Gonadorelin analogue used for advanced prostate cancer; given by subcutaneous injection for 7 days and then nasally; peptide hormone; metabolism plus some excreted in urine	May cause tumour 'flare' leading to spinal cord compression; ureteric obstruction and bone pain
Cyproterone acetate	2 days	Metabolism	Antiandrogen used for prostate cancer and to cover 'flare' of gonadorelin analogues; given orally; hydrolysed and conjugated with glucuronic acid and sulphate; metabolites eliminated in urine and bile	See bicalutamide
Flutamide	8	Metabolism	Antiandrogen used for advanced prostate cancer and to cover the 'flare' of gonadorelin analogues; given orally; complete bioavailability; rapid oxidation in the liver to an active hydroxy metabolite	See bicalutamide
Goserelin	4	Metabolism	Gonadorelin analogue used for prostate cancer and advanced breast cancer; potent LHRH agonist; given by subcutaneous implant into the anterior abdominal wall; metabolised by peptidase-mediated hydrolysis	See buserelin
Leuprorelin acetate (leuprolide)	3–4	Metabolism	Gonadorelin analogue used for advanced prostate cancer; given by subcutaneous or intramuscular injection; metabolised by proteases	See buserelin; plus muscle weakness, hypertension, palpitations
Triptorelin	3	Metabolism	Gonadorelin analogue used for advanced prostate cancer (and endometriosis); given by intramuscular injection; metabolised by proteases	See buserelin

Key AIDS, acquired immunodeficiency syndrome; AUC, area under the curve for plasma concentration versus time; CNS, central nervous system; FDA, US Food and Drug Administration; LHRH, luteinising hormone releasing hormone.

[a]The toxicity that is typical for a class of drug is described in the general text for that class; toxicity given in this table represents 'non-class' effects and/or severe dose-limiting toxicity.

General features: toxicity and prescribing

53 Drug toxicity and overdose

Most therapeutic drugs are developed for their ability to alter human homeostatic mechanisms in order to produce a beneficial response; only antimicrobial agents and parasiticides have the theoretical possibility of a therapeutic response without some direct action on human metabolic or physiological processes. Several therapeutic agents, for example atropine (belladonna), tubocurarine (curare), ergot alkaloids (causing St Anthony's fire), digoxin (digitalis) and dicoumarol (causing haemorrhagic disease in cattle) have effects that were first recognised as a result of either accidental or intentional poisonings. It is hardly surprising, therefore, that all drugs are capable of producing adverse effects. The relationship between a potentially beneficial drug and a poison was recognised five centuries ago when Paracelsus stated: 'all things are toxic and it is only the dose which makes something a poison'.

Many of the medicines prescribed today were first used as plant extracts, for example digitalis glycosides and opium extracts. It was the identification and isolation of the active chemical entities in plant extracts that allowed the dose and purity of the active ingredient to be controlled sufficiently to optimise the ratio between risk and benefit. The current vogue for 'natural, herbal remedies' may be considered to represent a backward step as far as controlling the safety and efficacy of drugs is concerned.

Drug toxicity can develop during the normal therapeutic use of a drug or as a result of an acute overdose. In some cases, toxicity occurs in the majority of treated individuals because of the nature of the drug, for example cytotoxic agents used for cancer chemotherapy. Significant toxicity is rare with the majority of commonly prescribed drugs when used at recommended dosages. There is considerable interindividual variability in the development of adverse reactions, and toxicity may be reduced by taking into account factors that are known to increase vulnerability prior to drug administration, such as age, concurrent disease or bodyweight, when selecting both the drug and the dosage. Usually, a reduction in dosage or a change of drug during chronic treatment will reduce the severity of adverse effects (but see immunological mechanisms discussed below).

Toxicity following an acute overdose usually produces predictable adverse reactions, which may be life threatening and/or prejudice long-term health. Rapid treatment is then required and this may be aimed at preventing further drug absorption, increasing drug elimination/inactivation and managing the adverse effects produced.

This chapter is, therefore, divided into two main sections:

- *drug toxicity*, which discusses mechanisms for adverse effects produced both during normal drug therapy and after an overdose
- *self poisoning and drug overdose*, which is concerned with the management of drug overdose.

Drug toxicity

This section provides a framework for classifying adverse effects, rather than an exhaustive catalogue of drugs and their toxicities. The adverse effects caused by different drugs are listed in the *British National Formulary* (BNF), and it is apparent that for most drugs, toxic effects are more numerous than beneficial properties. Prescribers should be alert to both predicted and unexpected reactions to medicines and should consider the risk–benefit ratio for the particular individual and the suitability of alternative drugs and/or treatments. People who are prescribed drugs should also be informed of the risk–benefit balance inherent in their treatment. Prescription information leaflets included with the dispensed medicine represent a useful way of providing such advice.

It should be appreciated that all drugs are associated with some risk of toxicity, although both the severity and incidence differ widely between drugs. The acceptability of a risk of toxicity is inversely related to the severity of the disease being treated; for example, serious idiosyncratic reactions with incidences of 1 in 10 000 have led to the withdrawal of some non-steroidal anti-inflammatory drugs (NSAIDs), whereas some cancer chemotherapeutic agents can cause significant toxicity in nearly all individuals. In addition 'one man's cure is another man's poison' because the beneficial effects of a drug in one situation (e.g. the antidiarrhoeal effect of opioids) may be an adverse effect in other circumstances (e.g. constipation, when an opioid is used for pain relief). Therefore, even classification of the nature of effect into beneficial or adverse may depend on the condition being treated.

A useful indication of the safety margin available for a drug is given by the therapeutic index (TI):

$$\text{Therapeutic index} = \frac{\text{Dose resulting in toxicity}}{\text{Dose giving therapeutic response}}$$

Drugs such as diazepam have a TI of about 50 and it is difficult for even the most inept doctor to cause serious adverse effects with diazepam. In contrast, digoxin has a TI of only about 2, and for such drugs, toxicity may be precipitated by relatively small changes in dosage regimen, bioavailability or the clearance of the drug from the body. The TI relates to serious adverse effects and does not indicate the potential for minor unwanted effects, which can inconvenience the patient enough for him or her to stop treatment.

Types of drug toxicity

Toxicity is frequently divided into two main types:

type A: these effects are dose-related and largely predictable

type B: these effects are not dose-related and are idiosyncratic and unpredictable.

Our understanding of the mechanisms involved in toxicity has increased greatly in recent years, and this provides a useful framework for students to integrate future knowledge:

- pharmacological: type A
- biochemical: type A and some type B
- immunological: type B
- unknown: mostly type B?

Pharmacological toxicity

In 'pharmacological toxicity', the toxic reaction is an extension of the known pharmacology of the drug at its site(s) of action (Table 53.1), and there are numerous examples in this book where the adverse effect is really an excessive therapeutic action.

Table 53.1

Drugs with adverse effects that are related to their primary therapeutic properties

Drug	Adverse effect
Warfarin	Haemorrhage
Insulin	Hypoglycaemia
β-Adrenoceptor antagonists (β-blockers)	Heart block when used as an antiarrhythmic
Loop diuretics	Hypokalaemia
General anaesthetics	Medullary depression
Acetylcholinesterase inhibitors	Muscle weakness

For many effects, the response increases with increase in dose, with low subtherapeutic doses giving an inadequate response, therapeutic doses giving the desired response, but very high doses giving an excessive response that can be regarded as a form of toxicity. A good example is warfarin (Ch. 11), where inadequate doses are associated with a lack of effect and a risk of thrombosis remains, whereas at excessive doses there is a risk of haemorrhage. The increase in response with increase in dose has given rise to the concept of a 'therapeutic window' within which most individuals should show a beneficial response with minimal risk of adverse effects (response 1 in Fig. 53.1). This concept is particularly valuable in the interpretation of measurements of drug concentrations in plasma, which can be used to monitor compliance and to assess likely response (Table 53.2).

In many other cases, the toxic reaction may be unrelated to the primary therapeutic effect (examples are given in Table 53.3), and may be caused by a secondary effect that is not the primary aim of the treatment given (response 2 in Fig. 53.1). This toxicity would usually be present to a limited extent at appropriate therapeutic doses.

The separation of therapeutic and toxic dose–response curves is a measure of the TI. If these are very close (e.g. response 2 in Fig. 53.1), then there is a low safety margin and most individuals will exhibit some degree of toxicity, for example myelosuppression with cytotoxic anticancer drugs.

A high TI occurs when the toxicity would not be seen with normal therapeutic doses (response 3 in Fig. 53.1), for example heart failure caused by myocardial depression in those with normal left ventricular function taking β-adrenoceptor antagonists. However, some individuals may be uniquely sensitive to the toxic effect because of their genetics or their physical condition, for example β-adrenoceptor antagonists may precipitate heart failure in those with pre-existing impaired left ventricular function.

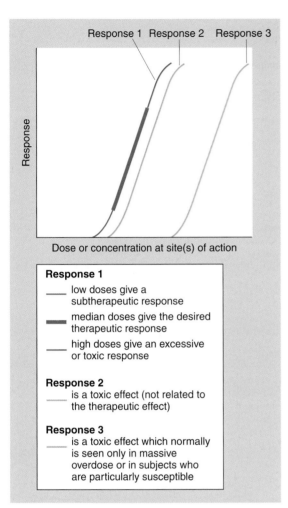

Response 1 Response 2 Response 3

Response 1

____ low doses give a
subtherapeutic response

____ median doses give the desired
therapeutic response

____ high doses give an excessive
or toxic response

Response 2

____ is a toxic effect (not related to
the therapeutic effect)

Response 3

____ is a toxic effect which normally
is seen only in massive
overdose or in subjects who
are particularly susceptible

Fig. 53.1
Dose–response relationships in relation to toxicity. Response 1 is
the primary therapeutic effect, which shows an increase in the
magnitude of response with increase in dose from sub-therapeutic,
through therapeutic, to potentially toxic. Response 2 is an undesired
effect seen at a dose only slightly greater than those producing the
therapeutic effect. Response 3 is an adverse effect normally seen only
in overdose.

Pharmacological toxicity is the most common cause
of adverse effects. Such toxicity can be minimised by an
assessment of the risk–benefit balance for the individual
to be treated. This should take into account factors that
may influence both pharmacokinetics and sensitivity,
including age, physiological status (e.g. renal function),
concurrent medication, disease processes, environmental
aspects (e.g. smoking), etc.

Because of the predictable nature of pharmacological
toxicity, it is possible to co-prescribe drugs that will
reduce the possibility of toxic effects; examples include
antiemetics given with cancer chemotherapy, vitamin B_6
given with isoniazid, and leucovorin (folinic acid) given
after methotrexate.

Biochemical toxicity

In 'biochemical toxicity', the toxicity or tissue damage is
caused by an interaction of the drug, or an active metabolite, with cell components, especially macromolecules
such as structural proteins and enzymes. A generalised
scheme is given in Figure 53.2. For most approved
drugs, this form of toxicity is characterised during both
preclinical studies in animals and early clinical trials
(Ch. 3), for example by monitoring changes in serum
enzyme levels.

In some situations, an understanding of the
mechanism of toxicity has allowed the development of
appropriate treatments. An example is the key observation that the thiol (-SH) group of the tripeptide
glutathione provides a cytoprotective mechanism for
preventing cell damage caused by highly reactive
chemical species, such as the toxic drug metabolite of
paracetamol (see below and Fig. 53.3). The nature of the
cell damage caused depends on the stability of the toxic
reactive chemical (metabolite); extremely unstable
metabolites may bind covalently to and inactivate the
enzyme that forms them; more stable species, however,
may be able to diffuse to a distant site, for example
DNA, and initiate changes, such as cancer. Examples of
biochemical toxicity are given below.

Paracetamol

Paracetamol-induced hepatotoxicity represents the
results of an imbalance between metabolic inactivation
of paracetamol via conjugation with glucuronic acid and
sulphate and activation to an unstable toxic metabolite
via oxidation by cytochrome P450. This metabolite binds
covalently to proteins and causes cell necrosis. Low doses
of paracetamol are safe because they are eliminated by
conjugation with little oxidation; however, in overdose,
the sulphate conjugation reaction is saturated and there
is increased cytochrome P450-mediated oxidation to the
toxic unstable quinone-imine metabolite (Fig. 53.3). Early
after an overdose, much of the toxic metabolite is inactivated by a cytoprotective pathway involving glutathione, but there is increased covalent binding and cell
death once the available glutathione has been depleted.
This biochemical mechanism explains the site of toxicity
(centrilobular necrosis in the liver because of the large
amounts of cytochrome P450 present) and the increased
toxicity seen in individuals treated with inducers of
cytochrome P450 (especially alcohol-related induction
of CYP2E1), and in those with low hepatic stores of
glutathione due to poor nutrition. An understanding of
the mechanism of toxicity of paracetamol led to the
development of treatment with N-acetylcysteine, which
enhances the cytoprotective processes by providing an
additional source of thiol groups for conjugation of the
active metabolite and protection of thiol groups in
proteins (see treatment of drug overdose, below).

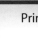

Table 53.2
Therapeutic windows based on plasma concentrations

Drug	Therapeutic concentration range[a]		Toxic response
	Minimum	**Maximum**[b]	
Aspirin (analgesia) ($\mu g\ ml^{-1}$)	20	300	Tinnitus, metabolic acidosis
Carbamazepine ($\mu g\ ml^{-1}$)	4	10	Drowsiness, visual disturbances
Digitoxin ($ng\ ml^{-1}$)	15	30	Bradycardia, nausea
Digoxin ($ng\ ml^{-1}$)	0.8	3	Bradycardia, nausea
Gentamicin ($\mu g\ ml^{-1}$)	2	12	Ototoxicity, renal toxicity
Kanamycin ($\mu g\ ml^{-1}$)	10	40	Ototoxicity, renal toxicity
Phenytoin ($\mu g\ ml^{-1}$)	10	20	Nystagmus, lethargy
Theophylline ($\mu g\ ml^{-1}$)	10	20	Tremor, nervousness

[a]The values given represent average values only; individuals will vary in their inherent sensitivity and response to particular concentrations. The concept of a therapeutic window also applies to situations where the response can be measured directly (e.g. blood clotting control with warfarin and hypoglycaemia with oral hypoglycaemics).
[b]The maximum concentration may be based on toxicity related to the primary therapeutic response (e.g. carbamazepine) or an unrelated effects (e.g. gentamicin).

Table 53.3
Examples of drugs with adverse effects unrelated to their primary therapeutic use

Drug	Adverse effects
Opioid analgesic	Respiratory depression when used for analgesia
β-Adrenoceptor antagonist	Reduction in heart rate when used for hypertension
Anticonvulsant	Sedation when used for epilepsy

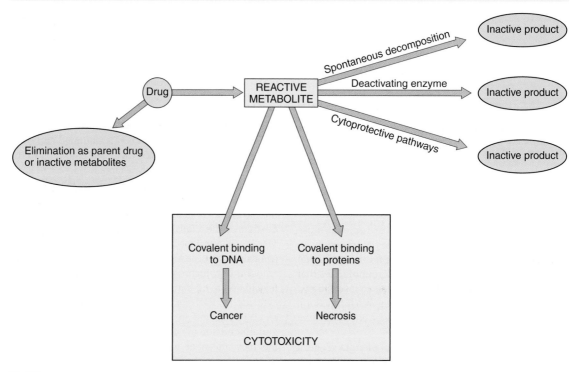

Fig. 53.2
Metabolism and cytotoxicity. The extent of cytotoxicity depends on (i) the balance between the activation process and alternative pathways of elimination of the parent drug to produce an inactive product, and (ii) the balance between inactivation of the reactive metabolite and the production of biochemically adverse effects. Therapeutic interventions are aimed at either increasing elimination of the parent drug or enhancing cytoprotective pathways to protect against the effects of cytotoxic products.

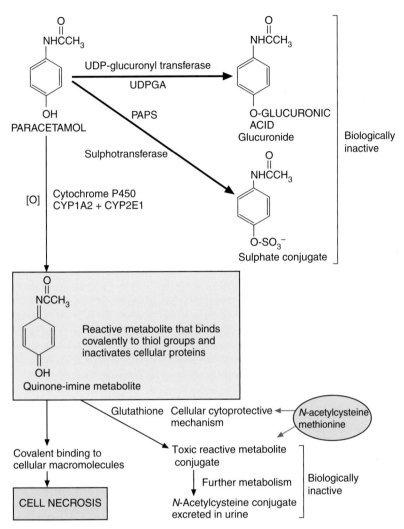

Fig. 53.3
Pathways of paracetamol metabolism. In overdose, the concentrations of 3′-phosphoadenosine 5′-phosphosulphate (PAPS) (for sulphation) and glutathione (for cytoprotection) are depleted, and extensive macromolecular binding leads to hepatocellular necrosis. UDPGA, uridine diphosphate glucuronic acid. N-acetylcysteine and methionine replenish glutathione in order to conjugate the toxic metabolite.

The sulphur-containing amino acid methionine can also prevent paracetamol-induced hepatotoxicity, and a combination of paracetamol plus methionine (co-methiamol) is available. Such a formulation may prove to be of particular value to high-risk groups such as children (because of the greater risk of accidental overdose) and alcoholics (because of the possibility of induction of CYP2E1 and depressed glutathione levels).

Cyclophosphamide

Cyclophosphamide is an anticancer drug that is converted to highly toxic metabolites, which are eliminated in the urine and cause haemorrhagic cystitis (Ch. 52). This can be prevented by prior treatment with mesna (mercaptoethane sulphonic acid), which possesses both a thiol group for cytoprotection and a highly polar sulphonic acid group, which results in high renal excretion and delivery of this cytoprotective molecule to the bladder epithelium. Because of its polarity, mesna is absorbed slowly and incompletely from the gut, but is eliminated rapidly; it is, therefore, given intravenously prior to cyclophosphamide in order to cover the period of maximum excretion of toxic cyclophosphamide metabolites. It is not yet known if mesna will also protect against bladder cancer, which can arise about 10–20 years after initial treatment with cyclophosphamide.

Isoniazid

Isoniazid, which is used for the treatment of tuberculosis (Ch. 51), causes hepatitis in about 0.5% of treated individuals. This is believed to result from the formation of a reactive metabolite, N-acetylhydrazine, which is

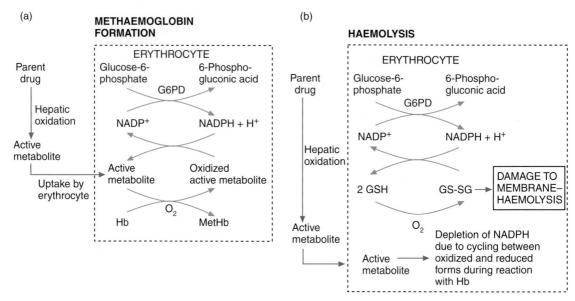

Fig. 53.4
Mechanisms of methaemoglobinaemia (a) and haemolysis (b). Hb, haemoglobin; G6PD, glucose 6-phosphate dehydrogenase; GS–SG, glutathione dimer (oxidised form); GSH, glutathione (reduced form), NADP, nicotinamide adenine dinucleotide phosphate. High concentrations of reduced glutathione are necessary for maintaining the erythrocyte cell membrane integrity; a build-up of oxidised glutathione is associated with haemolysis. The active metabolite may also react with glutathione directly to lower GSH concentrations.

produced by acetylation followed by oxidative metabolism. Fast acetylators (see Ch. 2) form more N-acetylhydrazine than do slow acetylators, but, unexpectedly, they are not more sensitive to isoniazid toxicity. The biochemical basis for the susceptibility of some individuals to the hepatotoxic metabolite is not known; it is possibly related to the balance between further activation of N-acetylhydrazine (by cytochrome P450-mediated oxidation) and detoxification of N-acetylhydrazine by further acetylation. Consequently, fast acetylators may produce more active metabolite and also inactive it more rapidly.

Spironolactone

Spironolactone (Ch. 14) is oxidised by cytochrome P450. The metabolite formed in the testes binds to and destroys testicular cytochrome P450 and this causes a decrease in the metabolism of progesterone to testosterone (which is also catalysed by a cytochrome P450). This effect, combined with an antiandrogenic action at receptor sites (pharmacological toxicity), results in gynaecomastia and decreased libido.

Aromatic amines and nitrites

Aromatic amines, such as the anti-leprosy drug dapsone and some antimalarials, are metabolised in the liver to toxic products, which are released into the circulation, where they can cause methaemoglobinaemia and/or haemolysis.

Methaemoglobinaemia. In the presence of oxygen, the active metabolite oxidises haemoglobin (Fe^{2+}) to methaemoglobin (Fe^{3+}) and is oxidised itself (Fig. 53.4a). Because of the large amounts of haemoglobin in the blood, compared with the amount of drug given, this would be inconsequential, except that the oxidised active metabolite can be recycled back to the active metabolite by reduction with NADPH (reduced nicotinamide adenine dinucleotide phosphate) in the erythrocyte. Consequently, one molecule of the metabolite is able to oxidise many molecules of haemoglobin. The recycling depends on the presence of NADPH, which is formed during the metabolism of glucose 6-phosphate via glucose 6-phosphate dehydrogenase (G6PD) (Fig. 53.4). The amounts of G6PD, and hence of NADPH, are determined genetically, and the incidence of G6PD deficiency is high in Black races and very high in Mediterranean races, such as the Kurds. Such subjects have limited NADPH reserves and, therefore, have a low ability to reduce the oxidised drug metabolite (Fig. 53.4) back to the active metabolite. In consequence, there is limited redox cycling of the active drug metabolite and such individuals are less susceptible to drug-induced methaemoglobinaemia.

Haemolysis. This arises from accumulation of oxidised glutathione (GS–SG in Fig. 53.4b) in the erythrocyte; oxidised glutathione accumulates because recycling of the drug metabolite, linked to the formation of methaemoglobin (Fig 53.4a), causes depletion of NADPH, which is the cofactor essential for the reduction of oxidised glutathione. Low endogenous levels of

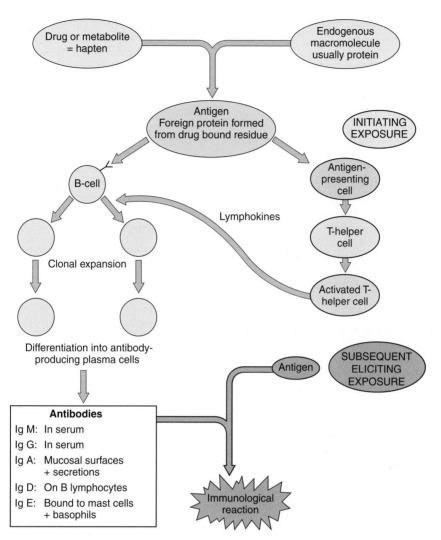

Fig. 53.5
Mechanisms of drug allergy. The initial exposure produces an antigen, which results in the production of antibodies via B-cell clonal expansion and differentiations; this is stimulated by cytokines from activated T-helper cells. The eliciting exposure occurs later (usually at least 3 days later, during which time therapy may or may not be continuing); antigen–antibody interaction then exposes a complement-binding site, which triggers the reaction. The nature of the immunological reaction depends on the nature of the antibody and/or localisation of the antigen. Treatment is with immunosuppressant drugs (Ch. 38).

NADPH, as found in the groups with G6PD deficiency (see above), means that NADPH reserves can be depleted rapidly and the oxidised glutathione cannot be reduced; therefore, individuals with G6PD deficiency are very susceptible to haemolysis. Given the geographical distribution of G6PD deficiency, it is ironic that the amino groups associated with this form of toxicity are often present in drugs used to treat tropical infections (primaquine for the treatment of malaria see Ch. 51 and Box 47.6).

Immunological toxicity

Immunological toxicity is frequently referred to as 'drug allergy' and is the form of toxicity with which people may be most familiar, for example penicillin allergy.

Immunological mechanisms are implicated in a number of common adverse effects, such as rashes and fever, but may also be involved in organ-directed toxicity. Although the term allergy may not be strictly correct for all forms of immunologically mediated toxicity, it is probably better than hypersensitivity, which has also been used to describe an elevated sensitivity to any mechanism or effect.

Low-molecular-weight compounds (<1100 Da) are not able to elicit an allergic response unless the compound, or a metabolite, forms a stable or covalent bond with a macromolecule. Covalent binding to a normal protein produces a 'novel protein' that is recognised as foreign by the immune system and acts as an antigen. The process has been recognised for many years and is summarised in Figure 53.5.

Immunologically mediated toxicity shows a wide range of characteristics.

- Toxicity is unrelated to pharmacological toxicity, but has been implicated in some forms of biochemical toxicity because immunological toxicity may arise if a reactive metabolite is formed which binds covalently to proteins.
- Toxicity is unrelated to dose: once the antibody has been produced, even very small amounts of antigen can trigger a reaction.
- There is normally a lag of at least 3 days between initial exposure and the development of symptoms; however, the first dose of a subsequent treatment may give an immediate reaction.
- Cross-reactivity is possible among different compounds that share the same antigen determinant or structural component that is involved in antibody recognition, such as the penicilloyl group of the penicillin family.
- The incidence varies between different drugs – for example, from about 1 in 10 000 for phenylbutazone-induced agranulocytosis to 1 in 20 for ampicillin-related skin rashes.
- The response is idiosyncratic but genetically controlled; individual responsiveness cannot be predicted, but individuals who have a history of atopic disease are more likely to develop a 'drug allergy'.

The effects produced may be subdivided into the classic four types of allergic reaction (see also Ch. 38).

- Type 1: immediate or anaphylactic reactions. These are mediated via IgE antibodies attached to the surface of basophils and mast cells; the release of numerous mediators, for example histamine, 5-hydroxytryptamine (5HT) and leukotrienes, produces effects that include urticaria, bronchial constriction, hypotension, oedema and shock. A skin-prick challenge test usually produces an acute inflammatory response. Examples of drugs having this type of effect are penicillins and peptide drugs such as crisantaspase.
- Type 2: cytotoxic reactions. The antigen is formed by the drug binding to a cell membrane; subsequent interaction of this antigen with circulating IgG, IgM or IgA antibodies activates complement and initiates cell lysis. Loss of the carrier cell can result in thrombocytopenia (e.g. digitoxin, cephalosporins, quinine), neutropenia (e.g. phenylbutazone, metronidazole), and haemolytic anaemia (e.g. penicillins, rifampicin [rifampin] and possibly methyldopa).
- Type 3: immune-complex reactions. The antigen–antibody interaction occurs in serum and the complex formed is deposited on endothelial cells, basement membranes, etc. to initiate a more localised inflammatory reaction, for example arteritis and nephritis. Examples include serum sickness (urticaria, angioedema, fever) with penicillins, lupus erythematosus-like syndrome with hydralazine and procainamide (especially in slow acetylators) and possibly NSAID-related nephropathy.
- Type 4: cell-mediated delayed-type reactions. Reaction to the eliciting exposure is delayed. The reactions occur mostly in skin through the formation of an antigen between the drug (hapten) and skin proteins. This is followed by an infiltration of sensitised T-lymphocytes, which recognise the antigen and release lymphokines to produce local inflammation, oedema and irritation, for example contact dermatitis.

In addition to true immunologically mediated toxicity, as described above, there are examples of so-called 'allergic' reactions, such as aspirin hypersensitivity, which show many of the characteristics given above (e.g. rashes, induction of asthma in susceptible individuals, cross-reactivity with other aromatic acids such as benzoates), but for which a true immunological basis has not been demonstrated.

It has been estimated that 'drug allergy' accounts for about 10% of adverse drug reactions but that severe reactions are rare. For example, only about 5 individuals in 10 000 develop an anaphylactic reaction to penicillins, but about one-half of these are sufficiently serious to warrant hospital treatment, which is aimed at blocking the effects on the airways and heart and preventing further mediator release (see Ch. 39). However, given the large numbers of subjects receiving drugs such as penicillins, 'drug allergy' is an important source of iatrogenic morbidity.

Self-poisoning and drug overdose

Self-poisoning can be either accidental or deliberate. Approximately a quarter of a million episodes are believed to occur each year in England and Wales, although less than 40% of these reach hospital. Deaths from self-poisoning still average about 2000 each year in England and Wales. Accidental poisoning is common in children under 5 years of age, when it often involves household products as well as medicines. A second peak of self-poisoning occurs in the teens and early twenties, when it is more frequent in girls. The incidence then progressively falls with increasing age. Most deliberate self-poisoning represents 'parasuicide' or attention-seeking behaviour. True suicide attempts comprise a minority of events, occurring most frequently in those over 45 years. However, it is important to recognise that the severity of poisoning bears little relationship to suicidal intent. About 30% of the deaths from deliberate overdose are in those over 65 years of age: self-poisoning at this age occurs most often in response to depression or specific life events such as bereavement.

The drugs most frequently used for self-poisoning are benzodiazepines, analgesics and antidepressants. Alcohol is often taken together with these drugs. It is important to attempt to identify the cause of the poisoning since it may influence treatment. However, it should be remembered that information from the patient about which drug was taken, how much, and the time of overdosing, is frequently unreliable.

Management principles

The emergency treatment of poisoning is described in the introduction to the BNF. Additional sources of information include Regional Medicines Information Centres and Poisons Information Centres; computer databases available to registered users include TOXBASE (which has information on household products and industrial and agricultural chemicals as well as drugs) and TICTAC (which provides computer-aided identification of tablets and capsules). The management of drug overdose, which is outlined below, has a number of principal aims (Fig. 53.6).

Managing adverse effects

Immediate measures

There are certain immediate measures required when someone presents with a possible drug overdose or poisoning:

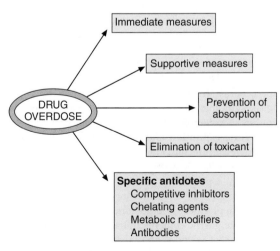

Fig. 53.6
Principles underlying the management of drug overdose.

- remove the person from contact with poison if appropriate, for example gases, corrosives
- assess vital signs: pulse, respiration and pupil size; inspect the person for injury
- ensure a clear airway; if breathing but unconscious, place in the coma position
- obtain a clear history if possible
- preserve any evidence, for example bottles, written notes, etc.

Supportive measures

Examples of unwanted effects seen in drug overdose are shown in Table 53.4. A number of the effects will require supportive measures (Fig. 53.7).

Cardiac or respiratory arrest. These may result from a toxic effect of the drug on the heart, from depression of the respiratory centre or from metabolic disturbance. Assisted ventilation, ranging from mouth-to-mouth, or Ambu-bag inflation, to the use of a ventilator, may be required. In some circumstances, recovery is possible even after prolonged resuscitation.

Hypotension. A low blood pressure is common in severe poisoning with central nervous system (CNS) depressants. It should be treated if accompanied by poor tissue perfusion or low urine output. Depression of the vasomotor centre can cause arterial dilation and peripheral venous pooling, producing a low central venous pressure. This should be raised to 10–15 cm H_2O (measured from the midaxillary line) by intravenous infusion of a colloid solution, such as dextran polymers. If hypotension occurs with a normal or raised central venous pressure, this suggests myocardial depression. Positive inotropic drugs such as the β_1-adrenoceptor agonist dobutamine (Ch. 7) should then be used.

Arrhythmias. Disturbances of cardiac rhythm should only be treated if they are severe. Ventricular arrhythmias causing hypotension often require intervention, but caution should be exercised if there is a long Q–T interval on the electrocardiogram (ECG), since the tachycardia often fails to respond to standard antiarrhythmic drugs. It is essential to correct metabolic derangements that predispose to arrhythmias, for example hypothermia, hypoxia, hypercapnia, hypokalaemia, hyperkalaemia and acidosis.

Convulsions. These may be caused by a treatable underlying change such as hypoxia, hypoglycaemia or hypocalcaemia, or they may be a direct toxic effect of the drug on neuronal function. Lorazepam or diazepam intravenously (or rectal diazepam if the intravenous route is unavailable) (Ch. 20) is the treatment of choice. Artificial ventilation with neuromuscular blockade (Ch. 27) is used if the siezures cannot be controlled.

Renal failure. Kidney damage is usually a consequence of prolonged hypotension. Other causes include a direct nephrotoxic effect of the drug and renal damage produced by the products of toxic muscle necrosis (rhabdomyolysis).

Table 53.4
Complications of acute poisonings

Cardiac arrest	Direct cardiotoxicity	Many
	Hypoxia	Many
	Electrolyte/metabolic disturbance	Many
Central nervous system depression		Many
Convulsions	Direct neurotoxicity	Tricyclic antidepressants, theophylline
	Hypoxia	Many
Hypotension	Myocardial depression	β-Adrenoceptor antagonists, tricyclic antidepressants (dextropropoxyphene*)
	Peripheral vasodilation	Many
Arrhythmia	Direct cardiotoxicity	β-Adrenoceptor antagonists, tricyclic antidepressants, verapamil, digoxin
	Hypoxia	Many
	Electrolyte/metabolic disturbance	Many
Renal failure	Hypotension	Many
	Rhabdomyolysis	Opioids, hypnotics, ethanol, carbon monoxide
	Direct nephrotoxicity	Paracetamol, heavy metals
Hepatic failure	Direct hepatotoxicity	Paracetamol, carbon tetrachloride
Respiratory depression	Direct neurotoxicity	Sedatives, hypnotics, opioids

*Dextropropoxyphene has recently been withdrawn in the UK

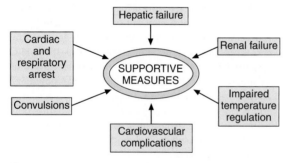

Fig. 53.7
Main effects of overdose requiring supportive measures.

Hepatic failure. This usually results from the direct toxic effects of specific agents, such as paracetamol.

Impaired temperature regulation. Hypothermia is common, and can be caused by depression of metabolic rate with reduced heat production and by increased heat loss from cutaneous vasodilation. It is common with phenothiazines and barbiturates, but is seen with any prolonged coma. Rewarming, preferably by wrapping in a 'space blanket', reduces the risk of serious ventricular arrhythmias. By contrast, CNS stimulants such as Ecstasy can produce hyperthermia, as does aspirin by uncoupling cellular oxidative phosphorylation.

Reducing toxicity

The adverse effects can be reduced by:

- minimising further drug absorption
- maximising drug elimination
- negating effects with antidotes, etc.

Prevention of absorption of poisons

There are three principal methods of preventing further absorption of the drug: emesis, gastric aspiration and lavage, and activated charcoal.

Emesis. Vomiting can be induced in a conscious person who has not ingested a corrosive agent. Stimulation of the pharynx can be tried in children but is often ineffective. Ipecacuanha is sometimes advocated to induce vomiting. It is a plant extract, containing emetine and cephaeline, which irritates the stomach and stimulates the medullary vomiting centre. Most people vomit within 30 min and prolonged vomiting can occur. There are doubts as to its effectiveness in removing drug from the stomach, and the unwanted effects of ipecacuanha (nausea, drowsiness and lethargy) may mask symptoms of the overdose; in consequence, the routine use of emetics is no longer recommended.

Gastric aspiration and lavage. This should not be considered in unconscious or drowsy persons without protection of the airways by a cuffed endotracheal tube to prevent aspiration of gastric contents into the lungs. It should never be used after ingestion of corrosives or petroleum products. A large-bore orogastric tube is used to aspirate gastric contents initially and then to lavage with doses of water at body temperature. Its effectiveness is unproven. Gastric lavage is normally only used for up to 1 h after ingestion of a significant amount of

Table 53.5
Drug adsorption onto activated charcoal

Drug/compounds not adsorbed	Drugs/compounds adsorbed
Acids	Aspirin
Alkalis	Carbamazepine
Cyanide	Dapsone
DDT (insecticide)	Digoxin
Ethanol	Ecstacy
Ethyleneglycol (antifreeze)	Paraquat (herbicide)
Ferrous salts	Phenobarbital
Lead	Quinine
Lithium	Sustained-release preparations
Mercury	Theophylline
Methanol	Tricyclic antidepressants
Organic solvents	

drug. There may be benefit for up to 4 h after aspirin and/or in unconscious persons, and for up to 4–6 h after a life-threatening overdose of tricyclic antidepressants, but activated charcoal is now preferred.

Activated charcoal. This formulation of charcoal has a large adsorbent area and is given as a suspension in water. Activated charcoal adsorbs, or binds, the drug and retains it in the gastrointestinal lumen. Not all drugs are adsorbed onto charcoal (see Table 53.5). About 10 g of charcoal is required for every 1 g of poison, which makes it impractical for poisons that are usually ingested in large quantities. An initial dose of 50 g of charcoal for adults can prevent drug absorption if given within 1 h of drug ingestion (later after poisoning with modified-release preparations, or drugs with anti-muscarinic properties that delay gastric emptying). Repeated administration of 50 g every 4 h over 24–36 h achieves further retention of adsorbed drug in the small intestine. Drug is continuously being transferred in both directions across the gut wall, with the concentration gradient normally favouring net absorption, owing to the high concentration free in solution within the gut lumen. If drug in the bowel is bound onto the charcoal, this lowers the free concentration and can result in net transfer from the body into the gut and enhanced elimination of the compound. This is useful for overdose with barbiturates, carbamazepine, dapsone, quinine and theophylline. Charcoal should not be given to drowsy or comatose persons, because of the risk of aspiration into the lungs. Constipation is the major unwanted effect of charcoal; charcoal should not be given in the absence of bowel sounds, because of the risk of obstruction.

Elimination of poisons

There are three principal methods of enhancing elimination of the drug: activated charcoal (see above), renal elimination and haemodialysis/haemoperfusion.

Renal elimination. Forced diuresis with intravenous infusion of large quantities of fluid was advocated in the past for drugs that are mostly eliminated unchanged by the kidney or if renally excreted metabolites are toxic. Major disadvantages of forced diuresis are serious disturbances of fluid or electrolyte balance, and therefore it is no longer recommended. Altering urine pH while maintaining normal urine flow can be effective in increasing the renal elimination of drugs that are weak electrolytes. This is achieved by increasing the ionisation of the drug, which reduces reabsorption from the renal tubule by lowering its lipid solubility (Ch. 2). Only a modest increase in urinary flow rate is required. Weak acids, such as salicylates, are excreted more readily in alkaline urine (alkaline diuresis – achieved by giving sodium bicarbonate), while the converse is true for weak bases (acid diuresis – achieved by giving ammonium chloride).

Haemodialysis or haemoperfusion. These are reserved for the most severely poisoned subjects. These techniques are successful only if a large proportion of the body burden of the drug is retained in the plasma and available for removal (i.e. the drug has a low apparent volume of distribution; see Ch. 2). Haemodialysis relies on diffusion of the drug across a semi-permeable membrane from blood to the dialysis fluid, and is used for salicylates, phenobarbital, methanol, ethylene glycol and lithium. Haemoperfusion involves adsorption of drug from blood as it passes down a column containing activated charcoal or a resin; it is used for short- or medium-acting barbiturates, chloral hydrate, meprobamate and theophylline.

Specific antidotes

Antidotes are only available for a minority of drugs commonly involved in poisonings. Some important examples are given below.

Competitive inhibitors

- Atropine acts at muscarinic receptors to block the parasympathetic effects of organophosphorus insecticides. It is given by intravenous or intramuscular injection.
- Naloxone acts at opioid receptors to reverse the effects of narcotic analgesics. Its short half-life, compared with those of most opioids, means that repeated injections or an infusion are usually needed.
- Flumazenil is an antagonist at benzodiazepine receptors. It is rarely needed for the treatment of intentional overdose, because fatalities are uncommon with this class of drug and flumazenil can cause convulsions in benzodiazepine-dependent subjects. It is of value in reversing the effects of benzodiazepines when toxicity occurs in those with chronic liver disease.

Chelating agents

Chelating agents act by forming a complex with the drug or chemical, which reduces the free (active) drug concentration:

- desferrioxamine for ferrous ions; given by intravenous infusion
- dicobalt edetate for cyanide; given by intravenous injection
- dimercaprol for antimony, arsenic, bismuth, gold and mercury; it is used with sodium calcium edetate for lead; given by intramuscular injection
- penicillamine for lead; given by regular oral dosing
- sodium calcium edetate for lead; given by intravenous infusion
- sodium nitrite, together with sodium thiosulphate, for cyanide; both given by intravenous injection.

Compounds that affect drug metabolism

- Ethanol is used in the treatment of methanol poisoning, because it acts as a competitive substrate for alcohol dehydrogenase, preventing formation of the toxic metabolites formaldehyde and formic acid.
- N-Acetylcysteine provides a substrate for conjugation of the cytotoxic metabolite of paracetamol when the natural conjugating ligand, glutathione, is depleted.

Antibodies

Digoxin can be neutralised in severe poisoning by specific antibody fragments. The antibodies are raised in sheep and cleaved to remove the antigenic crystalline (Fc) portion of the molecule while retaining the specific antigen-binding fragment (Fab).

Some specific common poisonings

Paracetamol

Paracetamol overdose can be fatal, with about 200 deaths occurring each year in England and Wales. Metabolism of paracetamol takes place in the liver, mainly producing non-toxic conjugates (Fig. 53.3). A small amount is oxidised by the cytochrome P450 system to a reactive intermediate, N-acetyl-p-benzoquinone imine (NAPBQI), which is inactivated by conjugation with the thiol group on glutathione. When hepatic glutathione is depleted (which occurs readily in overdose), oxidative stress, coupled with NAPBQI-mediated denaturation of protein, produces hepatic necrosis. Similar processes in the kidney can cause renal tubular necrosis.

In the first 24 h there are few symptoms apart from nausea, vomiting, abdominal pain and sweating; these usually resolve. Liver damage begins within 24 h after a large overdose, producing right upper quadrant pain and tenderness. Jaundice is apparent by 36–48 h and liver damage is maximal by 3–4 days. Severe liver failure, requiring transplantation for survival, can ensue. The most sensitive measures of liver damage are the prothrombin time, or the international normalised ratio (INR), and the plasma unconjugated bilirubin. Renal failure is seen in about a quarter of those with severe liver damage.

Activated charcoal in large doses is recommended within 1 h of a potentially serious paracetamol overdose. Because antidotes are most effective when given early, blood should be analysed for paracetamol if there is any suspicion of poisoning. Blood should be taken at 4 h or more after the suspected overdose, since a low plasma level before then could reflect incomplete absorption of a large overdose. Antidotes used in paracetamol poisoning, such as N-acetylcysteine and methionine, replace glutathione as a thiol donor in the liver; glutathione itself is not used, because it cannot enter liver cells from the blood.

Methionine can be given orally as an initial measure, but not with or after activated charcoal, because methionine can compete with paracetamol for adsorption. Methionine should not be used if there is vomiting, or started more than 10–12 h after ingestion of paracetamol, since the efficacy of methionine in late poisoning is unknown. Administration of intravenous acetylcysteine more than 4 h after the overdose is the preferred treatment for potentially serious poisoning, and should be started prior to the analysis of a plasma paracetamol concentration. A graph is available (Fig. 53.8) to indicate the risk of liver damage for a given plasma paracetamol concentration related to the time after ingestion. The plasma concentration before 4 h is unreliable because absorption and distribution may still be occurring, while

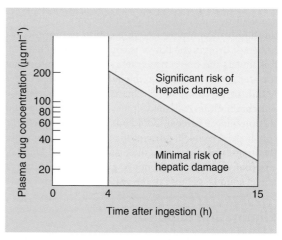

Fig. 53.8
Relationship between plasma paracetamol concentration and the risk of liver damage.

plasma concentrations after 15 h must be interpreted by extrapolation of the graph. Treatment is only necessary if potentially toxic paracetamol concentrations are detected. It is important to realise that toxicity can occur at much lower plasma paracetamol concentrations under certain circumstances:

- concurrent use of drugs such as alcohol or phenytoin that induce liver cytochrome P450 (Ch. 2) and hence increase the formation of the reactive metabolite
- pre-existing liver disease
- malnourished/anorexic persons
- infection with human immunodeficiency virus (HIV).

All such individuals should be treated if plasma paracetamol concentrations are only one-half of those shown in Figure 53.8.

Treatment used to be confined to the first 15 h after overdose, but recent evidence suggests that liver damage can be reduced even when the antidote is delayed for up to 20–30 h. It may be useful even later after ingestion to reduce the severity of established liver damage.

Salicylates

Although salicylate poisoning is becoming less common, there are still about 150 deaths each year in England and Wales. Aspirin is hydrolysed rapidly to salicylic acid after absorption, but further metabolism, by conjugation with glycine, is rate-limited. Symptoms of toxicity are nausea, vomiting, abdominal pain, tinnitus, deafness, hyperventilation and sweating. Agitation frequently occurs in adults, but children become comatose. The chain of metabolic events produced by aspirin is shown in Figure 53.9.

Activated charcoal is recommended for reducing absorption if given early. Correction of fluid, electrolyte and acid–base balance is fundamental to successful management; a fluid deficit of 3–4 l is not unusual in severe poisoning. Forced alkaline diuresis is no longer advocated to enhance salicylate elimination; simple alkalinisation of the urine with 1.26% sodium bicarbonate to raise the pH above 7.5 is effective and safer. Haemodialysis is the treatment of choice in severe poisoning, especially if there is severe metabolic acidosis.

Tricyclic antidepressants

Approximately 400 deaths per year occur in England and Wales from overdose with tricyclic antidepressants. Antimuscarinic effects delay gastric emptying and oral activated charcoal is used routinely for up to 4 h after the overdose. Drowsiness and confusion are followed by convulsions and coma in more severe poisoning. Cardiac depression can produce hypotension. Serious arrhythmias, such as ventricular tachycardia, can occur,

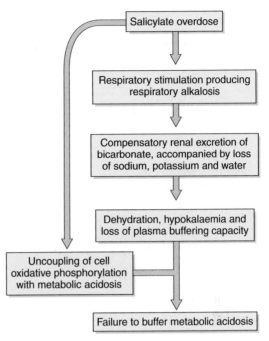

Fig. 53.9
The metabolic consequences of salicylate overdose.

and ECG monitoring is recommended for at least 24 h. Arrhythmias frequently respond to correction of acidosis or hypoxia; if this is not successful, phenytoin or direct current shock can be used. Antiarrhythmic drugs that depress cardiac contractility should be avoided.

Opioid analgesics

The triad of signs characteristic of opioid overdose are:

- respiratory depression
- pinpoint pupils
- impaired consciousness.

They can be reversed rapidly by administration of naloxone (Ch. 19), which is a competitive antagonist at opioid μ-receptors. After an initial intravenous bolus dose of naloxone, it is often necessary to give repeated boluses or a continuous infusion, because the half-life of naloxone is very short compared with those of most opioids. In poisoning with buprenorphine, the effect of naloxone is often incomplete, and assisted ventilation may also be needed. In poisoning with co-proxamol (dextropropoxyphene with paracetamol), especially if taken with alcohol, acute cardiovascular collapse can occur within 30 min of ingestion. For this reason co-proxamol has been withdrawn from the market in the UK. Acute poisoning with organophosphorus insecticides can produce signs that are similar to those with opioids, but naloxone will have no effect.

Ecstasy

Ecstasy (3,4-methylenedioxymethamphetamine; MDMA), toxicity is characterised by tachycardia, hyper-reflexia, hyperpyrexia, and initial hypertension followed by hypotension. In severe cases, delirium, convulsions, coma and cardiac dysrhythmias may occur. MDMA is metabolised by CYP2D6 (Ch. 2), and genetic differences in

this enzyme may result in wide interindividual differences in susceptibility to the toxic effects of MDMA. Some subjects may present with hyponatraemia, possibly as a result of drinking excessive water as a precaution to prevent dehydration. Treatments include activated charcoal – but only for up to 2 h post ingestion, since MDMA is absorbed rapidly – and diazepam for agitation or convulsions.

FURTHER READING

[No authors listed] 2003 Pharmaceutical drug overdose case reports. From the World Literature. *Toxicol Rev* 22, 191–197

Bateman DN (1994) NSAIDs: Time to re-evaluate gut toxicity. *Lancet* 343, 1051–1052

Buckley NA, Dawson AH, Whyte IM, Henry DA (1994) Greater toxicity in overdose of dothiepin than of other tricyclic antidepressants. *Lancet* 343, 159–162

Buckley NA, Dawson AH, Whyte IM, O'Connell DL (1995) Relative toxicity of benzodiazepines in overdose. *BMJ* 310, 219–221

Dargan PI, Jones AL (2003) Management of paracetamol poisoning. *Trends Pharmacol Sci*, 24, 154–157

Dawson AH, Whyte IM (2001) Therapeutic drug monitoring in drug overdose. *Br J Clin Pharmacol* 52(suppl 1), 97S–102S

Edwards JG (1995) Suicide and antidepressants. Controversies on prevention, provocation, and self poisoning continue. *BMJ* 310, 205–206

Hawton K, Ware C, Mistry H et al (1995) Why patients choose paracetamol for self poisoning and their knowledge of its dangers. *BMJ* 310, 164

Henry JA, Alexander CA, Sener EK (1995) Relative mortality from overdose of antidepressants. *BMJ* 310, 221–224

Jick SS, Dean AD, Jick H (1995) Antidepressants and suicide. *BMJ* 310, 215–218

Lee WM (1995) Drug-induced hepatotoxicity. *N Engl J Med* 333, 1118–1127

Park BK, Kitteringham NR, Pirmohamed M, Tucker GT (1996) Relevance of induction of human drug-metabolising enzymes: pharmacological and toxicological implications. *Br J Clin Pharmacol* 41, 477–491

Park BK, Kitteringham NR, Powell H, Pirmohamed M (2000) Advances in molecular toxicology – towards understanding idiosyncratic drug toxicity. *Toxicology* 153, 39–60

Roujeau JC, Stern RS (1994) Severe adverse cutaneous reactions to drugs. *N Engl J Med* 331, 1272–1285

Sung J, Russell RI, Yeomans N et al (2000) Non-steroidal anti-inflammatory drug toxicity in the upper gastrointestinal tract. *J Gastroenterol Hepatol* 15(suppl), G58–G68

Vale JA, Proudfoot AT (1995) Paracetamol (acetaminophen) poisoning. *Lancet* 346, 547–552

Waring RH, Emery P (1995) The genetic origin of responses to drugs. *Br Med Bull* 51, 449–461

Self-assessment

1. Case history questions

> A 70-year-old man with a history of depressive illness and alcohol abuse was prescribed a compound analgesic containing 500 mg paracetamol and 30 mg codeine phosphate (co-codamol 30/500). Eight hours after collecting his prescription, he was seen as an emergency by his GP, who considered the man had taken an overdose and he was admitted to hospital.

a. What features might be seen soon after the overdosage and during the subsequent 24–48 h?
b. Outline what suitable pharmacological treatments should be undertaken.
c. Would co-codamol have been a safer alternative to prescribe?

The answers are provided on page 746.

54 Drug abuse and dependence

Drug abuse is defined as self-administration of any drug in a manner that differs from the approved use in that culture. A number of therapeutic drugs are abused because of their effects on the nervous system. Examples in Western society include hypnotics, anxiolytics (Ch. 20) and opioid analgesics (Ch. 19). The effects of many drugs of abuse are often complicated by the impurity and multiple constituents of samples of the abused drug.

Most drugs with potential for abuse also produce dependence. This is a syndrome that exists when an individual continues compulsively to take a drug because of the pleasurable effect it produces, often despite adverse social consequences or medical harm that it might produce. Dependence produces varying degrees of need for the drug, from mild desire to a craving.

Dependence may be psychological, caused by the necessity to prevent the unpleasant psychological reaction (dysphoria) that occurs on drug withdrawal, or physical, when there are abnormalities of behaviour and autonomic symptoms on withdrawal. Physical dependence causes symptoms on drug withdrawal that can also be provoked by the use of a specific antagonist to the drug. Habituation to the use of a drug (shown by adverse psychological reactions on stopping use) is a far more powerful stimulus to drug-seeking behaviour than physical withdrawal symptoms.

The biological basis of dependence

Dependence is related to dopaminergic activity in the mesolimbic system of the brain. This system is involved in regulation of mood and affect, but also in motivation and reward processes (producing responses varying from slight mood elevation to intense pleasure or euphoria in response to food intake, sexual activity etc.).

The mesolimbic system is activated by impulses arising in the ventral tegmental area of the brain. These impulses are relayed through the medial forebrain bundle, via the nucleus accumbens, to the prefrontal cortex (see Ch. 21). Stimulation of postsynaptic dopamine D_2 receptors (possibly the D_4 subtype), acting via G_i (inhibitory) G-proteins to reduce the generation of the intracellular second messenger cyclic adenosine monophosphate (cAMP) in the nucleus accumbens, is central to reward and much drug-seeking behaviour.

Most drugs of abuse directly or indirectly release dopamine in the nucleus accumbens; supporting this concept are the findings that drug withdrawal leads to reduced dopaminergic function in the same area. For example, the acute effect of morphine is to enhance dopaminergic input to the nucleus accumbens by stimulating the ventral tegmental area; inhibition of adenylate cyclase and reduced intracellular generation of the second messenger cAMP ensues. The decrease in adenylate cyclase activity in the nucleus accumbens reduces the motivational response to normal rewards. This is probably critical to producing drug dependence, since the drug becomes essential to maintain a 'normal' level of pleasure. Drug cessation decreases dopamine release in the nucleus accumbens and precipitates the psychological withdrawal reaction. Other transmitters also have a role in the genesis of dependence. Animal studies show changes in the mesolimbic system during dependence that include reduced 5-hydroxytryptamine (5HT, serotonin), gamma-aminobutyric acid (GABA) and noradrenaline, as well as increased glutamate, opioid and acetylcholine-mediated neurotransmission. Overall this suggests that many neurotransmitter systems are involved.

Neuroadaptive changes that occur with repeated use of an addictive drug lead to sensitisation of the mesolimbic system to further drug administration. Drug craving may also be related to neural inputs to the mesolimbic pathway from the amygdala, which are involved in emotion and conditioned responses. By contrast, physical dependence on a drug is unrelated to activity in the mesolimbic system and arises from excessive noradrenergic output from the locus ceruleus, a structure in the base of the brain that is involved in arousal and vigilance.

The development of tolerance to dependence-inducing drugs may also be explained by the changes that occur in the nuclear accumbens on chronic drug use. For example, with chronic opioid use, inhibitory autoreceptor upregulation in the ventral tegmental area acts to reduce dopamine release in the nucleus accumbens; this results in loss of D_2 receptor-mediated inhibition and a compensatory increase in adenylate cyclase activity. This produces supersensitivity of D_1 excitatory receptors, and thus tolerance to further doses of the drug. Larger doses are then necessary to maintain normal function in the mesolimbic system, let alone achieve a pleasurable response.

This chapter covers other drugs that are encountered in clinical practice primarily because of their abuse, such as Ecstasy and cannabis, or because of their potential to cause dependence, such as nicotine and ethanol (Box 54.1).

Drugs of abuse

Psychomotor stimulants

Several drugs that have central stimulant properties are abused and produce dependence. Those more commonly encountered are considered here.

Cocaine

Cocaine is usually taken as the hydrochloride salt. 'Crack' cocaine is the free-base form, named after the crackling sound produced when it is smoked.

Mechanism of action and effects

The psychomotor effects of cocaine are due to inhibition of neuronal presynaptic catecholamine reuptake into nerve terminals. This in turn may activate opioid systems in the brain, with upregulation of μ-receptors

(Ch. 19). Cocaine binds strongly to the catecholamine reuptake transporters, particularly inhibiting dopamine and, to a lesser extent, noradrenaline reuptake. Reduced serotonin reuptake may contribute to wakefulness. Changes in various pituitary neuroendocrine functions occur with more prolonged use; in particular, release of corticotrophin and luteinising hormone (LH) is enhanced. Tolerance to the psychomotor effects of cocaine is limited. One of the metabolites of cocaine, norcocaine, has direct vasoconstrictor activity.

Effects of cocaine include:

- intense euphoria
- alertness and wakefulness
- increased confidence and strength
- heightened sexual feelings
- indifference to concerns and cares
- severe psychological, but not physical, dependence, through the reinforcing effect of the rapid onset, yet brief duration of action; this develops particularly rapidly with 'crack' cocaine
- despondency and despair rapidly follow withdrawal; after chronic use, withdrawal can produce a dysphoric mood with fatigue, vivid dreams, insomnia or excessive sleeping, increased appetite and either psychomotor retardation or agitation
- toxic psychosis, with delusions of great stamina, occurs with chronic use
- in overdose, excessive catecholamine concentrations produce convulsions, hypertension, cardiac rhythm disturbances and hyperthermia (due to excessive muscle activity and reduced heat loss); if severe, death can occur from respiratory depression and circulatory collapse; the cardiovascular toxicity can be treated with combined α- and β-adrenoceptor blockade, and seizures by intravenous diazepam
- cocaine snuff produces necrosis of the nasal septum through its vasoconstrictor action
- exposure in utero leads to impaired brain development and other teratogenic effects.

Pharmacokinetics

Cocaine, as the hydrochloride salt, is used orally, intranasally or by intravenous injection; the intravenous route gives an intense and rapid onset of effect. 'Crack' cocaine is prepared by mixing with sodium bicarbonate or ammonia and water, then heating to remove the hydrochloride. In this free-base form it is smoked, which produces an effect similar to intravenous use. Cocaine is metabolised by plasma esterases and its half-life is very short.

Management of cocaine dependence

There are no recognised drug treatments for cocaine dependence. Prolonged behavioural treatments remain the main approach. Tricyclic antidepressants (especially desipramine) are sometimes advocated for the severe depression that can occur on withdrawal.

Amfetamine and derivatives

Amfetamine, metamfetamine (methamphetamine) and 3,4-methylenedioxymethamphetamine (MDMA, 'Ecstasy') are all drugs of abuse.

Mechanism of action and effects

Amfetamine and related drugs have indirect sympathomimetic effects, releasing cytosolic monoamines from central nervous system (CNS) neurons (Ch. 4). This action (principally as consequence of dopamine release) produces CNS stimulation that is most marked in the reticular formation, but occurs in many other areas of the brain. The D-isomer (dexamfetamine) is twice as potent as the L-isomer of amfetamine in its central stimulant activity. Effects include:

- euphoria, similar to that experienced with cocaine; this is particularly intense after intravenous use
- reduced fatigue and increased alertness for repetitive tasks
- anorexia
- psychotic behaviour during repeated use over a few days or with acute intoxication, causing hallucinations, paranoia and aggressive behaviour and repetitive actions; acute intoxication can cause convulsions and death
- peripheral sympathomimetic effects can lead to hypertension and cardiac arrhythmias
- tolerance develops rapidly to some of the central effects of amfetamine, such as anorexia, presumably through central monoamine depletion; tolerance to the euphoric effects and motor stimulation is slower
- withdrawal leads to prolonged sleep, followed by fatigue, depression, anxiety, craving, and increased appetite.

MDMA (Ecstasy) produces euphoria similar to that of amfetamine but with less stimulant effect. Disturbance of thermoregulatory homeostasis occurs, leading to a syndrome resembling heat stroke with hyperthermia and dehydration, usually after exertion in hot environments. Stimulation of antidiuretic hormone release can cause thirst and water intoxication, a consequence of water retention and hyponatraemia. The toxic effects of MDMA include cardiac arrhythmias, convulsions, muscle damage and severe metabolic acidosis, which may be fatal. The long-term toxicity is unknown.

Pharmacokinetics

Although amfetamine is sometimes used intravenously or via nasal inhalation, absorption from the gut is rapid and complete. Amfetamine readily crosses the blood–brain barrier. About half is excreted unchanged in the urine, and the rest is metabolised in the liver. The half-life of amfetamine varies according to urine flow and pH; if the urine is acid, then greater ionisation increases excretion to produce a short half-life (Ch. 2). By contrast, if urine pH is high, then the half-life is long because of renal tubular reabsorption of the drug. Metabolites of amfetamine are believed to contribute to the psychotic effects seen with long-term use.

Ecstasy is usually taken orally. It undergoes hepatic metabolism via CYP2D6, and polymorphism of this enzyme may explain some of the serious intoxication that occurs with the drug. The half-life is short.

Nicotine and tobacco

Mechanism of action

Over 300 chemical compounds are present in tobacco smoke. However, the actions of nicotine are central to the pharmacological effects of smoking. Nicotine has dose-related peripheral actions. At low doses, stimulation of aortic and carotid chemoreceptors enhances sympathetic nervous system activity (Ch. 4). At higher doses, there is direct stimulation of the nicotinic N_1 receptors on autonomic ganglia (Ch. 4). At even higher doses, nicotine acts as a ganglion-blocking agent. Initial stimulation of autonomic nervous tissue is therefore followed by depression. Effects on the CNS are mediated by presynaptic nicotinic receptors structurally distinct from those in the periphery. Stimulation of CNS nicotinic receptors increases neuronal permeability to sodium and potassium, and enhances release of neurotransmitters such as dopamine and glutamate. These receptors are found in the mesocortical and mesolimbic dopaminergic systems, in projections from the ventral forebrain to the cortex that mediate arousal, and in hippocampal projections where stimulation enhances learning and short-term memory. Tolerance to the CNS effects of nicotine is rapid.

Effects of nicotine and tobacco

Tobacco components, including nicotine, have effects on a number of organ systems.

Respiratory effects. The lungs are the first area to be in contact with the chemical components of tobacco smoke and are also exposed to particles and gases. Tars and other irritants, rather than nicotine, are responsible for the chronic damage to the lungs.

- An increase in blood carboxyhaemoglobin concentration (from carbon monoxide in tobacco smoke) decreases oxygen-carrying capacity. This may be important in ischaemic heart disease, increasing the chance of provoking angina.
- Increased mucus secretion, with reduction of activity of bronchial cilia and consequent decreased clearance of lung secretions, leads to chronic bronchitis.
- Progressive destruction of the supporting tissue in the bronchioles produces emphysema and chronic obstructive lung disease. Smoking is now the major cause of this condition.

- The risk of lung cancer is increased to about 20 times that of a non-smoker. Inhalation of tobacco smoke is a major contributory factor and explains the greater risk in cigarette smokers. Giving up smoking reduces the risk progressively over about 10 years of abstinence. The constituent of tobacco smoke responsible for altering DNA structure and initiating the cancer process remains controversial, but the relationship between smoking and lung cancer has been confirmed by numerous epidemiological studies. Compared with non-smokers, passive smokers also have a 20–25% increased risk of lung cancer.

Cardiovascular effects

- Stimulation of the autonomic nervous system and sensory receptors in the heart increases heart rate, blood pressure and cardiac output.
- The risk of cardiovascular disease is increased by smoking cigarettes, but not by pipe and cigar smoking, and it occurs at a younger age. The overall risk of death from coronary artery disease is doubled in smokers compared with non-smokers, but the magnitude of the effect is related to the numbers of cigarettes smoked. Peripheral vascular disease and stroke are also increased. Even passive smokers have an excess risk of vascular disease of 25%. The major reason for the excess of events is accelerated formation of atheromatous plaques, although contributory effects include increased plasma fatty acids and enhanced platelet aggregability. The risk of vascular disease falls over the first 3–5 years after stopping smoking to a level close to that of non-smokers.

Psychological effects. The psychological effects of smoking are substantial, as indicated by the difficulties experienced by those 'giving up smoking'.

- Decreased appetite, with weight gain on stopping smoking.
- Emotional dependence on nicotine and the physical act of smoking is powerful. Physical withdrawal is less marked but includes restlessness, irritability, anxiety, depression, difficulty concentrating, sleep disturbance and increased appetite.

Other effects. Nicotine and smoking have a number of other effects.

- Peptic ulceration is twice as common in smokers.
- Smoking in pregnancy, especially during the second half, has several effects. The most important are an increased risk of a low-birthweight child, and increased perinatal mortality. The vasoconstrictor effects of nicotine are responsible. Physical and mental development is slowed in children born to mothers who smoked during pregnancy.
- Smoking induces several hepatic cytochrome P450 isoenzymes (Ch. 2), and increases the clearance of drugs such as theophylline (Ch. 12) and imipramine (Ch. 22).

Pharmacokinetics of nicotine

Nicotine is absorbed from the mouth in its un-ionised form, which is found in the less acidic environment of cigar and pipe tobacco smoke. Acid cigarette smoke ionises nicotine, which can then only be absorbed in significant amounts from the larger surface area of the lung. About 10% of the nicotine from a cigarette is absorbed, but at a faster rate than from cigars or a pipe, giving a higher, but less prolonged, peak plasma concentration. Nicotine can also be absorbed transdermally. It is metabolised in the liver and has a short half-life. The major metabolite, cotinine, has a longer half-life than nicotine and its plasma concentration can be used as a monitor of smoking behaviour.

Dependence on and withdrawal from nicotine

Withdrawal is often difficult to achieve unless motivation is high. Patients should be supported by counselling about health gains and advice on overcoming problems, such as weight gain. Behavioural therapy as an aid to quitting has a success rate of 20% at 1 year. Pharmacotherapy is often used to reduce the intensity of withdrawal symptoms.

Nicotine replacement therapy. Smokers adjust their smoking habit to maintain plasma nicotine concentrations just above a threshold that averts withdrawal symptoms. The plasma concentration falls rapidly within 1–2 h of the last cigarette, and rather more slowly after smoking a cigar or pipe. The resultant craving for nicotine can be reduced by nicotine replacement. This can be delivered from transdermal patches, by chewing gum, via an inhaler (with most absorption occurring in the mouth) or via a nasal spray. The delivery method determines the speed at which plasma nicotine concentration rises; this is most rapid after nasal spray. The individual can choose the most appropriate vehicle for his or her needs and preferences. Established cardiovascular disease is a caution for, but not a contraindication to, nicotine replacement therapy. Behavioural therapy enhances the success rate achieved by nicotine replacement therapy. Use of nicotine replacement therapy doubles the chance of achieving abstinence.

Bupropion. This is an atypical antidepressant. Most antidepressants are ineffective for smoking cessation, but the use of bupropion is associated with smoking cessation rates equal to, or slightly greater than, nicotine replacement therapy. Treatment should be started 1 week before a 'quit date'. Used together with nicotine replacement therapy, bupropion produces a modest increase in the chance of stopping. An additional benefit is that smokers who use bupropion as an aid to quitting are less likely to gain weight. Bupropion is a weak inhibitor of neuronal reuptake of noradrenaline and dopamine, and probably works by enhancing mesolimbic dopaminergic activity. It is given as a modified-release formulation and has a long half-life. Elimination is by hepatic metabolism, which also generates active metabolites. Unwanted effects include anxiety, headache, insomnia and dry mouth. There is an increased risk of epileptic seizures, and bupropion should be avoided if there is a past history of seizures. Recent evidence indicates that, in contrast to other antidepressants that have been studied, nortriptyline is as effective as bupropion for smoking cessation.

Psychotomimetic agents

Hallucinogens

Lysergic acid diethylamide (LSD), psilocybin ('magic mushrooms'), mescaline (from peyote cactus) and the synthetic drug dimethyltryptamine (DMT) are adrenergic hallucinogenics that have structural similarities to monoamine neurotransmitters. They share several properties, including cross-tolerance.

Mechanism of action and effects
The actions of hallucinogens on the brain are probably related to postsynaptic $5HT_2$ receptor stimulation in the cerebral cortex and locus ceruleus, a region of the midbrain that receives sensory signals. LSD also produces presynaptic $5HT_{1A}$ receptor blockade in the dorsal raphe neurons, inhibiting firing of neuronal projections to the forebrain. Tolerance to LSD occurs rapidly, and appears to be related to downregulation of these receptors. The actions of LSD, psilocybin and mescaline are similar. LSD is the most potent hallucinogen.

- Visual hallucinations are frequent, especially with high doses, and auditory acuity is accentuated. There may be an overlap of sensory impressions such that music is 'seen' or colours 'heard', which can produce severe anxiety. Time appears to pass slowly. Emotions are altered, with either elation or depression, and rapid mood swings can occur. The overall experience can produce a 'good' or a 'bad' trip, and can vary in the same individual on different occasions.
- Serious psychotic reactions can occasionally occur, and long-term psychotic disorders can be precipitated. The other unpleasant persistent effect in some individuals is 'flashback', seeing bright flashes, or halos or trails attached to moving objects.
- Physical consequences of CNS stimulation include dizziness, weakness, drowsiness and paraesthesiae.
- Excessive sympathetic nervous system stimulation with large doses produces nausea, salivation, lacrimation, dizziness, mydriasis, tremor, hyperthermia, tachycardia and hypertension.
- Tolerance can occur within 5 days.
- Emotional dependence is frequent, but physical dependence is not seen.

Pharmacokinetics
Oral absorption of these drugs is good. Physical effects begin after about 20 min, but psychoactive effects are delayed for 2–4 h and then last up to 12 h. DMT has a rapid onset of hallucinogenic action, within 15–30 min, but the duration is only 1–2 h. Elimination is by hepatic metabolism and the half-lives are short.

Cannabis

Cannabis can be smoked as marijuana, which consists of dried leaves or flowers of the *Cannabis sativa* (hemp) plant, or as resin extracted from the leaves of the plant and then dried, known as hashish. Solvent extraction of the resin produces cannabis oil, which can be added to tobacco. The hallucinogenic effects of cannabis are much less marked than those of the aminergic hallucinogens such as LSD.

Mechanism of action and effects
The constituent compounds (cannabinoids) interact with specific CB_1 receptors in the brain. These receptors are coupled to G_i proteins that reduce intracellular cAMP production, and inhibit cell membrane Ca^{2+} and K^+ channels; there is a natural ligand, called anandamide (an arachidonic acid derivative). CB_1 receptors are found in greatest density in areas of the brain involved in cognition and pain recognition (cerebral cortex), memory (hippocampus), reward (mesolimbic system) and motor coordination (substantia nigra and cerebellum).

- The psychomotor effects result largely from the cannabinoid tetrahydrocannabinol (THC) and one of its metabolites, 11-hydroxy-THC, which produce euphoria, heightened intensity of sensations, and relaxation. Occasionally, panic reactions, hallucinations and depersonalisation occur. Psychotic reactions are rare except in predisposed individuals, but recent evidence shows that use of cannabis substantially increases the risk of developing schizophrenia. Recent memory is markedly impaired and complex mental tests are less well executed, although the user may perceive that their performance is enhanced. Motor incoordination may affect driving ability.
- Effects on the cardiovascular system include tachycardia and increased systolic blood pressure with a postural fall.
- The tars inhaled during chronic use predispose to heart disease, chronic bronchitis and lung cancer.
- THC has an antiemetic action (Ch. 32), which may be useful during cancer chemotherapy.
- Tolerance to the psychomotor effects of cannabis occurs with regular use, and there is recent evidence of dependance.

Pharmacokinetics
Metabolism of THC is extensive, with some active metabolites being produced. The high lipid solubility of THC means that absorption from the lung or gut is high,

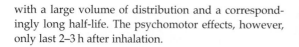
with a large volume of distribution and a correspondingly long half-life. The psychomotor effects, however, only last 2–3 h after inhalation.

Dissociative anaesthetics

Phencyclidine (PCP) and ketamine differ from adrenergic hallucinogens in their mode of action. Both drugs were developed as anaesthetics, but PCP was withdrawn because of adverse effects.

Mechanism of action and effects

Both drugs block the excitatory effects of glutamate at NMDA (*N*-methyl-D-aspartate) receptors. These receptors are abundant in the cortex, basal ganglia and sensory pathways of the CNS. PCP also releases dopamine from nerve terminals in a similar manner to amfetamine. The term dissociative anaesthetic refers to the feelings of detachment (dissociation) from the environment and self that are produced by the drugs. These are not true hallucinations.

- Acute effects include euphoria, decreased inhibition, a feeling of immense power, analgesia, altered perception of time and space, and depersonalisation. Ketamine creates a 'mellow, colourful wonderworld'.
- Catatonic rigidity can occur, followed by ataxia and slurring of speech.
- Adverse experiences include confusion, restlessness, disorientation and impaired judgement. Irritability, paranoia, depression and anxiety are also common. Psychotic reactions are precipitated in susceptible people.
- Ketamine can produce near-death experiences.
- Persistent abuse of PCP leads to memory loss, speech and thought difficulties, and depression that persist for months after the last use.
- Tolerance is unusual, but psychological dependence occurs.

Pharmacokinetics

PCP is rapidly absorbed from the gut, nose or lungs after smoking. Effects are seen within minutes of ingestion and usually last 4–6 h. It is a weak base that is excreted in the urine. It is also excreted into the stomach, and reabsorbed by the small intestine. The half-life is very long at 2–3 days. Ketamine is used intravenously. It is metabolised in the liver and has a short half-life.

CNS depressants

Alcohol (ethyl alcohol, ethanol)

Mechanism of action and effects

Alcohol has multiple actions on the CNS. Non-specific actions such as increased fluidity of neuronal cell membranes (cf. general anaesthetics) may be important

---

> **Box 54.2**
>
> **Possible mechanisms of action of alcohol**
>
> Inhibition of monoamine oxidase B in neurons
> Inhibition of Na⁺/K⁺-ATPase in neuronal membranes
> Increased neuronal adenylate cyclase activity
> Decreased intracellular phosphatidylinositol system activity, leading to reduced Ca²⁺ availability
> Enhanced opioid δ-receptor activation

by reducing Ca^{2+} flux across the cell membrane, but several other actions have been described (Box 54.2). Overall, alcohol facilitates central inhibitory neurotransmission, particularly enhancing the effects of GABA, and is therefore a general CNS depressant. There is an initial depression of inhibitory neurons, particularly in the mesolimbic system, which produces a sense of relaxation, but this is followed by progressive depression of all CNS functions. Mental processes that are modified by education, training and previous experience are affected first, while relatively 'mechanical' tasks are less impaired. Despite subjective impressions, there is no increase in mental or physical capabilities, unless anxiety has previously reduced performance. All effects are closely related to blood alcohol concentration (Table 54.1). In chronic alcoholics, tolerance to many of the psychological effects of alcohol is seen. Alcohol intake is usually measured in units (Box 54.3).

Other effects of alcohol

Alcohol has a range of effects.

Cardiovascular effects

- A modest alcohol intake may have protective effects on the circulation, by inhibiting platelet aggregation and increasing high-density lipoprotein cholesterol. The form in which the alcohol is taken is probably not important. The extent of this beneficial effect may have been overestimated; it is probably greatest at 1 unit per day and is lost when intake exceeds 3–4 units per day.
- Higher intake of alcohol has pressor effects that raise blood pressure, possibly through increased vascular sensitivity to catecholamines. This increases the risk of coronary artery disease and stroke.
- Cardiac arrhythmias can be provoked by high alcohol intake, particularly atrial fibrillation. This can occur after an alcoholic binge ('holiday heart') or following more chronic abuse (Ch 8).
- Alcoholic cardiomyopathy is a dilated cardiomyopathy that is only partially reversible with abstinence, and can lead to heart failure. An average intake of 10 units of alcohol daily for 8–10 years can produce this condition.

Table 54.1
The effects of alcohol at various plasma concentrations

Plasma concentration (mg 100 ml^{-1})	Effects
30	Mild euphoria owing to suppression of inhibitory pathways in the cortex; the individual is more talkative, emotionally labile with loss of self-control; the risk of accidental injury is increased
80	The legal limit for driving in the UK; the risk of serious injury in a road accident is more than doubled
100–200	Speech becomes slurred and motor coordination is impaired
>300	Often produces loss of consciousness
>400	Frequently fatal as a result of respiratory and vasomotor centre depression

---

Box 54.3

Alcoholic content of alcoholic drinks

1 unit alcohol is about 10 g and is found in:
- $1/2$ pint of normal strength beer, lager, cider
- $1\frac{1}{2}$ pints low-alcohol beer, lager, cider
- $1/3$ pint strong beer, lager, cider
- $1/5$ pint extra-strong beer, lager, cider
- 1 glass of wine (8 units per 75 cl bottle)
- 1 small measure of sherry (13 units per bottle)
- 1 standard measure of spirits (30 units per bottle)
- $2/3$ bottle of 'alcopop'

Liver

- Hypoglycaemia occurs as a consequence of the metabolism of alcohol in the liver. The metabolic process generates excess protons, which encourages the conversion of glucose, via pyruvate, to lactate and predisposes to lactic acidosis. Alcoholics often have a low-carbohydrate diet, which compounds the hypoglycaemia. Hypoglycaemia tends to occur several hours after heavy alcohol intake and can contribute to convulsions on alcohol withdrawal.
- The lactic acidosis created by alcohol metabolism in the liver impairs the renal excretion of uric acid, which predisposes to gout.
- Lactic acidosis also facilitates synthesis of saturated fatty acids, which accumulate in the liver, leading to a fatty liver, possibly with altered liver function. Plasma triglycerides are also increased.
- Alcoholic hepatitis is usually a consequence of short-term heavy alcohol abuse. It can be fatal.
- Cirrhosis occurs with prolonged alcohol abuse, but individual susceptibility varies widely. On average, consumption of more than 8 units per day for at least 10 years is required for cirrhosis to occur in men. About two-thirds of this amount creates the same risk for women. Established cirrhosis reduces the first-pass metabolism and clearance of drugs eliminated by the liver (Ch. 56).
- Chronic intake of alcohol induces hepatic drug-metabolising enzymes, especially CP2E1, which decreases the effectiveness of some therapeutic drugs, for example warfarin, phenytoin and carbamazepine.

Other gastrointestinal consequences

- Erosive gastritis can occur as a result of stimulation of gastric secretions.
- Pancreatitis is probably caused by raised triglycerides or by pancreatic duct obstruction by proteinaceous secretions induced by alcohol.

Sexual function

- Sexual desire is often increased by alcohol, but the ability to sustain penile erection is reduced, possibly because of the vasodilator actions of alcohol.
- Direct damage to the Leydig cells of the testis reduces the circulating testosterone, leading to reduced libido, infertility and a loss of the male distribution of body hair. Altered steroid metabolism in the liver leads to an increase in circulating oestrone in males, which causes gynaecomastia.

Neuropsychiatric effects

- A combination of alcohol toxicity with vitamin B_6 and thiamine deficiency in the diet of alcoholics predisposes to peripheral neuropathy and dementia. Specific mid-brain damage can result and produces the syndromes of Wernicke's encephalopathy and Korsakoff's psychosis.
- Alcohol has anticonvulsant properties and withdrawal predisposes to convulsions, even in individuals without a history of epilepsy.
- Alcohol can disturb sleep patterns, with decreased rapid eye movement (REM) sleep and increased stage 4 sleep during intoxication. Withdrawal increases REM sleep, with associated nightmares (Ch. 20).

- Dose-related memory impairment can be caused by suppressed hippocampal function.
- Subdural haematoma is more common after head injury in heavy drinkers, perhaps as a consequence of cerebral atrophy.
- Depression or anxiety states are more common in heavy drinkers.

Carcinogenesis and teratogenesis

- Cancer of the mouth, oesophagus and liver are more common with heavy alcohol use. Colon and breast cancer may also be increased.
- The fetal alcohol syndrome is believed to be caused by the effects of alcohol on neuronal adhesion molecules that regulate neuronal migration. Heavy maternal drinking during pregnancy leads to impaired learning and memory in the child. Genetic factors may be involved in the susceptibility of the fetus to these problems.

Pharmacokinetics

Although ethanol is absorbed from the stomach, the majority is absorbed from the small intestine, due to its larger surface area. High concentrations of alcohol (above 20%) and large volumes inhibit gastric emptying and delay absorption, as do foods high in fat or carbohydrate. Peak blood alcohol concentrations, therefore, depend on the dose and strength of the alcohol and on whether or not it was taken with food. Once absorbed, alcohol undergoes substantial first-pass metabolism in the liver. Distribution of alcohol is fairly uniform and the ready passage across the blood–brain barrier and high cerebral blood flow ensure rapid access to the CNS. The effects on the brain are more marked when the concentration is rising, indicating a degree of acute tolerance.

Metabolism occurs mainly in the liver (Fig. 54.1), more than 90% being oxidised, mainly by alcohol dehydrogenase, while the rest is removed unchanged in expired air in close proportion to the blood concentration (the basis of the alcohol breath test) or the urine. Alcohol metabolism shows saturation kinetics due to the limited supply of nicotine adenine nucleotide (NAD^+) cofactor for the oxidative process. The maximum rate of alcohol metabolism averages $8 \, g \, h^{-1}$. The extent of first-pass metabolism of alcohol is related to the speed of absorption; thus, with slower absorption, such as when alcohol is taken with food, less alcohol will reach the systemic circulation. The initial metabolic reaction is mediated by alcohol dehydrogenase, producing acetaldehyde. This is further metabolised by aldehyde dehydrogenase to acetic acid (Fig. 54.1). Accumulation of acetaldehyde in the circulation is responsible for many of the unpleasant effects of a hangover.

Small amounts of alcohol are metabolised via the microsomal ethanol oxidising system (CYP2E1), the activity of which is increased by enzyme inducers such as alcohol itself (which does not affect the activity of alcohol dehydrogenase) (Ch. 36).

Some drugs, such as metronidazole (Ch. 51) and chlorpropamide (Ch. 40), inhibit aldehyde dehydrogenase, leading to acetaldehyde accumulation if alcohol is taken with them. Typical 'hangover' effects of flushing, sweating, headache and nausea then occur after small amounts of alcohol. Genetic variability in alcohol and aldehyde dehydrogenases occur among ethnic groups, leading to variable levels of alcohol or aldehyde metabolism.

Alcohol abuse and dependence

There are no reliable estimates of the number of people in the UK with alcohol-related problems, although it has

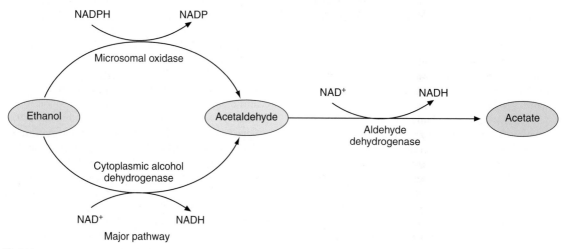

Fig. 54.1
The metabolism of alcohol. Alcohol dehydrogenase is responsible for 80–90% of the metabolism of ethanol.

anorexia, nausea and retching. Convulsions can occur through neuronal excitation. Insomnia, tachycardia and hypertension are common with more severe withdrawal reactions. The most severe form of withdrawal is *delirium tremens*, with confusion, paranoia, and visual and tactile hallucinations. Delirium tremens can cause death from respiratory and cardiovascular collapse.

If an individual is drinking excessively, controlled drinking may be an option. However, if there is alcohol dependence or alcohol-related problems, then abstinence is usually preferable.

Controlled detoxification is usually undertaken with a sedative agent, such as a benzodiazepine (Ch. 20), to attenuate withdrawal symptoms. Chlordiazepoxide is usually used, decreasing the dose over 7–10 days. Clomethiazole (Ch. 20) is sometimes used, but carries a greater risk of dependence. Clonidine (a presynaptic α_2-adrenoceptor agonist at the vasomotor centre in the brain; Ch. 6) can be useful, by reducing the excessive sympathetic stimulation that accompanies withdrawal. Beta-adrenoceptor antagonists (Ch. 5) may be helpful for the same reason. Multivitamin preparations containing an adequate amount of thiamine should be given for 1 month to prevent Wernicke's encephalopathy. Relapse is common after withdrawal from alcohol.

Two drugs are licensed in the UK to assist in the management of chronic alcoholism. Disulfiram, an inhibitor of acetaldehyde dehydrogenase, causes unpleasant hangover symptoms after small amounts of alcohol. Given alone, or with psychosocial rehabilitation, it can help to maintain abstinence. Acamprosate inhibits the excitatory amino acid glutamate by antagonism at the NMDA receptor, although several other contributory effects have been suggested. It has few unwanted effects, is non-addictive and can be used to reduce craving for alcohol.

been suggested that 1–2% of the population are affected. The distribution curve for alcohol consumption is continuous but skewed at higher alcohol intakes; the risk of alcohol-related problems rises with the average alcohol intake. Up to 30% of hospital admissions are for alcohol-related problems, although the contribution of heavy drinking is often unrecognised. Screening for alcohol abuse can be carried out by obtaining a complete history of alcohol intake and, if necessary, using the CAGE questions (Box 54.4). Abnormal measurements of both the mean corpuscular volume (MCV) of red cells (which is raised with increasing alcohol intake because of an effect of alcohol on the cell membrane) and the liver enzyme γ-glutamyl transpeptidase (γGT) will identify about 75% of people with an alcohol problem.

Psychological dependence on alcohol is common, but physical dependence also occurs. Withdrawal symptoms occur 6–24 h after the last drink in dependent persons. If mild, these are related to autonomic hyperactivity and include anxiety, agitation, tremor, sweating,

FURTHER READING

Balfour D, Benowitz N, Fagerström K et al (2000) Diagnosis and treatment of nicotine dependence with emphasis on nicotine replacement therapy. *Eur Heart J* 21, 438–445

Barlecchi CE, MacKenzie TD, Schrier RW (1994) The human cost of tobacco. *N Engl J Med* 330, 907–912, 975–980

DeGraff AC (2002) Pharmacologic therapy for nicotine addiction *Chest* 122, 392–393

Garbutt JC, West SL, Carey TS et al (1999) Pharmacological treatment of alcohol dependence. *JAMA* 281, 1318–1325

Hall W, Solowij N (1998) Adverse effects of cannabis. *Lancet* 352, 1611–1616

Hall W, Zador D (1997) The alcohol withdrawal syndrome. *Lancet* 349, 1897–1900

Leshner AI (1996) Molecular mechanism of cocaine addiction. *N Engl J Med* 335, 128–129

Mendelson JH, Mello NK (1996) Management of cocaine abuse and dependence. *N Engl J Med* 334, 965–972

O'Connor PG, Schottenfeld RS (1996) Patients with alcohol problems. *N Engl J Med* 338, 592–602

Raw M, McNeill A, West R (1999) Smoking cessation: evidence-based recommendations for the healthcare system. *BMJ* 318, 182–185

Rigotti A (2002) Treatment of tobacco use and dependence. *N Engl J Med* 346, 506–512

Schaffer A, Naranjo CA (1998) Recommended drug treatment strategies for the alcoholic patient. *Drugs* 56, 571–585

Sutherland G (2002) Current approach to the management of smoking cessation. *Drugs* 62(suppl 2), 53–61

Swift RM (1999) Drug therapy for alcohol dependence. *N Engl J Med* 340, 1482–1490

Tomkins DM, Sellers EM (2001) Addiction and the brain: the role of neurotransmitters in the cause and treatment of drug dependence. *CMAJ* 164, 817–821

Self-assessment

In the following questions, the first statement, in italics, is true. Are the following statements also true?

1. *Cocaine potently inhibits the uptake of noradrenaline into nerve terminals and this is the explanation for its mydriatic effect.*

   a. 'Crack' cocaine is the free-base form of cocaine.
   b. Cocaine can be given topically into the eye to test for Horner's syndrome.
   c. Prolonged cocaine use has little damaging effect on the cardiovascular system.
   d. Tolerance to the euphoric and anorexic effects of cocaine rapidly develops.

2. *MDMA (Ecstasy) causes release of 5HT from nerve endings while inhibiting 5HT uptake.*

   a. A toxic effect of taking Ecstasy in some individuals is hyperthermia and dehydration.
   b. Ecstasy suppresses appetite.
   c. Amfetamines are not banned in sporting events.

3. *Cannabis may impair driving ability and complex mental tasks, and psychotic reactions can occur in predisposed individuals.*

   a. The euphoria caused by cannabis lasts for 24 h.
   b. THC, the active ingredient of cannabis, causes nausea and vomiting.
   c. Cannabis acts on specific receptors in the brain.

4. *Nicotine induces very strong dependence.*

   a. Tolerance to the effects of nicotine develops very slowly.
   b. Nicotine causes tachycardia and reduced gut motility.

   c. Cotinine, a metabolite of nicotine, has a long half-life and can be measured in serum to determine smoking habits.
   d. Nicotine patches given alone are the optimum method for someone giving up smoking.
   e. A physical withdrawal symptom does not occur when giving up smoking.

5. *Ethanol is metabolised to a toxic substance, acetaldehyde, in the liver and then to acetic acid.*

   a. Chronic intake of alcohol induces hepatic drug-metabolising enzymes.
   b. A modest intake of alcohol increases the incidence of cardiovascular disease.
   c. Some individuals have a genetically determined low ability to metabolise ethanol.

6. *One part of a therapy to reduce alcohol intake is to inhibit acetaldehyde metabolism with disulfiram, causing sickness, headache and hangover symptoms following a small amount of alcohol intake.*

   a. Acamprosate, which is used to encourage abstinence, acts to reduce alcohol metabolism in a similar way to disulfiram.
   b. The severity of symptoms of withdrawal from ethanol consumption (detoxification) cannot be controlled by pharmacological means.

7. *Up to one-third of hospital admissions are for alcohol-related problems.*

   a. Ethanol can cause a macrocytosis.
   b. Ethanol enhances antidiuretic hormone secretion.
   c. The plasma level of the liver enzyme γ-glutamyl transpeptidase is depressed with heavy ethanol intake.

The answers are provided on page 747.

Drugs of abuse

Drug	Half-life (h)	Elimination	Comments
Alcohol (ethyl alcohol, ethanol)	Zero order	Metabolism + renal	Oxidation is saturated at normal intakes
Amfetamine	8–10	Renal + metabolism	*Dextro*-isomer (dexamfetamine) is the active form and is sometimes used for treatment of hyperactivity in children (especially in the USA); rapidly absorbed (within 3 h); half-life is dependent on the urine pH (basic drug)
Benzodiazepines	–	–	See Ch. 20
Cannabis	–	–	See Ch. 32
Cocaine	1–1.5	Metabolism + renal	Oxidised and hydrolysed in the liver; about 10% excreted unchanged in urine
Ecstasy (3,4-methylenedioxy-methamphetamine; MDMA)	6 (*R*), 4 (*S*)	Metabolism + renal	Peak plasma concentrations occur about 2 h after dosage; half-lives differ slightly between the enantiomers; oxidised by CYP2D6 (polymorphism of which may explain in part the idiosyncratic cases of intoxication); saturation of metabolism may contribute to the risk of overdose; the amfetamine analogue (MDA) and ethylamphetamine analogue (MDE or 'Eve') show similar properties
Lysergic acid diethylamide (LSD)	5	Metabolism + renal	Few data are available; LSD is detectable in urine after oral dosage; 2-oxo-3- hydroxy-LSD is a major urinary metabolite
Metamfetamine (methamphetamine)	10–12	Renal + metabolism	Rapidly absorbed after ingestion; about 40% excreted in urine unchanged; oxidised by CYP2D6; few data available; renal excretion is pH-dependent (methamphetamine is a metabolite of selegiline)
Nicotine	0.5–2	Metabolism + renal	Very rapidly absorbed after inhalation; the kinetics are absorption rate-limited when given as a patch, with peak plasma concentrations at 5–9 h; the main metabolite, cotinine, has a half-life of 10–40 h (and can be used to assess exposure)
Opioids	–	–	See Ch. 19
Psilocybin	? (minutes)	Metabolism	Oxidised very rapidly by dephosphorylation to psilocin and also in the intestine to 4-hydroxyindole-3-acetic acid; few data available

55

Prescribing, adherence and information about medicines

About 80% of medicines are prescribed in general practice (primary medical care). On average, men visit their general practitioners three and a half times each year and women visit five times. A little over two-thirds of consultations end with the issuing of a prescription. Prescribing is particularly frequent for elderly people, who are likely to continue treatment for long periods of time. For these reasons, regular review of prescribed treatment should take place to determine whether it is still appropriate or necessary, and to ensure that important drug interactions and unwanted effects are not overlooked. Some drugs also require regular monitoring of efficacy (e.g. warfarin, antihypertensive treatment), blood concentrations (e.g. lithium) or for unwanted effects (e.g. amiodarone, thiazide diuretics).

Duties of the prescriber

There are certain legal requirements that must be met when a medicine is prescribed. The minimum are:

- the name of the person for whom the drug is prescribed (surname and initial) and address; in the case of children up to 12 years, the patient's age must be specified
- drug name
- dose
- route of administration
- frequency of administration
- duration of therapy
- doctor's name, address and signature
- date.

Generic prescribing

In most situations, the generic name (the officially accepted chemical name) of the drug is preferred to the proprietary trade name (a 'brand' name approved for use by a specific pharmaceutical company). One ad-vantage of the generic name is that it is likely to indicate the nature of the drug. For example, all β-adrenoceptor antagonist drugs (β-blockers) end with either -olol or –alol, such as atenolol, labetalol, metoprolol and sotalol. Similarly, tricyclic antidepressants end with -tyline or -pramine, for example amitriptyline, nortriptyline, clomipramine, imipramine and lofepramine. By contrast, the trade names for these drugs give little idea of the active ingredient: Tenormin®, Trandate®, Lopressor® and Sotacor®; Tryptizol®, Allegron®, Anafranil®, Tofranil® and Gamanil®. Another problem with trade names is that they rarely give any indication when there is more than one active ingredient. For example, Tenoret-50® contains both atenolol and chlortalidone. The generic names for many compound preparations have this indicated by the term 'co-'; for example, co-tenidone is the generic equivalent of Tenoret-50®. Because different brand names can in fact describe the same medicine, a person who is given a repeat prescription may become confused if prescribed the same medicine under a different name. Moreover, the substitute brand may differ in its tablet size, colour and scoring.

Another advantage of generic prescribing is that pharmacists can dispense any product that meets the necessary specifications, rather than having to buy in a specific brand. This helps to simplify stock holding and avoids unnecessary delays when dispensing. Generic prescribing is sometimes cheaper than prescribing by trade name, although the difference depends very much on pack size and other commercial factors and is sometimes marginal.

In recent years, there has been an increasing tendency for doctors to prescribe by generic name. It is likely that economic arguments have been the chief factor leading to this change. Despite the advantages, generic prescribing can create difficulties. For drugs with a narrow therapeutic index, for example anticonvulsants, oral anticoagulants, oral hypoglycaemic agents and theophylline preparations (especially modified-release ones), this may present a theoretical problem. If repeat prescriptions are filled with a generic drug supplied from a different source, there is a possibility of variations in bioavailability or active ingredient. Recent stringent control has almost eliminated this problem, except for some modified-release formulations such as those for lithium or theophylline. In these situations, brand prescribing is recommended.

Dosage

The total treatment is related to the individual dose size, its frequency and the duration of therapy. The route of administration is also important.

Dose. This is an essential item on all prescriptions and should be written in grams (g), milligrams (mg) or micrograms (which should not be abbreviated).

The route of administration. The route should be identified: oral, rectal, or by various forms of injection, for example intravenous, intramuscular or subcutaneous. Considerable confusion can arise with intravenous administration of drugs since there are numerous systems for delivery. Drugs can be given by direct injection into a vein or can be infused, for example through the side-arm of a continuously running intravenous drip, via a motor-driven pump or added to the intravenous infusion fluid reservoir. It is particularly important when prescribing drugs for intravenous administration to make clear the precise intentions.

Frequency and times of administration. Sometimes, drugs are administered once only, while others must be given on a regular basis, in which case the frequency or times of administration should be specified, for example twice daily or 9 a.m. and 9 p.m.

Duration of therapy. Duration can be specified in a number of ways, one being to complete the box near the top of the prescription sheet. Alternatively, it can be written on the prescription or the total number of tablets/capsules can be specified. Medicines are now dispensed in original packs with tablets individually packed by the pharmaceutical company. Specifying the duration of therapy is essential in the case of controlled drugs (preparations that are subject to the prescription requirements of the Misuse of Drugs Regulations 2001), such as opioids, for which there is a legal requirement that the total amount to be dispensed must be written in both figures and words.

Other items on a prescription

Other essential items on prescriptions include the doctor's signature and the address of his or her place of work. The latter is effectively waived for hospital prescriptions since it is assumed that the medical practitioner is based at the hospital in question. The prescription must be dated. Increasing use is now made of computer-issued prescriptions. The specific requirements for these are essentially similar to those outlined above. Computer-issued prescriptions avoid handwriting problems and assist in record keeping and in data accumulation and analysis.

Abbreviations

Directions for prescribing should preferably be in English (rather than Latin) without abbreviation. However, there are a number of abbreviations that are widely accepted. They include the following for route of administration: o or p.o., oral; i.v., intravenous; i.m., intramuscular; s.c., subcutaneous; and p.r., per rectum. Others, such as intrathecal, must not be abbreviated, because of the potential seriousness of inappropriate administration: intrathecal vincristine, for example, has caused the death of several people. Besides the abbreviations already listed for quantities, ml or mL is acceptable. Quantities of less than 1 g should be written in milligrams (e.g. 400 mg, rather than 0.4 g), whereas quantities of less than 1 mg should be written in micrograms (e.g. 500 micrograms, rather than 0.5 mg). If decimals are unavoidable, a zero should precede the decimal point when there is no figure (e.g. 0.5 ml, not .5 ml).

Concerning timing of doses, od (*omni die*) is acceptable, but there is nothing wrong with saying once daily! The abbreviation om (*omni mane*) stands for in the morning, and on (*omni nocte*) for at night; ac is short for *ante cibum* (before food) and pc for *post cibum* (after food). Twice daily can be abbreviated to bd (*bis die*), thrice daily to tds (*ter die sumendus*) and four times daily to qds (*quater die sumendus*).

Adherence or concordance (formerly compliance)

The term 'compliance' is used to describe the extent to which a person takes his or her medicine. However, other terms such as 'adherence' or 'concordance' are now preferred, since they emphasise the partnership between the person and health professions in the process of taking medicines, rather than simply following instructions. It is frequently assumed that once a prescription has been given, the recipient will automatically comply with the doctor's instructions. There is, however, abundant evidence that this is often not the case. Indeed, many prescriptions are not even taken to the pharmacist for dispensing, and a very substantial proportion of those collected are not taken in the manner intended. Prescriptions are sometimes not presented to a pharmacist because of cost or because the doctor failed to discuss the 'hidden agenda' for which the presenting complaint was a front.

The degree of adherence is affected by many factors, which include the duration of treatment. Less than 50% of people comply fully with long-term therapy, such as that for high blood pressure or psychotic illness.

The frequency of dosing is a major influence. Few people like taking their medicines with them to work. Therefore, adherence with twice-daily regimens tends to be better than that for more frequent administration.

There is a further improvement in the extent of adherence with once- rather than twice-daily dosing.

Unwanted effects can reduce the likelihood of a person complying with therapy, but at times can be turned to advantage. For example, giving the entire dose of a tricyclic antidepressant at night means that the sedation can be used to aid sleep. Giving the person advanced warning of likely unwanted effects such as dry mouth with this compound may earn the person's trust and encourage him or her to continue therapy.

A proportion of non-adherence is caused by people forgetting whether or not they have taken their medicine on a particular day. Use of calendar packs can be helpful in this situation.

The person's health beliefs are also particularly important. Adherence can be improved by involving the person in monitoring his or her disease and its control by therapy, for example home monitoring of blood pressure, blood sugar in diabetes mellitus, or peak flow measurements in asthmatics. Supplying accurate information about medicines can improve the level of satisfaction, and satisfied people are more likely to take their medicines.

Informing people about their medicines

It is almost incredible to think that at one time doctors were reluctant to allow the name of a medicine to be shown on the container in which it was dispensed. However, paternalistic attitudes amongst the medical profession have been slow to disappear. Several surveys carried out in the early 1980s showed that most people felt that neither doctors nor pharmacists gave sufficient explanations about medicines. This situation was summarised by Leighton Cluff in the USA in his comment 'Better instructions are provided when purchasing a new camera or automobile than when a patient receives a life-saving antibiotic or cardiac drug.' More than 60% of people prescribed a medicine in the previous month remember being told only very little or nothing about it. People are particularly keen to know when and how to take their medicine; about unwanted effects and what to do about these; precautions to take, such as possible effects on driving; problems with alcohol or other drugs; the name of the medicine; the purposes of treatment; how long to take it and what to do if a dose is missed.

Manufacturers of pharmaceuticals now produce printed leaflets about medicines, which are included in original packs. People who receive leaflets about their medicines are better informed and more satisfied than those who have not been given this information. However, leaflets are complementary to, and not a substitute for, discussion with the medical practitioner, pharmacist, practice nurse, etc. The Internet provides an increasingly rich source for people about their medicines and the variety of treatments available for their conditions. However, advertising and lack of peer-review of websites reduces the value of the information in many cases.

Drug therapy in special situations

Prescribing in pregnancy

Guidelines for prescribing during pregnancy are set out in the *British National Formulary* (BNF) and only general points are made below. Pregnancy can be associated with medical problems that require treatment, but exposure of the fetus to any unnecessary drugs is undesirable, particularly in the first trimester, because of the risk of teratogenicity. The problem is illustrated by the fact that approximately 90% of women take medication during pregnancy, and an unrecorded number will take over-the-counter medication without guidance from a medical practitioner or a pharmacist.

Unequivocal teratogenic activity of drugs in humans is limited to a relatively small number of compounds, but their actions can be catastrophic. The list includes ethanol, thalidomide, some anticonvulsants, some chemotherapeutic drugs (e.g. alkylating agents and antimetabolites), warfarin, androgens, danazol, diethylstilbestrol, lithium and retinoids. Because of their long half-lives, some retinoids can result in teratogenesis even if the course of treatment in the mother is stopped before pregnancy occurs. Although teratogenesis is commonly thought of in terms of structural abnormalities or dysfunctional growth in utero, by definition it also refers to long-term functional defects. For example, maternal consumption of alcohol during pregnancy can cause behavioural and cognitive abnormalities in childhood, despite the birth of a seemingly unaffected infant. Some drugs may initially appear harmless yet exhibit a long latency period: diethylstilbestrol, which was given during pregnancy between the 1940s and early 1970s, resulted in abnormalities in the children when they reached adulthood.

Notwithstanding the limited list of drugs that are known to cause teratogenesis, there is a much larger number that should be avoided or used with caution in pregnancy, because of their pharmacologic potential to produce biochemical dysfunction leading to detrimental effects in the fetus. The reader is referred to Appendix 4 of the BNF for a detailed list of drug effects on the fetus. Examples of drugs that cause potentially serious pharmacological effects in the fetus following placental transfer of drug include:

- warfarin: warfarin-induced anticoagulation (Ch. 11) may predispose to cerebral haemorrhage in the fetus during delivery; by contrast, heparin is effective in the mother and does not cross the placenta
- non-steroidal anti-inflammatory drugs (NSAIDs; Ch. 29), which prevent closure of the ductus arteriosus after delivery; closure is a prostaglandin-mediated action and is impaired by inhibition of cyclo-oxygenase
- amiodarone (Ch. 8), which impairs iodine incorporation into thyroxine, and maternal use of which can cause neonatal goitre.

Drugs can be given during late pregnancy to affect uterine contraction. Calcium channel antagonists (Ch. 6) can inhibit or delay labour by reducing uterine contraction, whereas the prostaglandin analogue misoprostol (Ch. 33) can produce uterine contractions and lead to abortion.

Pharmacokinetics

The placenta provides a potential barrier to the transfer of drugs from the maternal circulation, but lipid-soluble drugs cross, particularly if they are of low molecular weight. Only limited metabolism of drugs can occur in the placenta, and this may further restrict fetal exposure. The fetal liver has only a modest ability to metabolise drugs. The fetus represents a slowly equilibrating maternal kinetic compartment, with transfer across the placenta being determined by the concentration gradient between fetal and maternal circulations.

Maternal pharmacokinetics are affected by a number of physiological changes, especially in late pregnancy. These include:

- increased hepatic drug metabolism
- increased renal blood flow and glomerular filtration rate
- decreased plasma concentrations of albumin.

These changes mean that maternal drug concentrations are often lower than those in a non-pregnant woman given the same dose. Care needs to be taken in the interpretation of data from therapeutic drug monitoring using plasma samples, because the total concentration may be decreased, which could be interpreted as needing an increase in dosage, but if this is due to decreased binding to plasma proteins, then the free, and active, concentration may be unaltered.

Drugs and breastfeeding

Appendix 5 of the BNF states, 'For many drugs insufficient evidence is available to provide guidance and it is advisable to administer only essential drugs to a mother during breast feeding.' In general, drugs licensed for use in children can be safely given to the nursing mother. Drugs known to have serious toxic effects in adults or known to affect lactation, such as bromocriptine, should be avoided. If drugs have to be used, compounds with short half-lives are preferred, since they are less likely to accumulate in neonates (who have lower drug clearance, see below). Neonatal exposure can be minimised if the feed is timed to coincide with the trough blood concentration in the mother, which is just before taking a dose.

The reader should refer to the up-to-date lists in the BNF. The American Academy of Pediatrics has published guidelines and categorised drugs into: (A) breastfeeding compatible; (B) breastfeeding compatible but with concern; (C) breastfeeding – no data available; (D) breastfeeding discouraged; (TX) breastfeeding temporarily discouraged after the drug; (X) breastfeeding contraindicated.

Pharmacokinetics

Several factors influence transfer from maternal circulation into breast milk, including the characteristics of the milk (which changes in the first few days of lactation), the physicochemical properties of the drug, and the amount of drug in the maternal circulation. Lipid-soluble compounds diffuse into breast milk and may concentrate because of the high fat content in milk. Water-soluble drugs diffuse from plasma into milk, and the concentrations in breast milk are similar to the non-protein-bound fraction in the maternal plasma. Most drugs penetrate into breast milk in quantities too small to be of concern.

Prescribing for children

Both the pharmacokinetics and responses to drugs may differ between neonates, infants and children compared with adults. There are considerable differences between neonates (<1 month), infants (1–12 months) and children, because many metabolic and physiological processes are immature at birth and develop rapidly in the first months of life. In neonates, inefficient metabolism and renal clearance mean that lower doses of all drugs are needed after allowing for bodyweight, and doses need to be calculated with special care.

Although medicines should be used within the terms of the product licence (see Ch. 3), many of the drugs given to children have not undergone formal clinical evaluation is this age group, and are not specifically licensed for paediatric use. It is recognised that 'off-label' use (strictly speaking, an unlicensed use) may be necessary, and the Medicines Act (1968) does not prohibit such use. There is an increasing recognition of the need for formal clinical trials in the paediatric population, but such studies raise significant ethical issues.

Pharmacokinetics

Absorption. Slow rates of gastric emptying and intestinal transit may reduce the rate of drug absorption in neonates, but total absorption of poorly absorbed drugs may eventually be more complete, because of longer contact with the intestinal mucosa.

Distribution. Neonates and young children have a lower body fat content and higher total body water compared with adults; this influences the distribution of both lipid- and water-soluble drugs. Neonates have a lower plasma albumin concentration, which also has a lower affinity for drug binding. In addition, the higher plasma concentrations of free fatty acids and bilirubin compete with drugs for plasma protein binding sites and vice versa (Ch. 2). The overall effect is reduced plasma protein binding, which not only increases the apparent volume of distribution of the drug but also increases the proportion of drug able to cross the blood–brain barrier and that available for metabolism. Drugs that are strongly bound to albumin should not be used during neonatal jaundice because the drugs may displace bilirubin (which is mostly in the unconjugated form) from protein binding sites, and increase the risk of kernicterus.

Metabolism. The liver drug-metabolising enzyme systems are immature in the neonate, and first-pass metabolism and hepatic drug clearance are low, especially for substrates of CYP1A2 and glucuronidation. When the enzyme systems mature, drug metabolism processes become more extensive, and clearance is higher in young children than in adults, because the relative liver mass and hepatic blood flow are higher.

Renal elimination. Renal function in the neonate and infant is much less developed than in children or adults. The glomerular filtration rate in the newborn is about 40% of the adult level, and tubular secretory processes are poorly developed. Elimination of drugs such as digoxin, gentamicin and penicillin will therefore be delayed.

In children, the larger volume of distribution and faster hepatic elimination mean that weight-related doses of metabolised drugs need to be higher than in adults. Prescribed doses are most accurately judged by considering both age and body surface area. In children, body surface area is a better guide to appropriate drug dosage than bodyweight (see Self-assessment section of Ch. 52). The dose for a child can be approximated as:

$$\frac{\text{Adult dose} \times \text{surface area of child (in m}^2)}{1.8}$$

where 1.8 is the average body surface area of a 70 kg adult.

Prescribing for the elderly

The elderly (usually taken to mean those over 70 years old) comprise a heterogeneous group who show considerable variation in 'biological' age. Changes occur in both the pharmacodynamics and pharmacokinetics of drugs with increasing age.

The density or numbers of receptors may be reduced with age; for example, β-adrenoceptors are decreased in number, reducing the response to agonist drugs. The elderly are often more susceptible to sedatives and hypnotics, possibly because of changes in receptor numbers and/or changes in the efficiency of the blood–brain barrier.

Altered structure and function of target organs can also influence the effects of drugs. For example, baroreceptor function is impaired in the elderly and vasodilator drugs are more likely to provoke postural hypotension. The high peripheral resistance and less distensible arterial tree found with increasing age also respond less well to arterial vasodilators.

These changes reflect the ageing process itself; however, they are often complicated by the presence of chronic disease (frequently involving multiple pathological processes) and variation due to both genetic and environmental influences. The risks of unwanted effects are higher in the elderly as a consequence of these changes, and of the frequent simultaneous use of several drugs. For all these reasons, it is usual to start drug treatment in the elderly with the smallest effective dose. Rational prescribing should also seek to minimise the numbers of drugs used.

Pharmacokinetics

Absorption. Drug absorption is unchanged by ageing, although bioavailability may be increased due to reduced first-pass metabolism.

Distribution. Older people have a lower lean body mass and a relative increase in body fat compared with young adults. The apparent volume of distribution of water-soluble drugs is therefore lower in the elderly and a smaller loading dose of a drug such as digoxin may be needed. Conversely, lipid-soluble drugs may be eliminated more slowly owing to their increased volume of distribution because of the relative increase in body fat (and slower hepatic metabolism).

Metabolism. The size of the liver and its blood flow decrease with age. Although enzyme activity per hepatocyte probably shows little change, the overall capacity for drug metabolism, particularly phase 1 reactions, is reduced. This is particularly important for lipid-soluble drugs, such as nifedipine or propranolol, which undergo extensive first-pass metabolism.

Renal elimination. Increasing age is also associated with a progressive reduction in glomerular filtration rate. Elimination of polar drugs and metabolites is therefore slower; this can produce toxicity when renally eliminated drugs with a low therapeutic index are prescribed, for example lithium, digoxin or gentamicin. Creatinine clearance is an estimate of glomerular filtration rate which usually correlates well with the clearance of drugs that are eliminated in the urine unchanged (as the parent drug). The elderly have a lower muscle mass than younger people, and so the plasma creatinine concentration (which is dependent on lean body mass) is a poor guide to renal glomerular function. Plasma creatinine in the elderly frequently remains within the 'normal' laboratory reference range even when renal function is substantially reduced. The Cockcroft and Gault equation, which relates plasma creatinine to creatinine clearance, contains elements reflecting sex- and age-dependent differences in muscle mass.

Creatinine clearance (ml min^{-1}) for males equals:

$$\frac{1.23 \times (140 - \text{age in years}) \times \text{weight (in kg)}}{\text{plasma creatinine (micromol l}^{-1})}$$

and for females equals:

$$\frac{1.04 \times (140 - \text{age in years}) \times \text{weight (in kg)}}{\text{plasma creatinine (micromol l}^{-1})}$$

Prescribing in renal failure

Individuals with renal failure show increased responses to many drugs, especially when the drug, or its active metabolite, is eliminated in the urine. There are also pharmacodynamic changes; for example, there are altered responses to drugs in people with uraemia, and drugs acting on the central nervous system (CNS) in particular produce enhanced responses, possibly because of increased permeability of the blood–brain barrier.

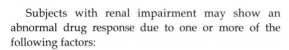

Subjects with renal impairment may show an abnormal drug response due to one or more of the following factors:

- failure to excrete the drug or its metabolites may produce toxicity
- there may be increased sensitivity, even if elimination is unaltered
- many unwanted effects are poorly tolerated in such individuals
- some drugs cease to be effective in such individuals.

Appendix 3 of the BNF gives advice on drug prescribing to those with renal impairment.

Pharmacokinetics

A reduction in drug dosage in renal failure is usually necessary only if a high proportion of the drug is eliminated by the kidney and also the compound has a low therapeutic index. Maintenance dosage may be lowered by either reducing the dose or increasing the dose interval (see Ch. 2, Equation 2.23); loading doses do not usually require any modification. Drugs that do not have dose-related unwanted effects rarely need large dose modifications. A further important consideration is the avoidance of drugs that have toxic effects on the kidney. Use of these in renal impairment can sometimes produce an irreversible decline in renal function.

The kidneys provide the major route of elimination for water-soluble drugs and water-soluble metabolites (see Ch. 2). Renal elimination of drugs can be affected indirectly by abnormal renal perfusion, such as might occur in shock, or directly by changes in the kidney, for example renal tubular necrosis. Reduced renal function may increase the risk of toxicity from the parent drug and/or its metabolites due to their accumulation in the body, although in some cases, sensitivity may be increased in renal failure in the absence of obviously impaired elimination of the drug per se. Impaired renal function does not affect the majority of drugs, because most drugs are eliminated by hepatic metabolism.

Elimination of drugs by the kidney is significantly impaired only when the glomerular filtration rate is reduced below 50 ml min^{-1}. For some drugs, clinically important accumulation does not occur until much lower filtration rates. Changes in renal tubular secretion of drugs in renal disease are less well established.

For the purposes of prescribing and dosage adjustment, renal impairment can be divided into three grades:

1. mild, with a glomerular filtration rate of 20–50 ml min^{-1}
2. moderate, with a glomerular filtration rate of 10–20 ml min^{-1}
3. severe, with a glomerular filtration rate of <10 ml min^{-1}.

The corresponding serum creatinine levels are 150–300, 300–700 and >700 mmol l^{-1}, respectively, although serum creatinine is not always a reliable indicator of renal function (see 'Prescribing for the elderly', above). For some drugs, only severe renal impairment needs to be considered (for example, a reduction in dosage is recommended for ampicillin), while for other drugs, even mild impairment may be important (for example, dosage reduction and haematological monitoring are recommended for carboplatin, whereas cisplatin should be avoided) (see Appendix 3 of the BNF for details).

There are several other ways in which renal impairment may influence the handling of drugs.

- Metabolism in the liver can be altered in uraemic patients; although most oxidative metabolism is unchanged, other processes such as reduction, acetylation and ester hydrolysis are impaired.
- Metabolism in the kidney is important for the 1-α hydroxylation of vitamin D and also for the degradation of insulin, both of which can be impaired in renal failure.
- The distribution of drugs can be affected by changes in fluid balances in renal failure, and more importantly by altered protein binding. Circulating concentrations of albumin are decreased in severe renal failure with proteinuria. In addition, retained endogenous metabolites, such as the tryptophan metabolite indican, may compete for drug-binding sites on plasma proteins. The increased concentrations of free drug can lead to an enhanced response.
- The greater concentration of free drug in the circulation can lead to increased elimination (by filtration and/or metabolism) so that the active unbound drug concentration may be unchanged (see 'Drug Interactions', below).
- Tissue binding of digoxin is reduced in renal failure, so a lower loading dose should be given to compensate for the reduced volume of distribution.

Prescribing in liver disease

Changes in both drug responses and pharmacokinetics can occur in liver disease. The severity of the liver disease is important, as is whether the disease is decompensated, for example jaundice, hypoproteinaemia or encephalopathy. Many of the pharmacodynamic and pharmacokinetic changes in liver failure arise from decreased hepatic synthesis of proteins that perform essential functions within the hepatocyte, or which are released into the blood, such as albumin and clotting factors.

CNS depressant drugs, such as morphine and chlorpromazine, have an enhanced effect in people with liver failure. This is caused by increased sensitivity of neuronal tissue (although the mechanism is not known) and can provoke encephalopathy in susceptible patients. Decreased plasma protein binding may contribute to the greater sensitivity by increasing the percentage of free drug so that more drug can cross the blood–brain barrier. Benzodiazepines may be used during investigational procedures, and the effects can be reversed by giving the benzodiazepine antagonist flumazenil.

Encephalopathy may be triggered by drugs that cause constipation (which increases the formation of potentially toxic metabolites, such as ammonia, by the intestinal bacteria). Diuretics that produce hypokalaemia can precipitate hepatic encephalopathy in chronic liver disease, and, therefore, potassium-sparing diuretics such as spironolactone are usually used (spironolactone also blocks the effects of circulating aldosterone, which may be increased in liver disease).

The reduced ability to synthesise vitamin K-dependent clotting factors makes people with chronic liver disease prone to clotting problems: they would be very sensitive to anticoagulant drugs, which are clearly contraindicated.

People with pre-existing liver disease are likely to be more susceptible to potentially hepatotoxic drugs. This raises a problem for pain relief, since paracetamol is hepatotoxic at high doses, whereas NSAIDs can increase the risk of gastrointestinal bleeding and cause fluid retention, and opioids can precipitate encephalopathy. In practice, lower doses of paracetamol are usually given, taking care that the amounts do not exceed the reduced threshold for hepatotoxicity shown by such individuals (see Ch. 53).

Pharmacokinetics

Prescribing in liver disease should be carried out with care, and drugs that are extensively metabolised by the liver should be given in smaller doses. The need for dose reduction arises primarily from an increase in bioavailability and a decrease in systemic clearance, both of which increase the average steady-state plasma concentration and the area under the plasma concentration–time curve for a single dose.

The rate of absorption of drugs from the gut is not greatly affected, but other aspects of drug handling may be altered. Distribution may be affected if protein synthesis is reduced, because the plasma albumin concentrations are decreased, resulting in a higher percentage of free drug in plasma and a greater apparent volume of distribution. An elevated plasma bilirubin may displace some drugs from their plasma protein binding sites, and this would also increase the apparent volume of distribution; examples of drugs that can be affected are lidocaine and propranolol.

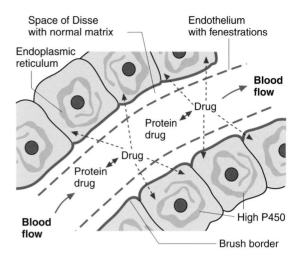

Fig. 56.1
Schematic for the uptake of a drug from the sinusoid of a normal healthy liver.

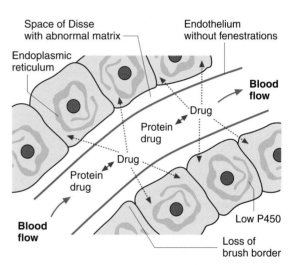

Fig. 56.2
Schematic for the uptake of a drug from the sinusoid of a liver showing the features characteristic of cirrhosis.

The liver has characteristics that facilitate the rapid and extensive uptake and metabolism of lipid-soluble drugs (Fig. 56.1). These include:

- fenestrations in the endothelium, allowing ready access to extracellular fluid
- rapid diffusion across the space of Disse (which is a matrix consisting primarily of type 4 collagen)
- a brush border on hepatocytes, allowing rapid uptake
- high intracellular enzyme activity for both phase 1 and phase 2 metabolism.

During chronic liver disease, a number of changes may occur which reduce the capacity of the liver to metabolise drugs (Fig. 56.2):

- fenestrations in the endothelium are lost
- diffusion across the space of Disse may be reduced in fibrosis/cirrhosis as type 4 collagen is replaced by type 1 and type 3 collagen (which can form dense fibrils)
- the brush border on hepatocytes is lost
- intracellular enzyme activity is reduced
- intrahepatic vascular shunts may reduce the perfusion of hepatocytes.

Reduced hepatic uptake and metabolism or biliary excretion of drugs may result in a greater proportion of the drug and/or metabolites being eliminated via other routes, such as the urine.

First-pass metabolism may be considerably reduced in conditions such as liver cirrhosis, and the consequences are most apparent with drugs that undergo extensive hepatic first-pass metabolism in patients with normal liver function. Bioavailability may increase considerably and approach 100%, such that the bioavailability could change fivefold or more (e.g. from <0.2 to 1.0).

Biliary excretion is impaired in conditions causing reduced formation of bile. A correlation between drug clearance and bilirubin would be expected for drugs eliminated unchanged in bile, such as rifampicin and fusidic acid. Reduced elimination of drug metabolites in bile could affect enterohepatic circulation (Ch. 2). Reduced bile production can affect the absorption of highly lipid-soluble molecules, such as the fat-soluble vitamins, that require micelle formation for effective absorption

Systemic clearance may be reduced for drugs eliminated by hepatic metabolism. This affects both high-clearance drugs, where the elimination rate is dependent on effective liver blood flow, and low-clearance drugs, where it is dependent on hepatic extraction and enzyme activity.

Drug interactions

Many people receive more than one drug during a course of treatment because:

- combination therapy is preferable or necessary for producing an adequate effect or response, such as the chemotherapy of malignant disease, or treatment of hypertension
- a single condition or pathology may give rise to a variety of symptoms that are controlled by different drugs
- the person may suffer from more than one condition or pathology requiring treatment with drugs that are unrelated pharmacologically.

The term 'interaction' implies that the response to the combination of drugs is different to that which could be predicted from a simple summation of the effects produced by each drug if given singly. Interactions may result in either a decrease in response (antagonism) or increase in response (synergism) compared with that predicted; this may be either beneficial, or potentially harmful because of a lack of clinical response or the risk of toxicity.

Beneficial interactions are usually well recognised – for example, combinations of different anticancer drugs, and levodopa plus carbidopa – and are part of prescribing recommendations. In consequence, the focus of this section, and of Appendix 1 of the BNF, is those interactions that may give rise to adverse effects, especially when the interaction would not be readily predicted based on a knowledge of the sites and mechanisms of action.

Interactions are of greatest importance for drugs that have a narrow therapeutic index and for groups at increased risk, such as the elderly (who are more likely or suffer multiple pathologies and may have decreased hepatic and renal function).

Drug interactions may arise from interference at the site or mechanism of action (pharmacodynamics) or from altered delivery of the drug to its site of action (pharmacokinetics).

Pharmacodynamic interactions

Pharmacodynamic interactions are usually predictable, based on the known actions of the drug. Interactions may relate to the principal site of action of the drug, or to secondary sites of action that are responsible for unwanted effects of the drug. In principle, drugs that are highly selective for a single site of action are less likely to produce pharmacodynamic interactions than are drugs that show low selectivity. An example of a serious synergistic interaction is between an angiotensin-converting enzyme (ACE) inhibitor, such as enalapril (Ch. 6), and spironolactone (Ch. 14); the ACE inhibitor reduces the production of aldosterone and the effect on the renal tubule, reducing the excretion of K^+, is exaggerated by the action of spironolactone, causing potentially life-threatening hyperkalaemia.

Pharmacokinetic interactions

Absorption. Co-administration of two drugs could give an interaction if one drug affected the rate or extent of absorption of the other drug. Changes in the rate of absorption, for example by increasing or decreasing gastric emptying or intestinal motility, will affect the peak concentration but not usually the extent of absorption. Interactions affecting the rate of absorption are less important than those that alter the extent of absorption. Examples of interactions affecting the extent of absorption include retention of the drug in the gut lumen (e.g. tetracycline antibiotics bind to divalent or trivalent metals, such as Ca^{2+} or Fe^{3+}, to form complexes that are not absorbed) and inhibition or induction of first-pass metabolism in the gut lumen, gut wall or liver.

Distribution. The main interaction affecting drug distribution arises from competition for the non-specific binding sites on plasma proteins, such as albumin (see Table 2.2). Interactions affecting plasma protein binding are of greatest importance when:

- the displaced drug is highly protein bound; for example, if competition for protein binding sites reduces binding from 98% to 96%, this will double the free drug concentration in plasma (from 2% to 4%); a 2% change in the binding of a drug which is 50% bound and 50% free would not be clinically or biologically significant
- the displaced drug has a narrow therapeutic index, so that a two- to threefold change in free drug concentration gives an increase in drug actions
- the displaced drug has a low apparent volume of distribution, such that the plasma contains a significant proportion of the body load; if the drug has a high apparent volume of distribution, the increase in free drug in the plasma volume (about 3 l) may be negligible after it has been distributed to (or 'diluted' in) a much higher apparent volume of distribution (for example 300 l)
- the displacing drug is of low potency, such that large doses (on a milligram basis) are given and protein binding sites become limiting.

In reality, such interactions are of limited clinical relevance even when the above criteria are fulfilled. For example, the potentially important interaction between warfarin and aspirin is due to their combined pharmaco-dynamic effects on haemostasis (Ch. 11) rather than the displacement of warfarin (which is 99% bound and has an apparent volume of distribution of $0.1 \, l \, kg^{-1}$) from its protein binding sites. One reason for this is that the additional free drug that has been displaced from protein binding sites may undergo rapid elimination by metabolism or glomerular filtration. When this occurs, a new 'steady state' will be established when the combination is given, with similar amounts of free drug but reduced amounts of bound drug. Therefore, the total (free and bound) plasma concentration of the drug (which is measured in most drug assays) will be lower. Measured total concentrations may be misleadingly low and indicate an inappropriate increase in drug dose. Examples of drugs displaying this problem are theophylline and phenytoin.

Metabolism. Interactions affecting metabolism could theoretically arise from simple competition for the same enzyme, but this would only be important if the combination resulted in saturation of the enzyme system. The doses of most drugs are such that the concentrations do not approach the K_m of the enzymes involved in their metabolism, so first-order kinetics (Ch. 2) apply. Under

these circumstances, the presence of two substrates is no different to the presence of increased amounts of a single substrate; in consequence, the clearance and half-lives of drugs given in combination are the same as when each is given alone. A clinically useful exception is the administration of ethanol to prevent the metabolism of methanol (in overdose) to formate, in order to reduce the risk of blindness (Ch. 53).

Important interactions can occur when one drug in a combination induces or inhibits the enzymes involved in the metabolism of the other drug. This has been well recognised for drugs affecting the cytochrome P450 enzyme system (Table 2.8), largely because of the importance of this enzyme system for the elimination of most drugs and the potential for induction of different isoenzymes. Enzyme inhibition occurs as soon as the drug concentration is sufficiently high, and inhibition can occur after a single dose (e.g. cimetidine). In contrast, enzyme induction requires the synthesis of additional enzyme and it takes a few days (or longer) for the elevated enzyme activity to reach a new equilibrium between synthesis and degradation. Induction or inhibition of hepatic enzymes can affect both systemic clearance and first-pass metabolism (bioavailability) after oral dosage.

Co-administration of two drugs, one of which is an enzyme inducer, will reduce the concentrations of the other drug. This may decrease the response to the second drug (if the parent compound is active), but could also increase the response to a prodrug, if the induced enzyme was responsible for this bioactivation. A problem can also arise when drug dosage has been optimised for the combination and treatment with the inducer is then stopped. Under such circumstances, the enzyme activity decreases (usually over a period of 2–3 weeks) and plasma levels of the still-prescribed drug will increase, possibly giving a risk of toxicity.

Excretion. Each of the three processes that are important in the renal elimination of drugs, i.e. glomerular filtration, pH-dependent reabsorption and renal tubular secretion, could be a site for a drug interaction.

- *Glomerular filtration* depends on renal perfusion and removes free or non-protein-bound drug only. In consequence, drugs affecting renal perfusion or plasma protein binding (see above) could give rise to interactions.
- *pH-dependent reabsorption* could be altered by drugs that affect urine pH, either directly or via metabolic effects; the pH changes associated with aspirin overdose could affect the excretion of drugs taken concurrently.
- *Renal tubular secretion* can give rise to interactions when there is competition for the transporter. Probenecid was co-administered with penicillins in order to inhibit their renal tubular secretion. Aspirin can interfere with the transport of both endogenous

compounds (e.g. uric acid) and drugs (e.g. methotrexate).

The biliary excretion of drugs is not an important site for drug interactions, but the enterohepatic cycling of drugs can be affected by the co-administration of poorly absorbed broad-spectrum antibacterials, which affect the hydrolysis of drug conjugates in the lower bowel (Fig. 2.13).

FURTHER READING

Bressler R, Bahl JJ (2003) Principles of drug therapy for the elderly patient. *Mayo Clin Proc* 78, 1564–1577

Briggs GG, Freeman RK, Yaffe SJ (1998) Drugs in pregnancy and lactation. A reference guide to fetal and neonatal risk, 5th edn. Baltimore, Williams and Wilkins

Dickinson BD, Altman RD, Nielsen NH, Sterling ML; Council on Scientific Affairs, American Medical Association (2001) Drug interactions between oral contraceptives and antibiotics. *Obstet Gynecol* 98, 853–860

Henderson L, Yue QY, Bergquist C, Gerden B, Arlett P (2002) St John's wort (Hypericum perforatum): drug interactions and clinical outcomes. *Br J Clin Pharmacol* 54, 349–356

Ito S (2000) Drug therapy for breast-feeding women. *N Engl J Med* 343, 118–126

Johnson TN (2003) The development of drug metabolising enzymes and their influence on the susceptibility to adverse drug reactions in children. *Toxicology* 192, 37–48

Koren G, Pastuszak A, Ito S (2000) Drugs in pregnancy. *N Engl J Med* 338, 1128–1137

Larimore WL, Petrie KA (2000) Drug use during pregnancy and lactation. *Primary Care* 27, 35–53

Patsalos PN, Froscher W, Pisani F, van Rijn CM (2002) The importance of drug interactions in epilepsy therapy. *Epilepsia* 43, 365–385

Patsalos PN, Perucca E (2003) Clinically important drug interactions in epilepsy: interactions between antiepileptic drugs and other drugs. *Lancet Neurol* 2, 473–481

Routledge PA, O'Mahony MS, Woodhouse KW (2004) Adverse drug reactions in elderly patients. *Br J Clin Pharmacol* 57, 121–126

Spina E, Scordo MG, D'Arrigo C (2003) Metabolic drug interactions with new psychotropic agents. *Fundam Clin Pharmacol* 17, 517–538

Strolin Benedetti M, Baltes EL (2003) Drug metabolism and disposition in children. *Fundam Clin Pharmacol* 17, 281–299

Thurmann PA, Steioff A (2001) Drug treatment in pregnancy. *Int J Clin Pharmacol Ther* 39, 185–191

Turnheim K (2003) When drug therapy gets old: pharmacokinetics and pharmacodynamics in the elderly. *Exp Gerontol* 38, 843–853

Self-assessment answers

Chapter 2

1. a. **False**. An increase in dose results in an increase in the concentrations of the drug in plasma and body tissues. A twofold increase in drug concentrations gives twofold higher concentrations available to elimination processes; consequently, the rate of elimination increases proportionately. Since clearance is given by the rate of elimination/plasma concentration, this ratio is not altered. A decrease in clearance with increase in dose occurs when the elimination process is saturated and an increase in concentration cannot give an increase in the rate of elimination. Few drugs show saturation kinetics (zero order) at therapeutic doses.

   b. **True**. This statement is true for all 'pre-systemic' sites of metabolism of the oral dose, e.g. gut lumen, gut wall and liver. Low bioavailability may also arise from poor absorption.

   c. **True**. If the liver is able to 'mop up' a high proportion of the drug as it is absorbed from the gastrointestinal tract, it will also clear a high proportion of drug from the blood after it has entered the general circulation. For example, if 80% of an oral dose undergoes first-pass liver metabolism during absorption, then 80% of all drug delivered to the liver via the systemic blood flow will also be cleared; systemic clearance will equal 80% of liver blood flow.

   d. **True**. A longer half-life can arise from a higher apparent volume of distribution or a lower clearance; babies (under 6–12 months) show lower systemic clearance because of both reduced hepatic metabolism and lower renal excretion.

   e. **False**. A decrease in renal function could affect systemic clearance, providing that renal clearance of the drug was a significant part of total plasma clearance. However, bioavailability is simply the fraction of the oral dose that reaches the general circulation, and the kidneys are not part of the route between gut lumen and general circulation. (Although the AUC of an oral dose may be increased in renal disease, the AUC of an intravenous dose will show a similar increase and bioavailability is not altered.)

   f. **False**. Benzathine benzylpenicillin is a depot injection of penicillin in which the prolonged half-life results from prolonged and sustained release from the site of injection. Once absorbed into the blood, the circulating penicillin is handled by the kidneys as normal.

   g. **False**. Nifedipine is metabolised by CYP3A4; no interaction would occur, because smoking induces CYP1A2. Our increased understanding of the cytochrome P450 isoenzymes has allowed more rational predictions of 'drug–drug' and 'drug–environmental chemical' interactions.

   h. **False**. Phenobarbital is a potent inducer of cytochrome P450 enzymes, which can increase the ability of the liver to extract the drug from the blood. This can increase the systemic clearance but decreases the oral bioavailability of co-administered drugs.

   i. **True**. A loading dose is designed to produce the body load that will be present during chronic treatment (at steady state) without the time delay while the drug accumulates during chronic treatment. Drugs with short elimination half-lives do not accumulate significantly and therefore the body load after the first normal (non-loading) dose will be the same as during chronic treatment (see also the answer to the data interpretation question 3d below).

   j. **False**. The influence of body composition on the apparent volume of distribution depends on the nature of the drug. Lipid-soluble drugs would show an increased apparent volume of distribution (V) in an obese patient (when expressed per kilogram body weight) but the converse would apply to water-soluble drugs. However, the V and clearance (CL) of drugs are independent variables; there is no reason why the different distribution in the body should affect the ability of the liver to extract the drug from the blood. Students sometimes can get confused about V and CL and think that if more drug enters the fat this will lower the blood concentration and hence must lower CL. It is important to appreciate that V and CL are independent variables. If more drug enters adipose tissue (because there is more of it), then plasma concentration (C_p) will tend to be lower and, therefore, V (V = the amount in the body/C_p), will be higher. Because the plasma concentration at any time is lower and CL is a constant for that drug, then the rate of elimination at any point in time will be lower (CL = rate of elimination/C_p). The elimination half-life is related to both V and CL (half-life is 0.693 V/CL) and an increase in V without a change in CL would result in an increase in half-life. Because the steady-state plasma concentration (C_{ss}) depends on CL but not on V ($C_{ss} = D \times F/\text{CL} \times t$, where D is administered dose, F is bioavailability and t is the interval between doses), there would not be any need to modify a chronic dosage regimen because of an increase in V. However, the steady-state body load ($Cp_{ss} \times V$) would be higher and, therefore, it could take longer to reach steady-state conditions (as indicated by the increase in half-life). [If you have understood this answer, then you have 'cracked' pharmacokinetics!]

k. **False**. This statement is true for some drugs but not for all drugs: it depends on the drug. Administration of drugs with food will generally decrease the rate of absorption (because of effects on gastric emptying and/or absorption rate) and this will often reduce the peak plasma concentration. This may, in some cases, reduce unwanted effects. Another advantage of taking medicines with meals is that it can increase compliance with a three times daily (tds) dosage schedule. Potential disadvantages are the delay in absorption and, in some cases, interference with absorption, giving a decrease in bioavailability; for example, the absorption of tetracycline antimicrobials is almost completely abolished if they are taken with milk.

2. Drug bioavailability

a. The *rate* of absorption is determined by the rate of increase after oral dosing (providing that the elimination rates or oral and intravenous doses are parallel). Drug A is absorbed very rapidly, while drug B takes about 6h to reach a peak concentration.

b. The *extent* of absorption (bioavailability or F) is determined by the $\text{AUC}_{oral}/\text{AUC}_{iv}$. For drug A, the AUC_{oral} is much smaller than AUC_{iv} and therefore F is much less than 1. In contrast, for drug B, the AUC_{oral} approximately equals the AUC_{iv} and so F is approximately 1.

c. The rate of distribution is given by the rate of decrease between the administration of the intravenous bolus dose (at time 0) and the establishment of the terminal elimination phase. The terminal phase for drug A starts at about 1 h, whereas that for drug B starts at about 4 h. Therefore, A distributes more rapidly. The *extent* of distribution is given by the apparent volume of distribution, V, which is indicated by the intravenous dose divided by the intercept (C_{p0}) obtained on back-extrapolation of the terminal phase of the plasma concentration–time curve (intravenous dose/C_{p0}). Both A and B give a similar intercept and, therefore, have similar apparent volumes of distribution.

d. The elimination half-life is given by 0.693/terminal slope (0.693/k or 0.693/β) and it is obvious that drug B has a longer half-life than drug A. The reason for the longer half-life of B is the lower clearance (CL) of B (since the volume of distribution is similar for A and B). This is also apparent by visual inspection of the graphs; CL = $\text{Dose}_{iv}/\text{AUC}_{iv}$ and the AUC_{iv} for B is much greater than that for A (the doses were the same).

e. The potential for accumulation depends on the difference between half-life and dose interval. It is clear that nearly all of drug A has been removed from the plasma (and therefore the body) by 24 h, whereas considerable amounts of B remain at 24 h. Therefore, B would show significant accumulation on daily dosage.

3. Parameter calculations

a. The extent of absorption (note units cancel to give a fraction)

$$F = \frac{\text{AUC}_{oral}}{\text{AUC}_{iv}} \times \frac{\text{Dose}_{iv}}{\text{Dose}_{oral}}$$

A $F = \dfrac{2}{16} \times \dfrac{20\,000}{20\,000} = 0.125$

B $F = \dfrac{995}{1000} \times \dfrac{20\,000}{20\,000} = 0.995$

C $F = \dfrac{26}{40} \times \dfrac{20\,000}{20\,000} = 0.65$

b. The extent of distribution is given by V, which equals clearance, CL (calculated from intravenous data), divided by k, the terminal elimination rate constant, i.e.

$$\text{CL} = \frac{\text{Dose}_{iv}}{\text{AUC}_{iv}} \quad \text{then} \quad V = \frac{\text{Dose}_{iv}}{\text{AUC}_{iv} \times k}$$

The units are

$$\frac{\mu g}{\mu g\ ml^{-1}\ min \times min^{-1}} = ml$$

A $V = \dfrac{20\,000}{16 \times 0.0063} = 198\,413\ ml = 198l$

B $V = \dfrac{20\,000}{1000 \times 0.00022} = 90\,909\ ml = 91l$

C $V = \dfrac{20\,000}{40 \times 0.014} = 35\,714\ ml = 36l$

c. The rate of elimination is reflected in $t_{1/2}$:

$$t_{1/2} = \frac{0.693}{k}$$

A $\quad t_{1/2} = \dfrac{0.693}{0.0063 \text{ min}^{-1}} \quad = \quad 110 \text{ min} = 2 \text{ h}$

B $\quad t_{1/2} = \dfrac{0.693}{0.00022 \text{ min}^{-1}} = 3150 \text{ min} = 53 \text{ h}$

C $\quad t_{1/2} = \dfrac{0.693}{0.014 \text{ min}^{-1}} \quad = 49.5 \text{ min} = 1 \text{ h}$

These values were calculated using the intravenous data. The terminal half-lives of A and B are the same after both oral and intravenous dosage; the half-life for C is $(0.693/0.003) = 231$ min (4 h) after oral administration, suggesting an absorption rate-limited terminal phase (i.e. absorption is slower than elimination).

The clearance (CL) is the volume of blood cleared per minute

$$CL = \frac{\text{Dose}_{iv}}{\text{AUC}_{iv}} \quad = \quad \boxed{\frac{\mu g}{\mu g \text{ ml}^{-1} \text{ min}} = \text{ml min}^{-1}}$$

A $\quad CL = \dfrac{20\,000}{16} = 1250 \text{ ml min}^{-}$

B $\quad CL = \dfrac{20\,000}{1000} = 20 \text{ ml min}^{-}$

C $\quad CL = \dfrac{20\,000}{40} = 500 \text{ ml min}^{-}$

The route of administration is indicated by the percentage dose in urine as the parent drug, after the intravenous dose. Drug A is cleared by non-renal routes and is all metabolised. Drug B is cleared mostly (95%) by metabolism, and drug C is cleared almost totally by renal elimination.

$$\text{Renal clearance (CL}_r) = \frac{\text{amount excreted in urine}_{(0-t)}}{\text{AUC}_{(0-t)}}$$

A $\quad CL_r = \dfrac{20\,000 \times 0.00}{16} = 0 \text{ ml min}^{-1}$

B $\quad CL_r = \dfrac{20\,000 \times 0.05}{1000} = 1 \text{ ml min}^{-1}$

C $\quad CLr = \dfrac{20\,000 \times 0.98}{40} = 490 \text{ ml min}^{-1}$

d. The potential for accumulation during chronic dosage is determined by comparison of the amount in the body during chronic dosage with that following a single dose.

$$\text{Accumulation} = \frac{\begin{array}{c}\text{Steady state}\\ \text{body load}\\ \hline \text{Single dose}\\ \text{body load}\end{array}} = \frac{C_{ss} \times V}{\text{Dose} \times F} = \frac{\text{Dose} \times F \times V}{\text{Dose} \times F \times CL \times t}$$

where t is dose interval during chronic intake and C_{ss} is Dose $= F/CL = t$. Since V/CL is $1/k$ or $t_{1/2}/0.693$ ($t_{1/2} = 1.44$), this equation is simply:

$$\text{Accumulation} = \frac{t_{1/2} \times 1.44}{t}$$

Therefore, the potential for accumulation with any proposed dose interval is directly proportional to the half-life, and the accumulation potential is $B \gg A > C$. (In reality, A and C would not show any significant accumulation on chronic dosage.)

e. To discuss factors that may influence the drugs, we need to be able to interpret what the numerical values mean in physiological terms. **Drug A** is eliminated by metabolism with no renal excretion of the parent drug. It is therefore very lipid soluble (hence the very high value for V). The short half-life results from the very high clearance, which approximates to liver blood flow. The low oral bioavailability is also consistent with high hepatic first-pass metabolism.

Absorption rate. This is probably very rapid because of the drug's high lipid solubility; a modified-release formulation may be required because of this rapid absorption and short half-life.

Bioavailability. If the liver is the main site of first-pass metabolism, then bioavailability could be greatly increased by liver disease. Enzyme inducers would decrease bioavailability still further; inhibitors would increase it.

Distribution. This would mainly be influenced by the proportion of body fat.

Elimination. Hepatic clearance will depend largely on effective liver blood flow; therefore, perfusion abnormalities (e.g. hepatic cirrhosis) would have a major influence. Age may affect liver function. Enzyme induction would have little effect (since clearance is largely determined by liver blood flow); inhibitors could decrease hepatic metabolism of the drug and hence clearance. Pharmacogenetic differences in metabolising enzymes could be important if poor metabolisers showed low clearance (this would depend on the importance of the genetically determined enzyme in the overall clearance). **Drug B** is eliminated mostly by metabolism but clearance is low and some is excreted in the urine as the parent drug.

Absorption rate. This is probably rapid (terminal phase is the same after oral and intravenous dose but elimination is very slow for both routes). Modified-release formulation would not be needed because of the long half-life.

Bioavailability. This would be high because of the drug's slow metabolism/low clearance; it is unlikely to be influenced by induction or inhibition of hepatic enzymes (even if first-pass metabolism doubled, the bioavailability would only decrease to 0.99).

Distribution. The slightly greater water solubility, compared with drug A, gives a lower volume of distribution.

Elimination. Renal function will not greatly influence total clearance. Renal clearance is only 1ml min^{-1}, which is negligible compared with glomerular filtration rate; therefore, nearly all filtered drug is reabsorbed from the tubule. Urine pH could affect this reabsorption, but renal clearance (1 ml min^{-1}) is only 5% of total clearance (20 ml min^{-1}). The main factor influencing the clearance of this drug will be the activity of the metabolising enzymes. Liver blood flow will not be important, since the metabolic clearance (19 ml min^{-1}) is only a very small fraction of liver blood flow. Factors influencing the enzyme activity could include inducers/inhibitors, age and pharmacogenetics.

Drug C is eliminated almost exclusively by renal excretion without metabolism. The pharmacokinetics of this drug are dominated by its high water solubility.

Absorption rate. The drug shows 'flip-flop' kinetics and the elimination rate after oral dosage is determined by the absorption rate of this polar drug. The half-life after oral dosage (4 h) means that a modified-release oral formulation is not really needed, despite the rapid elimination half-life (seen after intravenous administration).

Bioavailability. The low bioavailability is a reflection of the high water solubility and the slow rate of absorption from the gut. The non-bioavailable fraction of the oral dose is probably simply lost in the faeces. (Note, it is not likely to undergo first-pass metabolism, because the drug is not metabolised.)

Elimination. The renal clearance (490 ml min^{-1}) is greatly in excess of the glomerular filtration rate and approaches renal blood flow. The drug must therefore undergo renal tubular secretion. Factors influencing this drug will be renal blood flow (e.g. age and renal disease) and inhibitors of renal tubular secretion. Urine pH is unlikely to be a major influence (there is incomplete absorption from the gut despite the range of pH values in the gut lumen, which

suggests that the water solubility of the drug is not influenced by pH).

Chapter 4

1. **False**. Noradrenaline is the transmitter substance at the postganglionic nerve endings. Adrenaline is released only from the adrenal medulla and acetylcholine is the transmitter in sweat glands and hair follicles.

2. **False**. Although acetylcholine is the transmitter at all ganglia and the neuromuscular junction, at sensible doses ganglion-blocking drugs block the nicotinic N_1 receptors in autonomic ganglia but not N_2 receptors at the neuromuscular junction.

3. **True**. Plasma or pseudocholinesterase can also metabolise acetylcholine but does so more slowly. Plasma cholinesterase, however, has a broader spectrum of activity and can metabolise drugs such as suxamethonium (succinylcholine).

4. **True**. Dopamine is predominantly an important transmitter in the CNS but is also a transmitter in selected situations in the periphery, e.g. the renal vascular smooth muscle.

5. **True**. This is important, as selective inhibitors of MAO-A used in the treatment of depression leave MAO-B unaffected and it can metabolise tyramine in food, therefore avoiding the 'cheese reaction'.

6. **False**. Stimulation of α_1-adrenoceptors on resistance vessels causes constriction; therefore, their blockade lowers blood pressure. However, α_2-adrenoceptor (presynaptic) stimulation reduces noradrenaline release and blockade of these receptors would raise blood pressure.

7. **False**. Botulinum toxin inhibits acetylcholine release and can be used locally where there is skeletal muscle spasm or excessive sweating.

8. **False**. The β_3-adrenoceptor has been found in adipocytes, the heart, colon and some other tissues but is less widespread than the β_2-adrenoceptor. The β_3-adrenoceptor on adipocytes is being investigated to see if its stimulation will be effective to treat obesity.

9. **True**. Propranolol is a non-selective antagonist of β-adrenoceptors, and the role of the presynaptic β_2-adrenoceptor is to increase noradrenaline release.

10. **True**. Selective reversible inhibitors of the uptake of noradrenaline or 5HT (e.g. fluoxetine) are available and are used in the treatment of depression.

11. **False**. Sympathetic nervous stimulation releases noradrenaline and inhibits motility but increases the tone of the sphincters.

12. **False**. When the sympathetic supply to the radial muscle of the iris is stimulated, the muscle contracts and the pupil size increases. This effect can be used to facilitate retinal examination.

Chapter 5

1. a. **False**. Nitric oxide increases cGMP synthesis to bring about reduced intracellular free Ca^{2+} and vasodilation.
   b. **True**. Glyceryl trinitrate undergoes extensive first-pass metabolism after oral dosing, since initial entry into the systemic circulation is via the portal circulation and the liver. Transdermal patches or sublingual administration avoid the portal circulation and the drug gains direct access to the systemic circulation.
   c. **False**. Glyceryl trinitrate does not increase total coronary blood flow. It can, however, treat angina by increasing flow to the ischaemic areas by dilating collateral blood vessels or reducing coronary vasospasm.
   d. **False**. A major component of the benefit of glyceryl trinitrate is its peripheral vasodilator action, reducing preload and, to a lesser extent, peripheral vascular resistance, and afterload. These reduce workload on the heart. The reflex tachycardia that occurs through a fall in peripheral resistance can be reduced by concomitant treatment with a β-adrenoceptor antagonist.
   e. **False**. t-PA cleaves plasminogen to increase the formation of plasmin, which results in the degradation of the fibrin that forms the framework of the thrombus.

2. Answer **d**
   a. True and can therefore give a more predictable response.
   b. True. Unlike the short-acting dihydropyridines, verapamil also acts on the heart and reflex tachycardia does not occur. Modified-release formulations of dihydropyridines also reduce the incidence of reflex tachycardia.
   c. True. Platelet inhibition with an intravenous glycoprotein IIb/IIIa antagonist such as tirofiban reduces the risk of myocardial infarction or death in those at high risk. These agents are most effective when there is a raised plasma concentration of the markers of myocardial damage, troponin I or T.
   d. False. Cholesterol reduction to <4.0 mmol l^{-1} should be attempted. Statins reduce reinfarction and cardiac death by 25–30%. Fibrates are less effective, but may be useful if the total cholesterol is low but the HDL cholesterol is also low.
   e. True. Nifedipine and similar calcium channel antagonists do not improve prognosis after myocardial infarction. Verapamil and diltiazem produce a small reduction in reinfarction, but do not reduce mortality. They may be detrimental if there are signs of heart failure. These drugs should only be considered as an option for those at high risk who cannot tolerate a β-adrenoceptor antagonist and who do not have significant left ventricular dysfunction.

3. Case history answers

   a. For acute attacks, sublingual glyceryl trinitrate is the first-choice drug to give rapid relief, although protection is only short lived.
   b. For prophylaxis, a β-adrenoceptor antagonist is often the treatment of first choice, or a calcium channel antagonist if this is contraindicated. A combination of both, or addition of a long-acting nitrate (but tolerance is a problem), could be used if symptoms are not well controlled with a single agent, but the benefit of triple therapy is not convincing. For example, atenolol and verapamil or diltiazem given together significantly decrease the number of angina attacks compared with either used alone. These drugs will also lower blood pressure and heart rate, which are precipitating factors for angina. Their use together should be carefully monitored, however, because of the dangers of compounding bradycardia or heart failure. Antianginal drugs have not been shown to reduce the risk of subsequent myocardial infarction.
   c. Additional therapy to improve prognosis includes low-dose aspirin (75–150 mg), which has been shown to reduce the risk of subsequent myocardial infarction. Lowering plasma cholesterol concentration by diet or by drugs such as simvastatin can also reduce the risk of subsequent myocardial infarction.
   d. Smoking, lack of exercise and obesity are all risk factors for coronary heart disease. TK is exposed to these increased risks and should address these by lifestyle changes.
   e. In an 80-year-old person, there is likely to be reduced hepatic metabolism of calcium channel antagonists. Because they are significantly metabolised by first-pass metabolism, it is likely

that they will produce a greater reduction in blood pressure at smaller doses.

f. The most consistent evidence is for combined use of heparin and aspirin in unstable angina. Addition of a β-adrenoceptor antagonist produces a small additional benefit.

g. Coronary artery occlusion at the site of an atheroma, causing necrosis.

h. The benefit of thrombolytic therapy is strongly dependent upon the delay between symptoms and administration. The benefit is particularly great if thrombolytic therapy can be administered within 6 h from the onset of pain, but there is good evidence for benefit until at least 12 h.

i. Allergic reactions to streptokinase are extremely rare. TK had not had a previous myocardial infarction and had not previously been administered streptokinase, so would be unlikely to have high titres of streptokinase-neutralising antibodies. It would, therefore, be safe to give TK streptokinase unless he had severe symptomatic hypotension.

j. Aspirin and thrombolytic therapy have been shown to have additive benefit for treating acute myocardial infarction, reducing subsequent reinfarction or death.

k. Low doses of aspirin reduce the production of the platelet aggregating agent thromboxane A_2 by platelets, while having less effect on the production of the platelet disaggregating agent prostaglandin I_2 from endothelial cells. Large doses of aspirin do not produce any additional benefit, and the risk of gastric irritation or ulceration is increased.

l. This is incorrect. Streptokinase has a longer duration of action than rt-PA and it is generally unnecessary to administer heparin when streptokinase has been given. However, it is necessary after rt-PA, when it improves the long-term patency of the artery.

m. Low-dose aspirin, β-adrenoceptor antagonists and ACE inhibitors all reduce mortality and the risk of reinfarction. The β-adrenoceptor antagonist will need to be given under close observation, since it carries a risk of worsening heart failure. In people who have signs of heart failure, verapamil and diltiazem may also be detrimental. Warfarin reduces mortality and reinfarction to a similar extent as low-dose aspirin, so is not required unless aspirin is poorly tolerated.

Chapter 6

1. a. **False**. Thiazide diuretics cause growth retardation of the fetus and are not recommended.

Methyldopa, nifedipine and labetalol are most often used.

b. **True**. Calcium channel antagonists act by opening L-type voltage-gated Ca^{2+} channels and nifedipine is relatively selective for smooth muscle. Verapamil and diltiazem, which have intermediate selectivity, also have cardiodepressant properties that may contribute to their blood pressure-lowering actions.

c. **False**. Selective stimulation of imidazoline receptor type I_1 in the ventrolateral medulla is the principle mechanism of action of moxonidine, which lowers blood pressure in hypertension by decreasing sympathetic outflow and increasing vagal outflow.

d. **True** for (i) and (ii); **false** for (iii). Only β-adrenoceptor antagonists having partial agonist activity, e.g. pindolol, produce peripheral vasodilatation by stimulating $β_2$-adrenoceptors in skeletal muscle blood vessels.

e. **True**. Spironolactone blocks the aldosterone receptor, which stimulates the Na^+/K^+-ATPase pump, facilitating uptake of Na^+ into the interstitium from the tubule and, therefore, conserving K^+ and losing Na^+. Amiloride, however, directly blocks the Na^+ channel on the luminal side of the tubule.

f. **False**. Baroreceptor impulses to the vasomotor centre are inhibitory. Increased impulses, therefore, reduce sympathetic outflow, enhance vagal outflow and lower blood pressure.

g. **False**. Prazosin is a selective $α_1$-adrenoceptor antagonist and, therefore, dilates blood vessels. It does not block the presynaptic receptor, which is $α_2$-type, and, therefore, stimulation of this receptor to limit further noradrenaline release can still take place.

h. **True**. Longer-term vasodilation and blood pressure lowering may be because of inhibition of Ca^{2+} entry into vessel cells and synthesis of vasodilator prostaglandins.

i. **True**. ACE breaks down bradykinin, which is found in endothelial cells and is a potent vasodilator.

j. **False**. Minoxidil causes extrusion of K^+ from the cell, which results in the stabilisation of the membrane potential and vasodilatation.

k. **False**. Nitroprusside is converted to cyanide and then to thiocyanate. The toxicity of these limits its use to 3 days.

2. Answer **B**.

   A. **True,** due to the vasodilator actions of the diuretics.

   B. **False.** ACE contributes to bradykinin catabolism and the inhibitor therefore increases bradykinin levels, which results in cough.

C. **True.** Satisfactory lowering of blood pressure can only be achieved with a single drug in about 40% of hypertensives.

D. **True.** The AT_1 receptor is relevant to the vasoconstrictor and aldosterone secretory actions of angiotensin. The AT_2 receptor is involved in vascular growth and is less affected by the receptor antagonists such as losartan.

E. **True.** Nifedipine is less cardiodepressant than verapamil because of its greater arterial selectivity.

3. Case history answers

a. Option **D** (Fig. 6.11)

A. Thiazide diuretics can cause hyperglycaemia and are less suitable for diabetics. Both thiazides and propranolol increase plasma lipids.

B. Furosemide is a less effective hypotensive agent than the thiazides in uncomplicated hypertension but could be useful if there was evidence of renal impairment.

C. The potassium-sparing diuretics are less effective than thiazides in essential hypertension. They should not be used in combination with an ACE inhibitor.

D. A calcium channel antagonist plus atenolol is the most suitable of the choices described. Calcium channel antagonists do not affect lipid levels.

b. ACE inhibitors reduce angiotensin II formation and increase the formation of the vasodilator bradykinin, and improve survival after a myocardial infarction, especially if there is left ventricular impairment. They could be given together with a β-adrenoceptor antagonist, which shows additional benefit if there is left ventricular impairment. Calcium channel antagonists are not of significant benefit regarding long-term outcome when given after a myocardial infarction (Ch. 5). ACE inhibitors appear to protect the kidney in diabetic nephropathy and could be considered in this situation.

Chapter 7

1. a. **True.** In the healthy heart, to maintain cardiac output, contractility rises when there is an increase in afterload, which is, in turn, determined largely by peripheral resistance. In the failing heart, contractility cannot increase, so stroke volume falls.

b. **False.** The plasma osmotic pressure works to move fluid from the interstitium into the vessel, and the hydrostatic pressure in the other direction. Therefore, oedema occurs when the hydrostatic pressure is greater than the plasma osmotic pressure.

c. **False.** In cardiac failure, the baroreceptor reflex sensory input to the vasomotor centre is reduced, resulting in increased sympathetic outflow.

d. **False.** Although digoxin may be of benefit, the mainstay of treatment is diuretics such as furosemide. If diuretics are given concurrently with digoxin, K^+-sparing diuretics may also be required, as hypokalaemia resulting from urinary K^+ loss can increase the risk of digoxin-induced rhythm disturbances.

e. **False.** Potassium ions and digoxin compete for the pump; therefore, high extracellular K^+ inhibits the effect of digoxin, and low K^+ can increase the arrhythmic potential of digoxin.

f. **False.** The effect of low therapeutic doses of digoxin is to stimulate the vagus, sensitise baroreceptor outflow and thereby increase vagal outflow from the vasomotor centre; overall, this increases the refractory period of the atrioventricular node. This is the reason that digoxin is useful in some arrhythmias, such as atrial fibrillation.

g. **True.** Dobutamine acts through stimulation of $β_1$-adrenoceptors, which results in an increase in cAMP and thereby increased cardiac contractility. Desensitisation occurs because of downregulation of the receptors in response to prolonged stimulation by the drug. Desensitisation to milrinone does not occur, because it 'bypasses' the receptor and increases cAMP by preventing its breakdown (phosphodiesterase inhibitors are, however, of limited use).

h. **False.** Dobutamine is a selective $β_1$-adrenoceptor agonist and does not produce vasodilation.

i. **True.** Digoxin is eliminated unchanged by the kidney. Its half-life can be increased markedly in renal failure.

j. **True.** ACE inhibitors decrease angiotensin II and decrease aldosterone output. This results in less reabsorption of Na^+ in the collecting ducts in exchange for K^+ efflux into the tubules, resulting in increased K^+ retention. Spironolactone can produce additional clinical benefit but care must be taken to avoid dangerous hyperkalaemia, with regular monitoring of plasma K^+ concentration.

2. Case history answers

a. The main direct consequences of reduced cardiac output are increased fatigue and reduced muscle perfusion. The body's compensatory mechanisms of activation of the sympathetic nervous system and the renin–angiotensin system try to overcome the low cardiac output.

b. The place of digoxin is well established in heart failure associated with atrial fibrillation and a rapid ventricular rate, but its benefit in heart failure in sinus rhythm remained controversial until recently. However, evidence is now available for the use of small doses of digoxin combined with diuretics and ACE inhibitors when there is severe left ventricular systolic dysfunction and sinus rhythm. Beta-adrenoceptor antagonists used injudiciously may worsen heart failure by reducing cardiac output. Very careful administration of low doses of β-adrenoceptor antagonists can be useful, but only when the heart failure has been stabilised with diuretics and an ACE inhibitor. A β-adrenoceptor agonist such as dobutamine may be of use in symptomatic treatment of acute heart failure but is not usually used in chronic heart failure. The treatment of first choice for chronic heart failure fluid retention is a diuretic.

c. For mild symptoms, a thiazide diuretic may be adequate but in most patients a loop diuretic such as furosemide is used. The loss of renal function in the elderly and renal underperfusion in heart failure means that thiazide diuretics are less effective in older people with this condition.

d. The addition of K^+-sparing diuretics to furosemide or thiazide diuretics is the best way to prevent or treat the hypokalaemia. The adverse metabolic effects of thiazides are of less concern in people with a serious disorder such as heart failure.

e. ACE inhibitors slow the progression of heart failure and improve survival. There is a small risk of severe hypotension following the first dose, and omission of the diuretic immediately prior to this may be helpful.

f. The cough is thought to be caused by increased concentrations of bradykinin, as ACE inhibitors prevent the breakdown of bradykinin by kininase II, which is the same enzyme that converts angiotensin I to angiotensin II. An alternative strategy is to use an angiotension II receptor antagonist such as losartan. These drugs are well tolerated and can improve symptoms, and they reduce morbidity and mortality.

Chapter 8

1. a. **True**. Gradual pacemaker depolarisation in pacemaker cells results from an influx of Na^+ and Ca^{2+}, possibly against a background of slowing K^+ efflux. The maintenance of the resting potential depends heavily on K^+ current.

   b. **False**. Calcium influx also occurs from outside the cell in the plateau phase. The plateau is further stabilised even at rather small levels of

Ca^{2+} influx because the muscle cell membrane extrudes smaller amounts of K^+ from the cells.

c. **False**. Reducing the phase 4 slope certainly diminishes the pacemaker rate of firing, as it takes longer to reach the threshold potential. However, although β-adrenoceptor antagonists and vagal stimulation reduce phase 4 slope, adrenergic stimulation and hypokalaemia in particular increase the slope. This can also occur in cells that do not normally have pacemaker activity. This is part of the explanation for the arrhythmic effects of adrenergic stimulation and hypokalaemia.

d. **False**. Normally this is true, but if the intracellular Ca^{2+} concentration rises (e.g. under the influence of cardiac glycosides, noradrenaline [norepinephrine]), this can exchange with Na^+ passing inwards, causing membrane depolarisations. These are called afterdepolarisations or 'triggered activity'.

e. **False**. Class Ib Na^+ channel blockers (e.g. lidocaine) bind and dissociate rapidly to channels in their activated and refractory state – that is, in phase 0 and 2 – but dissociate from the channel in its resting state. They are, therefore, useful in those ventricular arrhythmias that have a long refractory period and would be particularly beneficial in arrhythmias where the myocardium is influenced by high-frequency excitation. The class Ic Na^+ channel blocking drug flecainide interacts slowly with Na^+ channels and does not show preference for channels in any particular state. It, therefore, causes a general reduction in excitation, blocking both Na^+ and K^+ channels. The class Ia blocking drugs seem to have intermediate actions between these two.

f. **True**. Beta-adrenoceptor antagonists reduce pacemaker depolarisation rate by indirectly (through β-adrenoceptors) blocking Ca^{2+} channels in SA and AV nodal tissue.

g. **True**. Although the type of Ca^{2+} channels utilised in the plateau phase 2 is different from those utilised in the pacemaker depolarisation during phase 4 of the action potential cycle, verapamil will act both to slow the rate of rise of the pacemaker depolarisation and to reduce the plateau phase, thus shortening the action potential. With these effects, verapamil is useful in supraventricular tachycardias but not in ventricular arrhythmias.

h. **False**. Adenosine has no beneficial effect on ventricular arrhythmias. Its main effect involves enhancing K^+ conductance and inhibition of Ca^{2+} influx. The result is reduced AV nodal conduction and an increase in the AV nodal refractory period. Adenosine is useful because it has a high efficacy and a short duration of action.

2. Case history answers

a. The aim at this stage is to restore and maintain sinus rhythm in this patient, who appears to have no structural heart disease. Since the arrhythmia is of short duration, pharmacological cardioversion may be successful. This could be achieved by flecainide, propafenone, sotalol or amiodarone. Amiodarone is usually reserved for patients with significant cardiac dysfunction or those refractory to other agents. Flecainide and propafenone should be avoided in those with significant cardiac dysfunction or concomitant ischaemic heart disease. However, they are probably suitable for this patient. Digoxin, calcium antagonists and β-adrenoceptor antagonists are ineffective for terminating atrial fibrillation. Synchronised DC cardioversion is successful in up to 90% of patients who have no structural heart disease or heart failure, who are aged less than 50 years and whose duration of atrial fibrillation is less than 1 year. It could be considered if drugs are unsuccessful. About 50% of the time, recent-onset atrial fibrillation (less than 48 h duration) spontaneously converts to sinus rhythm. In this man, the atrial fibrillation could have been brought on by excess alcohol (so-called 'holiday heart'). If this patient moderates his alcohol intake, then prophylaxis would not be necessary after a single attack.

b. Anticoagulation with warfarin is essential for at least 3–4 weeks before and 4 weeks after a DC cardioversion, to minimise the risk of a systemic embolus. For prophylaxis against recurrence, antifibrillatory drugs are usually given for 3–6 months following DC cardioversion, since this is the period of highest risk of recurrence. Digoxin, verapamil and β-adrenoceptor antagonists are not effective for prophylaxis. After 5 years of recurrence of atrial fibrillation, sinus rhythm could not be restored. Therefore, the aim in this man is to control ventricular rate. Digoxin suppresses AV nodal conduction and can reduce the ventricular response rate. This is mediated through potentiation of vagal effects on the heart and is less effective during exercise; therefore, the addition of a β-adrenoceptor antagonist or calcium channel antagonist (such as verapamil or diltiazem) may be necessary. However, β-adrenoceptor antagonists (in high doses), verapamil and diltiazem are negatively inotropic and if there is significant cardiac dysfunction or heart failure they are contraindicated. The positive inotropic action of digoxin might be helpful if there is coexisting left ventricular impairment. The major long-term consequence of atrial fibrillation is the risk of thromboembolism and this is greatest in those over 75 years of age.

For Mr GH, aspirin is sufficient as he is at a relatively low risk of stroke because of his age and lack of any coexisting hypertension, diabetes or significant left ventricular impairment.

Chapter 9

1. a. **False**. Aspirin has been shown to reduce the risk of a first embolic stroke in atrial fibrillation.
   b. **True**. The immediate risk of intracranial haemorrhage with t-PA is high and could be compounded by simultaneous administration of antiplatelet or anticoagulant agents. These should be considered later, when the effect of the thrombolytic has waned.
   c. **True**. The excitatory amino acid glutamate can cause a substantial rise in intracellular Ca^{2+}, causing Ca^{2+} overload. This causes cell death by generation of free radicals. However, trials of drugs that interfere with glutamate synthesis or effect have been disappointing.
   d. **False**. Aspirin alone or possibly together with dipyridamole reduces the risk of stroke but warfarin increases mortality and morbidity in patients with recurrent transient ischaemic attacks or strokes.

2. Answer **E**.
   A. **False.** Alzheimer's disease is associated with a lack of cholinergic transmission and an overactivity of glutaminergic transmission.
   B. **False.** NICE advises that the antcholinesterases should not be prescribed if the MMSE is below 12.
   C. **False.** Memantine inhibits the glutamate NMDA receptor.
   D. **False.** They can be useful co-prescribed.
   E. **True.**

3. Case history answers

a. There is no standard treatment for acute stroke. Although thrombolysis has been shown in some trials to be useful in the treatment of stroke, safe and effective use is determined by a rigid set of criteria as there is a significant risk of intracranial haemorrhage. Thrombolysis is inappropriate in this situation. His blood pressure is high and it is a considerable time since the onset of symptoms. Thrombolysis has been approved for use within 3 h of the onset of symptoms. The rapid resolution of signs indicates a TIA, for which thrombolysis is not given.

b. His blood pressure must be brought under control. Reduction in blood pressure has a major effect on the prevention of a recurrent stroke. He should be started on a low dose of aspirin.

c. Antiplatelet therapy should be continued. The antiplatelet drug dipyridamole may show some added benefit when given with aspirin and can be used if patients continue to have TIAs despite treatment with aspirin; definitive evidence of this is awaited from ongoing trials. Cholesterol reduction with statin is effective in secondary prevention of ischaemic stroke. However, an important reason for cholesterol reduction in this situation is prevention of ischaemic cardiac events, since coronary artery disease often coexists with atheromatous cerebrovascular disease. It may be worth treating this patient with a statin even if his cholesterol is not raised.

Chapter 10

1. a. **False**. There is a two- to fourfold increase in risk of developing coronary disease, stroke or heart failure compared with age-matched subjects who do not have intermittent claudication.

   b. **True**. By reducing cholesterol synthesis, simvastatin increases hepatic LDL receptors, which results in reduced LDL cholesterol in blood and a small accompanying increase in high density lipoprotein (HDL) cholesterol. The main potential benefit of lowered LDL cholesterol in these patients is a reduction in coronary artery disease events.

   c. **False**. Verapamil is ineffective in the treatment of Raynaud's phenomenon and the agent of choice is nifedipine.

2. Answer **A**.

   A. **True**. Cilostazol inhibits phosphodiesterase type III in vascular smooth muscle cells and in platelets, increasing the levels of cAMP.

   B. **False**. Unlike the other phosphodiesterase III inhibitors such as milrinone, cilostazol does not increase the incidence of arrhythmias. However, it is not recommended that cilostazol is used in patients with congestive heart failure.

   C. **False**. Cilostazol is extensively metabolised by CYP3A4 and CYP2C19 isoenzymes in the liver.

   D. **False**. Cilostazol inhibits platelet aggregation.

   E. **False**. Cilostazol increases plasma HDL cholesterol.

3. Case history answers

   a.
      i. The potential benefit of propranolol in lowering blood pressure is outweighed by blockade of β_2-adrenoceptors in the limb blood vessels, impairing vasodilation.

      ii. Cardioselective β-adrenoceptor antagonists such as atenolol do not cause deterioration in walking distance when used alone.

      iii. Vasodilators will lower blood pressure but do not improve walking distance. In some patients, they may redirect blood from the maximally dilated ischaemic tissues to healthy tissues (vascular steal). This can be particularly troublesome in critical limb ischaemia, or when the cardiac output is also reduced by concurrent use of a β-adrenoceptor antagonist.

      iv. Lowering LDL cholesterol can stabilise atherosclerotic plaques, perhaps reducing the consequences of coexistent heart disease; it is not known if walking distance or limb survival is improved.

      v. Low-dose aspirin inhibits platelet aggregation and reduces future cardiac events, which are common in this group of patients.

      vi. Cilostazol can increase walking distance by up to 35%.

   b. Intensive management of blood pressure, control of diabetes and antiplatelet therapy will reduce the risk of cardiac events. An exercise programme can improve walking distance. Smoking is a major contributory factor to impaired walking distance and cardiac events.

   c. Excessive warming of limbs may dilate normal arteries, 'stealing' blood from diseased tissues.

Chapter 11

1. a. **False**. Streptokinase is usually infused for 1 h and rt-PA for 3 h. rt-PA has a short duration of action but streptokinase has a longer half-life, permitting a shorter infusion time.

   b. **True**. Warfarin can cause fetal abnormalities and, unless essential, should not be given in early pregnancy.

   c. **False**. Clopidogrel prevents platelet aggregation induced by the release of ADP after platelet activation. Clopidogrel also inhibits thrombin-induced platelet aggregation.

   d. **True**. The increased expression of GPIIb/IIIa receptors on platelets is essential for aggregation as fibrinogen links adjacent platelets by binding to GPIIb/IIIa receptors, thereby initiating aggregation.

   e. **True**. Thromboxane A_2 (TXA$_2$) required for platelet aggregation is synthesised by the cyclo-oxygenase type 1 (COX 1) enzyme, whereas prostaglandins synthesised during inflammation are synthesised predominantly, but not exclusively, by cyclo-oxygenase type 2 (COX 2) enzymes. Aspirin is 160 times more active at inhibiting COX-1 than COX-2. Therefore, at the low doses required to inhibit TXA_2 synthesis, it has no anti-inflammatory effect.

f. **False**. Vitamin K is produced by gut bacteria. Alteration of gut flora by broad-spectrum antibacterials will reduce vitamin K formation and hence clotting factors. This will enhance the activity of warfarin.

g. **False**. Tranexamic acid inhibits plasminogen activation, reducing fibrin degradation and the risk of bleeding.

h. **False**. The action of unfractionated heparin but not LMWH can be reversed by the strongly basic protein protamine, which rapidly binds to it, forming an inactive compound.

2. Answer **C**.

A. **False**. Warfarin is less predictable and regular INR monitoring is required.

B. **False**. Heparin is inactive orally and must be given by intravenous or subcutaneous routes.

C. **True**. Warfarin but not ximelagatran is metabolised by liver cytochrome P450 metabolising isoenzymes. Omeprazole inhibits these isoenzymes.

D. **False**. Warfarin can be reversed with vitamin K_1 but there is no known antagonist (yet!) of ximelagatran.

E. **False**. Broad-spectrum antibacterials may suppress the production of vitamin K by gut bacteria and increase the activity of warfarin. This would not affect the activity of ximelagatran.

3. Case history answers

a. Postoperative venous thromboembolism occurs in 40–50% of people who undergo hip replacement, and fatal pulmonary embolism in 1–5%, if prophylactic anticoagulant therapy is not given. This woman is also at increased risk because of obesity.

b. This is controversial. Initiating prophylaxis postoperatively allows more effective haemostatic control during and immediately postsurgery and does not reduce the effectiveness of treatment.

c. Heparin is not active orally. The onset of action of heparin is rapid, whereas warfarin takes several days for full effectiveness but can be given orally. Heparin would, therefore, be chosen if started pre- or postoperatively.

d. The woman was obese, a risk factor for postoperative venous thrombosis. Daily self-administered subcutaneous prophylaxis with LMWH could be used. LMWH has a better bioavailability, a longer half-life and lower risk of producing thrombocytopenia. Unlike unfractionated heparin, its effect is predictable.

Chapter 12

1. a. **True**. This is particularly important and the T helper type 2 cells are involved in the generation of cytokines that promote activation of eosinophils and expression of IgE receptors on mast cells and eosinophils. The T helper type 2 cells also express endothelial adhesion molecules that attract eosinophils.

b. **False**. Leukotriene C_4 is a bronchoconstrictor, increasing mucus secretion and oedema.

2. **True**. Salbutamol is effective taken before exercise but the longer acting β_2-adrenoceptor agonists are slower in onset. Cromoglicate taken prophylactically may also be effective.

3. **False**. Hyper-reactivity of airways is seen but epithelial cells show variable damage.

4. **True**. There is evidence of tolerance to β_2-adrenoceptor agonists, which can be reduced by administration of corticosteroids.

5. a. **True**. Erythromycin and ciprofloxin inhibit liver cytochrome P450 enzymes, which metabolise theophylline.

b. **False**. The methylxanthines (present in coffee) increase alertness and can cause irritability and headache.

c. **True**. All methylxanthines have positive inotropic and chronotropic activity and a narrow therapeutic index.

6. a. **False**. Ipratropium is less effective against allergen challenge but can be useful as an adjunct and in the management of COPD.

b. **False**. Ipratropium can cause a modest tachycardia owing to blockade of muscarinic receptors in the heart.

c. **True**. Ipratropium has a quaternary structure and, therefore, is poorly absorbed.

7. a. **False**. Montelukast inhibits receptors for the cysteinyl leukotrienes (C_4, D_4, E_4).

b. **True**. The leukotriene antagonists need to be administered orally on a regular prophylactic basis to reduce asthmatic attacks. They are much less effective once an attack has started.

8. a. **True**. Glucocorticoids affect several steps in the inflammatory pathways involved in the genesis of asthma.

9. Extended-matching answers.

1. Answer **F**. This patient is being treated according

to the British Thoracic Society Guidelines. An appropriate add-on medication that has been added to the guidelines recently for use in life-threatening situations is intravenous magnesium sulphate.

2. Answer **D**. This patient should additionally be advised to use a spacer with all inhaled drugs. This improves the effectiveness of the medication and will reduce deposition of steroids in the mouth and oropharynx, reducing the occurrence of fungal growth and hoarseness.

3. Answer **A**. The antimuscarinic drug ipratopium provides equal or greater benefit to β_2-adrenergic receptor agonists in COPD and will reduce the volume of sputum produced. Corticosteroids are of modest benefit in only a small percentage of patients with COPD.

4. Answer **B**. This patient has a infection-related exacerbation of her COPD and should be treated with an appropriate antibiotic. Nebulised salbutamol and ipratropium should also be started.

5. Answer **C**. Approximately 80% of severe asthmatic attacks occur between midnight and 8 a.m. Salbutamol is a shorter-acting β_2-adrenergic receptor agonist, providing relief for 2–6 hours. A trial of salmeterol or formoterol, which are long-acting β_2-adrenergic receptor agonists providing brochodilation for 12 h or longer, could be tried. It is not recommended that the long-acting drugs are used for routine relief of acute asthmatic episodes.

10. Extended-matching answers

    1. Answer **D**. Salbutamol acts selectively on the β_2-adrenergic receptors in airways, which are coupled to G-protein-linked receptors, and its bronchdilator action results from the cellular events following the increase in cAMP.
    2. Answer **A**. theophylline inhibits the breakdown of cAMP by phosphodiesterases.
    3. Answer **F**. Aspirin can induce bronchoconstriction in a subset of sensitive asthmatics (as many as one in five). This results from inhibition of COX-1-generated prostaglandin E_2, which normally inhibits the formation of the bronchconstrictor leukotriene C_4/D_4. Celecoxib, which is a selective COX-2-inhibiting NSAID, does not have this effect, but should still be used with care in asthmatics.
    4. Answer **E**. Montelukast selectively inhibits receptors for the bronchoconstrictor cysteinyl leukotrienes $C_4/D_4/E_4$.
    5. Answer **C**. Prostaglandin $F_{2\alpha}$ is a bronchoconstrictor and asthmatics are more sensitive to its action.

Chapter 13

1. a. **True**. Diphenhydramine and chlorpheniramine are common constituents of compound cough mixtures.
   b. **True.** Dextromethorphan has the same cough-suppressant potency as codeine but is not analgesic.

2. a. **False**. Surfactant acts like a detergent and lowers the surface tension, enabling the alveoli to expand and retain an expanded shape.
   b. **False**. Doxapram is used in hospitals for postoperative respiratory failure. It stimulates the respiratory centre and the carotid chemoreceptors but its precise mode of action is unknown.
   c. **False**. Mecysteine breaks the disulphide cross bridges that maintain the polymeric gel-like structure of mucus.

3. Answer **B**.

   A. **False.** Inhibitors of the angiotensin II receptor do not cause cough. Inhibition of angiotensin-converting enzyme (ACE) which reduces the formation of angiotensin II also prevents the breakdown of bradykinin and this increases coughing. ACE inhibitors may also increase substance P and thromboxane, which are implicated in cough.
   B. **True.** Guaifenesin is included in many cough remedies and is particularly useful in the treatment of dry cough.
   C. **False.** Opioids vary widely in their abilities to suppress cough.
   D. **False.** Dextromethorphan has none of the analgesic, sedative, or respiratory depressive properties associated with the opioids.
   E. **False.** The Cochrane database states that there is no good evidence that antitussives are useful in acute cough.

Chapter 14

1. **False**. Much of the K^+ filtered at the glomerulus is reabsorbed in the proximal tubule and in the loop of Henle. Secretory loss into the urine is mainly in exchange for Na^+, occurring through specialised K^+ channels in the collecting ducts.

2. **True**. Impermeability to water and an active $Na^+/Cl^-/K^+$ cotransporter in the thick ascending limb are pertinent to the generation of the hyperosmotic interstitium and the counter-current mechanisms for concentrating urine.

3. **True**. These regions are permeable to water, where an osmotic effect can be exerted.

4. **True**. As a result of extracting water from intracellular compartments and expanding extracellular and intravascular fluid volume, they can precipitate pulmonary oedema.

5. **True**. Acetazolamide results in a mild metabolic acidosis and a reduced plasma HCO_3^- concentration which limits the H^+/Na^+ exchange at the luminal membrane.

6. **False**. By inhibiting the $Na^+/K^+/Cl^-$ cotransporter, the medullary interstitial hypertonicity falls. Because this hypertonicity provides the osmotic force for the absorption of water in the collecting ducts (in the presence of antidiuretic hormone, vasopressin), the reduced osmotic pressure results in less water reabsorption. Loop diuretics are highly protein bound and little is filtered at the glomerulus. The drugs reach the luminal membrane cotransporter by secretion into the proximal tubule via the organic acid transport mechanism.

7. a. **True**. Loop diuretics are widely used in the control of oedema in heart failure for the elimination of the excessive salt and water load. The direct venodilator activity of furosemide reduces central blood volume.
   b. **False**. A thiazide diuretic or metolazone can be added to a loop diuretic to act sequentially at different sites in the nephron, thus producing a marked diuresis and natriuresis.
   c. **False**. Delivery of greater concentrations of Na^+ to the collecting ducts increases the exchange for K^+ at that site, thus increasing K^+ loss.
   d. **False**. Once the cotransporter mechanism is maximally inhibited, no further water or salt excretion can occur
   e. **True**. When high doses are used, especially in the presence of renal damage, or when taken with an aminoglycoside antibiotic, ototoxicity can occur.

8. a. **False**. Like the loop diuretics, the thiazides have to act from the renal tubular lumen on the co-transporter that is on the luminal membrane. The thiazides are secreted by the proximal tubule transport mechanism into the lumen.
   b. **False**. The thiazide diuretics do not increase Ca^{2+} excretion, unlike the loop diuretics, which do cause urinary loss of Ca^{2+}.
   c. **True**. Metolazone is more potent than other thiazide diuretics and when given together with furosemide produces an intense diuresis. Its greater effect is possibly a result of additional actions in the proximal tubule. Unlike other thiazide diuretics, it also works in advanced renal failure.
   d. **True**. Thiazide diuretics could exacerbate diabetes mellitus. The mechanism may be through inhibition of insulin synthesis.

9. a. **False**. Although both drugs ultimately reduce activity of the Na^+ reuptake channel, amiloride blocks the channel directly, whereas spironolactone prevents the actions of aldosterone-induced proteins, which enhance the Na^+ channel numbers and activity.
   b. **True**. ACE inhibitors, by inhibiting aldosterone secretion, will increase K^+ concentration in the interstitium and blood by reducing K^+ excretion. Hyperkalaemia may result

10. a. **False**. Because the diuretics act at different sites, an additional natriuresis is produced.
    b. **False**. Canrenone is an active diuretic, responsible for most of the effects of spironolactone.

11. **True**. Some diuretics may act partly by the generation of prostaglandins. In addition, prostaglandins help to maintain renal blood flow. Therefore, NSAIDs can reduce diuretic activity.

12. Extended-matching answers

    1. Answer **A**. Amiloride is a K^+-sparing diuretic. Lisinopril can also increase plasma K^+ concentrations by increasing the levels of aldosterone. The raised K^+ levels may have been the cause of the severe bradycardia.
    2. Answer **C**. One component of the antihypertensive action of bendroflumethiazide is via prostaglandins, which promote sodium excretion by the kidney and cause vasodilation. Because NSAIDs such as naproxen will prevent prostaglandin formation by inhibiting cyclo-oxygenase, their administration will diminish the antihypertensive actions of bendroflumethizide at the vascular and renal levels.
    3. Answer **E**. Thiazide-like diuretics can worsen insulin resistance, resulting in increased glucose levels.
    4. Answer **B**. The loop diuretic may cause hypokalaemia. This enhances the toxicity of digoxin, resulting in arrhythmia.

Chapter 15

1. a. **False**. Atropine blocks muscarinic receptors, inhibiting the parasympathetic effects on the detrusor muscle. This results in urinary retention.

b. **True**. The tricyclics act to reduce detrusor instability, in part by their antimuscarinic actions.

c. **False**. Distigmine contracts detrusor muscle, which is undesirable in the presence of urinary outflow obstruction.

2. Case history answers

a. Drugs may be used in mild disease and while awaiting a transurethral resection of the prostate. Selective α_1-adrenoceptor antagonists increase urine flow to a limited extent but also decrease urgency, frequency and hesitancy. Antagonists selective for α_{1A}-adrenoceptors, such as tamsulosin, are claimed to have fewer unwanted effects. Finasteride, which inhibits conversion of testosterone to dihydrotestosterone, reduces prostate size slowly.

b. α_1-Adrenoceptor antagonists can cause postural hypotension, especially with the first dose. They cause dizziness and can interact with other drugs to lower blood pressure. Finasteride can reduce libido and cause impotence.

c. The outcome is variable; symptoms may not worsen appreciably for many years but moderate symptoms can lead to a poor quality of life. Complications include urinary retention, incontinence and renal insufficiency owing to hydronephrosis.

3. Extended-matching answers

1. Answer **B**. Finasteride inhibits the conversion of testosterone to dihydrotestosterone, which is a promoter of prostatic cell growth. Reduction in up to 30% of the prostate size can be obtained.

2. Answer **D**. Amitryptiline is an inhibitor of muscarinic receptors and inhibits the micturition reflex.

3. Answer **F**. Oxybutynin is a muscarinic receptor antagonist and inhibits the micturition reflex. Amitryptiline may be of use but has greater unwanted effects.

Chapter 16

1. a. **True**. Nitrates result in increased nitric oxide production and elevate cGMP. Sildenafil has a similar effect by preventing cGMP breakdown. This can lead to additive unwanted effects, particularly hypotension.

b. **False**. These two drugs can act together to cause hypotension.

c. **False**. Phosphodiesterase type V is found in other blood vessels and tissues, which can result in unwanted effects when sildenafil is given.

d. **False**. Parasympathetic stimulation enhances erection. Drugs known to inhibit the parasympathetic outflow, e.g. tricyclic antidepressants, can cause erectile failure.

e. **True**. Painful priapism with erections lasting many hours can occur.

f. **False**. Testosterone can be useful if the impotence is due to hypogonadism.

g. **True**. Probably through vascular dysfunction.

h. **False**. Although both are mainly metabolised in the liver, tadalafil has a much longer biological half-life than sildenafil.

i. **False**. Sildenafil inhibits the breakdown of cGMP.

2. Case history answers

a. The following points should be noted.

- The contribution of psychological factors in his erectile dysfunction need to be assessed and dealt with if they are present.
- Vascular disease, smoking and his level of alcohol consumption may all contribute to the erectile dysfunction, and Mr JA should be helped to manage these.
- Because of the evidence of coronary artery disease, it would be advisable to be more aggressive in treating his blood pressure and reducing his cholesterol levels. Although lowering his blood pressure and cholesterol alone are unlikely to restore the erectile function, they may improve the patient's wellbeing and have a psychological benefit. Coronary artery disease is a known indicator of erectile dysfunction.
- Beta-adrenergic blocking drugs and thiazide diuretics can contribute to erectile problems, and Mr JA could be changed to enalapril, which has not been shown to contribute to impotence.

b. Cimetidine is an inhibitor of the liver P450 isoenzymes that break down sildenafil. The initial dose of sildenafil should be reduced. Alternatively, Mr JA could use ranitidine, which does not inhibit the liver enzymes. Studies of sildenafil in patients with a history of cardiovascular disease have shown that sildenafil is safe but the use of nitrates is an absolute contraindication. Mr JA should be told about the possibilities of drug interactions and possible side-effects.

Chapter 17

1. a. **True**. It was thought for many years that there are not distinctive receptors at which general anaesthetics act, but rather they produce more general effects on constituents of the cell membrane such as lipids or proteins. However, it

is now considered that they have actions at a number of excitatory and inhibitory receptors.

b. **False**. Many inhalational anaesthetics are volatile liquids.

c. **False**. The main inhalational anaesthetics are halogenated compounds.

2. a. **False**. It causes cardiac arrhythmias, hepatotoxicity with repeated use, and hypotension. It also sensitises the heart to catecholamine. It is, however, a potent anaesthetic.

b. **True**. This is particularly true with highly lipid-soluble agents, which will accumulate in body fat stores and be slowly released after the operation.

c. **False**. Even at concentrations higher than 50%, nitrous oxide is not potent enough to produce effective surgical anaesthesia on its own.

d. **True**. Nitrous oxide and oxygen are used concurrently with fluorinated anaesthetics. The other attribute of nitrous oxide is that, unlike fluorinated compounds, it has analgesic activity.

3. **False**. Halothane undergoes substantial metabolism, but the other halogenated anaesthetics do not.

4. a. **False**. The half-life of the rapid distribution phase of thiopental is only about 3 min, hence its short duration of action. However, the elimination of thiopental from the body is much slower and the half-life is approximately 12 h. This partially accounts for the hangover effect seen with this drug.

b. **True**. Propofol is useful for short operations, where it has rapid elimination and little hangover effect. The hepatic clearance of propofol has a half-life of 1–2 h. It can also be given by continuous infusion in intensive care units.

c. **True**. Either extravascular injections of thiopental or intra-arterial injections can have damaging consequences, because its pH is approximately 9–10.

d. **False**. Ketamine does have analgesic action, unlike other available intravenous anaesthetics. It can be useful when pain is difficult to control.

5. **False**. Fentanyl is increasingly given for intra-operative analgesia. It is short acting and with rapid recovery; consequently, it has a low incidence of hangover effects.

6. a. **True**. This was true when slow-acting anaesthetics were given, but it is less problematic with rapidly acting inhalational anaesthetics.

b. **True**. Most are negatively inotropic and they depress myocardial function by interfering with Ca^{2+} fluxes. Halothane also sensitises the heart to catecholamines and can lead to arrhythmias.

c. **True**. Inhalational anaesthetics reduce the ventilatory response to carbon dioxide and hypoxia and increase the arterial partial pressure of carbon dioxide.

d. **True**. Sevoflurane is rapid in onset and also is more rapidly eliminated than halothane or isoflurane.

7. Answer **C**.

A. The MAC of nitrous oxide required for anaesthesia if given alone would be greater than 100%!

B. The major route of elimination is via the airways.

C. Unlike other intravenous anaesthetics, ketamine is analgesic.

D. Fentanyl is often used as an analgesic given together with many inhalational anaesthetics.

E. With modern anaesthetic practice, atropine is seldom given to dry bronchial and salivary secretions.

8. Case history answers.

a. Atropine or hyoscine block muscarinic receptors, blocking bronchial and salivary secretions. Modern anaesthetics have less irritant effect, thus reducing this problem. Muscarinic antagonists can reduce the bradycardia caused by some inhalation anaesthetics and suxamethonium.

b. Atropine can cause CNS excitation, whereas hyoscine causes sedation and has antiemetic properties.

c. Relatively minor but frequent complications occur with suxamethonium including bradycardia, postoperative myalgia, transient elevation of the plasma K^+ concentrations and raised intraocular, intracranial and intragastric pressures. A rare, but potentially fatal, complication is malignant hyperthermia, which is genetically determined. The short-acting non-depolarising blocking drug rocuronium has a short duration of action and does not cause these problems.

d. Pancuronium is probably not the ideal muscle relaxant to use. It does not cause histamine release, but it can cause tachycardia and hypertension and is long-acting (Ch. 27). An alternative would be vecuronium, which has an intermediate duration of action, does not release histamine and lacks cardiovascular effects. The short-acting rocuronium is more expensive but has rapid onset and short duration of action and a low risk of cardiovascular effects.

e. Opioid-induced apnoea. The use of pethidine followed by fentanyl may be generous for a short operation, resulting in respiratory depression. The patient could be treated by the administration of naloxone. The dose of neostigmine given may have been insufficient to reverse the competitive blocking effect of the long-acting pancuronium. The patient could have a genetically determined deficiency of pseudocholinesterase (plasma cholinesterase), which metabolises suxamethonium. This is present in about 1 in 2000 individuals. If respiratory depression is caused by suxamethonium (succinylcholine), administration of neostigmine would make it worse. Fresh frozen plasma containing pseudocholinesterase could be administered.

   f. Although mivacurium is a short-acting muscle relaxant, it is metabolised by pseudocholinesterase and its effect would be prolonged if there is a reduced level of this metabolising enzyme.

   g. Neostigmine inhibits acetylcholinesterase. It partially or fully reverses the actions of competitive neuromuscular blocking drugs acting at N_2 receptors at skeletal muscle but also enhances the activity of acetylcholine at muscarinic receptors, causing bradycardia and respiratory bronchoconstriction. Glycopyrronium selectivity blocks muscarinic receptors, thus reducing excess muscarinic stimulation.

Chapter 18

1. **a.** **False**. If absorbed, systemic high doses of local anaesthetics can produce cardiovascular collapse and CNS depression.

   b. **False**. Initial decline in local activity is due to removal into the systemic circulation. The anaesthetic is then metabolised.

   c. **True**.

   d. **False**. Prazosin is a vasodilator and would increase the removal of the local anaesthetic from its injection site: adrenaline (epinephrine) or other local vasoconstrictors are necessary.

2. **a.** **True**. It is a long-acting local anaesthetic similar to bupivacaine but may be less arrhythmogenic.

   b. **False**. Ropivacaine (levobupivacaine) is marketed and shows lower cardiotoxicity than the racemic bupivacaine.

3. Answer **A**.

   A. Most local anaesthetics are weak bases, pKa 7–9. Raising the pH will increase the relative amount of the non-ionised species and will therefore enhance lipid solubility and membrane penetration. (Increased pH may, however, reduce the water solubility of the drug in solution.)

   B. Uptake into the systemic circulation is the most important primary determinant in terminating their action **and** producing toxicity. Following

most regional anaesthetic procedures, maximum arterial plasma concentrations of anaesthetic develop within about 10 to 25 min. Avoidance of intravascular administration is essential.

   C. Altered local pH could change the ratio of cationic to non-ionised species of the local anaesthetic, affecting its potential to penetrate membranes and block Na^+ channels.

   D. With the exception of cocaine, local anaesthetics dilate blood vessels, hastening their removal from the site of injection.

   E. Adrenaline (epinephrine) should not given with a local anaesthetic injection in digits and appendages, because of the risk of ischaemic necrosis.

4. Extended-matching answers

   1. Answer **A**. Cocaine can be administered topically and, unlike other local anaesthetics, inhibits the reuptake of released noradrenaline, resulting in vasoconstriction.

   2. Answer **B**. Adrenaline (epinephrine) causes vasoconstriction and the administered local anaesthetic resides at its site of injection for a longer period.

   3. Answer **D**. Tetracaine is poorly absorbed and is used topically for conjunctival anaesthesia.

   4. Answer **E**. Lidocaine can be given intravenously for the treatment of ventricular arrhythmias.

Chapter 19

1. **a.** **True**. In patients with pain, analgesia is often associated with wellbeing (μ-receptors), whereas in pain-free patients, dysphoria can occur (κ-receptors).

   b. **False**. Tolerance to miosis and the constipatory effects of opioids develops much less than to the other biological effects, including analgesia and respiratory depression. Cross-tolerance to opioids is common.

   c. **False**. Because of its long half-life and less potential to cause euphoria, it is used in controlled withdrawal in patients with opioid dependence. It is orally well absorbed and has a slow onset of action. Patients exhibit slower and less intense withdrawal symptoms with methadone.

2. **a.** **True**. Because the opioid μ-opioid receptors subserve analgesia and the κ-receptors are involved in respiratory depression, it is claimed that meptazinol has less respiratory depressant action.

b. **False**. Naloxone is short-acting opioid antagonist acting at μ-, κ- and δ-receptors. It is used in opioid overdosage. Severe withdrawal symptoms can occur in addicts following naloxone administration.

3. a. **True**. Tricyclic antidepressants can be effective for the treatment of pain of neuropathic origin. They may act by enhancing amine levels in the descending inhibitory pathways that control the pain gate mechanism (see Fig. 19.3, p. 256).
   b. **False**. Phenytoin, carbamazepine and sodium valproate are useful analgesics in neuropathic pain, probably by stabilising neuronal membranes and inhibiting neurotransmitter release.

4. **True**. Because it is a partial agonist, it can actually reduce the effects of morphine.

5. Answer **D**.

   A. Constipation continues to be a problem with long-term morphine treatment, and laxatives are often required
   B. Chronic pain is usually less responsive to opioids, and non-opioid treatments (e.g. anticonvulsants) may be required.
   C. Naloxone is an antagonist used to treat opioid overdosage.
   D. This is correct. Miosis is one of the signs of opioid abuse.
   E. Fentanyl is not suitable. Methadone can be used as a substitute in the detoxification process.

6. Case history answers

   a. Morphine acts at specific opioid receptors at spinal and supraspinal sites to produce analgesia and unwanted effects. Morphine is a strong agonist at all μ-receptors that subserve analgesia, euphoria, respiratory depression and dependence.
   b. Morphine oral solution is used to control short-term breakthrough exacerbations of pain on a patient-initiated basis. Repeated use of this form of morphine should signal a reassessment of the dose of the long-acting morphine. When the patient is unable to take oral medication because of weakness or vomiting, rectal or continuous subcutaneous infusion may be required (see d). Normally, 80% of patients require less than 200 mg per day to control severe pain. With terminally ill patients having persistent severe pain, the dose is gradually increased over a period of 1–2 weeks until an appropriate level of control is achieved. The maximum level may be as high as 2–3 g per day. Unwanted effects can occur; therefore, close monitoring is needed when treatment is first initiated or dosage altered.

   c. For reasons that are not easily explained from a theoretical viewpoint, addiction seldom occurs in patients with a high degree of pain. Possible reasons may be a high natural opioid level or high catecholamine levels.
   d. Diamorphine can be used instead of morphine. It is more potent, but is no more efficacious. Its major advantage in practice is its high solubility, which reduces the volume of intramuscular injections or continuous subcutaneous infusion if these are required. Infrequently, an unusual response to morphine may require its replacement by other opioids. Fentanyl is a suitable replacement delivered via a transdermal patch and having fewer unwanted effects.
   e. Diclofenac is an aspirin-like NSAID often used in the treatment of arthritic conditions. Unlike opioids, it has both analgesic and anti-inflammatory actions. NSAIDs appear to have only a small central component to their actions.
   f. The pain from metastases is compounded by local inflammation: in this case, the bone metastases cause 'inflammatory pain', which may be reduced by diclofenac, thereby reducing the requirement for morphine.
   g. Inflammation increases local pressure (and hence pain) within the bone; dexamethasone is a potent corticosteroid, reducing inflammation and swelling.
   h. Nausea is an unwanted effect caused by morphine, occurring particularly during the first week of administration, but may also be a consequence of the cancer itself or related complications such as hypercalcaemia. Tolerance to the nausea induced by morphine occurs.
   i. Metoclopramide is a dopamine antagonist that acts on the chemoreceptor trigger zone (CTZ) to reduce chemical and radiation-induced nausea.
   j. A centrally acting antiemetic such as prochlorperazine can be used. They have the same mechanism of action as metoclopramide.
   k. Gastric and/or duodenal inflammation (which may cause considerable discomfort) or even ulceration may occur with prolonged use of diclofenac and a corticosteroid. Cimetidine in this patient relieved the gastric discomfort associated with oral administration of diclofenac.
   l. Cimetidine is a histamine H_2 receptor antagonist. Note, cimetidine inhibits the enzymes that convert codeine into morphine and may reduce its analgesic effect. (Diclofenac is available in a combined formulation with the prostaglandin analogue misoprostil, which has gastroprotective activity.)

m. Constipation is a feature of morphine therapy. Tolerance does not develop to opioid-induced constipation. Peristalsis is reduced, while the tone of the intestinal muscle is increased.

n. Docusate sodium has some faecal-softening properties and is a stimulant of intestinal smooth muscle, which restores peristalsis.

o. In practice, terminally ill patients are often given danthron, in combination with either docusate sodium (co-danthrusate) or poloxamer (co-danthramer). Danthron is a stimulant drug and stool softener and is particularly useful when 'bowel movements must be by strain'. The irritant properties of danthron and its carcinogenic potential restrict its general use. The alternatives in use include senna preparations (stimulants) and magnesium sulphate (a bulk purgative). Other agents do exist, but cost is a prime factor when cheap agents are as effective as their more expensive counterparts.

p. Temazepam is a short-acting benzodiazepine used to aid sleeping.

Note. Pain control must also take note of the psychological, social and spiritual condition of the patient. At all times, if pain control is inadequate, adjuvant treatments such as radiotherapy or transcutaneous electrical nerve stimulation should be considered. Where neuropathic pain is evident, tricyclic antidepressants or anticonvulsants should also be considered.

Chapter 20

1. a. **False**. Dependence, tolerance and withdrawal symptoms occur on long-term continuous usage.
   b. **True**. Additional CNS depression can occur.

2. a. **True**. Benzodiazepines are metabolised largely by the liver and rate of metabolism is reduced in the elderly; the elderly are also more sensitive to the effects of the drugs.
   b. **False**. Buspirone is not a benzodiazepine and has less sedative action than temazepam.

3. **False**. Benzodiazepines affect the structure of sleep, with loss of REM sleep. Zolpidem has less effect than some other benzodiazepines.

4. Answer **E**.
   A. An alternative hypnotic is unlikely to work and switching between hypnotics is not good practice.
   B. With long-acting benzodiazepines, withdrawal symptoms may take up to 3 weeks to appear.

C. Barbiturates are contraindicated as hypnotics because of unwanted effects, tolerance and dependance liability.

D. Buspirone acts at the $5HT_{1A}$ receptor. It is used in general anxiety disorders and is not sedative.

E. Benzodiazepines potentiate the entry of Cl^- through the receptor-operated channel which is part of the $GABA_A$ receptor.

5. Case history answers

a. Mrs FL's insomnia and anxiety are a response to bereavement and might present fewer long-term problems than chronic 'endogenous' anxiety. Benzodiazepines and the newer hypnotics are much safer as hypnotics than their predecessors (barbiturates and phenothiazines). Nevertheless, the central concept in benzodiazepine therapy is to use the minimal effective dose for the shortest possible period. A short-acting benzodiazepine (e.g. temazepam) taken at night should help to restore her sleep pattern and help Mrs FL cope with pressures at work. The relatively short half-life of temazepam (5–10 h) should minimise risk of sedation during the working day. However, if the daytime anxiety also warrants treatment, the long-acting diazepam given at night may be the drug to choose. The anxiolytic buspirone is not sedative but is ineffective against panic attacks. Short or intermittent courses of treatment only should be given.

b. Benzodiazepines are $GABA_A$ agonists that enhance $GABA_A$-mediated inhibition of neuronal activity in the brain and spinal cord. Benzodiazepines bind to $GABA_A$ receptors at a site separate from GABA itself and increase frequency of GABA-induced channel opening, causing Cl^- entry into the cell and neuronal hyperpolarisation. Benzodiazepines are *relatively* free of serious unwanted effects if used correctly (e.g. compared with barbiturates) and are safe in overdose, but sedation and psychomotor impairment may interfere markedly with driving and operating machinery (worsened by interaction with alcohol, barbiturates, and older sedative antihistamines). Rebound wakefulness may occur in the morning. Other unwanted effects include headache, dry mouth, hypotension, anterograde amnesia, skin rashes and blood dyscrasias. Psychotic reactions (hallucinations) have been reported with triazolam.

c. Rebound wakefulness may indicate a need for a longer-acting benzodiazepine such as nitrazepam or diazepam, which may also help to reduce Mrs FL's daytime anxiety and panic attacks. Conversely, daytime sedation may interfere with driving and work, exacerbated by long-acting metabolites of these drugs. An alternative may be to prescribe buspirone; however, this requires

1–2 weeks for a response. Switching to a newer hypnotic such as zolpidem is unlikely to make a difference (see NICE guidelines).

d. Long-term use of a benzodiazepine is associated with dependence, manifested mainly as a withdrawal reaction, which may include rebound anxiety, tremor, nausea, irritability, anorexia and dysphoria. Together with rapid development of tolerance (especially to hypnotic action), these contraindicate benzodiazepine treatment for more than 3 weeks. In the longer term, a course of antidepressants may be indicated. Mrs FL's recovery from bereavement may be aided by psychological counselling and support from family and employer.

6. Extended-matching answers

1. Answer **A**. Withdrawal from long courses of benzodiazepines is difficult. She is liable to show withdawal symptoms or return of the original complaints that determined the original prescription. Psychological and other forms of counselling may be advisable. Withdrawal should include gradual dosage reduction and anxiety management. Long-term psychological support is equally important for successful outcome, particularly for reducing the incidence and severity of post-withdrawal syndromes.

2. Answer **E**. Continuing with a benzodiazepine is unlikely to improve matters after a year of treatment. The use of anxiolytics may be masking depression. An option might be to assess for depression and to use an SSRI such as paroxetine. Some of the SSRIs are licensed for the treatment of anxiety and panic disorders. General assessment is also recommended, to rule out other disorders, and non-pharmacological treatments should be considered.

Chapter 21

1. a. **False**.
   b. **True**. Regular blood monitoring is required.
   c. **False**. Injections are at 1- to 3-month intervals.

2. a. **True**. Negative symptoms are more difficult to treat; 'atypical' antipsychotics may have greater activity against negative symptoms.
   b. **False**. The plasma levels of chlorpromazine are highly variable and do not correlate with clinical effect.

3. **True**. Their antimuscarinic activity may contribute to this.

4. Answer **B**.

A. It has a very low incidence of extrapyramidal side-effects.
B. Clozapine can cause agranulocytosis, and blood monitoring is necessary.
C. Thioridazine causes significant postural hypotension.
D. Antipsychotics do not cause nausea and some are used in the treatment of nausea and vomiting.
E. Lithium is reabsorbed through the proximal convoluted tubule in the kidney at the same site that Na^+ is absorbed.

5. Answer **D**.

A. The ability to block dopamine receptors in the substantia nigra will increase the extrapyramidal side-effects.
B. Blockade of muscarinic receptors will increase side-effects such as confusion, although it may reduce parkinsonism-like effects.
C. Block of α_1-adrenergic receptors will cause hypotension.
D. Serotonin receptor blocking activity could contribute to its antipsychotic potential.
E. Blockade of histamine receptors will contribute to its sedative effect.

6. Case history answers

a. Positive symptoms of schizophrenia are associated with overactivity of dopaminergic pathways in the mesolimbic area and median temporal lobe, e.g. hippocampus and amygdala, although evidence of biochemical or organic abnormalities is sparse. Pharmacologically, florid schizophrenia symptoms may be mimicked by dopamine agonists (e.g. amphetamines) and are improved by dopamine antagonists. Antipsychotic activity correlates most closely with antagonism of dopamine D_2 (and possibly D_3) receptors.

b. Distinct from their antipsychotic activity, drugs also block dopamine D_2 receptors in nigrostriatal pathways. This upsets the 'balance' between dopaminergic and cholinergic activity, leading to extrapyramidal movement disorders (e.g. tremor, akasthisia, tardive dyskinesia). The movement disorders thus mimic those seen in Parkinson's disease, where they are caused by a *neurological* deficit in dopaminergic activity. As with Parkinsonian patients, anticholinergic drugs are sometimes used in schizophrenia to ameliorate extrapyramidal side-effects. Mr PS's movement disorders (problems with writing/typing) appear relatively mild, possibly because chlorpromazine (an early phenothiazine) also has antimuscarinic activity. Paradoxically, newer phenothiazines (e.g. fluphenazine) often produce worse movement disorders than chlorpromazine. Mr PS's weight gain may be Cushingoid, caused by chlorpromazine antagonising the dopamine-dependent suppression of adrenocorticotrophic hormone (ACTH) release from the hypothalamus.

c. As well as the above caused by dopamine antagonism, many antipsychotic drugs (especially early ones) produce unwanted effects due to blockade of histamine receptors (sedation, tiredness), muscarinic receptors (dry mouth, blurred vision, impotence) and α_1-adrenoceptors (vasodilation and postural hypotension). Chlorpromazine may also produce 'yellowing' or darkening of vision because of idiosyncratic deposition in the cornea.

d. Approaches include the possible use of a long-acting depot preparation (decanoates, etc.), and the importance of support from the patient's GP and family in maintaining compliance. A principal cause of poor compliance is unwanted effects of antipsychotic therapy. Since adverse effects vary widely from drug to drug, the choice of drug may have major impact on compliance, e.g. a drug causing severe movement disorders may be least appropriate in elderly patient at risk from falls, a drug with strong antimuscarinic effect (e.g. sexual dysfunction) may be more resented in younger patients.

e. Mr PS may benefit from a different antipsychotic drug, like fluphenazine or flupentixol, which produce less antagonism of histamine receptors (less sedation) and muscarinic receptors (less dry mouth, blurred vision, etc.), even though movement disorders may be worse than with chlorpromazine. Negative symptoms (apathy, withdrawal) are relatively poorly controlled with most antipsychotics compared with 'positive' symptoms (delusions, hallucinations), and both types of symptoms may be particularly resistant in a proportion of patients. An 'atypical' antipsychotic drug (clozapine, sulpiride) may help with the apathy and withdrawal reported by Mr PS, with relatively little sedation and movement disorders. Clozapine can cause blood, disorders (agranulocytosis and aplastic anaemia), and blood monitoring is mandatory.

Chapter 22

1. a. **True**. Downregulation of $5HT_2$ receptors parallels the time course of improvement of clinical condition, whereas the time course of the increase in amine transmitters does not.

b. **False**. Different TCAs vary widely in their abilities to independently affect noradrenaline and serotonin reuptake.

c. **True**. TCAs have a greater potential to produce serious unwanted effects, e.g. causing cardiac arrhythmias in acute overdose. Interestingly, patient acceptability is similar with both drug classes.

2. a. **False**. Lofepramine is among the least cardiotoxic of the tricyclic and related antidepressants.

b. **True**. MAOI and SSRI should not be combined. The combination can cause CNS excitation, tremor and hyperthermia. An MAOI should not be started until 1–5 weeks after stopping the SSRI, depending upon which SSRI has been taken.

3. a. **True**. Trazodone is atypical since it blocks $5HT_2$ receptors

b. **False**. Although, like TCAs, venlafaxine inhibits both noradrenaline and 5HT reuptake, it lacks the sedative and antimuscarinic effects of TCAs.

c. **False**. Venlafaxine is claimed to produce improvement in about 1 week, whereas other antidepressants can take many weeks for their effects to be seen.

4. a. **True**. Alcohol should not be consumed by patients taking TCAs.

b. **False**. The half-life of lithium is long (about 24 h).

c. **False**. Although it is most commonly used in bipolar affective disorder, it is also used in patients with severe recurrent depressive episodes that do not respond to other treatment.

5. Answer **D**.

A. Many TCAs have antimuscarinic activity, which could exacerbate urinary retention.

B. This statement is false, as the antidepressant activity resides in the ability of the drugs to block serotonin receptors and not muscarinic receptors.

C. Moclobemide is a selective reversible inhibitor of MAO-A and has relatively little effect on MAO-B. As both MAO-A and MAO-B metabolise tyramine in cheese, which is the source of the hypertension in the 'cheese reaction', tyramine would be effectively metabolised.

D. Generally, an SSRI is more suitable than most TCAs in this situation because of the lower toxicity in overdose. The effectiveness of the drugs is not different. Some TCAs, however, such as lofepramine, have a low toxicity in overdose despite being a tricyclic structure.

E. This is false. The increase in brain monoamine levels occurs in hours to days following treatment with a TCA. However, the effect on behaviour, mood and the depression may take 4–6 weeks or longer to come into play.

6. Answer **B**.

A. **False,** as venlafaxine is predominantly an inhibitor of reuptake of noradrenaline and serotonin. It has little activity in blocking the serotonin receptors.

B. **True.** Venlafaxine is generally considered to be in the class of the serotonin and noradrenaline reuptake inhibitors, although it does have a greater effect on serotonin reuptake.

C. **False.** Venlafaxine has relatively little activity in blocking muscarinic receptors.

D. **False.** Venlafaxine increases monoamines in the synaptic clefts, as does an MAOI. These two drugs can, therefore, exacerbate each other's action on monoamine levels.

E. **False.** There is some suggestion that venlafaxine may be faster in onset than TCAs. However, this is an equivocal finding and remains to be confirmed.

7. Case history answers

a. The causes of depression are unknown. Although it can occur in reaction to a stressful situation, most cases do not have an obvious precipitant. It is a syndrome (a cluster of symptoms), several features of which DW was exhibiting. The symptoms had been developing for a long period of time.

b. Risk factors include gender (more frequent in women), age (peak age 20–40 years), family history of depression, marital status (higher rates in separated and divorced) and stress. Can we be certain that any of these were contributory? Exercise obsession, weight loss? Potential anorexia?

c. There is a biological association of depression with reduced CNS monoaminergic neurotransmission, notably noradrenaline and 5HT, but it is still unclear whether this is cause or effect. Drugs that deplete monoamines can induce depression, and when monoamines are repleted, symptoms decrease. Probably because of the depletion of monoamines, there is an upregulation of postsynaptic monoamine receptors. These include $5HT_2$ and α_1-adrenoceptors; β_1-adrenoceptors may also be upregulated. Drugs used to treat depression increase CNS 5HT and/or noradrenaline in the synaptic cleft, which eventually results in receptor downregulation and a return to normal in the postsynaptic receptor numbers.

d. TCAs may not be the most appropriate choice if DW was showing suicidal tendencies. Their therapeutic index is low and a better choice would be an SSRI.

e. Unwanted effects include muscarinic receptor blockade (dry mouth, blurred vision, constipation), cardiotoxicity, sedation (variable) and postural hypotension.

f. The onset of action is delayed for at least 2–4 weeks. Two-thirds of depressed people improve, one-third do not. One-third of depressed patients would have got better without drug therapy. Whether TCAs prevent recurrence is unknown. Alternative treatments include SSRIs such as fluoxetine. This has fewer unwanted effects such as cardiotoxicity and antimuscarinic actions, but causes nausea, insomnia and agitation in some patients. Its antidepressant action is no better than that of TCAs. Other possibilities are MAOIs, which have considerable unwanted effects and require dietary restriction of tyramine (cheese) intake; they are less used now. RIMAs (e.g. moclobemide) are selective for inhibition of the MAO-A isoenzyme, leaving type B unaltered, and this is able to metabolise tyramine. Drugs previously called atypical antidepressants act partially by blocking monoamine receptors. Trazodone blocks postsynaptic $5HT_2$ receptors and has only a small effect on the inhibition of 5HT reuptake.

Chapter 23

1. False. Absences, manifested by unawareness of surroundings without motor disturbance, occur in children.

2. False. In 'jacksonian epilepsy', jerking localised to a particular group of muscles may occur, which can then gradually involve many other muscles.

3. a. **False**. There are currently no glutamate antagonists that are useful in treatment of epilepsy.

b. **False**. GABA causes hyperpolarisation by increasing Cl^- influx into cells and cannot be given orally. However, several anti-epileptic drugs act by enhancing the effect of GABA.

4. False. Phenytoin exhibits 'use-dependent' blockade of Na^+ channels, i.e. the block increases with duration of contact with the receptors.

5. a. **False**. Salicylates and valproate displace phenytoin from plasma proteins, to which 80–90% of the drug is bound. This increases the free plasma concentration and the effect of phenytoin.

b. **False**. Phenytoin exhibits first-order kinetics up to the lower parts of the therapeutic dose range, but at higher doses the relationship switches to zero-order kinetics after the liver metabolising enzymes have become saturated.

6. False. Although vigabatrin is effective in all types of epilepsy, acting by specifically reducing the breakdown of GABA, it is reserved for patients resistant to other drugs.

7. Answer **B**.

A. Phenytoin is not used in treating absence seizures, and in a young person should be avoided if possible because it causes hirsuitism, gingival hyperplasia, acne and facial coarsening.

B. Ethosuximide is a first-line drug in absence seizures.

C. Valproate inhibits liver drug-metabolising enzymes, thus increasing the chance of ethosuximide toxicity.

D. T-type Ca^{2+} channels are blocked by ethosuximide.

E. The full benefit of sodium valproate may take several weeks to develop.

8. Answer **B**.

A. The risk of teratogenesis is increased if more than one drug is given.

B. Tolerance to the therapeutic effects and unwanted effects develops with time.

C. The pharmacokinetics of phenytoin can change from linear to zero order as the dose is increased.

D. Phenytoin is highly protein bound and can be displaced by salicylates, increasing the concentration of free phenytoin and thus the clinical effect and risk of unwanted effects.

E. Diazepam is used as an adjunct to other treatments for prophylaxis and in status epilepticus.

9. Case history 1 answers

a. Absence seizures usually respond well to sodium valproate or ethosuximide. Ethosuximide is effective only in absence seizures. Phenytoin and phenobarbital are ineffective in absences.

b. Sodium valproate causes nausea, reversible transient hair loss and weight gain. Uncommonly, liver damage can occur. Ethosuximide causes nausea, anorexia and headache.

c. Monotherapy with ethosuximide or sodium valproate should be tried before combining therapies. Compliance should also be checked before combining therapies. Sodium valproate reduces the clearance of ethosuximide and may cause toxicity.

10. Case history 2 answers

a. A variety of drugs could be used in this patient. First-line drugs usually include carbamazepine, phenytoin or sodium valproate.

b. Non-hormonal contraceptives such as barrier or intrauterine device are effective and do not carry the risk of drug interactions. However, many women will want to use a hormonal method.

c. Carbamazepine, phenytoin, phenobarbital and topiramate all induce liver enzymes that increase the metabolism of sex steroids and reduce efficacy of oral contraceptives.

d. Injected medroxyprogesterone acetate is affected less than sex steroids administered orally. The interval between injection of medroxyprogesterone acetate should, however, be reduced to 10 weeks. Medroxyprogesterone acetate may also reduce the incidence of epileptic attacks.

e. It is recommended that, at a minimum, pills containing a high concentration of estrogen (50 μg) should be given. Up to three pills per day, each containing 35 μg estrogen, may be required to prevent breakthrough bleeding. The pill-free period can also be reduced. If any change in medication for her epilepsy is made, additional barrier methods of contraception should be used until medication is stabilised.

f. No. The progestogen-only pill would be unsafe, as its metabolism is increased.

Chapter 24

1. a. **False**. Symptoms develop when more than 50% of neurons have been lost.

b. **True**. There is overactivity of glutaminergic neurons in parkinsonism and this exacerbates the excessive outflow of GABA nerves to the motor cortex.

c. **False**. Levodopa has a short half-life and this may contribute to end-of-dose movement disorders.

2. a. **True**. In clinical trials of up to 6 months' duration in early Parkinson's disease, ropinirole has been shown to be as effective as levodopa.

b. **False**. Trihexyphenidyl can cause minor unwanted effects but also can cause severe confusion, particularly in the elderly.

3. a. **True**. Bromocriptine stimulates dopamine receptors and its half life of 6–8 h is longer than that of levodopa.

b. **True**. Particularly tremor and rigidity may be partially because of other transmitter substances.

c. **True**.

d. **False**. Selegiline only inhibits MAO-B, leaving MAO-A intact to metabolise tyramine in cheese and some other foods.

e. **False**. Entacapone inhibits the enzyme catechol-*O*-methyl transferase, which breaks down about 10% of levodopa. It therefore helps to maintain concentrations of levodopa, which has a short half-life.

4. a. **False**. Baclofen is used in the treatment of spasticity by inhibiting excitatory synapses and stimulating responses of the inhibitory transmitter GABA.
   b. **True**. Botulinum toxin is used in spasticity by local injection and inhibits acetylcholine release for up to 3 months.

5. Answer **A**.

   A. Reduced dopaminergic and increased cholinergic function is present in parkinsonism.
   B. Selegiline is selective for MAO-B.
   C. Only 1–2% of an oral dose of levodopa enters the brain in the absence of a decarboxylase inhibitor.
   D. Most drugs stimulate the D_2 receptor family, although some have less activity on D_1 receptors.
   E. Carbidopa is a peripheral decarboxylase inhibitor, it does not cross the blood–brain barrier..

6. Case history 1 answers

   a. The cause of Parkinson's disease is a selective degeneration of dopaminergic neurons in the corpus striatum and the substantia nigra. The cause of this degeneration is unknown but hypotheses include actions of reactive oxygen metabolites, neurotoxins or immune disturbances. The basal ganglia of patients with Parkinson's disease generally have less than 10% of the normal amount of dopamine. This results in complex neurochemical disturbances. There is inadequate dopaminergic transmission. Cholinergic overactivity results from the removal of the inhibitory effect of dopamine on cholinergic neurons. There is also overactivity of glutamate neurons, and control of this may be a target for useful future drugs for the treatment of parkinsonism.
   b. Patients have akinesia, rigidity and tremor possibly from inhibition of the motor cortical system, whereas the descending inhibition of the brainstem locomotor areas may contribute to abnormalities of gait and posture. Patients have difficulty getting going and problems with fine movement, particularly in writing.
   c. Levodopa is the immediate precursor of dopamine and is transported into the CNS by an active transport mechanism. Dopamine does not gain access. Levodopa causes nausea and vomiting because of its effect on the chemoreceptor trigger zone (the blood–brain barrier is deficient in the area postrema). Co-beneldopa is a combination of levodopa and benserazide. Benserazide or another compound, carbidopa, are used because they inhibit peripheral dopa decarboxylase activity and, therefore, prevent the breakdown of levodopa to dopamine. They do not cross the blood–brain barrier, so levodopa is still converted to dopamine in the brain. Protection against peripheral unwanted effects can also be achieved with the peripheral-acting dopamine antagonist domperidone. Unwanted effects of levodopa are nausea and vomiting, postural hypotension, hallucinations and confusion, and unpredictable motor disturbances.
   d. Levodopa remains the most effective treatment for Parkinson's disease. However, there has been extensive debate about when to start therapy with levodopa. There is no convincing evidence that levodopa accelerates neurodegeneration, and survival is reduced if treatment is delayed until greater disability is present. In time, and despite long-term treatment with levodopa, there is an increasing incidence of dyskinesias and on–off fluctuations of effect, although most patients continue to derive benefit throughout the duration of their illness. At the end of 5 years of treatment, approximately 50% of patients will be experiencing reduced effectiveness with levodopa. In patients with young-onset disease at about the age of 40, almost all have developed dyskinesias and on–off problems after 5 years. These motor fluctuations can be as a result of unpredictable pharmacokinetic changes, such as unpredictable absorption across the blood–brain barrier or delayed gastric emptying, or because of progression of the disease process following further loss of dopaminergic neurons. Resolving these problems is highly individual, with dosage adjustments (either up or down) and shortening the interval between doses sometimes being helpful. The dyskinesia and on–off effects may be helped by smaller, more frequent doses of levodopa or perhaps by modified-release formulations. An antimuscarinic drug can be given with levodopa and is particularly useful in the treatment of tremor. However, they have the propensity to cause confusion and hallucinations, particularly in the elderly, so they are often reserved for patients suffering from severe tremor. Other drugs which inhibit dopamine metabolism can also be introduced. Selegiline is an inhibitor of MAO-B. Its use has been questioned after a study which showed an increase in mortality; however, a second large study has not confirmed this. The

catechol-*O*-methyl transferase inhibitors such as entacapone have also been developed as another way of reducing the breakdown of levodopa and dopamine. These agents seem to be able to prolong the benefits of levodopa therapy. A direct dopamine agonist could also be added to levodopa treatment for Mrs FT. The ergot derivatives, such as lisuride and pergolide, are used. A new non-ergot drug, ropinirole, has recently been licensed for the treatment of early Parkinson's disease. Its ability to stimulate D_3 receptors may contribute to its action. Apomorphine given subcutaneously can also be used to counteract the off periods in advanced disease.

e. Vitamin B_6 reduces the central effectiveness of levodopa as it is a cofactor for conversion to dopamine, and, therefore, dopamine formation in the periphery would be enhanced.

f. Beta-adrenoceptor antagonists have been found to be helpful to reduce tremor in some patients with Parkinsonism.

g. No currently available drug has been proven to reduce disease progression. Studies suggesting that selegiline may be protective have not been confirmed. It does not delay the onset of dyskinesias during levodopa treatment. An early study that requires confirmation is that ropinirole may delay disease progression.

7. Case history 2 answer

There is extensive debate about when to commence levodopa therapy. The goal should be to improve quality of life and limit long-term unwanted effects. If the degree of disability is not severe and the patient, carers and clinicians are in agreement, there may be no immediate need for therapy; however, this is controversial, as survival is reduced if treatment with levodopa is delayed until disability develops. If treatment is required, dopamine agonists could be started. These are less likely to produce dyskinesias and could delay the need for levodopa until progressive disabilities start to occur. The possibility of brain damage caused by boxing injury should also be considered. This responds poorly to standard treatments for Parkinson's disease.

Chapter 25

1. a. False. Interferon-β is used in multiple sclerosis and may diminish the production of inflammatory interferon-γ.

b. False. Multiple sclerosis is usually characterised by relapses and remissions over a number of years, although after about 10 years a steady decline sets in.

c. True. Glutamate is an excitatory amino acid neurotransmitter but can cause cell damage and death by a number of mechanisms, including an uncontrolled increase in intracellular Ca^{2+}.

d. False. Riluzole reduces glutamate release and action, thereby reducing its toxicity.

e. True. Possibly because of its immunosuppressive and anti-inflammatory actions.

2. Answer **B**.

A. Influenza-like symptoms can occur in about 50% of people.

B. NICE have been unable to recommend the use of glatiramer acetate because of its relative lack of effect.

C. **False**. Glatiramer acetate can cause flushing, chest tightness, palpitations, anxiety and breathlessness.

D. **False**.

E. Long-term disability is due to demyelination of nerves and consequent further damage. Demyelination of nerves results in disordered neuronal conduction.

Chapter 26

1. a. False. Because of habituation problems and unwanted effects, ergotamine should not be used more than twice a month for acute attacks.

b. False. Sumatriptan is more rapidly absorbed when given by subcutaneous or nasal routes of administration. It gives slower relief when given orally.

2. True. Plasma levels of 5HT fall but urinary levels of the 5HT metabolite increase dramatically.

3. a. True. By inhibiting $5HT_2$ receptors, there is reduced perivascular inflammation, vasodilation and pain.

b. False. Ergotamine causes vasoconstriction and should be avoided in patients with vascular diseases.

c. False. Although sumatriptan causes chest discomfort and is contraindicated in patients with ischaemic heart disease or angina, the chest discomfort and tightness in those without ischaemic heart disease is probably caused by oesophageal spasm, not myocardial ischaemia.

d. False. The prophylaxis of migraine is effective in only about 40% of individuals.

4. **True**. Metoclopramide is an antiemetic, increases gastric emptying and improves paracetamol absorption.

5. **False**. In some people, stress, chocolate, cheese, alcohol, etc. can provoke migraine attacks.

Chapter 27

1. a. **False**. The depolarising block is enhanced when body temperature is artificially lowered.
   b. **False**. Mivacurium and atracurium are the muscle relaxants with the greatest propensity to cause histamine release and haemodynamic effects.

2. a. **True**. Dantrolene relaxes skeletal muscle by preventing Ca^{2+} release from the sarcoplasmic reticulum.
   b. **True**. Contraction is an-all-or-none response of the fibre in response to nerve stimulation.
   c. **False**. The N_2 receptor at skeletal muscle is selectively blocked by non-depolarising and depolarising muscle relaxants. The N_1 receptor at ganglia is selectively blocked by ganglion-blocking drugs. Selectivity is lost if inappropriately large doses of these agents are administered.

3. a. **False**. Short-acting non-depolarising neuromuscular blockers such as rocuronium can be used for intubation.
   b. **False**. Because of the quaternary nature of their structure, they are not absorbed orally. They do not cross the blood–brain barrier or placenta.

4. a. **False**. Botulinum toxin contains two subunits that promote presynaptic binding and long-lasting block of ACh release.
   b. **True**. Botulinum toxin is extremely toxic on systemic absorption.
   c. **True**. Botulinum toxin only inhibits ACh release. Although sweat glands are sympathetically innervated, the postganglionic neurons are cholinergic and release ACh.

5. Answer **E**.

   A. All non-depolarising neuromuscular-blocking drugs have a quarternary ammonium in their structure and will not cross the blood–brain barrier.
   B. Pancuronium is a long-acting blocking drug and is used for procedures taking longer than 90 min.
   C. Short-acting non-depolarising blocking drugs such as rocuronium or mivacurium are viable alternatives.

   D. More than 90% of receptors need to be occupied to produce a complete block of skeletal muscle contractility.
   E. Atracurium is one of the most potent neuromuscular-blocking drugs for the release of histamine.

6. Case history – see the case history answers for Chapter 17, page 717.

Chapter 28

1. a. **False**. Respiratory depression is caused by blockade of nicotinic receptors by high doses of an anticholinesterase (AChE inhibitor) and is not treatable by atropine. Artificial ventilation may be required. Atropine-like drugs could, however, reduce muscarinic receptor-mediated bronchoconstriction.
   b. **False**. Breakdown of anticholinesterase is not affected. Lack of effect of the anticholinesterase may be due to an inadequate number of responsive nicotinic N_2 receptors.

2. a. **True**. The neuromuscular blockade with suxamethonium may be prolonged and an extended period of apnoea may result.
   b. **False**. The cholinergic crisis results from the excessive effects of an AChE inhibitor and would be exacerbated by the long-acting pyridostigmine. Assisted ventilation and withdrawal of the treatment should be performed or, if any AChE inhibitor was used to confirm the diagnosis, short-acting edrophonium should be given.

3. Answer **D**.

   A. About 15% have a thymoma and 60–80% have hyperplasia of the thymus.
   B. Neostigmine and pyridostigmine are the main anticholinesterases used in treating myasthenia gravis; they are quarternary amines and do not cross the blood–brain barrier.
   C. Glucocorticoids work by suppressing the nicotinic receptor antibodies.
   D. Muscarinic receptor blockers will prevent the parasympathomimetic effects of physostigmine (diarrhoea, urination, miosis, bradycardia, nausea, lacrimation, salivation).
   E. Plasmapheresis is carried out to reduce the levels of circulating nicotinic receptor antibodies.

4. Case history answers

   a. Electromyography (Jolly test), single muscle fibre electromyography, anti-acetylcholine receptor

(AchR) antibody titres, injection of a short-acting inhibitor of AchE (the Tensilon test, the proprietary name for edrophonium).

b. AchR antibody blocks nicotinic N_2 receptors, receptors are destroyed and receptors are cross-linked, which causes them to be destroyed more rapidly. The decrease in functional receptors reduces motor endplate potentials and reduces the likelihood of the muscle contracting.

c. It is short acting, giving an effect in 30–60 s and effects subsiding in 4–5 min.

d. Symptomatic treatment with an AchE inhibitor. Immunosuppression with a corticosteroid, using azathioprine or ciclosporin in addition if necessary.

Chapter 29

1. a. **False**. Although COX-2 can be induced by cytokines, endotoxins and other inflammatory mediators in many cells, it is present constitutively in other cells such as in blood vessels and can be induced with appropriate stimuli.

   b. **True**. PGE_2 generated by COX-2 sensitises the sensory pain neurons to bradykinin and other mediators but does not itself stimulate sensory pain fibres.

   c. **False**. There is a wide range in the ratios with which NSAIDs inhibit COX-1/COX-2. This relates approximately, but somewhat loosely, to the extent of their anti-inflammatory and gastrointestinal unwanted effects.

   d. **False**. Paracetamol is analgesic and antipyretic but has only a weak anti-inflammatory effect. The reasons for this are imperfectly understood but it may have an inhibitory effect on COX-3 enzymes in the brain.

2. a. **True**. Reduced blood flow contributes to the gastric damage caused by NSAIDs. They also inhibit bicarbonate and mucus secretion.

   b. **False**. An increase in the risk of haemorrhage can occur.

   c. **False**. The COX-2-selective inhibitor celecoxib is associated with less gastrointestinal side-effects than is the non-selective naproxen.

3. a. **False**. Long-term use of high doses of aspirin or paracetamol can result in renal ischaemia, sodium and water retention, papillary necrosis and chronic renal failure.

   b. **True**. Particularly in those over 75 years of age and in whom there is a history of peptic ulcer.

c. **False**. Ibuprofen is good in mild to moderate arthritis but other NSAIDs such as indometacin or diclofenac have greater anti-inflammatory potential, although a greater propensity to cause unwanted effects.

d. **False**. In a subgroup of asthmatics, aspirin induces an asthmatic response through formation of the bronchoconstrictor LTC_4. COX-1-generated prostaglandins are involved and COX-2-selective inhibitors have less potential to cause asthmatic attacks.

4. a. **False**. Inhibition of platelet aggregation is partly through generation of TXA_2 by COX-1 enzymes. Celecoxib is a selective COX-2 inhibitor. Although it requires further investigation, some studies have suggested that in susceptible individuals the use of selective COX-2 inhibitors is associated with an excess of cardivascular complications.

   b. **True**. Pyrexia is caused by elevation of PGE_2 levels under the influence of COX-2 enzymes.

5. Extended-matching answers

   1. Answer **D**. This man's hypertension and heart failure mean that you would not want to give him an NSAID that may result in salt and water retention. Both the COX-2-selective and non-selective NSAIDs contribute to salt and water retention.

   2. Answer **B**. The COX-2-selective celecoxib could be prescribed. COX-1 inhibitors such as aspirin or diclofenac may precipitate a hypersensitive asthmatic attack. Paracetamol would not be useful as it has little anti-inflammatory action.

   3. Answer **A**. This man should be given low-dose aspirin (75 mg daily). This is a relatively selective COX-1 inhibitor and prevents platelet aggregation by inhibiting TXA_2 synthesis while having a minimal effect on the production of the vasodilator PGI_2 (prostacyclin), which is generated in the vascular endothelium by COX-2. This low dose has been shown to have a beneficial long-term effect on the occurrence of another infraction.

Chapter 30

1. a. **False**. NSAIDs do not slow disease progress, indeed some evidence suggests they may hasten the disease progress.

   b. **True**. The second-line drugs take a long time to act (4–6 months) but they should be discontinued if there is no sign of improvement by that time.

2. a. **True**. Sodium aurothiomalate can be given intramuscularly and auranofin by mouth.

    b. **True**. Proteinuria occurs associated with immune-complex nephritis. Only 15% of patients continue with treatment after 5–6 years because of unwanted effects.

3. a. **False**. Methotrexate prevents reduction of folic acid to dihydrofolate and tetrahydrofolate (essential for DNA production). Folic acid can be given daily to prevent gastrointestinal and haematological complications.

    b. **True**. Although 5-aminosalicylic acid is the active moiety in the treatment of inflammatory bowel disease, it is less effective than sulfasalazine in treating rheumatoid arthritis.

    c. **True**. More than 50% of people with rheumatoid arthritis continue with methotrexate for 5 years or more, whereas with most other disease-modifying drugs 50% have to be stopped within 2 years.

4. **False**. The combination of methotrexate with ciclosporin, sulfasalazine or hydroxychloroquine has shown significant benefit; it is reserved for people with severe rheumatoid disease.

5. a. **False**. Although corticosteroids can give dramatic relief of symptoms in rheumatoid arthritis, there is no evidence that they slow progression of the disease.

    b. **True**. Adrenal atrophy can last for many months following treatment.

6. **False**. Chloroquine and hydroxychloroquine can cause remission of rheumatoid arthritis but do not slow the progression of joint damage.

7. Extended-matching answers

    1. Answer **A**. The brief duration of the symptoms and their mild nature warrant the administration of an NSAID such as ibuprofen and follow-up.

    2. Answer **G**. The persistence of the symptoms and their spread to the knees suggest that a DMARD should be started. Guidelines now advise that DMARDs should be considered for persistent inflammatory joint disease of more than 8 weeks' duration.

    3. Answer **D**. Methotrexate is a DMARD that requires folate supplements (see answer to 3a above). Methotrexate takes 4–6 weeks for its onset of action. Methotrexate and ibuprofen should be given to cover this interim period.

B. It is the uric acid in the joint that causes the symptoms.

C. Drugs like probenicid, not allopurinol, enhance the renal secretion of urate.

D. This is one of the anti-inflammatory mechanisms of colchicine.

E. Aspirin can inhibit the renal secretion of urate, exacerbating the gout.

2. Case history answers

    a. The treatment of choice for an acute attack is an NSAID *but not aspirin*. Indometacin is often used and is effective within 2 days. If patients cannot take an NSAID, colchicine or glucocorticoids can be used, but both have significant unwanted effects. Salicylates should be avoided as at low doses they reduce uric acid excretion, although at high doses they are uricosuric.

    b. Plasma uric acid will be raised. An arthrocentesis sample will show uric acid crystals. Infection should be excluded in an acutely inflamed joint.

    c. Uric acid crystals in the joint space. People who develop gout have had hyperuricaemia for years. Uric acid is a relatively insoluble metabolic product of purine metabolism. Sardines, liver and kidney are rich in purines, and a diet rich in purines can contribute to gout in some people. In most people, hyperuricaemia is caused by impaired renal clearance of uric acid. Overproduction of uric acid as a result of excessive alcohol consumption can also contribute. Joint trauma, lead toxicity and cool temperatures can decrease uric acid solubility.

    d. NSAIDs are drugs of choice in acute attacks (see a).

    e. Hyperuricaemia is treated after resolution of the acute attack. Allopurinol reduces plasma uric acid by inhibiting xanthine oxidase. This increases concentrations of hypoxanthine and xanthine, which are more water-soluble. Patients who overproduce uric acid are best treated with allopurinol.

    f. Those that have low renal excretion of uric acid may be treated with a uricosuric drug (probenecid, sulfinpyrazone). Both inhibit the reabsorption of uric acid in the proximal convoluted tubule.

    g. Untreated gout can lead to formation of kidney stones. A significant number of people with gout will have hypertension.

Chapter 31

1. Answer **D**.

    A. Hypoxanthine is more water-soluble than urate; this is the rationale for the use of allopurinol.

Chapter 32

1. a. **False**. The CTZ is outside the blood–brain barrier. Moreover, toxins can also cause vomiting by stimulating vagal afferents in the stomach.

b. **True.** Common antihistamines like promethazine have antimuscarinic activity and inhibit activity in the vomiting centre and in the vestibular nuclei. It is not certain whether the antihistamine component plays a role.

2. **False.** Metoclopramide increases stomach and intestinal motility (prokinetic activity) which can add to its antiemetic effects.

3. Answer **C**.

   A. The vagal afferents from the stomach are emetogenic and respond to toxins etc.
   B. Selective 5HT antagonists are not effective against motion sickness, where a drug with antimuscarinic actions, e.g. hyoscine or promethazine, should be used.
   C. **True.**
   D. The effect of stimulating NK_1 receptors in the CTZ is to cause vomiting.
   E. Digoxin stimulates nausea and vomiting.

4. Case history answers

   a. Cyclophosphamide induces nausea and vomiting in almost all people, but vincristine is much less emetogenic. The vomiting arises from stimulation of the CTZ.
   b. A selective $5HT_3$ receptor antagonist such as ondansetron, alone or together with a corticosteroid, would be beneficial.
   c. Ondansetron inhibits $5HT_3$ receptors in the CTZ and *also* $5HT_3$ and $5HT_4$ receptors in the stomach. In the stomach, some cancer chemotherapeutic agents can cause damage and release of 5HT, which stimulates vagal afferents to the vomiting centre. It is uncertain how corticosteroids work, but they have an antiemetic effect which is additive with ondansetron.
   d. Anticipatory nausea and vomiting is poorly treated with antiemetic drugs. Treatment with benzodiazepines prior to the course of treatment can be helpful.

Chapter 33

1. a. **True.** Although the organism only appears to live on gastric mucosa, it is known that gastric metaplasia develops in the duodenum in response to low pH and by this means duodenal colonisation can occur.
   b. **False.** Approximately 80% of duodenal ulcers recur if *H. pylori* is not eliminated.
   c. **True.** Although the relationship between *H. pylori* and gastric cancer is somewhat difficult to prove,

it has been estimated from epidemiological studies that this infection may increase the risk of developing gastric adenocarcinoma by five- to sixfold. It is possible that acquisition of the infection at a young age may be of relevance.

   d. **True.** The relevance of this to *H. pylori* is that when infection is associated with pangastritis, glandular atrophy and reduced gastric acid secretion occurs. This can then result in bacterial overgrowth and the formation of *N*-nitroso compounds that are mutagenic. Although *H. pylori* can resist acid transiently because of its ability to produce ammonia, it is destroyed by longer exposure.
   e. **False.** In some countries the resistance to metronidazole is as high as 90% and in some locations in France resistance to erythromycin is as high as 17%.
   f. **True.** Omeprazole has to be converted to its active sulphenamide form by protonation in acid. This is why it is active on the proton pump in the parietal cell but not other proton pumps in the body that operate at higher pH. This contributes to its selectivity.
   g. **False.** Histamine acts on H_2 receptors on parietal cells to stimulate acid secretion. This is the basis for the selective action of histamine H_2 receptor antagonists such as ranitidine and cimetidine.
   h. **True.** Acetylcholine stimulates muscarinic receptors, which, by increasing Ca^{2+}, causes increased acid secretion. Selective vagotomy is used to treat ulcer disease.

2. **False.** Antacids do heal peptic ulcers but their effects are slower than with proton pump inhibitors or histamine H_2 receptor antagonists.

3. a. **True.** Cimetidine causes gynaecomastia. This is because of its greater antiandrogenic effect.
   b. **False.** Histamine H_2 antagonists reduce acid secretion by about 60%. The action of other agents that promote acid secretion, for example gastrin and acetylcholine, are unaffected by histamine H_2 receptor antagonists.
   c. **False.** The active metabolite sulphenamide irreversibly inhibits the proton pump and fresh protein must be synthesised to replace the inhibited pump. This is the explanation for the very long duration of action of omeprazole.

4. **True.** Omeprazole can inhibit the metabolism of drugs such as warfarin or phenytoin. Lansoprazole, by contrast, is only a weak enzyme inhibitor.

5. a. **False.** Part of the way that prostaglandins protects the mucosa is by increasing gastric mucosal blood flow, removing back-secreted H^+

and providing HCO_3^-. Prostaglandins additionally increase mucus secretion, decrease acid secretion and increase HCO_3^- secretion.

b. **False.** Prostaglandin (particularly PGI_2) in large doses can increase gastrointestinal motility and increase gastrointestinal secretions.

c. **False.** Healing can be brought about by both of these anti-ulcer drugs. Omeprazole may produce more rapid healing since the rate of healing is probably related to the degree of acid suppression.

6. **True.** This is the mechanism for its usefulness in the treatment of oesophageal reflux disease. Metoclopramide and similar drugs are most effectively used as adjuncts to proton pump inhibitors and H_2 receptor antagonists.

7. Answer **C**.

A. *H. pylori* is found in the duodenum associated with colonisation by gastric metaplasia of the duodenal mucosa.

B. Increasingly, resistance of *H. pylori* to clarithromycin is developing.

C. Cimetidine inhibits the cytochrome P450 metabolising enzymes that break down warfarin, hence increasing the plasma levels of warfarin.

D. The solution contains urea not urease. The urease associated with *H. pylori* then converts the urea to ammonia, which causes a colour change in the pH indicator.

E. Although the plasma half-life of omeprazole is about 2 h, its biological half-life is much longer, as it is converted to a sulphenamide which irreversibly inhibits the parietal cell proton pump.

8. Case history answers

a. This man could be experiencing non-ulcer dyspepsia or have peptic ulceration. Whichever he has, if his symptoms are associated with *H. pylori* infection, they will return, as *H. pylori* has not been eradicated. Ranitidine for only 2 weeks of treatment is available without prescription. If ranitidine had been continued, the symptoms would probably have been suppressed for longer. Failure to eradicate *H. pylori* results in a recurrence of peptic ulcer disease in 80% of people within a year. At this stage, of course, it is not known if peptic ulcer disease is present. However, even if he has non-ulcer dyspepsia and is *H. pylori* positive, it is likely that he will develop peptic ulcer disease in the future.

b. No. If *H. pylori* is present, the symptoms will still recur in a high percentage of individuals.

c. It is recommended that any person over 45 years of age should be endoscopically examined, and

he should be referred for this procedure. The GP could assess for *H. pylori* infection serologically using a skin prick test; alternatively, this could be done in hospital with urea breath test or bacteriological culture on a gastric antral biopsy. Intake of any NSAIDs, smoking or alcohol intake should be assessed, as these are strongly contributory to ulcer disease. (An endoscopic examination revealed a duodenal ulcer.)

d. The answer to this is complex and imperfectly understood. If there is only antral inflammation and *H. pylori,* more gastrin is produced and excess acid, resulting in duodenal ulcers. If a pangastritis exists, it is associated with corporal atrophy, lower levels of acid secretion and gastric ulcers.

e. Numerous treatment regimens have being evaluated. Seven days therapy with a proton pump inhibitor or ranitidine plus two antimicrobials (either metronidazole or amoxicillin or clarithromycin in a combination dictated by local sensitivities) results in 70–90% eradication rate.

f. It is possible that the strain of *H. pylori* was resistant to metronidazole and clarithromycin. In some places, metronidazole resistance is 90% and clarithromycin 17%. Tests should be carried out to see if *H. pylori* is still present.

g. Culture sensitivities of the *H. pylori* in a biopsy specimen could be sought. Resistance to tinidazole is currently less than that to metronidazole. Quadruple therapy, which has 93–98% success, could be used – for example, a proton pump inhibitor or ranitidine plus tinidazole plus amoxicillin plus bismuth. Ranitidine bismuth substrate could replace a separate proton pump inhibitor or ranitidine plus bismuth, providing the benefits of quadruple therapy but in triple formulation.

Chapter 34

1. a. **True.** Sulfasalazine consists of sulfapyridine and 5-ASA linked by an azo bond. The azo bond is cleaved by bacteria to release the active 5-ASA. Sulfapyridine probably produces many of the unwanted effects of sulfasalazine.

b. **True**. Modified-release formulations are available for rectal administration to deliver the drug to distal colonic mucosa. About 20% of the mesalazine administered in this way is absorbed into the circulation.

2. a. **True.** There is increased risk of Crohn's disease in smokers but a slightly decreased risk of ulcerative colitis.

b. **False**. Although mesalazine may be of some benefit in colonic Crohn's disease, it is less effective than for ulcerative colitis. Mesalazine is not very effective for small-bowel Crohn's disease.

c. **False**. Although they are effective for inducing remission, there is little evidence that corticosteroids prevent relapse.

d. **False**. People with chronic Crohn's disease can become corticosteroid-dependent, and immunosuppressants such as azathioprine can be useful in reducing this dependence. Many months of treatment are required before they are fully effective.

3. Answer **E**.

A. Crohn's disease is transmural but can affect any part of the gastrointestinal tract.

B. Sulfasalazine is formed from 5-ASA, which is the active constituent, linked by an azo bond to sulphaphyridine, which is responsible for many of the unwanted effects.

C. Azathioprine is usually given in corticosteroid-refractory disease or when people are having frequent courses of steroids for treatment (more than two 6-week courses per year).

D. Infliximab is a TNFα antibody given systemically for the treatment of refractory disease.

E. Antibiotics such as metronidazole can be useful in treating Crohn's disease, particularly if there is perianal disease.

4. Case history answers

a. The cause of Crohn's disease is unknown. Several hypotheses have implicated a number of risk factors, including infection, altered immune state, combined measles, mumps and rubella (MMR) vaccine, and local ischaemia. None of these has been confirmed.

b. Initial treatment is with corticosteroids. In this man, the Crohn's disease is confined to the distal colon. Topical treatment with corticosteroids such as budesonide could be used to limit systemic unwanted effects. If, however, there was involvement of the proximal large bowel or small bowel, it would be necessary to give an oral corticosteroid such as prednisolone.

c. Corticosteroids have a variety of actions. They can alter the release of inflammatory mediators such as arachidonic acid metabolites, kinins and cytokines. They can alter cell mediated cytotoxicity, antibody production, adhesion molecule expression, phagocytic function, leucocyte chemotaxis and leucocyte adherence.

d. Corticosteroids should be given until remission occurs. If possible, the corticosteroid should be administered locally to keep the plasma concentration low, but for individuals who experience systemic symptoms (such as fatigue, anorexia or weight loss) oral therapy is indicated.

e. Systemic corticosteroids suppress the hypothalamic–pituitary–adrenal axis and can reduce the circulating levels of endogenous adrenal glucocorticoids. Gradual reduction of the dose of therapeutically administered glucocorticoid allows recovery of the production of endogenous corticosteroids.

f. If the colitis is restricted to the distal colon, topical administration of mesalazine or an oral formulation that delivers 5-ASA to the colon could be used. 5-ASA is, however, less effective in Crohn's disease, particularly if it involves the small bowel.

g. Continuous corticosteroid therapy for periods of 6 months or longer is eventually required in 40–50% of people with Crohn's disease. If more than two 6-week courses of corticosteroid per year are required to miantain control of symptoms, immunosuppressive therapy should be considered. Immunosuppressive therapy is usually with azathioprine or 6-mercaptopurine: prolonged treatment with these drugs is usually required (up to 6 months) before a clinical response occurs. TNFα antibody treatment is also of benefit in severe disease that is not responsive to other therapies.

Chapter 35

1. a. **False**. Defecation once every 3 days or three times a day is not abnormal.

b. **True**. Increased fibre intake and exercise will help in the majority of cases of 'simple' constipation.

c. **False**. Chronic use is associated with deterioration of colonic function, with damage to the myenteric plexus (cathartic colon). It was long considered that this condition was caused by the inappropriate prolonged use of stimulant laxatives; however, it is now thought that it is probably due to the refractory constipation rather than to drug use.

2. a. **True**. Aluminium salts cause constipation, as do many other drugs, including some antidepressants, opioid analgesics and calcium antagonists.

b. **False**. Some laxatives (magnesium salts) can act within 6 h, whereas lactulose and docusate take considerably longer to exert their activity.

3. a. **False**. Viral gastroenteritis is a major cause of infant diarrhoea and rotavirus predominates.

b. **True**. Overgrowth of the anaerobe *Clostridium difficile* following usage of broad-spectrum antimicrobials can occur and is increasingly resistant to metronidazole treatment.

c. **True**. However, the clinical importance of this is debated.

4. a. **False**. There are now frequent epidemics of cholera that are resistant to tetracycline.

b. **False**. A hypertonic solution will have an osmotic action drawing water into the bowel; the formulated solution should be isotonic or slightly hypotonic.

5. Answer **A**.

A. Adequate water intake is necessary when constipation is treated with bulk laxatives.

B Magnesium sulphate is an osmotic laxative but also stimulates cholecystokinin release, which stimulate enteric nerves.

C. Lactulose is an osmotic laxative.

D. Aluminium hydroxide causes constipation.

E. Sterculia is a bulking laxative and takes more than 24 h to act.

6. Answer **D**.

A. Rotavirus causes diarrhoea in young children but is a very uncommon cause in adults.

B. *Campylobacter jejuni* is a Gram-negative microaerophilic bacterium.

C. *Campylobacter jejuni* is the commonest cause of gastroenteritis in adults in developed countries.

D. Loperamide inhibits gut contractility and may increase the residence of invasive organisms.

E. In otherwise healthy individuals, oral rehydration is all that is required; in the very young or elder, intravenous rehydration may be required.

Chapter 36

1. Answer **D**.

A. In the UK, paracetamol poisoning is the most common cause of acute liver failure.

B. **True.**

C. Mannitol is an osmotic diuretic (Ch. 14). It has few uses, but one is for the reduction of cerebral oedema.

D. The coagulopathy which occurs is inadequate clotting due to a reduction in vitamin K-dependent clotting factors. Vitamin K should be given, not warfarin, which will make the problem worse.

E. Terlipressin is an analogue of varopressin; it causes vasoconstriction and can be given to treat shock.

2. Answer **B**.

A. Interferon alfa prevents virus replication (Ch. 52) and can augment the immune system.

B. The polyethylene glycol conjugated with interferon alfa (pegylated interferon alfa) has a plasma half life of about 80 h compared with 3–4 h for the non-conjugated form.

C. It is ineffective orally and is given by subcutaneous injection.

D. Lamivudine is converted to its active triphosphate form by phosphorylation with viral enzymes.

E. Combined ribavarin and interferon alfa is recommended by NICE for the treatment of hepatitis C, giving better results than either treatment alone.

3. Case history answers

a. Spironolactone would be a reasonable choice as any changes in serum K^+ should be avoided because such people are easily tipped into encephalopathy/coma by electrolyte imbalances; therefore avoid furosemide/thiazides initially, although after a few days they could be cautiously given. There is an increase in circulating aldosterone, probably because of decreased metabolism and renin stimulation secondary to low plasma volume. This probably contributes to fluid retention; therefore, spironolactone or amiloride is usually chosen.

b. Diminished hepatic reserve is indicated by four factors: (i) increased plasma bilirubin, which will be a combination of unconjugated bilirubin (because of impaired glucuronidation) plus conjugated bilirubin (because of impaired biliary excretion); (ii) decreased plasma albumin, caused by decreased synthesis, which will lower the osmotic pressure of blood and, therefore, draw less water back out of tissues, leading to oedema/ascites; (iii) decreased clotting factors caused by decreased synthesis, which may contribute to oesophageal bleeding (note, a proton pump inhibitor, such as omeprazole, is often used to reduce risk of a gastrointestinal bleed); (iv) increased oestrogenic activity, as evidenced by gynaecomastia and testicular atrophy, probably caused by decreased inactivation of oestrogenic steroids in the liver.

c. The long-acting diazepam is probably not a good choice. The shorter-acting midazolam would be preferred. People with cirrhosis are more susceptible to all CNS depressant drugs and diazepam is likely to give an increased response. The general mechanism is not known (may be change in blood–brain barrier). The metabolism of diazepam by cytochrome P450 will be reduced and, therefore, there will be an increased plasma concentration. (Note: there will be decreased formation of the active desmethyl metabolite.) A short-acting benzodiazepine without active metabolites would be better, e.g. midazolam.

d. If diazepam was administered, a much lower dose than usual should be given and slower recovery would be expected.

e. These will be decreased albumin and α_1-acid glycoprotein in the plasma; therefore, less protein binding of propranolol can occur and there will be more free drug in blood, leading to an increased response. Decreased first-pass metabolism means that bioavailability will increase from about 30% up to 70–80%. This is because of decreased cytochrome P450 activity and increased portocaval shunting of blood. The elimination half-life is independent of bioavailability but it will be longer because of reduced cytochrome P450.

f. Colestyramine is a non-absorbed anion exchange resin that adsorbs bile acids in gastrointestinal lumen. In liver cirrhosis, fibrosis reduces outflow from bile cannaliculi and there is decreased bile flow. This leads to a build-up of bile salts in blood and deposition in the skin, which causes itching. Adsorption of bile salts in the gut by colestyramine lowers blood bile salts by reducing enterohepatic circulation. Lactulose is used to modify the gut flora. A possible cause of encephalopathy is the failure of the liver to detoxify bacterial products formed in the large bowel. (Encephalopathy is more common during constipation.) Possible bacteria metabolites of importance are ammonia and tyramine. Lactulose is not absorbed in upper gastroinestinal tract but is fermented in lower bowel; the metabolic product (Ch. 35) lowers lumen pH and may act by altering the microbial metabolism, with decreased formation of ammonia and tyramine. It also prevents constipation.

g. Analgesia in cirrhosis is a problem, and there is no ideal answer. Opioids should usually be avoided because of risk of encephalopathy but reduced doses could be given. NSAIDs are best avoided, to reduce the risk of haemorrhage from oesophageal varices. Paracetamol is a possible risk because it is hepatotoxic: however, it is well tolerated in people with cirrhosis, probably because the decreases in effective perfusion of hepatocytes and reduced activity of cytochrome P450 outweigh the decrease in conjugation with glucuronic acid, sulfate and glutathione.

Chapter 37

1. **True**. This is the expert advice given by NICE.

2. **True**.

3. **False**. Sibutramine inhibits the reuptake of released noradrenaline.

4. **False**. The hypothalamus controls appetite, and naturally occuring appetite suppressants and stimulants have been identified.

5. **False**. Leptin is produced in adipose tissue and reduces the production of the appetite-stimulant neurotransmitter neuropeptide Y.

6. Answers **B**.

   A. Depression and other psychosocial problems have been shown to be associated with obesity in some people.
   B. This is the expert advice given to prescribers in the British National Formulary.
   C. Combination therapy with more than one anti-obesity drug is contraindicated.
   D. Sibutramine can cause headaches, hypertension and other unwanted effects, and blood pressure should be monitored.
   E. Orlistat inhibits pancreatic lipase in the gut, reducing triglyceride absorption.

Chapter 38

1. a. **True**.
   b. **True**. Ciclosporin is nephrotoxic.

2. **True**. This enhances the formation of anti-inflammatory proteins by actions in the nucleus; a corticosteroid-sparing effect is possible.

3. **True**. Azathioprine has a toxic action on cells and proliferation of antibody-producing cells is inhibited. Proliferation of cells involved in cell-mediated immunity is also inhibited.

4. Answer **A**.

   A. Glucocorticoids decrease the expression of genes involved in the production of some inflammatory mediators.
   B. Glucocorticoids inhibit the production of leukotrienes.
   C. Glucocorticoids can cause increased blood sugar levels.

D. Glucocorticoids will inhibit growth in children.

E. Glucocorticoids inhibit macrophage activation in delayed hypersensitivity.

5. Case history answers

a. Basiliximab given before and 4 days after surgery has been shown to reduce acute rejection by 35%. Reduction of acute rejection is also achieved with combination therapy and corticosteroids; a calcineurin inhibitor such as ciclosporin and an antiproliferative immunosuppressant such as azathioprine can be used. When used in combination, lower doses of the drugs can be administered than when giving the drugs alone. Intensive monitoring of liver and renal functions are important.

b. Oversuppression of the immune response brings with it problems of opportunistic infections associated with reduced immunity. Additional 'steroid effects' as described for iatrogenic Cushing's-like syndrome may be apparent.

Chapter 39

1. a. **False**. The parent drug, terfenadine, is associated with ventricular arrhythmias in high doses. Fexofenadine retains the parent drug's antihistamine activity without having unwanted effects on the heart.

   b. **False**. The histamine receptors on the parietal cell are H_2 subtype and are not affected by these antihistamines, which act on H_1 receptors. H_2 receptor antagonists such as cimetidine are used.

   c. **False**. Fexofenadine acts only on the H_1 receptors.

2. a. **False**. Nasal corticosteroids are very effective.

   b. **False**. Prostaglandins and leukotrienes can also be released from mast cells and contribute to symptoms.

3. Answer **D**.

   A. In atopy there is a predominance of a Th2 response profile which is partially genetically determined.

   B. The Th2 response leads to increased production of IgE.

   C. Mast cell degranulate following allergen cross-linking of IgE on mast cells.

   D. Although the main effect of histamine in allergy is on the H_1 receptor, actions on H_2 receptors also contribute to the allergic symptoms.

   E. Leukotriene synthesis in mast cells increases, contributing to the allergic response.

4. Answer **B**.

   A. First-generation drugs such as promethazine are more sedating than second-generation drugs such as fexofenadine.

   B. **True.**

   C. Antihistamines can be effective in motion sickness but not vomiting caused by cancer chemotherapeutic agents.

   D. Second-generation antihistamines cross the blood–brain barrier less readily than the first-generation antihistamines.

   E. Antihistamines reduce vasodilation induced by the action of histamine at the H_1 receptor which contributes to the wheal and flare response.

5. Case study answers

   a. The family history of atopy and the child's atopic dermatitis as an infant increase the likelihood that he would have had allergies. He is likely to have had seasonal allergic rhinitis but he may also have had sensitisation to cat and/or dust mite or other allergens. His fitness and lack of current drug intake suggest that it is not non-allergic rhinitis, which may arise because of infections, drugs etc.

   b. Yes. As many as 50% of children older than 3 years with recurrent otitis media have confirmed allergic rhinitis.

   c. It was important to carry out sensitivity testing, and sensitivity to cat dander and house-dust mite was identified in this boy. Avoidance of exposure to allergens is advisable and should be actively pursued in the home and school environment. If pharmacological treatment is required, a non-sedating oral antihistamine should reduce rhinorrhoea, sneezing and itching but will have little effect on nasal congestion. A short course of nasal inhaled corticosteroids can be effective in controlling symptoms of allergic rhinitis, including congestion. Nasal cromoglicate may also offer symptom relief but is not preferred treatment.

Chapter 40

1. a. **False**. Glibenclamide stimulates insulin secretion from the beta cells of the islets and would be ineffective in the absence of any insulin-secreting ability.

   b. **True**. Sulphonylureas cause weight gain partly by stimulating appetite: metformin might be a better choice.

   c. **True**. Glibenclamide has a long duration of action and active metabolites can increase when renal

Self-assessment answers

function declines. Hypoglycaemia is a greater problem in the elderly.

2. **True**. These drugs act in part by different mechanisms. Additionally, metformin does not stimulate appetite, indeed, it may suppress appetite.

3. a. **True**. Neonates born to diabetic mothers who were taking oral hypoglycaemics in pregnancy have problems with hypoglycaemia.
   b. **True**. Sulphonylureas have some structural similarities to the sulphonamides and trimethoprim and can produce severe hypoglycaemia when given together.

4. **False**. Isophane insulin is complexed with protamine and has a duration of action of 20 h, whereas synthetic insulin lispro is modified structurally and has a faster onset of action and shorter duration.

5. Answer **A**.

   A. **True**. A trial of this for 3 months should be tried before suggesting other treatments.
   B. **False**. Treatment, support and advice should take place over many months.
   C. **False**. Sulphonylureas can stimulate appetite by increasing insulin secretion and causing further weight gain.
   D. **False**. NICE has advised (August 2003) that the use of a thizolidinedione (pioglitazone or rosiglitazone) as second-line therapy added to either metformin or a sulphonylurea is not recommended, except for: people who are unable to tolerate metformin and sulphonylurea combination therapy, or people in whom either metformin or a sulphonylurea is contraindicated; in such cases, the thiazolidinedione should replace whichever drug in the combination is poorly tolerated or contraindicated.
   E. **False**. Metformin has a cardioprotective effect which can only in part be explained by its effects on glucose and may be due to improvements in the lipid profile.

6. Case history answers

   a. Type 1.
   b. An upper respiratory infection can be all that is necessary to tip someone into ketoacidosis. Aggravating factors: candidiasis in the throat, overbreathing causing dryness.
   c. There is a familial tendency, although neither type 1 nor type 2 diabetes mellitus is a single gene disorder, so there is no classic pattern of inheritance.

   d. Once tubular maximum for glucose reabsorption in the kidneys is exceeded, the glucose in the distal tubules causes an osmotic diuresis, leading to polyuria, and then to thirst.
   e. Insulin, fluids and salts to correct dehydration, glucose levels, ketoacidosis and electrolyte imbalances. Ketoacidosis can lead to coma.
   f. A dietary regimen should be agreed to create a stable pattern of eating habits commensurate with his lifestyle. Diets low in animal fat and high in fibre are recommended, ideally with carbohydrate intake distributed throughout the day.
   g. Initiate a stable pattern of eating habit and activity, twice-daily subcutaneous insulin injections before breakfast and evening meal. The insulins would contain a mixture of short- and long-acting insulins, the ratios of which vary depending upon his glucose levels. Insulins frequently used are soluble insulin and isophane insulin.
   h. The time to onset of activity of neutral soluble insulin is 30 min, with peak activity at 1–3 h.
   i. The percentage of glycosylated haemoglobin can be measured. High concentrations are indicative of increased risk for microvascular and neuropathic complications.
   j. Newer, rapid-acting monomeric insulin lispro may be helpful. This has a time to onset of only 15 min and a time to peak plasma levels of 0.5–0.75 h. It should, therefore, be given immediately before a meal. A possible altered regimen may involve insulin lispro during the day with insulin isophane given in the evening. However, overall education about eating and lifestyle would probably provide greater benefit than a change of insulin regimen.

Chapter 41

1. a. **False**. T_3 and T_4 are largely bound to thyroxin-binding globulin (TBG).
   b. **True**. Thyroxine is cleared in about 6 days.
   c. **True**. The T_3–receptor complex activates transcription and protein synthesis.
   d. **False**. Iodine is converted to iodide and inhibits T_3 and T_4 release.

2. a. **True**.
   b. **True**. Levothyroxine is the standard treatment.
   c. **True**. Thyroxine has a very long half-life.

3. Answer **D**.

   A. The long half-life of T_4 (about 7 days) means that it takes 5–6 weeks to reduce thyroid hormone levels to normal.

B. The metabolite methimazole is the active component.

C. The Committee on Safety of Medicines warns that signs of bone marrow suppression should be watched for; these include symptoms and signs suggestive of infection, especially sore throat. A white blood cell count should be performed if there is any clinical evidence of infection. Carbimazole should be stopped promptly if there is clinical or laboratory evidence of neutropenia.

D. Carbimazole inhibits the action of thyroxine peroxidase.

E. Carbimazole accumulates in the thyroid and needs to be given only once a day.

4. Answer **B**.

A. If T_4 levels were low, then thyrotrophin levels would be raised, as the negative feedback effect of T_4 on thyrotrophin release would be reduced.

B. Normal treatment is with T_4 (levothyroxine).

C. The half-life of levothyroxine is 6–7 days; therefore, steady state would not be reached until 5–7 weeks of administration.

D. Special care is required, as a rapid increase in metabolic activity can cause excessive heart stimulation.

E. Levothyroxine stimulates oxygen consumption in metabolically active tissues.

5. Case history answers

a. An autoimmune disease in which antibodies to TSH are generated and bind to and activate TSH receptors on the thyroid, promoting thyroid hormone release.

b. TSH (thyrotrophin) levels could be measured. It will be low due to the negative feedback effect of elevated T_3 and T_4.

c. Bound T_3 and T_4 levels may be high due to increased binding capacity of binding proteins or increased levels of binding proteins rather than actual elevated levels of free T_3 and T_4.

d. Drugs of choice for controlling symptoms are β-adrenoceptor antagonists, although they do not improve fatigue and muscle weakness. Digoxin should be given for the atrial fibrillation (Ch. 8), and anticoagulation with warfarin to prevent thromboembolism, which has an increased incidence in people with atrial fibrilliation and thyrotoxicosis.

e. Carbimazole is the drug of choice, given in a high dose, then reducing over 4–6 weeks.

f. The clinical state should be stabilised with carbimazole and a β-adrenoceptor antagonist. Carbimazole is stopped 3–4 days before radioiodine is given, as it can prevent the uptake of iodine by thyroid cells.

g. It can take several months for maximum benefit of ^{131}I to occur.

Chapter 42

1. a. **False**. Vitamin D deficiency leads to hyperparathyroidism, which may assist in reducing the worst excesses of vitamin D deficiency. PTH increases calcitriol formation and calcitriol has a negative feedback effect on PTH.

b. **True**. Calcitonin reduces Ca^{2+} resorption and inhibits bone turnover.

c. **False**. Bisphosphonates inhibit bone dissolution, and effects occur slowly; plasma concentrations fall slowly, with a maximum effect after about a week.

2. a. **False**. Oestrogens inhibit the cytokines that recruit the bone-resorbing osteoclasts. Oestrogens also inhibit the actions of PTH.

b. **False**. Raloxifene has been licensed to reduce bone density loss in postmenopausal women. It is an oestrogen receptor stimulant selective for its actions on oestrogen receptors in bone and without stimulant effects on oestrogen receptors in breast and uterus.

3. Answer **B**.

A. Glucocorticoids can reduce the number of bone-froming cellular units (osteoclasts/osteoblasts), decrease calcium absorption even at low doses, increase renal calcium excretion, decrease gonadal hormone levels, and increase bone resoprtion.

B. Raloxifene is oestrogenic on bone but anti-oestrogenic on receptors in the breast and uterus.

C. Bisphosphonates reduces bone calcium mobilisation aned are particularly useful in corticosteroid-induced osteoporosis.

D. The anti-oestrogenic effects of raloxifene can result in hot flushes and thromboembolism in some women.

E. **True**.

4. Answer **D**.

A. Sunlight is involved in the formation of cholecalciferol in the skin, which is then converted to active vitamin D compounds in the liver and kidneys.

B. Ergocalciferol is hydroxylated in the kidney to calcitriol before it can exert its biological activity. In renal failure, if 1α-hydroxylase activity is defective, calcitriol may have to be substituted.

C. Because of the lack of vitamin D compounds, less calcium and phosphate will be absorbed from the gut.

D. Low levels of calcium and lack of vitamin D may result in higher levels of parathyroid hormone (secondary hyperparathyroidism).

E. Vitamin D promotes bone mineralisation laying down hydroxyapatite on the collagen organic matrix.

Chapter 43

1. a. **False**. Somatostatin is an inhibitor of GH release.
    b. **False**. Somatostatin is also produced from intestinal and pancreatic cells.
    c. **True**. Because dopamine is a stimulant of GH release in healthy individuals and bromocriptine is a dopamine receptor agonist.
    d. **True**. Octreotide is a long-acting analogue of somatostatin.

2. a. **True**. It can be used to improve fertility in women with high levels of prolactin.
    b. **False**. On continued administration, gonadotrophin receptors are downregulated and steroid synthesis declines.
    c. **False**. Gonadorelin will inhibit testosterone synthesis in prostate cancer and reduce the size of the prostate.
    d. **True**. Gonadorelin, a gonadotrophin analogue, reduces oestrogen synthesis, which inhibits endometriosis.
    e. **True**.

3. a. **True**. Vasopressin is a nonapeptide released from the hypothalamus.
    b. **False**. In nephrogenic diabetes insipidus, the kidney is unresponsive to vasopressin.
    c. **False**. Paradoxically, in diabetes insipidus, the response to thiazide diuretics is a reduction in polyuria.

4. Answer **A**.

    A. GH is released in a pulsatile manner and is high particularly during deep sleep in children.
    B. GH stimulates IGF-1 release from the liver; it then acts on receptors in many tissues and in concert with other hormones.
    C. Although in normal individuals dopamine and its analogues stimulate GH release, in acromegaly they paradoxically inhibit release.
    D. IGF-1 inhibits GH release and also stimulates somatostatin release from the hypothalamus, which further inhibits GH release.

E. GH is now obtained by recombinant DNA techniques to avoid transmission of Creutzfeldt–Jakob disease.

5. Answer **A**.

    A. GnRH is given in a pulsatile manner to stimulate FSH and LH release. If given continuously, there is soon a downregulation of gonadotrophin receptors and inhibition of gonadotrophin release.
    B. **True**. Given continuously, testosterone will be inhibited, although an initial stimulation of release may precede this. This effect is used to shrink prostate cancers.
    C. **True**. As mentioned in part A, gonadotropin secretion is inhibited by high-dose continuous GnRH.
    D. **True**. Early in the menstrual cycle, low levels of oestrogen inhibit gonadotrophin secretion.
    E. **True**. Downregulation of receptors is preceded by stimulation of gonadotrophin release.

6. Case history answers

    a. No. Epiphyseal closure occurs much later, so treatment at this age can dramatically increase height.
    b. Biosynthetic GH (somatropin) has a half-life of only 25 min and levels fluctuate widely. However, high protein binding of the IGF-1 that is released under the action of GH means that three injections a week are sufficient to maintain IGF-1 at required levels.
    c. Insulin-like effects can produce hypoglycaemia and there is pain at the site of injection. Headache and oedema can also occur.

Chapter 44

1. a. **False**. Fludrocortisone is a synthetic mineralocorticoid with a salt-retaining: anti-inflammatory ratio of about 12.5:1. The glucocorticoid prednisolone should be used orally.
    b. **True**. Beclometasone is used by inhalation for its local effects on the airways in the treatment of asthma.

2. a. **False**. Corticosteroids lead to reduced tissue uptake of glucose and increased gluconeogenesis, leading to 'steroid diabetes'.
    b. **True**. After prolonged administration it is possible that the hypothalamic–pituitary–adrenal axis (both secretion of CRF and ACTH) will be suppressed (Fig. 44.3), i.e. endogenous cortisol levels are low. Slow withdrawal allows the adrenals to recover their normal cortisol secretion and avoids corticosteroid deficiency.

3. a. **False**. Reduced plasma sodium results in stimulation of renin secretion, which is converted to angiotensin II. This then stimulates aldosterone release from the adrenal cortex, which acts to increase Na^+ reabsorption in the distal part of the distal tubule.

b. **True**. ACTH stimulates both cortisol and aldosterone secretion by the adrenal cortex.

4. a. **False**. Dexamethasone can inhibit vomiting and will add to the antiemetic actions of agents such as ondansetron in vomiting caused by cancer chemotherapy (Ch. 32).

b. **True**. Because of their catabolic effect on proteins, they delay the healing of wounds.

c. **True**. Immunosuppressive effects of glucocorticoids can exacerbate an underlying infection.

5. Case history 1 answers

a.
  (i) A tumour of the adrenal cortex secreting cortisol.
  (ii) Excess secretion of ACTH by a pituitary tumour.
  (iii) Excess secretion of ACTH by a non-pituitary tumour (commonly small-cell carcinoma of the lung, medullary or thyroid carcinoma).
  (iv) Iatrogenic, from therapeutic administration of glucocorticoids or ACTH.

b. The cause could not be a primary cortisol-secreting adrenocortical tumour or glucocorticoid administration, as the ACTH levels would be low due to negative feedback of glucocorticoid on the anterior pituitary and hypothalamus. The possibility is an ACTH-secreting pituitary adenoma or ACTH-secreting non-pituitary tumour.

c. The dexamethasone suppression test is not definitive; it can suppress ACTH of pituitary origin but not from ectopic ACTH-producing tumours or adrenocortical tumours.

d. Control by inhibitors of adrenal corticosteroid synthesis, e.g. trilostane or metyrapone. (Note: she would probably also be showing signs of excess mineralocorticoid activity, which should also be treated in parallel with spironolactone.)

6. Case history 2 answers

a. Beclometasone, budesonide and fluticasone are all available for inhalation. They are systemically absorbed, but, with low doses, amounts reaching the systemic circulation are insufficient to have significant systemically mediated effects. This does not apply with high doses, where systemic unwanted effects may sometimes be evident.

b. Although systemic unwanted effects may be few with low doses, local problems such as oral candidiasis or other fungal infections may arise, but this could be managed with a spacer and good oral hygiene. High doses may lead to iatrogenic Cushing-like symptoms (see below).

c. Hydrocortisone intravenously. This is a lipid-soluble corticosteroid; giving it intravenously would minimise the time to onset of action, which can still, however, take hours. The objective is to reduce both the acute and chronic inflammation accompanying this acute exacerbation of asthma.

d. Oral prednisolone is often used.

e. A short course of high-dose prednisolone would be given and then gradually tail off the dose over the following 1–2 weeks in order to allow the return of normal hypothalamic–pituitary–adrenal axis function, which may have been suppressed by the high-dose prednisolone.

f. Systemic unwanted effects are less with inhaled corticosteroids than with oral corticosteroids.

g. A high concentration of drug is needed at target cells, and poor technique, inflammation, mucus, etc. might prevent inhaled drugs reaching their target. Systemic prednisolone following oral administration reaches the target cells more effectively than following inhalation of a corticosteroid.

h. For long-term oral treatment, use the lowest possible dose of corticosteroid to prevent unwanted effects. The dose may vary with the severity of the asthma. Therefore, monitor peak expiratory flow rate (usually done at home each morning). Relatively frequent dose adjustments may be needed.

i. Corticosteroids have a wide range of metabolic effects in addition to their anti-inflammatory and immunomodulatory actions. The cushingoid symptoms described can all be attributed to actions on carbohydrate, protein and lipid metabolism and suppression of the hypothalamic–pituitary–adrenal axis.

Chapter 45

1. a. **False**. Until the late part of the follicular phase, oestrogens do have a negative feedback effect, but at a level of approximately 200 pg ml^{-1} oestradiol, there is a switch to positive feedback and the mid-cycle LH and FSH surge results.

b. **True**. Although the LH levels fall precipitously after the mid-cycle surge, they are high enough to support the secretion of progesterone.

2. a. **False**. The inhibition of ovulation is seen in between 25% and 40% of women. In women given medroxyprogesterone acetate by injection, however, the percentage in whom inhibition of ovulation occurs is almost 100%.

b. **False**. Progesterone inhibits the motility of the fallopian tube, whereas oestrogens have the opposite action. An imbalance of either may alter the chances of fertilisation and implantation.

c. **True**. Removal of the corpus luteum before 6–8 weeks of pregnancy results in abortion, whereas after that time the placental production of steroids under the influence of HCG is sufficient to maintain the pregnancy.

3. a. **False**. Although the progestogens in the second-generation pills have variable androgenic activity, the progestogens gestodene and desogestrel have weak or no androgenic activity.

b. **False**. Although there are some small variations, overall the biphasic and triphasic patterns of application mimic more closely the steroidal changes in the menstrual cycle. However, they do not reduce the steroid load overall.

c. **False**. The fact that ethinylestradiol undergoes enterohepatic cycling serves to maintain plasma concentrations.

d. **False**. With the progesterone-only contraceptive, if there is a delay of only 3 h or more after the normal time of taking the pill, then contraceptive protection may be reduced.

4. **True**. By inducing liver microsomal enzymes, the effective concentrations may be reduced as metabolism is enhanced.

5. a. **True**. The excess risk of thromboembolic disease in women taking the combined contraceptive pill is significantly greater in those who smoke over the age of 35 years.

b. **True**. However, there is little evidence for a lesser effect of the third-generation progestogens on carbohydrate metabolism when compared with second-generation progestogens such as levonorgestrel.

6. a. **False**. Particularly in the first 6 months of treatment, breakthrough bleeding frequently occurs.

b. **True**. Both sex steroids undergo first-pass metabolism and this can be avoided by absorption through the skin.

c. **True**. Raloxifene stimulates oestrogen receptors in bone and liver but not breast and reproductive tissue.

d. **True**. Tibolone has weak oestrogenic and progestogenic activity and has been shown to reduce bone loss.

7. a. **False**. Oxytocin is less effective in earlier pregnancy compared with term. In this case it is probable that an intravaginal pessary of prostaglandin would be used, as this causes uterine contractility and also softens the cervix. This may be followed by oxytocin.

b. **False**. Oestrogens increase the gap junctions in the uterus, thus facilitating the transmission of the uterine contractility from the fundal region through the body of the uterus. Progesterone prevents the action of oestrogens.

c. **False**. The source of the prostaglandins during labour is the uterine amnion membranes and the decidua.

8. a. **False**. In some women, uterine hypertonus occurs with the administration of prostaglandins.

b. **False**. Ergometrine is given alone or together with oxytocin at the time of delivery to reduce postpartum haemorrhage. It should not be given for labour induction.

9. **False**. The reason is not known but the combined oral contraceptive does relieve dysmenorrhoea in some women.

10. **True**. Magnesium sulfate inhibits Ca^{2+} availability and uterine contractility and can delay pre term delivery for a short period of time.

11. Answer **D**.

A. In a woman of 35 years of age who smokes, it has been shown that the combined oral contraceptive results in a significant increase in cardiovascular complications. It would therefore not be a good choice.

B. The combined contraceptive pill reduces the risk of endometrial cancer.

C. The IUCD is as effective as the oral contraceptive.

D. The increase in risk of thromboembolic complications is related to the oestrogen content of the pill.

E. Medroxyprogesterone acetate given intramuscularly is effective for 8–12 weeks.

12. Answer **C**.

A. Mifepristone is a progesterone receptor antagonist; inhibition of the actions of progesterone results in abortion, although the precise mechanisms are uncertain.

B. Expert advice is that all women with intact membranes should be initially administered intravaginal prostaglandins to soften the cervix prior to rupture of the membranes, giving intravenous oxytocin if required.

C. **False,** as both oxytocin and prostaglandins can cause uterine hypertonus and potentially fetal anoxia if given in inappropriate amounts.

D. Although β_2-adrenoceptor agonists may delay labour for 48 h, overall they have not been shown to decrease morbidity or mortality in the preterm newborn child.

E. **True,** it can also cause uterine hypertonus, reducing uterine blood loss postpartum.

Chapter 46

1. a. **True.** Testosterone is well absorbed orally but degraded by first-pass metabolism to inactive metabolites.

   b. **True.** Other treatments are required, including the administration of HCG and other gonadotrophins.

   c. **True.** Nandrolone has fewer androgenic effects than testosterone, but has many other unwanted effects.

2. **True.**

3. Answer **D.**

   A. 5α-Reductase converts testosterone to the active dehydrotestosterone.

   B. Cyproterone is an antiandrogen; it inhibits spermatogenesis and is used as a form of chemical castration.

   C. Nandrolone is an androgen and promotes an increase in muscle mass.

   D. Danazol has antiandrogen, anti-oestrogen and antiprogesterone activity and is used in treatment of endometriosis.

   E. Testosterone is markedly anabolic, increasing turnover and growth in many tissues and cells.

Chapter 47

1. a. **False.** Vitamin B_{12} is absorbed with the aid of intrinsic factor in the distal ileum.

   b. **True.** It is given by intramuscular injection every 2–3 months for life.

   c. **True.** Macrocytes (large red cells) are seen.

2. a. **True.**

   b. **True.** Methotrexate, trimethoprim and phenytoin inhibit the enzymes that convert folic acid to dihydrofolate in the DNA synthesis pathway.

   c. **False.** Folic acid is given daily orally for up to 4 months to replenish stores.

3. **True.** The main cause of erythropoietin deficiency is renal failure.

4. **False.** CSFs are used to enhance blood cell development, for example where damage to cell-producing systems has occurred due to cytotoxic drugs.

5. Answer B.

   A. The kidneys are the main producers of erythropoetin.

   B. Anaemia associated with renal disease is commonly treated with erythropoetin.

   C. Adequate iron stores are necessary for erythropoetin to be successful.

   D. Erythropoetin is sometimes abused by athletes to increase their red cell count and enhance performance.

   E. It is inactive orally and must be given by intravenous or subcutaneous routes.

6. Answer **C.**

   A. Tetrahydrofolate is utilised in the synthesis of the purine and pyrimidine bases in DNA.

   B. Treatment is required for 4 months to correct deficiences and replenish stores.

   C. Folate is absorbed in the proximal jejunum, and absorption is deficient in coeliac disease.

   D. Methotreaxate inhibits dihydrofolate reductase which converts dihydrofolate to tetrahydrofolate. Giving folinic acid (synthetic tetrahydrofolate) bypasses this block.

   E. **True.**

7. Case history answers

   a. The haemoglobin was low; it was less than 115 g l⁻¹ and in a woman this indicates anaemia. The MCV was 61 fl (normal 76–96). The common cause for low MCV is iron-deficiency anaemia. Iron-deficiency anaemia is common in menstruating women. The other common cause is gastrointestinal bleeding, including haemorrhoids.

   b. Serum ferritin should be low and iron-binding capacity elevated.

   c. Oral ferrous salts (e.g. sulphate, the form most easily absorbed).

   d. Gastrointestinal distension and loose bowel movements are common.

   e. From the duodenum and upper jejunum.

   f. It is optimally absorbed as haem.

   g. No. The rise in haemoglobin should be about 10 g l⁻¹ each week.

   h. Lack of compliance; continued bleeding, malabsorption.

   i. Intramuscular iron sorbitol injection. 10–20 injections required over 2–3 weeks.

Self-assessment answers

Chapter 48

1. a. **False**. The relationship is between high LDL cholesterol and coronary risk of atherosclerosis. High LDL cholesterol is associated with lipid peroxidation, take-up into macrophages and formation of fatty streaks.
   b. **True**. One in 500 of the population has a single recessive gene disorder causing reduced synthesis of LDL receptors.
   c. **False**. The resins sequester bile acids that contain cholesterol. This decreases absorption of ingested cholesterol and also increases bile acid–cholesterol synthesis in liver, leading to further elimination of cholesterol.

2. a. **False**. Reducing cholesterol synthesis results in increased LDL receptors in the liver and hence increased LDL clearance from plasma.
   b. **False**. Serum LDL cholesterol falls by 20–35%.
   c. **False**. The two classes of drugs act by different mechanisms and act synergistically. The combination of two drugs can be used where the response to the statins is inadequate.

3. Answer **A**.

   A. The outer coat is phospholid; cholesterol and triglycerides together with the phospolipid and apoliprotein constituents comprise a structure to carry the water-insoluble lipids in plasma.
   B. VLDL carries 20% cholesterol, whereas HDL has 40%.
   C. Increasing concentrations of statin reduce cholesterol dose-dependently.
   D. Cholesterol has a negative feedback effect on cholesterol synthesis.
   E. Fibrates act to enhance liver uptake of LDL.

4. Case history answers

   a. General advice would include avoidance of smoking, and have a low-fat diet and take exercise. Determine if there are problems of obesity, diabetes or hypertension. Consider the use of aspirin where appropriate.
   b. A statin would be recommended as first-choice drug in preventing cardiovascular events in peoples at increased risk. This man is at increased risk. Statins are of proven benefit using data from extensive investigations; they are also well tolerated (see f).
   c. The reduction would depend upon dosage of statins, but a reduction in the region of 25% should be aimed for. This could take more than a month to achieve.
   d. Statins inhibit HMG-CoA reductase and increase LDL receptors (Fig. 48.1).
   e. The target total cholesterol recommended is 5 mmol l^{-1} and an LDL cholesterol concentration of less than 3 mmol l^{-1}.
   f. Gastrointestinal upsets. Use of statins is not recommended in people with liver disease or in pregnancy. Liver function tests need to be performed.
   g. In addition to the statins, use fibrates, ezetimibe or anion-exchange resins. Because the sites of action are different to those of the statins, an additive effect should be expected.
   h. Fibrates decrease VLDL production, increase hepatic LDL uptake and stimulate lipoprotein lipase. Ezetimibe is a specific cholesterol absorption inhibitor. Anion-exchange resins sequester bile acids in the intestine and reduce cholesterol uptake.

Chapter 49

1. a. **False**. Topical corticosteroids (e.g. hydrocortisone cream) are the mainstay of treatment of atopic dermatitis, used for up to 4 weeks.
   b. **True**. One of the sedative antihistamines (e.g. promethazine) may be of value, although direct effect on itching may be limited. Topical antihistamines and topical doxepin (an antidepressant) are also available.

2. a. **False**. In severe psoriasis, ciclosporin or methotrexate can be used.
   b. **True**. Oral retinoids such as vitamin A and derivatives reduce cell growth and can be used in psoriasis, but they can be teratogenic. Oral and topical retinoids are also useful in acne.

3. a. **True**.
   b. **False**. Resistance is increasing. There is cross-resistance between erythromycin and clindamycin, and, when possible, non-antibiotic antibacterials (benzoyl peroxide or azelaic acid) should be used.

4. Answer **D**.

   A. **False.** β-Adrenoceptor antagonists can exacerbate psoriasis.
   B. **False**. Regular short daily exposure doses of sunlight may benefit psoriasis. It increases production of vitamin D in the skin and ultraviolet rays fight psoriasis by slowing down the rapid proliferation of the skin cells. Sunburn should be avoided. Ultraviolet exposure is a treatment for psoriasis.

C. **False**. Methotrexate can produce bone marrow depression and hepatoxicity and regular monitoring is required.

D. **True**. Calcipotriol has several beneficial actions, including inhibition of T-cell proliferation and the release of inflammatory cytokines.

E. **False**. Etanercept and infliximab have been shown to be of benefit in treatment of resistant psoriasis.

5. Case history answers

a. Atopic dermatitis is possible because of the appearance of the rash and the child's atopy and the previous history of her mother.

b. The following are the initial management approaches:

- good skin hygiene with regular bathing but avoidance of soaps
- emollients in bath water and topically applied to moisturise the skin and reduce water loss
- short courses of topically applied hydrocortisone as the mainstay of treatment
- if necessary, topically applied antihistamine or oral sedative antihistamine if the itch is severe, although there is not a consensus that antihistamines are beneficial; topical doxepin may also help reduce itch.

c. Assessment of contributory factors such as food allergies and other allergens, psychological factors and removal of irritants and allergens. Severe acute exacerbations may require rigorous topical measures and antibacterial treatment.

Chapter 50

1. a. **False**. Adrenaline (epinephrine) may cause mydriasis, which serves to narrow even further the angle between the iris and the cornea.

b. **True**.

c. **True**. Tropicamide blocks the muscarinic receptors in the circular muscle of the iris, causing mydriasis, which narrows the anterior angle and may reduce aqueous draining in angle-closure glaucoma.

2. a. **False**. Cocaine causes mydriasis as well as having a local anaesthetic effect. It prevents the reuptake of released noradrenaline, which contracts the radial muscle, narrowing the drainage angle.

b. **True**. Cyclopentolate acts for 12–24 h, whereas tropicamide has a duration of action of about 3 h.

c. **True**. Pilocarpine is a muscarinic receptor stimulant; it contracts the ciliary muscle, causing

the lens to shorten and bulge and accommodate for near vision.

3. Extended-mtching answers

1. Answer **G**. A β-adrenoceptor antagonist such as timolol reduces aqueous production but does not affect the pupil size, which is controlled by muscarinic and α_1-adrenergic receptors on the circular and radial muscles, respectively, of the iris.

2. Answer **C**. A selective α_2-adrenoceptor agonist such as aproclonidine reduces aqueous production but does not affect the pupil size, which is controlled by muscarinic and α_1-adrenergic receptors on the circular and radial muscles, respectively, of the iris.

3. Answer **D** and **A**. Phenylephrine will dilate the pupil (α_1-adrenoceptor stimulation of the iris) but not the ciliary muscle (muscarinic receptors). Cocaine will also dilate the pupil by preventing reuptake of released noradrenaline.

4. Answer **F**. Tropicamide is a relatively short-acting muscarinic antagonist with only a relatively weak blocking action on muscarinic receptors on the ciliary muscle. Atropine is very long-acting.

5. Answer **H**. Atropine is a long-acting mydriatic that can be used to prevent adhesions but has a marked effect to block accommodation for near vision (cycloplegia).

4. Case history answers

a. Reduced drainage of aqueous humour through the trabecular meshwork into the canal of Schlemm and the episcleral veins.

b. Beta-adrenoceptor antagonists are the drugs of first choice. α_2-adrenoceptor stimulants, prostaglandin analogues, inhibitors of carbonic anhydrase enzymes and muscarinic agonists could also be used.

c. Beta-adrenoceptor antagonists: avoid if asthma, bradycardia, heart block, heart failure. Alpha$_2$-stimulants: avoid if severe cardiovascular disease. Muscarinic agonists: avoid if conjuctival or corneal damage, cardiac disease, asthma. Carbonic anhydrase inhibitors: can cause hypokalaemia and electrolyte imbalance. They should be avoided in pregnancy. Prostaglandin F_2-analogue: avoid in pregnancy and asthma.

Chapter 51

1. a. **True**. Benzylpenicillin is actively secreted into the proximal tubule. This can be inhibited by probenecid or by other drugs that use the same secretory mechanism, such as aspirin.

b. **False**. Broad-spectrum penicillins in particular can cause diarrhoea.

c. **False**. Azlocillin is broken down by β-lactamase.

d. **False**. Penicillins bind to penicillin-binding proteins and disrupt cell membrane peptidoglycans.

2. a. **True**. Cefotaxime is a third-generation cephalosporin antibacterial that penetrates the CNS and is resistant to β-lactamases.

b. **False**. But cephalosporins should be given carefully. Between 8% and 16% of patients who are allergic to penicillins will exhibit allergy to cephalosporins.

3. a. **True**. Imipenem is rapidly metabolised by dihydropeptidases in the kidney and is given in combination with cilastin, which inhibits the metabolising enzyme.

b. **False**. Like all β-lactams given in correct doses, imipenem is bactericidal.

4. a. **True**. The quinolones have good activity against *Pseudomonas* species.

b. **False**. Ciprofloxacin inhibits the hepatic metabolism of theophylline and can increase its toxicity.

5. a. **True**. Erythromycin often causes nausea and diarrhoea. Azithromycin is better tolerated.

b. **False**. Gentamicin is nephrotoxic and ototoxic, and its plasma levels should be monitored.

c. **True**. Gentamicin is poorly absorbed from the gastrointestinal tract and is given parenterally.

6. a. **True**. Most sore throats are caused by viruses; those with bacterial causes usually resolve without antibacterials. The selection of increasingly resistant organisms relates to unnecessary use of antibiotics.

b. **True**. Tetracyclines can chelate with Ca^{2+} and form permanent yellow–brown deposits on developing teeth.

c. **True**. It is reserved for MRSA and metronidazole-resistant *Clostridium difficile*, which causes pseudomembranous colitis.

7. a. **True**. Rifampicin is a broad-spectrum antibiotic and can be utilised in some serious diseases caused by Gram-negative bacteria such as *Legionella* and mycobacteria and also for MRSA.

b. **False**. Isoniazid has a highly selective action to inhibit the production of mycolic acids, which are unique to the cell wall of *Mycobacterium* species.

c. **False**. There is a high degree of resistance to co-trimoxazole in the bacteria causing hospital urinary tract infections.

d. **True**. Trimethoprim inhibits the conversion of folate to products used in the construction of DNA. Deficiency can result in megaloblastic anaemia and this can be prevented by giving additional folinic acid.

8. **Case history 1 answers**

a. The most common cause of community-acquired infection is *Streptococcus pneumoniae*, but other 'atypical' organisms could be involved. In JW, who was previously well, a recent stay in a hotel abroad might indicate the involvement of *Legionella*, which multiplies in warm water, for example in the tanks of air-conditioning systems. (The incubation time is 5–10 days.) Co-amoxiclav (amoxicillin + clavulanic acid) plus erythromycin or another macrolide should be given before the diagnosis is confirmed. If his condition is severe, rifampicin should also be given. The treatment should be reviewed immediately the microbiology sensitivities are known.

b. Amoxicillin is bactericidal and acts by interfering with bacterial cell wall peptidoglycan synthesis. It also allows greater activity of enzymes that lyse bacterial cells. Clavulanic acid inhibits β-lactamase, thus extending the spectrum of activity of amoxicillin. Erythomycin inhibits bacterial protein synthesis by acting on the bacterial ribosome. Rifampicin, perhaps better known for its role in treating tuberculosis, inhibits DNA-dependent RNA polymerase in many Gram-positive and Gram-negative bacteria.

9. **Case history 2 answers**

a. *Staphylococcus aureus* is a likely cause of acute pneumonia following an attack of influenza. Although the treatment must be guided by the sensitivity tests, most *S. aureus* strains are sensitive to flucloxacillin and this is the most appropriate antibiotic to start with. In the circumstances, it may be combined with fusidic acid or gentamicin. *S. aureus* commonly produces abscesses in the lungs. Pulmonary infection with *S. aureus* may also occur in people with cystic fibrosis. A Gram stain of the sputum demonstrates Gram-positive cocci in clusters – typical of staphylococci. The production of coagulase and DNAase identifies the organism as *S. aureus*. Many different species of coagulase-negative staphylococci exist and are found as part of the normal skin flora. The coagulase-negative staphylococci are typical causes of prosthetic valve endocarditis, joint prostheses and infected venous catheters. Of concern is the large number of antibiotic-resistant staphylococci (MRSA), which pose a threat to people who are frail or immunocompromised.

b. A range of other second-choice antibacterials effective against β-lactamase-producing *S. aureus* might be useful. For example, fusidic acid, gentamicin, a cephalosporin, a quinolone or erythromycin may be effective. There are increasing concerns about MRSA. Vancomycin is a glycopeptide. It is bactericidal and acts by inhibiting cell wall synthesis. It is effective against some MRSA. A new group of drugs, the streptogramins, have recently become available, and quinupristin with dalfopristin is effective against MRSA.

10. Case history 3 answers

   a. Clinically, the man is likely to have *Pneumocystis carinii* pneumonia (PCP), which is the predominant respiratory illness in people with AIDS. This organism, which is a protozoan, is believed to be acquired at a young age and reactivates with waning immunity. The organism is endemic in the community and multiplies within the lungs and causes symptoms. There is often a seasonal prevalence of PCP. Symptoms can be scant, and, if present, consist of breathlessness and cough. Induced sputum or bronchoalveolar lavage specimens should be sent to laboratory for detection of PCP and routine culture.

   b. PCP can be detected in sputum or lavage by staining with methenamine silver stain for typical casts. It can also be detected by use of the polymerase chain reaction, and on lung biopsy.

   c. The treatment of choice is high-dose co-trimoxazole. Many people with AIDS have hypersensitivity reactions to sulphonamides and are on multiple drug combinations. Alternative treatments for PCP are aerosolised or parenteral pentamidine, dapsone and trimethoprim, primaquine, etc.

   d. Long-term treatment with corticosteroids or other immunosuppressives.

   e. After an attack of PCP, a prophylactic regimen should be taken, for example nebulised pentamidine or oral trimethoprim 3 days per week.

11. Case history 4 answers

   a. *Salmonella, Shigella, Proteus* and *Pseudomonas* species are non-lactose fermenting and produce pale-coloured colonies on this medium. All were contenders. (The last three were excluded on biochemical screening. *S. enteritidis* phage type 4 was eventually identified.)

   b. Antibacterials have *no* role to play in the management of the majority of cases of *Salmonella* gastroenteritis. Exceptions are if the gastroenteritis occurs in an individual who is immunocompromised or if there is evidence of systemic invasion. Ciprofloxacin would be the antibiotic of choice; it can be given orally and is cheaper than intravenous preparations. Dehydration and electrolyte imbalance should be corrected by fluid replacement. Control of the diarrhoea by antidiarrhoeal drugs is contraindicated because of the risk of inducing paralytic ileus and causing septicaemia.

   c. Food poisoning, as this case would seem to be from the history, is a notifiable condition and should be reported to the consultant in Communicable Disease Control. Because the man has attended a convention, it is very likely that this is part of an outbreak and all persons attending the convention should be contacted to find out if they have been symptomatic and to collect faecal specimens for culture. Specimens of food, if still available, should also be collected for culture. (*S. enteritidis* phage type 4 has been epidemiologically linked to the use of contaminated hens' eggs.)

Chapter 52

1. The criteria for combination therapy in cancer treatment are:

   ● each drug should be active as a single agent (ethics of clinical trials means that new drugs are not usually tested for this criterion in clinical studies)
   ● each drug should have a different target within the cell (increases cell kill and decreases drug resistance)
   ● each drug should show different unwanted effects (ideally this will give additivity for effect [previous criteria] but not of toxicity, and hence an increase in therapeutic index.)

   For each of the three drug regimens, the first criterion can be assumed to be met because all the agents are well-used drugs. Table A1 summarises the sites of action and side-effects of the drugs in each regimen. As can be seen, all three use drugs that have different actions, although regimen (c) is targeted only at DNA function. Regimen (b) contains drugs that all have bone marrow toxicity. This will need careful monitoring during therapy.

2. Because many of the drugs used in cancer therapy have a therapeutic index of 1 (i.e. toxic dose is the therapeutic dose), it is important to tailor the dosage

Table A1
Effects of three treatment regimens

	Site of action	Principal toxicity
(a) Acute lymphoblastic leukaemia		
Vincristine	Binds to tubulin/metaphase arrest	BMS + peripheral neuropathy
Asparaginase	Depletes asparagine in blood	↓ Clotting factors/insulin/albumin
Prednisolone	DNA transcription of cytokines (etc.)	Steroid actions
(b) Hodgkin's lymphoma (MOPP regimen)		
Chlormethine	Alkylates DNA	BMS + nausea/vomiting
Vincristine	Binds to tubulin/metaphase arrest	BMS + peripheral neuropathy
Procarbazine	Inhibits synthesis of DNA, RNA and protein	BMS + nausea
Prednisolone	DNA transcription of cytokines (etc.)	Steroid action; therefore monitor BMS + toxicity
(c) Testicular teratoma		
Etoposide	↑ DNA cleavage by topoisomerase II	BMS, nausea, alopecia
Bleomycin	Oxidative damage to DNA	Pulmonary fibrosis 'allergy'
Cisplatin	Cross-links DNA	Nausea, BMS, nephrotoxicity, ototoxicity

BMS, bone marrow suppression.

to the individual patient. Children have a higher cardiac output and greater hepatic and renal blood flows than adults on a bodyweight basis. (Such parameters are related to bodyweight to the power 0.65–0.75 [$W^{0.7}$].) Therefore, the clearance of drugs tends to be faster in children than in adults and a proportional higher dose is necessary to give the same blood levels. Surface area also correlates to $W^{0.7}$; therefore, it is usual to correct the doses to surface area (calculated by the formula given or by nomogram). For example, if an adult male (W = 72.1 kg) is given 100 mg of a drug, how much would you give a 1-year-old child (W = 9.9 kg)? Simple correction for W would suggest 13.7 mg (100 × 9.9/72.1), but correction for surface area using a nomogram would give 23.2 mg (100 × 0.434/1.874). If the relation to $W^{0.7}$ was used, the calculated dose would be $100 \times 9.9^{0.7}/72.1^{0.7}$ = 100 × 4.98/19.98 = 24.9 mg. Interestingly, this goes against what you may have assumed, i.e. that children would be 'more sensitive' and be given lower doses. The organs of elimination are essentially mature by about 6–9 months of age.

Chapter 53

1. Case history answers

a. Initial features would be those of opioid overdosage caused by the codeine with possible symptoms of respiratory depression, pinpoint pupils, coma and cardiovascular collapse. The opioid antagonist naloxone is a rapid reversible antagonist of opioids at μ-, κ- and δ-receptors. It has a short half-life and may have to be given repeatedly. Naltrexone is an alternative opioid antagonist with a longer half-life than naloxone. Later developing symptoms of nausea, abdominal pain and sweating, and, if untreated, jaundice, are those owing to liver damage caused by the toxic metabolite of paracetamol.

b. *N*-Acetylcysteine is given, which conjugates with the hepatotoxic metabolite of paracetamol, and is most effective when given early after overdosage; the risk of liver damage is related to the time of ingestion before treatment and the plasma paracetamol concentrations. Alcohol consumption would increase the toxic effects of codeine and paracetamol. It enhances the central depressant actions of the opioid. Alcohol also induces cytochrome P450 enzymes, increasing formation of the toxic metabolite of paracetamol and causing toxicity at lower levels of paracetamol ingestion. The toxicity of paracetamol would also be increased by intake of drugs such as carbamazepine or rifampicin, which would enhance P450 metabolising enzymes and increase formation of the toxic metabolite.

c. Co-codamol also contains the opioid codeine together with paracetamol. The benefit of the opioid component of these compound analgesics is uncertain in comparison with giving paracetamol alone. Paracetamol with methionine could be considered as an alternative.

Chapter 54

1. a. **True**. Unlike the salt form of cocaine, the free base can be illicitly smoked.
   b. **True**. In the absence of sympathetic supply to the iris in Horner's syndrome, cocaine will not cause mydriasis.
   c. **False**. Acute actions are cardiac arrhythmias, and chronic use can lead to heart failure.
   d. **True**. In only a few days, tolerance develops to euphoria and appetite suppression.

2. a. **True**. Malignant hyperthermia is observed in some individuals after ingesting Ecstasy. This resembles heat stroke and dehydration.
   b. **True**. Like other amfetamines, Ecstasy has a short-term effect to suppress appetite.
   c. **False**. They produce increases in performance and are banned substances.

3. a. **False**. The euphoric effects last only 2–3 h.
   b. **False**. THC is used to inhibit nausea and vomiting in patients taking cytotoxic drugs.
   c. **True**. Cannabis acts on cannabinoid receptors in the brain and periphery. The natural ligand for these receptors is anandamide.

4. a. **False**. Tolerance develops rapidly.
   b. **True**. These effects are caused by stimulation of autonomic ganglia.
   c. **True**. Cotinine is stable and inactive, and can be measured.

   d. **False**. Nicotine patches and counselling are required.
   e. **False**. Irritability, sleep disturbances reduced psychomotor test performance occurs on giving up smoking.

5. a. **True**. The induction of enzymes can decrease the effectiveness of some drugs such as warfarin and phenytoin.
   b. **False**. Modest ethanol intake can increase high-density lipoprotein concentrations, which has cardiovascular protective effects. This is lost if consumption is greater than 3–4 units per day.
   c. **True**. Some individuals have a genetically determined variant of alcohol dehydrogenase that has reduced ability to metabolise ethanol. This incidence is low in Caucasians but high in some Asian races.

6. a. **False**. Acamprosate acts to reduce craving for alcohol and not by inhibiting its metabolism.
   b. **False**. Benzodiazepines or clomethiazole can attenuate withdrawal symptoms but there is a risk of dependence to these agents.

7. a. **True**. Ethanol intake is a common cause of macrocytosis (increased red cell volume) in the absence of anaemia.
   b. **False**. The diuresis resulting from ethanol intake is partly caused by inhibition of release of antidiuretic hormone.
   c. **False**. Plasma γ-glutamyl transpeptidase is elevated.

Index

Page numbers in *italic* refer to figures, tables, boxed material and drug compendia.

749

753

Index

Index